Clinical Anesthesia Fundamentals

Clinical Anesthesia Fundamentals

SECOND EDITION

EDITED BY

Bruce F. Cullen, MD
Emeritus Professor
Department of Anesthesiology and Pain Medicine
University of Washington School of Medicine
Seattle, Washington

M. Christine Stock, MD, FCCM, FCCP
Professor Emerita
Department of Anesthesiology
Northwestern University, Feinberg School of Medicine
Chicago, Illinois

Rafael Ortega, MD
Professor and Chair
Department of Anesthesiology
Boston University School of Medicine
Boston, Massachusetts

Sam R. Sharar, MD
Professor
Vice-Chair for Faculty Affairs and Development
Department of Anesthesiology and Pain Medicine
University of Washington School of Medicine
Seattle, Washington

Natalie F. Holt, MD, MPH
Adjunct Assistant Professor
Department of Anesthesiology
Yale School of Medicine
New Haven, Connecticut
Deputy Chief Medical Officer
Great Plains Area Indian Health Service
Aberdeen, South Dakota

Christopher W. Connor, MD, PhD
Assistant Professor
Department of Anesthesiology
Brigham and Women's Hospital, Harvard Medical School
Research Associate Professor in Physiology & Biophysics
Boston University School of Medicine
Boston, Massauchsetts

Naveen Nathan, MD
Associate Professor
Cover Editor, *Anesthesia & Analgesia*
Associate Chair of Education
Department of Anesthesiology
Northwestern University, Feinberg School of Medicine
Northwestern Memorial Hospital
Chicago, Illinois

Clinical Anesthesia Founding Editors

Paul G. Barash, MD
Professor
Department of Anesthesiology
Yale School of Medicine
Attending Anesthesiologist
Yale-New Haven Hospital
New Haven, Connecticut

Bruce F. Cullen, MD
Emeritus Professor
Department of Anesthesiology and Pain Medicine
University of Washington School of Medicine
Seattle, Washington

Robert K. Stoelting, MD
Emeritus Professor and Past Chair
Department of Anesthesia
Indiana University School of Medicine
Indianapolis, Indiana

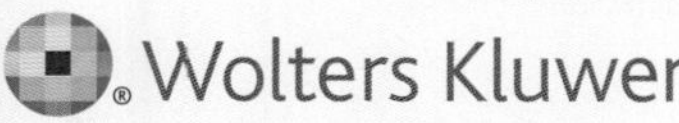

Philadelphia • Baltimore • New York • London
Buenos Aires • Hong Kong • Sydney • Tokyo

Senior Acquisitions Editor: Keith Donnellan
Senior Development Editor: Ashley Fischer
Editorial Coordinator: Ann Francis
Marketing Manager: Kirsten Watrud
Production Project Manager: Kirstin Johnson
Design Coordinator: Stephen Druding
Art Director, Illustration: Jennifer Clements
Manufacturing Coordinator: Beth Welsh
Prepress Vendor: TNQ Technologies

2nd edition

9 8 7 6 5 4 3 2 1

Printed in China

Library of Congress Cataloging-in-Publication Data

ISBN-13: 978-1-975113-01-8

Cataloging in Publication data available on request from publisher.

shop.lww.com

CCS0721

Contributors

Ron O. Abrons, MD
Associate Professor
Department of Anesthesia
Roy J. and Lucille A. Carver College of Medicine
University of Iowa Healthcare
Iowa City, Iowa

Pudkrong Aichholz, MD
Acting Assistant Professor
Department of Anesthesiology and Pain Medicine
University of Washington School of Medicine
Seattle, Washington

Shamsuddin Akhtar, MD
Professor
Department of Anesthesiology
Yale School of Medicine
New Haven, Connecticut

Abbas Al-Qamari, MD
Assistant Professor
Department of Anesthesiology
Northwestern University, Feinberg School of Medicine
Chicago, Illinois

Trefan Archibald, MD
Acting Assistant Professor
Department of Anesthesiology and Pain Medicine
University of Washington School of Medicine
Seattle, Washington

Lovkesh Arora, MBBS, MD, FASA
Clinical Associate Professor
Department of Anesthesia
Roy J. and Lucille A. Carver College of Medicine
Divisions of Anesthesiology and Critical Care
University of Iowa Healthcare
Iowa City, Iowa

Yogen Girish Asher, MD
Assistant Professor
Department of Anesthesiology
Northwestern University, Feinberg School of Medicine
Chicago, Illinois

Christopher R. Barnes, MD
Assistant Professor
Department of Anesthesiology and Critical Care Medicine
University of Washington School of Medicine
Harborview Medical Center
Seattle, Washington

John F. Bebawy, MD
Associate Professor
Departments of Anesthesiology and Neurological Surgery
Northwestern University, Feinberg School of Medicine
Chicago, Illinois

Itay Bentov, MD, PhD
Associate Professor Anesthesiology and Pain Medicine
Department of Anesthesiology and Pain Medicine
University of Washington School of Medicine
Seattle, Washington

Honorio T. Benzon, MD
Professor Emeritus of Anesthesiology
Department of Anesthesiology
Northwestern University, Feinberg School of Medicine
Chicago, Illinois

Wendy K. Bernstein, MD, MBA
Department of Anesthesiology and Perioperative Medicine
University of Rochester Medical Center
Rochester, New York

Sanjay M. Bhananker, MD, FRCA
Professor
Department of Anesthesiology and Pain Medicine
University of Washington School of Medicine
Seattle, Washington

Jessica R. Black, MD
Assistant Clinical Professor
Department of Anesthesiology
University of California San Diego School of Medicine
La Jolla, California

Brent T. Boettcher, DO, FASA
Assistant Professor
Department of Anesthesiology
Director, Transplant Anesthesia
Medical College of Wisconsin
Milwaukee, Wisconsin

Robert Canelli, MD
Assistant Professor
Department of Anesthesiology
Boston University School of Medicine
Boston, Massachusetts

Louanne M. Carabini, MD, MA
Associate Professor of Anesthesiology
Northwestern University, Feinberg School of Medicine
Chicago, Illinois

Vanessa M. Cervantes
Clinical Assistant Professor
Department of Anesthesiology and Pain Medicine
University of Washington School of Medicine
Seattle, Washington

Niels Chapman, MD
Clinical Professor
Department of Anesthesiology
University of New Mexico School of Medicine
Albuquerque, New Mexico

Christopher W. Connor, MD, PhD
Assistant Professor
Department of Anesthesiology
Brigham and Women's Hospital, Harvard Medical School
Research Associate Professor in Physiology & Biophysics
Boston University School of Medicine
Boston, Massachusetts

Matthew A. Dabski, MD, MPH
Assistant Professor of Anesthesiology
Department of Anesthesiology
Upstate University Hospital
Syracuse, New York

Arman Dagal, MD, FRCA, MHA
Professor
Department of Anesthesiology and Pain Medicine
University of Washington School of Medicine
Seattle, Washington

Chad T. Dean, MD
Assistant Professor
Department of Anesthesiology and Critical Care
University of Chicago Medicine,
Chicago, Illinois

Alexander Dekel, MD
Department of Anesthesiology
Boston Medical Center
Boston, Massachusetts

Alexander M. Deleon, MD
Assistant Professor
Department of Anesthesiology
Northwestern University, Feinberg School of Medicine
Chicago, Illinois

Nicholas Flores-Conner, MD
Voluntary Clinical Instructor
Department of Anesthesiology
Boston Medical Center
Boston, Massachusetts

Julie K. Freed, MD, PhD
Associate Professor
Department of Anesthesiology
Medical College of Wisconsin
Milwaukee, Wisconsin

Jorge A. Gálvez, MD, MBI
Division Chief, Division of Pediatric Anesthesiology
Children's Hospital and Medical Center
Omaha, Nebraska
Kugler Vonderfecht Professor
Vice Chair of Pediatric Anesthesiology
University of Nebraska Medical Center
Omaha, Nebraska

R. Mauricio Gonzalez, MD
Clinical Associate Professor of Anesthesiology
Boston University School of Medicine
Vice Chair of Clinical Affairs
Department of Anesthesiology
Boston Medical Center
Boston, Massachusetts

Andreas Grabinsky, MD
Associate Professor
Department of Anesthesiology and Pain Medicine
University of Washington School of Medicine
Seattle, Washington

Matthew Grunert, MD
Instructor in Anesthesia
Department of Anesthesiology and Pain Medicine
Brigham and Women's Hospital
Boston, Massachusetts

Matthew R. Hallman, MD
Associate Professor
Department of Anesthesiology and Pain Medicine
University of Washington School of Medicine
Seattle, Washington

Thomas R. Hickey, MS, MD
Assistant Professor of Anesthesiology
Yale School of Medicine
New Haven, Connecticut
VA Connecticut Healthcare System
West Haven, Connecticut

Louise Hillen, MD
Acute Pain and Regional Anesthesiology Fellow
Department of Anesthesiology
Northwestern University, Feinberg School of Medicine
Chicago, Illinois

Natalie F. Holt, MD, MPH
Adjunct Assistant Professor, Department of Anesthesiology
Yale School of Medicine
New Haven, Connecticut
Deputy Chief Medical Officer
Great Plains Area Indian Health Service
Aberdeen, South Dakota

Robert S. Holzman, MD, MA (Hon), FAAP
Professor of Anaesthesia
Harvard Medical School
Senior Associate in Perioperative Anesthesiology
Department of Anesthesiology, Critical Care and Pain Medicine
Boston Children's Hospital
Boston, Massachusetts

Peter Von Homeyer, MD, FASE
Associate Professor
Department of Anesthesiology and Pain Medicine
University of Washington School of Medicine
Seattle, Washington

Rebecca S. Isserman, MD
Assistant Professor
Department of Anesthesiology and Critical Care
Perelman School of Medicine at the University of Pennsylvania
The Children's Hospital of Philadelphia
Philadelphia, Pennsylvania

Aaron M. Joffe, DO, MS, FCCM
Professor, Vice Chair for Clinical Affairs
Department of Anesthesiology and Pain Medicine
University of Washington School of Medicine
Harborview Medical Center
Seattle, Washington

Kyle E. Johnson, MD
Vice-Chairman, Department of Anesthesiology
Cardiothoracic Anesthesiology
Riverside Regional Medical Center
Newport News, Virginia

Rebecca L. Johnson, MD
Associate Professor of Anesthesiology
Department of Anesthesiology and Perioperative Medicine
Mayo Clinic College of Medicine and Science
Rochester, Minnesota

Dost Khan, MD
Assistant Professor
Department of Anesthesiology
Northwestern University, Feinberg School of Medicine
Chicago, Illinois

Antoun Koht, MD
Professor of Anesthesiology, Neurological Surgery and Neurology
Department of Anesthesiology
Northwestern University, Feinberg School of Medicine
Chicago, Illinois

Sundar Krishnan, MBBS
Associate Professor
Department of Anesthesiology
Duke University School of Medicine
Durham, North Carolina

Howard Lee, MD
Assistant Professor
Department of Anesthesiology
Northwestern University, Feinberg School of Medicine
Chicago, Illinois

James P. Lee, MD
Assistant Professor
Department of Anesthesiology
University of Utah School of Medicine
Salt Lake City, Utah

Joseph Louca, MD
Assistant Professor
Department of Anesthesiology
Boston University School of Medicine
Boston Medical Center
Boston, Massachusetts

Jonathan B. Mark, MD
Professor of Anesthesiology
Duke University School of Medicine
Staff Anesthesiologist
Veterans Affairs Medical Center
Durham, North Carolina

Katherine Marseu, MD, FRCPC
Assistant Professor
Department of Anesthesiology and Pain Management
Toronto General Hospital
University Health Network, University of Toronto
Toronto, Ontario, Canada

Grace C. McCarthy, MD
Assistant Professor
Department of Anesthesiology
Duke University School of Medicine
Duke University Health System
Veteran Affairs Anesthesiology Service
Durham, North Carolina

Najma Mehter, MD
Assistant Professor
Department of Anesthesiology and Pain Medicine
University of Washington School of Medicine
Seattle, Washington

Sara E. Meitzen, MD
Assistant Professor of Anesthesiology
Department of Anesthesiology
University of California San Diego School of Medicine
San Diego, California

Ashleigh Menhadji, MD
Assistant Professor
Department of Anesthesiology
Boston University School of Medicine
Boston Medical Center
Boston, Massachusetts

Candice R. Montzingo, MD
Associate Professor
Department of Anesthesiology
University of Utah Hospital
Salt Lake City, Utah

Naveen Nathan, MD
Associate Professor
Cover Editor, Anesthesia & Analgesia
Associate Chair of Education
Department of Anesthesiology
Northwestern University, Feinberg School of Medicine
Northwestern Memorial Hospital
Chicago, Illinois

Mark C. Norris, MD
Clinical Professor of Anesthesiology
Department of Anesthesiology
Boston University School of Medicine
Boston Medical Center
Boston, Massachusetts

Rafael Ortega, MD
Professor and Chair
Department of Anesthesiology
Boston University School of Medicine
Boston, Massachusetts

Paul S. Pagel, MD, PhD
Anesthesiology Service
Clement J. Zablocki Veterans Affairs Medical Center
Professor of Anesthesiology
Medical College of Wisconsin
Milwaukee, Wisconsin

Louisa J. Palmer, MBBS
Instructor of Anesthesia
Department of Anesthesiology
Brigham and Women's Hospital, Harvard Medical School
Boston, Massachusetts

Sujatha Pentakota, MD
Instructor
Department of Anesthesiology
Brigham and Women's Hospital, Harvard Medical School
Boston, Massachusetts

Bridget P. Pulos, MD
Assistant Professor
Department of Anesthesiology
Mayo Clinic College of Medicine and Science
Rochester, Minnesota

Ramesh Ramaiah, MD
Associate Professor
Department of Anesthesiology and Pain Medicine
University of Washington School of Medicine
Seattle, Washington

Glenn Ramsey, MD
Professor
Department of Pathology
Northwestern University, Feinberg School of Medicine
Chicago, Illinois

Meghan E. Rodes, MD
Associate Professor
Department of Anesthesiology
Northwestern University, Feinberg School of Medicine
Chicago, Illinois

Gerardo Rodriguez, MD
Clinical Associate Professor of Anesthesiology and Surgery
Department of Anesthesiology
Boston University School of Medicine
Associate Medical Director SICU
Staff Anesthesiologist
Boston Medical Center
Boston, Massachusetts

Douglas A. Rooke, MD, PhD
Resident Physician
Department of Anesthesiology and Pain Medicine
University of Washington School of Medicine
Seattle, Washington

G. Alec Rooke, MD, PhD
Professor
Department of Anesthesiology and Pain Medicine
University of Washington School of Medicine
Seattle, Washington

William H. Rosenblatt, MD
Professor of Anesthesiology
Department of Anesthesiology
Yale School of Medicine
New Haven, Connecticut

Francis V. Salinas, MD, FASA
Clinical Assistant Professor of Anesthesiology
Department of Anesthesiology and Pain Medicine
University of Washington School of Medicine
Attending Anesthesiologist
Swedish Medical Center
Seattle, Washington
Medical Director, Interventional and Surgical Services
Swedish Issaquah Hospital
Issaquah, Washington
Seattle, Washington

Barbara M. Scavone, MD
Professor, Department of Anesthesia and Critical Care
Professor, Department of Obstetrics and Gynecology
The University of Chicago Pritzker School of Medicine
Chicago, Illinois

Alan Jay Schwartz, MD, MSEd
Professor of Clinical Anesthesiology and Critical Care
Department of Anesthesiology and Critical Care
Perelman School of Medicine at the University of Pennsylvania
The Children's Hospital of Philadelphia
Department of Anesthesiology and Critical Care Medicine
Philadelphia, Pennsylvania

Archit Sharma, MD, MBA, FASE
Clinical Associate Professor
Department of Anesthesia
Roy J. and Lucille A. Carver College of Medicine
University of Iowa Healthcare
Iowa City, Iowa

Sasha Shillcutt, MD, MS, FASE
Professor
Department of Anesthesiology
University of Nebraska Medical Center College of Medicine
Omaha, Nebraska

Ian Slade, MD
Assistant Professor
Department of Anesthesiology and Pain Medicine
University of Washington School of Medicine
Seattle, Washington

Peter Slinger, MD, FRCPC
Professor of Anesthesia
Department of Anesthesiology and Pain Medicine
Toronto General Hospital
University Health Network, University of Toronto

Karen J. Souter, MB, BS, FRCA, MACM
Professor
Department of Anesthesiology and Pain Medicine
University of Washington School of Medicine
Seattle, Washington

Nicole Z. Spence, MD
Assistant Professor
Director of Acute Pain Service
Department of Anesthesiology
Boston University School of Medicine
Boston, Massachusetts

Lalitha Vani Sundararaman, MD
Department of Anesthesiology, Perioperative and Pain Management
Harvard Medical School
Massachusetts General Hospital
Brigham and Women's Hospital
Boston, Massachusetts

James E. Szalados, MD, JD, MBA, MHA, FCCM, FCCP, FNCS, FCLM, FACHE
Director, Surgical Critical Care and Surgical and Trauma ICUs
Neurointensivist and Director, Neurocritical Care and Neurocritical Care Unit
Director, ICU Telemedicine Outreach Program
Departments of Anesthesiology, Surgery, and Neurology
Rochester General Hospital and Rochester Regional Health
Attorney and Counselor at Law, Consulting Attorney
The Szalados Law Firm
Rochester, New York

Justin N. Tawil, MD
Assistant Professor of Cardiothoracic Anesthesiology and Critical Care Medicine
Associate Program Director Critical Care Medicine
Department of Anesthesiology
Medical College of Wisconsin
Milwaukee, Wisconsin

Stephan R. Thilen, MD
Associate Professor
Department of Anesthesiology and Pain Medicine
University of Washington School of Medicine
Seattle, Washington

Theodora Valovska, MD
Department of Anesthesiology, Pain Management and Perioperative Medicine
Henry Ford Health Systems
Detroit, Michigan

Eduard Vaynberg, MD
Assistant Professor of Anesthesiology
Boston University School of Medicine
Director of Pain Management
Department of Anesthesiology
Boston Medical Center
Boston, Massachusetts

Amy E. Vinson, MD, FAAP
Assistant Professor of Anaesthesia
Harvard Medical School
Senior Associate in Perioperative Anesthesia
Boston Children's Hospital
Department of Anesthesiology
Critical Care & Pain Medicine
Boston, Massachusetts

Andrew M. Walters, MD
Assistant Professor
Department of Anesthesiology and Pain Medicine
University of Washington School of Medicine
Seattle, Washington

Mary E. Warner, MD
Professor of Anesthesiology
Department of Anesthesiology
Mayo Clinic College of Medicine and Science
Rochester, New York

Wade A. Weigel, MD
Anesthesiologist
Department of Anesthesiology
Virginia Mason Franciscan Health
Seattle, Washington

Ian Yuan, MD
Assistant Professor
Department of Anesthesiology and Critical Care
Perelman School of Medicine at the University of Pennsylvania
The Children's Hospital of Philadelphia
Philadelphia, Pennsylvania

Preface

Published in 2015, the inaugural first edition of *Clinical Anesthesia Fundamentals* was the brainchild of Paul Barash—one of the founding editors (along with Bruce Cullen and Robert Stoelting) of the *Clinical Anesthesia* textbook series that has been in continuous publication since 1989—and was intended to be a complementary text to the larger and more comprehensive *Clinical Anesthesia* compendium (currently in its eighth edition). In contrast to this compendium that targets the seasoned trainee and veteran practitioner, *Clinical Anesthesia Fundamentals* was specifically designed to fill the void in anesthesia and perioperative care education exemplified by the early trainee's question "Where can I go to most efficiently learn the fundamentals of anesthesia care?". The book's primary goal was to provide a complete, yet succinct introduction to the essential clinical principles and practices for early learners of anesthesia, including medical students, junior anesthesiology residents, anesthesiology assistants, and student registered nurse anesthetists. The book's second goal was to incorporate novel formats that target the cognitive needs and learning tools demanded by "digital native" learners of the millennial generation, including a manageable print book size, liberal use of graphic and tabular presentations that facilitate trainees to thoughtfully apply their basic science knowledge to the clinical setting, and an extensive, "immediately at hand" companion eBook with digital teaching tools designed both to appeal to millennial learners and to reinforce content acquisition through complementary methods of content delivery.

Did the first edition of *Clinical Anesthesia Fundamentals* achieve its goal? You, the readers, are the final arbiters of that query—however, we are encouraged by reader reviews that not only support continued editions, but also offer specific suggestions for improvement. As a result, this second edition relies even more heavily on a fully interactive digital resource, including colorful and meticulously designed infographics in almost every chapter. These infographics serve as visual representations of the book's contents and provide an easy-to-understand overview of a variety of pertinent topics. The information is displayed succinctly and clearly to present learners with an alternative resource to study the material. Additionally, the electronic version of the book includes a collection of interactive questions based on each one of the infographics; all questions provide feedback expanding on the correct answer and explaining all incorrect choices. This learning innovation provides the opportunity to review the infographics and then engage in a challenging question and answer exercise intended for knowledge consolidation. All of the videos have been refreshed and the interactive lectures have been streamlined to facilitate broadcasting them swiftly over the internet.

As in the first edition, all components of the eBook are viewable through any web browser, and also as a download to one's smartphone or tablet, thus providing immediate and ubiquitous access for the reader. A new chapter on "Anesthesia for the Older Patient" brings the chapter total to 45. Finally, the book concludes with a series of Appendices, carefully selected for their reference value and clinical relevance to early anesthesia trainees, including essential physiologic formulas/definitions, an electrocardiography atlas, pacemaker/defibrillator protocols, and key standards/algorithms from the American Society of Anesthesiologists, American Heart Association, and Anesthesia Patient Safety Foundation.

In a reflective and somber note, we are saddened to share that since publication of the first edition, two of our long-time editorial colleagues have passed away—Michael K. Cahalan in 2019 and Paul G. Barash in 2020. Both men were highly committed and tireless contributors to the *Clinical Anesthesia* series—Paul since its first edition in 1989 and Mike since its fifth edition in 2009—and are universally recognized in our field as consummate clinicians, dedicated educators, and invaluable mentors to both trainees and peers. Moreover, they were role models of professionalism and interpersonal relationships whose teachings, spirits, and senses of humor are legendary and will live on in each of us. We mourn their loss and keep them and their families in our hearts.

We wish to express our appreciation to both our new and returning contributors who not only provided fundamental content in a novel, yet highly concise format, but did so despite the unexpected and concurrent personal and professional demands of the COVID pandemic. Finally, we owe a debt of gratitude to Ashley Fischer, Senior Development Editor at Wolters Kluwer, whose day-to-day management of this endeavor resulted in a publication that exceeded the Editors' expectations.

Bruce F. Cullen, MD
M. Christine Stock, MD, FCCM, FCCP
Rafael Ortega, MD
Sam R. Sharar, MD
Natalie F. Holt, MD, MPH
Christopher W. Connor, MD, PhD
Naveen Nathan, MD

Contents

SECTION III: Clinical Practice of Anesthesia

SECTION IV: Appendices

Digital Contents

For access to digital contents and interactivities, please see eBook bundled with this text. Access instructions are located in the inside front cover.

I Introduction

1 History and Future

Rafael Ortega and Robert Canelli

Introduction

Most medical textbooks begin by discussing the history of the subject. Why? Succinctly stated, we only learn from the past. Although modern anesthesiology is practiced in today's future-driven environment, there is much to learn by analyzing the historical evolution of the specialty.

The field of anesthesiology is at a turning point that will define the future course of the profession. Today, anesthesiologists face new challenges, from utilizing new drugs and sophisticated instrumentation, to expanding their roles in perioperative medicine and critical care, to confronting professional competition and health care reform.

Understanding how and why anesthetics came into use, how they have evolved, and how the profession has grown is essential for a true understanding of the specialty and anticipating new forays into the future.

In the 2020 Covid-19 pandemic, anesthesiologists were at the forefront of patient care and the specialty's contributions to medicine were reaffirmed. Serendipitously, Dr John Snow, considered by many to be the father of epidemiology, and Dr Jerome Adams, the Surgeon General of the United States during the pandemic, are both anesthesiologists. This coincidence provides the historical framework for many of the details presented in this chapter.

I. Pain and Antiquity

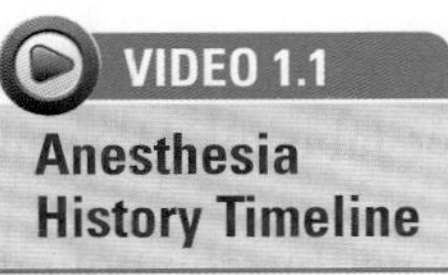

From early Mesopotamian and Egyptian cultures to Asian and Central American cultures, practices for the relief of pain have existed for centuries. For instance, the Greek physician Dioscorides reported on the analgesic properties of the mandrake plant, 2000 years ago. With the advent of surgical medicine, various combinations of substances, including opium, alcohol, and marijuana, were inhaled by diverse cultures for their mind-altering and analgesic effects. The "soporific sponge," which was popular between the 9th and 13th centuries, became the primary mode of delivering pain relief to patients during surgical operations. The sponges were saturated with a solution derived from the combination of poppies, mandrake leaves, and various herbs. Before the surgical procedure, the sponge was moistened with hot water to reconstitute the ingredients and then placed over the mouth and nose so the patient could inhale the anesthetic vapors. ***Laudanum***, an opium derivative prepared as a tincture in the 16th century by Paracelsus (1493-1541) was used as an analgesic. However, like other medications of the time, it was also prescribed for a variety of diseases such as meningitis, cardiac disease, and tuberculosis. In Indian culture, avatars such as Dhanwantari used anesthetics for surgical pain and severed nerves for relief of neuralgia. Chinese physicians have used acupuncture and various herbal substances to ease surgical pain for centuries. In 1804, ***Seishu Hanaoka*** (1760-1835), a surgeon from Japan, induced general anesthesia with a herbal combination containing anticholinergic alkaloids capable of inducing unconsciousness. Hanaoka developed an enteral formulation called ***tsusensan***. His patients would ingest this concoction before Hanaoka would begin the surgical procedure.[1]

II. Inhaled Anesthetics

A. Nitrous Oxide

Joseph Priestley (1733-1804), an English chemist and clergyman known for his isolation of oxygen in its gaseous form, was also the first to isolate ***nitrous oxide***. Although he did not report on nitrous oxide's possible medical applications, it was his discovery and isolation of this and various other gases that would allow for modern methods of inhaled anesthesia. Sir Humphry Davy (1778-1829) described nitrous oxide's effect on breathing and the central nervous system. In 1800, he stated, "As nitrous oxide in its extensive operation appears capable of destroying physical pain, it may probably be used with advantage during surgical operations in which no great effusion of blood takes place." Despite his insight, Davy did not employ nitrous oxide as an anesthetic, but his lasting legacy to history was coining of the phrase ***"laughing gas,"*** which describes nitrous oxide's ability to trigger uncontrollable laughter.

> **? Did You Know?**
>
> By 1800, Sir Humphry Davy was aware that nitrous oxide had analgesic properties and that it had potential to be used during surgical procedures. However, it was Horace Wells who, 45 years later, first attempted to use nitrous oxide as a general anesthetic.

Horace Wells (1815-1848) was the first individual to attempt a public demonstration of general anesthesia using nitrous oxide. Wells, a well-known dentist from Hartford, Connecticut, had used nitrous oxide for dental extractions. In 1845, he attempted to publicly perform the painless extraction of a tooth using nitrous oxide. However, possibly due to inadequate administration time or dilution of the gas with air, the patient was not fully insensible to pain and was said to have moved and groaned. Because of this, Wells was discredited and became deeply disappointed at his failed demonstration. Wells spent the better part of his remaining life in self-experimentation and unsuccessfully pursuing recognition for the discovery of inhaled anesthesia.[2]

B. Diethyl Ether

Although the origin of diethyl ether's discovery is debated, it may first have been synthesized by the eighth-century Arabian philosopher Jabir ibn Hayyan or 13th-century European alchemist Raymundus Lully.

> **? Did You Know?**
>
> Physicians and chemists were familiar with the compound, diethyl ether, for centuries before it was used as a general anesthetic.

By the 16th century, Paracelsus and others were preparing this compound and noting its effects on consciousness. Paracelsus documented that diethyl ether could produce drowsiness in chickens, causing them to become unresponsive and then wake up without any adverse effects. In the 17th and 18th centuries, ether was sold as a pain reliever, and numerous famous scientists of the time examined its properties. Because of its effects on consciousness, it also became a popular recreational drug in Britain and Ireland as well as in America, where festive group events with ether were called "ether frolics."

Although many were aware of the effects of inhaled ether, it was a physician from Georgia who first administered ether with the deliberate purpose of producing surgical anesthesia. ***Crawford Williamson Long*** (1815-1878) administered ether as a surgical anesthetic on March 30, 1842, to James M. Venable for the removal of a neck tumor. However, his results were not published until

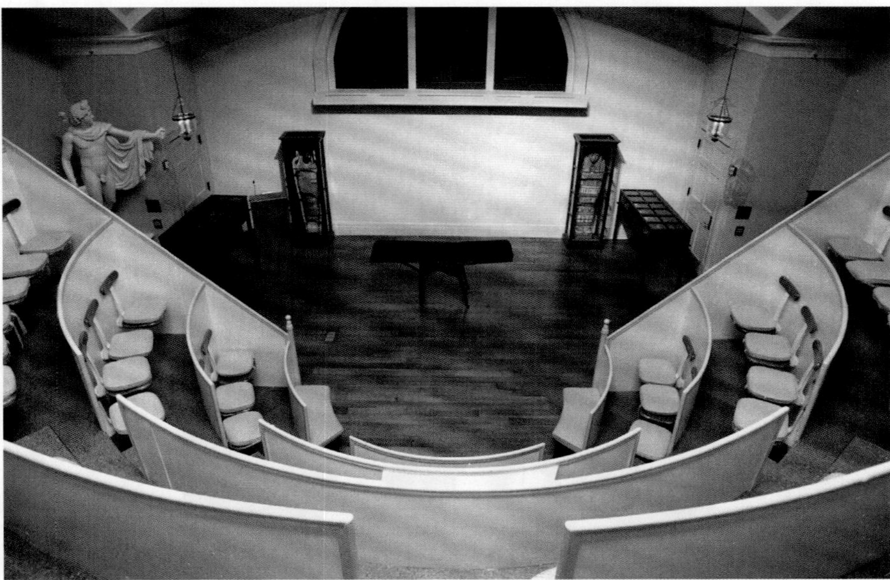

Figure 1.1 The surgical amphitheater at the Massachusetts General Hospital, today known as the Ether Dome, where Morton's demonstration took place on October 16, 1846.

1849, 3 years after William T. G. Morton's famous public demonstration. This was not from a lack of insight, but rather a lack of desire for recognition. When he finally did publish his experiments with ether, he stated he did so at the bequest of his friends who felt he would be remiss not to state his involvement in the history of inhalation anesthesia.

On October 16, 1846, William T. G. Morton (1819-1868) induced general anesthesia with ether, which allowed surgeon John Collins Warren (1778-1856) to remove a vascular tumor from Edward Gilbert Abbott. The anesthetic was delivered through an inhaler consisting of a glass bulb containing an ether-soaked sponge and a spout at the other end through which the patient could breathe. The glass bulb was open to room air, allowing the patient to breathe in fresh air that mixed with the ether inside the bulb before passing through the spout and into the patient's lungs. The event occurred in a surgical amphitheater at the Massachusetts General Hospital, known today as the ***Ether Dome*** (**Figure 1.1**). News of the demonstration spread quickly, and within a matter of months, the possibility of painless surgery was known around the world.

C. The Ether Controversy

In all, Morton completed three trials at the Massachusetts General Hospital before the hospital deemed it safe for use. Although today Morton is usually credited with this discovery, at the time, those involved were aware that Charles T. Jackson was the intellectual discoverer of this process and Morton was simply its executor. Charles Jackson (1805-1880), a notable Boston physician, chemist, and Morton's preceptor, stated that he counseled Morton on the use of inhaled ether for insensibility to pain.[3]

Shortly after Morton's demonstration, Henry Jacob Bigelow (1818-1890), professor emeritus in the Department of Surgery at Harvard Medical School, described his famous account of the events that transpired at Massachusetts General Hospital, proclaiming that Morton and Jackson had discovered how

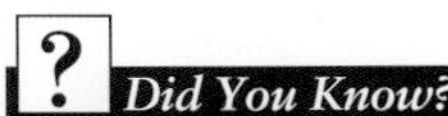

The ether controversy refers to the acrimonious arguments that ensued among the various individuals who believed they deserved the credit for having introduced inhalation anesthesia.

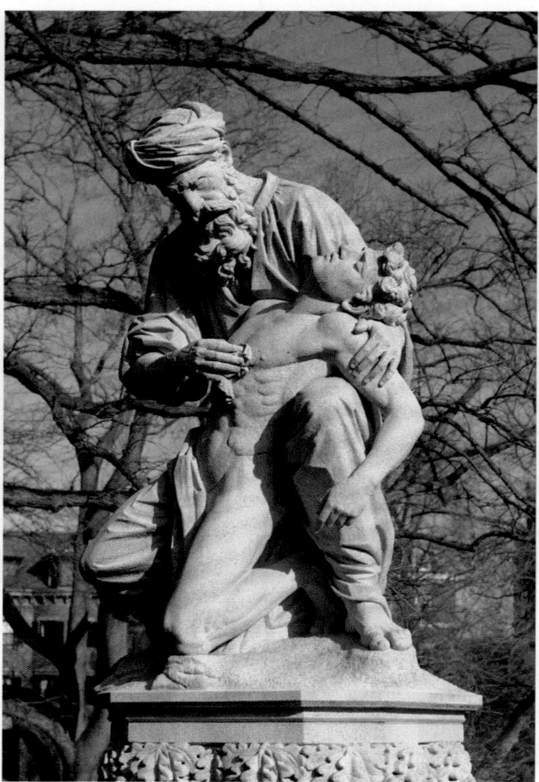

Figure 1.2 The sculpture atop the Ether Monument in the Public Garden in Boston symbolizing the relief of human suffering.

to render patients insensible to pain. The article, published in the ***Boston Medical and Surgical Journal*** (the predecessor to the ***New England Journal of Medicine***), was widely distributed.[4] The news reached Horace Wells, who contended that he had discovered inhaled anesthetics through his use of nitrous oxide. It was these assertions that would lead to what is now called the ***"ether controversy."*** The debate was made worse by what was most likely an attempt for monetary reward, with Morton's subsequent denial of Jackson's share in the discovery, leading to all three being pitted against one another.[5]

The controversy would destroy both the reputations and lives of those involved, and to this day, it lives on through various monuments throughout New England and other areas of the nation avowing credit to those depicted. It should be noted that, although not usually cited as being involved in the ether controversy, Crawford Long did publish his accounts of his use of ether. As such, there are various monuments asserting his place in the history of anesthesia (**Figure 1.2**).

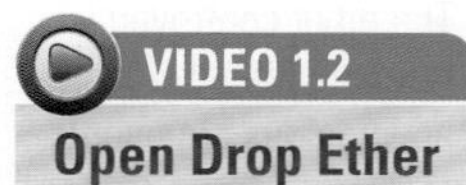

D. Spread of Ether

After Morton's famous demonstration, Henry Jacob Bigelow and his father Jacob Bigelow wrote letters to English physicians Francis Boott and Robert Liston, respectively. Boott, a general practitioner, and Liston, a surgeon, conducted Europe's first successful administration of surgical anesthesia with ether in December 1846, leading to Liston's famous words, "Well gentlemen, this Yankee Dodge sure beats ***mesmerism*** hollow." News traveled fast, and use of ether anesthesia swiftly found its way throughout the European continent.

E. Chloroform

Although ***chloroform*** had been discovered nearly 2 decades earlier, it was not used as a surgical anesthetic until a year after Morton's demonstration in 1847. James Young Simpson, a Scottish obstetrician, had learned of ether's effects after Liston's successful operation and had employed it with some of his patients. Although it did relieve some of the suffering associated with childbirth, Simpson was not satisfied and began to search for a better solution. Through the advice of a chemist, he became aware of chloroform and its anesthetizing effects. On November 4, 1847, he and two friends imbibed the contents of a bottle containing chloroform. Needless to say, they were satisfied by their self-experimentation and Simpson began using chloroform to relieve the pain of childbirth.

F. Critics of Anesthesia

The anesthetic use of chloroform and ether was not without its skeptics, and arguments against its use were made on moral, religious, and physiologic grounds. However, unlike ether, in Europe, chloroform use was more easily legitimized through the scientific logic of ***John Snow***, who proclaimed its safety over ether and would eventually administer it to Queen Victoria during the birth of Prince Leopold. Perhaps because of the widespread use of chloroform and the effect a monarch can have on its citizens, the use and study of surgical anesthesia prospered in the 19th-century Europe, while in the United States it remained comparatively stagnant.

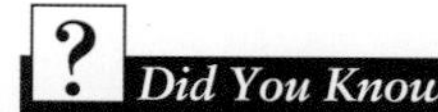

The scientific study of surgical anesthesia prospered in the 19th-century Europe, while in the United States it remained comparatively stagnant for decades.

G. The Birth of Modern Surgical Anesthesia

The aforementioned London physician John Snow (1813-1858), best known for his epidemiologic work on cholera showing that the source was a public water pump, could also be called the first true anesthetist (the British equivalent of an anesthesiologist). As was his manner, he delved deeply into the study and understanding of volatile anesthetics. Unlike Morton, Wells, and Jackson, Snow was not worried about his role and potential legacy in medicine, but rather with the safe and proper administration of anesthesia. His calm and attentive attitude in the operating theater and focus on the patient's well-being, rather than his self-pride, is a model to be emulated.

H. Modern Inhaled Anesthetics

Perhaps Snow's intense study of the mechanism of action and possible side effects of inhaled anesthetics inspired the quest for an ideal inhalation anesthetic. Throughout the 20th century, various drugs such as ethyl chloride, ethylene, and cyclopropane were used for surgical anesthesia. But these were eventually abandoned due to a variety of drawbacks such as their pungent nature, weak potency, and flammability. The discovery that ***fluorination*** contributed to making anesthetics more stable, less toxic, and less combustible led to the introduction of halothane in the 1950s. The 1960s and 1970s would bring about various fluorinated anesthetics such as methoxyflurane and enflurane. These were eventually discontinued due to untoward side effects. Although initially more difficult to synthesize and purify, isoflurane, an isomer of enflurane, had fewer side effects than previous agents. It has been used since the late 1970s and is still a popular inhalation anesthetic today. There were no further advances in inhaled anesthetics until the introduction of desflurane in 1992 and sevoflurane in 1994. Both of these agents, along with isoflurane and nitrous oxide, are the most widely used inhaled agents today.

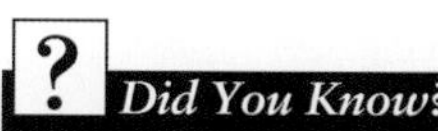

Inhaled anesthetics such as cyclopropane and ether were abandoned due to their high flammability, among other reasons.

III. Intravenous Anesthetics and Regional Anesthesia

In 1853, Alexander Wood administered intravenous morphine for the relief of neuralgia through a hollow needle of his invention. This extraordinary accomplishment allowed for the administration of intravenous agents for both anesthesia and analgesia.

A. Intravenous Anesthesia

Phenobarbital was the first drug to be used for the intravenous induction of anesthesia. It was synthesized in 1903 by Emil Fischer and Joseph von Mering. Because it was long acting, it caused prolonged periods of unconsciousness followed by slow emergence and as such was not an ideal anesthetic. However, its success in producing anesthesia and the promotion and study of intravenous anesthetics by men such as John Lundy opened new possibilities in anesthesia. In 1934, Ralph Waters (1883-1979) from the University of Wisconsin and John Lundy (1894-1973) from the Mayo Clinic administered thiopental (a potent short-acting barbiturate) as a successful intravenous induction agent. Lundy emphasized the approach, referred to as "***balanced anesthesia,***" that consisted of a combination of several anesthetic agents and strategies to produce unconsciousness, neuromuscular block, and analgesia. Through use of this approach, Lundy allowed for a safer and more complete administration of anesthesia. Thiopental's popularity led to the introduction of several other types of intravenous hypnotics including ketamine (1962), etomidate (1964), and propofol (1977). Since that time, other intravenous agents such as benzodiazepines and new opioids have been added to the specialty's armamentarium.

> **? *Did You Know?***
>
> The barbiturates were the first drugs to be administered intravenously for induction of anesthesia.

B. Regional Anesthesia

Cocaine, originally described by Carl Koller in 1884 as a local anesthetic, became a mainstay for regional anesthesia through the early 1900s. During this time period, various nerve and plexus blocks were described, as was the technique of spinal anesthesia, all using cocaine as a local anesthetic. However, early cases of regional anesthesia were not without incident. Adverse effects, including postdural puncture headache, vomiting, and cocaine's addictive quality, necessitated the development of local anesthetics such as procaine in 1905 and lidocaine in 1943, which were much safer.

Throughout the 1940s, advances continued in the field of regional anesthesia with the advent of continuous spinal anesthesia by William T. Lemmon in 1940 and Edward Tuohy's eponymous needle in 1944. Tuohy's modification of the spinal needle allowed a catheter to pass into the epidural space and administer doses of local anesthetics. From that point to the present, subarachnoid and epidural administration methods of local anesthetics and opioids are commonly employed for analgesia during labor and delivery as well as for managing postoperative pain. Innovations such as ultrasound imaging and nerve stimulators are now used to facilitate locating and identifying nerves, thus improving the quality of the block.

IV. Neuromuscular-Blocking Agents

Curare has been used for centuries by Amerindians of South America. Applied to arrows and darts, its paralyzing effects were originally employed for hunting and warfare. Through accounts from Spanish exploration of the area, news of curare and its effects reached Europe. Initially, medical applications for curare were limited; however, with the introduction of endotracheal intubation and mechanical ventilation, curare could be used to prevent laryngospasm during laryngoscopy and relax abdominal muscles during surgical procedures. In 1942, Griffith and Johnson introduced the first drug form of curare called intocostrin. Intocostrin facilitated both tracheal intubation and abdominal muscle relaxation, allowing for a more optimized surgical patient. Although other muscle relaxants were studied, they were subsequently discarded due to undesirable autonomic nervous system effects. The next great step in neuromuscular-blocking agents came in 1949 with the synthesis of the depolarizing neuromuscular-blocking agent ***succinylcholine*** by Nobel Laureate Daniel Bovet (1907-1992). Nondepolarizing neuromuscular-blocking agents such as vecuronium and rocuronium, as well as atracurium and cis-atracurium, were introduced into clinical practice in the late 20th century.

? *Did You Know?*

The first pharmaceutical form of curare was introduced in 1942, marking the beginning of the use of neuromuscular-blocking agents during surgical procedures.

V. Anesthesiology as a Medical Specialty

Anesthesiology as a medical specialty developed gradually in the United States during the 20th century. For decades after Morton's demonstration, there was no formal instruction in anesthesia. In the first part of the 20th century, Ralph Waters advocated for dedicated anesthesia departments and training programs. Later, anesthesiologists such as Thomas D. Buchanan and John Lundy established formal anesthesia departments in the New York Medical College and the Mayo Clinic, respectively, and Waters at the University of Wisconsin–Madison established the first anesthesiology postgraduate training program in 1927.

VI. Modern Anesthesiology Practice

In the early 1900s, Sir Robert Macintosh and Sir Ivan Magill made significant contributions to airway management, primarily by facilitating endotracheal intubation through the development of simple laryngoscopes. Anesthesiology further evolved in the second half of the 20th century with a proliferation of residency training programs and a strong emphasis on safety. In 1985, the ***Anesthesia Patient Safety Foundation*** was established with a mission "to ensure that no patient is harmed by anesthesia." Additional monitoring tools such as blood gas analysis, pulse oximetry, and capnometry notably decreased mortality rates during anesthetic procedures. In the 21st century, there have been significant refinements in anesthesia delivery systems, such as with microprocessor-controlled anesthesia machines and mechanical ventilators, and real-time data collection with an electronic medical record.

Presently, the ***American Society of Anesthesiologists*** provides ***guidelines*** for anesthesiology. The stated goals of this professional organization are to establish "an educational, research, and scientific association of physicians organized to raise and maintain the standards of anesthesiology and to improve the care of patients."

The history of nurses administering anesthesia in the United States is intertwined with the rapid development of the country after the 1840s and the relative scarcity of physicians. It is known that nurses provided anesthesia as early as the Civil War, but it was not until 1956 that the term ***certified registered nurse anesthetist (CRNA)*** was introduced. In 2013, the Emery Rovenstine Memorial Lecture, considered by many the main event during the American Society of Anesthesiologists' annual meeting, addressed the competition between anesthesiologists and nurse anesthetists to provide anesthesia care.

The American Society of Anesthesiologists supports a physician-led model for anesthesia care known as the ***anesthesia care team.*** On the other hand, the ***American Association of Nurse Anesthetists***, the organization representing nurse anesthetists, promotes independent practice and is aggressively lobbying in legislative and regulatory arenas to achieve their goal. In 2001, Medicare allowed states to opt out of a regulation that required CRNAs to administer anesthetics under the supervision of a physician, and today there are several federal and state jurisdictions allowing CRNAs to practice independently. The controversy over who can administer anesthesia independently, which may have financial and quality of care implications, continues to be debated.

The current economic environment will test anesthesiology as a service to patients and as an area of specialization for physicians. The diversity in the composition of the anesthesia care team varies across the country and will continue to change as economic pressures evolve. Although some may view the current challenges as a menace for this medical specialty, many find opportunities for improvement.

Three different approaches to the delivery of anesthesia care in the United States are currently used. Most anesthetics are delivered by a team typically comprising an anesthesiologist, a CRNA, and an anesthesiologist assistant or a resident. However, there are anesthesiologists delivering anesthesia care themselves in a "physician-only" model, and in some areas of the country, there are CRNAs working alone. In recent years, individual practices have merged into large groups, and anesthesia practice management has become more demanding and complex.

Today, anesthesiologists act as perioperative physicians capable of coordinating pre-, intra-, and postoperative care. The versatility and skills of anesthesiologists were tested during the Covid-19 pandemic, during which they served as specialized airway and mechanical ventilator management teams. Many anesthesiologists act as part- or full-time providers of intensive care, pain management, or other nonoperating room services. Students interested in pursuing a career in anesthesiology must be passionate about the specialty, excel academically, and have a unique predisposition blending a calm and poised attitude with the ability to make swift decisions and take immediate action. Considering the aging population and the ever-increasing need for health care, including surgical procedures, anesthesiology as a profession has a bright future.

For further review, please see the associated Interactive Video Lectures accessible in complimentary eBook bundled with this text. Access instructions are located on the inside front cover.

References

1. Ortega RA, Mai C. History of anesthesia. In: Vacanti CA, Sikka PK, Urman RD, et al, eds. *Essential Clinical Anesthesia*. Cambridge University Press; 2011:1-6.
2. Haridas RP. Horace Wells' demonstration of nitrous oxide in Boston. *Anesthesiology*. 2013;119(5):1014-1022. PMID: 23962967.
3. Zeitlin GL, Charles Thomas Jackson, "The Head Behind the Hands." Applying science to implement discovery in early nineteenth century America. *Anesthesiology*. 2009;110(3):687-688.
4. Bigelow HJ. Insensibility during surgical operations produced by inhalation. *Boston Med Surg J*. 1846;16:309-317.
5. Ortega RA, Lewis KP, Hansen CJ. Other monuments to inhalation anesthesia. *Anesthesiology*. 2008;109(4):578-587. PMID: 18813035.

Questions

1. **The first successful public demonstration of the use of ether anesthesia during a surgical procedure is generally credited to whom?**

A. Joseph Priestley
B. William Morton
C. Charles Jackson
D. Henry Bigelow

2. **Advantages of fluorinating anesthetic agents include all of the following EXCEPT:**

A. Greater potency
B. Greater stability
C. Less pungent
D. Less combustibility

3. **Which of the following neuromuscular-blocking agents (NMBAs) was first used in clinical practice?**

A. Vecuronium
B. Succinylcholine
C. Pancuronium
D. Curare

4. **The term "balanced anesthesia" refers to which of the following?**

A. A combination of anesthetic agents to produce unconsciousness, neuromuscular block, and analgesia
B. The combined use of spinal anesthesia and sedation
C. General anesthesia with a barbiturate and morphine
D. Total intravenous anesthesia

5. **The correct historical order of introduction of the following local anesthetics is:**

A. Lidocaine, procaine, bupivacaine
B. Procaine, cocaine, lidocaine
C. Cocaine, procaine, lidocaine
D. Cocaine, bupivacaine, procaine

Answers

1. B

On October 16, 1846, William T. G. Morton induced general anesthesia with ether, which allowed surgeon John Collins Warren to remove a vascular tumor from Edward Gilbert Abbott. This demonstration is considered the first successful public administration of anesthesia for a surgical procedure. Charles Jackson, a notable Boston physician, chemist, and Morton's preceptor, stated that he counseled Morton on the use of inhaled ether for insensibility to pain, but was not the first to publicly demonstrate its use as a surgical anesthetic. Priestley lived in the 1700s and was known for his isolation of oxygen in its gaseous form and his isolation of nitrous oxide. Bigelow observed Morton's demonstration and wrote about it in the ***Boston Medical and Surgical Journal.***

2. C

Various anesthetics, such as ethyl chloride, ethylene, and cyclopropane, had a variety of drawbacks such as their pungent nature, weak potency, and flammability. The discovery that fluorination contributed to making anesthetics more stable, less toxic, and less combustible led the introduction of halothane in the 1950s. The 1960s and 1970s would bring about various fluorinated anesthetics such as isoflurane, which is still widely used today.

3. D

The first medically used NMBA, intocostrin, was based on the drug curare. Applied to arrows and darts, its paralyzing effects were originally employed for hunting and warfare. Pancuronium and vecuronium belong to the class of NMBAs known as nondepolarizing and were introduced into clinical practice much later. Succinylcholine was developed in 1949 by Nobel Laureate Daniel Bovet and is a depolarizing NBMA.

4. A

In 1926, Lundy introduced the term balanced anesthesia to describe a combination of several anesthetic agents and strategies to produce unconsciousness, neuromuscular block, and analgesia, which included an opioid and an inhalant anesthetic.

5. C

Cocaine, originally described by Austrian ophthalmologist Carl Koller in 1884 as a local anesthetic, became a mainstay for regional anesthesia through the early 1900s. However, adverse effects, including postdural puncture headache, vomiting, and its addictive quality, necessitated the development of local anesthetics such as procaine in 1905 and lidocaine in 1943, which were much safer. Bupivacaine was synthesized in 1957.

II Scientific and Technical Foundations of Anesthesia

PART A Core Organ Functions: Anatomy & Physiology

2 The Respiratory System

Howard Lee and Abbas Al-Qamari

An understanding of the basic concepts of the respiratory system and the mechanics of ventilation and gas exchange is essential to the practice of anesthesiology. The principles described in this chapter are used every day in operating rooms and intensive care units around the world. Understanding these principles can help guide clinical decision-making and allows for informed discussions with other consulting services in the perioperative management of patients.

I. Muscles of Ventilation

A. Diaphragm

> **? Did You Know?**
>
> During nonstrenuous breathing, the diaphragm does most of the work inspiration and that exhalation is mainly passive.

The diaphragm, the main muscle of ventilation, completes the majority of the work of breathing. The diaphragm is anchored by a mobile central tendon that originates from the vertebral bodies, lower ribs, and sternum. During inspiration, the diaphragm contracts and negative pressure is generated in the intrapleural space causing inflow of gas into the lungs. As the diaphragm relaxes, exhalation ensues and the volume within the thoracic cavity decreases forcing gas to leave the lungs. During nonstrenuous breathing, exhalation is mainly passive. Approximately 50% of the diaphragm's musculature is composed of fatigue-resistant, slow-twitch muscle fibers,[1,2] allowing the diaphragm to maintain normal respiration without developing fatigue.

B. Accessory Muscles

As the work of breathing increases, accessory skeletal muscles in addition to the diaphragm are utilized. The external intercostal muscles assist in inhalation, while the internal intercostal muscles to some degree provide support for exhalation. The most important expiratory accessory muscles are the abdominal muscles that assist in depressing the ribs and producing forced exhalation through an increase in intra-abdominal pressure. Additionally, abdominal muscles play a pivotal role in generating the propulsive expiratory force involved with coughing and maintaining adequate bronchial hygiene. The cervical strap muscles are the most important inspiratory accessory muscles, and they help to elevate the sternum and upper chest to increase thoracic cavity dimensions. The scalene muscles help prevent inward motion of the ribs, while the sternocleidomastoid muscles help to elevate the upper part of the rib cage. As the work of breathing continues to increase, the large back and paravertebral muscles become involved. Importantly, as the accessory muscles are skeletal muscles, they are prone to fatigue.[1,2]

II. Structures of the Lung

A. Thoracic Cavity and Pleura

The lungs are contained within the bony thoracic cage, consisting of the 12 thoracic vertebrae, 12 rib pairs, and the sternum. The intercostal muscles lie between the ribs. The diaphragm makes up the inferior border of the thoracic cavity and the mediastinum separates the lungs medially.

Each lung weighs approximately 300 to 450 g. The right lung is slightly larger than the left. Fissures separate the right lung into three lobes and the left lung into two lobes. Each lung is composed of 10 segments, the anatomic divisions of which correspond to the branching of the proximal conducting airways. The lung parenchyma is invested by a layer of visceral pleura, which also covers the surfaces of the interlobar fissures. As this visceral layer is reflected upon itself at the level of the hilum and pulmonary ligament, it becomes the parietal pleura. This pleura covers the entirety of the thoracic cage and diaphragm. A 20-μm-thick fluid layer separates the two layers, allowing for the smooth movement of the lung against the thoracic cavity.[1-3]

B. Airways

Immediately distal to the larynx begins the trachea. A series of C-shaped cartilaginous rings support the trachea anteriorly and laterally. The posterior, or membranous, portion of the trachea lacks this rigid support structure, thereby allowing flexibility for food boluses that traverse the esophagus.

At the distal end of the trachea is the carina, the first branch point in the respiratory tree, beyond which left and right main stem bronchi begin. The right main bronchus has a significantly less acute angle of branching. This "straight shot" allows for a less circuitous path for aspirated material and is the primary reason aspiration events occur more often in the right lung.

The right main stem bronchus then divides into the right upper lobe bronchus and bronchus intermedius. The bronchus intermedius divides almost immediately into the right middle and right lower lobe bronchi. The left main bronchus divides into the left upper and left lower lobe bronchi. It is at this lobar level that the cartilage rings are replaced proximally by platelike islands of cartilage within the wall of the airway.

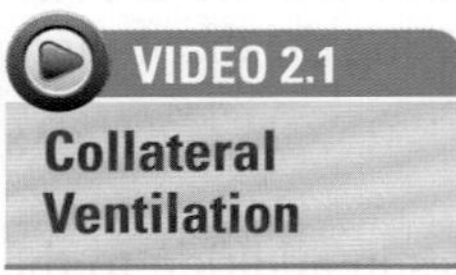

Each lobar branch then further divides into segmental branches. The airways continue to divide for another 5 to 25 generations depending on their position within the lung. As branching progresses, the amount of cartilage contained within the wall continues to decrease. The point at which cartilage is totally absent from the airway wall is termed the ***terminal bronchiole*** and is the final conducting airway before reaching the functional unit of the lung known as the ***acinus***.

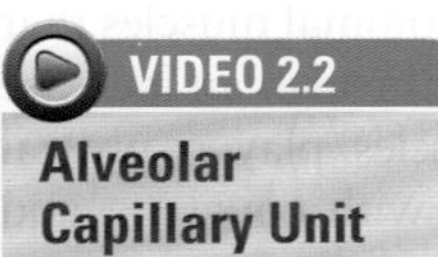

Each acinus comprises respiratory bronchioles, alveolar ducts, alveolar sacs, and grapelike clusters of alveoli. The alveolus serves as the main point of gas exchange between lung parenchyma and the pulmonary vasculature. Approximately 300 million alveoli are present in an average adult male. Each alveolus comprises type I cells, which form the majority of the epithelial surface of the alveolus, and type II cells, which produce surfactants and function as reserve precursor cells for type I cells.[1-3]

C. Vasculature

Within the pulmonary system, there exist two types of vascular supply. Bronchial circulation, which arises from the aorta and the intercostal arteries, supplies oxygenated blood to the tissues of the bronchi, visceral pleura, and pulmonary vasculature. It is not involved with alveolar gas exchange.

The second vascular supply is the pulmonary circulation, which delivers deoxygenated systemic blood to the pulmonary capillaries for interface with the alveoli. It is here that alveolar gas exchange occurs, allowing oxygen to be absorbed and carbon dioxide to be excreted. The newly oxygenated blood is then sent back into the systemic circulation for distribution to the rest of the body.

The pulmonary arterial trunk arises directly from the right ventricle. It very quickly bifurcates into the left and right main pulmonary arteries. These pulmonary arteries further divide into separate lobar arteries that enter the hilum of their respective lungs.

After entering the lung, the pulmonary vasculature divides along with its corresponding airway. They subdivide into arterioles and then finally into capillaries at the level of the alveolus. As one moves past the alveolus, the vessels become venules. These venules eventually coalesce into lobular veins, then further on to the four pulmonary veins, two each from left and right lung. These pulmonary veins drain into the left atrium, where the oxygenated blood is then circulated systemically until it returns to the right atrium and ventricle for recirculation through the pulmonary system. It should be noted that blood in the pulmonary arteries is typically deoxygenated and the pulmonary venous blood is oxygenated. This arrangement is opposite of the systemic circulation as the vascular nomenclature is based on the direction of blood flow in relation to the heart.[1,2]

III. Breathing and Lung Mechanics

The generation of a breath, which allows for the inflow of atmospheric air into the lungs and outflow of carbon dioxide–rich air from the alveoli, is a function of periodic changes in partial pressure gradients. The manner in which pressure gradients are achieved depends on whether a breath is spontaneously or mechanically generated.

A. Spontaneous Ventilation

Except in the case of alveolar collapse, the pressure within the alveoli is greater than the intrathoracic pressure surrounding the lung parenchyma. This alveolar pressure is generally atmospheric at end expiration and end inspiration. Intrapleural pressure is approximately −5 cm water (H_2O) at end expiration and can be approximated with an esophageal balloon. Using zero as a reference for atmospheric pressure during a no-flow state at end expiration, the end-expiratory transpulmonary pressure (TPP) can be calculated:

$$P_{transpulmonary} = P_{alveolar} - P_{intrapleural}$$
$$P_{transpulmonary} = 0 \text{ cm } H_2O - (-5 \text{ cm } H_2O)$$
$$P_{transpulmonary} = 5 \text{ cm } H_2O$$

When the diaphragm and intercostal muscles contract and inspiration occurs, the intrathoracic volume increases and a new intrapleural pressure is generated, approximately −8 to −9 cm H_2O. Alveolar pressure also decreases to −3 to −4 cm H_2O, maintaining the TPP at 5 cm H_2O, but generating a pressure gradient between the alveoli and upper airway. This change allows for air to flow down the gradient into the alveoli leading to expansion of alveoli and participation in gas exchange.

When the diaphragm and intercostals relax, the intrapleural pressure returns to −5 cm H_2O. TPP does not support the expanded alveoli at these intrathoracic volumes, and they begin to collapse. The air flows from the alveoli out toward the upper airway, and the previous end-expiratory pressures and alveolar size are reestablished.

B. Mechanical Ventilation

Most mechanical ventilation modes involve the application of positive pressure with each breath. As positive pressure is delivered, the alveoli expand, and gas flows to the alveoli until alveolar pressure equals that in the upper airway. When the positive pressure breath is stopped, expiration occurs passively until another positive pressure breath is delivered[2,3] (Chapter 42: Critical Care).

C. Movement of the Lung Parenchyma

The movement of the lung tissue itself is passive and depends on overcoming two types of resistance: elastic resistance of the lung parenchyma, chest wall, and gas-liquid interface in the alveoli and nonelastic resistance of the airways to gas flow. The work necessary to overcome these two resistances is the physiologic work of breathing.

D. Elastic Resistance

Both the lung parenchyma and thoracic cavity have their own elastic recoil properties. The tendency of the lungs to collapse is due to the high number of elastin fibers within the tissue as well as the surface tension at the air-fluid interface of the alveoli. The tendency of the chest wall is to move outward due to its structural makeup and muscle tone.

E. Surface Tension

Alveoli are lined by a thin surface fluid layer. This fluid layer creates surface tension favoring collapse of the alveolus. In order for the alveolus to remain inflated, the pressure keeping the alveolus open must be greater than the surface tension created by the surface fluid layer. Laplace law helps to quantify the pressure within the alveolus with a given surface tension:

$$\text{Pressure} = \frac{2 \times \text{Surface tension}}{\text{Radius}}$$

As demonstrated by the equation, the higher the surface tension, the greater the propensity of the alveolus to collapse. To overcome this tendency to collapse, the lung produces surfactant at the gas-fluid interface. Surfactant reduces surface tension, allowing the alveolus to more readily stay expanded. The higher the concentration of surfactant in an alveolus, the more the surface tension is reduced. Conversely, as the concentration decreases, the effect on surface tension decreases. This relationship helps to stabilize the alveoli. As the alveolus decreases in size, the concentration of surfactant increases, helping to prevent collapse. As the alveolus begins to over distend, the surfactant concentration decreases and alveolar shrinkage is favored.[2,3]

F. Compliance

Compliance is a useful measure of elastic recoil. It is defined as a change in volume divided by the change in pressure:

$$C = \Delta V / \Delta P$$

The higher the pressure needed to produce a specific change in volume, the lower the compliance of the system and the higher the elastic recoil of that same system.

Compliance can be calculated for both the lung and the chest wall separately. Normal lung compliance is 150 to 200 mL/cm H_2O and is defined as

$$C_{\text{Lung}} = \frac{\text{Change in lung volume}}{\text{Change in transpulmonary pressure}}$$

Chest wall compliance is normally 100 mL/cm H_2O and is defined as

$$C_{\text{Chest wall}} = \frac{\text{Change in chest volume}}{\text{Change in transthoracic pressure}}$$

where transthoracic pressure equals atmospheric pressure minus intrapleural pressure.

Total respiratory compliance of chest wall and lung compliance is normally 80 to 100 mL/cm H_2O. It is defined mathematically as

$$1/C_T = (1/C_{\text{Lung}}) = (1/C_{\text{Chest well}})$$
$$C_T = \text{total compliance}$$

Compliance can be affected by the presence of secretions, inflammation, fibrosis, fluid overload, and a host of other factors. It is a useful measure, especially in the setting of mechanical ventilation, to demonstrate worsening or improvement of lung mechanics.[2,3]

G. Transpulmonary Pressure

Transpulmonary pressure (TPP) is the true distending pressure within the alveoli. Calculation of the TPP requires the measurement of intrapleural pressure, but this is rarely done directly. Rather, esophageal pressure, a surrogate marker of pleural pressure, can be measured with an esophageal balloon catheter. Titration of positive end-expiratory pressure (PEEP) to maintain a zero to positive TPP can improve alveolar overdistention/collapse leading to improved lung recruitment. TPP = alveolar pressure − esophageal pressure.[4] Plateau pressure is a surrogate of alveolar pressure. For example, if a patient continues to be hypoxemic with a plateau pressure of 20 cm H_2O, the PEEP should be titrated up to where the measured esophageal pressure is 20 cm H_2O to maintain a TPP of zero (**Figure 2.1**).

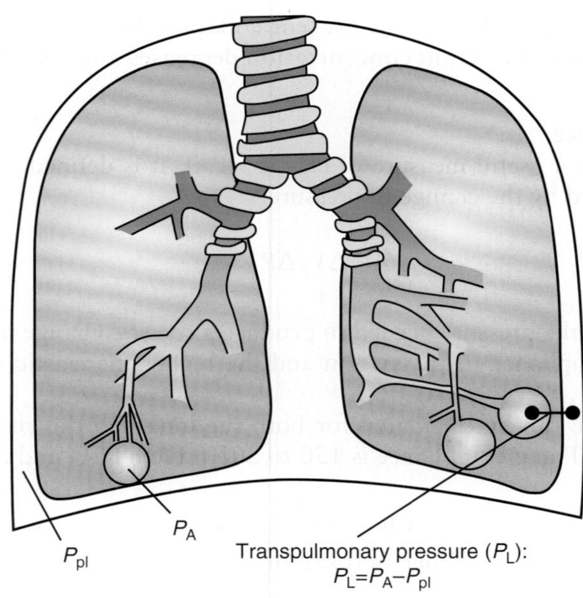

Figure 2.1 Transpulmonary pressure (P_L), alveolar pressure (P_A), and pleural pressure (P_{pl}). This figure shows $P_L = P_A - P_{pl}$. When placing an esophageal balloon, the esophageal pressure would be a surrogate of the P_{pl} allowing for the calculation of the P_L.

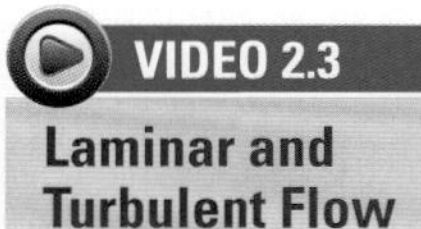

IV. Resistance to Gas Flow

Airway resistance to gas flow must also be overcome by the respiratory system. Normal airway resistance is 1-3 cm H_2O/L/sec.[5] During a respiratory cycle, gas simultaneously flows both in laminar and turbulent patterns. The physics of the two gas flow patterns are markedly different, altering the airway resistance presented to the respiratory system.

A. Laminar Flow

In laminar gas flow, the velocity of gas decreases away from the center of gas flow. In other words, maximal gas flow velocity is in the centermost area of gas flow. This type of flow is usually inaudible on physical examination. Resistance to laminar flow is described by the following equation:

$$R = \frac{8 \times \text{length} \times \text{viscosity}}{\pi \times (\text{radius})^4 \text{ flow}}$$

In laminar flow, airway radius influences resistance to gas flow by a power of 4. Viscosity increases resistance, but density has no effect on resistance in laminar gas flow. Less dense gases such as helium will not improve gas flow in the setting of laminar flow.

B. Turbulent Flow

Flow through branched or disordered tubes often produces a disruption of laminar flow resulting in turbulent flow. At high flow rates, turbulent flow can occur even in an unbranched system. In contrast to laminar flow, where the centermost gas has the maximum velocity, turbulent flow advances at

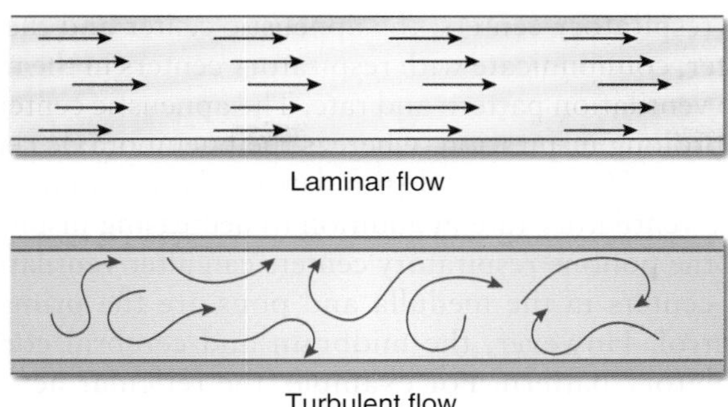

Figure 2.2 Illustration of laminar and turbulent flow.

the same velocity throughout the gas stream. The mathematical computation of turbulent flow is complex. Resistance to gas flow is proportional to the flow rate of gas in turbulent flow in contrast to laminar flow where resistance is inversely proportional to flow rate. Although laminar flow is sensitive to changes in radius, turbulent flow is even more so sensitive to changes in radius. Changes in airway radius result in a change in resistance to a power of five in turbulent flow, whereas in laminar flow, the change in resistance is to a power of four. Lastly, resistance to turbulent flow is directly proportional to gas density rather than viscosity. As gas density decreases, resistance decreases as well. It is in cases of turbulent flow and increased airway resistance that less dense gases such as helium are useful[2,3] (**Figure 2.2**).

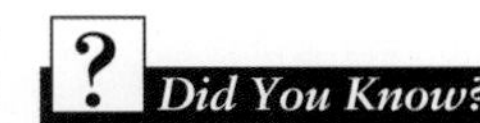

Helium is useful to decrease resistance to flow only if flow is turbulent—as one might observe during asthma.

V. Ventilation

Arguably, the central function of the pulmonary system is oxygen and carbon dioxide gas exchange. Ventilation, movement of gas in and out of the lungs, is essential for continued exchange to occur at the level of the alveolus and pulmonary capillary membrane. Respiratory centers in the brain normally control ventilation. As anesthetic management often alters normal ventilation, a thorough understanding of ventilatory physiology is essential to the practice of anesthesiology and critical care medicine.

A. Respiratory Centers

Basal ventilation is controlled by respiratory centers located in the brain stem, particularly the medulla and the pons. They process an array of information to determine a ventilation rate and pattern and can function independent of an intact cerebrum.[6]

The medulla oblongata contains the most basic ventilation control centers, the dorsal respiratory group (DRG) and the ventral respiratory group (VRG). The DRG provides for a ventilation rate by rhythmically stimulating inspiration. The VRG, conversely, coordinates exhalation. The DRG stimulates inspiration, which is followed by a signal by the VRG to extinguish the stimulation from the DRG, halting active inspiratory effort and allowing for passive exhalation. Without the VRG, DRG activity results in an irregular breathing pattern characterized by maximum inspiratory efforts and bouts of apnea. In this manner, the DRG and VRG work in combination, resulting in rhythmic ventilation.

The pontine respiratory centers, the apneustic center and the pneumotaxic respiratory center, communicate with respiratory centers in the medulla oblongata to alter the ventilation pattern and rate. The apneustic center sends signals to the DRG to prolong inspiration, whereas the pneumotaxic center functions to limit inspiration. With increased stimulation, the pneumotaxic center will also increase the ventilatory rate in addition to decreasing inspiratory volume. In this fashion, the pontine respiratory centers can alter ventilation.

Respiratory centers in the medulla and pons are the primary centers of ventilation control. However, the midbrain and cerebral cortex may also affect the ventilatory pattern. For example, the reticular activating system in the midbrain increases rate and volume of inspiration with activation. Reflexes can also alter ventilation. Both the swallowing and vomiting reflex result in a cessation of inspiration to avoid aspiration. The cough reflex is stimulated by irritation of the trachea and requires a deep inspiration followed by a forced exhalation against momentarily closed vocal cords to create an expulsive maneuver to be effective at clearing irritants and secretions. Smooth muscle spindles in the airways of lungs likely react to pressure changes from pulmonary edema or atelectasis, providing proprioception for the lung and resulting in ventilatory alterations. Golgi tendon organs, tendon spindles primarily located in intercostal muscles, are stimulated when stretched, inhibiting further inspiration. The Hering-Breuer reflex, although weakly present in humans, may also alter ventilation by inhibiting inspiration during lung distention. In this manner, reflexes and higher brain centers affect ventilation patterns established by respiratory centers in the brain stem.

B. Chemical Ventilatory Control

The respiratory centers regulate ventilation based on the relative chemical content of oxygen and carbon dioxide. Central and peripheral chemoreceptors provide chemical environmental data to the respiratory centers.[7]

Central chemoreceptors are located in the medulla and relay information on ventilation needs based on pH. Despite not being directly sensed, carbon dioxide has a potent effect on central chemoreceptors by conversion to hydrogen ions altering the pH:

$$CO_2 + H_2O \rightarrow H_2CO_3 \rightarrow H^+ + HCO_3^-.$$

As carbon dioxide readily passes the blood-brain barrier, it is converted into hydrogen ions, stimulating the central chemoreceptors in the medulla. The response to elevations in carbon dioxide is rapid, resulting in increases in tidal volume and ventilation rate within 1 to 2 minutes. Over several hours, the response to sustained elevations in carbon dioxide diminishes as bicarbonate ions are likely transported into the cerebrospinal fluid, neutralizing the stimulating hydrogen ions formed by elevated carbon dioxide levels. The ability of the cerebrospinal fluid to alter and neutralize its hydrogen ions over time explains the respiratory center's response to chronic versus acute elevations in carbon dioxide levels. Of note, central chemoreceptors will also decrease ventilation secondary to hypothermia, but most importantly, they respond to changes in hydrogen ion concentrations secondary to carbon dioxide concentrations.

Carotid body chemoreceptors deliver signals to the respiratory centers based on oxygen and carbon dioxide content from the periphery. These peripheral chemoreceptors are found at the bifurcation of the common carotid artery and communicate to the respiratory centers via the afferent glossopharyngeal nerve. Carotid body chemoreceptors also deliver signals of acidosis, both from metabolic and elevated carbon dioxide causes, although signals of increased acidosis from peripheral chemoreceptors have minimal effects on ventilation. Aortic body chemoreceptors found around the aortic arch also deliver signals regarding partial pressure of oxygen via the vagus nerve. This signal leads primarily to changes in circulation with minimal effects on ventilation.

Breath holding and the ventilatory response to altitude aptly illustrate chemoreceptor signal integration by respiratory centers. Knowing that central carbon dioxide–sensing chemoreceptors override peripheral oxygen-sensing chemoreceptors aids in understanding the process of chemoreceptor ventilatory control. With significant altitude elevation, the arterial partial pressure of oxygen (Pao_2) decreases, thereby stimulating the peripheral carotid body chemoreceptor to acutely increase ventilation. The increased ventilation in turn lowers carbon dioxide levels, decreasing the hydrogen ion concentration, resulting in inhibition of ventilation from the central chemoreceptors. The increased signal from the peripheral chemoreceptors coupled with the decreased drive from the central chemoreceptors results in a new equilibrium. These changes cause increased ventilation but continued hypoxemia, likely the cause of the headache associated with altitude sickness. With time, renal compensation allows bicarbonate ions to be removed from the cerebrospinal fluid to normalize hydrogen ion concentration. The normalization removes inhibition of ventilation from the central chemoreceptors, allowing the respiratory centers to comply with the ventilatory signal transmitted by the peripheral chemoreceptors responding to hypoxemia. Mountain climbers routinely practice acclimatization to allow chemoreceptors to function with physiologically appropriate outcomes.

Breath holding, a common childhood game, also clearly demonstrates chemoreceptor ventilatory physiology. The combination of stimulating signals from the central chemoreceptors, at arterial carbon dioxide partial pressure ($Paco_2$) of 50 mm Hg and peripheral chemoreceptors at Pao_2 of 65 mm Hg, compels adults to breathe. With breath holding, the Pao_2 decreases to approximately 65 mm Hg within 1 minute, while the $Paco_2$ increases 12 mm Hg in the first minute and then 6 mm Hg per minute thereafter.[8] Most adults can hold their breath for a minute, reaching $Paco_2$ levels of 65 mm Hg and Pao_2 levels of 50 mm Hg. If one inhales supplemental oxygen, minimizing ventilatory signals from the peripheral chemoreceptors, ventilation does not occur until $Paco_2$ levels reach 60 mm Hg or in 2 to 3 minutes. Hyperventilation with supplemental oxygen can depress $Paco_2$ to 20 mm Hg, allowing breath holding to continue for approximately 5 minutes. Notably, hyperventilation without supplemental oxygen can be deleterious and result in unconsciousness as the hypoxemic ventilatory drive from peripheral oxygen-sensing chemoreceptor is outweighed by central carbon dioxide–sensing chemoreceptors. Thus, hyperventilating room air prior to a prolonged underwater swim is highly inadvisable!

Graphic representation of carbon dioxide and oxygen response curves allows for quantitative understanding of ventilation control. The $Paco_2$ and Pao_2 ventilation response curves represent resultant ventilation at different levels of $Paco_2$ and Pao_2, respectively. The $Paco_2$ ventilation response curve is fairly linear in the normal range (**Figure 2.3**). The change in ventilatory

? Did You Know?

Signaling to the respiratory centers is initiated at arterial partial pressure of oxygen (PaO_2) <100 mm Hg, but ventilation is not altered until oxygen partial pressure falls below 65 mm Hg, at which point tidal volume and ventilation rate are increased.

? Did You Know?

Peripheral carotid body chemoreceptors respond primarily to lack of oxygen, while central chemoreceptors react to elevations in carbon dioxide.

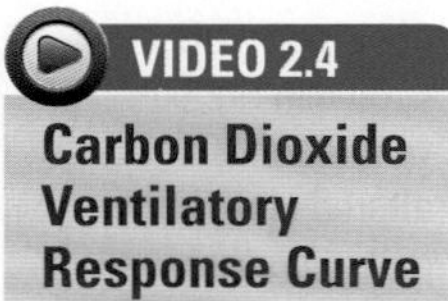

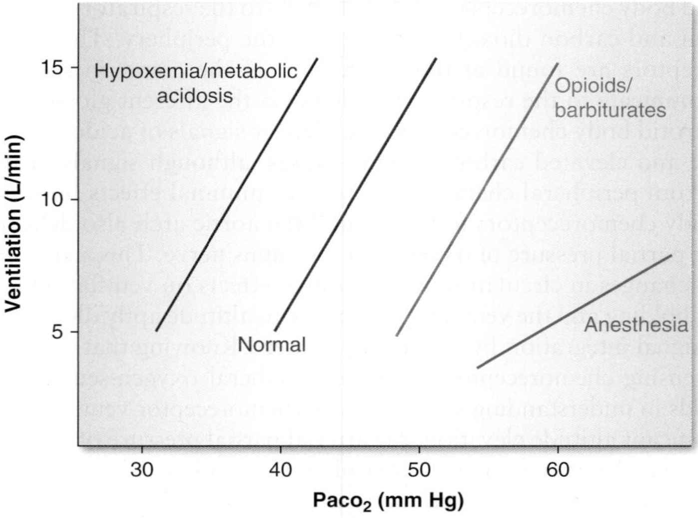

Figure 2.3 Carbon dioxide ventilatory response curve. The linear ventilatory response to carbon dioxide in the normal physiologic range is illustrated by the blue curve. Ventilation response is increased with hypoxemia and metabolic acidosis and decreased with respiratory depressants as depicted by the red and green curves, respectively. Anesthesia results in a decreased rate of ventilatory response, as seen with the yellow curve.

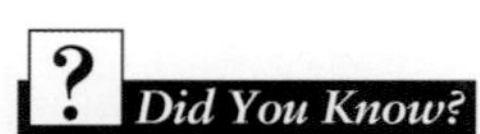

With $PaCO_2$ levels >80 mm Hg, CO_2 acts as a ventilatory depressant and hypnotic.

response increases at $Paco_2$ > 80 mm Hg, resulting in a parabolic graph, and peaks at about 100 mm Hg, the point at which carbon dioxide becomes a ventilatory depressant. The $Paco_2$ response curve may be shifted left with arterial hypoxemia, the peripheral chemoreceptor response, metabolic acidosis, or a central nervous system etiology. The left shift will result in an increase in minute ventilation at constant $Paco_2$ levels. The response to $Paco_2$ may be decreased with opioids or barbiturates, which act as ventilatory depressants, shifting the response curve to the right. Opioids result in decreased minute ventilation with decreased respiratory rates and increased tidal volumes, while barbiturates and inhaled anesthetics initially result in increased ventilatory rates with decreased tidal volumes. Continued administration of barbiturates or inhalational anesthetics will eventually depress the ventilatory response to $Paco_2$, resulting in a flatter curve.

The Pao_2 ventilation response curve depends on the concurrent $Paco_2$ level.[9] Holding $Paco_2$ levels constant illustrates the sole effect of Pao_2 on ventilation (**Figure 2.4**). At normocarbic levels, peripheral chemoreceptors will stimulate ventilation at levels of Pao_2 below 65 mm Hg. With hypercarbia, the signals from peripheral chemoreceptors lead to increased ventilation only when Pao_2 levels are below 100 mm Hg, the level at which peripheral chemoreceptors begin to send impulses to the respiratory centers. Normally, however, as humans increase ventilation, $Paco_2$ levels decrease. As $Paco_2$ levels decrease, the ventilatory impulse from central chemoreceptors is decreased to the point where ventilation signals from the peripheral chemoreceptors are muffled, leading to a decreased ventilatory response. This phenomenon results in depressed oxygen-mediated ventilatory response compared to situations where $Paco_2$ levels are normal.

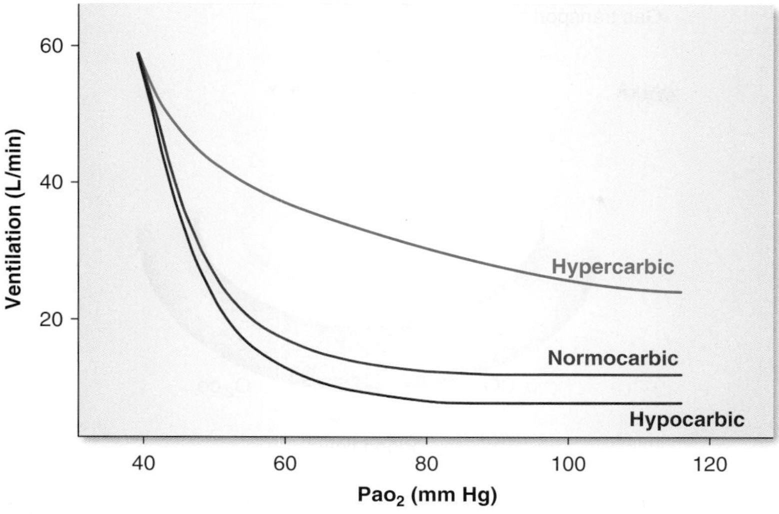

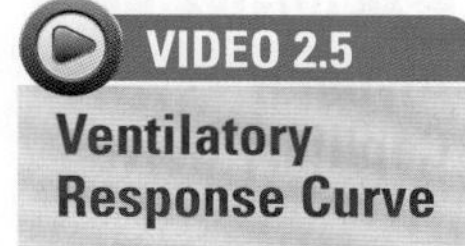

Figure 2.4 Oxygen ventilatory response curve. At normocarbic and hypocarbic levels, ventilation is stimulated at arterial carbon dioxide partial pressure (Pao_2) of 60 mm Hg, as illustrated by the blue and red curves, respectively. With hypercarbia, ventilation is stimulated at Pao_2 levels below 100 mm Hg, as seen with the green curve. Importantly, note that carbon dioxide levels are constant along curves in this figure.

Oxygen at supratherapeutic levels may be detrimental. In patients who depend on peripheral chemoreceptors for hypoxic ventilatory drive (of which there are very few), $Pao_2 > 65$ mm Hg will likely suppress ventilation and result in hypercarbia. Supratherapeutic oxygen delivery may also lead to free radical injury, resulting in acute lung injury.

A low level of carbon dioxide leads to suppression of ventilatory drive, cerebral vasoconstriction, and lowered plasma calcium ion concentration secondary to alkalosis. Conversely, elevated carbon dioxide may result in increased sympathetic output, causing tachycardia and hypertension, and will independently cause cerebral vasodilation. Elevated carbon dioxide can also act to cause disorientation with further increases leading to unconsciousness. Thus, the respiratory centers rely on impulse generation from chemoreceptors to maintain carbon dioxide and oxygen at physiologic levels.

VI. Oxygen and Carbon Dioxide Transport

Introduction of oxygen and removal of carbon dioxide are essential to normal cellular metabolism. Movement of these gases between the environment and tissue is complex, relying on both simple diffusion and carrier molecules.

A. Oxygen and Carbon Dioxide Transport in Lungs

Oxygen is first inhaled from the environment and travels down the airways as a component of air by convection secondary to the force generated from the energy of inspiration. As air reaches the distal airways, diffusion becomes the predominant mode of gas transport (**Figure 2.5**). Diffusion allows for movement of molecules across a distance to an area of lower concentration in an energy-independent manner. The pulmonary capillaries transport blood to alveoli, which has a lower partial pressure of oxygen than the air entrained into the alveoli. The lower partial

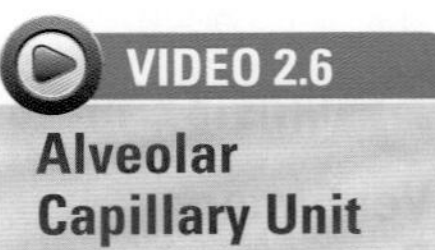

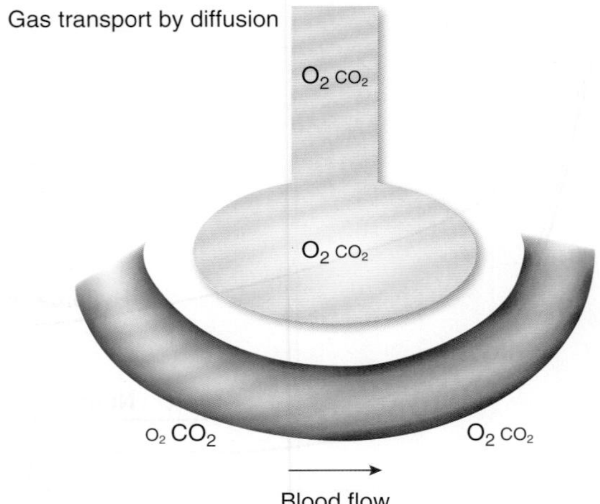

Figure 2.5 The transport of oxygen and carbon dioxide in terminal airways and across the alveolar-capillary membrane is dependent on diffusion. A larger font indicates a relative higher partial pressure of carbon dioxide or oxygen compared with a smaller font. Carbon dioxide and oxygen molecules move along a diffusion gradient from higher to lower partial pressures.

pressure of oxygen in blood creates a diffusion gradient, allowing oxygen to diffuse across the alveolar membrane into the pulmonary capillary bed. Relative concentrations of oxygen drive the movement of oxygen into the blood. This phenomenon also allows oxygenation in the absence of ventilation, apneic oxygenation, provided a diffusion gradient is present. Similarly, pulmonary capillary blood arrives at the alveoli with a relatively rich carbon dioxide concentration, allowing carbon dioxide to diffuse from the blood into the alveoli. The pulmonary diffusion capacity or the ability of carbon dioxide to pass between the alveoli to blood is 20 times greater than oxygen, allowing for it to diffuse across the alveolar membrane with greater efficiency. After oxygen diffuses from the alveoli to the pulmonary capillary bed, oxygen from terminal airways will then diffuse into the alveoli. Concurrently, carbon dioxide newly introduced into the alveoli is transported along a diffusion gradient in a reverse pathway until it reaches the upper airways for exhalation by ventilation. The pulmonary capillary blood, which has now absorbed oxygen from and released carbon dioxide to the alveoli, propagates forward. This exchange allows for new oxygen-poor and carbon dioxide–rich blood to interact with the alveoli. By this process, diffusion allows for oxygen and carbon dioxide to be exchanged at the alveoli–pulmonary capillary interface. Note that diffusion is a passive process. Oxygen and carbon dioxide are not actively selected. If the partial pressure of oxygen in the alveoli is decreased by significantly elevated carbon dioxide levels, diffusion hypoxia may result as the diffusion gradient for oxygen is diminished. Diffusion allows gas exchange to occur along a concentration gradient from the airways across the alveolar-capillary membrane to the blood.

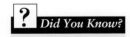

? *Did You Know?*

The diffusing capacity of carbon dioxide is 20 times greater than that of oxygen.

B. Oxygen and Carbon Dioxide Transport in Blood

The transport of oxygen and carbon dioxide in the blood depends on hemoglobin.[10] Oxygen is transported in the blood both bound to hemoglobin and dissolved in blood. Oxygen dissolved in blood is a small fraction of the amount bound to hemoglobin. Hemoglobin is a complex molecule consisting of four heme subunits, with each subunit binding a molecule of oxygen. The binding of oxygen to hemoglobin is illustrated by the oxygen-hemoglobin dissociation

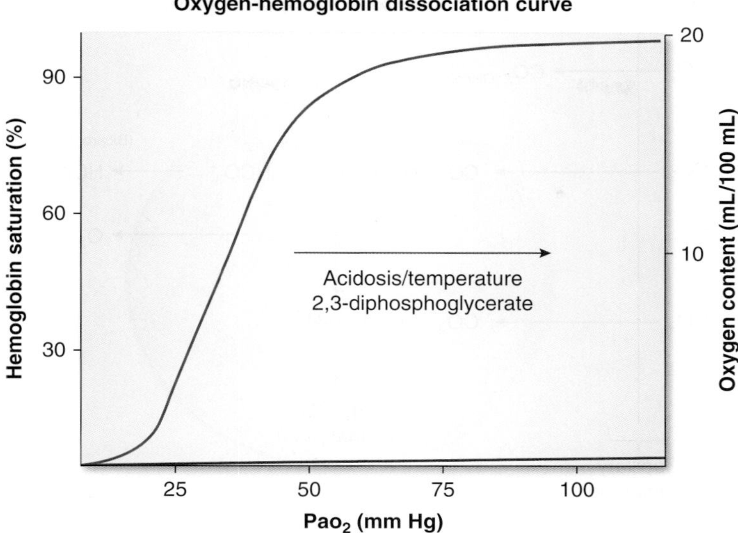

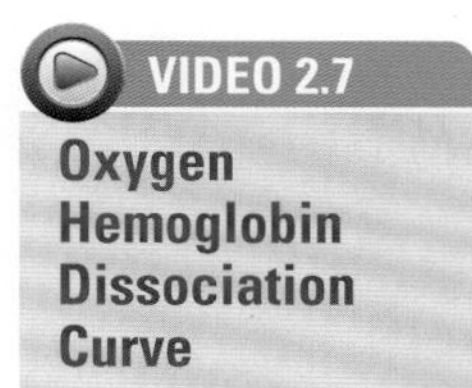

Figure 2.6 The oxygen-hemoglobin dissociation curve (blue curve) demonstrates that a majority of oxygen content is bound to hemoglobin at partial pressures of 60 mm Hg. The linear portion of the curve allows for oxygen unloading at partial pressures of oxygen found in the peripheral systemic capillary beds, the site of tissue oxygenation. Furthermore, increases in acidosis, temperature, and 2,3-diphosphoglycerate decrease hemoglobin's affinity for oxygen, allowing for increased oxygen supply to areas with increased metabolic needs as evidenced by increase temperature, acidosis, and deoxygenated hemoglobin. Of note, the majority of oxygen content is found bound to hemoglobin, as seen by the small portion of oxygen content supplied by oxygen dissolved in blood (*red curve*).

curve (**Figure 2.6**). The curve demonstrates two important concepts. First, it demonstrates that hemoglobin allows the blood to carry a large content of oxygen, even at the low partial pressure of 60 mm Hg of oxygen. Second, the linear part of the curve allows for delivery of a significant amount of oxygen with just a slight change in partial pressures of oxygen, allowing for oxygen unloading to tissues. The affinity of hemoglobin for oxygen is altered under certain conditions. Affinity for oxygen by hemoglobin is decreased by acidosis, elevation in temperature, and increased levels of 2,3-diphosphoglycerate (a by-product of red blood cell metabolism), which aids partially deoxygenated hemoglobin to release further oxygen. This decreased affinity, however, is beneficial as it allows for unloading of oxygen from hemoglobin in tissues with higher metabolic requirements, as evidenced by increased acidosis, temperature, and deoxygenated hemoglobin. The Bohr effect specifically describes hemoglobin's decreased affinity for oxygen in environments with carbon dioxide elevation or acidosis.

Carbon dioxide is transported in the blood in three different forms (**Figure 2.7**). It is either dissolved in blood, transported as bicarbonate, or exists a carbamino compound. The solubility of carbon dioxide is much greater than oxygen, accounting for approximately 10% of the carbon dioxide transported in venous blood. Bicarbonate, the form in which the bulk of carbon dioxide is transported, is formed by carbonic anhydrase enzymes in the red blood cells. The formation of bicarbonate results in hydrogen ions as a by-product. As hemoglobin releases oxygen, it becomes deoxygenated and readily accepts hydrogen ions, acting as a buffer and favoring the formation of further

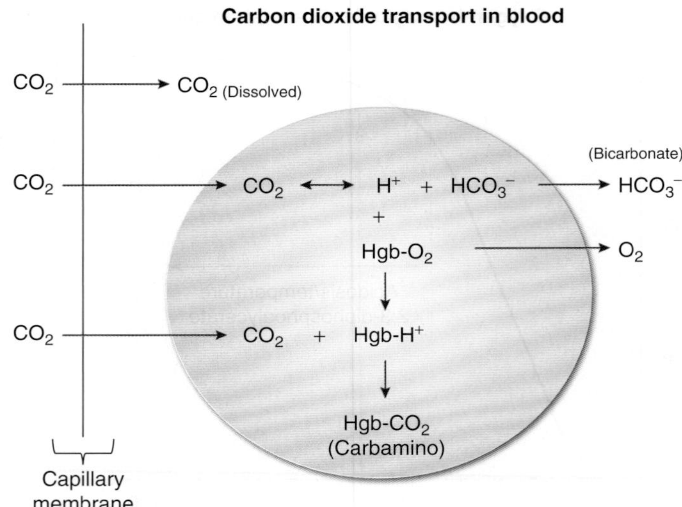

Figure 2.7 Three forms of carbon dioxide (CO_2) transport in blood are illustrated. CO_2 enters the capillary and a portion is dissolved in blood. A majority of CO_2 enters the red blood cells and is converted to bicarbonate (HCO_3^-), which is transported in the blood. The conversion of CO_2 to HCO_3^- results in hydrogen ions (H^+), which are stabilized by deoxyhemoglobin as depicted by Hgb-H^+. Stabilization of the H^+ favors the formation of more HCO_3^- and allows Hgb-H^+ to form a carbamino compound, the third form taken by carbon dioxide.

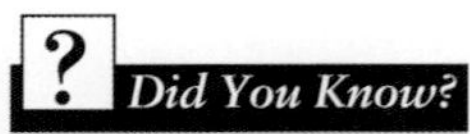

Ten percent of carbon dioxide in blood is dissolved, and the bulk of carbon dioxide is transported and stored as bicarbonate.

bicarbonate. Additionally, deoxygenated hemoglobin buffered with hydrogen ions can bind carbon dioxide, allowing transport in the form of a carbamino compound. The ***Haldane effect*** is the ability of deoxygenated hemoglobin to transport carbon dioxide by facilitating the formation of bicarbonate and acting as a buffer for formed hydrogen ions and as a carbamino compound. Basically, the ability of blood to transport carbon dioxide is increased with lower oxygen concentrations.

VII. Ventilation and Perfusion

In order for gas exchange to occur, ventilated alveoli must be exposed to blood within pulmonary capillaries. Physiologically, lungs are heterogeneous. Alveoli are exposed to varying amounts of ventilation and perfusion.[11] However, the matching of ventilation and perfusion is paramount to oxygen and carbon dioxide exchange.

A. Ventilation and Perfusion Distribution

Ventilation distribution within the lung depends on the compliance of alveoli and the relative distending pressure. Theoretically, the pressure within all the alveoli in the lung is constant, but the pressure outside the alveoli is heterogeneous throughout the lung, resulting in different-sized alveoli (**Figure 2.8**). In the upright position, alveoli are resting at larger inflated volumes at the apex compared with the base of the lung secondary to greater compression from gravitational pressure of alveoli at the base. The alveoli at the base are relatively less inflated; however, at rest, they are more compliant. As the lungs are inflated, the basal alveoli receive more ventilation because they are at a more compliant point than apical alveoli and the distending pressure is greater.

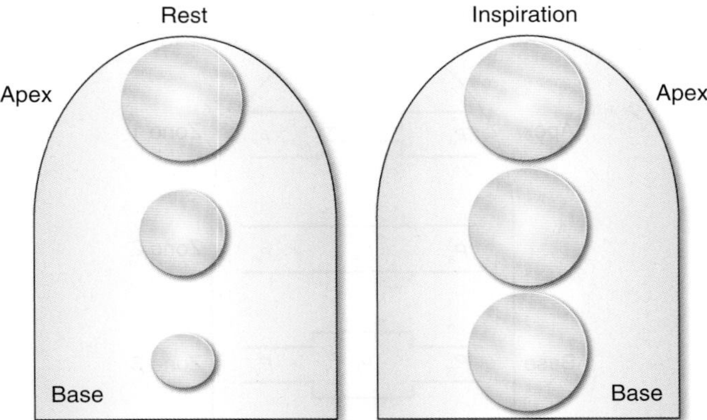

Figure 2.8 Ventilation distribution. Apical alveoli are distended compared with basal alveoli at rest secondary to greater compressive force at the base of the lung, as depicted by the three different alveolar positions at rest. The less distended basal alveoli are therefore resting at a more compliant position than the distended apical alveoli. With inspiration, the basal alveoli are exposed to greater ventilation, while the apical alveoli see minimal ventilation, as illustrated by the change in distention between the alveoli from rest to inspiration.

Ventilation distribution is also affected by anatomy and flow rates. Central regions of the lung are preferentially ventilated, but as flow rates are increased, this ventilatory difference is minimized. Simply stated, during spontaneous ventilation, more gas is distributed to gravity-dependent areas.

Alveolar perfusion is also heterogeneous in the lung and depends mainly on gravity (**Figure 2.9**). Gravity increases the flow of blood to dependent areas. West et al[12] divided the lung into three zones based on relative alveolar pressure (P_A), pulmonary artery pressure (P_a), and pulmonary venous pressure (P_v). Physiologically, the pulmonary artery pressure must always exceed pulmonary venous pressure; the zones are described by the degree of alveolar pressure in relation to pulmonary artery and venous pressure. Perfusion depends on the relative resistance to the pulmonary artery pressure in each of the zones. Zone 1 is the area of the lung in which $P_A > P_a > P_v$ and is found in the least gravity-dependent area of the lung. The pulmonary artery pressure is low enough that the alveolar pressure can result in pulmonary capillary compression, limiting perfusion. Zone 2 occurs where $P_a > P_A > P_v$. Fortunately, this zone comprises most of the lung, allowing for matching of perfusion and ventilation. Perfusion in zone 2 is determined by the relative pressure difference between pulmonary artery and alveolar pressure. Zone 3 exists in the most gravity-dependent area where $P_a > P_v > P_A$. In zone 3, perfusion depends on the pulmonary artery and venous pressure gradient. Anatomy also affects the perfusion of the lung. Areas of the lung exposed to greater pulmonary pressures tend to be anatomically closer to the source of pulmonary perfusion, the pulmonary artery. Again, like ventilation, perfusion is greater at gravity-dependent areas.

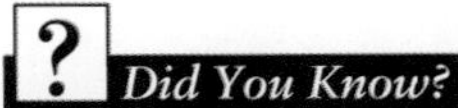

During spontaneous ventilation, both ventilation and perfusion are greater in gravity-dependent areas.

B. Ventilation and Perfusion Relationship

Matching ventilation with perfusion is vital to ensuring carbon dioxide and oxygen gas exchange. Ideally, ventilation would be perfectly matched with perfusion, optimizing the possibility for gas diffusion across the alveolar and

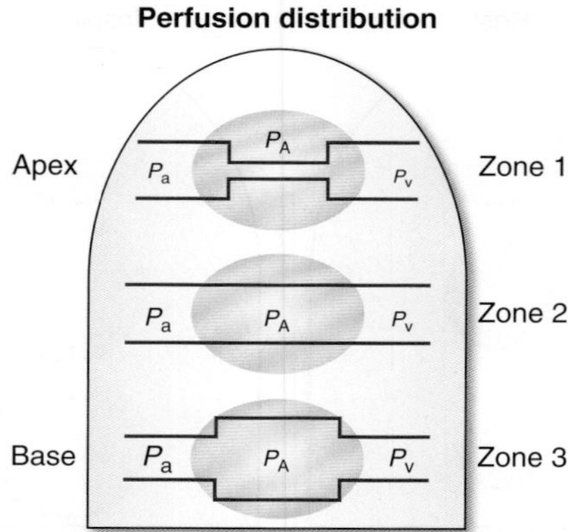

Figure 2.9 Perfusion distribution is heterogeneous throughout the lung. Font size indicates the relative alveolar pressure (P_A), pulmonary arterial pressure (P_a), and pulmonary venous pressure (P_v). At the apex, P_A is greater than P_a and P_v, limiting perfusion as illustrated by the compression of the red capillary resulting in zone 1. At the base, P_a and P_v are greater than P_A, resulting in increased perfusion as depicted by the dilated red capillary resulting in zone 3. P_A is between P_a and P_v in zone 2.

pulmonary capillary membranes. The distribution of ventilation and perfusion, however, is heterogeneous in the lung, resulting in mismatches of ventilation and perfusion (**Figure 2.10**). Mismatches in ventilation and perfusion routinely occur along a continuum.

Ventilation in the excess of perfusion is termed ***dead space***. Dead space is the portion of ventilation inadequately exposed to perfusion, primarily altering carbon dioxide elimination. Dead space can be absolute if the ventilation

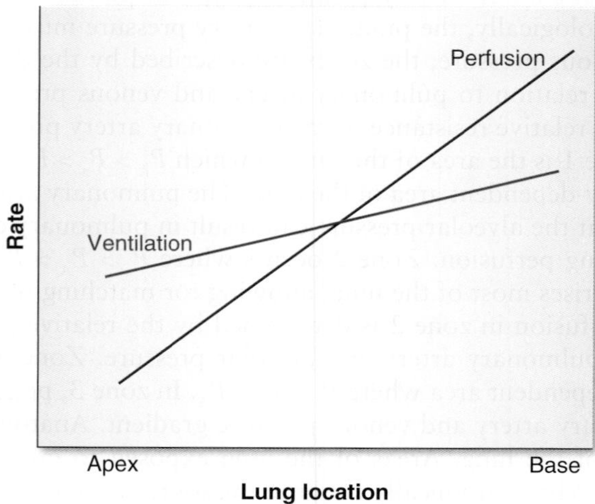

Figure 2.10 Ventilation perfusion matching. Both ventilation and perfusion of alveoli increase at the base compared with the apex, but the rate of increase is greater for perfusion than for ventilation, with progression to the base of the lung. The intersection point indicates where ventilation and perfusion are evenly matched. The area to the right of the intersection point is relative dead space, and the area to the left of the intersection point is relative shunt.

is exposed to no perfusion or relative when the ventilation is exposed to poor perfusion. Dead space is a combination of anatomical and alveolar dead space. ***Anatomical dead space***, an absolute dead space, is the portion of ventilation to structures that are incapable of gas exchange, such as the pharynx, trachea, and large airways. Typically, anatomical dead space is approximately 2 mL/kg. Anatomically, ventilation must first supply anatomical dead space as it is a conduit for gas travel to the alveoli, resulting in an increased proportion of dead space ventilation with decreases in tidal volume. ***Alveolar dead space***, which can be both absolute and relative, consists of ventilation to alveoli with suboptimal perfusion exposure. Approximately one-third of minute ventilation in spontaneously ventilating individuals is dead space. With positive pressure ventilation, dead space ventilation may further increase.

Increased dead space ventilation is a result of either increased ventilation in poorly perfused alveoli, decreases in perfusion locally or globally, or both. Dead space ventilation most often is increased secondary to decreased cardiac output, which results in decreased pulmonary perfusion. Pulmonary perfusion can also be decreased by embolic phenomenon in the pulmonary vasculature. A routine assessment of dead space ventilation is a comparison of end-tidal carbon dioxide and arterial carbon dioxide. If ventilation and perfusion were perfectly matched, end-tidal carbon dioxide and arterial carbon dioxide would, for clinical purposes, be equal as all the ventilated gas would equilibrate with the arterial carbon dioxide. As some of the ventilated gas are not exposed to capillaries carrying carbon dioxide, dead space gas picks up negligible carbon dioxide. This gas returning from under/nonperfused alveoli dilutes the carbon dioxide from the perfusion-exposed ventilation and results in a gradient between alveolar and end-tidal carbon dioxide. As the gradient between end-tidal carbon dioxide to arterial carbon dioxide increases, concerns for pulmonary perfusion are raised. Dead space ventilation is most often a consequence of decreased perfusion when ventilation is stable. Thus, changes in dead space ventilation should be evaluated for changes in cardiac output and pulmonary perfusion.

Perfusion in excess of ventilation is termed ***shunt***. Shunt is the portion of perfusion inadequately exposed to ventilated alveoli and primarily affects oxygenation. Like dead space, shunt may be absolute if the capillary blood flow is exposed to no ventilation or relative if exposed to inadequate ventilation. Relative shunt is also referred to as venous admixture. Normal absolute anatomical shunt is approximately 5% of cardiac output. This results from pleural and bronchial, veins that drain structures of the lung, and Thebesian veins that drain the endocardium, but do not participate in gas exchange with the alveoli. Shunt, both absolute and relative, may also be secondary to pathologic states, such as atelectasis, pulmonary edema, and pneumonia. Shunt is the most common cause of poor oxygenation. Arterial oxygen saturation, however, cannot be used as an assessment for shunt. It does not incorporate the effect of mixed venous blood, the blood that leaves the right heart for gas exchange. If blood leaving the right heart has high oxygen saturation, shunt could be underestimated as this blood would need minimal oxygenation to appear normal. Shunt is better assessed by comparing arterial oxygen and mixed venous saturation levels, requiring a pulmonary artery catheter. Placement of a pulmonary artery catheter is not without consequence. Health care providers often rely on clinical acumen to determine the cause of poor oxygenation, realizing that shunt is often the causative pathophysiology.

Ventilation and perfusion matching is critical. Physiologic mechanisms help to optimize matching. Hypocapnic pulmonary bronchoconstriction is provoked by low carbon dioxide. Dead space ventilation results in low carbon dioxide levels. Bronchoconstriction of dead space airways diverts ventilation to areas with better perfusion, decreasing dead space ventilation. Hypoxic pulmonary vasoconstriction is triggered by low oxygen levels as seen with shunt. Vasoconstriction of shunt pulmonary vasculature diverts blood to better-ventilated regions, decreasing shunt. Hypocapnic pulmonary bronchoconstriction decreases dead space ventilation by decreasing ventilation in lung regions with poor perfusion. Pulmonary hypoxic vasoconstriction decreases shunt by decreasing perfusion to lung areas with poor ventilation. These processes help to improve ventilation and perfusion matching.

VIII. Tissue Oxygenation Assessment

Appropriate tissue oxygenation is a central tenet of anesthetic practice. Quantitative evaluations of oxygenation allow for a better understanding of the etiology of hypoxia or poor tissue oxygenation. The alveolar gas equation calculates the highest possible alveolar partial pressure of oxygen. Also, of importance, the equation demonstrates how increased carbon dioxide concentration will result in decreased arterial oxygenation. As described by the equation, increasing the inspired concentration of oxygen can overcome the deficiency in the oxygen gradient caused by hypoventilation. The equation also allows comparisons of alveolar and arterial oxygen partial pressures. Significant differences between alveolar and arterial partial pressure of oxygen may indicate ventilation-perfusion mismatch or alveolar-pulmonary capillary diffusion impairment. Fortunately, alveolar-pulmonary capillary diffusion impairment is rarely clinically significant and can be overcome with supplemental oxygen except for the most extreme situations.

Ventilation-perfusion mismatch in the form of shunt is the most common cause of poor oxygenation. The amount of shunt can be calculated using the shunt fraction equation or ventilation-perfusion ratio but requires a pulmonary artery to measure mixed venous saturation. If arterial oxygenation is adequate and tissue oxygenation is still poor, the ability to deliver oxygen is investigated. Assuming delivery of blood is adequate with normal cardiovascular function, the oxygen-carrying capacity of blood is analyzed with the oxygen content equation. The oxygen content equation highlights the reliance on hemoglobin to meet tissue oxygen needs. If tissue oxygenation is poor despite adequate arterial oxygenation and hemoglobin content, abnormal hemoglobin or tissue metabolism should be considered. Tissue oxygenation requires complex physiologic processes, which may be better elucidated quantitatively when problems arise.

IX. Lung Volumes

Lung volume varies by the size of the individual, and as such, normal values are generally based on height. Combinations of two or more lung volumes are known as ***capacities*** (**Figure 2.11**).

A. Functional Residual Capacity

The functional residual capacity (FRC) is the amount of air left in the lungs at the end of passive exhalation after a normal breath. It is the combination of the residual volume and expiratory reserve volume. One of its main purposes

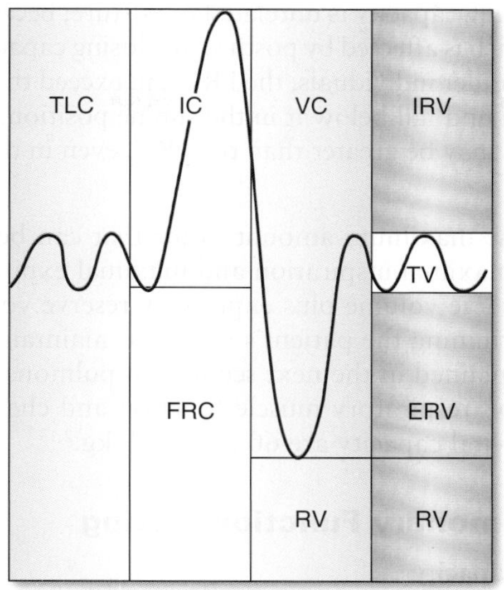

Figure 2.11 Graphical representation of lung volumes and capacities; the four volumes on the right side combine to form total lung capacity. The remainder of the boxes demonstrates the various lung capacities and their relationship to the overlying spirograph. ERV, expiratory reserve volume; FRC, functional residual capacity; IC, inspiratory capacity; IRV, inspiratory reserve volume; RV, residual volume; TLC, total lung capacity; TV, tidal volume; VC, vital capacity. (From Tamul PC, Ault ML. Respiratory function in anesthesia. In: Barash P, Cullen B, Stoelting R, et al, eds. *Clinical Anesthesia*. 7th ed. Wolters Kluwer/Lippincott Williams & Wilkins; 2013:263-285, with permission.)

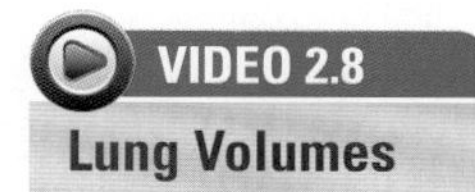

is to serve as an oxygen reservoir during periods of apnea. During apnea, there is still perfusion to the lungs. It is the stored oxygen within the FRC that is obtained by the pulmonary circulation. For this reason, arterial hypoxemia does not occur instantaneously during apnea but rather over a longer period. Reductions in FRC can result in a much shorter period to arterial hypoxemia during apnea.

There are several reasons that FRC can be reduced. Conditions that affect the lung parenchyma directly are pulmonary edema, atelectasis, pulmonary fibrosis, and acute lung injury. Mechanical or functional causes include posture (erect to supine position decreases FRC by 10%), pregnancy, obesity (due to a decrease in chest wall compliance), and abdominal compartment syndrome. These conditions lead to cephalad displacement of abdominal contents. Ventilatory muscle weakness and pleural effusion are also functional causes of hypoxemia.

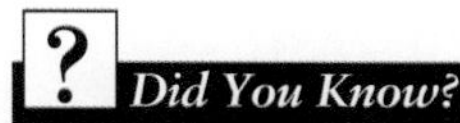

Arterial hypoxemia does not occur instantaneously during apnea because the capillary blood that continues to perfuse the alveoli extracts oxygen from within the FRC.

B. Closing Capacity

Small distal airways with little or no cartilaginous support depend on traction from the elastic recoil of surrounding tissue to remain open. Along with this, small airway patency is dependent on lung volume. The lung volume at which these small airways begin to close is known as the ***closing capacity***.

In young individuals, the FRC far exceeds the closing capacity. As one ages or with obesity, however, the closing capacity steadily increases until it equals or even surpasses that of the FRC. When the closing capacity is reached, alveoli in the affected portions of lung are perfused but not ventilated, which leads to intrapulmonary shunting. This intrapulmonary shunt in combination with a low oxygen reserve in the setting of a low FRC can lead to significant arterial hypoxemia.

Unlike FRC, closing capacity is unrelated to posture; because of this, the relation of the FRC (which is affected by posture) to closing capacity can change with patient position. In older individuals, the FRC can exceed the closing capacity in the upright position and fall below it in the supine position. In elderly patients, the closing capacity may be greater than the FRC, even in the upright position.

C. Vital Capacity

Vital capacity is the maximum amount of air that can be expelled from the lungs after both a maximal inspiration and maximal expiration: tidal volume plus inspiratory reserve volume plus expiratory reserve volume. This value is important for determining the patient's ability to maintain bronchial hygiene by coughing, as explained in the next section on pulmonary function testing. It is dependent upon respiratory muscle function and chest wall compliance. Normal values for vital capacity are 60 to 70 mL/kg.[2,13]

X. Pulmonary Function Testing

A. Forced Vital Capacity

The forced vital capacity (FVC) test is performed by having the patient inhale maximally and then forcefully exhaling as rapidly and thoroughly as possible into a spirometer. The overall volume should be equal to the vital capacity. The value of the FVC is that the measurement is done at maximal expiratory effort over a certain amount of time. As a result, maximal flows can be calculated at particular lung volumes. Because the flow cannot be increased above a maximum rate for a given lung volume at maximal effort, the test results are generally very reproducible with adequate patient cooperation. Normal values of this test are dependent on the patient's height, age, sex, and race.

B. Forced Expiratory Volume

The forced expiratory volume in 1 second (FEV_1) test is performed by measuring the volume of air expired at maximal effort in the first 1 second of exhalation at maximal effort after a maximal inhalation. Because it is a measurement of volume over a specific period, it is a measure of flow. The FEV_1 can be decreased by both obstructive conditions and restrictive conditions, and by poor patient cooperation or poor effort.

C. FEV_1/FVC Ratio

One of the more useful calculations is the ratio of the FEV_1 to the FVC. It helps to elucidate whether a patient has a restrictive or obstructive etiology of decreased FEV_1 and is expressed as a percentage. A normal patient is able to expel 75% to 85% of his or her FVC in the first second of maximal expiratory effort. In patients with a predominantly obstructive process, the FEV_1/FVC ratio is reduced. In restrictive lung processes, the FEV_1 and FVC are generally reduced proportionally to each other, so the ratio is normal to even slightly elevated due to increased elastic recoil of the lung.

D. Forced Expiratory Flow

Another common measurement is the forced expiratory flow (FEF). There are a few different types of FEF measurements. They are differentiated by the point during exhalation of the FVC at which they are measured. One of the more common values is the $FEF_{25\%-50\%}$. It is an average FEF of the middle 50% of the FVC. It is thought to be more sensitive for detection of early, mild obstructive pulmonary processes and it is not effort dependent. Other measures are the $FEF_{50\%}$ and $FEF_{75\%}$, which are the flows present after 50% of

Table 2.1 Pulmonary Function Tests in Restrictive and Obstructive Lung Disease

Value	Restrictive Disease	Obstructive Disease
Definition	Proportional decreases in all lung volumes	Small airway obstruction to expiratory flow
FVC	↓↓↓	Normal or slightly ↑
FEV_1	↓↓↓	Normal or slightly ↓
FEV_1/FVC	Normal	↓↓↓
$FEF_{25\%-75\%}$	Normal	↓↓↓
FRC	↓↓↓	Normal or ↑ if gas trapping
TLC	↓↓↓	Normal or ↑ if gas trapping

FEV, forced expiratory volume; FRC, functional residual capacity; FVC, forced vital capacity; TLC, total lung capacity; ↓↓↓, ↑↑↑, large decrease or increase, respectively; ↓, ↑, small/moderate decrease or increase, respectively.

From Tamul PC, Ault ML. Respiratory function in anesthesia. In: Barash P, Cullen B, Stoelting R, et al, eds. *Clinical Anesthesia*. 8th ed. Wolters Kluwer/Lippincott Williams & Wilkins; 2013:361-383, with permission.

the FVC has been exhaled and 75% has been exhaled, respectively. All these values are decreased in the setting of obstructive pulmonary disease.

E. Maximal Voluntary Ventilation

Maximal voluntary ventilation (MVV) is a pulmonary function test that is used to evaluate a patient's exercise capacity as well as his or her ability to tolerate major surgery. The patient is asked to breathe as hard and as fast as he or she can for 10 to 15 seconds. The total volume over this time is measured and then extrapolated to 1 minute. Numerous conditions can cause a reduction in MVV. These include obstructive and restrictive lung conditions, heart disease, neuromuscular impairment, and lack of patient cooperation or understanding (**Table 2.1**).[2,13]

F. Flow-Volume Loops

Flow-volume loops are graphic representations of the respiratory cycle. The gas flow rate is represented on the x-axis and lung volume on the y-axis (**Figure 2.12**). Notice that expiratory flow in **Figure 2.12** is above zero on the x-axis and inspiratory flow is below. These graphic representations were previously very commonly used to ascertain whether obstruction of large airways was intrathoracic or extrathoracic. With the advent of modern imaging modalities, this method has become less useful, although it is important to note the change in morphology of the curve with different types of obstruction (**Figure 2.13**). As demonstrated in **Figure 2.13**, a variable nonfixed extrathoracic obstruction will produce a flattened curve in the inspiratory part of the cycle. A variable nonfixed intrathoracic obstruction will result in a flattened expiratory portion of the loop. A fixed obstruction produces flattened curves in both parts of the cycle regardless of its position.[2,13]

G. Carbon Monoxide Diffusing Capacity

The transfer of oxygen from the alveolus to erythrocyte is done through diffusion. Three main variables affect the diffusion of oxygen into the bloodstream. They are as follows:

1. Area of the interface between alveolus and capillary—the greater the area, the greater the capacity for diffusion.

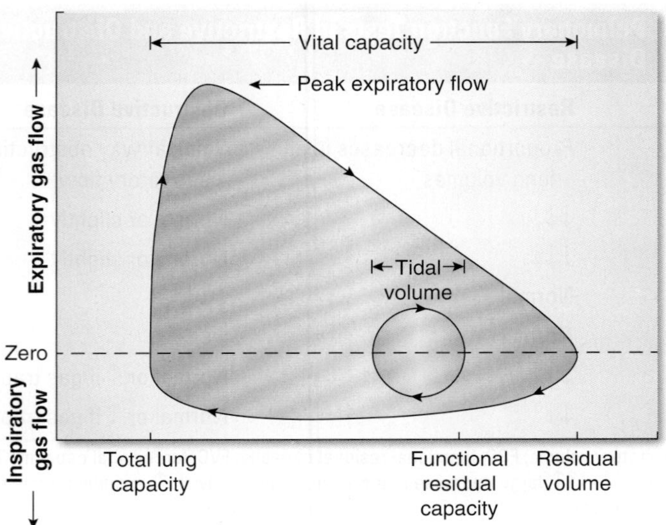

Figure 2.12 **Flow-volume loop in a normal patient.** (From Tamul PC, Ault ML. Respiratory function in anesthesia. In: Barash P, Cullen B, Stoelting R, et al, eds. *Clinical Anesthesia*. 7th ed. Wolters Kluwer/Lippincott Williams & Wilkins; 2013:263-285, with permission.)

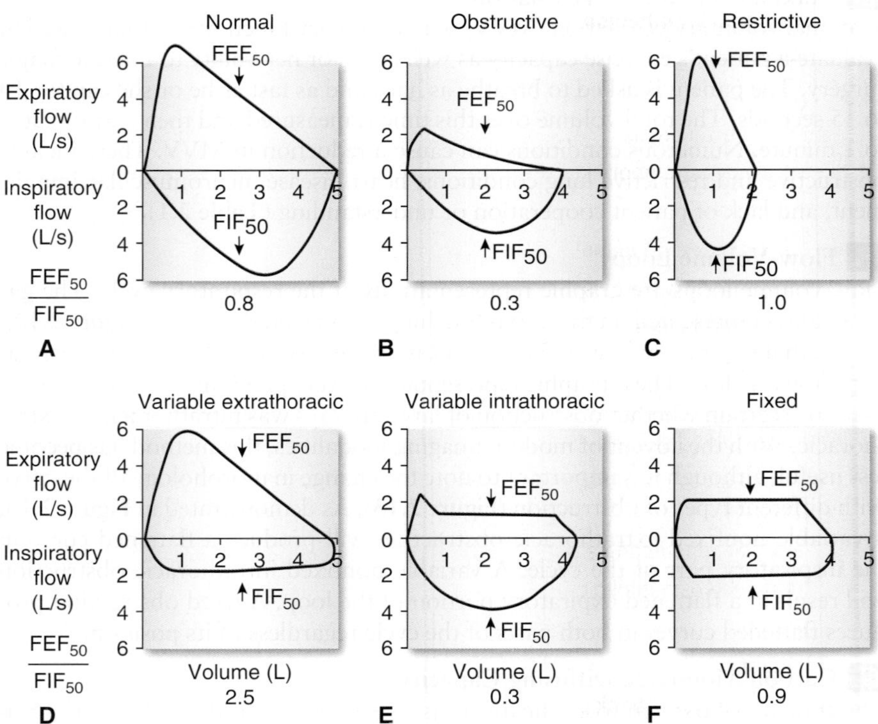

Figure 2.13 **Flow-volume loops in various disease states. FEF, forced expiratory flow; FIF, forced inspiratory flow.** (Redrawn from Spirometry: Dynamic lung volumes. In: Hyatt R, Scanlon P, Nakamura M, eds. *Interpretation of Pulmonary Function Tests: A Practical Guide*. 3rd ed. Philadelphia: Lippincott Williams & Wilkins, 2009:5–25.)

2. Thickness of the membrane between the two—the thicker the membrane, the lower the amount of diffusion.
3. The difference in oxygen tension between alveolar gas and venous blood—the greater the difference, the greater the amount of oxygen diffused.

It is very difficult to measure the diffusing capacity of oxygen because the partial pressure of oxygen varies so greatly over time within the pulmonary vascular system. An ideal surrogate is carbon monoxide whose normal partial pressure within the circulation approaches zero. It has an affinity for hemoglobin that is 20 times stronger than that of oxygen. Therefore, its level throughout the pulmonary circulation remains relatively constant for the purposes of measurement.

The most widely used test to determine the diffusing capacity of the lungs for carbon monoxide (DLCO) is the single breath method. The patient is asked to exhale completely, followed by inhalation to total lung capacity of a gas mixture containing a low concentration of carbon monoxide and an inert gas such as helium. After reaching total lung capacity, the patient is asked to hold his or her breath for 10 seconds, then exhale completely again to residual volume. The concentration of carbon monoxide is then measured in the exhaled sample.

Decreases in the DLCO can be caused by a variety of reasons. These can be divided mainly into conditions that affect the area available for diffusion or increase the thickness of the alveolar-capillary membrane (**Table 2.2**).[14]

Table 2.2 Causes of a Decreased Diffusing Capacity

Decreased *area* for diffusion:
Emphysema
Lung/lobe resection
Bronchial obstruction, as by tumor
Multiple pulmonary emboli
Anemia
Increased *thickness* of alveolar-capillary membrane:
Idiopathic pulmonary fibrosis
Congestive heart failure
Asbestosis
Sarcoidosis involving parenchyma
Collagen vascular disease—scleroderma, systemic lupus erythematosus
Drug-induced alveolitis or fibrosis—bleomycin, nitrofurantoin, amiodarone, methotrexate
Hypersensitivity pneumonitis, including farmer lung
Histiocytosis X (eosinophilic granuloma)
Alveolar proteinosis
Miscellaneous:
High carbon monoxide back pressure from smoking
Pregnancy
Ventilation-perfusion mismatch

From Hyatt R, Scanlon P, Nakamura M. Diffusing capacity of the lungs. In: *Interpretation of Pulmonary Function Tests: A Practical Guide*. 3rd ed. Lippincott Williams & Wilkins; 2009:41-49, with permission.

XI. Preoperative Pulmonary Assessment

Much of the preoperative assessment regarding pulmonary function is aimed at identifying patients who may be at greater risk for postoperative pulmonary complications (PPCs). It is also an opportunity to assess the baseline pulmonary characteristics of the patient that may guide clinical decision-making intra- and postoperatively. For any patient, the most important part of the preoperative evaluation is the history and physical examination. Beyond this, ancillary tests that can be considered are as follows:

- Chest radiography
- Arterial blood gas
- Spirometry

The decision to pursue further testing and the specific tests one orders should be tailored both to the individual patient's condition as well as the operation or procedure the patient is about to undergo. The American Society of Anesthesiologists guidelines on preoperative pulmonary evaluation state that clinicians should "balance the risks and costs of these evaluations against their benefits. Clinical characteristics to consider include type and invasiveness of the surgical procedure, interval from previous evaluation, treated or symptomatic asthma, symptomatic COPD, and scoliosis with restrictive function."[15]

Some conditions that predispose to derangements in pulmonary function are as follows:

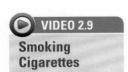

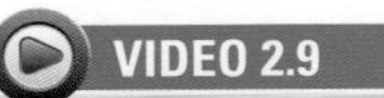

- Chronic lung disease
- Smoking history, persistent cough, or wheezing
- Chest wall and spinal deformities
- Morbid obesity
- Requirement for single-lung ventilation or lung resection
- Severe neuromuscular disease

Again, the most important part of any evaluation regarding pulmonary status is the history and physical examination. Any test that is ordered should be done with a specific purpose in mind, for example, knowing the baseline $Paco_2$ or Pao_2 of a patient with severe chronic obstructive pulmonary disease in order to help guide the decision to extubate at the conclusion of the anesthetic course.[2]

XII. Anesthetic Considerations in Obstructive and Restrictive Lung Disease

A. Obstructive Lung Disease

Patients with obstructive lung disease are predisposed to having more reactive airways that could potentially lead to bronchoconstriction and significant wheezing. Because of this, one should consider administering preoperative bronchodilators and a dose of intravenous corticosteroids. The patient should also be at a relatively deep plane of anesthesia before instrumenting the airway to help lessen the chance of bronchoconstriction; opioids and lidocaine preintubation are also helpful in this regard.

During mechanical ventilation, it is advisable to avoid high respiratory rates and excessive tidal volume to prevent gas trapping and to allow for a longer expiratory time. Longer expiratory time may result in a lower rate of mechanical ventilation, and thus may also require that the selected tidal volume may need to be higher. If tracheal extubation is planned at the conclusion of the procedure, care must be taken to prevent bronchoconstriction and the resultant increase in airway resistance. Extubating the patient at a deep plane of anesthesia and using mask ventilation for emergence is a useful strategy.

B. Restrictive Disease

Patients with restrictive disease have a decrease in all measured lung volumes, including the FRC. These patients typically breath with small tidal volumes at increased rates. As discussed previously, the FRC acts as an oxygen reservoir during periods of apnea. With this reservoir reduced in capacity, patients with restrictive disease tolerate much shorter periods of apnea than normal patients. Rapid desaturation during apnea is common.

These patients will also require smaller tidal volumes and may have elevated peak inspiratory pressures during mechanical ventilation due to reduced lung compliance. They will likely require higher respiratory rates as well. Care must be taken during mechanical ventilation to not allow inspiratory pressures to become elevated > 30-35 cm H_2O in an effort to prevent barotrauma.

XIII. Postoperative Pulmonary Function and Complications

A. Postoperative Pulmonary Function

The main alteration in postoperative lung mechanics is a restrictive defect. This change occurs in nearly all patients, and as a result, patients tend to breathe faster and shallower. With any type of operation under general anesthesia, the FRC does not return to its preoperative level for up to a week, perhaps even a few weeks for operations involving a sternotomy.[2]

B. Postoperative Pulmonary Complications

Two significant postoperative complications specifically related to the respiratory system are atelectasis and pneumonia. PPCs lead to not only increased cost and patient length of stay but also significant morbidity and mortality.[16] The incidence of these two complications is related to the site of surgery. Open upper abdominal operations have a much higher rate, lower abdominal and thoracic have a slightly lower rate than upper abdominal surgery, and all other peripheral operations have the lowest risk. There are a number of strategies to consider preventing pulmonary complications. Smoking cessation is an adjustable preoperative modifiable risk factor that should ideally be addressed 8 weeks prior to elective surgery. If patients stop smoking within 4 weeks of surgery, they may benefit from improved mucociliary function; however, sputum production may increase leading to the development of PPCs. When able, providers should consider regional techniques instead of general anesthesia, but if general anesthesia is needed, anesthesiologists should consider lung protective ventilation, use of PEEP, use of recruitment maneuvers and assure adequate reversal of neuromuscular blocking agents.[16] Postoperative strategies used to avoid PPCs focus on improving lung expansion. The use of incentive spirometry is widespread and very helpful when used appropriately. Many patients use the device incorrectly or not often enough, so training and monitoring by the staff caring for the patient is crucial. Early patient ambulation is vital to prevent PPCs. Having adequate analgesia is also helpful so that the above strategies can effectively be used. Adequate analgesia can be achieved with a multimodal approach using parenteral or intravenous medications, neuraxial analgesics, or regional techniques. The analgesic techniques employed depend on the surgical site and individual patient characteristics.[2]

For further review and interactivities, please see the associated Interactive Video Lectures and "A Closer Look" infographic accessible in the complimentary eBook bundled with this text. Access instructions are located in the inside front cover.

References

1. Tomashefski JF, Farver CF. Anatomy and histology of the lung. In: Tomashefski JF, Cagle PT, Farver CF, et al, eds. *Dail and Hammar's Pulmonary Pathology*. Vol 2. 3rd ed. Springer; 2008:20-48.
2. Tamul PC, Ault ML. Respiratory function in anesthesia. In: Barash P, Cullen B, Stoelting R, et al, eds. *Clinical Anesthesia*. 8th ed. Wolters Kluwer/Lippincott Williams & Wilkins; 2017:361-383.
3. Butterworth JF IV, Mackey DC, Wasnick JD. *Respiratory Physiology & Anesthesia. Morgan & Mikhail's Clinical Anesthesiology*. 6th ed. McGraw-Hill; 2018.
4. Talmor D, Sarge T, Malhotra A, et al. Mechanical ventilation guided by esophageal pressure in acute lung injury. *N Engl J Med*. 2008;359(20):2095-2104. PMID: 19001507.
5. Bigatello L, Pesenti A. Respiratory physiology for the anesthesiologist. *Anesthesiology*. 2019;130(6):1064-1077. PMID: 30998510.
6. Guz A. Regulation of respiration in man. *Annu Rev Physiol*. 1975;37:303-323.
7. Berger AJ, Mitchell RA, Severinghaus JW, et al. Regulation of respiration. *N Engl J Med*. 1977;297(2,3,4):92-97, 138-143, 194-201. PMID: 865581.
8. Stock MD, Downs JB, McDonald JS, et al. The carbon dioxide rate of rise in awake apneic humans. *J Clin Anesth*. 1988;1:96. PMID: 3152423.
9. Weil JV, Byrne-Quinn E, Sodal IE, et al. Hypoxic ventilatory drive in normal man. *J Clin Invest*. 1970;49:1061-1072. PMID: 5422012.
10. Tyuma I. The Bohr effect and the Haldane effect in human hemoglobin. *Jpn J Physiol*. 1984;34(2):205-216 PMID: 6433091.
11. Galvin I, Drummond GB, Nirmalan M. Distribution of blood flow and ventilation in the lung: gravity is not the only factor. *Br J Anaesth*. 2007;98(4):420-428. PMID: 17347182.
12. West JB, Dollery CT, Naimark A. Distribution of blood-flow and pressure-flow relations of the whole lung. *J Appl Physiol*. 1965;20:175-183.
13. Hyatt R, Scanlon P, Nakamura M. *Spirometry: dynamic lung volumes*. In: *Interpretation of Pulmonary Function Tests: A Practical Guide*. 3rd ed. Lippincott Williams & Wilkins; 2009:5-25.
14. Hyatt R, Scanlon P, Nakamura M. *Diffusing capacity of the lungs*. In: *Interpretation of Pulmonary Function Tests: A Practical Guide*. 3rd ed. Lippincott Williams & Wilkins; 2009:41-49.
15. American Society of Anesthesiologists Task Force on Preanesthesia Evaluation. Practice advisory for preanesthesia evaluation: an updated report by the American Society of Anesthesiologists task force on preanesthesia evaluation. *Anesthesiology*. 2012;116:522-539. PMID: 22273990.
16. Miskovic A, Lumb AB. Postoperative pulmonary complications. *Br J Anaesth*. 2017;118(3):317-334. PMID: 28186222.

POSITIVE PRESSURE VENTILATION

A CLOSER LOOK

The airway pressure waveform during volume-controlled ventilation has distinct features as seen below. Changes in this waveform can imply certain conditions.

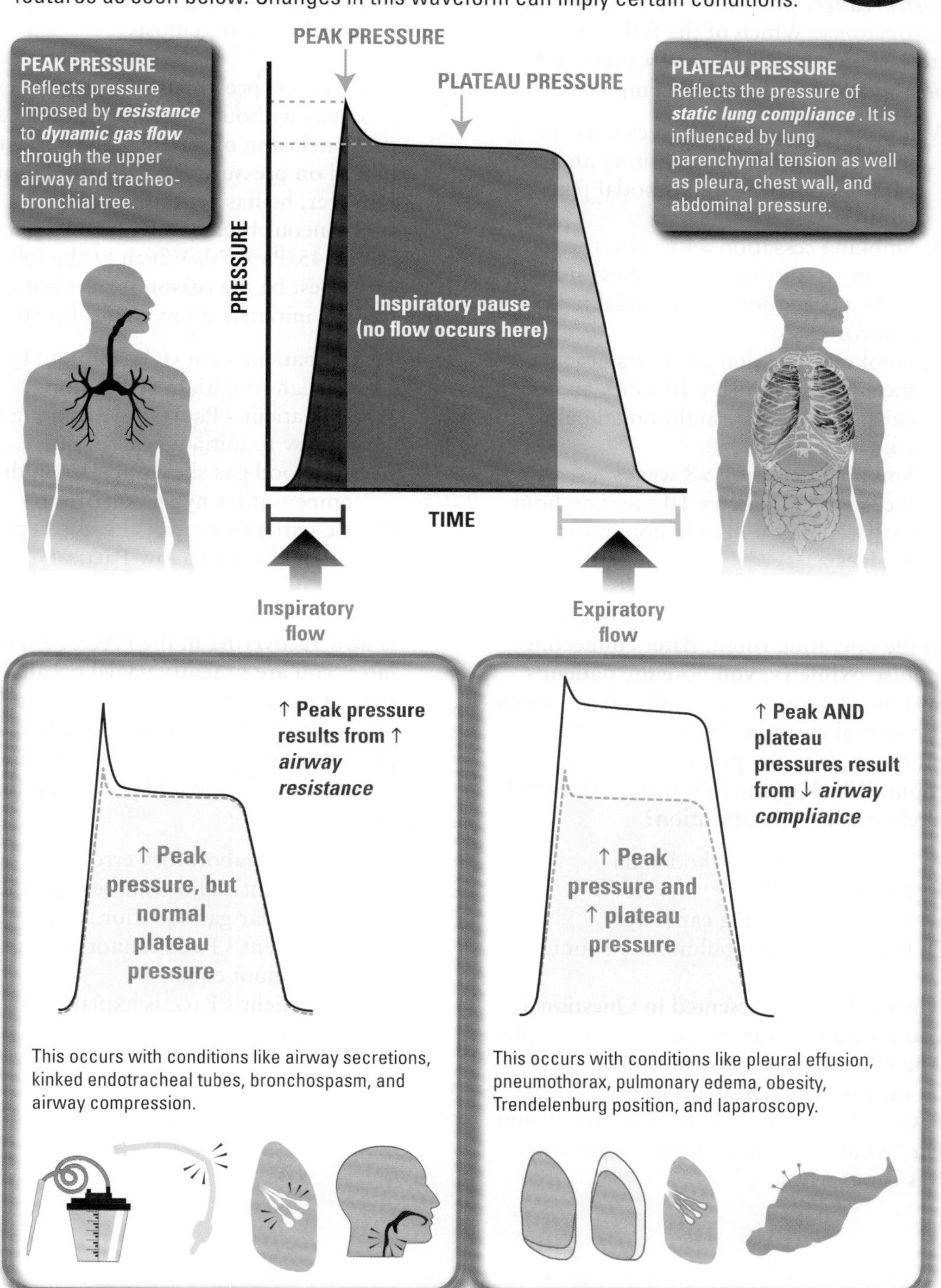

PEAK PRESSURE
Reflects pressure imposed by ***resistance*** to ***dynamic gas flow*** through the upper airway and tracheo-bronchial tree.
PEAK PRESSURE
PLATEAU PRESSURE
PLATEAU PRESSURE
Reflects the pressure of ***static lung compliance***. It is influenced by lung parenchymal tension as well as pleura, chest wall, and abdominal pressure.
PRESSURE
Inspiratory pause (no flow occurs here)
TIME
Inspiratory flow
Expiratory flow
↑ Peak pressure results from ↑ *airway resistance*
↑ Peak pressure, but normal plateau pressure
This occurs with conditions like airway secretions, kinked endotracheal tubes, bronchospasm, and airway compression.
↑ Peak AND plateau pressures result from ↓ *airway compliance*
↑ Peak pressure and ↑ plateau pressure
This occurs with conditions like pleural effusion, pneumothorax, pulmonary edema, obesity, Trendelenburg position, and laparoscopy.

Infographic by: Naveen Nathan MD

Questions

1. *A 72-year-old man with significant 100 pack-year smoking history and gastric cancer presents for an open total gastrectomy.* **Which of the following steps should be taken to best prevent postoperative pulmonary complications?**

   A. Smoking cessation >8 weeks, use of incentive spirometry 10 times an hour, early ambulation, multimodal pain control
   B. Smoking cessation >4 weeks, use of incentive spirometry 10 times an hour, early ambulation, multimodal pain control
   C. Smoking cessation 24 hours, use of incentive spirometry 10 times an hour, early ambulation, multimodal pain control
   D. Smoking cessation >8 weeks, use of incentive spirometry 10 times an hour, early ambulation, only nonopioid analgesia

2. **The patient in Question 1 is brought to the operating room. After connecting a pulse oximetry, you note the patient's Spo_2 is 88% on room air after lying supine for several minutes. His Spo_2 was 91% on room air in the preoperative waiting room. Which of the following is the most likely cause of desaturation?**

   A. The patient has orthodeoxia.
   B. Increase in FRC.
   C. Increase in closing capacity.
   D. Decrease in intrapulmonary shunt.

3. **During the case presented in Question 1, you note an upward slope in capnography. The $ETCO_2$ is 46 mm Hg. The arterial blood gas demonstrates a pH of 7.28, a $PaCo_2$ of 64 mm Hg and a Pao_2 of 65 mm Hg. What is the most likely reason why this is occurring?**

   A. Intrapulmonary shunt
   B. Dead space
   C. Poor systemic perfusion
   D. Renal tubular acidosis

4. **The case (as presented in Question 1), proceeds without any complications. At the conclusion of the case, the patient is placed on pressure support ventilation; however, he has yet to initiate a spontaneous breath. ABG shows pH 7.52/$PaCo_2$ 45/Pao_2 70. Which of the following is the best be the reason for the patient not to have initiated spontaneous breaths?**

   A. The patient's $Paco_2$ is 45 mm Hg and too high to initiate ventilation.
   B. The patient's $Paco_2$ is 45 mm Hg and too low to initiate ventilation.
   C. The blood gas shows alkalemia due to compensatory hyperventilation.
   D. The patient's central chemoreceptor will only react to low Pao_2.

5. **The patient in Questions 2.1 through 2.4 is now recovering in the PACU. An hour later, you are urgently paged because the patient has an Spo_2 of 88% while getting an Fio_2 of 0.24 with time, ABG that shows pH 7.42/$PaCo_2$ 75/Pao_2 56 while on room air. What is the most likely reason for the low Pao_2?**

   A. There is a laboratory error.
   B. The patient's Pao_2 can be explained by the alveolar gas equation.
   C. The patient's Pao_2 cannot be explained by the shunt equation.
   D. The patient's Pao_2 is explained by carbon monoxide.

Answers

1. A

Postoperative pulmonary complications (PPCs), such as atelectasis and pneumonia, are related to the site of surgery. Having an open upper abdominal surgery has a high rate for developing PPCs. Advocating smoking cessation for greater than 8 weeks, using incentive spirometry (correctly) 10 times an hour, promoting early ambulation, and using multimodal pain control are all crucial in preventing PPCs. Answer B is not the best answer as 4 weeks of smoking cessation is inferior to 8 weeks. Four weeks of smoking cessation may lead to improvement of a patient's mucociliary function, but they still may have increased sputum production leading to PPCs. Answer C is not the best answer as patients who have stopped smoking for 24 hours will have their carbon monoxide levels returned to baseline, but do not gain all the other benefits. Answer D is not the best answer as pain control is essential in preventing PPCs. Use of multimodal analgesia is preferred in order to minimize splinting and improve pulmonary hygiene.

2. C

FRC is related to posture and decreases upon supine positioning. Closing capacity (CC) is when lung volume in small airways begins to close and is unrelated to patient positioning. It increases with age and can equal or surpass FRC. When this occurs, affected alveoli are perfused but not ventilated, which leads to intrapulmonary shunt and arterial hypoxemia. Answer C is the best choice. The patient is aged 72 years and his CC is greater than FRC, which is also decreased when laying supine, leading to intrapulmonary shunt. Answer B is incorrect because FRC decreases in the supine position. Answer A is incorrect as orthodeoxia is a phenomenon in which oxygen saturation improves in the supine position secondary to arteriovenous shunts. Answer D is incorrect as typically an increase in intrapulmonary shunt leads to hypoxemia.

3. B

The patient has a respiratory acidosis with renal compensation. Answer B is the best answer. Some of the ventilated gas is not exposed to capillaries carrying CO_2, and dead space gas picks up negligible carbon dioxide. This dilutes the CO_2 from the perfusion-exposed ventilation and results in a gradient between $Paco_2$ and $ETCO_2$. Answer A is incorrect as intrapulmonary shunt will not influence ventilation. Answer C is not the correct answer as the patient does not have poor systemic perfusion leading to a respiratory acidosis. Poor systemic perfusion would rather lead to the development of a metabolic acidosis. Renal tubular acidosis can occur; however, this would not explain the patient's ABG. Answer D is not correct.

4. B

Typically, $Paco_2 > 80$ mm Hg leads to respiratory depression; however, this patient has COPD and his resting $Paco_2$ is higher. The ABG shows alkalemia secondary to a metabolic cause. CO_2 needs to rise to trigger ventilation; thus, answer B is incorrect. Answer D is incorrect as central chemoreceptors typically react to CO_2, while peripheral chemoreceptors react to low Pao_2. At normocarbic levels, peripheral chemoreceptors will stimulate ventilation at levels of Pao_2 below 65 mm Hg. With hypercarbia, the signals from peripheral chemoreceptors lead to increased ventilation only when Pao_2 levels are below 100 mm Hg, the level at which peripheral chemoreceptors begin to send impulses to the respiratory centers. Answer D is not the correct answer.

5. B

The patient is eucapnic. He has COPD and is expected to have a lower Spo_2. Based on the ABG, there is renal compensation. Patients with COPD tolerate lower Pao_2 before initiating drive. Additionally, given that the patient is expected to have renal compensation as he is a chronic CO_2 retainer. The patient's Spo_2

can be explained by the alveolar gas equation ($PaO_2 = FIO_2 (P_{atm} - P_{H_2O}) - PaCO_2/RQ$). P_{atm} is atmospheric pressure. P_{H_2O} is the partial pressure of water, which is ~47 mm Hg. RQ is the respiratory quotient, which is typically 0.8 (assuming normal diet). $PaO_2 = 0.24 (760 - 47) - 75/0.8 \rightarrow PaO_2 = 0.24(713) - 75/0.8 \rightarrow PaO_2 = 56$. Normally A-a gradient = (Age + 10)/4. As this patient is aged 72 years, the expected A-a gradient would be approximately 20. The patient's ABG can be explained by the increase in $PaCO_2$. Answer D is incorrect as the patient's SpO_2 does not reflect a patient with elevated carbon monoxide.

3 Cardiovascular Anatomy and Physiology

Christopher R. Barnes and Peter von Homeyer

I. Cardiac Anatomy

The normal adult heart is about the size of a fist, weighs approximately 300 g, and has a trapezoid shape with its apex oriented leftward and anterior in the chest (**Figure 3.1**).[1] The anterior thoracic surface projections of the heart and great vessels, relative to the bony ribs, sternum, and xiphoid process, are shown in **Figure 3.2**. As the central "pump" of the human body, it contracts about 100,000 times per day and propels blood into the pulmonary and systemic circulations. The right and the left chambers are anatomically separated by septa. Only in the fetal circulation or in the setting of certain pathologies (eg, atrial or ventricular septal defects) is there direct communication of blood flow between the right and left sides. On each side, blood first returns from the venous circulation into a thin-walled atrium. It then flows through an ***atrioventricular*** (AV) ***valve*** into a muscular ventricle, and finally through a ***semilunar valve*** into the great arteries—the **aorta** on the left and the ***pulmonary artery*** (PA) on the right (**Figure 3.3**).

The ***heart wall*** has three layers: the thin, inner endocardium; the thick, middle myocardium; and the outer epicardium (ie, the visceral pericardium). The myocardium is anchored to the cardiac ***fibrous skeleton***, a system of dense collagen forming two rings and connective trigones that separate the atria and ventricles to prevent uncontrolled conduction of electrical impulses and also serve as anchors for the AV valves.

The ***right atrium*** (RA), ***superior vena cava*** (SVC), and ***inferior vena cava*** (IVC) form the right lateral border of the heart. Venous return from the heart itself enters the RA through the ***coronary sinus*** (CS), which collects blood from the major cardiac veins. The internal wall of the RA includes the right-sided wall of the ***interatrial septum*** (IAS). The center of the IAS features the fossa ovalis, a small groove that is a remnant of the foramen ovale. In the fetal circulation, it allows for oxygenated blood to flow from the right-sided to the left-sided circulation. It usually closes after birth, but remains patent in 25% to 30% of the population.

The ***right ventricle*** (RV) forms most of the anterior surface of the heart and some of its inferior surface and has about a sixth of the muscle mass of the ***left ventricle*** (LV). The muscular ***interventricular septum*** (IVS) functions as a contractile wall for both the RV and the LV.

The ***tricuspid valve*** (TV) has three distinct leaflets (anterior, septal, and posterior) that are attached to tendinous cords. It connects to papillary muscles

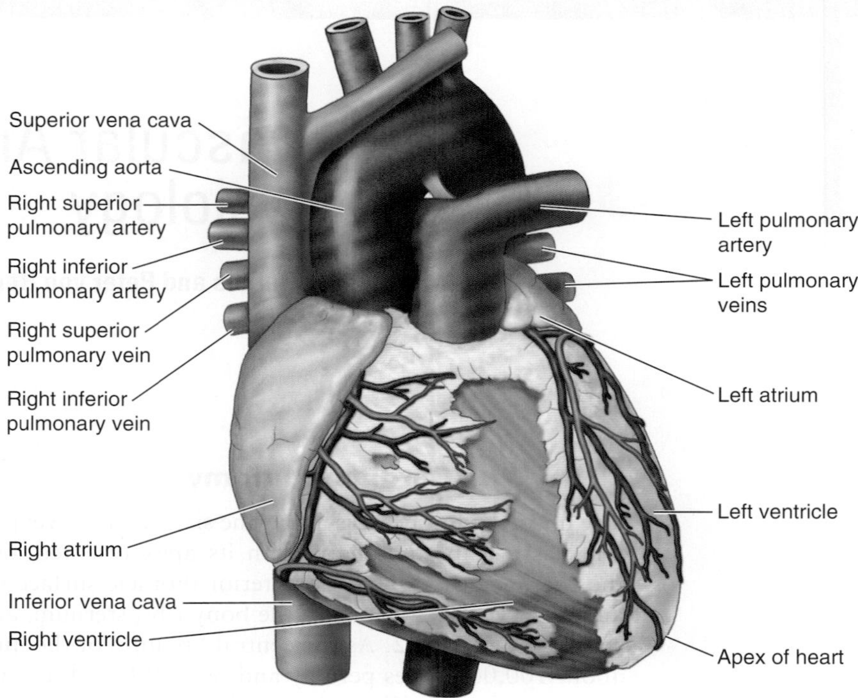

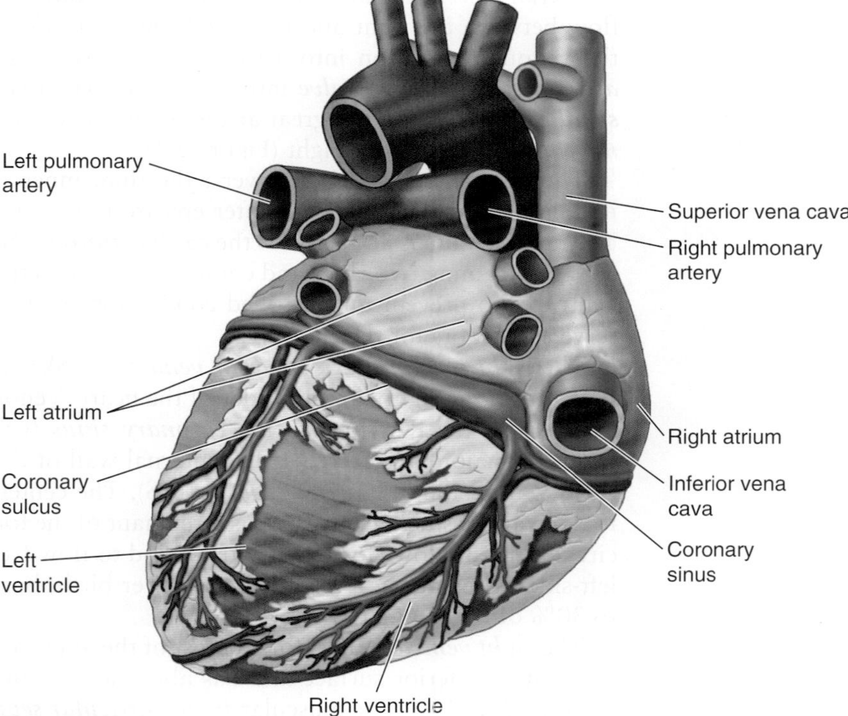

Figure 3.1 Key anatomic features of the heart from the anterior view (A) and posteroinferior view (B). (From Thorax. In: Moore KL, Agur AMR, Dalley II AF, eds. *Clinically Oriented Anatomy*. 8th ed. Wolters Kluwer; 2018:290-403, Figure 4.53B and 4.53C.)

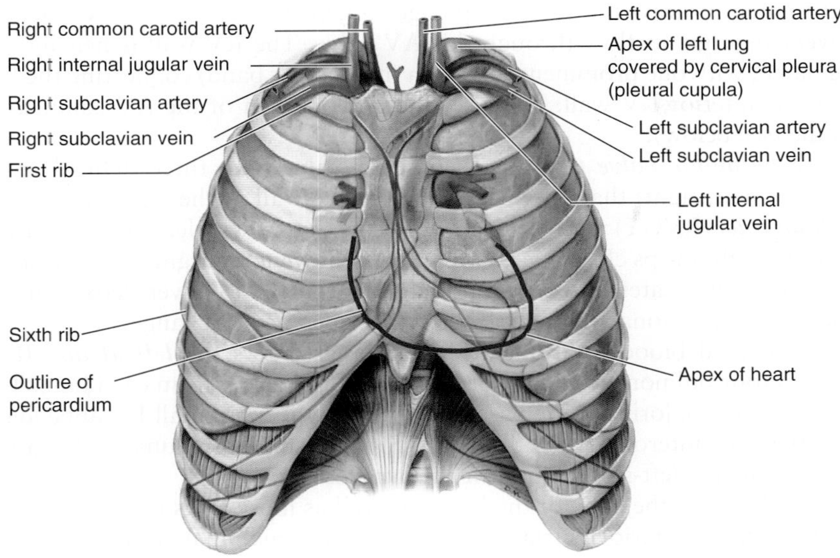

Figure 3.2 Anterior surface projections of the heart and great vessels relative to the lungs and ribs. Note the close relation of the lung apices to the internal jugular and subclavian veins (relevant to placement of central venous catheters) and the bare area of the pericardium that can be accessed for pericardiocentesis with needle placement under and to the left of the xiphoid process of the sternum. (From Thorax. In: Moore KL, Agur AMR, Dalley II AF, eds. *Clinically Oriented Anatomy*. 8th ed. Wolters Kluwer; 2018:290-403, Figure 4.31A.)

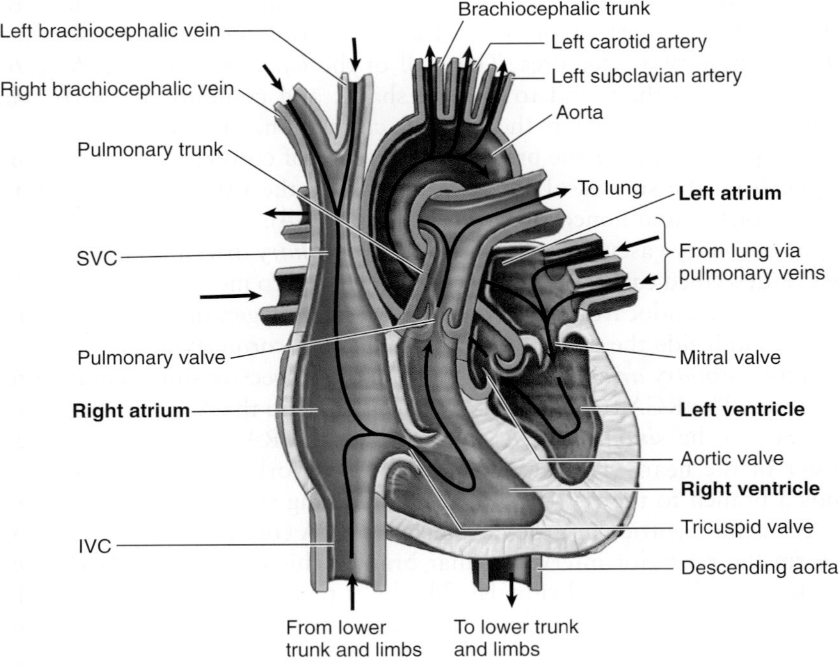

Figure 3.3 The course of normal blood flow from the great venous vessels through the right and left heart chambers to the systemic aorta. IVC, inferior vena cava; SVC, superior vena cava. (From Thorax. In: Moore KL, Agur AMR, Dalley II AF, eds. *Clinically Oriented Anatomy*. 8th ed. Wolters Kluwer; 2018:290-403, Figure 4.49A.)

that tighten to draw the valve cusp edges together in ventricular systole and prevent regurgitant flow through this AV valve. The RV wall is heavily trabeculated, with one prominent trabecula (moderator band) connecting the IVS with the anterior RV wall. It houses the right branch of the AV conduction bundle (see below).

The ***pulmonic valve*** (PV) is a semilunar valve with three defined cusps (anterior, left, right) that are pushed toward the wall of the ***right ventricular outflow tract*** (RVOT) with ventricular contraction in systole. After relaxation in diastole, the cusps close like an umbrella to prevent regurgitation. The main PA quickly bifurcates into right and left branches that deliver deoxygenated blood to the pulmonary circulation for subsequent gas exchange.

Oxygenated blood returning from the lungs enters the ***left atrium*** (LA) through four pulmonary veins, normally two originating from each lung. The LA forms the majority of the base of the heart, with the small LA appendage as part of its anterolateral wall. The IAS has a small semilunar indentation representing the left-sided aspect of the oval fossa.

The LV forms the apex of the heart, as well as most of its left (lateral) and diaphragmatic (inferior) surfaces, and its normal maximal wall thickness is 10 mm (compared with 3 mm in the RV). The IVS is concave to the highly trabeculated LV wall, resulting in an almost circular LV chamber on anatomic cross-section.

Unlike the right-sided TV, the left-sided AV ***mitral valve*** (MV) is bicuspid, with anterior and posterior leaflets that are connected to anterolateral and posteromedial papillary muscles by tendinous cords similar to those of the TV. Both MV leaflets receive cords from papillary muscles that keep this valve shut in the setting of high intraventricular pressure during systole.

> **? *Did You Know?***
>
> Coronary artery anatomy is termed either right dominant or left dominant, depending on which main coronary artery feeds the posterior descending branch (in the interventricular groove) to the posteroinferior surface of the heart. Right-dominant circulation is most common, found in 70% of the population.

The inflow and outflow tracts of the LV lie almost parallel to each other, with the anterior leaflet of the mitral valve forming a natural separation between these two structures. The wall of the ***left ventricular outflow tract*** (LVOT) is smooth, round to oval in shape, and contains the ***aortic valve*** through which blood enters the systemic circulation. This valve has three distinct cusps named after the presence or absence of coronary artery ostia originating from the sinuses of Valsalva just above the valve: the left coronary, right coronary, and noncoronary cusps (**Figure 3.4**).

The coronary vasculature consists of the ***coronary arteries*** (**Figure 3.5**) and the CS (described earlier). The arteries carry blood to most of the myocardium except the subendocardial layers, which receive oxygen directly via diffusion from blood inside the cardiac chambers. The ***left coronary artery*** (LCA) and the ***right coronary artery*** (RCA) arise from the respective sinuses in the proximal aorta. The RCA travels to the right of the PA in the AV groove and sends branches to the ***sinoatrial*** (SA) ***node*** (inside the RA wall) and to the right border of the heart. The RCA continues posteriorly in the AV groove and sends a branch to the AV node of the conducting system before entering the posterior interventricular groove. When the RCA continues down that groove to form the posterior interventricular branch, this is termed ***right-dominant*** circulation (~70% of individuals). The LCA travels between the PA and the LA appendage and splits early in its course into the ***left anterior descending*** (LAD) artery and the circumflex branch. The LAD continues in the anterior interventricular groove all the way to the LV apex and around the inferior aspect of the heart where it often forms anastomoses with the branches of the posterior interventricular branch. The LAD also sends many septal branches to the IVS throughout its course, as well as prominent diagonal branch to

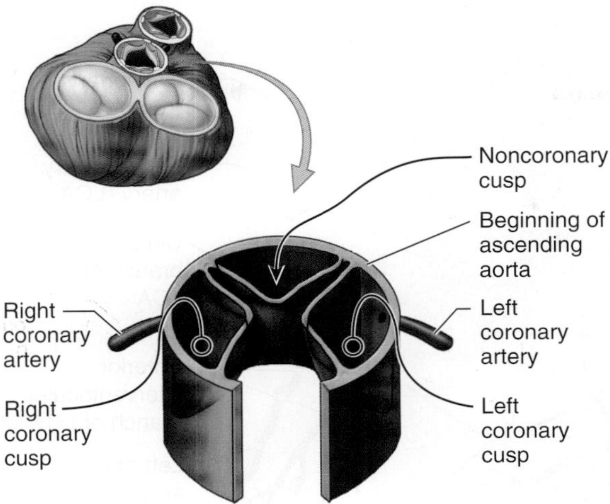

Figure 3.4 Relation between the aortic valve cusps and the coronary arteries. Like the pulmonary valve, the aortic valve has three semilunar cusps: right, posterior, and left. During systole, ejected blood forces the cusps apart. During diastole, the cusps close and coronary artery flow occurs. (From Thorax. In: Moore KL, Agur AMR, Dalley II AF, eds. *Clinically Oriented Anatomy*. 8th ed. Wolters Kluwer; 2018:290-403, Figure 4.59A.)

the lateral wall. When the circumflex branch gives rise to the posterior interventricular branch, this is termed ***left-dominant*** circulation (~30% of individuals). Such variable coronary artery anatomy is important when trying to understand the relation between coronary artery disease and regional dysfunction of ischemic myocardium.

Normal ***electrical conduction*** is initiated by an electrical impulse generated in the SA node, a locus of specialized cardiac cells in the RA wall that have no contractile function. As the pacemaker center of the heart, the SA node autonomically generates an impulse at about 60 to 80 beats per minute. From the SA node, bundles of cells lead to the AV node located above the right fibrous trigone of the heart at the AV border. From the AV node, the impulse is conducted via the AV bundle, also known as the ***bundle of His***, that pierces the fibrous skeleton of the heart and splits just above the muscular IVS into right and left bundles. The right bundle continues toward the apex of the heart and then splits into smaller subendocardial RV branches. The left bundle splits close to its origin into a left anterior and a left posterior branch, which then further split into subendocardial LV branches near the apex of the heart (**Figure 3.6**).

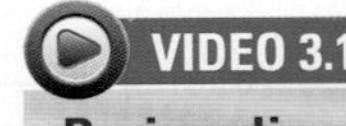

Pericardium

The ***pericardium*** is a double-layered sac around the heart. The visceral serous layer (epicardium) covers most of the heart's surface. It extends to and reflects at the proximal portion of the great vessels and turns into the parietal pericardial sac. Between the two layers, a small amount of fluid is considered physiologic. The pericardium protects and restrains the heart, reduces friction associated with its constant movement within the mediastinum, and separates the heart and origin of the great vessels from other structures inside the mediastinum. Abnormal pericardial fluid collections (eg, pericardial tamponade) can be accessed and withdrawn as described in **Figure 3.2**.

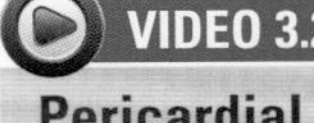

Pericardial Effusion

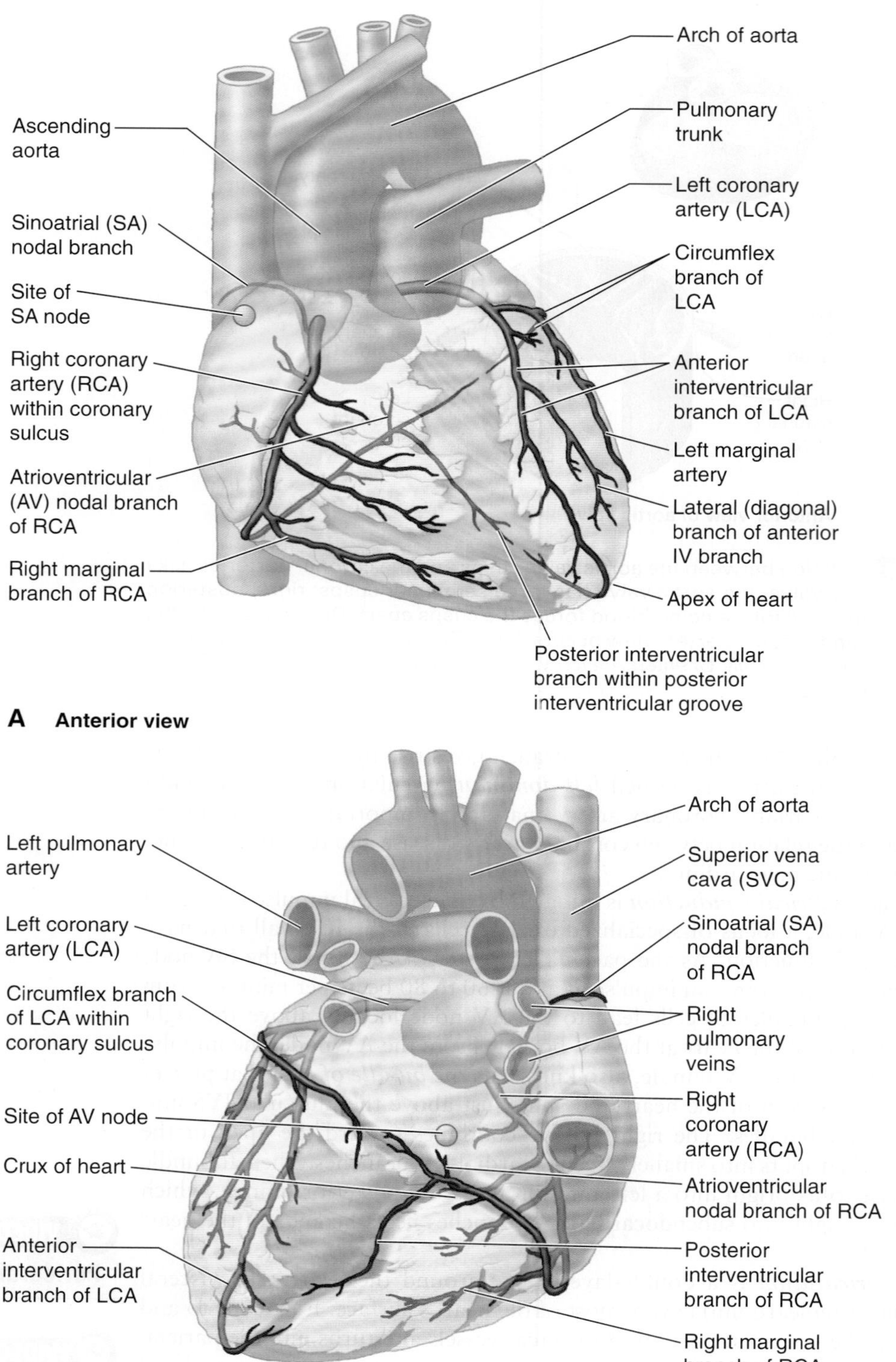

Figure 3.5 Coronary artery anatomy for the typical right-dominant pattern (see text for details) is shown from the anterior view (A) and the posterior view (B). (From Thorax. In: Moore KL, Agur AMR, Dalley II AF, eds. *Clinically Oriented Anatomy*. 8th ed. Wolters Kluwer; 2018:290-403, Figure 4.60A and 4.60B.)

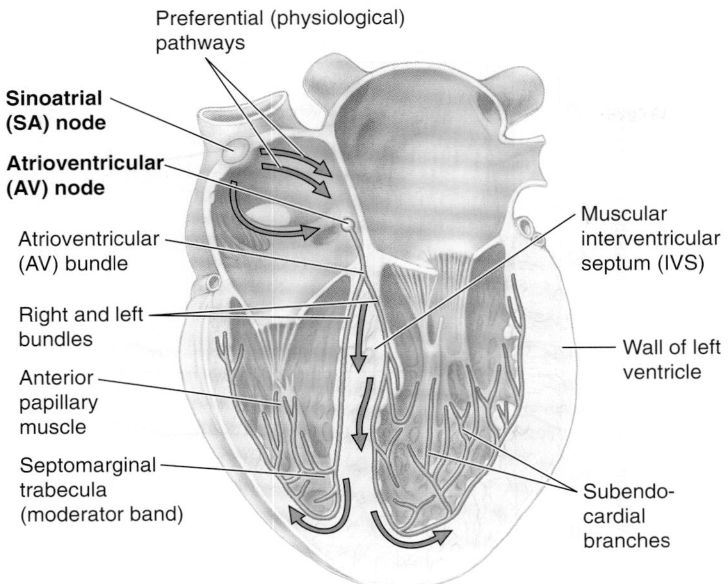

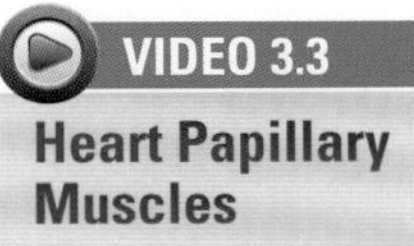

Figure 3.6 Impulses initiated at the sinoatrial (SA) node are propagated through the atrial musculature to the atrioventricular (AV) node, followed by conduction through the AV bundle and its right and left branches in the intraventricular septum (IVS) to the myocardium. (From Thorax. In: Moore KL, Agur AMR, Dalley II AF, eds. *Clinically Oriented Anatomy*. 8th ed. Wolters Kluwer; 2018:290-403, Figure 4.63B.)

II. The Cardiac Cycle

The *cardiac cycle* consists of an orchestrated sequence of spontaneous electrical and contractile events occurring simultaneously in both the right and left sides of the heart. When combined with the flow-directing influence of the four unidirectional heart valves, a sequential rise and fall of fluid pressures within each of the four heart chambers results in a predictable pattern of chamber volumes and pressures that produces forward cardiac output and accompanying heart sounds associated with valve closure.[2] These synchronized electrical and mechanical events are depicted under normal anatomic and physiologic conditions in **Figure 3.7**. Anatomic or physiologic abnormalities in any of these components can alter events of the cardiac cycle and ultimately impact cardiac performance.

VIDEO 3.4
Animated Cardiac Cycle

Focusing on the left heart, depolarization of the LV associated with the QRS complex of the electrocardiogram (ECG) initiates LV contraction and begins the period of *systole* with closure of the mitral valve contributing to the first heart sound (S_1). During early systole, both the mitral and aortic valves are closed; the mitral valve due to the positive LV → LA pressure gradient and papillary muscle contraction, and the aortic valve due to the positive aortic root → LV pressure gradient. Because LV volume is fixed during early systole, LV contraction results in a brief, yet rapid isovolumic elevation in LV pressure. The maximum rate of rise in LV pressure (+dP/dt) occurs during this brief *isovolumic contraction period* and is commonly used as the index of LV contractility (as discussed later).

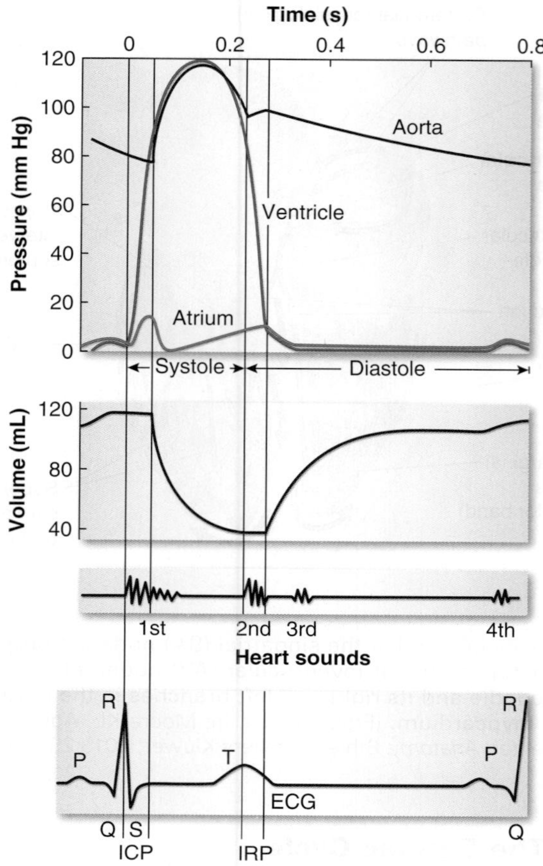

Figure 3.7 Mechanical and electrical events of the cardiac cycle also showing the left ventricular (LV) volume curve and the heart sounds. Note the LV isovolumic contraction period (ICP) and the relaxation period (IRP) during which there is no change in LV volume because the aortic and mitral valves are closed. The LV decreases in volume as it ejects its contents into the aorta. During the first third of systolic ejection (the rapid ejection period), the curve of emptying is steep. ECG, electrocardiogram. (From Pagel PS, Kampine JP, Stowe DF. Cardiac anatomy and physiology. In: Barash PG, Cullen BF, Stoelting RK, et al, eds. *Handbook of Clinical Anesthesia.* 7th ed. Lippincott Williams & Wilkins; 2013:239-262, Figure 10.3.)

Once the rapidly rising LV pressure exceeds aortic root pressure, the aortic valve passively opens and pulsatile aortic flow begins. Both the LV and aortic pressures continue to rise and then quickly peak and fall during the remainder of systole as ventricular contraction ceases and the LV repolarizes. The stroke volume ejected during systole is approximately two-thirds of the end-diastolic LV volume.

Systole ends when the slowly declining aortic root pressure exceeds the more rapidly falling LV pressure, resulting in passive closure of the aortic valve and its contribution to the second heart sound (S_2). As ***diastole*** begins, both the mitral and aortic valves are briefly closed. During this short-lived, ***isovolumic relaxation period***, LV pressure rapidly falls, while LA pressure slowly rises due to pulmonary inflow. When LA pressure exceeds LV pressure, the MV passively opens and diastolic filling of the LV begins. Diastole consists of four phases—isovolumic relaxation, early diastolic filling, diastasis, and atrial systole (LA contraction)—until the cardiac cycle is repeated with LV depolarization and contraction.

Similar parallel events occur in the right heart during the cardiac cycle with corresponding chamber volumes (ie, right and left ventricular stroke volumes are equal under normal anatomic conditions) and tricuspid/pulmonic valve movements mirroring the mitral/aortic movements. As a result of peristaltic inflow, lesser cardiac muscle mass, and lesser contractile strength of the RV, there is no isovolumic contraction period in the RV. The RV and PA pressures are significantly lower than corresponding left-sided pressures. Right-sided systolic ejection time may exceed the left-sided time, resulting in later closure of the pulmonic valve (compared with the aortic valve) and a split S_2. During spontaneous inspiration, ***venous return*** is increased to the right ventricle and decreased to the left ventricle, resulting in prolongation of the splitting of S_2, referred to as ***physiologic splitting***.

? *Did You Know?*

With spontaneous inspiration, venous return to the right ventricle is increased, resulting in prolonged ejection time compared with the left ventricle. This causes the pulmonic valve to close later than the aortic valve, producing respiration-induced variation in splitting of S_2 (physiologic splitting).

III. Control of Heart Rate

Heart rate is determined by the constantly and often instantaneously changing balance between multiple intrinsic and extrinsic factors. Key intrinsic factors include autonomic efferent innervation (both ***sympathetic nervous system*** [SNS] and ***parasympathetic nervous system*** [PNS]) (see Chapter 4), neural reflex mechanisms, humoral influences, and cardiac rhythm. Extrinsic factors include direct- and indirect-acting pharmaceutical and recreational drugs, fear, hyper- or hypothermia, and others that affect heart rate through modulation of intrinsic factors.

Efferent autonomic tone to the heart is initiated in the anterior (PNS) and posterior (SNS) hypothalamus and is modulated by the cardiac acceleration and cardiac slowing centers in the medulla prior to peripheral distribution. Sympathetic preganglionic fibers arising from T1 to T4 spinal levels enter the nearby paravertebral sympathetic chain, inferior cervical (stellate) ganglion, and middle cervical ganglion. They synapse with postganglionic SNS neurons that directly innervate the SA node, AV node, and myocardium via β_1-adrenergic norepinephrine receptors. PNS preganglionic fibers to the heart arise from the brainstem and are carried in the vagus nerve. Both the right and left vagus nerves exit their respective jugular foramina, traverse the neck within the carotid sheath posterior to the carotid arteries. They course directly to the heart where they synapse with short postganglionic PNS neurons that moderate the SA and AV nodes via muscarinic acetylcholine receptors. The opposing effects of the SNS (tachycardia) and PNS (bradycardia) on the SA node normally favor vagal inhibition. As a result of this vagal predominance, load-induced increases in heart rate are first achieved by release of PNS tone and thereafter by SNS activation. Several neural reflex mechanisms can also affect heart rate, including the ***baroreceptor response, atrial distention response (Bainbridge reflex), carotid chemoreceptor reflex, Cushing reflex***, and ***oculocardiac reflex*** (**Table 3.1**).

Humoral factors (eg, circulating catecholamines) also influence heart rate independent of the SNS and PNS. For example, the denervated heart following orthotopic heart transplantation still responds to exercise load with tachycardia, as a result of increased circulating catecholamine levels. Myocardial β_1-adrenergic receptors can also be activated, and heart rate is increased by direct pharmacologic agonists (isoproterenol, epinephrine), agents that indirectly cause release of endogenous catecholamines (ephedrine), or drugs that impair catecholamine metabolism or reuptake (cocaine).

Table 3.1 Cardiac Reflexes That Affect Heart Rate

Reflex	Afferent Sensor	Efferent Response
Baroreceptor	Baroreceptors sense blood pressure in carotid sinus (CN IX) and aortic arch (CN X)	*Low blood pressure* → increased SNS tone → increased heart rate, inotropy, and vasoconstriction *High blood pressure* → increased PNS tone (CN X) → reduced heart rate and inotropy
Atrial Receptor (Bainbridge)	Stretch receptors in the right atrium sense CVP (CN X)	*High CVP* → increased SNS tone and decreased PNS tone (CN X) → increased heart rate
Chemoreceptor	Pao_2 and pH sensors in carotid bodies (CN IX) and aortic bodies (CN X)	*Low Pao_2 and pH* → increased ventilation and PNS tone → decreased heart rate and inotropy
Oculocardiac	Stretch receptors in extraocular muscles sense pressure on globe (ciliary nerves and CN V)	*High globe pressure* → increased PNS tone (CN X) → decreased heart rate
Cushing	Increased ICP	*High ICP* → increased SNS tone → increased inotropy and vasoconstriction → low heart rate (baroreceptor reflex)

CN, cranial nerve; CVP, central venous pressure; ICP, intracranial pressure; Pao_2, arterial partial pressure of oxygen; PNS, parasympathetic nervous system; SNS, sympathetic nervous system.

IV. Coronary Physiology

Resting ***coronary blood flow*** is approximately 250 mL/min (~5% of total cardiac output) and can be increased up to 5-fold during strenuous physical exercise. Coronary blood flow is influenced by physical, neural, and metabolic factors. The primary physical factor is ***coronary perfusion pressure***—the difference between aortic pressure and either LV pressure (left coronary artery) or RV pressure (right coronary artery). Extravascular coronary artery compression (due to contracting myocardium), heart rate (altering the duration of diastole), vessel length, and blood viscosity also impact coronary perfusion. The primary neural factor is SNS tone to the heart, which increases coronary blood flow when increased aortic pressure outweighs reduced coronary flow associated with stronger myocardial contraction and shortened diastolic filling time (tachycardia). Active vasodilation of coronary arteries is limited because vagal stimulation has no apparent effect on vessel caliber, and unlike skeletal muscle vasculature, sympathetic cholinergic innervation is not present in coronary arteries. However, β_2-adrenergic receptor–mediated vasodilation can occur in small coronary arterioles and accounts for ~25% of coronary vasodilation observed during exercise-induced hyperemia. Lastly, increased myocardial metabolism is associated with the bulk of coronary vasodilation through the action of yet-to-be-defined local metabolic factors.

? *Did You Know?*

Because the subendocardium is exposed to higher pressures during systole than the subepicardial layer, the former is more susceptible to ischemia, particularly in settings of coronary stenosis, ventricular hypertrophy, or tachycardia.

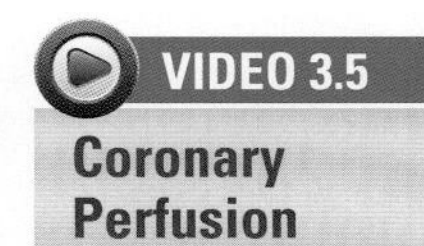

Coronary blood flow varies with the cardiac cycle and is determined by the difference between aortic pressure and tissue (wall) pressure. LCA flow is highly variable—it peaks during early diastole when perfusion pressure is highest and approaches zero in early systole when LV contraction (and coronary compression) is greatest. In contrast, RCA flow is more constant throughout the cardiac cycle and peaks during systole due to the lesser muscle mass and contraction load of the normal RV. Because the subendocardium is exposed to higher pressures during systole compared to the subepicardial layer, the former is more susceptible to ischemia, particularly in settings of coronary stenosis, ventricular hypertrophy, or tachycardia. However, ***subendocardial ischemia*** is partially offset by enhanced capillary anastomoses and local metabolic vasodilation in this layer.

The heart has the highest ***oxygen extraction ratio*** of any organ (~70%); as a result, under normal conditions, the venous oxygen saturation of blood in the coronary sinus (~30%) is lower than that in the right atrium (~70%). ***Myocardial oxygen consumption*** is determined by heart rate, myocardial contractility, and ventricular wall stress (including preload and afterload), with the major determinants being the heart rate and the magnitude of LV pressure developed during the isovolumic contraction period. Because of this high extraction ratio, increased myocardial oxygen demand can only be met through increased coronary blood flow. Thus, the dominant controller of coronary blood flow is myocardial oxygen consumption. The coronary circulation is ideally constructed for this purpose, as its myocardial capillary density is approximately eight times greater than that of skeletal muscle (approximately one capillary for each cardiac muscle fiber). When myocardial oxygen supply is unable to meet increases in myocardial oxygen demand (eg, coronary artery stenosis), ***myocardial ischemia*** occurs. Ischemia is first clinically manifested by increased LV end-diastolic volume and decreased LV compliance and can progress to wall motion abnormalities, decreased ejection fraction, ECG abnormalities (ST-segment changes), ***congestive heart failure*** (CHF), and ultimately ***cardiogenic shock***.

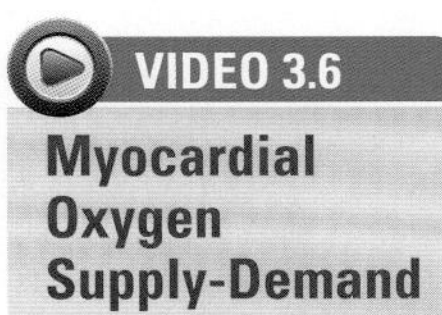

V. The Pressure-Volume Diagram

The mechanical events in the LV cardiac cycle depicted in **Figure 3.7** can also be presented graphically as the LV ***pressure-volume*** (P-V) ***diagram***, shown in **Figure 3.8**. With pressure plotted on the vertical axis and volume on the horizontal axis, a near-rectangular "loop" is formed in a counterclockwise path beginning in the lower right at end diastole (low LV pressure and high LV volume). It consists of four phases of the cardiac cycle: isovolumic contraction period (vertical right line), systole (horizontal top line), isovolumic relaxation period (vertical left line), and diastole (horizontal bottom line). The line drawn from the origin to the end-systolic "corner" of the P-V loop defines the ***end-systolic pressure-volume relation*** (ESPVR), with the slope of this line being an index of myocardial contractility. Similarly, the line drawn from the origin to the end-diastolic corner of the P-V loop defines the ***end-diastolic pressure-volume relation*** (EDPVR), the slope that can be used to quantify LV compliance.

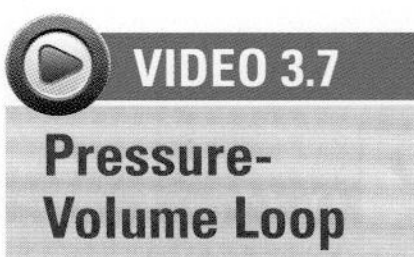

The size and shape of the P-V diagram, as well as the slopes of the ESPVR and EDPVR lines, allow recognition of various cardiac events without ECG correlation and will change predictably across a range of pathologic states such as ventricular dysfunction or valvular heart disease.[2,3] For example, the area of the P-V diagram defines LV ***stroke work*** for the cardiac cycle, whereas a right shift in the vertical right portion of the diagram indicates an increase in LV preload. Examples of P-V diagrams indicating impaired

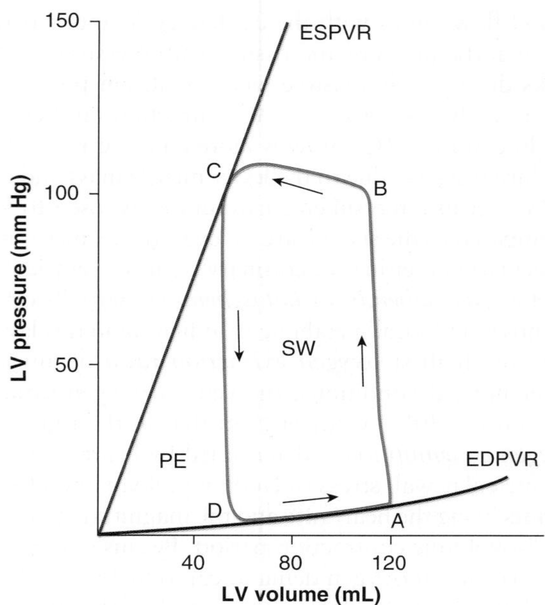

Figure 3.8 A steady-state left ventricular (LV) pressure volume diagram. The cardiac cycle proceeds in a time-dependent counterclockwise direction (*arrows*). Points A, B, C, and D correspond to LV end diastole (closure of the mitral valve), opening of the aortic valve, LV end systole (closure of the aortic valve), and opening of the mitral valve, respectively. Segments AB, BC, CD, and DA represent isovolumic contraction, ejection, isovolumic relaxation, and filling, respectively. The LV is constrained to operate within the boundaries of the end-systolic and end-diastolic pressure-volume relations (ESPVR and EDPVR, respectively). The area inscribed by the LV pressure-volume diagram is stroke work (SW) performed during the cardiac cycle. The area to the left of the LV pressure-volume diagram between ESPVR and EDPVR is the remaining potential energy (PE) of the system. (From Pagel PS, Kampine JP, Stowe DF. Cardiac anatomy and physiology. In: Barash PG, Cullen BF, Stoelting RK, et al, eds. *Handbook of Clinical Anesthesia*. 7th ed. Lippincott Williams & Wilkins; 2013:239-262, Figure 10.4.)

LV contractility and diastolic dysfunction associated with decreased LV compliance are shown in **Figure 3.9**.

? *Did You Know?*

In isolated cardiac muscle, contractile tension increases with stimulation frequency to a maximum of 150 to 180 contractions per second (Bowditch effect). However, such high heart rates reduce diastolic filling time in the intact heart and are only seen in special settings (dysrhythmias, strenuous exercise).

VI. Factors That Determine Systolic Function

A. Left Ventricular Pump

Each ventricle essentially operates as a hydraulic pump whose performance is defined by its ability to collect blood (diastolic function) and eject blood (systolic function), which is determined by the factors summarized in **Figure 3.10**. The key determinants of systolic function are the blood volume ejected (***stroke volume***), the volume efficiency of blood ejection (***ejection fraction***), the pumping frequency (***heart rate***), the volume of blood filling the pump (***preload***), the downstream resistance the ejected blood must overcome (***afterload***), and the contractile ability of the ventricle (***myocardial contractility***).

B. Cardiac Output and Ejection Fraction

The performance of the LV is practically measured as the *cardiac output* (CO), defined as the stroke volume (SV) times the heart rate (HR). The SV is the difference between the *end-diastolic volume* (EDV) and *end-systolic volume* (ESV). As shown in **Figure 3.8**, a normal EDV of ~120 mL and ESV of ~40 mL would yield

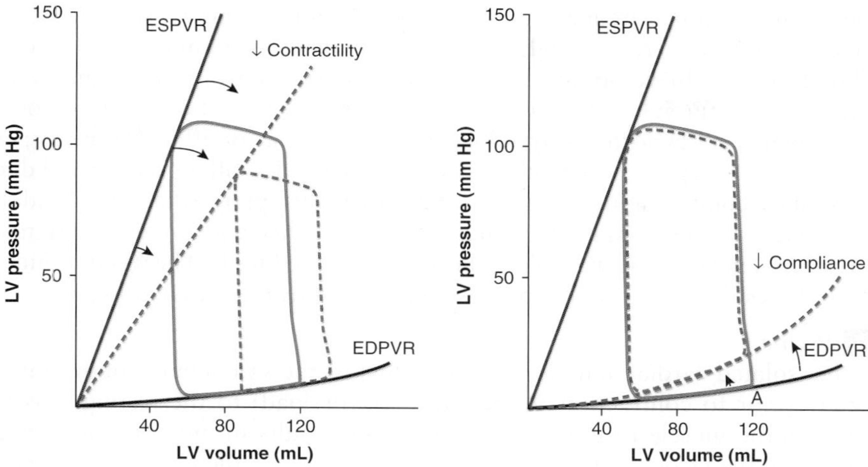

Figure 3.9 These schematic illustrations demonstrate alterations in the steady state left ventricular (LV) pressure-volume diagram produced by a reduction in myocardial contractility as indicated by a decrease in the slope of the end-systolic pressure-volume relation (ESPVR; *left*) and a decrease in LV compliance as indicated by an increase in the position of the end-diastolic pressure-volume relation (EDPVR; *right*). These diagrams emphasize that heart failure may result from LV systolic or diastolic dysfunction independently. (Reproduced with permission from Kaplan JA, Reich DL, Savino JS. *Kaplan's Cardiac Anesthesia: The Echo Era.* 6th ed. Elsevier Saunders; 2011:109, Figure 5-11.)

a SV of ~80 mL. The normal LV ejection fraction (SV/EDV) is therefore 67%. Thus, pump efficiency is impaired (ie, low ejection fraction) in settings such as a dilated LV with elevated EDV and normal SV (eg, dilated cardiomyopathy) or a normal-sized LV with poor contractility and low SV (eg, myocardial infarction).

C. Heart Rate

In the isolated cardiac muscle, contractile tension increases with stimulation frequency due to an increase in intracellular calcium content. This effect is known as the Bowditch or staircase phenomenon and results in maximal

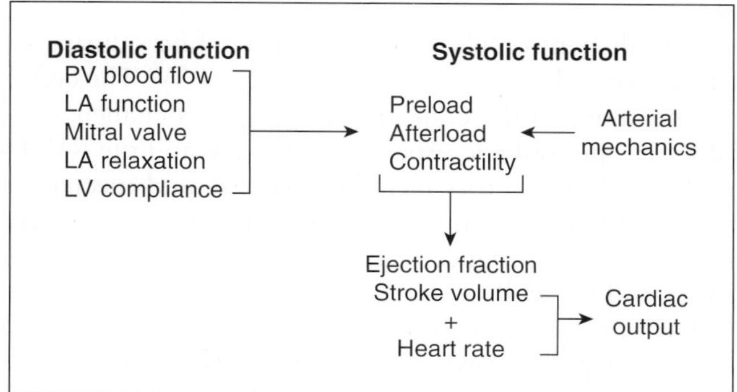

Figure 3.10 The major factors that determine left ventricular (LV) diastolic (*left*) and systolic (*right*) function. Note that pulmonary venous (PV) blood flow, left atrial (LA) function, mitral valve integrity, LA relaxation, and LV compliance combine to determine LV preload. (From Pagel PS, Kampine JP, Stowe DF. Cardiac anatomy and physiology. In: Barash PG, Cullen BF, Stoelting RK, et al, eds. *Handbook of Clinical Anesthesia.* 7th ed. Lippincott Williams & Wilkins; 2013:239-262, Figure 10.5.)

contractile tension at frequencies of 150 to 180 contractions per second. In the intact heart, however, such high heart rates do not allow for adequate diastolic filling time to achieve optimal EDV and therefore result in insufficient SV to maintain meaningful CO. Thus, the Bowditch effect is of little physiologic consequence in the normal physiologic heart rate range of 50 to 150 beats per minute. The exception is with clinical settings where LV filling is impaired due to extrinsic compression (eg, constrictive pericarditis, pericardial tamponade), where elevated heart rates may augment contractility and preserve systemic perfusion. Furthermore, pathologic heart rates exceeding 150 beats per minute typically result in profound hypotension and cardiovascular collapse.

D. Preload

In the isolated cardiac muscle, preload refers to the sarcomere length immediately prior to contraction. Applying force (preload) to the resting muscle stretches the muscle to the desired length and results in increases in resting tension, initial velocity of contraction, and peak contractile tension. This relation between preload (resting myocardial length) and contractile performance is termed the ***Frank-Starling relationship***. In the intact ventricle, this relation is between preload (EDV) and systolic ventricular pressure and SV, both of which influence cardiac output (SV × heart rate [HR]) and ventricular stroke work (SV × mean arterial pressure [MAP]).

Because EDV influences both systolic pressure and SV, preload is an important determinant of cardiac output and is moderated by circulating blood volume, venous tone, and posture. Furthermore, when afterload is held constant, the effects of preload on SV and cardiac output are strongly influenced by ventricular performance. For example, the failing LV is less preload sensitive than the normal LV; as a result, increases in EDV produce a lesser response in SV, resulting in pulmonary congestion, for example, during an exacerbation of congestive heart failure (CHF). Conversely, when contractility is enhanced by circulating or endogenous catecholamines, the LV is more preload sensitive, with increases in EDV leading to an amplified SV response. Preload is most reliably assessed by echocardiographic measurement of EDV.[4] In clinical practice, however, a variety of surrogates for EDV may also be considered indicators of preload, each of which can potentially be affected by specific anatomic and physiologic conditions that can introduce inaccuracies in preload assessment (**Figure 3.11**).

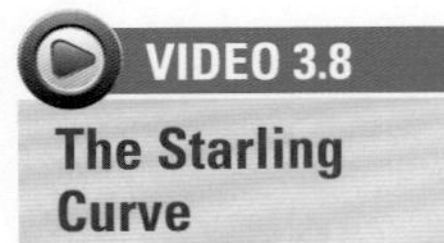

E. Afterload

Afterload refers to the tension placed on myocardial fibers during systole and is the force that the ventricle must overcome to eject its SV. The concept of afterload can seem nebulous in the clinical setting, as it is challenging to measure and reflects different physiologic processes in the LV and the RV. LV afterload is determined by multiple factors including the size and mechanical behavior of large arterial conduits (eg, atherosclerosis) and the aortic valve (eg, stenosis), terminal arteriolar impedance (eg, hypoxia-induced vasodilation, varying autonomic tone), and LV wall stress. RV afterload is determined by the size and mechanical behavior of large pulmonary arteries (eg, pulmonary embolism) and the pulmonic valve (eg, stenosis), pulmonary arteriolar impedance (hypoxia- and hypercarbia-induced vasoconstriction), and RV wall stress.

The important relation between ventricular volume, wall stress, and myocardial work is based on the balance of opposing forces that help maintain a spherical shell at a certain size, which is described by ***Laplace law*** (**Figure 3.12**). As an idealized spherical shell, the LV maintains any given size due to the balance between ventricular pressure (acting to enlarge the LV) and wall stress (acting to

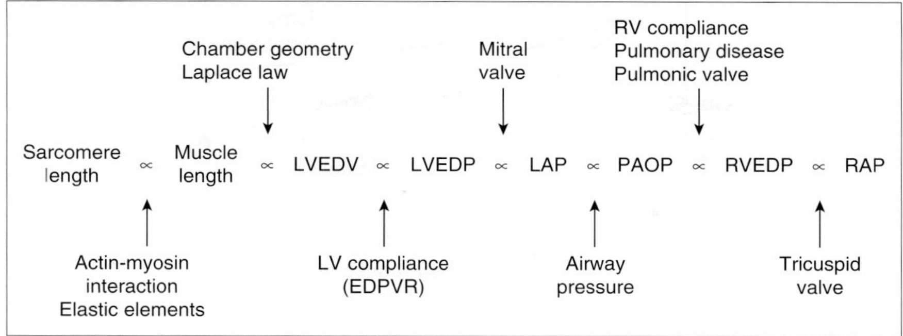

Figure 3.11 This schematic diagram depicts factors that influence experimental and clinical estimates of sarcomere length as a pure index of the preload of the contracting left ventricular (LV) myocyte. EDPVR, end-diastolic pressure-volume relation; LAP, left atrial pressure; LVEDP, LV end-diastolic pressure; LVEDV, LV end-diastolic volume; PAOP, pulmonary artery occlusion pressure; RAP, right atrial pressure; RV, right ventricle; RVEDP, RV end-diastolic pressure. (Reproduced with permission from Kaplan JA, Reich DL, Savino JS. *Kaplan's Cardiac Anesthesia: The Echo Era.* 6th ed. Elsevier Saunders; 2011:112.)

resist LV enlargement). Laplace's law relates LV pressure (p) and wall stress (σ) in the equation [$p = (2 * \sigma * h)/r$], where r is the sphere's radius and h is the LV wall thickness. Thus, increases in either LV pressure (eg, essential hypertension) or LV size (eg, chronic mitral insufficiency) result in increased wall stress and increased afterload. In order for myocardial cells to generate greater tension and wall stress in these settings, greater energy expenditure is required, thereby increasing both myocardial oxygen consumption and the risk of myocardial ischemia.

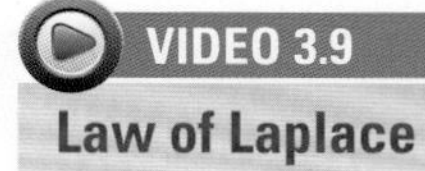

As with preload, changes in afterload can significantly influence SV and therefore cardiac output, particularly when ventricular performance is

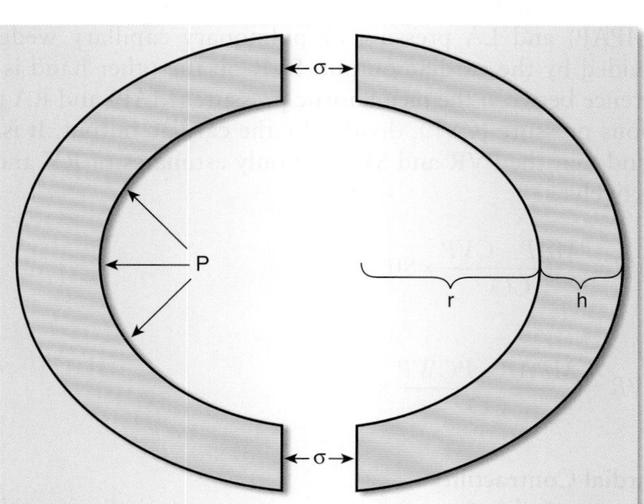

Figure 3.12 This schematic diagram depicts the opposing forces within a theoretical left ventricular (LV) sphere that determines Laplace law. LV pressure (P) pushes the sphere apart, whereas wall stress (σ) holds the sphere together. h, LV thickness; r, LV radius. (Reproduced with permission from Kaplan JA, Reich DL, Savino JS. *Kaplan's Cardiac Anesthesia: The Echo Era.* 6th ed. Elsevier Saunders; 2011:105, Figure 5-6.)

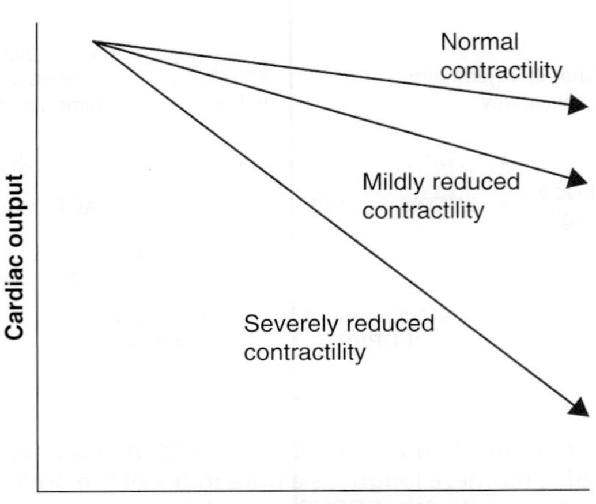

Figure 3.13 The effects of increasing afterload (systemic vascular resistance) on ventricular performance (cardiac output) are shown for three different states of contractility. Under normal conditions, increases in afterload reduce left ventricle (LV) performance. However, the failing LV is more afterload sensitive than the healthy LV; thus, a greater decrease in cardiac output occurs as myocardial contractility is progressively impaired.

abnormal. For example, the failing LV with reduced contractility is more afterload sensitive than the healthy LV and will demonstrate a proportionately greater decrease in cardiac output when afterload is increased (**Figure 3.13**).

As with preload, direct measurement of afterload in the clinical setting is challenging. The most common surrogate assessment of afterload is the calculation of vascular resistance using measurements of cardiac output and pressure changes across either the pulmonary vasculature (***pulmonary vascular resistance*** [PVR]) or the systemic vasculature (***systemic vascular resistance*** [SVR]). PVR is calculated as the difference between mean pulmonary artery pressure (MPAP) and LA pressure or pulmonary capillary wedge pressure (PCWP) divided by the cardiac output. SVR on the other hand is calculated as the difference between the mean aortic pressure (MAP) and RA pressure or central venous pressure (CVP), divided by the cardiac output. It is important to understand that the PVR and SVR are only estimates of RV and LV afterload, respectively.

$$SVR = \frac{MAP - CVP}{CO} \times 80$$

$$PVR = \frac{MPAP - PCWP}{CO} \times 80$$

F. Myocardial Contractility

Myocardial contractility is an intrinsic property of cardiac muscle. It refers to the force and velocity of muscular contraction of the ventricle under conditions of load and represents the systolic myocardial work done for a given preload and afterload. Also termed the inotropic state, contractility can be influenced by a number of intrinsic and extrinsic factors that increase inotropy (autonomic SNS activity, endogenous catecholamines, exogenous catecholamines, calcium, digitalis) or decrease inotropy (autonomic PNS activity,

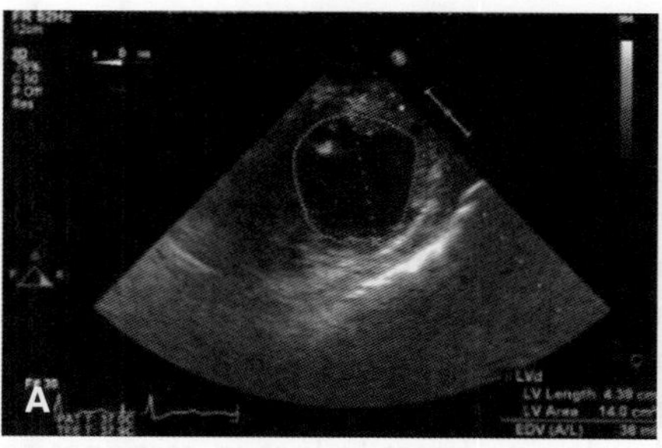

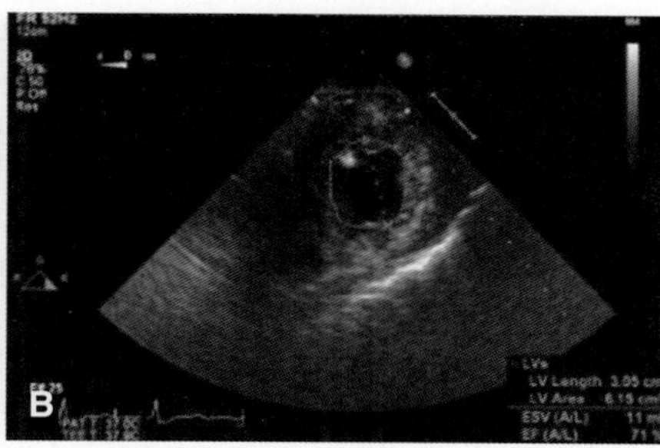

Figure 3.14 Calculation of fractional area change from left ventricle (LV) midpapillary short-axis images obtained at end diastole (A) and end systole (B). The LV endocardial border surrounding the black LV chamber is manually traced (excluding the papillary muscles), and the inscribed area is calculated by integrating software. The LV ejection fraction is determined as the difference between the end-diastolic area and the end-systolic area, divided by the end-diastolic area. (Reproduced with permission from Kaplan JA, Reich DL, Savino JS. *Kaplan's Cardiac Anesthesia: The Echo Era*. 6th ed. Elsevier Saunders; 2011:119, Figure 5-27.)

myocardial ischemia, hypoxia, hypercarbia, cardiomyopathy, hypocalcemia, β_1-adrenergic blocking drugs).

Contractility is difficult to measure in vivo because the strength of cardiac contraction is also determined by preload and afterload. As noted earlier, the maximum rate of rise in LV pressure (+dP/dt) that occurs during the brief isovolumic contraction period is one useful indirect index of LV contractility, in part because it is largely afterload independent. In contrast, the Frank-Starling relationship dictates that +dP/dt is highly dependent on preload. LV pressure (and hence +dP/dt) can only be directly measured invasively during cardiac catheterization but can be estimated by transesophageal echocardiography (TEE). The two most practical surrogate assessments of contractility by TEE are the ejection fraction (**Figure 3.14**) and P-V diagram analysis of the ESPVR (**Figures 3.8** and **3.9**).

VII. Factors That Determine Diastolic Function

A. Heart Chambers

In addition to its ability to eject blood during ventricular systole, pump performance of the heart is also dependent on its diastolic function—the ability to fully and efficiently relax allowing for blood collection prior to ventricular contraction. The atria contribute to this process as thin-walled, low-pressure chambers that function more as large reservoir conduits, in contrast to their respective thick-walled, high-pressure ventricles that function as forward propelling pumps.

B. Left Ventricular Response to Load

Diastolic loading of the ventricle generally occurs by adding volume (preload) to the chamber or by increasing resistance (afterload) to outflow. The ventricle responds to load by lengthening its myocardial fibers, increasing wall stress, or both, thereby modulating ventricular relaxation, filling, and compliance. Because such changes in load are dynamic and occur frequently both in daily activities (eg, exercise) and in the perioperative setting (eg, blood loss, fluid resuscitation, volatile anesthetics), the ability of the ventricle to rapidly adjust to such changes and ultimately maintain cardiac output (termed ***homometric autoregulation***) defines diastolic function.

For the LV, ***diastolic dysfunction*** occurs when the ventricle cannot rapidly adjust to increases in load, resulting in persistently elevated LV volumes or pressures that precipitate LV failure. Diastolic dysfunction occurs when LV relaxation or filling is impaired or when the LV becomes less compliant. This can occur as an isolated abnormality (with intact systolic function) or in association with systolic dysfunction.[5] Diastolic dysfunction is more common in the elderly and often associated with conditions that increase ventricular wall stiffness or afterload (eg, LV hypertrophy). Because prior knowledge of patients' diastolic function can affect clinical management, an understanding of its assessment strategies is vital. Unfortunately, no single index of diastolic function completely characterizes this portion of the cardiac cycle or accurately predicts those at greatest risk of developing heart failure in response to changing load conditions. Thus, both invasive and noninvasive assessments of ventricular relaxation, filling, and compliance may be needed.

C. Invasive Assessment of Diastolic Function

Complete and rapid ***LV relaxation*** is necessary to facilitate efficient passive ventricular filling and maximize EDV during diastole. Because LV relaxation is an active, energy-dependent process involving dissociation of contractile proteins in myocardial cells, myocardial ischemia is a frequent cause of impaired LV relaxation. Thus, ischemia can impair cardiac output and precipitate CHF through both diastolic and systolic mechanisms. Invasive assessment of LV relaxation is performed during cardiac catheterization by directly measuring the time course of LV pressure decline (−dP/dt) during the isovolumic relaxation period. The two most commonly calculated indices of LV relaxation from this method are the maximal rate of LV pressure reduction (smaller values of −dP/dt indicate impaired LV relaxation) and the time constant of LV relaxation (prolonged time constants indicate impaired LV relaxation). Although these indices have prognostic value, noninvasive techniques have largely supplanted them.

D. Noninvasive Assessment of Diastolic Function

As noted earlier, P-V diagram analysis of the EDPVR by echocardiography is one common method for assessing LV compliance (**Figures 3.8** and **3.9**). Also, because the isovolumic relaxation period for the LV is defined as the portion of the cardiac cycle between when the aortic valve closes and the mitral valve opens (**Figure 3.7**), the length of this period is related to LV relaxation. Impaired LV relaxation results in a prolonged ***isovolumic relaxation time*** (IVRT). The IVRT can be measured by observing aortic and mitral valve closure by echocardiography and, in the absence of aortic or mitral valve disease, is inversely proportional to LV relaxation.

A second method of assessing LV relaxation uses Doppler echocardiographic measurement of blood flow velocities across the mitral valve. During diastole, two distinct flow patterns occur at this location: an early E peak associated with early LV filling and a later A peak corresponding to LA contraction. When LV relaxation is prolonged, the E wave deceleration time is prolonged, the A wave velocity is increased, and the ratio of these two flow velocities decreases (E/A < 1). As diastolic function worsens and LA pressures increase, the E wave velocities increase, first to an E/A ratio in the normal range (E/A > 1) and then to higher ratios (E/A > 2).[6]

VIII. Blood Pressure

A. Systemic, Pulmonary, and Venous

Cardiac output enters the systemic and pulmonary circulations from the LV and RV, respectively, each of which contain serial arterial, microcirculatory, and venous components. Systemic blood pressures exceed pulmonary blood pressures due to differing anatomic structures and pump capabilities of the RV and LV, significantly lower vascular impedance of the pulmonary circulation compared with the systemic circulation, and nearly identical cardiac outputs in both circulations, the fluid mechanics analogue of ***Ohm law*** (pressure = flow × resistance).

The typical aortic ***pressure waveform*** is shown in **Figure 3.15**. The peak of the wave is the ***systolic blood pressure*** (SBP), and the nadir is the ***diastolic blood pressure*** (DBP), with the difference between the two termed the ***pulse pressure*** (PP). As the pressure wave moves distally in the arterial tree, the sharp dicrotic notch becomes more scooped, the SBP increases, the DBP decreases, and the PP increases due to the combination of elastic properties of the large artery walls, partial wave reflection at large artery branch points, and decreasing vessel compliance in smaller arteries. The ***mean arterial pressure*** (MAP) is the average pressure over the entire period and can be estimated from sphygmomanometer measurements of the SBP and DBP (MAP = DBP + [0.33 × PP]). Perfusion pressure refers to the driving pressure required to perfuse a specific tissue or organ and is defined as the difference between the MAP and the resistance pressure that must be overcome to affect perfusion. For example, the cerebral perfusion pressure is the MAP minus the intracranial pressure. Because the large arteries have elastic components and properties, the arterial system is distensible and able to maintain positive pressure throughout the cardiac cycle. Thus, only a portion of the energy of cardiac contraction results in forward capillary flow, with the remainder stored as potential energy in the elastic recoil of the arteries, a property known as the ***Windkessel effect***. Thus, this elastic property attenuates pulse pressure during systole, and as a result, its elastic recoil during diastole allows for forward flow and end organ perfusion throughout the entire cardiac cycle.

Because of lower vascular impedance in the pulmonary circulation, the RV accomplishes pulmonary perfusion with lower systolic pressures and less oxygen consumption and generates significantly lower arterial outflow pressures compared with the LV. Under normal anatomic conditions, the cardiac output of the RV is slightly lower than that of the LV due to bronchial blood flow from the systemic circulation (~1% of the total cardiac output) that returns deoxygenated blood directly to the left atrium. A very small portion of the cardiac output is returned directly to the LV from coronary arterial luminal shunts and coronary veins (Thebesian veins).

B. Vascular Resistance

For the systemic circulation, the blood pressure, cross-sectional area, and volume capacitance vary widely across its arterial, microcirculatory, and venous components. The arterioles serve as the principal points of resistance to blood flow in the systemic circulation, producing roughly 95% reduction in mean intravascular pressure. In the absence of mechanical obstruction in more proximal arteries, the modulation of arteriolar vascular smooth muscle tone is therefore the principal determinant of SVR and serves three important functions: (1) regulation of differential tissue blood flow to specific vascular beds; (2) modulation of systemic arterial blood pressure; and (3) converting pulsatile to nonpulsatile blood flow to facilitate consistent capillary perfusion.

VIDEO 3.10

Circulatory System Blood Flow and Pressures

Resting vascular smooth muscle exerts mild tonic arteriolar vasoconstriction that can be modulated by autonomic SNS activity, circulating hormones, drugs, ambient temperature, local metabolic activity, and autoregulation to achieve further vasoconstriction or vasodilation. For example, autonomic

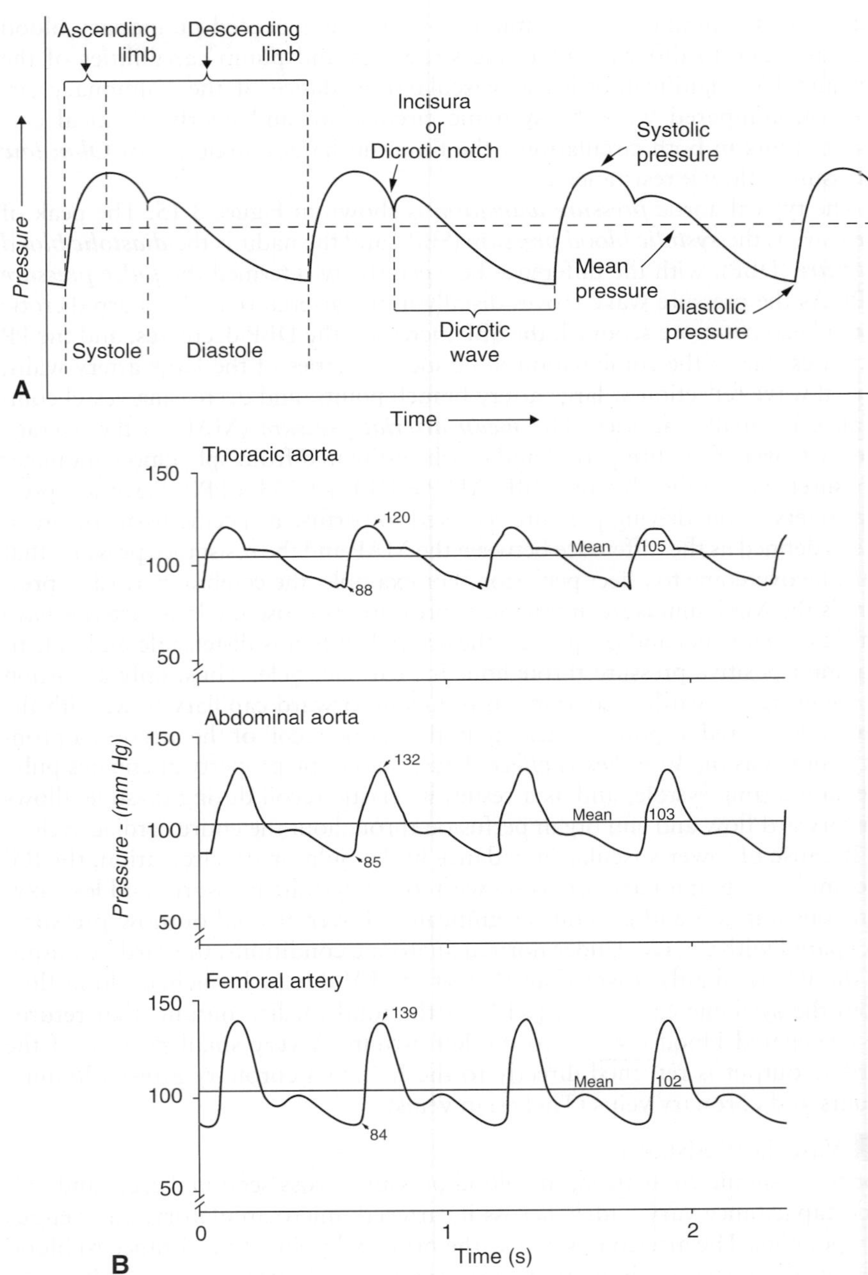

Figure 3.15 The typical aortic pulse pressure waveform is shown (A), with each pulse consisting of a brief, sharp ascending limb, followed by a more prolonged descending limb. Each pulse is easily separated into systole and diastole by the dicrotic notch, with the peak pressure corresponding the systolic pressure and the lowest pressure being the diastolic pressure. Mean arterial pressure is the average pressure over the entire pulse period (B). The pulse pressure waveform changes as one moves distally in the systemic arterial tree due to arterial branching and changes in vessel elasticity.

SNS stimulation results in norepinephrine release that activates β-adrenergic receptors in vascular smooth muscle to augment resting vasoconstriction. In vascular beds containing both α- and β_2-adrenergic receptors (eg, skeletal muscle), exogenous epinephrine at low doses will selectively activate β_2-adrenergic receptors and cause vasodilation, whereas high doses will result in predominate activation of α-adrenergic receptors and lead to enhanced vasoconstriction. Local metabolic activity plays an important role in regional control of vascular resistance because arterioles lie within the organ itself and are exposed to the local environment. When blood flow to tissue is inadequate to meet metabolic needs, local factors (eg, high carbon dioxide [CO_2], low pH) result in vasodilation in an attempt to increase blood flow to meet metabolic demand.

? Did You Know?

In the elderly, age-related autonomic nervous system dysfunction interferes with the baroreceptor reflex arc, such that hypotension-induced compensatory increases in heart rate and blood pressure are less pronounced compared to young adults.

Autoregulation refers to the intrinsic tendency of a specific organ or tissue bed to maintain constant blood flow despite changes in arterial pressure, independent of hormonal or neural mechanisms. Autoregulation is typically active within a specific range of arterial pressures, within which constant flow is achieved by changes in vascular resistance (**Figure 3.16**). Outside this range, blood flow varies proportionately to arterial pressure, with clinical consequences of ischemia (low pressure) or hyperemia (high pressure). The human organs with the most clinically significant autoregulation features are the brain, kidneys, and heart.[7]

C. Baroreceptor Function

In addition to the immediate regulation of blood flow by autoregulation at the tissue level, more widespread and short-term adjustments in systemic arterial pressure are also regulated by the baroreceptor reflex (**Table 3.1; Figure 3.17**). This

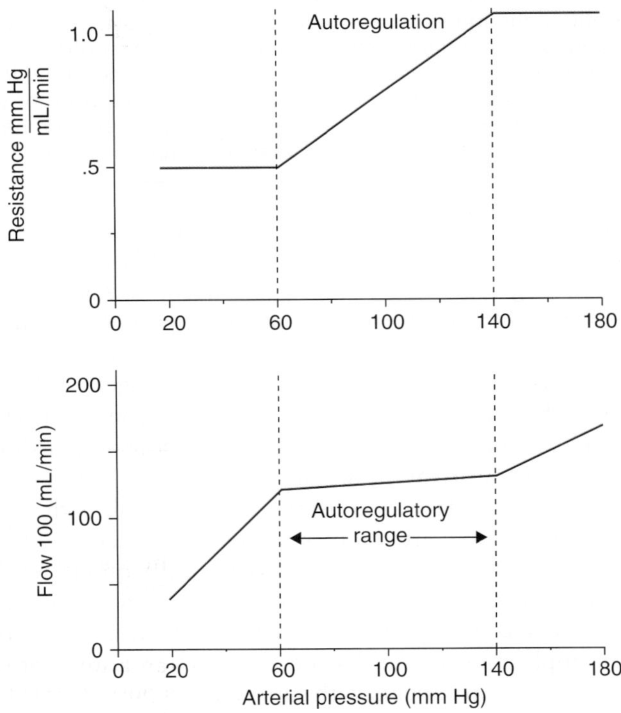

Figure 3.16 Autoregulation occurs when blood flow (*lower panel*) is maintained relatively constant over a wide range of mean arterial pressures (in this case 60-140 mm Hg). This process is accomplished by changes in vascular resistance (*upper panel*) that are independent of neural and hormonal influence.

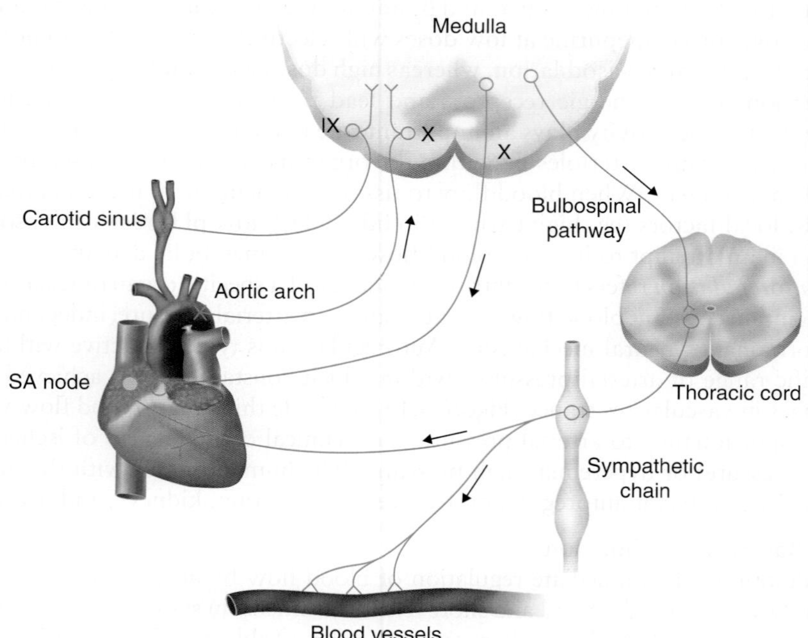

Figure 3.17 The afferent limb of the baroreceptor reflex is initiated by baroreceptors in the carotid sinus (glossopharyngeal nerve) and aortic arch (vagus nerve) with transmission to the medulla. Elevated blood pressure results in efferent vagal nerve traffic to the heart that slows heart rate and reduces contractility (to reduce blood pressure). In contrast, low blood pressure results in efferent sympathetic tone via the spinal cord and sympathetic chain that increases both heart rate and contractility, and also results in peripheral vasoconstriction. SA, sinoatrial.

inverse relation between arterial blood pressure and heart rate was first described by Etienne Marey in 1859 and serves to preserve cardiac output and arterial pressure under varying conditions such as postural changes, exercise, and hypovolemia. The afferent limb of the reflex is initiated by pressure-sensitive stretch receptors in the carotid sinus and the aortic arch that relay sensory information to the medullary vasomotor center via the glossopharyngeal and vagus nerves. The efferent limb of the reflex includes two possible responses: (1) elevated arterial pressure results in increased vagal PNS tone and decreased SNS tone, which modifies heart rate downward at the SA and AV nodes and reduces both myocardial contractility and arteriolar vasoconstriction to diminish both cardiac output and arterial pressure; (2) low arterial pressure results in increased SNS traffic at various levels of the sympathetic chain to modify heart rate upward at the SA node and augment ventricular contractility to enhance cardiac output, as well as increase arteriolar vasoconstriction to rapidly increase arterial pressure.

One clinical application of the baroreceptor reflex is the performance of external carotid massage in patients with supraventricular tachycardia. This will stimulate afferent glossopharyngeal nerve traffic and enhance reflex PNS vagal tone to slow pathologic tachycardias. The baroreceptor reflex also underlies the typical observation of compensatory tachycardia in patients with hypovolemic hypotension. Conversely, abnormal baroreceptor reflex responses can occur in patients with neurologic impairments at any point along the reflex arc. For example, age-related autonomic dysfunction in the elderly is often manifest by postural syncope due to reductions in cerebral perfusion pressure and flow.

IX. Venous Return

A. Vascular Compliance, Capacitance, and Control

As blood exits the capillary bed, it passes first through venules and then a steadily decreasing number of veins of increasing size. The vascular system cross-sectional area in the small and large veins is similar to that in the small and large arteries. Compared with their corresponding arterial structures, however, venous structures are generally slightly larger in diameter, have thinner walls containing less vascular smooth muscle, and possess far greater capacitance (lower vascular resistance). This 10 to 20 times higher compliance means that veins can accommodate large changes in blood volume with only a small change in pressure. Venous smooth muscle receives SNS innervation, which when activated decreases venous compliance and promotes venous return to the RA.

B. Muscle Action, Intrathoracic Pressure, and Body Position

Venous return to the RA contributes to ventricular preload and is primarily determined by extravascular factors. These include skeletal muscle contraction in the limbs (***muscle pump***), intrathoracic pressure changes associated with respiratory activity (***thoracoabdominal pump***), external vena cava compression, and forces of gravity associated with postural changes.[8,9] Skeletal muscle contractions in the arms and legs, in combination with pressure-passive one-way venous valves in peripheral veins, augment venous return, particularly during exercise. Muscle contraction compresses veins within large muscle groups and forces venous blood centrally, whereas skeletal muscle relaxation decompresses veins and draws in blood from the distal limb and adjacent veins. Repeated compression-decompression cycles rapidly propel venous blood centrally and enhance venous return. Patients with incompetent venous valves are unable to augment their venous return with exercise or postural changes and may experience syncope under these conditions.

Spontaneous respiration changes the transmural pressure in veins passing through the intrathoracic cavity and modifies venous return. During inspiration, diaphragmatic descent and thoracic cage expansion create negative intrathoracic pressure, while at the same time elevating intra-abdominal pressure. These combined forces increase the pressure gradient favoring increased venous return from the subdiaphragmatic vena cava to the RA. Additionally, negative intrathoracic pressure also reduces thoracic vena cava and RA pressures and further enhances venous return from the head, neck, and upper extremities. Conversely, spontaneous expiration increases intrathoracic pressure and impairs venous return. The overall effect of spontaneous ventilation is to enhance venous return compared with apneic conditions because mean intrathoracic pressures are slightly negative over the entire respiratory cycle. In contrast, positive-pressure ventilation increases mean intrathoracic pressures, impairs venous return, and can negatively impact cardiac output, especially in settings where high levels of positive end-expiratory pressure (PEEP) are being utilized.

C. Blood Volume and Distribution

Total body water constitutes ~60% of body weight (42 L in a 70-kg person), with ~40% (28 L) in the intracellular space and ~20% (14 L) in the extracellular space. Plasma volume accounts for one-fifth (3 L) of the extracellular volume, and erythrocyte volume (2 L) is part of the intracellular volume; therefore, blood volume is ~ 5 L in a 70-kg person. Blood volume is nonuniformly distributed throughout the circulatory tree, with approximately 65% in the systemic venous system, 15% in the systemic arterial system, 10% in the pulmonary circulation, and the remainder in the heart and systemic microcirculation.

X. Microcirculation

A. Capillary Diffusion, Oncotic Pressure, and Starling Law

The ultimate purpose of the cardiovascular system is to deliver oxygen and nutrients to tissues and to remove CO_2 and metabolic waste products from the cellular level. This process occurs in the rich network of capillaries that are only 5 to 10 μm in diameter, yet so overwhelming in number that the overall surface area of the network is 20 times greater than that of all the small and larger arteries. Capillary density is greatest in metabolically active tissues (eg, myocardium, skeletal muscle) and lowest in less active tissues (eg, fat, cartilage).

Water and solutes diffuse in both directions across the capillary wall, with water and water-soluble molecules (eg, sodium chloride, glucose) traversing the wall through clefts between adjacent endothelial cells, lipophilic molecules (oxygen, CO_2) moving directly across the endothelial cells, and large molecules traversing through large clefts or by pinocytosis within endoplasmic vesicles. Thus, the capillary wall acts as a semipermeable membrane across which water, gases, and small substrates move primarily by diffusion according to concentration gradients.[10] In addition, when there is a difference between hydrostatic forces and osmotic forces across the capillary wall, water movement also occurs by filtration. In the microvasculature, osmotic pressure is largely determined by protein concentration (particularly albumin) and is termed ***oncotic pressure***. According to the ***Starling hypothesis***, fluid filtration across the porous capillary wall is determined by the balance between the hydrostatic and oncotic pressure gradients across the wall, as well as by the size and number of intercellular clefts. The hydrostatic pressure gradient favors water movement out of the capillary and is slightly greater than the oncotic pressure gradient that favors water movement into the capillary. The relation between these factors is governed by the ***Starling equation***:

$$F = Kf * ([Pc - Pt] - \sigma[\pi c - \pi i]),$$

where F is the fluid movement across the capillary wall, Kf is the filtration constant of the capillary membrane (reflecting its permeability), Pc is the capillary hydrostatic pressure (higher on the arteriolar side of the capillary than on the venular side of the capillary), Pt is the tissue hydrostatic pressure (typically near zero), σ is the reflection coefficient (a correction factor for protein permeability of the capillary wall), pc is the plasma oncotic pressure, and pi is the interstitial oncotic pressure.

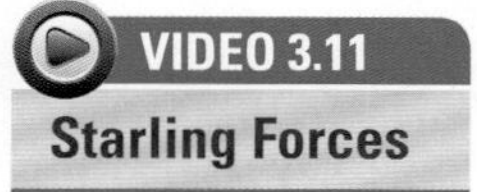

A high Kf indicates a highly water permeable capillary, such as in the presence of histamine (eg, airway edema that occurs during anaphylaxis), whereas a low Kf indicates low capillary permeability. The factors in the Starling equation including typical pressure values are illustrated in **Figure 3.18**.

The bulk flow of water and proteins across the capillary membrane is generally in the direction from the intravascular to the interstitial space. Highly permeable lymphatic capillaries collect this bulk flow in tissues and return the

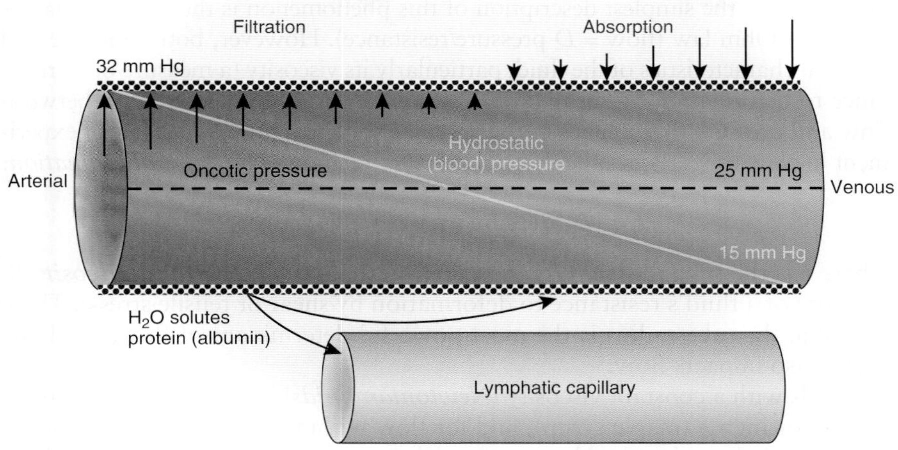

Figure 3.18 Fluid movement across the capillary membrane is determined by the permeability of the membrane to water, solutes, and protein; the hydrostatic pressure difference across the membrane; and the oncotic pressure difference across the membrane, and it is summarized by the Starling equation (see text). The hydrostatic pressure gradient varies across the length of the capillary, favoring fluid movement out of the capillary to a greater degree on the arterial end. The oncotic pressure gradient is uniform and favors fluid movement into the capillary. Net fluid movement is toward the interstitium, with lymphatic capillaries collecting the excess filtrate and returning it to the circulation.

fluid and proteins (predominately albumin) through lymphatic vessels of progressively increasing size, facilitated by intermittent skeletal muscle activity, smooth muscle in the lymphatic walls, and one-way valves. The volume of fluid returned to the circulation (largely through the thoracic duct) in 24 hours is approximately equal to the total plasma volume.

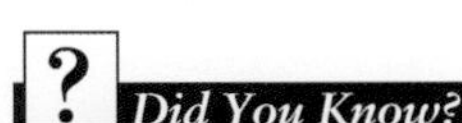

Unlike vasoconstriction in systemic arteriolar beds that adjust but do not abolish tissue blood flow, precapillary sphincters can completely occlude the vessel lumen and direct flow away from selected capillary beds (eg, shunting of blood away from the cutaneous circulation in cold environments).

B. Precapillary and Postcapillary Sphincter Control

Capillary blood flow in any given tissue bed is highly variable and is controlled by the precapillary and postcapillary sphincters. Transmural pressure (intravascular minus extravascular pressure) and contraction/relaxation of the precapillary and postcapillary sphincters are the primary determinants of capillary flow, with the latter mediated by both neural and local humoral factors. Unlike vasoconstriction in more proximal arteriolar beds that adjust but do not abolish tissue blood flow, precapillary sphincters can fully occlude the vessel lumen, directing flow away from capillary beds into nearby arteriovenous shunts. For example, in cold environments precapillary sphincter tone is increased to shunt blood away from cutaneous beds to retain heat. Abnormal perioperative thermoregulation occurs when this tone is impaired by various anesthetic agents. In addition, by reducing capillary flow, precapillary sphincter contraction also reduces fluid filtration due to a reduction in *Pc*. Postcapillary sphincter contraction also reduces capillary flow, but increases fluid filtration due to an increase in *Pc*.

C. Viscosity and Rheology

The flow of any fluid in any tube is always dependent on the pressure difference between ends of the tube; in the absence of a gradient, no flow will occur. As noted earlier, the simplest description of this phenomenon is the fluid mechanics analog of Ohm law (flow = *D* pressure/resistance). However, both tube size and physical characteristics of the fluid, particularly its viscosity (a measure of its resistance to deformation by shear forces), require a more detailed relation between flow and pressure that applies to the vascular system. Through a series of experiment in glass tubes, Poiseuille described such a relation—the ***Poiseuille equation***:

$$F = \left(\Delta \text{ pressure} \times \pi \times r^4\right) / \left(8 \times L \times \eta\right),$$

where r is the tube radius, L is the tube length, and η is the ***fluid viscosity*** (a measure of a fluid's resistance to deformation by shear or tensile stress). Thus, although the tube radius is the most powerful determinant of flow, fluid viscosity also impacts flow.

Fluids with a constant viscosity (***Newtonian fluids***) include those with low η (water) or high η (maple syrup), and for flow within any given tube geometry, their flow is linearly related to pressure difference. However, for fluids whose viscosity is variable (***non-Newtonian fluids***), flow varies not only with pressure difference, but also with factors that affect viscosity. Blood has a variable viscosity that is affected by several factors, including blood constituents and blood shear rate (the velocity gradient of blood as it moves from vessel wall [low velocity] to the vessel lumen [high velocity]). Because blood is rheologically a suspension of erythrocytes in plasma, increasing the concentration of erythrocytes (hematocrit) causes the blood viscosity to increase. For example, increasing the hematocrit from 45% to 70% (polycythemia) doubles the blood viscosity, with a proportionate reduction in blood flow for any given tube diameter and pressure difference (by Poiseuille equation), with potential clinical consequences of decreased oxygen delivery to tissues. In addition, in the ventricle, high shear rates occurring during systole decrease blood viscosity and facilitate flow, in contrast to low shear rates occurring during diastole increase blood viscosity.

For further review and interactivities, please see the associated Interactive Video Lectures and "At a Glance" infographic accessible in the complimentary eBook bundled with this text. Access instructions are located in the inside front cover.

References

1. Moore KL, Agur AMR, Dalley AF II. Thorax. In: Moore KL, Agur AMR, Dalley AF II, eds. *Clinically Oriented Anatomy*. 7th ed. Lippincott Williams & Wilkins; 2013:131-249.
2. Pagel PS, Kampine JP, Stowe DF. Cardiac anatomy and physiology. In: Barash PG, Cullen BF, Stoelting RK, et al, eds. *Clinical Anesthesia*. 7th ed. Lippincott Williams & Wilkins; 2013:239-262.
3. Grossman W. Diastolic dysfunction and congestive heart failure. *Circulation*. 1990;81(2 suppl):III1-III7. PMID: 2137051.
4. Schober P, Loer SA, Schwarte LA. Perioperative hemodynamic monitoring with transesophageal Doppler technology. *Anesth Analg*. 2009;109(2):340-353. PMID: 19608800.
5. Borlaug BA, Kass DA. Invasive hemodynamic assessment in heart failure. *Heart Fail Clin*. 2009;5(2):217-228. PMID: 19249690.
6. Cohen GI, Pietrolungo JF, Thomas JD, et al. A practical guide to assessment of ventricular diastolic function using Doppler echocardiography. *J Am Coll Cardiol*. 1996;27:1753-1760. PMID: 8636565.

7. Dagal A, Lam AM. Cerebral autoregulation and anesthesia. *Curr Opin Anaesthesiol.* 2009;22(5):547-552. PMID: 19620861.
8. Funk DJ, Jacobsohn E, Kumar A. The role of the venous return in critical illness and shock: part I—physiology. *Crit Care Med.* 2013;41(1):255-262. PMID: 23269130.
9. Funk DJ, Jacobsohn E, Kumar A. Role of the venous return in critical illness and shock: part II—shock and mechanical ventilation. *Crit Care Med.* 2013;41(2):573-579. PMID: 23263572.
10. Parker JC, Guyton AC, Taylor AE. Pulmonary transcapillary exchange and pulmonary edema. *Int Rev Physiol.* 1979;18:261-315. PMID: 361606.

CARDIOVASCULAR PHYSIOLOGY

AT A GLANCE

The functions of the cardiovascular system can be defined by a central pump which promotes blood flow that delivers oxygen to tissues at a sufficient perfusion pressure. Illustrated below are some of the most important equations that characterize this physiology.

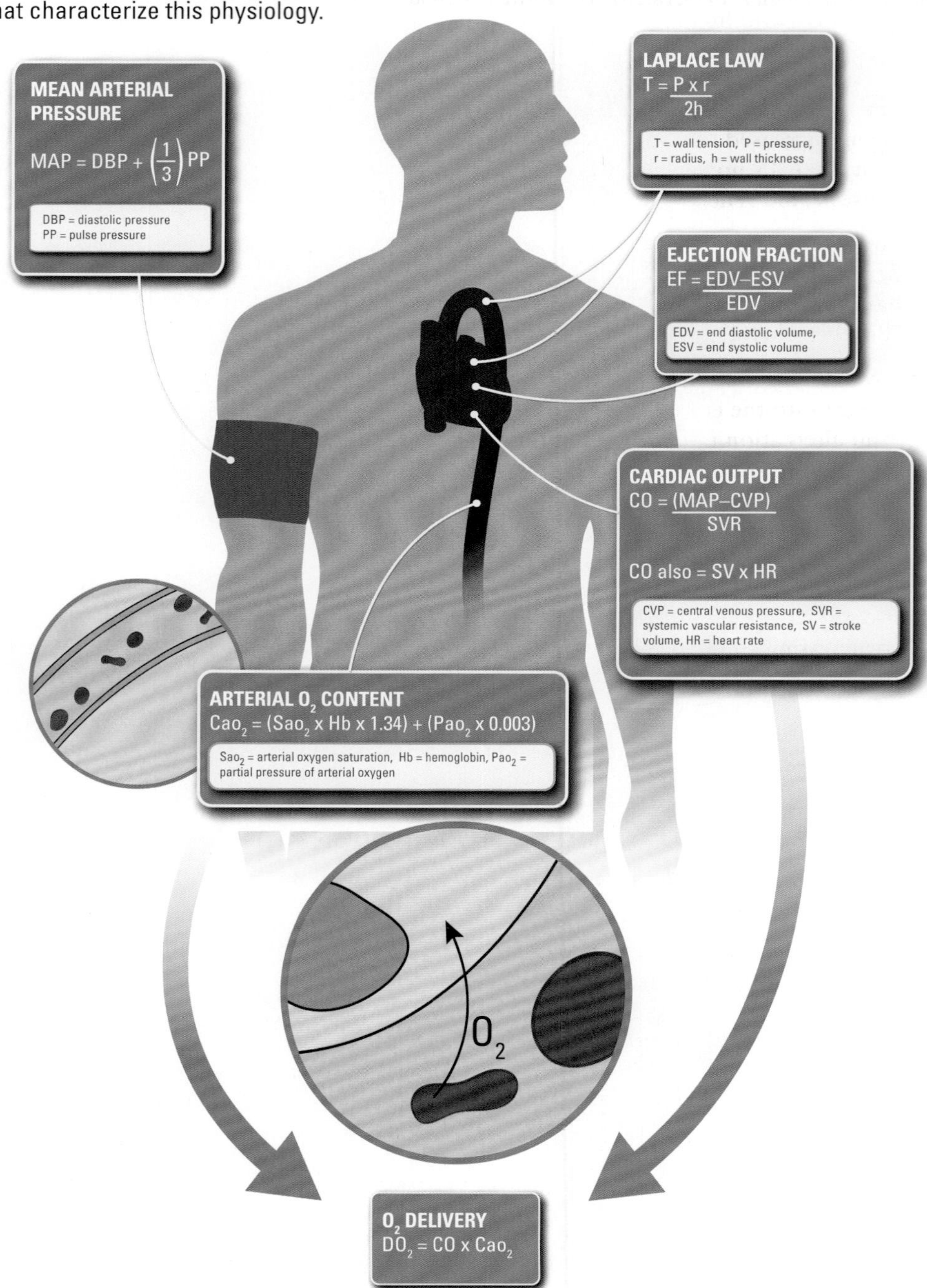

MEAN ARTERIAL PRESSURE
$MAP = DBP + \left(\frac{1}{3}\right) PP$
DBP = diastolic pressure
PP = pulse pressure
LAPLACE LAW
$T = \frac{P \times r}{2h}$
T = wall tension, P = pressure, r = radius, h = wall thickness
EJECTION FRACTION
$EF = \frac{EDV - ESV}{EDV}$
EDV = end diastolic volume, ESV = end systolic volume
CARDIAC OUTPUT
$CO = \frac{(MAP - CVP)}{SVR}$
CO also = SV x HR
CVP = central venous pressure, SVR = systemic vascular resistance, SV = stroke volume, HR = heart rate
ARTERIAL O_2 CONTENT
$Cao_2 = (Sao_2 \times Hb \times 1.34) + (Pao_2 \times 0.003)$
Sao_2 = arterial oxygen saturation, Hb = hemoglobin, Pao_2 = partial pressure of arterial oxygen
O_2
O_2 DELIVERY
$DO_2 = CO \times Cao_2$

Infographic by: Naveen Nathan MD

Questions

1. **A 43-year-old man involved in a motor vehicle collision with resultant open femur fracture is scheduled for open repair. After induction, he is found to be tachycardic into the 110s and hypotensive with SBPs in the 80s. Given your suspicion for ongoing hypovolemic hypotension, you administer 1L crystalloid bolus which results in increased tachycardia with heart rates in the 130s now. What physiologic response would reflect this?**

   A. Bowditch effect
   B. Bezold-Jarisch reflex
   C. Bainbridge reflex
   D. Windkessel effect

2. **A 21-year-old previously healthy woman is brought into the emergency department after an altercation in which she was stabbed. On examination, she is found to have a single 2-cm incision lateral to sternum on her left chest wall at approximately the fourth intercostal space. What cardiac structure are you most concerned about being violated by this penetrating trauma?**

   A. Right atrium
   B. Right ventricle
   C. Left atrium
   D. Left ventricle

3. **In a patient with left ventricular hypertrophy presenting with symptoms consistent with myocardial ischemia, which region of the heart would be at greatest risk for ischemia?**

   A. Endocardium
   B. Myocardium
   C. Epicardium
   D. Pericardium

4. **Lung-protective ventilation with an escalating PEEP ladder is a mainstay in the treatment of ARDS. What foreseeable changes in hemodynamics do you anticipate with higher levels of PEEP?**

   A. Improvement in systemic blood pressure with increased preload
   B. New or worsening hypotension as a result of decreased preload
   C. No difference in current hemodynamics
   D. None of the above

5. **Your patient with a prior history of orthotopic heart transplant undergoing noncardiac surgery acutely develops new bradycardia with a heart rate of 50 and associated hypotension intraoperatively. What would be the medication of choice to improve their hemodynamics?**

   A. Atropine
   B. Phenylephrine
   C. Ephedrine
   D. Epinephrine

Answers

1. C

The right atrial stretch receptors activated by a fluid bolus, interpret this as state of newly increased central venous pressure which results in increased sympathetic nervous system tone and a decrease in parasympathetic tone, thus resulting in increase this patient's tachycardia. A. Bowditch effect: Results in contractile tension as the frequency of contraction increases to a maximum of 150 to 180 contractions/s. B. Bezold-Jarisch reflex: Triad of hypotension, bradycardia, and coronary vasodilation that is the result of a surge in parasympathetic tone. D. Windkessel effect: Given the elastic components found in large arteries, this allows for vessel caliber dilation which functions effectively as stored potential energy, that when the vessels recoil during diastole, there is still forward pulsatile flow perfusing end organs.

2. B

The right ventricle is the anterior most chamber of the heart and thus is most susceptible to penetrating chest wall trauma.

3. A

The left ventricle is dependent on the left coronary artery which flow can be highly variable throughout the cardiac cycle. Peak blood flow occurs during diastole when perfusion pressure is greatest, and can be reduced to nearly zero flow as a result of vessel compression during systole as the LV contracts. Left ventricular hypertrophy further worsens this process as the hypertrophied myocardium is reliant on the same caliber arterioles that are more susceptible to be fully compressed by increase myocardial muscle mass, especially in clinical settings with increased oxygen consumption or demand.

4. B

Positive-pressure ventilation is associated with increased intrathoracic pressure which results in decreased venous return and therefore a decrease in cardiac preload. With increasing levels of PEEP, one should anticipate further increases in intrathoracic pressure and therefore a larger negative impact on venous return, which may result in new or more notable clinical hypotension.

5. D

As the denervated heart does not respond to vagal stimulation, or more broadly parasympathetic nervous system responses, the resting heart rate of patients is often slightly elevated in the 90 to 110s region. Additionally, the denervated heart will not respond to anticholinergic medications, like atropine, that result in an increase in heart rate as a result of inhibition of the PNS. While indirect acting sympathomimetics, like ephedrine, may work, the effects are likely to be blunted in the denervated heart. Thus, direct acting sympathomimetics, such as epinephrine, isoproterenol, and norepinephrine, should be used preferentially as the transplanted heart's β1 receptors will reliably still respond with an appropriate increase in cardiac output (increased inotropy and chronotropy).

4 Central and Autonomic Nervous System

Eduard Vaynberg

I. The Central Nervous System

The human nervous system is an evolutional wonder that governs all body processes serving both sensorium, executive functions, and processing the world around us. The nervous system is built from 10^{10} neurons connected into a vast functional network. The human central nervous system consists of the brain and the spinal cord (**Figure 4.1**).

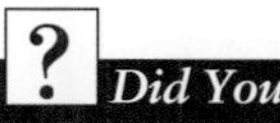

The olfactory nerve is the only cranial nerve whose input reaches the cerebral cortex without going through the thalamus.

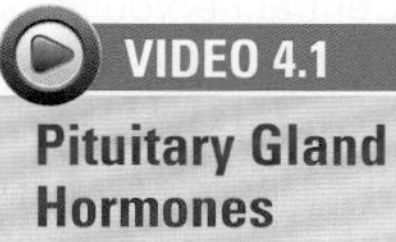

The brain (encephalon) is protected by the cranium and serves as a central processor for the information coming from the trunk and limbs, conducted by the spinal cord, peripheral nerves, and autonomic nervous system. There are also twelve pairs of cranial nerves connected directly to the brain serving head and neck functions.

The mature brain consists of four parts: brainstem, midbrain, diencephalon, and cerebrum. The brainstem (rhombencephalon) is divided into the medulla oblongata (connected directly to the spinal cord), pons, and cerebellum. The brainstem is protected by basal portions of occipital and sphenoid bones.

The medulla (***center, quintessence*** in Latin) conducts all signals between the spinal cord and the brain. It also contains the cardiovascular center that processes rate and force of cardiac contraction and the diameter of the blood vessels, and the respiratory center responsible for the basic rate of breathing. The medulla also controls vomiting, sneezing, coughing, and hiccupping.

The pons (***bridge*** in Latin) lies directly superior to the medulla and anterior to the cerebellum. As the name suggests, the pons serves as a connector between different parts of the brain. The pons is responsible for coordinating voluntary movement throughout the body, helps the medulla to control breathing, and serves as an origin of cranial nerves V (trigeminal), VI (abducens), VII (facial), and VIII (vestibulocochlear).

The cerebellum (***small brain*** in Latin) is the second largest part of the brain after the cerebrum lies in the inferior/posterior part of calvarium. The main function of the cerebellum is coordination of voluntary movements, and maintenance of posture and balance thus enabling all goal-directed muscular activities.

The midbrain (mesencephalon) extends from the pons to the diencephalon and is about 2.5 cm (1 in) long. The midbrain transmits nerve signals from motor areas in the cerebral cortex to the medulla, pons, and spinal cord. It also contains visual centers and auditory centers governing a variety of visual and auditory reflexes. The midbrain also secretes dopamine from substantia nigra neurons and is the origin of two pairs of cranial: III (oculomotor) and IV (trochlear).

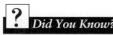

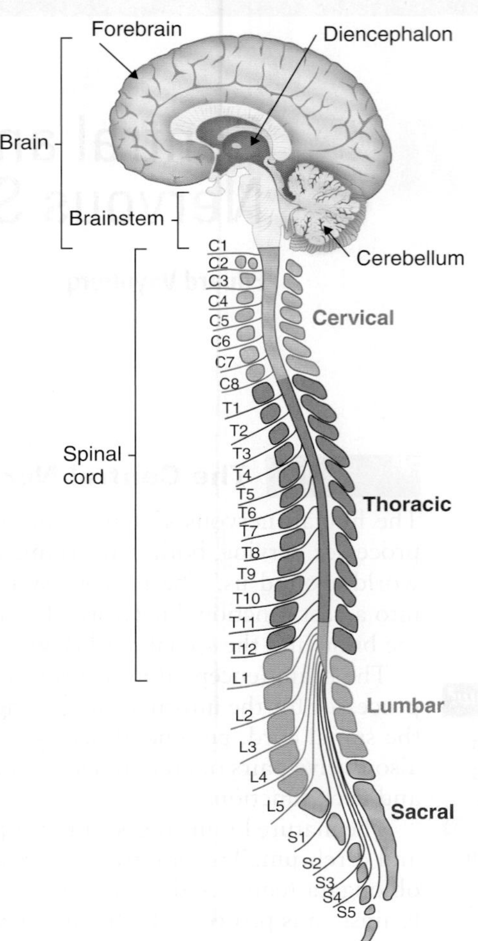

Figure 4.1 **Components of the central nervous system.** (From Central nervous system. In: Preston RR, Wilson TE, eds. *Lippincott® Illustrated Reviews: Physiology.* 2nd ed. Wolters Kluwer; 2019:66-76, Figure 6.1.)

The diencephalon forms a central core of the brain superior to the midbrain, and contains multiple nuclei responsible for a wide variety of sensory and motor processing: the thalamus, hypothalamus, and epithalamus. The pituitary gland is attached to the hypothalamus and secretes multiple hormones.

The thalamus is a major relay station for most sensory signals reaching the cerebral cortex from the brainstem. It also processes cerebellar motor information to motor areas of the cerebral cortex and plays a role in maintenance of consciousness.

The hypothalamus (***hypo*** means ***under*** in Latin) controls multiple body activities and is a major regulator of homeostasis of our bodies. Somatic and visceral senses arrive to the thalamus, as well as sensory input for vision, taste, and smell. Hypothalamic receptors also monitor blood glucose, osmotic pressure in the blood, and a variety of hormonal levels. The hypothalamus has multiple important functions: control of the autonomic nervous system, production of hormones, behavioral regulation (pain, pleasure, aggression, arousal, appetite, thirst), control of body temperature, and state of consciousness.

The cerebrum (triencephalon) is a center of intelligence enabling humans to learn, write, speak, remember, and work as physicians and nurses. The cerebrum consists of an outer cerebral cortex (outer region of gray matter) and deep nuclei (deeper regions of gray and white matter).

A. Cerebrospinal Fluid

Cerebrospinal fluid is clear, colorless liquid serving as a cushion to protect the brain and spinal cord from chemical and physical injuries and is contained by a combination of three meninges (pia, arachnoid, and dura mater) and bony structures of the skull and the spine.

Main components of spinal fluid are water, oxygen, glucose, and small amounts of proteins, urea, lactic acid, and white blood cells. Cerebrospinal fluid is secreted by choroid plexus epithelial cells in the roofs of the third and fourth ventricles at a rate of 0.4 mL per minute, thereby replacing total volume every 5 to 6 hours. Cerebrospinal fluid total volume is around 150 mL and is in constant flow with each heartbeat, circulating through first, second, and third cerebral ventricles, through the cerebral aqueduct in the midbrain into the fourth ventricle, and then into subarachnoid space. Gradual reabsorption into the blood through arachnoid villi eventually occurs at the same rate at which it is formed.

B. Spinal Cord

The spinal cord contains several sensory and motor pathways (**Figure 4.2**) while also serving as a relay and processing station for a variety of peripheral and central inputs. The adult spinal cord is 42 to 45 cm long with a diameter of 1.5 cm at the widest location (cervical enlargement spanning the C4-T1 vertebral levels).

The spinal cord is surrounded by cerebrospinal fluid, which is itself contained by three meninges (pia, arachnoid, and dura) within the vertebral canal. It is oval in cross-sectional shape, extending in adults from medulla oblongata to the superior border of the L2 vertebra (L4 in newborns), and ending distally in the conus medullaris. Arising from the conus is the filum terminale, an extension of pia, arachnoid, and dura mater that anchors the spinal cord to the coccyx.

The spinal cord has thirty-one segments from which thirty-one pairs of spinal nerves emerge through right and left intervertebral foramen. There are no internal divisions in the spinal cord, so as a matter of convention spinal nerves are named according to the vertebral levels where they arise: there are 8 pairs of cervical nerves (C1-C8), 12 pairs of thoracic nerves (T1-T12), 5 pairs of lumbar nerves (L1-L5), 5 pairs of sacral nerves (S1-S5), and 1 pair of coccygeal nerves (Co1). As the spinal cord ends at the L2 vertebra multiple spinal nerves (L3-Co1) must traverse the spinal canal to reach their exiting foramen, thus forming the cauda equina (***horse tail*** in Latin).

Two nerve roots connect each spinal nerve to the spinal cord. Dorsal (posterior) roots contain only sensory axons conducting nerve impulses from sensory receptors of the skin, muscles, and organs to the spinal cord. In contrast, ventral (anterior) roots a contain axons of motor neurons conducting signals from the central nervous system to the periphery. Neuronal cell bodies of these peripheral nerves are located in the dorsal and ventral root ganglia.

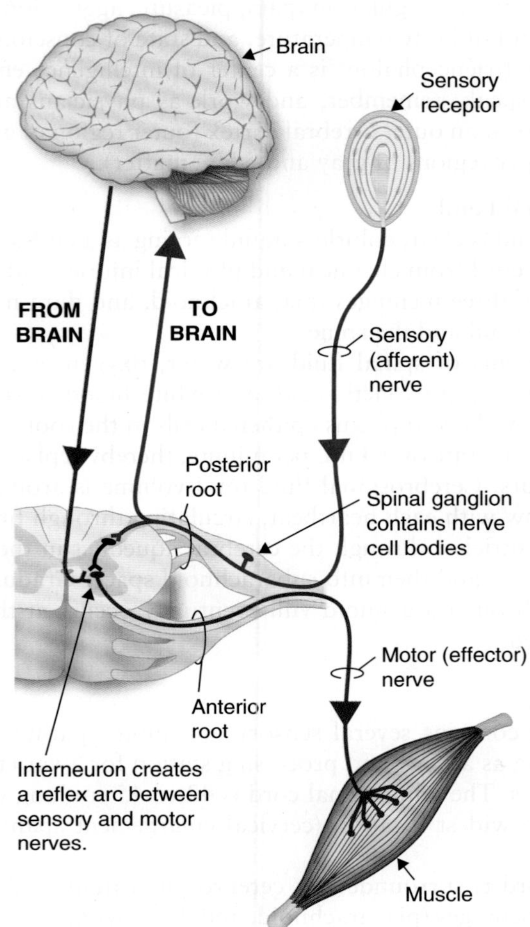

Figure 4.2 **Typical sensory and motor pathways.** (From Central nervous system. In: Preston RR, Wilson TE, eds. *Lippincott® Illustrated Reviews: Physiology.* 2nd ed. Wolters Kluwer; 2019:66-76, Figure 6.2.)

A transverse section of the spinal cord resembles a dark butterfly (gray matter) surrounded by white matter (**Figure 4.3**). The gray matter consists of dendrites and cell bodies of neurons, unmyelinated axons, and neuroglia. The white matter consists of bundles of myelinated axons of neurons. Two grooves (anterior median fissure and posterior median sulcus) separate white matter into right and left sides. Gray matter of the spinal cord contains neuronal cell bodies combined by functions into nuclei: sensory nuclei process input from receptors, and motor nuclei provide output to effector tissues (eg, skeletal muscle). White matter of the spinal cord is organized into three columns: ventral (anterior), dorsal (posterior), and lateral. Each column contains bundles of myelinated axons (ascending sensory and descending motor) that carry similar information from the common origin to a common destination within central nervous system. Sensory and motor tracts of the spinal cord connect to sensory and motor tracts in the brain. Eventually both sensory and motor fibers cross the midline such that the left side of our bodies is innervated by the right side of our brains, and conversely.

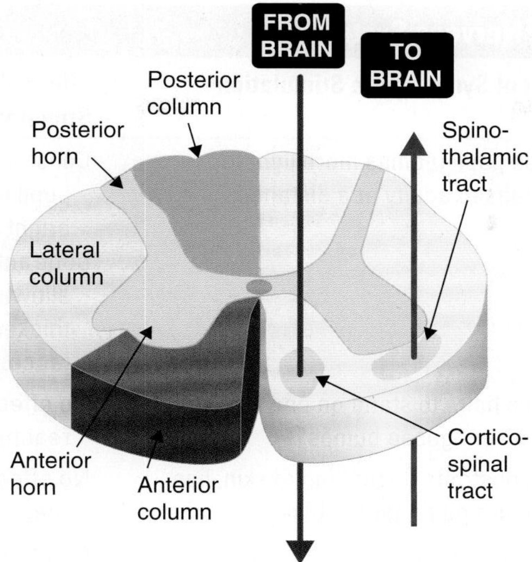

Figure 4.3 **Organization of the spinal cord.** (From Central nervous system. In: Preston RR, Wilson TE, eds. *Lippincott® Illustrated Reviews: Physiology.* 2nd ed. Wolters Kluwer; 2019:66-76, Figure 6.3.)

II. The Autonomic Nervous System

As is apparent from its name, the autonomic nervous system functions independent of our conscious efforts. The system controls smooth muscles, heart muscle, endocrine/exocrine glands, heart rate, blood pressure, respiratory rate, temperature, and other functions related to our body's homeostasis.

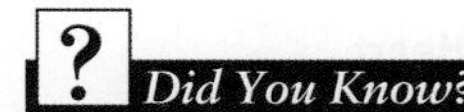

The total volume of cerebral spinal fluid is 150 mL, of which 50 mL is in the subarachnoid space of the spinal cord.

The autonomic nervous system has two output divisions. The sympathetic division (sympathetic nervous system [SNS]) is adrenergic and mediates our body's fight-or-flight response, among others. The parasympathetic division (parasympathetic nervous system [PNS]) is cholinergic and mediates our body's rest-and-digest actions, among others (**Table 4.1**).

The output neurons of the autonomic nervous system are motor neurons. Unlike motor pathways of the peripheral nervous system where one neuron connects the central nervous system with the target organ (skeletal muscle), each autonomic pathway has two motor neurons connected in series. The cell body of the first neuron (preganglionic neuron) is located in the brain or spinal cord, with its myelinated axon connecting to a second neuron (postganglionic neuron) within an autonomic ganglion. The unmyelinated axon of a second neuron (extends to the visceral target organ) (**Figures 4.4-4.6**). Alternatively, in some autonomic pathways, the preganglionic neuron connects to specialized cells within the adrenal medulla (chromaffin cells) instead of to a postganglionic neuron.

The main afferent input to the autonomic nervous system comes from autonomic (visceral) sensory neurons. Mostly these neurons transmit input from interoceptors, a set of sensory receptors located in the blood vessels, visceral organs, muscles, and the nervous system, and monitor internal environmental conditions of our bodies. For example, chemoreceptors monitor oxygen levels in our blood and mechanoreceptors monitor stretch in organ walls. Angina pectoris is a specific example of a visceral sensation: that is, a sensation of pain triggered by heart muscle suffering from ischemia.

Table 4.1 Functions of the Autonomic Nervous System

Organ, Tract, or System		Effect of Sympathetic Stimulation[a]	Effect of Parasympathetic Stimulation[b]
Eyes	Pupil ciliary body	Dilates pupil (admits more light for increased acuity at a distance)	Constricts pupil (protects pupil from excessively bright light) Contracts ciliary muscle, allowing lens to thicken for near vision (accommodation)
Skin	Arrector muscles of hair	Causes hairs to stand on end ("goose-flesh" or "goose bumps")	No effect (does not reach)[c]
	Peripheral blood vessels	Vasoconstricts (blanching of skin, lips, and turning fingertips blue)	No effect (does not reach)[c]
	Sweat glands	Promotes sweating[d]	No effect (does not reach)[c]
Other glands	Lacrimal glands	Slightly decreases secretion[e]	Promotes secretion
	Salivary glands	Secretion decreases, becomes thicker, more viscous[e]	Promotes abundant, watery secretion
Heart		Increases the rate and strength of contraction; inhibits the effect of parasympathetic system on coronary vessels, allowing them to dilate[e]	Decreases the rate and strength of contraction (conserving energy); constricts coronary vessels in relation to reduced demand
Lungs		Inhibits effect of parasympathetic system, resulting in bronchodilation and reduced secretion, allowing for maximum air exchange	Constricts bronchi (conserving energy) and promotes bronchial secretion
Digestive tract		Inhibits peristalsis, and constricts blood vessels to digestive tract so that blood is available to skeletal muscle; contracts internal anal sphincter to aid fecal continence	Stimulates peristalsis and secretion of digestive juices Contracts rectum, inhibits internal anal sphincter to cause defecation
Liver and gallbladder		Promotes breakdown of glycogen to glucose (for increased energy)	Promotes building/conservation of glycogen; increases secretion of bile
Urinary tract		Vasoconstriction of renal vessels slows urine formation; internal sphincter of bladder contracted to maintain urinary continence	Inhibits contraction of internal sphincter of bladder, contracts detrusor muscle of the bladder wall causing urination

Table 4.1 Functions of the Autonomic Nervous System (Continued)

Organ, Tract, or System	Effect of Sympathetic Stimulation[a]	Effect of Parasympathetic Stimulation[b]
Genital system	Causes ejaculation and vasoconstriction resulting in remission of erection	Produces engorgement (erection) of erectile tissues of the external genitals
Suprarenal medulla	Release of adrenaline into blood	No effect (does not innervate)

[a]In general, the effects of sympathetic stimulation are catabolic, preparing body for the fight-or-flight response.

[b]In general, the effects of parasympathetic stimulation are anabolic, promoting normal function and conserving energy.

[c]The parasympathetic system is restricted in its distribution to the head, neck, and body cavities (except for erectile tissues of genitalia); otherwise, parasympathetic fibers are never found in the body wall and limbs. Sympathetic fibers, by comparison, are distributed to all vascularized portions of the body.

[d]With the exception of the sweat glands, glandular secretion is parasympathetically stimulated.

[e]With the exception of the coronary arteries, vasoconstriction is sympathetically stimulated; the effects of sympathetic stimulation on glands (other than sweat glands) are the indirect effects of vasoconstriction.

From Overview and Basic Concepts. In: Moore KL, Agur AMR, Dalley II AF. *Clinically Oriented Anatomy.* 8th ed. Wolters Kluwer; 2018:1-70, Table 1.2.

A. Sympathetic Division

The classic SNS action is the fight-or-flight response—it is a series of immediate activities leading to increased alertness and metabolic activities to prepare the body for an emergency by increasing alertness, heart and breathing rate.

Preganglionic fibers of the SNS take origin from the gray matter of the spinal cord, travel through ventral roots of spinal nerves from the first thoracic to the second lumbar segments of the spinal cord, and comprise "thoracolumbar outflow." These small diameter myelinated fibers quickly leave the spinal nerves and synapse with the postganglionic neurons located at the chains of paravertebral sympathetic ganglia running in two parallel columns anterolateral to the vertebrae. The unmyelinated axons of the postganglionic neurons usually return to the spinal nerves to travel peripherally to connect to their visceral effectors (**Figure 4.5**).

The sympathetic ganglia are the sites of synapses between pre- and postganglionic sympathetic neurons. There are two major types of sympathetic ganglia: sympathetic trunk ganglia and the prevertebral ganglia. Sympathetic trunk ganglia extend from the base of the skull to the coccyx. Postganglionic axons from sympathetic trunk ganglia innervate organs above the diaphragm. Sympathetic trunk ganglia in the neck have specific names: superior cervical, middle cervical, and inferior cervical. Anatomic fusion of the first thoracic and inferior cervical ganglia is called a stellate ganglion. It carries sympathetic fibers from the face and upper extremity and is frequently blocked with local anesthetic as a treatment for complex regional pain syndrome of the upper extremity. In contrast, the prevertebral (collateral) ganglia lie anterior to the vertebral column and close to major abdominal arteries. Postganglionic axons from prevertebral ganglia innervate organs of the abdominal cavity below the diaphragm. There are five major prevertebral ganglia: celiac, superior mesenteric, inferior mesenteric, aorticorenal, and renal.

B. Parasympathetic Division

The PNS is often referred to as the rest-and-digest division because one of its primary activities is to conserve and restore body energy. The majority of its

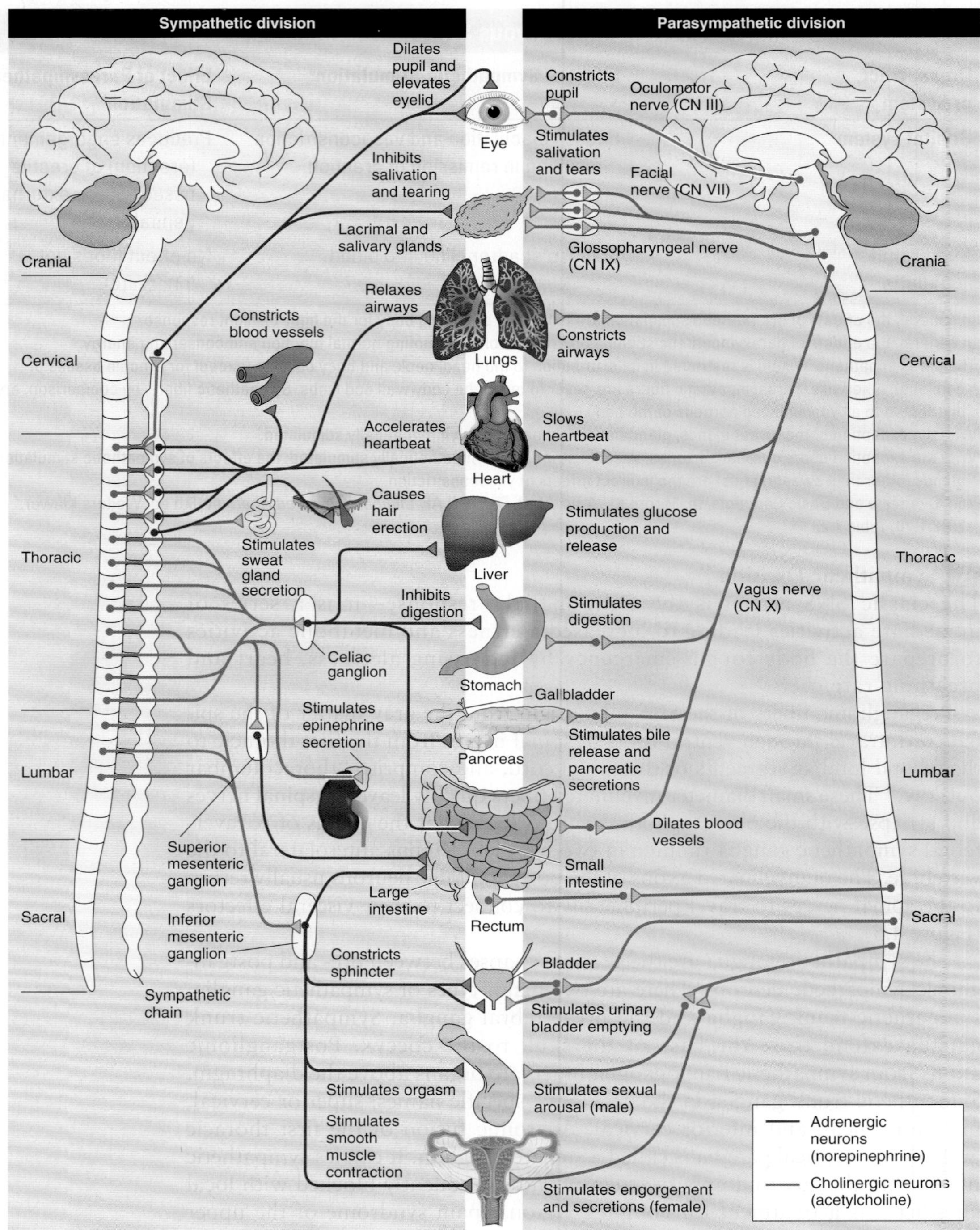

Figure 4.4 **Organization of the autonomic nervous system.** (From Automatic nervous system. In: Preston RR, Wilson TE, eds. *Lippincott® Illustrated Reviews: Physiology*. 2nd ed. Wolters Kluwer; 2019:77-90, Figure 7.4.)

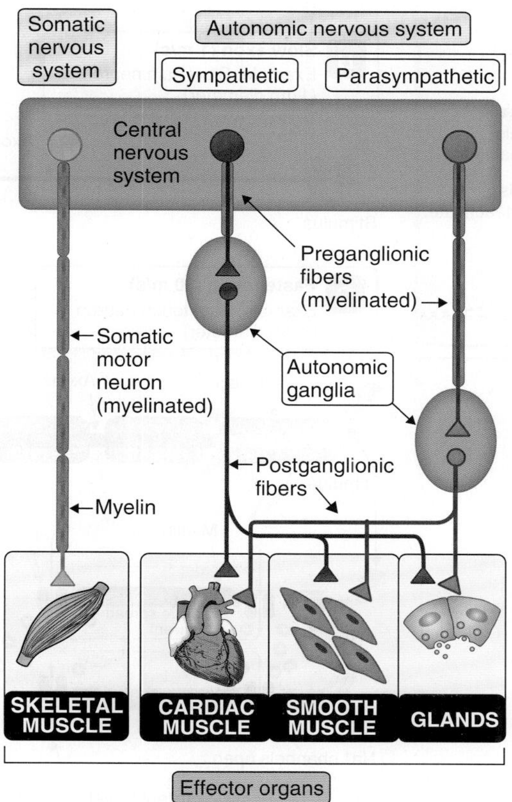

Figure 4.5 Efferent pathways of somatic and autonomic nervous systems. (From Automatic nervous system. In: Preston RR, Wilson TE, eds. *Lippincott® Illustrated Reviews: Physiology*. 2nd ed. Wolters Kluwer; 2019:77-90, Figure 7.3.)

output is directed to the smooth muscles and glands of the gastrointestinal and respiratory tracts. Preganglionic neurons of the PNS take origin from the cranial nerves III, VII, IX, and X in brainstem, as well as lateral gray matter of the second, third, and fourth sacral segments of the spinal cord conus medullaris, and comprise "craniosacral outflow." These fibers travel in the cranial and sacral nerves to the neuronal bodies of the postganglionic neurons that are located in ganglia near or inside the effector organ. The secondary neuron's postganglionic axons are usually very short and continue to specific muscles or glands within the target viscera.

C. Autonomic Nervous System Transmission Process

Generation of an action potential in the autonomic neuron starts the nerve conduction cascade and signal transmission. There are multiple factors affecting the speed of signal conduction: nerve fiber diameter, number of synapses, presence of myelin, and presence of nodes of Ranvier enabling salutatory conduction. The signal between neurons is transmitted at the ganglia across the synaptic cleft by release of special substances (neurotransmitters) from the terminal end of the preganglionic neuron. These neurotransmitters attach to a receptor of the postganglionic neuron or the effector cell and leads to a physiologic response (**Figure 4.7**).

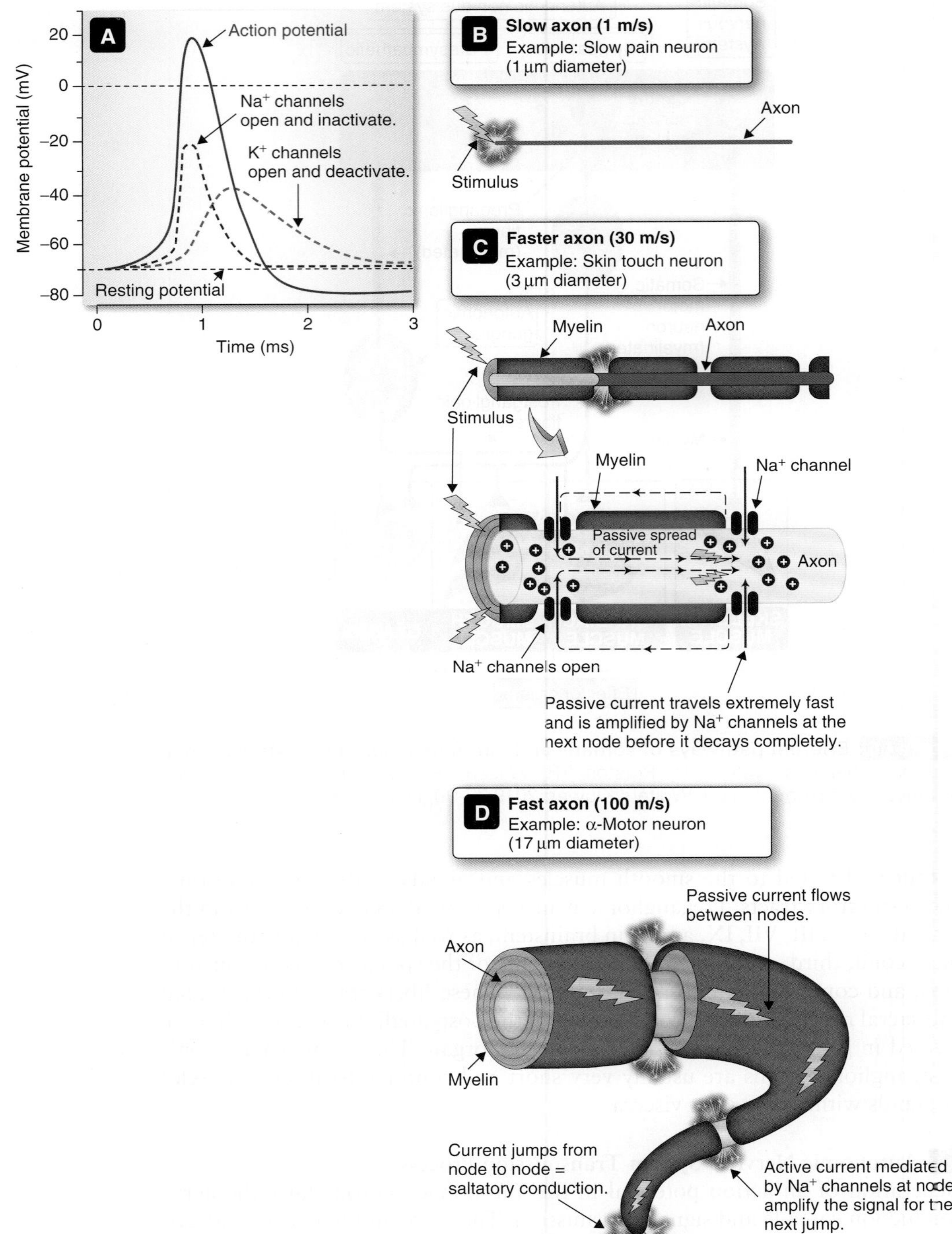

Figure 4.6 A, Time sequence of channel events during an action potential. B-D, Axonal conduction velocity related to myelin sheath and diameter neuronal fiber diameter. (From Nervous system organization. In: Preston RR, Wilson TE, eds. *Lippincott® Illustrated Reviews: Physiology*. 2nd ed. Wolters Kluwer; 2019:53-55, Figures 5.3 and 5.4.)

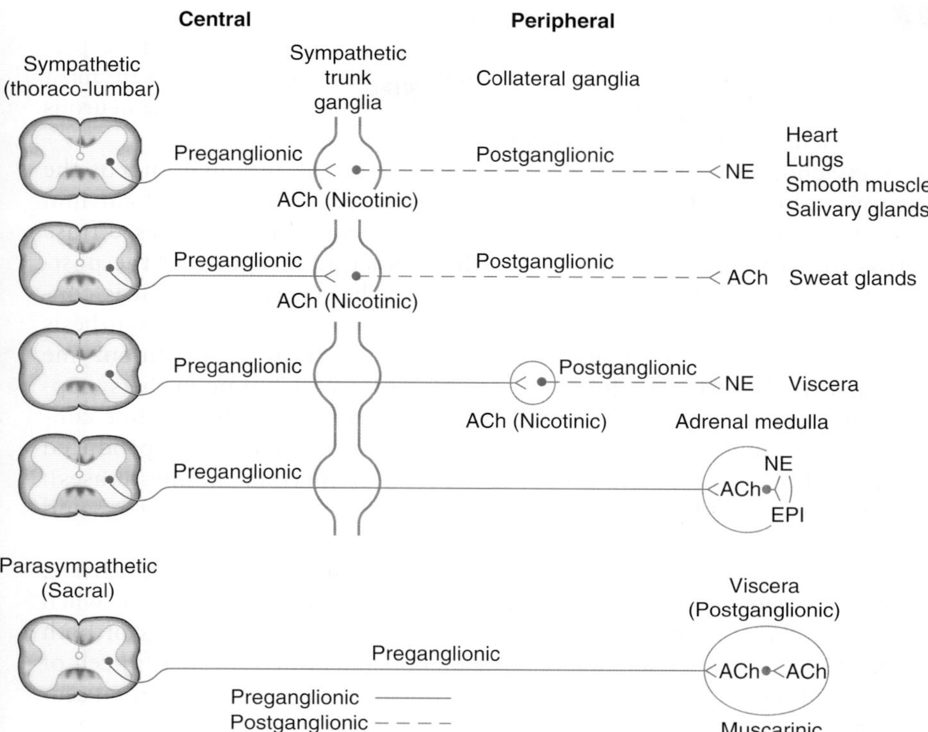

Figure 4.7 Schematic diagram of the efferent autonomic nervous system. Afferent impulses are integrated centrally and sent reflexively to the adrenergic and cholinergic receptors. Sympathetic fibers ending in the adrenal medulla are preganglionic, and acetylcholine (ACh) is the neurotransmitter. Stimulation of the chromaffin cells, acting as postganglionic neurons, releases epinephrine (EPI) and norepinephrine (NE). (From Grecu L. Autonomic nervous system: physiology and pharmacology. In: Barash PG, Cullen BF, Stoelting RK, et al, eds. *Clinical Anesthesia*. 7th ed. Lippincott Williams & Wilkins; 2013:362-407, Figure 15.22.)

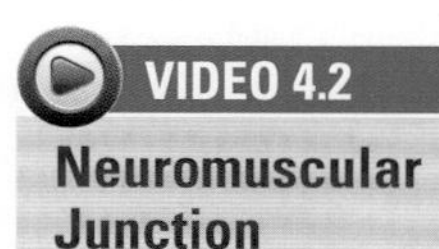

D. Autonomic Neurotransmitters

The nerve terminals of both sympathetic and parasympathetic preganglionic fibers secrete acetylcholine, and are therefore termed "cholinergic." Parasympathetic postganglionic fibers are cholinergic as well. In contrast, most sympathetic postganglionic fibers secrete norepinephrine (except those in sweat glands) and are therefore termed "adrenergic" (**Figure 4.5**).

The different postganglionic neurotransmitters used by sympathetic and parasympathetic postganglionic fibers explain the different effects the SNS and PNS have on effector organs. Most organs are innervated by both divisions, usually with opposing actions (**Table 4.1**). For example, the heart receives dual innervation that balances an increase in heart rate (SNS) against a decrease in heart rate (PNS). However, some organs are predominantly controlled by one of the divisions. For example, the SNS continuously stimulates smooth muscles in the walls of the arteries, maintaining them partially constricted (sympathetic tone). Decreasing sympathetic stimulation of the blood vessels leads to vasodilation and a reduction in the blood pressure.

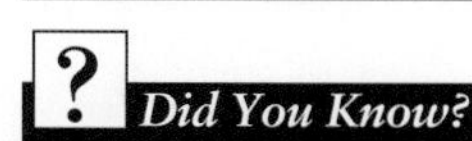

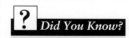

Neurotransmitters norepinephrine and epinephrine released into the circulation from the adrenal medulla are called hormones.

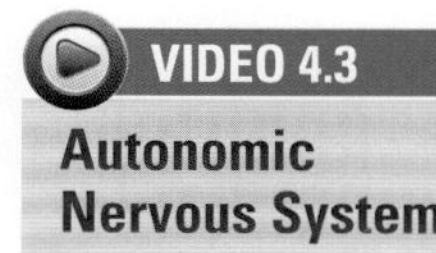

E. Cholinergic Neurons and Receptors

The cholinergic neurons include all sympathetic and parasympathetic preganglionic neurons, sympathetic postganglionic neurons that innervate most sweat glands, and all parasympathetic postganglionic neurons. These neurons use acetylcholine as a neurotransmitter.

Acetylcholine is stored in synaptic vesicles at the terminal end of the neuron and released by exocytosis when triggered by a release of calcium ions from the interstitial space. Acetylcholine containing vesicles diffuse across the synaptic cleft and bind with cholinergic receptors in the postsynaptic cell membrane. Acetylcholine cannot be recycled; thus, it is continuously synthesized in the presynaptic nerve terminal. The synthesis (acetylation of choline by acetyl coenzyme A) is catalyzed by an enzyme choline acetyltransferase. Rapid destruction of acetylcholine in the synaptic cleft is essential for rapid return of the effector organs to baseline condition. The rapid destruction of acetylcholine in the synapse is produced by acetylcholinesterase and pseudocholinesterase (plasma cholinesterases). These enzymes hydrolyze acetylcholine, ester-type local anesthetics, and succinylcholine, among others.

There are two types of cholinergic receptors: nicotinic and muscarinic. Nicotinic receptors (nicotine mimics the action of the acetylcholine when binding to these receptors) are present in dendrites and cell bodies of both sympathetic and parasympathetic postganglionic neurons, chromaffin cell of the adrenal medulla, and in the motor end plate at the skeletal neuromuscular junction. Muscarinic receptors (the mushroom poison muscarine mimics action of acetylcholine when binding to these receptors) are present in the membranes of all effector organs (smooth and cardiac muscles and glands) innervated by parasympathetic postganglionic fibers. Sweat glands receive most of their innervation from cholinergic sympathetic postganglionic neurons and possess muscarinic receptors.

Binding of acetylcholine to nicotinic receptors results in depolarization (excitation) of the postsynaptic cell (eg, postganglionic neuron, autonomic effector cell, or skeletal muscle cell). Binding of acetylcholine to muscarinic receptors can result in either depolarization (excitation) or hyperpolarization (inhibition) depending on the type of a neuron. For example, smooth muscles in the iris of the eye will contract, whereas smooth muscle in gastrointestinal sphincters will relax, once acetylcholine binds their muscarinic receptors.

1. Adrenergic Neurons and Receptors

The sympathetic postganglionic neurons predominately use norepinephrine as a neurotransmitter (epinephrine plays a minor role). Like acetylcholine, norepinephrine is stored in presynaptic vesicles and is released by exocytosis into the synaptic cleft where it binds to specific adrenergic receptors causing either excitation or inhibition of the effector cell. Adrenergic receptors can bind both epinephrine (released as a hormone) and norepinephrine (released as a neurotransmitter or as a hormone secreted directly into the blood by chromaffin cells of adrenal medulla).

The two main types of the adrenergic receptors found on viscera innervated by most sympathetic postganglionic neurons are alpha (α) and beta (β) (**Table 4.2**). There are further subtypes of the receptors based on either their activation response or anatomic distribution: α_1 and β_1 are generally excitatory, α_2

Table 4.2 Adrenergic Receptors

Receptor	Synaptic Site	Anatomic Site	Action	LV Function and Stroke Volume
α_1	Postsynaptic	Peripheral vascular smooth muscle	Constriction	Decreased
		Renal vascular smooth muscle	Constriction	
		Coronary arteries, epicardial	Constriction	
		Myocardium 30%-40% of resting tone	Positive inotropism	Improved
		Renal tubules	Antidiuresis	
α_2	Presynaptic	Peripheral vascular smooth muscle release	Inhibit NE	
			Secondary vasodilation	Improved
		Coronaries	?	
		CNS	Inhibition of CNS activity Sedation	
			Decrease MAC	
	Postsynaptic	Coronaries, endocardial CNS	Constriction	Decreased
			Inhibition of insulin release	
			Decreased bowel motility Inhibition of antidiuretic hormone	
			Analgesia	
		Renal tubule	Promotes Na^{2+} and H_2O excretion	
β_1	Postsynaptic NE sensitive	Myocardium	Positive inotropism and chronotropism	Improved
		Sinoatrial (SA) node		
		Ventricular conduction		
		Kidney	Renin release	
		Coronaries	Relaxation	
β_2	Presynaptic	Myocardium	Accelerates NE release	Improved
	NE sensitive	SA node ventricular conduction vessels	Opposite action to presynaptic α_2 agonism	
			Constriction	
	Postsynaptic (extrasynaptic) (EPI sensitive)	Myocardium	Positive inotropism and chronotropism	Improved
		Vascular smooth muscle	Relaxation	Improved

(Continued)

Table 4.2 Adrenergic Receptors (Continued)

Receptor	Synaptic Site	Anatomic Site	Action	LV Function and Stroke Volume
		Bronchial smooth muscle	Relaxation	Improved
β_3		Adipose tissue	Enhancement of lipolysis	
		Renal vessels	Relaxation	
DA_1	Postsynaptic	Blood vessels (renal, mesentery, coronary)	Vasodilation	Improved
		Renal tubules	Natriuresis Diuresis	
		Juxtaglomerular cells	Renin release (modulates diuresis)	
		Sympathetic ganglia	Minor inhibition	
DA_2	Presynaptic	Postganglionic sympathetic nerves	Inhibit NE release	Improved
	Postsynaptic	Renal and mesenteric vasculature	Secondary vasodilation Vasoconstriction	

CNS, central nervous system; EPI, epinephrine; LV, left ventricle; NE, norepinephrine.

From Grecu L. Autonomic nervous system: physiology and pharmacology. In: Barash PG, Cullen BF, Stoelting RK, et al, eds. *Clinical Anesthesia*. 7th ed. Lippincott Williams & Wilkins; 2013:362-407, Table 15.2.

and β_2 are generally inhibitory, and β_3 are present only on brown adipose tissue and lead to thermogenesis when activated. Most effector cells have either α or β receptors; a minority has both. Norepinephrine has higher affinity to α receptors, while epinephrine stimulates both α and β equally.

The primary mechanism of norepinephrine termination in the synaptic cleft is via reuptake into presynaptic neuronal terminals, where they undergo enzymatic destruction by either catechol-O-methyltransferase (COMT) and monoamine oxidase (MAO) to form vanillylmandelic acid that is excreted in urine. The metabolism of norepinephrine takes longer then acetylcholine; thus, norepinephrine effects last longer then acetylcholine.

Multiple medications are used to activate or block specific adrenergic and cholinergic receptors to modulate the desired effects of norepinephrine and epinephrine on human tissues. For example, phenylephrine is an adrenergic agonist at α_1 receptors that is frequently used intraoperatively to increase mean arterial pressure by induced vasoconstriction (ie, increased afterload). Esmolol is a selective β_1 blocker that is frequently used to rapidly decrease in heart rate and blood pressure through its inhibitory effects on cardiac chronotropy and inotropy, respectively.

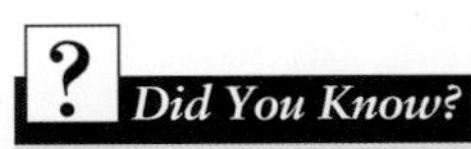

In general, the number of adrenergic receptors is inversely proportional to the concentration of circulating catecholamines.

2. Autonomic Nervous System Reflexes

The primary role of the autonomous nervous system is to rapidly modulate the balance between sympathetic and parasympathetic responses to changes in our homeostatic environment. The balance between sympathetic and parasympathetic activity is termed "sympathetic tone" and is regulated by the hypothalamus—increasing sympathetic activity and decreasing the parasympathetic activity as needed to maintain the proper tone.

During times of physical or emotional stress, the sympathetic division of the autonomous nervous system predominates. High sympathetic tone supports body functions needed for the fight-or-flight response: pupils dilate, heart rate and contractility increase, airways dilate, and blood flow is redirected to organs involved in a fight response (eg, skeletal muscle). In contrast, during periods of inactivity, the parasympathetic division predominates, prioritizing rest-and-digest activities (eg, gastrointestinal tract actions allowing us to better digest food).

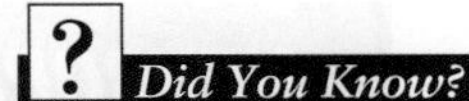

Orthostatic hypotension is a harbinger of an increase in perioperative morbidity and mortality and should be considered an additional risk factor for a given patient.

Not surprisingly, the sympathetic effects are more widespread and longer lasting than parasympathetic ones. Afterall, one's survival depends on how quickly and for how long the sympathetic division's responses can be activated and sustained. Three physiologic mechanisms allow that to happen: sympathetic postganglionic fibers diverge more extensively allowing for simultaneous activation of many organ systems; norepinephrine inactivation mechanisms allow it to remain much longer than acetylcholine in the synaptic cleft; and the adrenal medulla supplements neuronal supply of norepinephrine and epinephrine by secreting both substances directly into the circulation.

If autonomic pathways are disrupted either by a pathologic condition or as a side effect of medications, a loss of normal function is expected. An example of such a condition is pharmacologic disruption of the cervical sympathetic ganglia with local anesthetic following a stellate ganglion block or a brachial plexus block done via interscalene approach. This disruption results in development of Horner syndrome: the combination of ptosis, myosis, and anhidrosis due to unopposed action of parasympathetic fibers in these anatomic distributions.

A common example of naturally occurring autonomic dysfunction is orthostatic hypotension—a sustained decrease of systolic blood pressure by 20 mm Hg or of diastolic blood pressure by 10 mm Hg upon rapidly changing position from a supine or sitting position to a standing position. When functioning normally, SNS activity is quickly enhanced upon standing (as carotid baroreceptors sense the initial, gravity-induced fall in blood pressure), leading to a rapid compensatory increase in both vasoconstriction and cardiac output, thereby augmenting blood pressure and minimizing the clinical effects of orthostatic hypotension. With aging and/or use of beta-blocker medications, this compensatory SNS reflex is impaired, which can result in lightheadedness or even transient syncope when rapidly assuming a standing position.

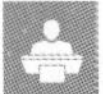

For further review and interactivities, please see the associated Interactive Video Lectures and "At a Glance" infographic accessible in the complimentary eBook bundled with this text. Access instructions are located in the inside front cover.

References

1. Tortora GJ, Derrickson B. *Principles of Anatomy and Physiology*. 14th ed. Wiley; 2014.
2. Moore KL, Dalley AF, Agur AMR. *Moore Clinically Oriented Anatomy*. 7th ed. Lippincott; 2013.
3. Standring S. *Gray's Anatomy the Anatomical Basis of Clinical Practice*. 40th ed. Churchill Livingston; 2008.
4. Shier D, Butler J, Lewis R. *Hole's Essentials of Human Anatomy and Physiology*. 10th ed. McGraw Hill; 2009.
5. Barash PG, Cahalan MK, Cullen BF, et al. *Clinical Anesthesia Fundamentals*. Wolters Kluwer; 2015.

NEUROPHYSIOLOGY

AT A GLANCE

Understanding cerebral physiology is critical to managing patients with central nervous system disease. The illustration below summarizes important elements of cerebral pressures, flows, and metabolism. Other factors that influence intracranial physiology are also depicted.

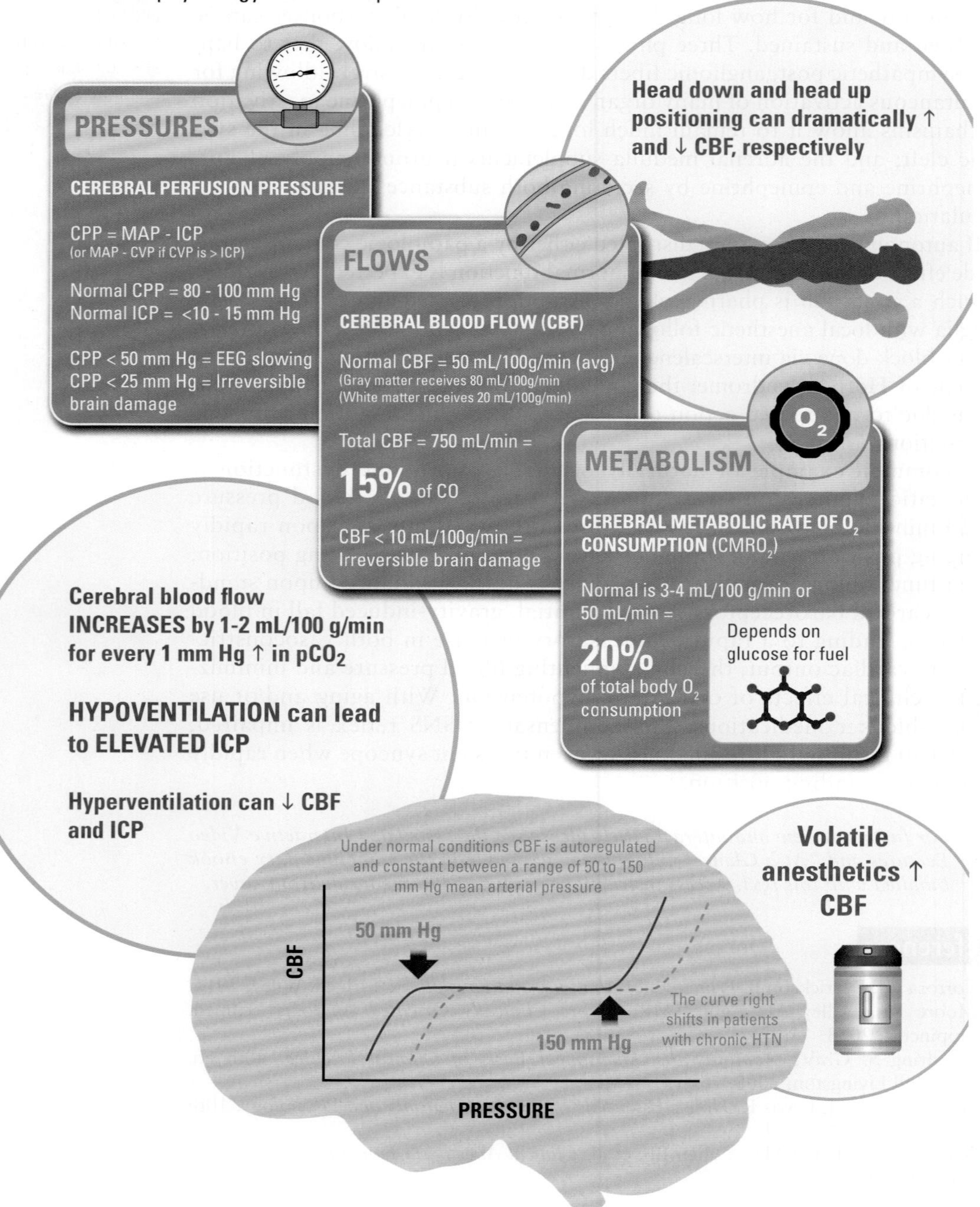

PRESSURES
CEREBRAL PERFUSION PRESSURE
CPP = MAP - ICP
(or MAP - CVP if CVP is > ICP)
Normal CPP = 80 - 100 mm Hg
Normal ICP = <10 - 15 mm Hg
CPP < 50 mm Hg = EEG slowing
CPP < 25 mm Hg = Irreversible brain damage
FLOWS
CEREBRAL BLOOD FLOW (CBF)
Normal CBF = 50 mL/100g/min (avg)
(Gray matter receives 80 mL/100g/min
(White matter receives 20 mL/100g/min)
Total CBF = 750 mL/min =
15% of CO
CBF < 10 mL/100g/min =
Irreversible brain damage
Head down and head up positioning can dramatically ↑ and ↓ CBF, respectively
METABOLISM
O2
CEREBRAL METABOLIC RATE OF O2 CONSUMPTION (CMRO2)
Normal is 3-4 mL/100 g/min or 50 mL/min =
20%
of total body O2 consumption
Depends on glucose for fuel
Cerebral blood flow INCREASES by 1-2 mL/100 g/min for every 1 mm Hg ↑ in pCO2
HYPOVENTILATION can lead to ELEVATED ICP
Hyperventilation can ↓ CBF and ICP
Under normal conditions CBF is autoregulated and constant between a range of 50 to 150 mm Hg mean arterial pressure
50 mm Hg
CBF
150 mm Hg
The curve right shifts in patients with chronic HTN
PRESSURE
Volatile anesthetics ↑ CBF

Infographic by: Naveen Nathan MD

Questions

1. **After a successful right stellate ganglion block is performed with local anesthetic, which of the following physical findings would be observed?**

    A. Myosis of the right eye
    B. Ptosis of the left eye
    C. Mydriasis of the right eye
    D. Increase in the heart rate

2. **Sympathetic nervous system effects usually last longer than parasympathetic effects for which of the following reasons?**

    A. Norepinephrine remains longer in the neuronal synaptic cleft than does acetylcholine
    B. Acetylcholine remains longer in the neuronal synaptic cleft than does norepinephrine
    C. The adrenal medulla secrets acetylcholine directly into the circulation
    D. Acetylcholine is rapidly deactivated by adrenal medulla

3. **In the human autonomous nervous system, norepinephrine is the neurotransmitter released from which of the following neurons?**

    A. Parasympathetic postganglionic neurons
    B. Parasympathetic preganglionic neurons
    C. Sympathetic postganglionic neurons
    D. Sympathetic preganglionic neurons

4. **The primary function of the cerebellum is which of the following?**

    A. Regulation of sympathetic tone
    B. Secretion of the cerebrospinal fluid
    C. Coordination of voluntary movements
    D. Secretion of dopamine

5. **Which of the following statements regarding acetylcholine is most accurate?**

    A. It is released by adrenal medulla.
    B. It is destroyed in the synaptic cleft by acetyl coenzyme A.
    C. It is synthesized by pseudocholinesterase.
    D. It is released into the synaptic cleft by exocytosis from the presynaptic terminal.

Answers

1. A

A stellate ganglion block eliminates sympathetic input to the cervical ganglia and their anatomic distributions, including the ipsilateral eye, face, and arm. The contralateral side is not affected by the block. Mydriasis is a parasympathetic response and is unaffected by a stellate ganglion (ie, sympathetic) block. Heart rate will either not change or will decrease due to unopposed parasympathetic stimulation to the heart.

2. A

Acetylcholine is eliminated faster than norepinephrine from the neuronal synaptic cleft. The adrenal medulla does not secrete nor deactivates acetylcholine.

3. C

Of these four autonomic system neurons, acetylcholine is released from all except the sympathetic postganglionic neuron. The only neuron using norepinephrine as a neurotransmitter is the sympathetic postganglionic neuron.

4. C

The cerebellum coordinates voluntary movements, maintains posture and balance, and enables goal-directed muscular activities. Sympathetic tone is regulated by the hypothalamus. Cerebrospinal fluid is secreted by choroid plexus epithelial cells in the third and fourth ventricles. Dopamine is secreted by cells in the substantia nigra of the midbrain.

5. D

Acetylcholine is stored in presynaptic vesicles and released by exocytosis. Acetylcholine containing vesicles diffuse through the synaptic cleft and bind with cholinergic receptors on the postsynaptic cell membrane. Its synthesis (acetylation of choline by acetyl coenzyme A) is catalyzed by the enzyme choline acetyltransferase. Its rapid destruction in the synaptic cleft is essential for prompt return of the effector organs to baseline condition and is affected by acetylcholinesterase and pseudocholinesterase (plasma cholinesterases). Acetylcholine is not released by the adrenal medulla.

5 The Renal System

Thomas R. Hickey and Natalie F. Holt

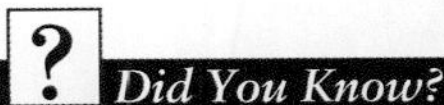

The kidneys receive the largest percentage of core organ cardiac output and account for about 7% of total body oxygen consumption, although their combined weight is only about 0.5% of total body weight.

I. Renal Anatomy and Physiology

A. Anatomy

The kidneys are paired retroperitoneal organs that lie at the T12 to L4 vertebral levels (**Figure 5.1**). The kidneys receive about 20% to 25% of the cardiac output. Blood supply is via a single renal artery to each side. The renal veins receive venous drainage from the kidneys as well as from the suprarenal glands, gonads, diaphragm, and body wall. Lymphatic drainage is to the lumbar nodes. Sympathetic innervation to the kidney arises from the celiac and intermesenteric plexuses and travels with the renal arteries. Parasympathetic innervation to the kidneys is via the vagus nerve and to the ureters is via the splanchnic nerves. Renal pain sensation travels back to spinal segments T10 to L1 via sympathetic fibers.

With the exception of the hilum, the renal parenchyma is enclosed by a tough but thin fibrous membrane and is divided into two distinct regions: the cortex and the medulla (**Figure 5.1**). The ***cortex*** is the outer portion of the kidney and contains alternating bands of cortical labyrinth (glomeruli and convoluted tubules) and parallel arrays of straight tubules (medullary rays). The ***medulla*** is the deeper part of the parenchyma and is divided into an outer region, which contains the thick ascending limb of the loop of Henle, and an inner region, which does not. The outer region of the medulla is itself divided into outer and inner stripes, which are defined by the presence (outer) or absence (inner) of proximal tubules (**Figure 5.1**). Tubules in the medulla are arranged into pyramids, which are oriented with the base toward the cortex and the tip (papilla) toward a minor calyx to where urine drains.

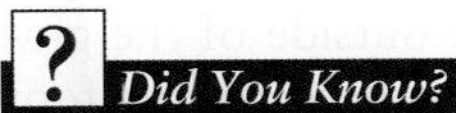

The renal medulla is the part of the kidney most vulnerable to hypoxia because it contains the thick ascending loops of Henle, which have high metabolic activity.

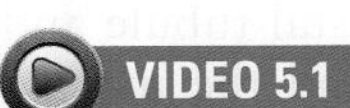

Renal Regulation of Water

B. Physiology: Correlation of Structure and Function

The Nephron

The ***nephron*** is the structural and functional unit of the kidney and is responsible for urine formation. There are about 1.2 million nephrons in the kidney. Nephrons play a dominant role in water and electrolyte homeostasis, acid-base balance, and blood pressure control. Each nephron comprises a glomerulus and a tubule (**Figure 5.2**). The ***glomerulus*** is a capillary tuft encased in a fibrous structure called Bowman capsule, together known as the ***renal corpuscle***. This is where blood filtration occurs. Absorption and secretion occur in the renal tubules, which are divided into three main segments—the proximal convoluted tubule, loop of Henle, and distal convoluted tubule. Filtrate from each nephron drains into the collecting system and passes through the papillary ducts toward the renal calyces.

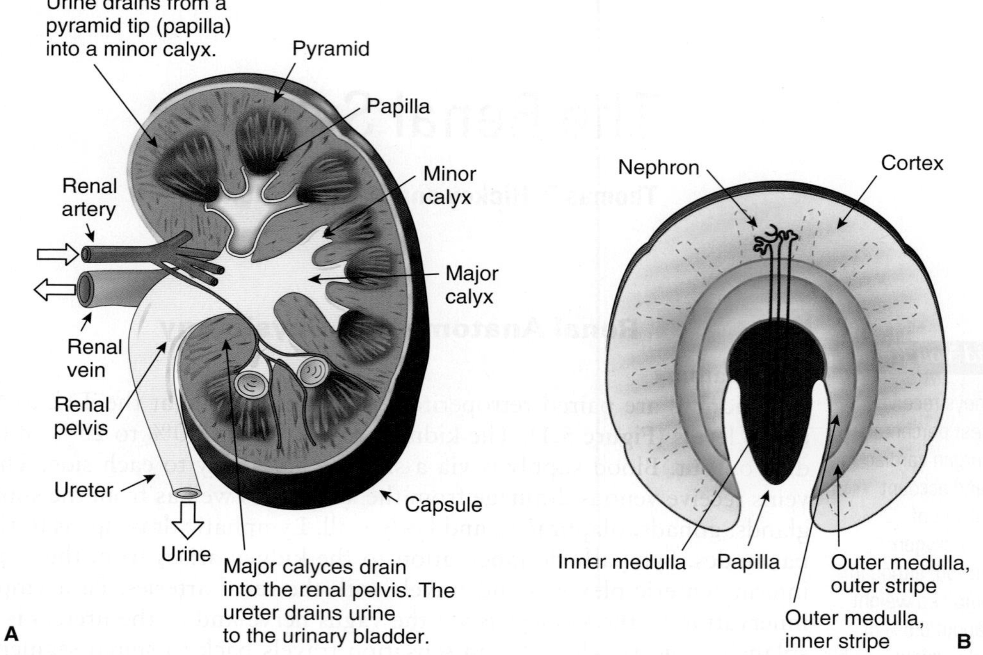

Figure 5.1 **A, Gross anatomy of the kidney. B, Medullary inner and outer stripes.** (From Filtration and micturition. In: Preston RR, Wilson TE, eds. *Lippincott® Illustrated Reviews: Physiology.* 2nd ed. Wolters Kluwer; 2019:323-338, Figures 25.2 and 25.3.)

The Glomerulus

Each nephron is associated with a glomerulus, which is a tuft of capillaries supplied by an afferent arteriole and drained by an efferent arteriole. Glomeruli are divided into two subtypes: ***superficial glomeruli*** (80%-85% of glomeruli; located near the renal capsule and associated with short loops of Henle) and ***juxtamedullary glomeruli*** (15%-20% of glomeruli, which have long loops of Henle extending deep into the medulla) (**Figure 5.3**).

Podocytes are specialized epithelial cells that cover the outside of the glomerular capillary and have extensions called foot processes. Between the foot processes are slit diaphragm. The glomerular filtration barrier is composed of three layers: the endothelium, basement membrane, and foot processes of the podocytes. This complex provides for selective permeability. Normally, selective permeability permits only about 25% of plasma elements to pass into Bowman capsule; proteins larger than ~65 kDa are unable to cross. However, in certain disease states, including nephrotic syndrome and glomerulonephritis, large proteins and/or red blood cells are able to penetrate Bowman capsule.

The Juxtaglomerular Apparatus

The juxtaglomerular apparatus is located at the end of the distal tubule and comprises afferent and efferent arterioles, the mesangium, and the macula densa (**Figure 5.4**). The mesangium consists of an extracellular matrix and specialized cells called mesangial cells. The macula densa is a region of the specialized, distal, thick ascending limb of the ***loop of Henle*** of the parent nephron. It is formed from low columnar cells that have their apical membranes exposed to the tubular fluid and the basilar aspect in contact with cells of the mesangium and the afferent arteriole. Gap junctions exist between the

Figure 5.2 The nephron: Structure and function.

mesangial cells, serving as a functional link between the macula densa, glomerular arterioles, and mesangium. The juxtaglomerular apparatus plays a key role in blood pressure regulation.

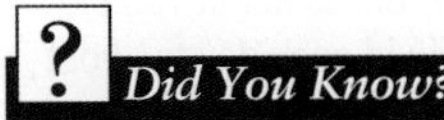

IgA nephropathy (also called Berger syndrome) is the most common cause of primary glomerulonephritis in developed countries. It is characterized by the presence of IgA antibodies to components of the renal mesangium.

Proximal Tubule and Loop of Henle

The cellular structure of the ***proximal tubule*** is highly specialized, reflecting the high energy demands required for a range of complex transport functions. Virtually no active transport occurs in the descending part of the loop of Henle (**Figure 5.4**). Rather, urine concentration occurs in this part of the loop through passive urea transporters and simple water channels. The thick ascending limb is where sodium and potassium adenosine triphosphatase (Na^+/K^+ ATPase)–driven active transport resorbs sodium and chloride. The macula densa is the modified part of the thick ascending limb of the loop of Henle, which forms part of the juxtaglomerular apparatus.[1]

The Distal Tubule

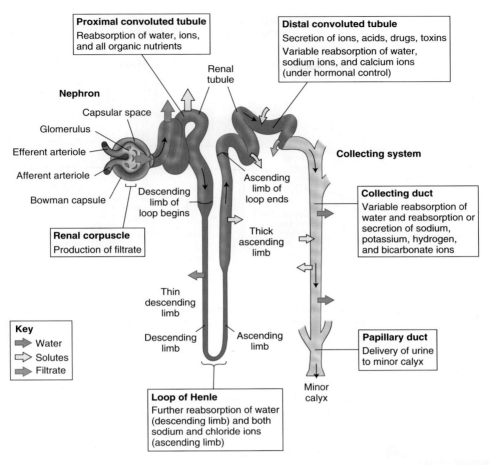

The ***distal tubule*** is composed of the distal convoluted tubule, the connecting tubule, and the initial collecting duct (**Figure 5.3**). The cells of the distal convoluted tubule actively transport sodium and have calcium ATPase, which is important in the reabsorption of divalent cations. The connecting tubules lie

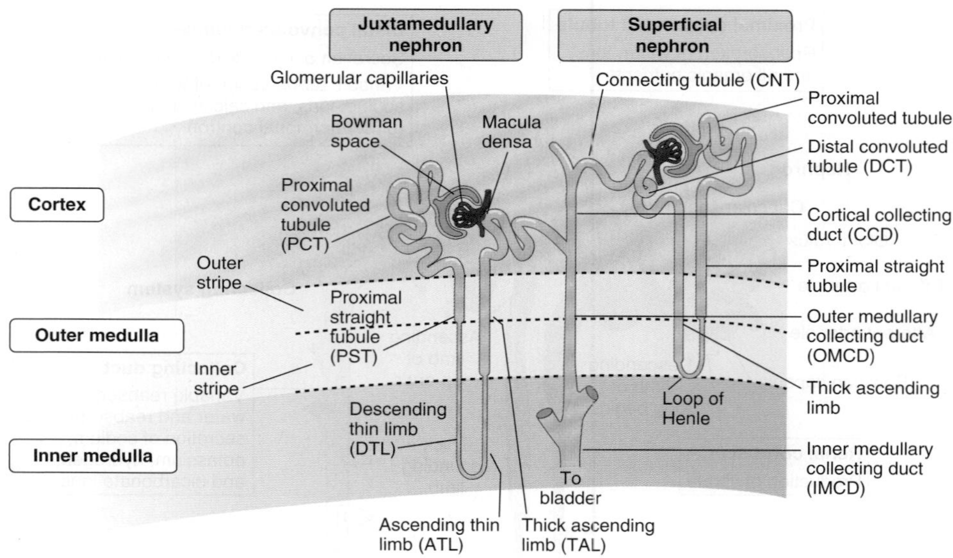

Figure 5.3 **Nephron types and the collecting duct system.** (From Filtration and micturition. In: Preston RR, Wilson TE, eds. *Lippincott® Illustrated Reviews: Physiology*. 2nd ed. Wolters Kluwer; 2019:323-338, Figures 25.5.)

within the cortical labyrinth, where several tubules join together to form the collecting duct. Cells of the connecting tubule are similarly involved in sodium and cation transport but, unlike the distal convoluted tubule cells, they have water channels.

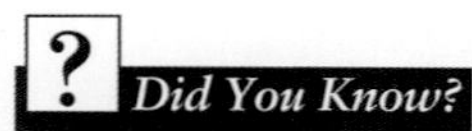

Tubular filtration reduces about 180 L of fluid each day to about 1 L/d of fluid that is excreted as urine.

C. Glomerular Filtration Rate

The glomerular filtration rate (GFR) is the volume of filtrate formed by both kidneys per minute. This is approximately 125 mL/min in an average patient with normal renal function. Fluid and solutes are forced under pressure from the glomerulus (afferent arteriole) into the capsular space of the renal corpuscle. A filtration membrane allows for passage into the capsular space of fluid and small solutes based on their physical size and charge. Filtration occurs by bulk flow driven by the hydrostatic pressure of the blood; small molecules pass rapidly through the filtration membrane, while larger molecules are retained within the arteriole. The relatively large diameter of the afferent arterioles and small diameter of the efferent arterioles result in a high capillary pressure (~60 mm Hg). This driving pressure is opposed by capsular hydrostatic pressure (~15 mm Hg) and colloid osmotic pressure with the glomerular capillaries (~32 mm Hg). Although the concentration of small solutes is the same across the filtration membrane, large proteins are retained and the osmotic pressure of the blood increases as the fluid moves out of the glomerulus. This results in a net filtration pressure of approximately 10 to 15 mm Hg. There is a direct relationship between the net filtration pressure and the GFR. If either the hydrostatic or osmotic pressure of the glomerular capillaries or the hydrostatic pressure of the capsular space changes, the GFR will also change.

D. Autoregulation of Renal Blood Flow and Glomerular Filtration

Autoregulation of renal blood flow and GFR are intimately related. In healthy individuals, renal blood flow is maintained nearly constant with changes in

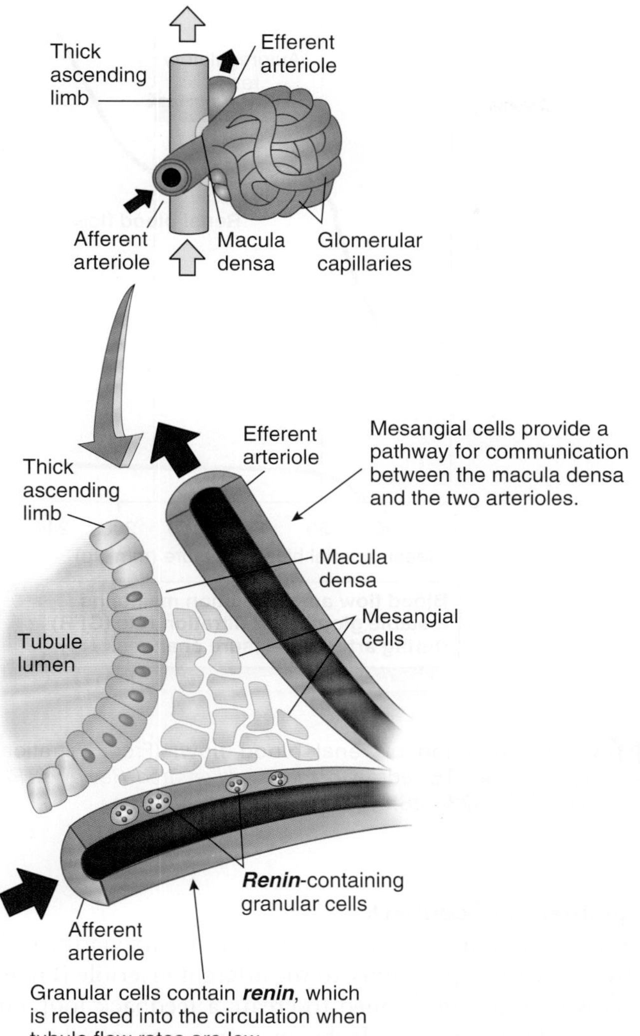

Figure 5.4 **Juxtaglomerular apparatus.** (From Filtration and micturition. In: Preston RR, Wilson TE, eds. *Lippincott® Illustrated Reviews: Physiology.* 2nd ed. Wolters Kluwer; 2019:323-338, Figures 25.10.)

systolic blood pressure from about 80 to 200 mm Hg (**Figure 5.5**). There are three main mechanisms whereby renal blood flow (and thus GFR) is regulated: myogenic response, tubuloglomerular feedback, and sympathetic nervous system stimulation.

Myogenic Response

The myogenic response is an intrinsic property of vascular smooth muscle, whereby arterioles constrict in response to increased transmural pressure and relax in response to decreased transmural pressure. This allows for relatively constant blood flow and GFR over a wide range of pressures.[2]

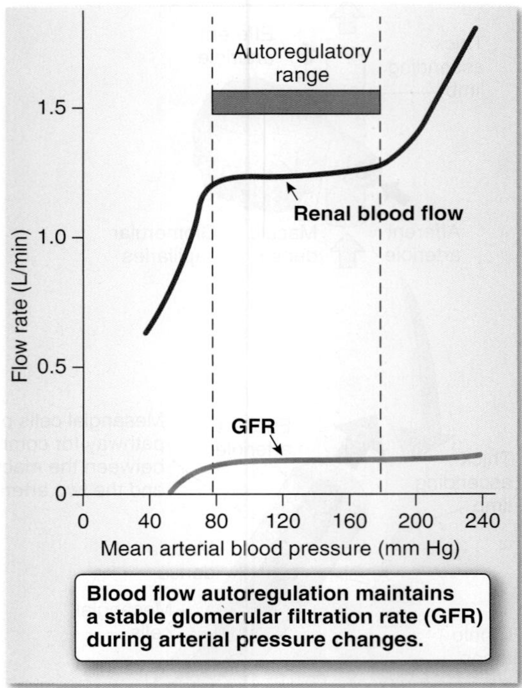

Figure 5.5 Autoregulation of renal blood flow. (From Filtration and micturit on. In: Preston RR, Wilson, TE, eds. *Lippincott® Illustrated Reviews: Physiology*. 2nd ed. Wolters Kluwer; 2019:323-338, Figures 25.9.)

Tubuloglomerular Feedback

The tubuloglomerular feedback mechanism occurs via the cells of the macula densa. By virtue of its proximity to the afferent arteriole (**Figure 5.4**), the macula densa is perfectly positioned to create a feedback loop controlling blood flow through the glomerulus. If the myogenic response does not fully regulate blood flow through the glomerulus, increased capillary pressure results in an increase in the GFR. The increased delivery of sodium chloride in the tubular fluid reaching the macula densa in the distal tubule results in vasoconstriction of the afferent arteriole (tubuloglomerular feedback). Increased sodium transport in the distal tubule is not the only mechanism triggering tubuloglomerular feedback. Tubular fluid flow, independent of sodium concentration, is sensed by primary cilia located on the apical (luminal) aspect of the macula densa cells and also trigger tubuloglomerular feedback.

Sympathetic Nervous System

During periods of stress, such as hypotension or hemorrhage, sympathetic stimulation overrides autoregulation. Increased renal sympathetic activity decreases sodium and water excretion by (1) increasing tubular water and sodium reabsorption throughout the nephron; (2) decreasing renal blood flow and GFR by vasoconstriction of the arterioles; and (3) increasing activity of the renin-angiotensin-aldosterone system (RAAS) by releasing renin from the juxtaglomerular granular cells.[3]

E. Tubular Reabsorption of Sodium and Water

Sodium moves freely from the glomerulus across the filtration membrane into Bowman capsule and has the same concentration in the tubular fluid as it has in the plasma. Approximately two-thirds of the filtrate reaching the proximal tubule is reabsorbed. This process is regulated both acutely and chronically by blood pressure, extracellular fluid volume, the RAAS, the sympathetic nervous system, and an intrarenal dopamine natriuretic system.[4] The bulk of sodium chloride, bicarbonate, phosphate, glucose, water, and other substrates is reabsorbed into the tubular cells as they move ***passively*** down their concentration gradients (**Figures 5.5** and **5.6**). Sodium-potassium ATPase in the basolateral membrane then ***actively*** pumps sodium out of the cell into the interstitial fluid, maintaining a low intracellular concentration. This maintains the driving force for sodium entry from the tubular fluid at the luminal side. The ***colloid oncotic pressure*** in the capillaries accompanying the proximal tubules is high because large molecules are retained by the filtration membrane of Bowman capsule. Sodium and water are reabsorbed from the interstitial fluid into the capillaries by bulk flow mediated by both hydrostatic and osmotic forces. The fraction of sodium reabsorbed in the proximal tubule varies according to prevailing conditions (**Table 5.1**). Water reabsorption occurs passively in the proximal tubule by osmosis and is coupled with sodium transport through the cells. Water also passes through the tight junctions between cells, which allows for diffusion of water and small ions.

The loop of Henle has three distinct regions: the thin descending segment, the thin ascending segment, and the thick ascending segment. The thin segments have thin membranes with no brush borders and few mitochondria (**Figure 5.3**) because of low metabolic requirements. There is little active reabsorption of water or solutes within these segments. However, the thin descending segment is highly permeable to water, but not to solutes. Therefore, as water diffuses passively out of the cells, the osmolarity of the tubular fluid increases to a maximum at the very tip of the loop of Henle. In contrast, both the thin and thick parts of the ascending limb are impermeable to water (**Figures 5.5** and **5.6**). Sodium moves into the cell along its gradient, which is maintained by basolateral Na^+/K^+ ATPase. At the same time, sodium cotransports potassium into the cell against its gradient.

The remainder of the ***distal nephron*** includes the connecting tubule and collecting duct (**Figures 5.2** and **5.3**). Only a small percentage of the original filtrate reaches these segments, but the reabsorption of water and solutes is highly regulated here and accounts for the fine tuning of fluid and electrolyte homeostasis by the kidney. There are distinct cell populations in the distal nephron. The connecting tubule consists of connecting cells and intercalated cells, while the collecting duct consists of principal cells and intercalated cells. Sodium reabsorption in the connecting tubule and collecting duct is mediated by the connecting cells and principal cells via hormone-sensitive (aldosterone) apical epithelial sodium channels.

Aldosterone forms a complex with receptors on the cell member of principal cells to promote the formation of sodium channels and enhances the activity of Na^+/K^+ ATPase pumps. The ***intercalated cells*** are of two types: type A, which secrete protons and reabsorb potassium, and type B, which secrete bicarbonate and reabsorb chloride. Water reabsorption, which occurs to a much greater extent in the collecting duct than the connecting tubule, is under the influence of antidiuretic hormone (ADH; aka arginine vasopressin). ADH

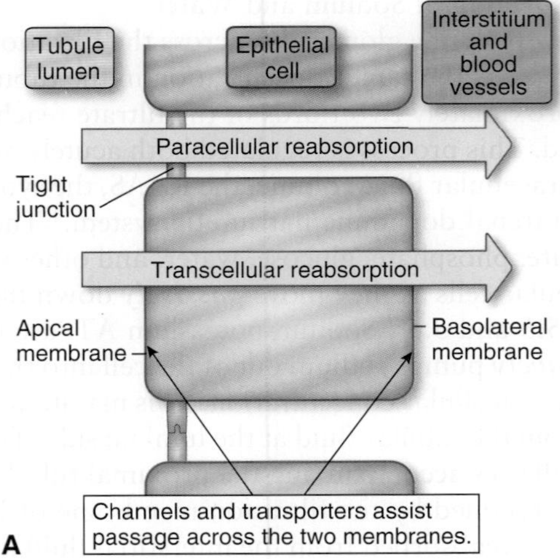

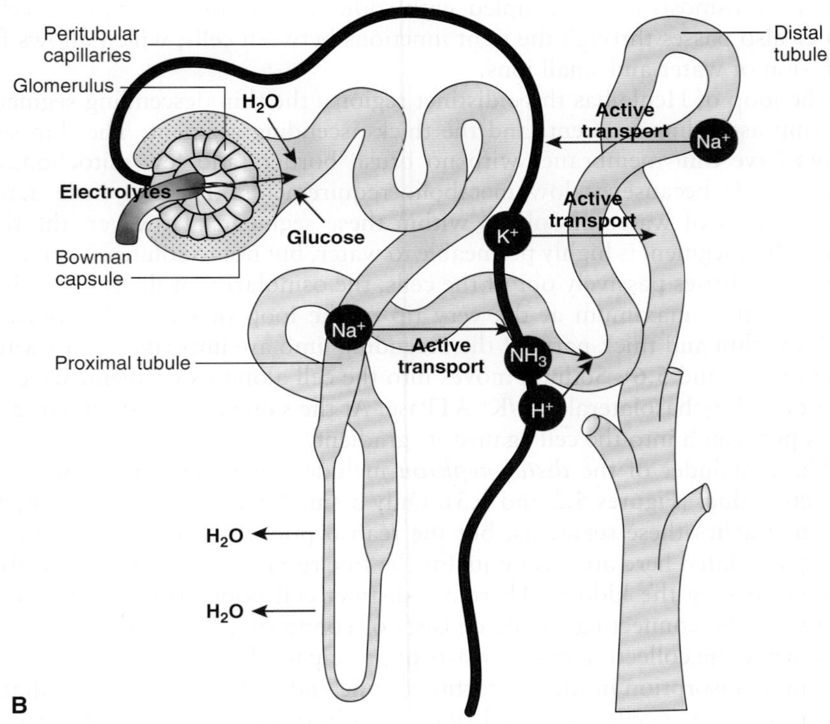

Figure 5.6 **A, Reabsorption from tubular lumen. B, Transport of substances across glomerulus.** (A, Derived from Filtration and micturition. In: Preston RR, Wilson, TE, eds. *Lippincott® Illustrated Reviews: Physiology.* 2nd ed. Wolters Kluwer; 2019:323-338 and B, Derived from *Straight A's in Anatomy and Physiology.* Lippincott Williams & Wilkins; 2007:313.)

Table 5.1 Factors Affecting Sodium Reabsorption by the Renal Tubule

Factors Decreasing Sodium Reabsorption	Factors Increasing Sodium Reabsorption
Increased blood pressure	Reduced blood pressure, hemorrhage
High salt intake	Low-salt diet
Increased extracellular volume	Sympathetic stimulation
Inhibition of angiotensin II	Angiotensin II

is produced in the posterior pituitary gland and released in response to hypovolemia and (to a less extent) hyperosmolality. ADH causes vasoconstriction in the kidney, especially of the efferent arteriole, which preserves glomerular filtration pressure even in the face of hypotension. ADH also binds to specific receptors on the medullary collecting ducts and enhances the expression of aquaporin channels on the principal cells, which increases water reabsorption. The collecting duct is normally relatively impermeable to water. However, it becomes highly permeable to water in the presence of ADH.

? *Did You Know?*

Fanconi syndrome is a disorder of proximal renal tubule function that causes substantial losses of water as well as many electrolytes, including potassium, bicarbonate, phosphate, amino acids, and glucose.

F. The Renin-Angiotensin-Aldosterone System

The RAAS is a complex hormonal system that regulates systemic blood pressure and fluid and electrolyte balance through local effects in the kidney and via systemic effects in other parts of the body. Renin is released by cells of the macula densa and collecting ducts in response to adrenergic stimulation, hypovolemia, or reduced perfusion. Renin converts ***angiotensinogen*** generated by the liver into ***angiotensin I (Ang I)***. Ang I is further cleaved by ***angiotensin-converting enzyme (ACE)*** produced by the lungs to form the active hormone ***angiotensin II (Ang II)*** (**Figure 5.7**). Recent studies have demonstrated that there are several Ang II receptor subtypes. However, the angiotensin type-1 receptor is by far the most common; through this receptor, angiotensin produces profound vasoconstriction at the level of the efferent arteriole, as well as promotes tubular sodium reabsorption, and secretion of aldosterone, vasopressin, and endothelin. Ang II also produces systemic vasoconstriction, but with only about one-tenth the potency of its renal effect.

Aldosterone is produced in the zona glomerulosa of the adrenal cortex in response to Ang II, adrenocorticotropic hormone, hyperkalemia, and hyponatremia. The net effect is increased sodium reabsorption. A feedback loops allows for precise control of the RAAS. Ang II feeds back to the juxtaglomerular apparatus to inhibit renin secretion from the macula densa and collecting duct cells. In addition, prostaglandins produced in the renal medulla are released in response to sympathetic nervous system stimulation and act to modulate the vasoconstrictive effects of the RAAS.

G. Renal Vasodilator Response

Exposure to stressors, of which surgery is one, results in the activation of ***vasopressor factors*** (RAAS, sympathetic discharge, vasopressin release), which maintain or increase systemic blood pressure but at the expense of renal circulation. The kidney is able to preserve its blood flow to some extent by the paracrine effects of several intrarenal vasodilators, including nitric oxide, prostaglandins, natriuretic peptides, and bradykinin (**Table 5.2**).[5]

The proximal tubule also produces dopamine from L-dopa via the enzyme L-amino acid decarboxylase. Circulating and locally formed dopamine

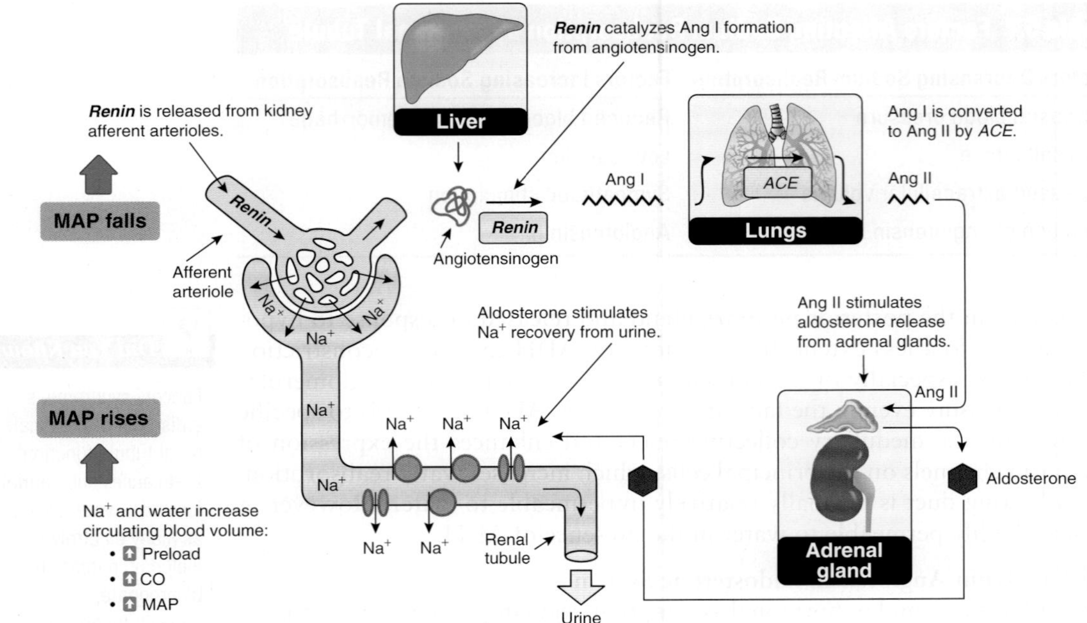

Figure 5.7 The renin-angiotensin-aldosterone system. ACE, angiotensin-converting enzyme; Ang I, angiotensin I; Ang II, angiotensin I; CO, cardiac output; MAP, mean aortic pressure. (Derived from Filtration and micturition. In: Preston RR, Wilson, TE, eds. *Lippincott® Illustrated Reviews: Physiology.* 2nd ed. Wolters Kluwer; 2019:323-338.)

activates ***dopamine receptors*** on arterioles and tubules via adenylyl cyclase, phospholipase C, and phospholipase A_2. Activation of dopamine receptors affects both sodium excretion and renal hemodynamics (**Table 5.3**). Sodium reabsorption is reduced in the proximal tubule, producing diuresis and natriuresis. Although dopamine is an effective diuretic, it has other effects on the cardiovascular system, which may include tachycardia and increased blood pressure even at so-called renal doses (1-3 µg/kg/min). Dopamine has not been shown to protect against or ameliorate either acute kidney injury (AKI) or chronic kidney disease (CKD) and is no longer recommended in the management of either condition.[6] The selective dopamine

Table 5.2 Renal Vasodilators

Factor	Comment
Nitric oxide	Main contributor to renal vasodilation
Prostaglandins	Released in response to stress, renal ischemia, and hypotension Oppose the RAAS and ADH
Natriuretic peptides (ANP, BNP)	Released in response to volume expansion Oppose the RAAS
Bradykinin	Also stimulates nitric oxide release

ADH, antidiuretic hormone; ANP, atrial natriuretic protein; BNP, brain natriuretic protein; RAAS, renin-aldosterone-angiotensin system.

Table 5.3 Effects of Dopamine on Renal Blood Flow and Tubular Function

Effects on Renal Blood Flow	Tubular Effects
Renal vasodilation by increasing prostaglandin production	Reduces activity of Na^+/H^+ exchanger in luminal membrane of proximal tubule
Increased renal blood flow, which causes increased GFR	Inhibits Na^+/K^+ ATPase pump on basolateral membrane of proximal tubule
	Inhibits renal renin expression and release in macula densa by inhibiting COX-2

COX-2, cylooxygenase-2; GFR, glomerular filtration rate; Na^+/H^+, sodium hydrogen ion; Na^+/K^+ ATPase, sodium potassium adenosine triphosphatase.

1 agonist fenoldopam is also an efficient diuretic, and there are some data suggesting that it may be effective in preventing cardiac surgery–associated AKI. It is, however, not in widespread use as a renoprotective agent and is only approved by the U.S. Food and Drug Administration as an antihypertensive in hypertensive crises.

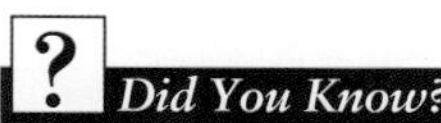

Aspirin and nonsteroidal anti-inflammatory drugs, including ketorolac, indirectly enhance catecholamine-induced renal vasoconstriction by reducing the production of renal prostaglandins, which normally exert a modulating vasodilatory effect.

II. Clinical Assessment of the Kidney

There are a number of tests that are used to evaluate renal function. Identifying preoperative kidney dysfunction is important, as perioperative kidney injury is a major source of morbidity and mortality.

A. Glomerular Filtration Rate

The GFR is a measure of plasma volume filtered per unit time. It represents an aggregate of the function of all the nephrons. GFR may be calculated from timed urine volumes plus urinary and plasma creatinine concentrations (creatinine clearance) or from measuring the clearance of exogenous substances such as inulin, which is filtered by the kidneys but not reabsorbed. GFR may also be estimated from the ***Cockcroft-Gault equation*** or the ***Modification of Diet in Renal Disease*** equation (**Table 5.4**).[7,8] GFR is about 125 mL/min in a healthy adult, but values vary by age, gender, and body weight.

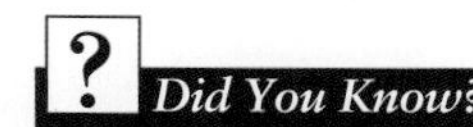

GFR decreases by approximately 8 mL/min/y after the age of 30 years.

Table 5.4 Calculations Used to Estimate Glomerular Filtration Rate

Cockcroft-Gault Equation
$\text{GFR}(\text{mL/min}) = \left[\left[(140 - \text{age}) \times \text{lean body weight (in kg)}\right] / (P_{Cr} \times 72)\right] \times 0.85 (\text{for women})\right]$
Modification of Diet in Renal Disease
$\text{GFR}(\text{mL/min/1.73 m}^2) = 170 \times P_{Cr}^{-0.999} \times \text{Age}^{-0.176} \times P_{BUN}^{-0.170} \times P_{Albumin}^{0.318} \times 0.762 (\text{for women}) \times 1.180 (\text{for blacks})$
Urine and plasma concentrations of creatinine and BUN measured in mg/dL. Plasma albumin concentration measured in g/dL. Urine volume measured in mL.

BUN, blood urea nitrogen; Cr, creatinine; GFR, glomerular filtration rate; P, plasma; U, urine.

Table 5.5 Factors That May Affect Serum Creatinine Levels

Physiologic Factors Affecting Serum Creatinine	Drugs Affecting Serum Creatinine
Age, gender, ethnicity—related to difference in muscle mass	Cimetidine, ranitidine, trimethoprim, salicylates, fibric acid derivatives—decrease tubular secretion
Muscle mass, rhabdomyolysis—increase creatinine production	Some cephalosporins, fluoxetine, acetoacetate (in DKA)—interfere with assay
Protein intake—increases creatinine production	Corticosteroids, vitamin D metabolites—affect production and release

DKA, diabetic ketoacidosis.

B. Serum Creatinine and Creatinine Clearance

Creatinine is a product of muscle metabolism that is freely filtered but not reabsorbed in the kidney. Normal serum creatinine concentrations range from 0.6 to 1.3 mg/dL. Although serum creatinine offers a reasonable estimate of GFR, creatinine values vary based on a number of physiologic factors and certain drug effects (**Table 5.5**). The relationship between serum creatinine and GFR is inverse and exponential (**Figure 5.8**). However, in AKI, a reduction in GFR will not be reflected in serum creatinine values for several days. In addition, serum creatinine will not increase until about 40% of nephrons are damaged.

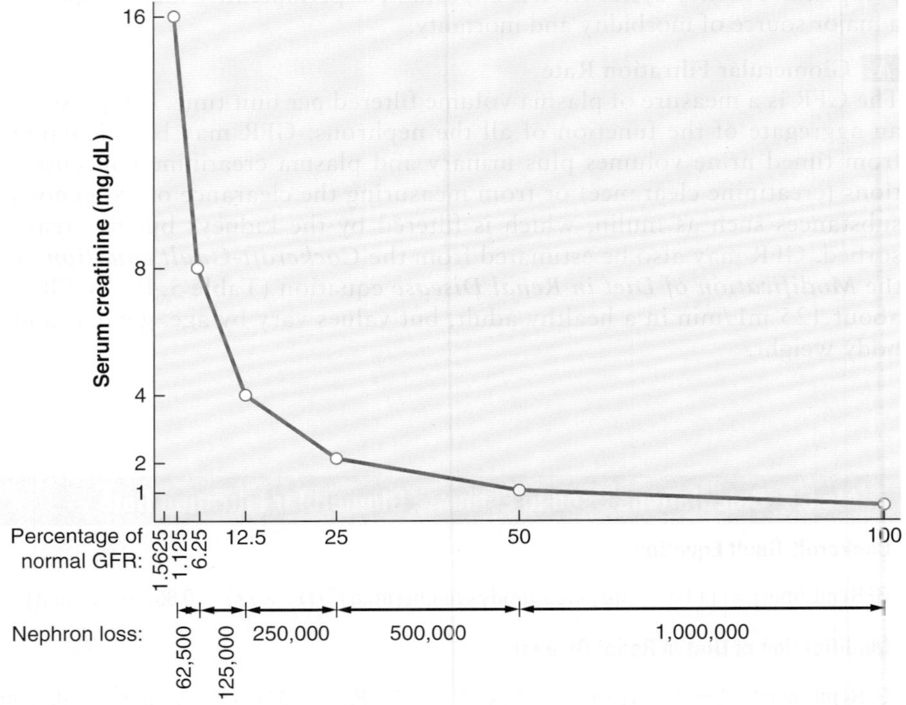

Figure 5.8 **Relationship between glomerular filtration rate (GFR) and serum creatinine.** (Modified from Faber MD, Kupin WL, Krishna G, et al. The differential diagnosis of ARF. In: Lazarus JM, Brenner BM, eds. *Acute Renal Failure.* 3rd ed. Churchill Livingstone; 1993:133.)

Table 5.6 Interpretation of Urine Findings

Finding	Condition
Renal Tubular Cells	Acute Tubular Injury
Red cell casts	Glomerular disease
Leukocytes	Urinary tract inflammation
White cell casts	Renal infection
Hyaline or granular casts	Any type of renal disease
Crystals	Metabolic disorders; medication-related
Bacteria	Urinary tract infection

C. Urinalysis and Urine Characteristics

Examination of the urine can reveal characteristics suggestive of renal disease. Inability to produce a concentrated urine—measured by specific gravity—given appropriate physiologic stimuli is a marker of renal tubular dysfunction. The presence of substances not ordinarily found in the urine—red or white blood cells, casts, crystals, microorganisms, large amounts of protein or glucose—can also provide clues to renal disease (**Tables 5.5** and **5.6**). Fractional excretion of sodium (FE_{Na}) can be estimated from a spot sample of blood and urine and can be used to differentiate between hypovolemia and intrinsic renal injury. A urinary sodium <20 mEq/L and an FE_{Na} <1% are suggestive of prerenal failure, while a urinary sodium >40 mEq/L and an FE_{Na} >2% are suggestive of renal tubular injury (**Table 5.7**).

Although routinely measured during surgery, urine output per se is neither a marker of renal function nor a predictor of postoperative AKI. Nevertheless, urine output <400 mL/24 h is often suggestive of kidney injury.

D. Novel Markers of Kidney Injury

There is significant interest in identifying markers that may detect kidney injury earlier than conventional methods and may also provide information about the underlying etiology of kidney disease. Cystatin C is produced in all nucleated cells and freely filtered but not reabsorbed by the tubules. It has been suggested as superior to creatinine as a measure of glomerular filtration because it is less affected by age, gender, and muscle mass and more likely to be elevated in mild kidney disease. Other markers that exhibit renal tubular damage have been identified. These include

Table 5.7 Laboratory Indices in Renal Failure

	Prerenal	Renal	Postrenal
Creatinine (mg/dL)	↑	↑	↑
BUN (mg/dL)	↑↑	↑	↑
Spot urine Na^+ (mEq/L)	<20	>40	>20
Urine osmolality (mOsm/L)	>500	<400	<350
FE_{NA} (%)	<1	>2	>2

BUN, blood urea nitrogen; FE_{NA}, fractional excretion of sodium in urine; Na, sodium.

Table 5.8 Markers of Renal Function

Factor	Pros	Cons
Creatinine	Easily measured Exponential inverse relationship with GFR	Late indicator of kidney dysfunction Varies by age, gender, muscle mass, and other factors
Urea	Easily measured Poor indicator of GFR	Blood urea nitrogen:creatinine ratio useful for differentiating prerenal vs intrinsic renal disease
Cystatin C	Endogenous marker of GFR Especially useful in detecting early kidney impairment	Assay is more expensive and less common than creatinine May be confounded in certain disease states, such as chronic inflammation
Proteinuria	Early sign of kidney impairment Helps to differentiate between tubulointerstitial and glomerular diseases	Not a marker of GFR
Urine specific gravity	Ability to concentrate urine to specific gravity >1.018 is indicative of preserved renal concentrating ability	Not a marker of GFR

GFR, glomerular filtration rate.

insulin-like growth factor–binding protein 7, tissue inhibitor metalloproteinase-2, neutrophil gelatinase–associated lipocalin, kidney injury molecule-1, and interleukin-18.

Table 5.8 summarizes the various markers of renal function used in clinical practice.[9,10]

III. Acute Kidney Injury

Perioperative AKI is a complication associated with significant morbidity and mortality. Recent studies suggest the incidence of AKI after noncardiac surgery is about 6%; after cardiac surgery, the incidence approaches 30%. Mortality among patients who experience postoperative AKI is up to three times higher than those who do not. Furthermore, only about half of patients who experience AKI will have a return to baseline renal function. Prevention and management of perioperative AKI is therefore vital.[10-12]

According to the Kidney Disease: Improving Global Outcomes, AKI is defined as an increase in serum creatinine of 0.3 mg/dL or more within 48 hours or a 1.5-fold or greater increase from baseline within 7 days (**Figure 5.9**).

Although overly simplistic, the etiology of AKI has historically been divided into prerenal, intrarenal (or intrinsic), and postrenal causes (**Table 5.9**). Prerenal AKI is the most common form of hospital-acquired AKI. When renal ischemia is prolonged, tubular injury ensues and the clinical picture is suggestive of intrinsic AKI. Urinary indices are helpful in distinguishing the etiology of AKI (**Tables 5.5 and 5.6**). Postrenal AKI is caused by an obstruction distal to the nephron. It is the least common form of AKI, but the most preventable. Renal ultrasonography is often the test of choice for ruling out the presence of obstructive nephropathy.

RIFLE (7 days)	AKIN (48 h)	KDIGO
Risk Increased sCr × 1.5 or GFR decrease > 25% OR urine output < 0.5 ml · kg^{-1} · h^{-1} for 6 h	**Stage 1** Increased sCr × 1.5–2 or sCr increase ≥ 0.3 mg dl^{-1} OR urine output < 0.5 ml · kg^{-1} · h^{-1} for > 6 h	**Stage 1** Increased sCr × 1.5–1.9 within 7 days OR sCr increase ≥ 0.3 mg dl^{-1} within 48 h OR urine output < 0.5 ml · kg^{-1} · h^{-1} for H 6–12 h
Injury Increased sCr × 2 or GFR decrease > 50% OR urine output < 0.5 ml · kg^{-1} · h^{-1} for 12 h	**Stage 2** Increased sCr × 2–3 OR urine output < 0.5 ml · kg^{-1} · h^{-1} for > 12h	**Stage 2** Increased sCr × 2–2.9 OR urine output < 0.5 ml · kg^{-1} · h^{-1} for ≥ 12 h
Failure Increased sCr × 3 or GFR decrease > 75% or sCr ≥ 4 mg dl^{-1} with an acute rise in sCr (≥ 0.5 mg dl^{-1}) OR urine output < 0.3 ml · kg^{-1} · h^{-1} for 24 h or anuria for 12 h	**Stage 3** Increased sCr × 3 or more or sCr ≥ 4 mg dl^{-1} with an acute rise in sCr (≥ 0.5 mg dl^{-1}) OR urine output < 0.3 ml · kg^{-1} · h^{-1} for > 24 h or anuria for 12 h	**Stage 3** Increased sCr × 3 or more or sCr ≥ 4 mg dl^{-1} or initiation of RRT or GFR decrease to < 35 ml min^{-1} (1.73 m)$^{-2}$ in patients < 18 yr old OR urine output < 0.3 ml · kg^{-1} · h^{-1} for ≥ 24 h or anuria for ≥ 12 h
Loss Persistent acute renal failure = complete loss of kidney function > 4 weeks		
End-stage renal disease End-stage kidney disease > 3 months		

Comparison of the three most notable and historic classification systems used to diagnose acute kidney injury. The initial system was the RIFLE (Risk, Injury, Failure, Loss of kidney function, End-stage renal failure), which was developed by an international consensus in 2004.[8] It defined five stages of renal injury: risk-end stage disease. A short time later, the Acute Kidney Injury Network (AKIN) developed its own diagnostic criteria that uses a smaller creatinine change to define acute kidney injury .This was based on studies showing that even small changes in serum creatinine resulted in adverse outcomes.[2–6] In 2012, the KDIGO (Kidney Disease: Improving Global Outcomes) classification system was produced and has been the main system in use since.[14]

GFR, glomerular filtration rate; sCr, serum creatinine.

Figure 5.9 **Acute kidney injury classification systems.** (From Gumbert SD, Kork F, Jackson ML, et al. Perioperative acute kidney injury. *Anesthesiology.* 2020;132:180-204, with permission.)

Patient-associated risk factors for the development of AKI include preexisting renal disease, advanced age, African American race, preexisting hypertension, congestive heart failure, pulmonary disease, insulin-dependent diabetes mellitus, peripheral vascular disease, the presence of ascites, and high body mass index. Procedure-associated risk factors include emergency surgery,

Table 5.9 Etiology of Acute Kidney Injury
Prerenal Azotemia
Hemorrhage
Burns
Cardiogenic shock
Sepsis
Aortic/renal artery clamping
Thromboembolism
Renal Azotemia
Acute glomerulonephritis
Acute interstitial nephritis (drug related, infectious, malignancy, autoimmune)
Acute tubular necrosis
Postrenal Azotemia
Nephrolithiasis
Benign prostatic hyperplasia
Clot retention
Malignancy

cardiac or major vascular surgery, prolonged aortic cross-clamp time, the use of cardiopulmonary bypass, intraoperative blood transfusions, episodes of intraoperative hypotension, and the use of vasopressors and diuretics.

Pharmacologic interventions to treat and prevent perioperative AKI have remained elusive. Neither dopamine nor the dopamine analogue fenoldopam has shown benefit in the prevention or management of AKI. Renal replacement therapy (RRT) is the only treatment for severe AKI. Indications for RRT include metabolic acidosis, severe electrolyte abnormalities, fluid overload, and signs or symptoms of severe uremia. There is no indication that the timing of RRT—early versus late—significantly affects outcomes, so the decision to initiate RRT is best made based on a patient-to-patient basis on symptom severity.

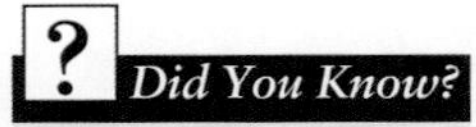

Renal replacement therapy is typically necessary when GFR is <10 mL/min.

IV. Chronic Kidney Disease

CKD is defined by the International Society of Nephrology and Kidney Disease Improving Global Outcomes as abnormalities of kidney structure or function present for more than 3 months (**Table 5.10**). CKD is classified based on cause, GFR, and albuminuria.[13] Grades of CKD have been established according to GFR and albuminuria, and risk can be apportioned according to these grades (**Figure 5.10**). Hypertension and diabetes are the leading causes of CKD, accounting for >70% of cases. The National Kidney Foundation's (NKF) Kidney Disease Outcomes Quality Initiative provides evidence-based clinical practice guidelines for all stages of CKD and their related complications, including the management of hyperglycemia, hyperlipidemia, and anemia.[13]

The kidneys exhibit various compensatory mechanisms to the loss of nephron volume that accompanies CKD. While effective in the short term, these mechanisms can contribute to long-term exacerbation of kidney injury. For example, there is accelerated filtration in the normally functioning nephrons—a process known as hyperfiltration. This occurs as a result of glomerular hypertension through activation of the RAAS and increased glomerular permeability. Over the long term, this leads to glomerulosclerosis and chronic tubulointerstitial ischemia.

Changes in bone structure and mineralization are nearly universal in patients with CKD, a complication known as renal osteodystrophy. The precipitating factor is decreased vitamin D activation in the kidney, which in turn leads to impaired gastrointestinal calcium absorption. Hypocalcemia stimulates parathyroid hormone secretion in an effort to restore serum calcium concentrations at the expense of increased bone resorption. Furthermore, as GFR decreases, phosphate clearance also decreases. An increase in serum phosphate concentration results in a reciprocal decrease in serum calcium concentration. Not only does this exacerbate hyperparathyroidism but also leads to calcium phosphate crystal deposition in joints that can lead to joint pain and increased fracture risk. Anemia occurs as a result of decreased erythropoietin—a hormone normally secreted by the kidneys—and decreased red cell survival time. The anemia is usually normochromic and normocytic. The current NKF guidelines for the treatment of anemia is to maintain a hemoglobin >13 mg/dL; this is accomplished by the administration of recombinant human erythropoietin or the synthetic analogue darbepoetin. Both platelet and white blood cell functions are impaired in patients with kidney disease. The most common laboratory abnormality is increased bleeding time.

Table 5.10 Effects of Chronic Kidney Disease on Other Organ Systems

System	Derangement	Causes
Cardiac	Hypertension Myocardial dysfunction Pericarditis Tamponade Congestive heart failure	Hypervolemia, activation of RAAS Activation of SNS Uremia, dialysis
Respiratory	Pulmonary edema Restrictive lung disease	Reduced oncotic pressure Uremic pleuritis
Metabolic	Metabolic acidosis Hyperkalemia Hypoglycemia Hyperphosphatemia Hypocalcemia	Inability to conserve bicarbonate and excrete titratable acids Reduced clearance of insulin/other hypoglycemic drugs; reduced renal gluconeogenesis Impaired calcium absorption due to reduced vitamin D activation
Hematologic	Anemia Platelet dysfunction	Loss of erythropoietin Action of uremic toxins, abnormal nitric oxide production, von Willebrand factor abnormalities and drugs
Immunologic	Cell-mediated defects Humoral immunity defects	Reduced clearance of cytokines
Gastrointestinal	Nausea and vomiting Delayed gastric emptying Anorexia	Uremia, drug therapy, dialysis
Neuromuscular	Encephalopathy Seizures, tremors, and myoclonus Autonomic dysfunction Polyneuropathy	Electrolyte and fluid abnormalities

RAAS, renin–angiotensin-aldosterone system; SNS, sympathetic nervous system.

Cardiovascular diseases occur more frequently in patients with CKD and are the most common causes of death in this population; however, sepsis and infectious-related deaths are also more common. Systemic hypertension contributes to the development of left ventricular hypertrophy, congestive heart failure, and cardiac ischemia. The etiology is multifactorial—volume and sodium overload, anemia, and hypertension are among the relevant factors. Uremic pericarditis is a unique complication of severe renal disease and may precipitate life-threatening cardiac tamponade.

Patients with ***end-stage renal disease*** require dialysis for survival. These patients have added physiologic derangements because of the dialysis therapy itself and the means of delivering that dialysis (**Tables 5.11** and **5.12**). Complications associated with chronic dialysis include an increased risk of infection, protein calorie deficiency malnutrition, amyloidosis, and uremia.

Prognosis of CKD by GFR and albuminuria categories

Prognosis of CKD by GFR and albuminuria categories: KDIGO 2012				Persistent albuminuria categories Description and range		
				A1	**A2**	**A3**
				Normal to mildly increased	Moderately increased	Severely increased
				<30 mg/g <3 mg/mmol	30–300 mg/g >30 mg/mmol	>300 mg/g >30 mg/mmol
GFR categories (mL/min/1.73 m^2) Description and range	**G1**	Normal or high	≥90			
	G2	Mildly decreased	60–89			
	G3a	Mildly to moderately decreased	45–59			
	G3b	Moderately to severely decreased	30–44			
	G4	Severely decreased	15–29			
	G5	Kidney failure	<15			

Green: Low risk (if no other markers of kidney disease, no CKD); Yellow: Moderately increased risk; Orange: High risk; Red: Very high risk; CKD: Chronic Kidney Disease; GFR: Glomerular filtration rate; KDIGO: Kidney Disease Improvement for Global Outcome.

Figure 5.10 Prognosis of chronic kidney disease by glomerular filtration rate and albuminuria categories. (From Kidney Disease: Improving Global Outcomes (KDIGO) CKD Work Group. KDIGO 2012 clinical practice guideline for the evaluation and management of chronic kidney disease. *Kidney Inter Suppl.* 2013;3:1-150.)

A. Drug Prescribing in Renal Failure

Many factors contribute to the altered drug pharmacokinetics seen in patients with CKD. In addition to reduced clearance, increased volume of distribution, decreased plasma protein binding, acidemia, coexisting liver disease, and changes in gastrointestinal uptake are all factors. Knowledge of a drug's pharmacokinetics will assist in modifying dose and interval timing and may help predict and prevent unwanted side effects[14,15] (Chapter 7) When possible, choosing drugs that do not rely on the kidneys for excretion is optimal. Drugs with active or toxic metabolites (eg, meperidine, morphine) are best avoided, as these metabolites can accumulate in patients with renal disease. For the most part, drug doses rarely require modification until the GFR is less than 30 mL/min. For medications with a wide therapeutic index, the interval between doses is often increased. For those who a narrow therapeutic index, reduced doses at normal intervals typically provide more predictable steady-state concentrations. Avoidance of known nephrotoxins, including contrast dye, nonsteroidal anti-inflammatories, aminoglycosides, and vancomycin, is

Table 5.11 Complications of Dialysis or Hemofiltration Access

Access Route	Complications
Temporary venous access (usually internal jugular vein, subclavian vein)	Bleeding, hypotension, hematoma (increased BUN, pigmenturia), thrombosis, stricture (SVC syndrome), pneumothorax, chylothorax, nerve injury
Peritoneal	Ileus, increased abdominal pressure, increased risk of aspiration, raised diaphragm, reduced lung volumes, restrictive respiratory pattern
Upper limb arteriovenous fistula	Restricted limb access, thrombosis, interference with blood sampling and pulse oximetry, shunting, reduced vascular resistance

BUN, blood urea nitrogen; SVC, superior vena cava.

also important. Though not renal toxins, per se, ACE inhibitor and angiotensin receptor blockers may compromise renal blood flow; therefore, they should be used cautiously in patients with compromised renal function.

B. Anesthetic Drugs in CKD

All volatile anesthetics reduce renal blood flow via their ability to decrease systemic arterial pressure and cardiac output. The pharmacokinetics of volatile anesthetics are not dependent on renal function, protein binding, or volume of distribution. Nephrotoxicity has been attributed to the ***fluoride ion*** released during the metabolism of the older anesthetics methoxyflurane and possibly enflurane in patients who have had long exposure to these agents. A similar association has not been observed with sevoflurane, despite the fact that it too produces the fluoride ion when during metabolism. In the presence of some carbon dioxide absorbents (soda lime, Baralyme), sevoflurane undergoes nonenzymatic degradation to an alkene known as compound A, which has been shown to be a dose-dependent nephrotoxin in animals. While no study has demonstrated clinically significant nephrotoxicity in humans, the U.S. Food and Drug Administration recommends that sevoflurane be used with fresh gas flow rates of at least 1 to 2 L/min.

Drugs eliminated unchanged by the kidneys (some nondepolarizing muscle relaxants, cholinesterase inhibitors, many antibiotics) have increased elimination half-times in patients with CKD, inversely related to GFR. Many

Table 5.12 Acute Complications of Dialysis

Hypotension	Ultrafiltration-induced volume depletion; osmolar shifts across the dialysis membrane; myocardial ischemia; arrhythmias, pericardial effusion
Arrhythmia	Acute potassium flux; rapid pH changes
Hypersensitivity reaction	Exposure to polyacrylonitrile surfaces of dialysis membrane, residual ethylene oxide from sterilization of equipment
Dialysis disequilibrium	Characterized by nausea, vomiting, seizures, and even coma due to rapid changes in pH and solutes across CNS membranes

CNS, central nervous system.

anesthetic drugs are protein bound to varying degrees. As a result of the hypoproteinemia that accompanies CKD, the free (active) fraction of many drugs is increased. Of the induction agents, thiopental is most extensively protein bound and therefore most affected in CKD, with ketamine and etomidate being less affected. Propofol is not affected by changes in kidney function because it is rapidly biotransformed by the liver into inactive metabolites, which are then excreted by the kidneys. Benzodiazepines are highly protein bound; therefore, the free fraction of benzodiazepines is increased in patients with CKD. In addition, diazepam and midazolam should be used with caution because active metabolites may accumulate in the presence of kidney dysfunction.

The use of fentanyl or ultrashort-acting narcotics is preferable in patients with kidney disease. The pharmacokinetics of remifentanil is unaffected by kidney disease, as remifentanil degrades rapidly by ester hydrolysis in the blood. Morphine and meperidine undergo metabolism to potentially neurotoxic compounds (morphine-3-glucuronide and normeperidine, respectively) that rely on renal clearance and are therefore best avoided in patients with CKD. Morphine-6-glucuronide, a morphine metabolite more potent than its parent compound, may also accumulate in patients with CKD and result in profound respiratory depression. Hydromorphone also has an active metabolite, hydromorphone-3-glucuronide, that may accumulate in patients with CKD; however, hydromorphone is better tolerated than morphine. The most important considerations are cautious dosing and careful monitoring for respiratory depression.

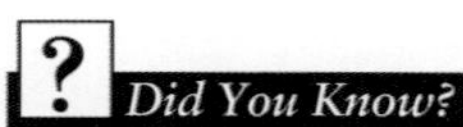

Repeated dosing or chronic use of meperidine, morphine, and hydromorphone in renal disease is associated with accumulation of excitatory neurotoxic metabolites.

Short-acting muscle relaxants are preferable in patients with renal disease; atracurium and cisatracurium, which are metabolized by spontaneous, organ-independent, nonenzymatic degradation, are the drugs of choice. Nevertheless, these two drugs have a toxic metabolite, laudanosine, which may accumulate during infusion of the parent drug and has been shown to be epileptogenic in animals. Succinylcholine is generally safe in patients with CKD who are not severely hyperkalemic. The potassium release after succinylcholine administration is not exaggerated in patients with kidney disease; an increase of 0.5 mEq/L is typical. Both vecuronium and rocuronium have been reported to have prolonged action in patients with severe kidney disease. Sugammadex is a muscle relaxant reversal agent that inactivates by encapsulation the steroidal neuromuscular blocking agents (NMDAs) vecuronium and rocuronium. The sugammadex-NMDA complex is excreted unchanged in the urine. Although the complex can be removed by dialysis, use of sugammadex is not advised in patients with estimated GFRs less than 30 mL/min.

C. Management of Anesthesia for Patients With Renal Disease

There is reasonable evidence to suggest that neuraxial anesthesia in the context of abdominal or cardiac surgery is associated with a reduced risk of AKI. Presumably, this is related to reduced systemic and renovascular sympathetic tone.

Dexmedetomidine, a selective alpha 2-adrenergic agonist, has been shown to reduce the incidence of cardiac surgery–associated AKI, although its impact on long-term outcomes remains controversial.[16,17] Presumably, this effect is due to intrinsic anti-inflammatory properties. As previously discussed, there is no evidence that dopamine administration preserves kidney function, despite the presence of vasodilatory dopamine receptors in the kidney. While some studies suggest the dopamine agonist fenoldopam may exert renoprotective effects, this finding is yet to be confirmed in large clinical trials.

Table 5.13 Properties of Commonly Used Diuretics

Drug	Site of Action	Effects	Side Effects
Carbonic anhydrase inhibitors (acetazolamide)	Proximal convoluted tubule	Inhibits Na^+ reabsorption and H^+ excretion	Hyperchloremia Hypokalemia
Loop diuretics (furosemide, bumetanide)	Thick ascending limb of the loop of Henle	Inhibits Cl^- reabsorption Renal vasodilation	Hypovolemia Hypokalemia Metabolic alkalosis Hypocalcemia
Thiazides (hydrochlorothiazide)	Between the ascending limb of the and distal convoluted tubule	Inhibits Na^+ reabsorption	Hypokalemia Hypochloremia Metabolic alkalosis Hypercalcemia
Potassium-sparing diuretics (spironolactone, triamterene)	Distal convoluted tubule	Inhibits aldosterone	Hyperkalemia
Osmotic diuretics (mannitol)	Filtered at the glomerulus, but not reabsorbed; increases water excretion via osmosis	Accelerates free water excretion Renal vasodilation	May precipitate congestive heart failure by increasing intravascular fluid volume

Goal-directed intraoperative fluid therapy appears to be the strategy of choice, with balanced salt solutions being preferred to 0.9% normal saline.[18-21] Hydroxyethyl starch should be avoided, as evidence from large randomized trials suggests its use is associated with an increased risk of AKI.[22,23]

? Did You Know?

Excessive increases in intrathoracic pressure caused by controlled ventilation or intra-abdominal hypertension caused by surgery or fluid overload can compromise renal blood flow.

V. Diuretic Drugs: Effects and Mechanisms

A. The Physiologic Basis of Diuretic Action

Diuretic drugs act on the mechanism that moves sodium ions from the tubular lumen into the cell where they can then be pumped across the basolateral surface by NA^+/K^+ ATPase and reabsorbed. Diuretics are typically classified according to their site of action in the nephron (**Table 5.13**). Diuretics are used in the management of several conditions, most notably hypertension and congestive heart failure. Choice of agent is based on underlying comorbities.

For further review and interactivities, please see the associated Interactive Video Lectures and "A Closer Look" infographic accessible in the complimentary eBook bundled with this text. Access instructions are located in the inside front cover.

References

1. Sipos A, Vargas A, Peti-Peterdi J. Direct demonstration of tubular fluid flow sensing by macula densa cells. *Am J Physiol Renal Physiol*. 2010;299(5):F1087-F1093.
2. Burke M, Pabbidi MR, Farley J, et al. Molecular mechanisms of renal blood flow autoregulation. *Curr Vasc Pharmacol*. 2014;12:1-14.
3. DiBona GF. Nervous kidney: interaction between renal sympathetic nerves and the renin-angiotensin system in the control of renal function. *Hypertension*. 2000;36(6):1083-1088.

4. McDonough AA. Mechanisms of proximal tubule sodium transport regulation that link extracellular fluid volume and blood pressure. *Am J Physiol Regul Integr Comp Physiol.* 2010;298(4):R851-R861.
5. Carey RM. The intrarenal renin-angiotensin and dopaminergic systems: control of renal sodium excretion and blood pressure. *Hypertension.* 2013;61:673-680.
6. Sadowski J, Badzynska B. Intrarenal vasodilator systems: NO, prostaglandins and bradykinin. An integrative approach. *J Physiol Pharmacol.* 2008;59(suppl 9):105-119.
7. U.S. Department of Health and Human Services. *National Kidney Disease and Education Program.* Estimating GFR. Accessed September 9, 2020. http://nkdep.nih.gov/lab-evaluation/gfr/estimating.shtml
8. MD+CALC. *Creatinine Clearance (Cockcroft-Gault Equation).* Accessed September 8, 2020. http://www.mdcalc.com/creatinine-clearance-cockcroft-gault-equation/
9. Chen LX, Koyner JL. Biomarkers in acute kidney injury. *Crit Care Clin.* 2015;31:633-648.
10. Gumbert SD, Kork F, Jackson ML, et al. Perioperative acute kidney injury. *Anesthesiology.* 2020;132:180-204.
11. Ostermann M, Joannidis M. Acute kidney injury 2016: diagnosis and diagnostic workup. *Crit Care.* 2016;20:299.
12. Hobson C, Ruchi R, Bihorac A. Perioperative acute kidney injury: risk factors and predictive strategies. *Crit Care Clin.* 2017;33:379-396.
13. Kidney Disease: Improving Global Outcomes (KDIGO) CKD Work Group. KDIGO 2012 clinical practice guideline for the evaluation and management of chronic kidney disease. *Kidney Int Suppl.* 2013;3(1):1-150. Accessed September 20, 2020. www.kdigo.org/clinical_practice_guidelines/pdf/CKD/KDIGO_2012_CKD_GL.pdf
14. Griffiths RS, Olyaei AJ. *Drug dosing in patients with chronic disease.* In: *Nephrology Secrets.* 3rd ed. Wolters Kluwer; 2012:197-206.
15. Gabardi S, Abramson S. Drug dosing in chronic kidney disease. *Med Clin North Am.* 2005;89(3):649-687.
16. Xue F, Zhang W, Chu HC. Assessing perioperative dexmedetomidine reduces the incidence and severity of acute kidney injury following valvular heart surgery. *Kidney Int.* 2016;89:1164.
17. Shi R, Tie HT. Dexmedetomidine as a promising prevention strategy for cardiac surgery-associated acute kidney injury: a meta-analysis. *Crit Care.* 2017;21:198.
18. Myles PS, Bellomo R, Corcoran T, et al. Restrictive versus liberal fluid therapy for major abdominal surgery. *N Engl J Med.* 2018;378:2263-2274.
19. Young P, Bailey M, Beasley R, et al. Effect of a buffered crystalloid solution vs saline on acute kidney injury among patients in the intensive care unit: the SPLIT randomized clinical trial. *J Am Med Assoc.* 2015;314:1701-1710.
20. Self WH, Semler MW, Wanderer JP, et al. Balanced crystalloids versus saline in noncritically ill adults. *N Engl J Med.* 2018;378:819-828.
21. Semler MW, Self WH, Wanderer JP, et al. Balanced crystalloids versus saline in critically ill adults. *N Engl J Med.* 2018;378:829-839.
22. Perner A, Haase N, Guttormsen AB, et al. Hydroxyethyl starch 130/0.42 versus Ringer's acetate in severe sepsis. *N Engl J Med.* 2012;367:124-134.
23. Myburgh JA, Finfer S, Bellomo R, et al. Hydroxyethyl starch or saline for fluid resuscitation in intensive care. *N Engl J Med.* 2012;367:1901-1911.

RENAL PROTECTION

A CLOSER LOOK

Understanding kidney physiology is critical to managing patients at risk of acute kidney injury. Surgery is the second leading cause of acute kidney injury in hospitalized patients after sepsis. The mechanism involves a combination of renal hypoperfusion and inflammation, which overwhelms the autoregulatory capacity of the kidneys.

URINE OUTPUT

It is important to monitor both the output of urine over time and its perceived color. Darker urine may indicate renal concentration of urine in the setting of hypovolemia. Urine output is influenced by mutliple factors (volume status, diuretics, ADH, stress response).

Renal blood flow (RBF) is autoregulated and constant between a range of 80 to 180 mm Hg mean arterial pressure in healthy patients.

RBF

80 mm Hg

180 mm Hg

MEAN ARTERIAL PRESSURE

CREATININE

Serum creatinine concentration rises during acute kidney injury. GFR has to ↓ by 50% before Cr increases.

AVOID NEPHROTOXINS

IV contrast, aminoglycosides, vancomycin, piperacillin-tazobactam, NSAIDs

MAINTAIN BLOOD PRESSURE

Avoid hypoperfusion of the kidneys

MAINTAIN EUVOLEMIA

Use balanced isotonic fluid, not normal saline or hydroxyethyl starch.

DIURETICS are NOT preventative and should only be used to regulate fluid balance. Mannitol and bicarbonate have NOT been proven to be renoprotective.

AVOID HYPO- and HYPERGLYCEMIA

Insulin relies on renal clearance; thus, patients receiving this drug with renal disease may develop hypoglycemia.

Although sevoflurane can theoretically produce a nephrotoxic product called compound A, it has been safely used in patients with renal disease.

Infographic by: Naveen Nathan MD

Questions

1. **The normal human GFR is approximately:**

   A. 25 mL/min
   B. 50 mL/min
   C. 125 mL/min
   D. 200 mL/min

2. **According to the Kidney Disease Improving Global Outcomes, which of the following meets the criteria for AKI?**

   A. An increase in serum creatinine of 0.3 mg/dL or more within 48 hours
   B. A decrease in urine output to <400 mL/d
   C. An increase in serum blood urea nitrogen by more than 1.5 times in 1 week
   D. An increase in serum cystatin C of 0.5 mg/dL or more within 24 hours

3. **Which of the following urinary index is MOST suggestion of AKI due to hypovolemia?**

   A. Spot urine Na^+ >20 mEq/L
   B. Urine osmolality <500 mOsm/L
   C. Serum creatinine 2× baseline
   D. FE_{Na} <1%

4. **Nephrotic syndrome is marked by massive proteinuria due to abnormal filtration of proteins. A lesion in which part of the kidney is most likely to account for this pathology?**

   A. Glomerular basement membrane
   B. Juxtaglomerular apparatus
   C. Ascending limb of the loop of Henle
   D. Proximal convoluted tubule

5. **The compound with the greatest contribution to renal vasodilation is:**

   A. Atrial natriuretic protein
   B. Bradykinin
   C. Nitric oxide
   D. Prostaglandin

6. **The action of which of the following agents is inhibited by spironolactone?**

   A. Bradykinin
   B. Aldosterone
   C. Antidiuretic hormone
   D. Angiotensin II

7. **Alport syndrome is a genetic disorder marked by hematuria and chronic glomerulonephritis caused by a collagen mutation. Based on the symptoms, this collagen is MOST likely a component of which of the following renal structures?**

   A. Proximal tubule
   B. Loop of Henle
   C. Distal convoluted tubule
   D. Glomerular basement membrane

8. **Which of the following is MOST related to the hypocalcemia that accompanies end-stage renal disease?**

   A. Reduced secretion of parathyroid hormone
   B. Reduced activation of vitamin D
   C. Increased renal phosphate clearance
   D. Impaired renal calcium reabsorption

9. **A 56-year-old patient with CKD due to hypertension is presenting for partial colectomy. Owing to its lack of active metabolites, which of the following narcotics is preferred for intraoperative pain management?**

   A. Fentanyl
   B. Hydromorphone
   C. Meperidine
   D. Morphine

10. **A 76-year-old man is undergoing on-pump coronary artery bypasss graft surgery. The intraoperative use of which of the following agents is MOST likely to reduce his risk of postoperative renal failure?**

    A. Dopamine
    B. Phenylephrine
    C. Vasopressin
    D. Dexmedetomidine

Answers

1. C

The glomerular filtration rate (GFR) is the volume of filtrate formed by both kidneys per minute. This is approximately 125 mL/min in an average patient with normal renal function, but values vary by age, gender, and body weight. GFR is an important component of chronic kidney disease (CKD) classification and its progression. A GFR below 60 mL/min defines CKD, which increases in severity as GFR decreases. Renal replacement therapy is typically required when GFR drops below 10 mL/min.

2. A

Acute kidney injury (AKI) is defined as an increase in serum creatinine of 0.3 mg/dL or more within 48 hours or a 1.5-fold or greater increase from baseline within 7 days.

3. D

Fractional excretion of sodium (FE_{Na}) can be estimated from a spot sample of blood and urine and can be used to differentiate between hypovolemia and intrinsic renal injury. A urinary sodium <20 mEq/L and an FE_{Na} <1% are suggestive of prerenal failure, while a urinary sodium >40 mEq/L and an FE_{Na} >2 % are suggestive of renal tubular injury.

4. A

The glomeruli are the filtering units of the kidney. The glomerular basement membrane (GBM) is a barrier to the filtration of large plasma molecules including proteins. Glomerular injury, including GBM lesions, is commonly the underlying pathology in nephrotic syndrome.

5. C

While all these substances are thought to be renal vasodilators, nitric oxide plays a central and multifaceted role. NO produced in the macula densa and secreted locally in the setting of increased renal blood flow blunts both the tubuloglomerular feedback and myogenic response to allow increased distal NaCl delivery.

6. B

Spironolactone is categorized as a mineralocorticoid receptor antagonist and potassium sparing diuretic. Aldosterone is the principle mineralocorticoid. It is a relatively weak diuretic and rarely used as a first-line antihypertensive. Potassium levels should be monitored, as this class of drugs can cause hyperkalemia.

7. D

The glomerular basement membrane (GBM) is a barrier to the filtration of large plasma molecules including proteins. Glomerular disease, often including GBM lesions, underlies glomerulonephritis and can manifest as hematuria. The various known mutations identified in Alport syndrome are in genes that encode collagens normally expressed in the GBM.

8. B

The kidney is a major site of conversion of vitamin D to its active metabolite by the action of enzyme 1-alpha-hydroxylase. This conversion decreases as GFR decreases. Decreased activated vitamin D leads to decreased gastrointestinal calcium absorption, which results in increased parathyroid hormone secretion. Meanwhile, increased inorganic phosphate in the setting of decreased phosphate clearance both drives down calcium levels and reduces vitamin D activation by decreasing 1-alpha-hydroxylase activity.

9. A

While nonopioid analgesia including regional and neuraxial techniques should be employed to the extent possible, opioids may be required. The use of fentanyl or ultrashort-acting narcotics is preferable in patients with kidney disease. Fentanyl undergoes hepatic metabolism, while remifentanil degrades rapidly by ester hydrolysis in the blood. Morphine and meperidine undergo metabolic conversion to potentially neurotoxic compounds that rely on renal clearance; for this reason, they are best avoided in patients with chronic kidney disease (CKD). Morphine-6-glucuronide, a morphine metabolite more potent that its parent compound, may also accumulate in patients with CKD and result in profound respiratory depression. Hydromorphone also has an active metabolite, hydromorphone-3-glucuronide, that may accumulate in patients with CKD.

10. D

Dexmedetomidine, a selective alpha 2-adrenergic agonist, has been shown to reduce the incidence of cardiac surgery–associated acute kidney injury. Unfortunately, other agents that have generated excitement for their potential renoprotective properties, such as dopamine, have failed to be proven clinically.

6 Liver Anatomy and Physiology

Niels Chapman

I. Gross Anatomy

The human liver is the largest solid organ, comprising 2% of total body mass and weighing approximately 1500 g. Anatomically, the liver has *four lobes* (*right, left, caudate, and quadrate*) and can be further subdivided into eight segments, according to Couinaud classification. Residing behind the rib cage in the right upper quadrant of the abdomen, the liver is covered in a thin connective tissue layer *(Glisson's capsule)* and is attached to the anterior abdominal wall by the falciform ligament and round ligament of the liver (umbilical cord remnant) and to the diaphragm by the coronary ligament (**Figure 6.1**).

Key related structures of the hepatobiliary system include the *gallbladder* and its *cystic duct* outflow tract, which combines with the common hepatic duct to form the ***common bile duct***. More distally, the common bile duct joins the pancreatic duct to form the *hepatopancreatic ampulla (ampulla of Vater)*, which then drains bile and pancreatic secretions into the second portion of the duodenum through the *sphincter of Oddi* (**Figures 6.1** and **6.2**).

II. Microscopic Anatomy

Hepatocytes are arranged within *hepatic sinusoids* surrounding a central hepatic vein and are bordered by interlobular *portal triads* consisting of a biliary duct, hepatic artery, and portal vein (**Figures 6.3** and **6.4**). This functional anatomy results from a complicated embryologic ballet in which the growing organ forms around portal veins, with bile ducts originating out of precursor ductal plates situated on the portal veins. Hepatic sinuses run from the peripheral portal triads to the centrilobular hepatic veins and are lined with fenestrated endothelial cells, featuring intracytoplasmic pores and loose intercellular junctions. In addition to the endothelial cells, other resident cell populations of the sinusoidal wall include *Kupffer cells* (macrophages), *stellate cells* (responsible for extracellular matrix production and capable of contractile function to regulate sinusoidal blood flow), and *pit cells* (lymphocytes). The space separating the sinusoids from hepatocyte bars is known as the *perisinusoidal*

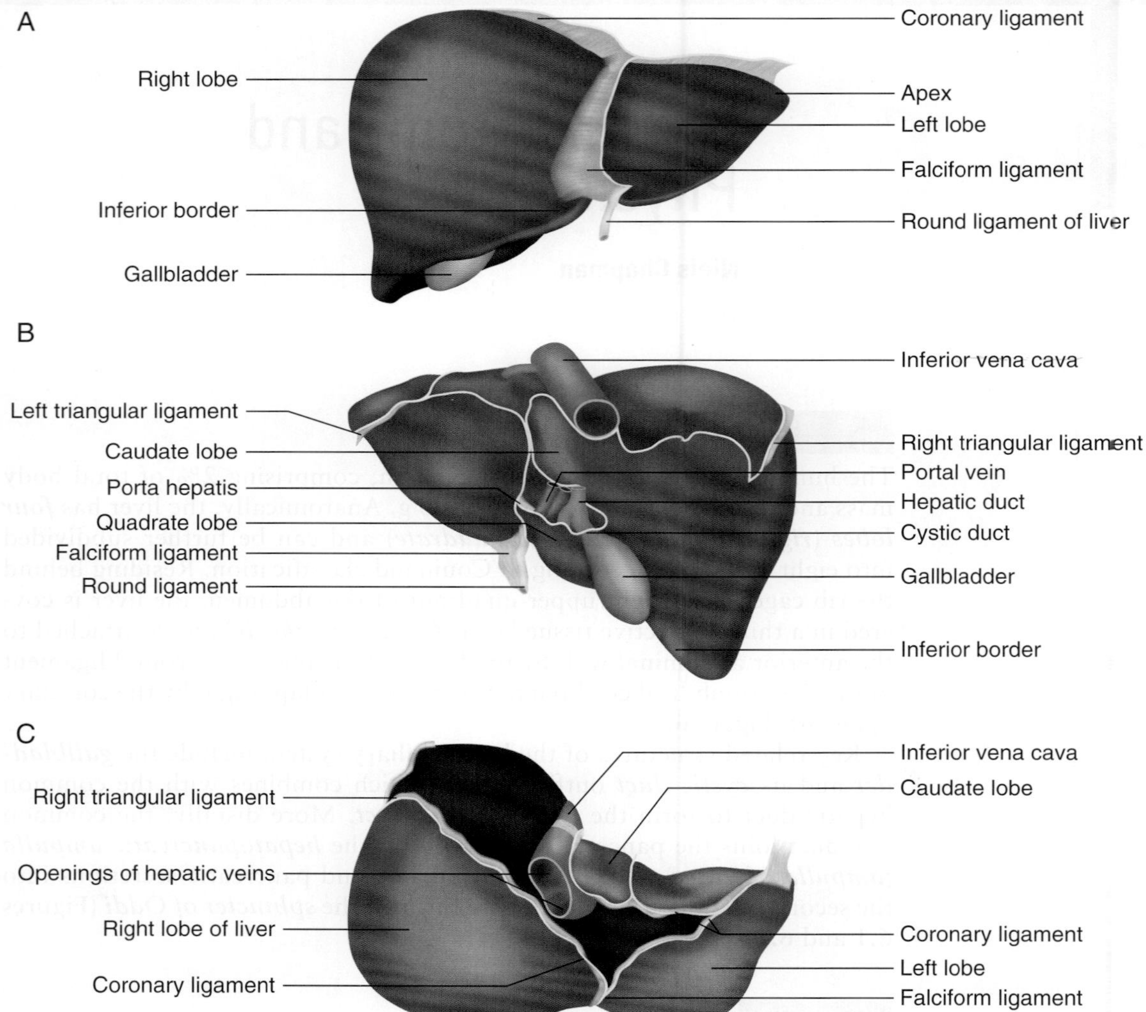

Figure 6.1 **Gross anatomy of the liver. A, Anterior view, diaphragmatic surface. B, Posteroinferior view, visceral surface. C, Superior view.** (Redrawn from Moore KL, Agur AMR, Dalley AF. *Clinically Oriented Anatomy*. 7th ed. Philadelphia: Wolters Kluwer; 2013. Figures 2.65A-C.)

space of Disse, and it contains extracellular matrix generated by stellate cells, Kupffer cells, and dendritic cells. These latter two cell types are involved in microbial and antigen host defense and contribute to the significant immune function of the liver as well as to the fibrosis observed with hepatic cirrhosis. (See **Table 6.1**.)

Bile is produced by hepatocytes and secreted into biliary canaliculi via *canals of Hering*, which are trough-like structures bordered by both hepatocytes and cholangiocytes that then drain into bile ducts.

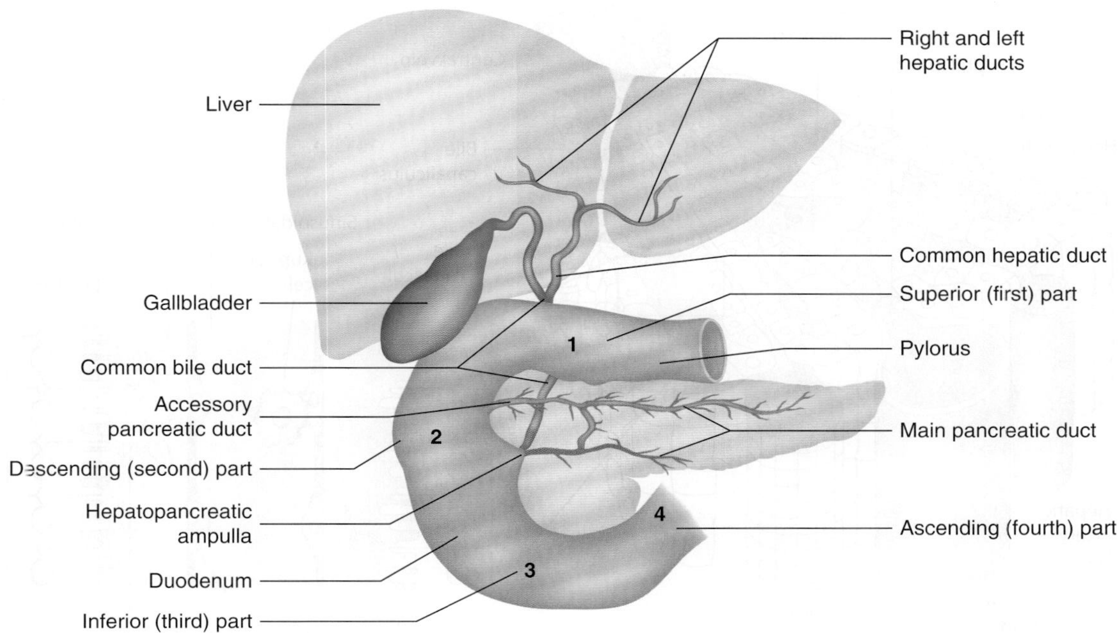

Figure 6.2 **Gallbladder, bile, and pancreatic ducts (anterior view).** (From Practice guidelines for preoperative fasting and the use of pharmacologic agents to reduce the risk of pulmonary aspiration: application to healthy patients undergoing elective procedures: an updated report by the American Society of Anesthesiologists Committee on Standards and Practice Parameters. *Anesthesiology.* 2011;114:495-511, with permission.)

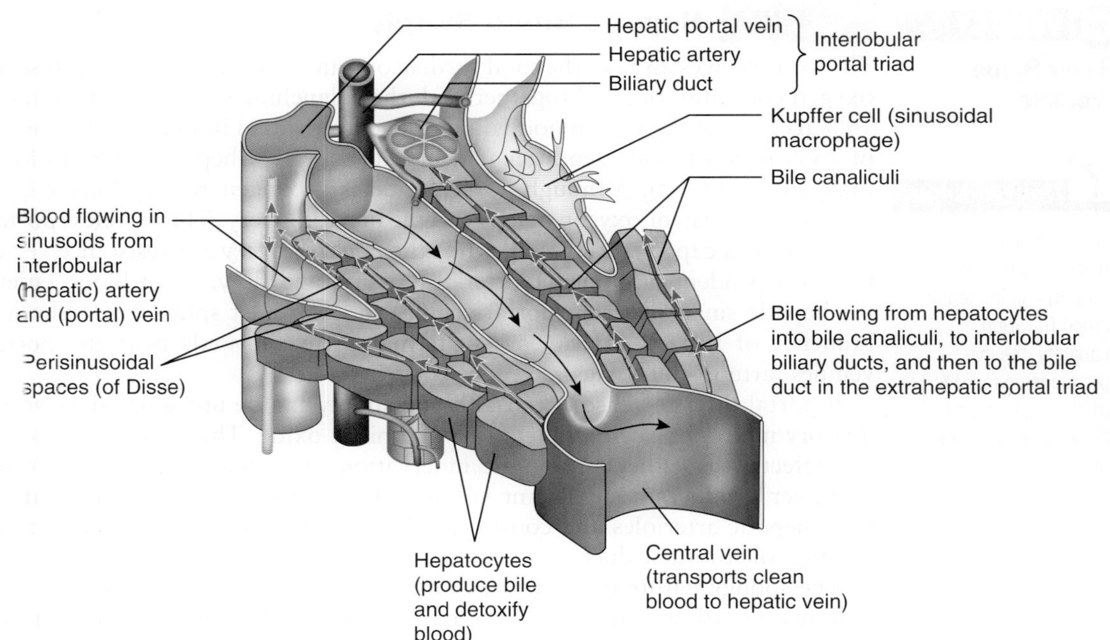

Figure 6.3 **Section of hepatic lobule with functional diagram of bile and blood flow.** (Modified from Starmer AJ, Spector ND, Srivastava R, et al. I-PASS, a mnemonic to standardize verbal handoffs. *Pediatrics.* 2012;129:201-205.)

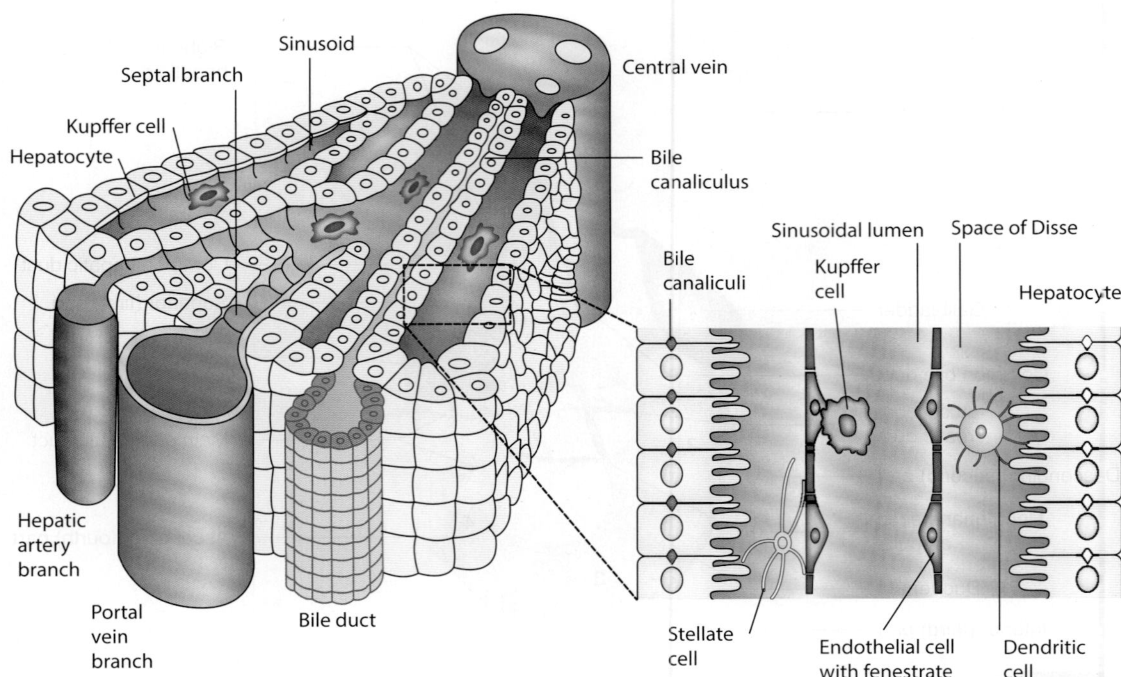

Figure 6.4 **Portion of hepatic lobule: Microanatomy.** (From Adams DH, Eksteen B. Aberrant homing of mucosal T cells and extra-intestinal manifestations of inflammatory bowel disease. *Nature Rev Immunol.* 2006;6:244-251, with permission.)

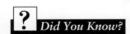

Liver Blood Volume

? *Did You Know?*

Due to its high blood flow (25% of cardiac output) and immense blood filtration capacity, the liver produces up to 50% of all lymph volume flowing in the thoracic duct.

III. Hepatic Blood Supply

The liver receives 25% of the total cardiac output, accounts for 20% of resting oxygen consumption, and together with the splanchnic vascular bed contains 10% to 15% of the total blood volume. The liver's dual blood supply consists of 75% portal blood (deoxygenated blood) and 25% hepatic arterial blood (oxygenated blood). Although portal blood is deoxygenated, its higher flow results in equivalent oxygen delivery to the hepatic artery. The valveless ***portal vein*** acts as a capacitance vessel, while the ***hepatic artery*** is a resistance vessel that is dependent on systemic arterial pressure and flow. Most blood enters the hepatic sinusoids from portal venules through inlet sphincters, although branches of hepatic arterioles also terminate in sinusoids near the portal venules (arteriosinus twigs).

If portal flow decreases, arterial blood supply can be upregulated by vasodilatory molecules such as adenosine and nitric oxide. These mechanisms are not affected by either autonomic innervation or systemic humoral factors. The liver produces a significant volume of lymph through direct exudation from hepatic arterioles and constitutes 25% to 50% of the total lymph flow through the thoracic duct.

The spongy nature of the liver, combined with the contractile potential of stellate cells, allows this organ to function as an autologous reservoir that can augment blood volume in hypovolemic states and can store blood in hypervolemic states. This latter phenomenon can be observed in conditions of right heart failure (congestive hepatopathy), hypervolemia (renal failure), and iatrogenic overresuscitation (**Figures 6.5** and **6.6**).

Table 6.1 Cellular Constituents of Microscopic Anatomy

Cell Type	Anatomic Location	Descriptive Function
Liver Sinusoidal Endothelial Cells	Low-shear, sinusoidal capillary channels	Receive blood from portal vein and hepatic artery. Most powerful scavenger system of the body. Remove and recycle blood-borne proteins, lipids, and xenobiotics. Unique features: No basement membrane, rapidly adaptable fenestrae organized into sieve plates, very "promiscuous" scavenger receptors, highly potent endocytic capacity. Strong similarities to lymphatic endothelial cells. Regulate immune and inflammatory response to antigens taken up from the gastrointestinal (GI) tract.
Liver Macrophages: Kupffer Cells (KCs) Liver Capsular Macrophages Recruited, monocyte-derived macrophages	Kupffer cells: sinusoidal blood Capsular macrophages: Perihepatic capsule Recruited macrophages: Variable, including replacement of KCs	Most liver macrophages are sessile, self-renewing. Collaborate with liver sinusoidal endothelial cells in pathogen uptake and elimination. Former terminology: Reticuloendothelial system. Current term: Mononuclear phagocyte system.
Hepatic Stellate Cells/ Pericytes	Subendothelial in the space of Disse. Long cytoplasmic processes run parallel to endothelium, second-order branches ramify and form meshwork	Store the majority of vitamin A/Retinol in the human body; store other lipids and assume phenotype of Lipocytes; contractile properties mediated through actin permit contraction and sinusoidal blood flow control. Act as progenitor cells in liver regeneration, are chiefly responsible for fibrotic degeneration (cirrhosis) and act as autocrine and paracrine cells.
Hepatocytes	Arranged in single-cell columns in hepatic sinusoids, surrounded by space of Disse and canals of Hering. Apical basal membrane studded with microvilli faces the space of Disse and sinusoids; smooth lateral membrane connects with other hepatocytes via occludins between which bile canaliculi collect and transport bile	Bipolar cells, simultaneously absorbing plasma, prepare heme, cholesterol, and xenobiotics for elimination, synthesize glycogen, fatty acids, albumin, and vitamin K–dependent coagulation factors, metabolize and secrete bile acids, lipids, cholesterol species absorbed via enterohepatic recirculation, and are critically involved in iron metabolism. The cytochrome system facilitates elimination of pharmaceuticals. Bile secretion is accomplished by osmotic effects following energy-dependent bile salt secretion and bile salt–independent flow.

(Continued)

Table 6.1 Cellular Constituents of Microscopic Anatomy (Continued)

Cell Type	Anatomic Location	Descriptive Function
Cholangiocyte	Canals of Hering, bile ducts; small, cuboidal cells centrally, higher cytoplasm to nucleus ratio peripherally	Respond to duodenal secretin and somatostatin signaling. Secretin causes alkalinization of canalicular (original hepatocytic) bile, with somatostatin having an opposing effect. Cholangiocytes absorb water, glucose, glutamate urate. Bile acids can be reabsorbed and reenter the system via cholehepatic shunting.
Lymphatic endothelial cells and lymphatic muscle cells	Periportal structures in the space of Mall	Passive uptake of hepatic sinusoidal transudate into single-layer lymph capillaries, which drain into valved lymphatic vessels. These are surrounded by lymphatic smooth muscle cells, which actively pump this fluid into portal and celiac lymph nodes. This process generates approximately 50% of total body lymph volume. Lymph flow is ipsidirectional with bile flow.
Pit Cells	Hepatic sinusoids	Nonsessile killer cells, acting in conjunction with Kupffer cells. Among other functions, pit cells adhere to and kill cancer cells.

A. Hepatic Autonomic System

While liver transplant recipients live well with a completely denervated donor organ, elevated rates of diabetes, dyslipidemia, hypertension, and obesity may underscore the effects of hepatic innervation. Food intake stimuli are modified through vagal sensing of portal vein glucose and lipid levels; insulin sensitivity and skeletal muscle glucose uptake are influenced by autonomic control of hepatic insulin sensitizing substance; hepatic glycogen storage is equally affected by autonomic control. Serum osmolality sensing in the sinusoidal system triggers a hepatorenal reflex with modulation of Na+ retention. Sinusoidal blood flow is affected by sympathetic effects on the hepatic artery and hepatic nerve efferent control of sinusoidal contraction. The biliary tree is densely innervated by parasympathetic nerve branches, with some nerve endings actually reaching the ductal lumen.

B. Lymphatic System

The liver produces a large volume of lymph amounting to 25% to 50% of volume transported in the thoracic duct. Lymphatic vessels are associated to three categories according to location: portal, sublobular, and capsular. The collected fluid contains approximately 80% of proteins measured in plasma. Bile constituents are found in hepatic lymph during biliary obstruction. Lymph vessels are primarily present along the portal vasculature, the hepatic artery, and the bile ducts. These valved capillaries increase in complexity from single-cell, permeable capillaries without basement membranes to larger collecting vessels with lower permeability. Most hepatic lymph appears to be derived from hepatic sinusoids or hepatic vasculature. The liver capsule has no intrinsic blood supply, but the organ surface is only separated from the parenchyma by

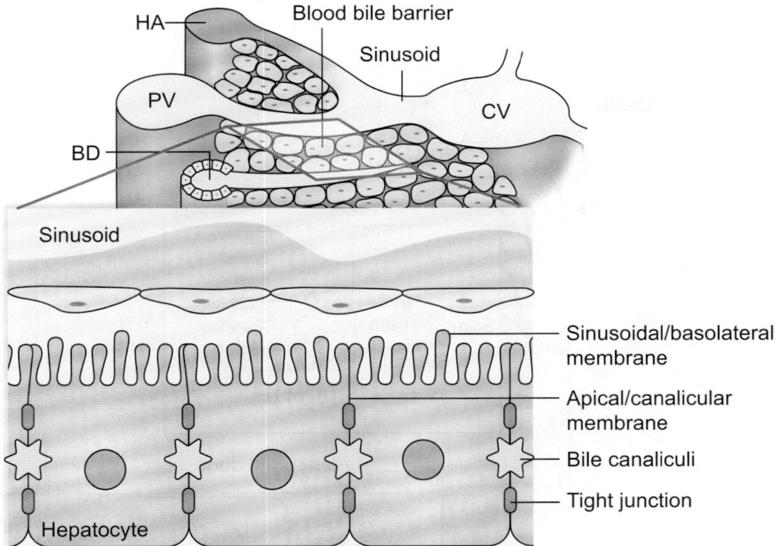

Figure 6.5 Barriers of the liver. Schematic depiction of the blood-bile barrier (BBIB) in the liver. The BBIB is composed of mainly tight junctions present at the apical membrane domain of the hepatocytes, which restricts the mixing of sinusoidal blood and bile. The hepatocytes polarize along the apical and basolateral membrane; the basolateral membrane faces the sinusoids, whereas the apical membrane faces the bile canaliculi. BD, bile duct; CV, central vein; HA, hepatic artery; PV, portal vein. (From Pradhan-Sundd T, Monga SP. Blood-bile barrier: morphology, regulation, and pathophysiology. *Gene Expr.* 2019;19(2):69-87.)

a single-cell layer suggesting a sinusoidal origin of capsular lymph. Lymphatic vessels combine to 12 to 15 vessels running along hepatic arteries and the bile duct and are bundled in multiple, regional lymph nodes (**Figures 6.7** and **6.8**).

IV. Hepatic Metabolic, Synthetic, and Excretory Functions

Bile formation is an essential, hepatic function enabling the elimination of lipids, cholesterol, and metabolic end products of hemoglobin metabolism and the absorption of fat-soluble vitamins and lipids. Bile secretion by hepatocytes into the canaliculi encompasses the energy-dependent transport of bile acids and organic anions as well as glutathione, bilirubin glucuronide, thyroid and steroid hormones, and xenobiotics. This canalicular bile amounts to 75% of the approximately 600 mL secreted per day. Cholangiocytes secreting HCO_3^- and H_2O as well as paracellular water influx constitute the remainder and render bile both isotonic and neutral to slightly alkaline. Bile flow ranges from 1.5 to 15 µL/kg/min and reaches the cystic and bile ducts via the hepatic duct. Passive and active resistance at the sphincter of Oddi facilitate gallbladder filling. Duodenal signaling following meal consumption triggers 80% to 100% emptying of the gallbladder. Primary bile acids (chenodeoxycholic acid and cholic acid) are acted on by resident bacteria to form secondary bile acids (lithocholic acid and deoxycholic acid), with a small fraction of ursodeoxycholic acid also detected.

The liver performs a remarkable spectrum of metabolic and excretory functions, ranging from nutritional substance uptake from the portal and systemic circulations, to synthesis of various proteins and bile components,

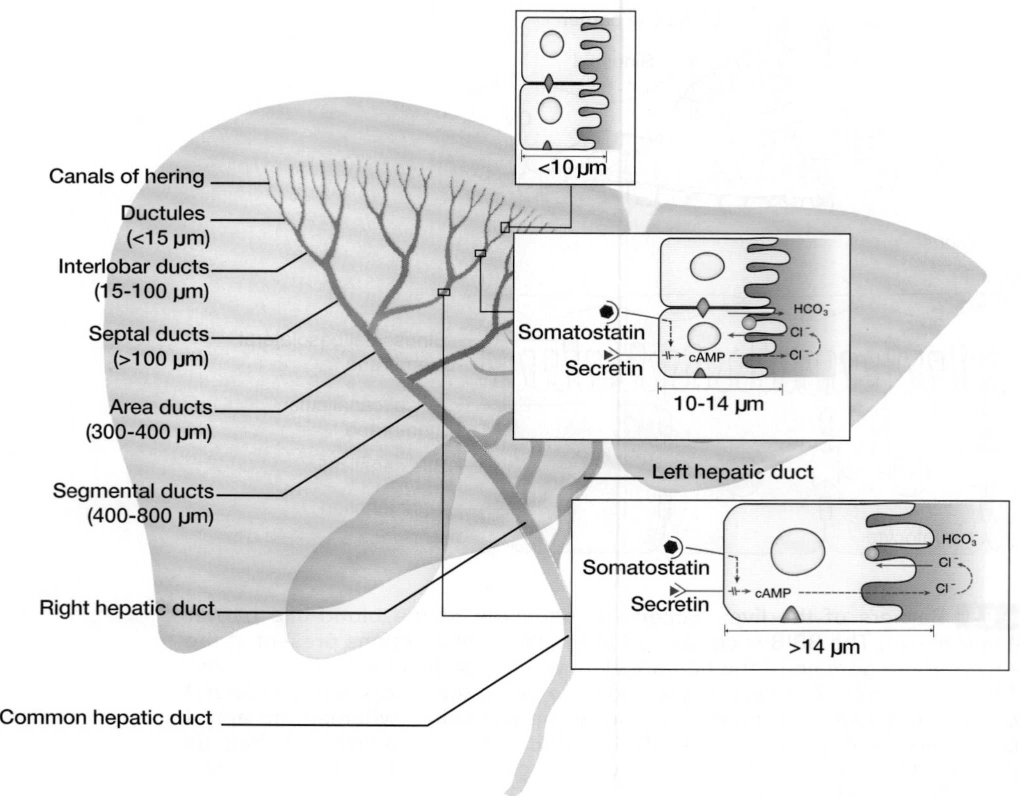

Figure 6.6 The figure illustrates the heterogeneity of the structure and function of the biliary tree and bile duct epithelial cells. Canalicular bile secreted by hepatocytes enters the biliary tree by joining upstream with the canals of Hering. As branches of the biliary tree join, the luminal diameter increases (values in parentheses) and the bile duct epithelial cells become larger. The range of receptors and transporters on medium and large bile duct cells is similar although secretin receptor expression and Cl^-/HCO_3^- exchange activity is greater in the median and large size bile duct cells. (Redrawn from Boyer JL. Bile formation and cholestasis. In: Schiff ER, Sorrell MF, Maddrey WC, eds. *Schiff's Diseases of the Liver.* Lippincott, Williams & Wilkins; 2002:135-165.)

to regulation of circulating nutrients and toxins, to immune host defense.[1] Examples of these functions include the following:

- ***Protein synthesis:*** Most blood proteins (except antibodies) are synthesized in and secreted by the liver, including albumin, the ***vitamin K–dependent coagulation factors (II, VII, IX, and X)***, and the ***vitamin K–independent factors (V, XI, XII, and XIII and fibrinogen)***. These can be assessed clinically as indirect indicators of hepatic synthetic function. Amino acid synthesis and breakdown also occur in the liver, the latter by transamination and oxidative deamination, with formation of keto acids, ammonia, and glutamine. Disruption of these synthetic functions can be observed in extreme starvation or liver failure, leading to hypoproteinemia, ascites formation, and bleeding disorders.
- ***Production of cholesterol and lipoproteins:*** The liver transforms ingested ***cholesterol*** and synthesizes various lipoprotein species that act as blood-borne, transportable, emulsified packages that allow transport of essential cell metabolism elements around the body.

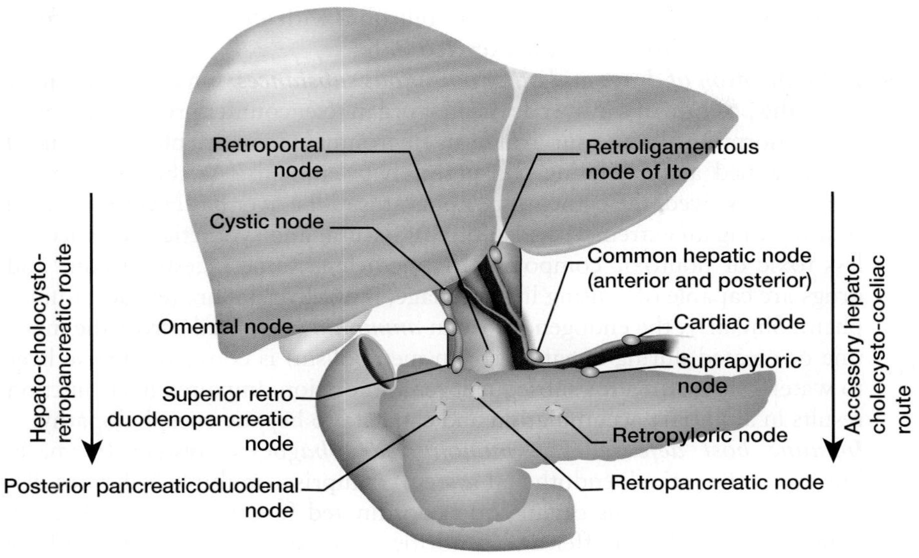

Figure 6.7 Schematic of extrahepatic lymph nodes.

- ***Nutrient storage:*** The liver converts excess glucose into ***glycogen*** for storage and blood glucose regulation and also stores ***fat-soluble vitamins (A, D, E, and K)*** and minerals. As a result, liver failure is often accompanied by profound hypoglycemia.
- ***Hemoglobin metabolism:*** The liver processes iron-containing heme (in the form of unconjugated ***bilirubin*** generated by erythrocyte destruction and hemoglobin release in the spleen) so that its iron content can by recycled

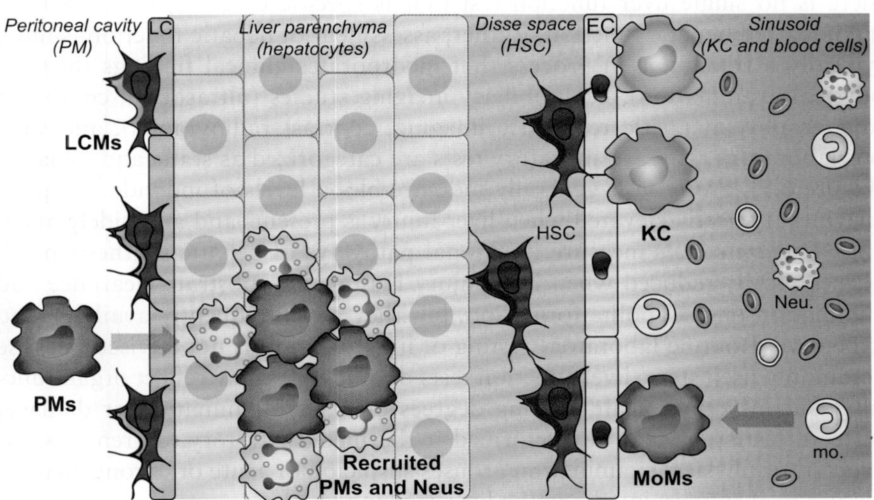

Figure 6.8 Liver macrophage heterogeneity. The liver is populated by different macrophage populations. The most abundant one is composted by embryonically derived Kupffer cells (KCs) which reside in liver sinusoids and interact mainly with HSC and EC. Monocyte-derived macrophages (MoMs) can also acquire a KC-like phenotype after inflammation. Liver capsular macrophages (LCMs) are present at the level of the liver capsule (LC). Finally, mature peritoneal macrophages (PMs) can also be recruited in the liver, notably in case of injuries in the parenchyma. EC, endothelial cell; HSC, hepatic stellate cell; Neu, neutrophils. (From Blériot C, Ginhoux F. Understanding the heterogeneity of resident liver macrophages. *Front Immunol.* 2019;10:2694.)

for various uses. The liver conjugates bilirubin with glucuronic acid to form water-soluble bilirubin that is excreted in bile.

- ***Detoxification of drugs and other poisonous substances:*** On an evolutionary basis, the position of the liver as the first organ to encounter products of intestinal absorption allowed survival in an environment in which plants produced toxins aimed at prohibiting consumption by animals. As the biochemical arms race evolved, the cytochrome apparatus in the liver has become capable of processing an extremely wide array of natural and synthetic substances to less toxic or nontoxic compounds. Nonetheless, some ingested toxins and drugs are capable of causing liver damage, if not liver failure (eg, acetaminophen). Similarly, the endogenous toxin ***ammonia*** (absorbed across the intestine or created during hepatic protein metabolism) is converted in the liver to water-soluble urea for subsequent renal excretion. Impaired liver function results in ammonia accumulation and can lead to hepatic encephalopathy.
- ***Immune host defense:*** The ***mononuclear phagocyte system*** (formerly known as the reticuloendothelial system) comprises multiple cell types distributed across various organs in a coordinated function of host defense, which includes the Kupffer and dendritic cells noted above. Impaired liver function can result in more frequent or severe systemic infections (eg, spontaneous bacterial peritonitis). Kupffer cells also lyse erythrocytes into heme and globin components, thereby augmenting splenic release of unconjugated bilirubin into the circulation, where it combines with circulating albumin, eventually returning to the liver for hemoglobin metabolism, as described in the previous section.

V. Assessment of Hepatic Function

Due to the multiple "functions" of the liver and its sizable metabolic capacity, there is no single liver function test that is specific or accurate in identifying impaired hepatic function. Rather, assessment of hepatic function is more typically a triangulation process that incorporates clinical findings (history, physical examination), hepatobiliary imaging studies (ultrasound, computed tomography, magnetic resonance imaging, contrast radiography), and various laboratory tests.[2,3] Laboratory tests are categorized as static and dynamic (**Figure 6.9**). ***Static tests*** generally measure blood levels of individual hepatic enzymes (typically elevated when liver injury is present) and are widely available. ***Dynamic tests*** measure functional pathways of hepatic synthesis products (typically reduced when liver injury is present), substrate clearance and elimination or metabolite formation, but they are infrequently available and expensive. Routine laboratory testing of liver function is not advised because commonly used static liver function tests do not accurately reflect organ function, but instead indicate varying degrees of liver inflammation or damage. Instead, testing should be performed if the medical history, current disease process, or physical examination arouses suspicion of acute or chronic hepatic disease or if surgery involving the liver is planned.

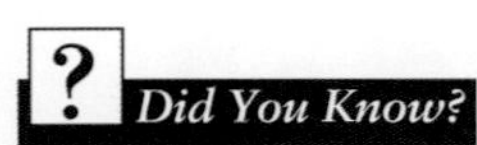

Much like the combination of cardiac imaging and cardiac enzyme measurements used to assess heart function and cardiac injury, the combination of hepatic imaging (computed tomography, ultrasound) and hepatic enzyme measurements (transaminases) is used to assess liver function and hepatic injury.

Standard laboratory assays can potentially indicate organ injury (transaminases, bilirubin), impaired synthetic function (serum albumin, prothrombin time, fibrinogen), or systemic effects of advanced organ dysfunction (platelet count). Specific static laboratory tests include the hepatic transaminases aspartate aminotransferase (AST), alanine aminotransferase (ALT), alkaline phosphatase (AP), and γ-glutamyl transpeptidase (GGT). The AST enzyme is also found in muscle and other nonhepatic tissues, and AP is also found in

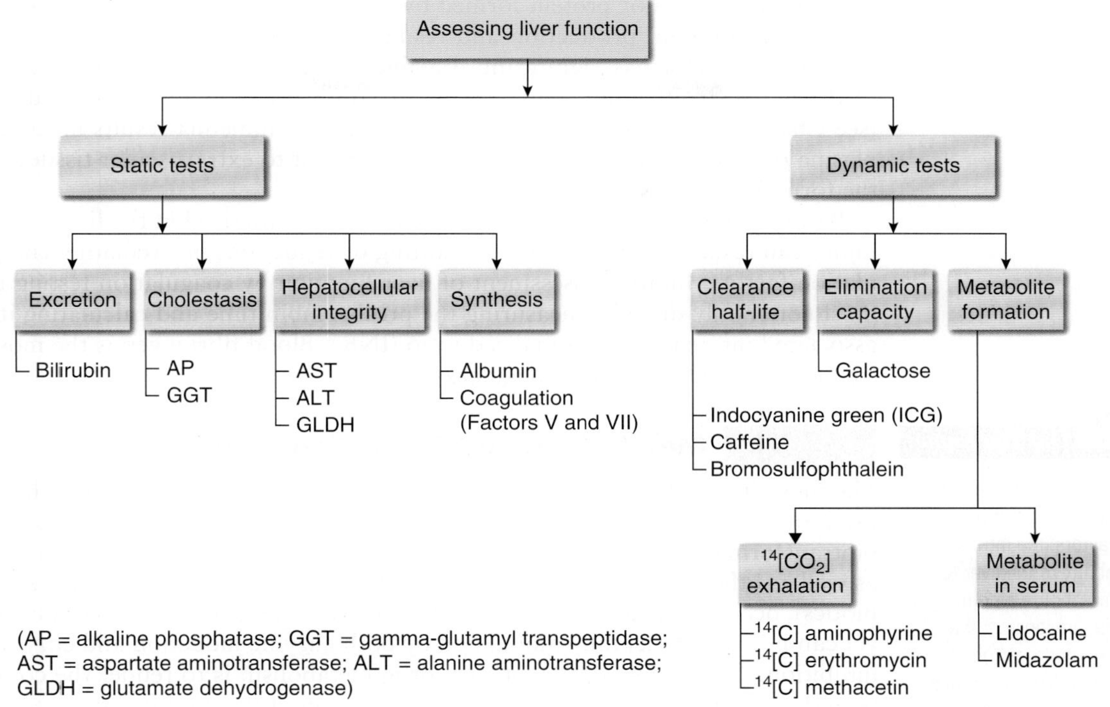

Figure 6.9 Laboratory tests of hepatic function. Laboratory tests of hepatic function generally fall into two categories: the commonly used static tests of circulating blood compounds, proteins, and coagulation factors, and the infrequently used dynamic tests of liver metabolism, elimination, and clearance functions. (From Beck C, Schawrtges I, Picker O. Perioperative liver protection. *Curr Opin Crit Care.* 2010;16:142-147, with permission.)

bone, placenta, and intestine. In contrast, ALT and GGT are almost exclusively found in the liver; therefore, ALT and GGT are felt to be more specific indicators of liver pathology. Both AST and ALT can be elevated in settings of acute liver damage when the enzymes leak out of injured hepatocytes into the blood. In chronic liver disease, elevations in AST and ALT may not be present; however, the AST/ALT ratio is typically elevated in patients with alcoholic hepatitis or cirrhosis. An AST/ALT ratio >2 is present in ~70% of these patients compared with 26% of patients with postnecrotic cirrhosis, 8% with chronic hepatitis, 4% with viral hepatitis, and none with obstructive jaundice. If AP or GGT levels are elevated, a problem with bile flow is most likely present. Bile flow problems can be due to a bile duct pathology within the liver, the gallbladder, or the extrahepatic ducts.

As noted previously, unconjugated bilirubin is a breakdown product of heme from erythrocytes and is then conjugated with glucuronic acid in the liver for excretion in the bile. Elevated blood levels of "indirect bilirubin" (unconjugated bilirubin) indicate excessive hemoglobin breakdown (eg, hemolysis) or impaired hepatic conjugation function. Elevated blood levels of "direct bilirubin" (conjugated bilirubin) occur when hepatic function is normal but bilirubin excretion is impaired (eg, common bile duct obstruction). Bilirubin elevation is associated with abnormal physical examination findings of scleral icterus and cutaneous jaundice.

Albumin is a major protein formed by the liver; thus, chronic liver disease can impair albumin production and result in reduced blood albumin levels. Hypoalbuminemia has significant systemic effects on both protein binding of drugs (eg, hypoalbuminemia results in larger fractions of unbound drug [see Chapter 7]) and oncotic pressure (eg, hypoalbuminemia results in lower plasma oncotic pressure, favoring water movement to extravascular tissues in the form of edema and ascites [see Chapter 3]).

Because many protein coagulation factors are synthesized in the liver, liver injury can result in abnormal blood clotting or reductions in circulating coagulation factors. Indirect assessment of liver function by coagulation testing is most commonly done by measuring the prothrombin time and calculating its associated international normalized ratio (INR). Blood fibrinogen is the most frequently tested individual coagulation factor.

? Did You Know?

Hepatic drug clearance depends on three factors: the intrinsic ability of the liver to metabolize a drug (ie, presence of the appropriate drug metabolizing enzyme), hepatic blood flow, and the extent of binding of the drug to blood components (eg, albumin).

VI. Metabolism and Drug Disposition

The majority of all pharmaceuticals used in medical practice, including those used routinely in the perioperative period and the critical care setting, undergo biotransformation or elimination in the liver. Liver metabolism of such drugs, as well as other natural and synthetic substances (collectively known as xenobiotics), occurs by drug metabolizing enzymes that are genetically determined, yet can be environmentally modulated by both enzyme induction and enzyme inhibition.[4,5] The general goal of such drug metabolism is to render the compounds more hydrophilic so that renal elimination of the modified drug or its metabolites can occur.

Hepatic drug metabolism occurs through two enzyme systems, either alone or in combination. ***Phase 1 enzymes*** generally alter existing functional groups to make the molecule more polar, thereby increasing its water solubility. Phase 1 enzymes consist of the ***cytochrome P450*** (CYP superfamily) class of enzymes that hydrolyze, oxidize, or reduce the parent compound (see Chapter 7). ***Phase 2 enzymes*** act primarily to conjugate polar compounds, thereby further increasing their hydrophilicity. Both phase 1 and phase 2 enzymes are inducible but can also be inhibited (usually by other drugs).

A more functional description of hepatic drug disposition of pharmaceuticals draws a distinction between substances cleared rapidly (essentially on the first pass through the liver from the portal or systemic venous circulations) and those that require considerable time for metabolism. Substances that undergo significant ***first-pass elimination*** are said to have a ***high extraction ratio***. Elimination of these drugs is largely determined by hepatic blood flow. Drugs that require a prolonged time for biotransformation are said to have a ***low extraction ratio***. Such drugs are often protein bound in the circulation and therefore are not readily available to drug metabolizing enzymes in the liver. Intermediate between these two extremes are substances that do not clearly fall into either category are said to have an intermediate extraction ratio. Elimination of these drugs is equally dependent on blood flow and metabolic activity. Examples of drugs commonly used in the practice of anesthesiology and pain medicine are listed for each of these three categories in **Table 6.2**.

Table 6.2 Examples of Hepatic Clearance Patterns of Common Pharmaceuticals

High Clearance (High Extraction Ratio, ie, Blood Flow Dependent)	Intermediate Clearance	Low Clearance (Low Extraction Ratio, ie, Blood Flow Independent)
Morphine	Aspirin	Warfarin
Lidocaine	Quinine	Phenytoin
Propofol	Codeine	Rocuronium
Propranolol	Nortriptyline	Methadone
Fentanyl	Vecuronium	Diazepam
Sufentanil	Alfentanil	Lorazepam

For further review and interactivities, please see the associated Interactive Video Lectures and "A Closer Look" infographic accessible in the complimentary eBook bundled with this text. Access instructions are located in the inside front cover.

References

1. Steadman RH, Braunfeld MY. The liver: surgery and anesthesia. In: Barash PG, Cullen BF, Stoelting RK, et al, eds *Clinical Anesthesia*. 8th ed. Wolters Kluwer; 2017:1298-1326.
2. Beck C, Schawrtges I, Picker O. Perioperative liver protection. *Curr Opin Crit Care*. 2010;16:142-147. PMID: 22534730.
3. Hoetzel A, Ryan H, Schmidt R. Anesthetic considerations for the patient with liver disease. *Curr Opin Anesthesiol*. 2012;25:340-347. PMID: 22450699.
4. Sweeney BP, Bromilow J. Liver enzyme induction and inhibition: implications for anaesthesia. *Anaesthesia*. 2006;61:159-177. PMID: 16430569.
5. Gupta DK, Henthorn TK. Basic principles of clinical pharmacology. In: Barash PG, Cullen BF, Stoelting RK, et al, eds. *Clinical Anesthesia*. 8th ed. Wolters Kluwer; 2017:156-188.

HEPATIC BLOOD FLOW AND DRUG CLEARANCE

A CLOSER LOOK

Both blood flow and metabolic function play important roles in the hepatic clearance of drugs as shown below.

At rest, the liver receives 25% of cardiac output and contains 10% of circulating blood volume

The **HEPATIC VEIN** drains blood into the IVC

Since portal venous blood is poorly oxygenated, it only meets **50%** of the liver's O_2 demand.

75% of incoming blood flow is derived from the **PORTAL VEIN**

The remaining 25% is from the **HEPATIC ARTERY**

***Clearance* is the volume of blood completely cleared of drug per unit time. For the liver, it is calculated as follows...**

HEPATIC DRUG **CLEARANCE** = HEPATIC **BLOOD FLOW** X HEPATIC **EXTRACTION RATIO**

$$\text{EXTRACTION RATIO} = \frac{C_i - C_o}{C_o}$$

C_i = concentration of drug coming into the liver
C_o = concentration of drug coming out of the liver

HIGH extraction ratio drugs

The majority of drugs used in anesthetic practice fall into this category. The liver enzymes that process these drugs are extremely efficient, thus there is very little drug left in the hepatic venous effluent. Changes in **hepatic blood flow will affect the clearance** of these drugs. However, changes in *hepatic metabolic function have little to no effect.*

LOW extraction ratio drugs

Drugs such as benzodiazepines, barbiturates and alfentanil have low extraction ratio. The liver enzymes that process these drugs are less efficient. Changes in **hepatic metabolic function will affect the clearance** of these drugs. However, changes in *hepatic blood flow have little to no effect.*

Infographic by: Naveen Nathan MD

Questions

1. **The dual blood supply to the liver can best be described by which of the following statements?**

   A. Liver blood supply is 75% from the hepatic artery and 25% from the portal vein.
   B. Liver blood supply is 50% from the hepatic artery and 50% from the portal vein.
   C. Liver blood supply is 25% from the hepatic artery and 75% from the portal vein.
   D. Liver blood supply is 10% from the hepatic artery and 90% from the portal vein.

2. **A 55-year-old man with end-stage liver disease from alcoholic cirrhosis would be expected to demonstrate all of the following abnormalities EXCEPT:**

   A. Increased susceptibility to bacterial infection
   B. Ascites
   C. Hyperglycemia
   D. Increased susceptibility to bruising

3. **Dynamic laboratory tests are more accurate measures of liver function than static laboratory tests, and both are easily obtained in most medical settings. TRUE or FALSE?**

   A. True
   B. False

4. **A 47-year-old woman with acute right upper quadrant pain and scleral icterus undergoes a series of static laboratory blood tests, demonstrating elevated levels of AST and ALT, with an AST/ALT ratio of 2.9. Which of the following clinical or diagnostic findings is also likely to be present?**

   A. Ultrasound examination showing a 7-mm common bile duct stone with proximal bile duct dilation
   B. Elevated blood alcohol content
   C. Computed tomography scan showing a 7-cm mass in the head of the pancreas
   D. Serology indicating acute hepatitis A

5. **Drug X has a high extraction ratio and is given by mouth to two different, yet otherwise healthy, adult patients: one with a normal cardiac output (Patient NL) and one in hypovolemic shock (Patient HS). Which of the following statements is most likely to be TRUE?**

   A. Drug X will be rapidly cleared by both patients.
   B. Drug X will be slowly cleared by both patients.
   C. Drug X will be cleared more rapidly by Patient NL.
   D. Drug X will be cleared more rapidly by Patient HS.

Answers

1. C

The liver receives 25% of total cardiac output, with 25% of the blood supply coming from the hepatic artery (oxygenated blood) and 75% from the portal vein (deoxygenated blood). Because of the differences in blood flow and oxygenation, each blood supply delivers a similar amount of oxygen content to the liver.

2. C

Because hepatic Kupffer cells and dendritic cells comprise part of the mononuclear phagocyte system, liver failure increases the frequency and severity of systemic infections. Because impaired hepatic protein synthesis reduces both plasma oncotic pressure and the production of various coagulation factors, liver failure results in increased extravascular fluid accumulation (edema, ascites) and impaired coagulation, respectively. However, impaired glycogen storage in patients with liver failure is more likely to result in hypoglycemia, rather than hyperglycemia.

3. B

Dynamic laboratory tests of liver function include measure of substrate half-life, elimination capacity, and metabolite formation (**Figure 6.9**); thus, they are likely more indicative of liver function than static tests (eg, blood AST, ALT). However, dynamic tests require specialized facilities and procedures and are not widely available.

4. B

An elevated AST/ALT ratio (>2) is most likely associated with alcoholic hepatitis or cirrhosis. Biliary obstruction due to gallstones or pancreatic masses is unlikely to result in an elevated AST/ALT ratio, although the AP and GGT would likely be elevated. Acute viral hepatitis may result in elevated AST and ALT, but the AST/ALT ratio is unlikely to be elevated.

5. C

Drugs with a high extraction ratio are cleared quickly, with significant first-pass liver metabolism. However, elimination of such drugs is highly dependent on hepatic blood flow. Therefore, in the case of hypovolemic shock, drug X will be cleared rapidly by Patient NL, but more slowly by Patient HS.

PART

B Pharmacology

7 Principles of Pharmacokinetics and Pharmacodynamics

Sujatha Pentakota

Pharmacokinetics and pharmacodynamics define the basic tenets of pharmacology. Pharmacokinetics (PK) describes what the body does to the drug, that is absorption, distribution, metabolism, and elimination. Pharmacodynamics (PD) deals with what the drug does to the body, that is the effects and side effects of drugs. PK relates the dose to concentration, and PD relates concentration to effect.

I. Principles of Pharmacokinetics

A. Drug Absorption and Routes of Drug Administration

Irrespective of the route of administration, all drugs must cross one or more cell membranes to exert their action. There are three kinds of transport processes by which drugs enter a cell:

- *Passive diffusion*: Drugs move across the cell membrane along a concentration gradient, and hence, the process does not consume energy.
- *Active transport*: Drugs are moved against a concentration gradient from a region of lower concentration to a region of higher concentration. This requires cellular energy, and the process is specific and saturable. It is not a common mode of transport for drug molecules, but examples include levodopa and propylthiouracil.
- *Facilitated diffusion*: This is passive diffusion across cell membrane involving a membrane protein. As drug molecules are moving along a concentration gradient, energy is not consumed. However, the process is carrier-mediated, specific, and saturable like active transport.

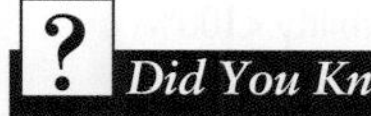

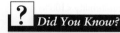

Fentanyl can be administered via intravenous, intrathecal, epidural, intranasal, per rectal, subcutaneous, and transdermal routes.

See **Table 7.1**, routes of drug administration using opioids as prototypes for additional details.

B. Drug Distribution, Elimination, and Biotransformation

1. Drug Distribution

Drug distribution is determined by cardiac output and the blood flow to individual organs. The vessel-rich organs, which receive most of the cardiac output (brain, lungs, heart, liver, and kidneys), quickly equilibrate with the drug concentration in plasma in a matter of minutes. Organs with lower perfusion, such as muscles, are the next group to equilibrate. The last organs to reach equilibrium are those with very poor perfusion, such as adipose tissue and vessel-poor organs such as bone. In all organs, the uptake of the drug is primarily limited by perfusion flow rather than local transport.[1]

Table 7.1 Routes of Drug Administration Using Opioids as a Prototype

Formulation	Bioavailability	Time to Maximum Plasma Concentration	Comments
Intravenous	100%	<1 min	• Gold standard
Oral (gastrointestinal)	0%-50%	1-3 h	• Hepatic first-pass metabolism reduces bioavailability in high hepatic extraction ratio drugs • Intestinal metabolism contributes to decreased bioavailability
Oral (transmucosal)	65%-75%	15-30 min	• Bypasses hepatic first-pass metabolism • Requires high lipophilicity, otherwise passes to gastrointestinal tract
Sublingual	75%	30-45 min	• Bypasses hepatic first-pass metabolism • Requires high lipophilicity, otherwise passes to gastrointestinal tract
Intranasal	90%	10-20 min	• Bypasses hepatic first-pass metabolism • Limited for low lipophilicity
Rectal (transmucosal)	20%-70%	0.75-2 h	• Partially bypasses hepatic first-pass metabolism
Subcutaneous	>75%	15-30 min	• Not limited by lipophilicity compared to transmucosal, transdermal, or intranasal routes
Transdermal	>90%	10-20 h	• Limited by permeability through skin • Constant concentration from 10 to 48 h
Intramuscular	100%	5-30 min	• Not limited by lipophilicity compared to transmucosal, transdermal, or intranasal routes
Inhalational	>90%	5-30 min	• Ventilation-perfusion mismatch results in some delayed uptake and bioavailability <100%
Intrathecal	Not reported	0.5-4 h	• Spinal and supraspinal sites of action
Epidural	100%	15-45 min	• Bolus opioids act at spinal sites, despite plasma absorption

After intravenous injection, most lipophilic drugs undergo redistribution to vessel-rich organs, such as the brain, and equilibrate with the brain in a few minutes. Further drug uptake organs like muscle then lowers the plasma drug concentration. This causes a reverse gradient relative to the drug concentration in the brain, and some drug diffuses back out of the brain into plasma. The plasma concentration continues to fall as the vessel-poor organs continue to take up the drug. For most anesthesia induction agents, the action of the drug is primarily terminated by this process of redistribution of the drug from the brain, rather than by elimination of the drug from the body.

Drug absorption plays a vital role in determining plasma drug concentrations for all routes of drug administration other than intravenous injection. Rapid absorption of a drug results in rapid onset of action and slow absorption allows a long duration of action. The rate of absorption depends on solubility and concentration of the drug. Incomplete absorption limits the amount of the drug that can become present at the drug's effect site.

2. Drug Elimination

The process of elimination entails either primary renal elimination or biotransformative reactions in the liver followed by renal excretion. Elimination or clearance describes the rate at which a drug is eliminated from the body, expressed as being equivalent to the volume of blood from which the drug is completely and irreversibly removed within a unit period of time. Elimination Clearance therefore has dimensions of volume/time.

Hepatic drug clearance is the volume of the blood flowing through the liver that is cleared of the drug in unit time. It is determined by the amount of drug delivered to the liver, which in turn is determined by hepatic blood flow and the intrinsic ability of the liver to metabolize the drug. The factors affecting hepatic clearance are hepatic artery blood flow, portal vein blood flow, intrinsic ability to metabolize the drug, and protein binding of the drug. Hepatic extraction ratio (HER) is the volume of blood from which the drug is irreversibly removed during one pass of blood through the liver. It is the ratio of hepatic clearance to hepatic blood flow. For drugs with low intrinsic clearance, HER is determined by hepatic blood flow.

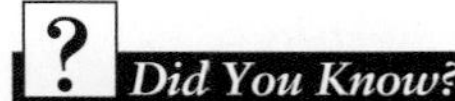

The decrease in plasma concentration and the termination of effect of intravenous anesthetic induction agents is primarily caused by redistribution.

HER >0.7 is considered high; 0.3 to 0.7 is intermediate; and <0.3 is low. Rowland equation[2] defines the hepatic clearance CL_H as follows:

$$CL_H = Q_H \cdot \frac{f_u CL_i}{Q_H + f_u CL_i}$$

where:

Q_H—hepatic blood flow
f_u—fraction of free drug
CL_i—intrinsic capacity of hepatocytes to metabolize the drug

These relationships are depicted in **Figure 7.1**. The relative HERs of some commonly used drugs in the perioperative period are as follows:

- ***Drugs with low HER***: Diazepam, lorazepam, methadone, rocuronium, phenytoin.
- ***Drugs with intermediate HER***: Midazolam, alfentanil, vecuronium.
- ***Drugs with high HER***: fentanyl, ketamine, propofol, morphine, naloxone, lidocaine, bupivacaine.

It follows that when changes in the cardiac output result in changes in hepatic and renal blood flow, the metabolism of drugs with high hepatic extraction ratio and subsequent renal clearance are adversely affected. In states of decreased cardiac output (eg, heart failure), the hepatic clearance of drugs with high HER is decreased.[3,4] In contrast, renal autoregulation tends to maintain renal perfusion pressure and so a relatively constant renal elimination clearance is seen until the capacity for autoregulation is exceeded.

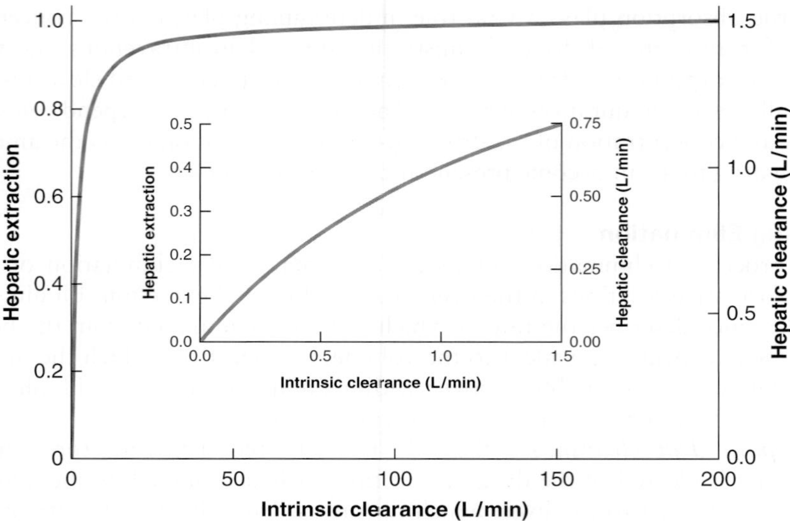

Figure 7.1 The relationship between hepatic extraction ratio (E, right y-axis), intrinsic clearance (CL_i, x-axis), and hepatic clearance (CL_H, left y-axis) at the normal hepatic blood flow (Q) of 1.5 L/min. For drugs with a high intrinsic clearance ($CL_i > Q$), increasing intrinsic, clearance has little effect on hepatic extraction, and total hepatic clearance approaches hepatic blood flow. In contrast, if the intrinsic clearance is small ($CL_i \leq Q$), the extraction ratio is similar to the intrinsic clearance (inset). (Adapted from Wilkinson GR, Shand DG. A physiologic approach to hepatic drug clearance. *Clin Pharmacol Ther.* 1975;18:377.)

3. Biotransformation

Drug molecules may undergo biotransformation by enzymatic reactions in the body. Most of these reactions occur in the liver and can result in any of the following outcomes:

- Inactive compounds for elimination
- A less active compound
- Transformation of a prodrug to an active drug molecule
- Formation of toxic metabolites

Hydrophilic compounds are excreted unchanged into urine and stool. Less hydrophilic compounds need to be metabolized into more hydrophilic compounds to enable their excretion in urine. This metabolism occurs via phase I and phase II reactions.

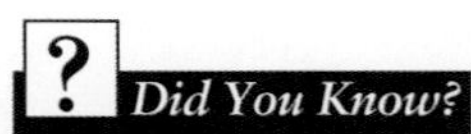

CYP3A accounts for 40% to 45% of all CYP-mediated drug metabolism. Phenytoin shortens the action of nondepolarizing muscle relaxants by inducing CYP3A and hence increasing the elimination clearance of the muscle relaxants.

Phase I reactions include hydrolysis, oxidation, and reduction, which make the drug molecules more susceptible to phase II reactions. Hydrolysis is the process of insertion of a water molecule into the drug, enabling the cleavage of the drug into two molecules. Amide local anesthetics and esters undergo metabolism by hydrolysis. Oxidation involves reactions where electrons are removed from a compound. This is an enzymatically mediated reaction where a hydroxyl group (−OH) is inserted into the drug molecule. The hydroxylated compound is usually unstable and splits into separate molecules. Reductions are reactions wherein electrons are added to a compound. The cytochrome P450 family of enzymes in the liver are predominantly involved in biotransformation reactions and catalyze most Phase I reactions. CYP3A4 is the most important of these, accounting for 40% to 45% of all CYP-mediated drug metabolism. High concentrations of these enzymes are found in the smooth endoplasmic reticulum of hepatocytes and on the membranes of upper intestinal enterocytes. These enzymes can in turn be induced or inhibited by other drugs. The phase II reactions produce conjugates that are polar, water-soluble compounds which can be easily excreted via kidneys or hepatobiliary secretion.

Enzymes involved in phase I and phase II reactions have several isoforms. Genetic variability affects the expression of these isoforms, affecting the rate of these biotransformation reactions. For example, different genotypes result in either normal, low, or absent plasma cholinesterase activity, accounting for the differences in response to succinylcholine (metabolized by plasma cholinesterase) among individuals. Genetic polymorphism is exhibited by the CYP-P450 enzyme system and various transferases involved in phase II reactions.[5]

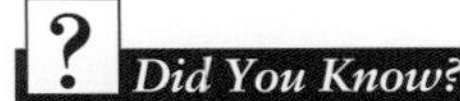

Genetic mutations on the chromosome coding for pseudocholinesterase may prolong the effect of succinylcholine from 2 to 4 minutes, up to 4 to 6 hours.

4. Renal Elimination

The kidneys excrete hydrophilic compounds and the hydrophilic metabolites of lipophilic compounds into urine. This occurs by passive glomerular filtration or by active secretion into the renal tubules. The effective renal clearance of the drug is the sum of the drug filtered by the glomeruli and actively excreted into renal tubules, minus the amount of drug that gets resorbed from the renal tubules. Drugs with significant renal excretion in perioperative practice are penicillin, cephalosporins, pancuronium, rocuronium, aminoglycosides, and neostigmine.

C. Pharmacokinetic Concepts

1. First Order, Zero Order, and Nonlinear Processes

A pharmacokinetic process whose rate is directly proportional to the concentration of the drug present is said to have ***first-order kinetics***. As the concentration of the drug increases, the rate of the process increases. The usual terminology used to define the rapidity of pharmacokinetics is "half-lives" ($t_{1/2}$)

$$t_{1/2} = 0.693\frac{V_d}{CL}$$

where V_d is the volume of distribution and CL is the clearance. As the rate of elimination increases, $t_{1/2}$ decreases. Half-life is the time required for the plasma concentration of a drug to decrease by 50%. For the process of elimination, most of drug is therefore removed from the plasma in 4 to 5 half-lives. The half-life of a first order kinetic process is constant and does not depend on the plasma concentration of the drug itself. The disposition of most drugs follows first order kinetics (**Figure 7.2**).

In contrast, a process with ***zero-order kinetics*** is a reaction whose rate is independent of the concentration of the drug undergoing the reaction. A constant amount of the drug is removed in a unit time.

Nonlinear kinetics describes a drug clearance process in which at low concentrations a drug is cleared by first order kinetics, but at high concentrations by zero order kinetics (eg, phenytoin or ethanol). This happens when the enzyme system involved becomes saturated[6] by the amount of drug present. These processes are also known as Michaelis-Menten processes.

Consequently, there are three factors that at any given time control the current plasma concentration of the drug: the dose of the drug administered intravenously, the distribution in and out of body tissues (diffusion), and the elimination of effective drug (clearance).

? *Did You Know?*

For a first-order reaction, the concentration of the drug decreases by a constant with each half-life and is independent of its concentration in plasma.

? *Did You Know?*

For a zero-order reaction, a plot of the concentration of any reactant versus time is a straight line with a slope of −k. For a first-order reaction, a plot of the natural logarithm of the concentration of a reactant versus time is a straight line with a slope of −k. For a second-order reaction, a plot of the inverse of the concentration of a reactant versus time is a straight line with a slope of k.

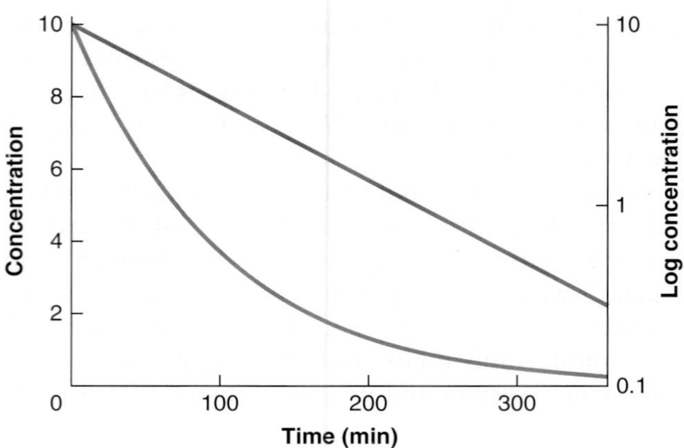

Figure 7.2 The plasma concentration versus time profile plotted on both linear (blue line, left y-axis) and logarithmic (red line, right y-axis) scales for a hypothetical drug exhibiting one-compartment, first-order pharmacokinetics. Note that the slope of the logarithmic concentration profile is equal to the elimination rate constant (k_e) and related to the elimination half-life ($t_{1/2,\beta}$). (From Gupta DK, Henthorn TK. Basic principles of clinical pharmacology. In: Barash PG, Cahalan MK, Cullen BF, et al, eds. *Clinical Anesthesia*. 8th ed. Wolters Kluwer; 2018:241-275, Figure 11.5.)

D. Mathematical Concepts in Pharmacokinetics

1. Volume of Distribution

In compartmental pharmacokinetic models, drugs are imagined to be distributed into one or more "boxes," or compartments. These compartments cannot be equated directly with specific tissues, but instead represent the collective activity of organs with similar rates of equilibration.

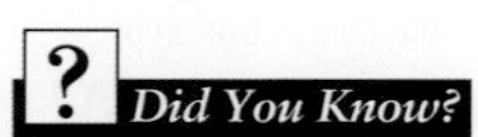

The volume of distribution is the ratio of the total amount of drug present in the body to plasma concentration.

The volume of distribution, V_d, relates the total amount of drug present to the concentration observed in the central compartment, such that V_d equals the amount of drug administered divided by the initial drug concentration in plasma. This is an ***apparent*** volume of distribution and has no relationship with the actual volume of any tissue. Indeed, the mathematical value of V_d can be larger than the actual physical volume of the patient. V_d is large for lipophilic drugs because of their extensive tissue uptake, and low and closer to plasma volume for hydrophilic drugs.

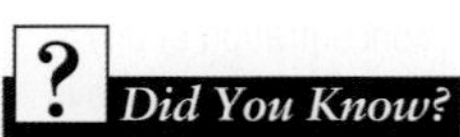

Drug elimination is dependent on volume of distribution of the drug and its clearance.

When injected intravenously (ie, bioavailability being 100%), the concentration of drug in plasma is the amount of the drug injected (mg) divided by the plasma volume (mL). If all the drug initially stays in plasma, the volume of distribution of the injected drug is equal to the plasma volume. However, drugs with a high V_d enter multiple extravascular compartments, and therefore, a higher dose of the drug is required to achieve a given plasma concentration (eg, propofol). Conversely, a drug which tends to stay in the intravascular compartment will have a low V_d (eg, neuromuscular blockers), and so a lower dose is adequate to achieve a given plasma concentration.

2. Effects of Hepatic or Renal Disease on Pharmacokinetic Parameters

In order to understand the effect of hepatic and renal disease on drug disposition, it is important to understand the concept of systemic clearance (CL_{SYS}) defined as:

$$CL_{SYS} = CL_R + CL_{NR}$$

where CL_R is renal clearance and CL_{NR} is nonrenal clearance.

Renal clearance is given by CL_R = (U.V/P), where U is the concentration of the drug in urine, P is the free plasma concentration of the drug, and V is the urine flow rate. Hepatic clearance CL_H, which is the primary contributor to nonrenal clearance, is given by Rowland equation, as above.

In patients with hepatic disease, the elimination half-life of drugs metabolized or excreted by the liver is often increased because of decreased clearance and possibly increased volume of distribution caused by ascites and altered protein binding.[7] Drug concentration at steady-state is inversely proportional to elimination clearance. Therefore, when hepatic drug clearance is reduced, repeated bolus dosing or continuous infusion of such drugs as benzodiazepines, opioids, and barbiturates may result in excessive accumulation of these drug and hence excessive and prolonged pharmacologic effects.[8] However, recovery from small doses of drugs such as thiopental and fentanyl occurs largely as a result of redistribution, and so recovery from conservative doses will be only minimally affected by reductions in elimination clearance.

? *Did You Know?*

In hepatic disease states, elimination of drug may be prolonged both due to increased volume of distribution and decreased hepatic clearance.

E. Physiologic Versus Compartmental Models

Perfusion-based physiologic pharmacokinetic models are realistic models of drug pharmacokinetics. Individual organ blood flow and metabolic rates are modeled in order to understand the disposition of drugs in these organs, thus helping to understand the effect of various physiologic and pathologic states on drug distribution and elimination.[9] Establishing these models requires the measurement of drug concentrations in many different tissues, which is technically challenging, invasive, and time consuming. Therefore, compartmental models, which are both mathematically and practically simpler, were developed.

In ***compartmental pharmacokinetics,*** the body is assumed to be a series of simple communicating compartments, arranged either in series or in parallel. Each compartment comprises organs with similar blood flow. It is assumed that the drug under consideration gets completely mixed in each compartment. The rate of movement between compartments is assumed to follow first-order kinetics and to be dependent only on passive movement in response to concentration gradients between the compartments. Rate constants are used to describe the rates of equilibration between these various compartments, but these can also be converted in half-life form.

A single compartment model is the simplest of these compartmental pharmacokinetic models. The administered drug is assumed to completely mix with the single compartment, that is plasma. The concentration of the drug in various pertinent tissues is assumed to correspond directly to the plasma drug concentration. So as the concentration of the drug increases in the plasma, the modeled concentration in various tissues increases similarly (see **Figure 7.2**). This single compartment model is too rudimentary for most anesthetic drugs, and so multicompartmental models are employed.

F. Multicompartmental Models

Many drugs exhibit three distinct pharmacokinetic phases after intravenous administration. These phases can be satisfactorily modeled with the three-compartment model.[10]

- ***Rapid distribution phase.*** After initial administration, there is redistribution from the plasma to a rapidly equilibrating tissue group (eg, a fast compartment or vessel rich group).
- ***Steady-state.*** A period of "dynamic equilibrium" in which the drug has completed distribution between the central and peripheral compartments.

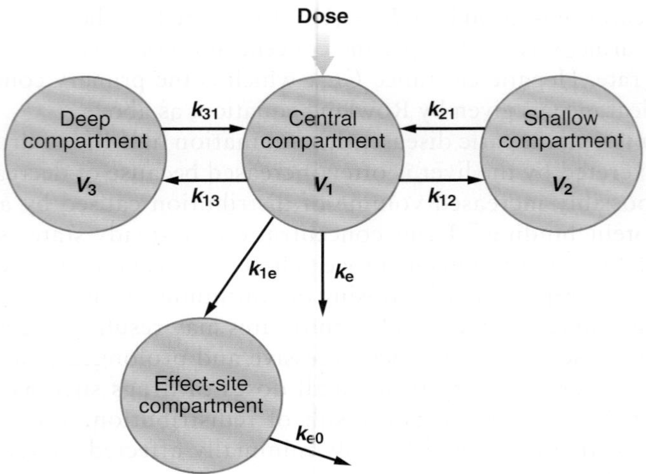

Figure 7.3 A schematic of a three-compartment pharmacokinetic model with the effect site linked to the central compartment. The rate constant for transfer between the plasma (central compartment) and the effect site, k_{1e}, and the volume of the effect site are both presumed to be negligible to ensure that the effect site does not influence the pharmacokinetic model. (From Gupta DK, Henthorn TK. Basic principles of clinical pharmacology. In: Barash PG, Cahalan MK, Cullen BF, et al, eds. *Clinical Anesthesia*. 8th ed. Wolters Kluwer; 2018:241-275, Figure 11.12.)

- ***Terminal phase/elimination phase.*** A decrease in plasma drug concentration due to elimination of drug from the body. During this phase, drug returns from sites at higher concentration (eg, fast and slow-distribution compartments) to the plasma from where it is subsequently eliminated.

Each of these three phases has its own half-life or rate constant. They are distribution half-life (α), elimination half-life (β), and terminal half-life (γ).

Figure 7.3 shows the standard representation of a multicompartment model. Drug transfer between the central compartment and the more rapidly equilibrating ("fast" or "shallow") peripheral compartment is characterized by the first-order rate constants k_{12} and k_{21}.

Transfer in and out of the more slowly equilibrating ("slow" or "deep") compartment is characterized by the rate constants k_{13} and k_{31}. In this model, there are three compartmental volumes: V_1, V_2, and V_3, whose sum equals V_{ss}; and three clearances: the rapid intercompartmental clearance, the slow intercompartmental clearance, and elimination clearance. k_{12}, k_{21}, k_{13}, k_{31}, and k_{10} represent the first-order fractional rate constants for distribution, redistribution, and elimination. Equations exist to convert back and forth between these multicompartmental model k rate constants (known as micro-constants) and the experimentally observable macroscopic rate constants α, β, and γ described above.

II. Principles of Pharmacodynamics

A. Modeling From Concentration to Effect

Pharmacodynamics focuses on the quantitative analysis of the relationship between the plasma drug concentration and effect. The mathematical models for pharmacodynamics are created by measuring the plasma drug concentrations that are required to generate defined drug effects.

1. Combined PK-PD Models

Even though the distribution of any administered drug is a complex biological process, plasma and organ concentrations can often be estimated accurately with simplified models. These models express the time course of drug in the body using a small number of mathematically computed pharmacokinetic parameters. By designing a pharmacokinetic model that also predicts the concentration of the drug at its effect site, it becomes possible to apply the model to address clinically important questions, such as the following:

- Understanding the distribution of the drug from the central compartment (plasma) to various organs.
- Estimating the time to onset and offset of drug effect.
- Correlating plasma drug concentration and response.
- Predicting the concentration of the drug in various tissues and body fluids.
- Determining the optimum drug dosing to avoid side effects or toxicity in a particular patient population.
- Designing a device dosing algorithm for an infusion regimen using an infusion pump.
- Determining the effect of altered physiologic states and disease processes on drug absorption, distribution, metabolism, and elimination, so improving safety profile of drug dosing in these conditions.
- Understanding drug interactions when multiple drugs are coadministered.

Combined PK-PD models fully characterize the relationships between time, dose, plasma concentration, and pharmacologic effect. This is achieved by adding an "effect compartment" to the standard compartmental PK model.[9] (See Figure 11.3).

The rate constant for drug removal from the effect site, which relates the concentration in the central compartment to the pharmacologic effect, is k_{e0}. The rate of equilibration between the plasma and the effect site, k_{e0}, can also be characterized by the half-life of effect site equilibration ($t_{1/2,ke0}$) using the formula:

$$t_{1/2,ke0} = 0.693/k_{eo}$$

$t_{1/2,ke0}$ is the time for the effect site concentration to reach 50% of the plasma concentration when the plasma concentration is held constant. For anesthetics with a short $t_{1/2,ke0}$ (ie, high k_{e0}), equilibration between the plasma and the effect site is rapid, and therefore, there is little delay before an effect is reached when a bolus of drug is administered, or an infusion of drug is initiated.

2. Drug-Receptor Interactions

Drugs produce their effect by binding to receptors, affecting a change in cellular function. These receptors can be on the cell membrane, in the cytoplasm, or in the nucleoplasm. The binding of drugs to receptors, like the binding of drugs to plasma proteins, is usually reversible and follows the Law of Mass Action:

$$(\text{Drug}) + (\text{receptor}) \leftrightarrow (\text{Drug-receptor complex})$$

The higher the concentration of free drug or unoccupied receptor, the greater the tendency to form the drug-receptor complex. The relation between drug concentration and the intensity of the response is most often characterized by a curvilinear relation (**Figure 7.4**). For most drugs, there is a minimum concentration that needs to be achieved before an effect can be observed (therapeutic

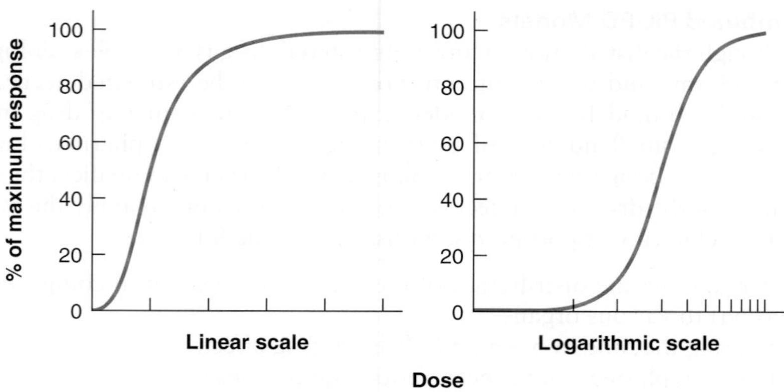

Figure 7.4 A schematic curve of the effect of a drug plotted against dose. In the left panel, the response data are plotted against the dose data on a linear scale. In the right panel, the same response data are plotted against the dose data on a logarithmic scale yielding a sigmoid dose-response curve that is linear between 20% and 80% of the maximal effect. Plotting the percentage of receptors occupied by a drug against the logarithm of the concentration of the drug yields a sigmoid curve. (From Gupta DK, Henthorn TK. Basic principles of clinical pharmacology. In: Barash PG, Cahalan MK, Cullen BF, et al, eds. *Clinical Anesthesia*. 8th ed. Wolters Kluwer; 2018:241-275, Figure 11.9.)

threshold). Once a pharmacologic effect is produced, small increases in drug concentration usually produce relatively large increases in drug effect. As the drug effect reaches near maximum, increases in concentration produce minimal changes in effect.

Drugs that combine to their receptor and produce maximal effect are termed "full agonists"; those which produce less than the maximum effect are called "partial agonists"; and those that do not produce any effect at all are termed "antagonists."

Competitive antagonists bind reversibly to receptors, and their blocking effect can be overcome by high concentrations of an agonist (ie, competition). They produce a parallel shift in the dose-response curve, but the maximum effect is not altered (**Figure 7.5**, curves A and B). Noncompetitive antagonists bind irreversibly to receptors and shift the dose-response curve downward and to the right, decreasing both the slope and the maximum effect (**Figure 7.5**, curves A and C). The effect of noncompetitive antagonists is reversed only by synthesis of new receptor molecules. As shown in **Figure 7.5**, drug A produces a maximum effect, E_{max}, and a 50% of maximal effect at dose or concentration $E_{50,A}$. Drug B, a full agonist, can produce the maximum effect, E_{max}; however, it is less potent ($E_{50,B} > E_{50,A}$). Drug C, a partial agonist, can only produce a maximum effect of approximately 50% E_{max}. If a competitive antagonist is given to a patient, the dose response for the agonist would shift from curve A to curve B—although the receptors would have the same affinity for the agonist, the presence of the competitor would necessitate an increase in agonist in order to produce an effect. The agonist would still be able to produce its maximal effect if a sufficient overdose was given to displace the competitive antagonist. However, the competitive antagonist would not change the binding characteristics of the receptor for the agonist and so curve B is simply shifted to the right but remains parallel to curve A. In contrast, if a noncompetitive antagonist binds to the receptor, the agonist

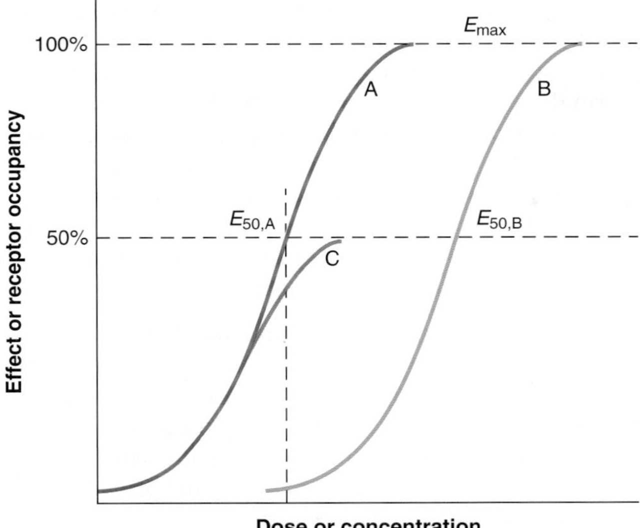

Figure 7.5 Schematic pharmacodynamic curves, with dose or concentration on the x-axis and effect or receptor occupancy on the y-axis, that illustrate agonism, partial agonism, and antagonism. (From Gupta DK, Henthorn TK. Basic principles of clinical pharmacology. In: Barash PG, Cahalan MK, Cullen BF, et al, eds. *Clinical Anesthesia*. 8th ed. Wolters Kluwer; 2018:241-275, Figure 11.10.)

would no longer be able to produce a maximal effect, no matter how much of an overdose is administered (curve C).

An inverse agonist is a drug that binds to the same receptor as an agonist but induces a pharmacological response opposite to that of the agonists (negative intrinsic activity). A neutral antagonist has no activity in the absence of an agonist or inverse agonist but can block the activity of either. Consequently, the efficacy of a full agonist is 100%, a neutral antagonist has 0% efficacy, and an inverse agonist has <0% (ie, negative) efficacy.

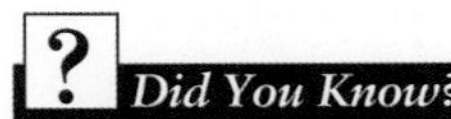

Naloxone-induced withdrawal syndrome in opioid dependent patients is due to inverse agonism.

B. Dose-Response Relationships

Potency is an expression of the activity of the drug, that is, the concentration of the drug required to produce a defined effect. The concentration of the drug that produces 50% of its maximum effect is termed C_{50}. The lower the C_{50}, the greater the potency of the drug.

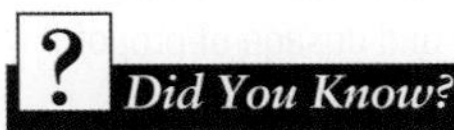

The potency of fentanyl is 100 times that of morphine.

Efficacy is an expression of the therapeutic effectiveness of the drug at its effector site. The efficacy of various drugs of the same class varies depending on their affinity to the receptor.

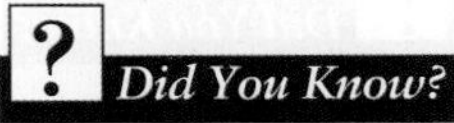

Drugs of the same class, acting at the same receptor, differ in their efficacy.

1. Concentration-Response Relationships

To estimate the drug effect, we need to know the concentration of the drug at the effect site which, for most anesthetic agents, is usually the brain. Measuring drug concentration in the brain directly is challenging, and hence, drug concentration in plasma is used as a surrogate. For all anesthetic agents, there is a distribution delay for the drug to be transported from the central compartment, that is, plasma, to the site of action. For example, after intravenous injection, propofol needs to be transported to the brain and bind to receptors there in order to cause its effect. After a few minutes, the concentration at the effect site at the neurons in the brain will equilibrate with the plasma propofol

? Did You Know?

The same drug effect may be seen at two significantly different plasma concentrations, which is termed "hysteresis," because the concentration in the brain may significantly lag the concentration in the plasma.

concentration, but this is a noninstantaneous event. Consequently, the effect of sedation or unconsciousness will be produced, depending on the dose of propofol that was administered. This causes a decrease in the bispectral index, which is commonly used to assess the depth of anesthesia. With time, even though the concentration of propofol in the plasma is decreasing, the BIS will continues to remain low as the brain concentration of propofol will still be high. Then propofol will begin to diffuse out of the brain back into plasma because of a reversal in the concentration gradient, and the BIS will start to increase. This mathematically translates into a reverse hysteresis loop, dependent both on the dose and route of administration.[11]

C. Therapeutic Thresholds and Therapeutic Windows

Therapeutic threshold is the minimum concentration of the drug that produces a desired drug effect. It depends on the required magnitude of the desired effect. For example, melanoma excision is less painful than knee replacement, and hence, the dose of fentanyl required to provide satisfactory analgesia is different for the two procedures. The dose of fentanyl providing analgesia after melanoma excision is not adequate to provide pain relief after knee surgery (ie, below the therapeutic threshold). Conversely, the dose of fentanyl providing pain relief after knee surgery will provide faster pain relief after melanoma excision because it will reach the therapeutic threshold faster. However, this might also result in a fentanyl plasma concentration above the toxic threshold for melanoma excision and result in obvious opioid side effects like respiratory depression. Plainly, the required target plasma concentration of fentanyl is different for the two procedures.

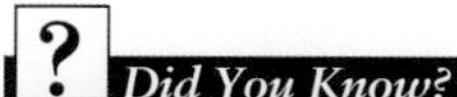

The effect site of drug action for anesthetic agents is usually the brain. Clinicians should be aware of the time to peak effect site concentration in order to time noxious procedures such as laryngoscopy.

The range between the therapeutic threshold and the toxic threshold is termed the "therapeutic window." The dosage of the drug at which there is a 50% probability of effect is termed the ED_{50}, and the dose at which there is a 50% probability of death is the LD_{50}.

The therapeutic index (TI) of a drug is the ratio of LD_{50} to ED_{50}.

$$TI = LD_{50}/ED_{50}.$$

The higher the TI, the safer the drug.

? Did You Know?

Propofol has a narrow therapeutic index. Hence, it is important to titrate the timing and dosage of propofol to effect during induction to avoid excessive myocardial depression.

III. Anesthetic Drug Interactions

The perioperative period is characterized by the administration of varying doses of multiple drugs to induce, maintain, and antagonize anesthetics along with antibiotics, antiepileptics, and each patient's preoperative medications. So there exists the potential for multiple drug interactions, some of which are part of the anesthetic plan (ie, coadministration of an opioid with a volatile anesthetic to decrease the minimum alveolar concentration), and others which are inadvertent consequences of the polypharmacy of the perioperative period.

? Did You Know?

These drugs have a narrow therapeutic index: aminoglycosides, cyclosporine, carbamazepine, digoxin, digitoxin, flecainide, lithium, phenytoin, phenobarbital, rifampicin, theophylline, and warfarin.

Drug interactions[12] may occur as either in vitro or in vivo processes. In vitro interactions are due to physical or chemical incompatibility. For example, ceftriaxone should not be reconstituted or mixed with lactated ringer's solution as it tends to precipitate in calcium-containing solutions.

In vivo interactions are due to induced changes in drug pharmacokinetics or pharmacodynamics. For example, one drug may interact pharmacokinetically with another by causing alterations in its absorption, distribution, metabolism, or elimination. Pharmacodynamic interactions result from the action of multiple drugs on at the same receptors or physiological system.

A. Pharmacokinetic Interactions

1. Absorption

With the increasing use of preoperative oral medications to attenuate cardiovascular risk (eg, β-receptor antagonists) or decrease opioid requirements after surgery (eg, cyclooxygenase inhibitors, gabapentinoids, sustained release opioids, etc.), anesthesiologists can no longer ignore drugs that alter absorption. For example, grapefruit juice inhibits CYP3A4 in jejunal cytochrome P450 enzyme activity and increases the absorption of nonmetabolized drugs such as statins, resulting in higher than expected systemic drug concentrations. Conversely, fexofenadine may block the transporters in the intestinal epithelium and decrease drug absorption. Drugs that alter the gastric pH (eg, ranitidine) or alter gastric emptying and intestinal transit time (eg, metoclopramide) can also alter drug dissolution and drug absorption.

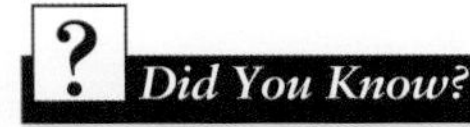

Cytochrome P450 in both the intestines and liver is vulnerable to inducement and inhibition by drugs.

2. Distribution

Drug displacement from protein binding sites by competing drugs increases the unbound concentration of a drug and potentially produces exposure to supratherapeutic concentrations and potential toxicity. This is not generally clinically important for anesthetic drugs because (1) for the most part, anesthetic drugs have a tremendous number of unoccupied binding sites and (2) the hepatic metabolism of most anesthetic drugs is flow limited rather than limited by enzymatic capacity. The liver will therefore rapidly normalize the excess free concentration to predisplacement concentrations.

The more common mechanism by which drug-drug interactions affect the distribution of anesthetic drugs is by changing cardiac output and hence the distribution of cardiac output.[13] These alterations in the tissue distribution of a drug will change the amount of drug delivered to the effect site. Volatile anesthetics and propofol can alter the distribution of regional blood flow and therefore alter the plasma drug concentration profile.

3. Metabolism

Many commonly used drugs induce (or inhibit) cytochrome P450 isozymes, which increase (or decrease) hepatic drug metabolism and consequently decrease (or increase) drug exposure. Antiepileptics may increase drug metabolism by the induction of cytochrome P450 3A4. Fortunately, it is relatively easy to increase the dose or dosing frequency of affected drugs to titrate to this effect. It may be more difficult to avoid a drug overdose when there is a decrease in drug metabolism. For example, with the concomitant administration of protease inhibitors that inhibit opioid metabolism, it is necessary to start with lower doses and then slowly increase the dose or dosing frequency to avoid prolonged exposure to supratherapeutic concentrations and toxicity. An additional therapeutic challenge is when the conversion of a prodrug to its active drug is inhibited by another drug. Because of the variability of the amount of CYP 2D6 inhibition by selective serotonin reuptake inhibitors, it may be easier to avoid opioids that require CYP 2D6 conversion (ie, codeine, oxycodone, and hydrocodone) rather than attempt to predict adequate analgesia in patients taking these drugs.[14]

B. Pharmacodynamic Interactions

The interaction between drugs may be additive, synergistic, or antagonistic. When additive, the effect of the drug combination is equal to the sum of their individual effects. When synergistic, the effect of the drug combination is greater than the sum of their individual effects. When antagonistic (or subadditive), the effect of the combination is less than the sum of the individual drug effects. The easiest pharmacodynamic drug-drug interactions to understand are the methods anesthesiologists use routinely and intentionally to antagonize the clinical effects of opioids and nondepolarizing neuromuscular blocking agents. The opioid antagonist naloxone is a direct antagonist of the μ-opioid receptor. It displaces the opioid from the μ-opioid receptor and reverses opioid-induced ventilatory depression and decreases the pain threshold. This antagonism is described as "competitive," that is, if there more opioid molecules in comparison to naloxone molecules, the later are displaced by the opioid molecules. Hence when naloxone is given to reverse opioid induced ventilatory depression, repeat dosing or an infusion may be required in order to maintain the clinical effect of the naloxone. When given in the absence of an opioid, naloxone binds to the μ-opioid receptor but does not activate it.

In contrast, the cholinesterase inhibitors (eg, neostigmine) increase the amount of acetylcholine available at the neuromuscular junction. Therefore, they are indirect antagonists of the nondepolarizing neuromuscular junction blocking agents.

1. Isobolograms

One method of quantify drug-drug interactions is Loewe isobologram. A curve is generated from the dose-response data of the individual drugs. An isobole curve defines the different dose combinations that yield the same effect. The isobole allows for a comparison with actual combination effects, making it possible to determine whether the interaction is synergistic, additive or antagonistic (subadditive) as depicted in **Figure 7.6**. The isobole is linear when the two drugs being studied have a constant potency ratio and curved when the potency ratio is variable.[15]

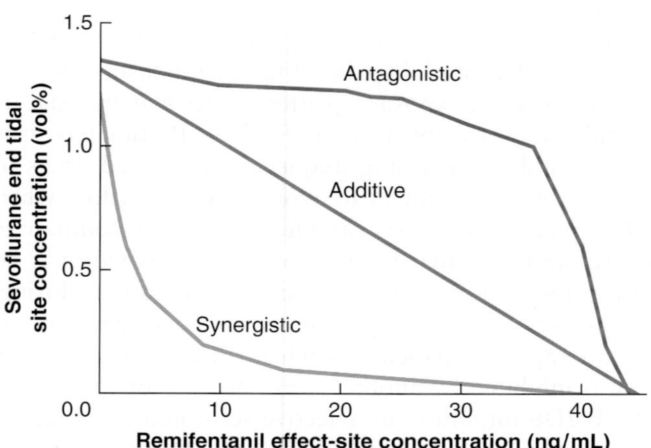

Figure 7.6 Isoboles to demonstrate additive (blue line), synergistic (green line), and antagonistic (red line) interactions between Drug A and Drug B. (From Gupta DK, Henthorn TK. Basic Principles of Clinical Pharmacology. In: Barash PG, Cahalan MK, Cullen BF, et al, eds. *Clinical Anesthesia*. 8th ed. Wolters Kluwer; 2018:241-275, Figure 11.27.)

2. Response Surface Models

Although it is possible to produce the clinical state of general anesthesia solely with the administration of high-effect site concentrations of a volatile anesthetic or an IV anesthetic, the unintended consequences of these include a prolonged time for emergence and undesired hemodynamic side effects (hypotension due to myocardial depression, and arterial and venous dilation). The combination of an opioid and a hypnotic is synergistic and produces a clinical anesthetic state while enabling faster emergence. Analysis of the combinations of an opioid and a hypnotic that produce the same clinical anesthetic state generates a three-dimensional surface that, when projected onto the concentration-effect plane, produces a family of concentration-response curves. These mathematical models are termed ***response surface models***. They include effect-site concentrations for each drug and the probability estimate of the overall effect. These models characterize the entire dose-response relation between combinations of anesthetic drugs and are mathematically consistent with the concentration-response curves of individual drugs (**Figure 7.7**).[16]

These models have been adapted to enable real-time clinical display. With manual entry of patient demographics and the drugs administered, combined with automated data collection from the anesthesia machine (such as end tidal of volatile anesthetic and infusion pump information), such display devices provide predictions of drug concentrations and estimated combined drug effects. Automatic control of drug infusions in order to attain a desired effect has led to the concept of target-controlled infusions (TCIs).

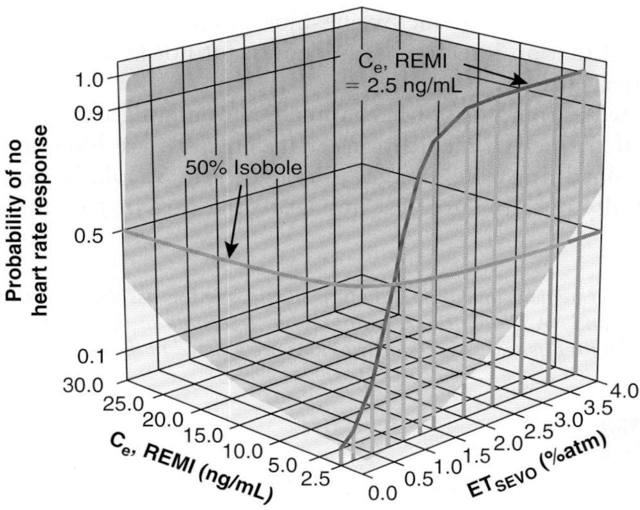

Figure 7.7 A response surface model characterizing the remifentanil-sevoflurane interaction for analgesia to electrical tetanic stimulation. The projection of the response surface onto the 50% probability horizontal plane results in the 50% effect isobole while the projection of the response surface onto the 2.5 ng/mL remifentanil effect site concentration vertical plane results in the sevoflurane concentration-response curve under 2.5 ng/mL of remifentanil. (Adapted from Manyam SC, Gupta DK, Johnson KB, et al. Opioid-volatile anesthetic synergy: a response surface model with remifentanil and sevoflurane as prototypes. *Anesthesiology.* 2006;105:267-278.)

Some devices will also display context-sensitive half time (CSHT), either graphically or numerically. CSHT is the predicted time that it will take for a given drug plasma concentration to fall by 50% after stopping the infusion. "Context" refers here to the dosage and duration of the infusion of the drug up to the current time. CSHT gives an estimate of the duration of remaining drug effect as a single combined function of the PKPD of the drug and the amount given so far. As the duration of an infusion increases, the CSHT increases and will eventually asymptotically approach a maximum half-time at steady state. However, some limitations of CSHT are as follows:

- CSHT is not a fixed kinetic parameter and cannot easily be extrapolated backward or forward to lesser or greater drug concentrations.
- For a given drug, the most relevant concentration decrease may not be 50% and the times for different percentage decreases in plasma concentration are not linear.
- Effect site concentration is more important than plasma concentration.

? *Did You Know?*

The increased use of medications that modulate the serotonergic pathways of the central nervous system can potentially produce serotonin syndrome (confusion, hyperactivity, memory problems, muscle twitching, excessive sweating, shivering, or fever).

C. Unintended Toxicity

While most outpatient medications have very little pharmacodynamic interaction with common perioperative medications, a few significant exceptions exist. Antidepressants that inhibit the CNS monoamine oxidase (to inhibit the degradation of serotonin) or that decrease the reuptake of serotonin can result in toxic serotonin CNS concentrations if they are combined with other monoamine oxidase inhibitors (eg, methylene blue) or other serotonin reuptake inhibitors (eg, methadone, meperidine, and tramadol). Unfortunately, washout of these antidepressants can take over 4 weeks and cause worsening pain or depression. When methylene blue administration is required, it is recommended that an interacting antidepressant not be restarted for at least 24 hours afterward.[17]

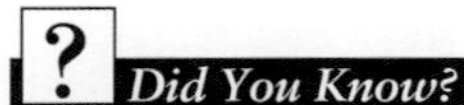

Garlic can increase the risk of bleeding when taken along with other antiplatelet agents and must be stopped 7 days before surgery.

There is widespread use of herbal medicines among the presurgical population.[18] Of the herbal medications that clinicians are likely to encounter, echinacea, ephedra, garlic, ginkgo, ginseng, kava, St John's wort, and valerian potentially pose the greatest impact to the care of patients undergoing surgery.

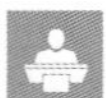

For further review and interactivities, please see the associated Interactive Video Lectures and "A Closer Look" infographic accessible in the complimentary eBook bundled with this text. Access instructions are located in the inside front cover.

References

1. Stanski DR, Greenblatt DJ, Lowenstein E. Kinetics of intravenous and intramuscular morphine. *Clin Pharmacol Ther*. 1978;24:52-59.
2. Rowland M, Tozer TN. *Clinical Pharmacokinetics. Concepts and Applications*. Lippincott Williams & Wilkins; 1995:161-167. ISBN 13: 978-0-6830-7404-8.
3. Nies AS, Shand DG, Wilkinson GR. Altered hepatic blood flow and drug disposition. *Clin Pharmacokinet*. 1976;1:1351-1355.
4. Wilkinson GR. Pharmacokinetics of drug disposition: hemodynamic considerations. *Annu Rev Pharmacol*. 1975;15:11-27.
5. Manikandan P, Nagini S. Cytochrome P450 structure, function and clinical significance: a review *Curr Drug Targets*. 2018;19(1):38-54. doi:10.2174/1389450118666170125144557. PMID: 28124606.
6. Bachmann KA, Belloto RJ Jr. Differential kinetics of phenytoin in elderly patients. *Drugs Aging*. 1999;15(3):235-250.

7. Patwardhan RV, Johnson RF, Hoyumpa A Jr, et al. Normal metabolism of morphine in cirrhosis. *Gastroenterology*. 1981;81:1006-1011.
8. Klotz U. Pharmacokinetics and drug metabolism in the elderly. *Drug Metab Rev*. 2009;41(2):67-76.
9. Thompson CM, Johns DO, Sonawane B, et al. Database for physiologically based pharmacokinetic (PBPK) modeling: physiological data for healthy and health-impaired elderly. *J Toxicol Environ Health B Crit Rev*. 2009;12(1):1-24.
10. Sahinovic MM, Struys MMRF, Absalom AR. Clinical pharmacokinetics and pharmacodynamics of propofol. *Clin Pharmacokinet*. 2018;57(12):1539-1558. doi:10.1007/s40262-018-0672-3.
11. Louizos C, Yáñez JA, Forrest ML, Davies NM. Understanding the hysteresis loop conundrum in pharmacokinetic/pharmacodynamic relationships. *J Pharm Sci*. 2014;17(1):34-91.
12. Olkkola KT, Ahonen J. Drug interactions. *Curr Opin Anaesthesiol*. 2001;14(4):411-416.
13. Henthorn TK, Krejcie TC, Avram MJ. Early drug distribution: a generally neglected aspect of pharmacokinetics of relevance to intravenously administered anesthetic agents. *Clin Pharmacol Ther*. 2008;84:18-22.
14. Crews KR, Gaedigk A, Dunnenberger HM, et al. Clinical pharmacogenetics implementation consortium guidelines for cytochrome p450 2d6 genotype and codeine therapy: 2014 update. *Clin Pharmacol Ther*. 2014;95:376-382.
15. Tallarida RJ. Drug combinations: tests and analysis with isoboles. *Curr Protoc Pharmacol*. 2016;72:9.19.1-9.19.19. doi:10.1002/0471141755.ph0919s72.
16. Manyam SC, Gupta DK, Johnson KB, et al. Opioid-volatile anesthetic synergy: a response surface model with remifentanil and sevoflurane as prototypes. *Anesthesiology*. 2006;105:267-278.
17. Boyer EW, Shannon M. The serotonin syndrome. *N Engl J Med*. 2005;352:1112-1120.
18. Ang-Lee MK, Moss J, Yuan CS. Herbal medicines and perioperative care. *J Am Med Assoc*. 2001;286(2):208-216.

PHARMACOKINETICS

A CLOSER LOOK

The liver plays a central role in terminating the effect of drugs. The majority of administered pharmaceutical agents will undergo hepatic metabolism. Some drugs are processed through phase 1 reactions while others undergo phase 2 metabolism. Many drugs will be biotransformed through both types of reactions.

Aspirin is an example of a drug that undergoes both phase 1 and phase 2 reactions

Phase 1 reactions

These reactions typically deactivate the function of a drug through oxidation, reduction, hydoxylation, or hydrolysis. In some cases, phase 1 reactions may in fact convert a prodrug into an active drug. The cytochrome P450 enzyme system is largely responsible for the majority of these reactions.

Phase 2 reactions

These reactions typically deactivate a drug through conjugation to another, polar molecule. The addition of this molecule renders the drug susceptible to elimination by the kidneys as it is now hydrophyllic. The uridyl-glucuronyltransferase enzyme system is largely responsible for the majority of these reactions.

Fentanyl is an example of a drug that only undergoes Phase 1 metabolism by CYP3A4 into inactive metabolites like norfentanyl.

Morphine is an example of a drug that only undergoes Phase 2 metabolism into morphine-3 (90%) and morphine-6 glucoronides (10%). The latter retains significant opiate activity.

73%

of hepatic biotransformation enzymes are part of the cytochrome P450 family

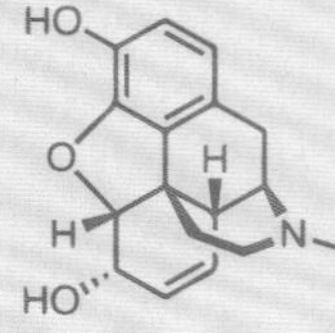

Infographic by: Naveen Nathan MD

Questions

1. **Regarding first-order kinetics, all of the following are true except:**
   A. Is concentration-dependent process
   B. Is saturable and, when saturated, reverts to zero-order kinetics
   C. Applicable to metabolism of methanol in methanol intoxication
   D. More common than zero-order kinetics

2. **Which of the following will NOT alter the volume of distribution of a drug?**
   A. Cardiac failure
   B. Clearance
   C. Age
   D. Burns
   E. Pleural effusion

3. **After stopping the infusion of propofol, CSHT of the propofol is:**
   A. The time taken for the concentration of the propofol to decrease by 50% at its effect site, the brain
   B. The time taken for 50% elimination of the propofol from the body
   C. The time taken for the plasma concentration of the propofol to decrease by 50%
   D. The taken for the propofol to have 50% of the peak effect

4. **Which of the following are the concepts related to pharmacokinetics?**
   A. Absorption, distribution, metabolism, and excretion
   B. Affinity, efficacy, potency, and distribution
   C. Agonist, partial agonist, and antagonist
   D. Protein binding, half-life, and context-sensitive half time

5. **Which statement about partial agonists is true?**
   A. Partial agonists are molecules that can cause a maximal response irrespective of the presence of antagonists.
   B. Partial agonists are molecules that have affinity but no efficacy at the target receptor.
   C. Partial agonists are molecules that have affinity and efficacy to the target receptor.
   D. Partial agonists are molecules that have an affinity to the target receptor, but only achieve a submaximal response.

Answers

1. C

First-order kinetics is a concentration-dependent process. Hence, the higher the concentration, the faster the clearance. The toxicity of methanol stems from the metabolites. As methanol follows a zero-order kinetic elimination, the real danger lies in the time from ingestion, not the total amount.

2. B

Volume of distribution is not affected by clearance. Although changes in tissue binding will affect partition coefficient and apparent volume of distribution, such changes will have no effect on average steady-state blood levels of the drug or clearance of the drug. The total body volume is affected by the other factors listed—cardiac failure, age, burns, and pleural effusion, which hence affect the available volume into which the drug may get distributed into.

3. C

CSHT is the time taken for the plasma drug concentration to decrease by 50%, when the infusion of the drug is stopped. It does not reflect the fall in drug concentration at the effect site, which is usually the brain, for anesthetic agents.

4. A

Pharmacokinetics deals with the what the body does to the drug—hence involves the concepts of absorption, distribution, metabolism, and excretion. These factors help determine plasma drug concentration of the administered drug.

5. D

Agonists are molecules that bind to receptors and initiate a physiological response. Antagonists, however, are molecules that bind to receptors and prevent the agonist-induced physiological response from occurring. They are both described in the context of their receptor affinity and efficacy.

8 Inhaled Anesthetics

Ramesh Ramaiah and Sanjay M. Bhananker

The value of inhaled gases as effective pain relievers was discovered in the 1840s. Nitrous oxide was effective for analgesia and sedation, whereas diethyl ether could produce general anesthesia. On October 16, 1846, William T. G. Morton successfully demonstrated the anesthetic effects of ether at a public gathering in Massachusetts General Hospital, which was the beginning of the era of anesthesia. Since then, several pure gases and volatile anesthetics (liquids that have been vaporized to be inhaled) have been synthesized, studied, and used in clinical practice.

I. Pharmacologic Principles

A. Terminology

The behavior of administered drugs is best described in terms of ***pharmacodynamics*** (what the drug does to the body) and ***pharmacokinetics*** (what the body does to the drug). Pharmacodynamics describes the effects of drugs on organ systems, tissues, and specific receptors. Pharmacokinetics describes the way in which drugs are absorbed upon their administration, their distribution within various body compartments, their metabolism, and their elimination or excretion.

B. Classification of Inhaled Anesthetics

Some inhaled anesthetics are in a gaseous state at room temperature and are stored in tanks. Examples of such anesthetic gases include nitrous oxide, xenon, and an explosive gas, cyclopropane, which is no longer in use. Most inhaled anesthetics in current use are termed volatile anesthetics because they are liquids at room temperature. These are stored in bottles and converted to a gas phase using special agent-specific vaporizers that can deliver a precise concentration of the drug into the anesthetic circuit. Outdated examples of volatile anesthetics include diethyl ether, halothane, and enflurane. Current volatile anesthetics include sevoflurane and isoflurane. Desflurane is an inhaled anesthetic that has characteristics of both a pure gas and a volatile anesthetic. That is, because its boiling point is 24 °C, it changes from a liquid to a gas at a temperature very near normal room temperature. Vaporization of desflurane requires a vaporizer that is more complex than is necessary for the other volatile anesthetics. For example, the desflurane vaporizer requires electrical power to operate, and the desflurane liquid within is kept pressurized in order to prevent spontaneous boiling.

C. Physical Characteristics of Inhaled Anesthetics

Table 8.1 describes some of the properties of inhaled anesthetic agents currently in use. A ***partition coefficient*** (eg, blood:gas or brain:blood) is expressed in various media as the solubility of these anesthetics. If a container with equal

Table 8.1 Physical Properties of Commonly Used Inhalational Anesthetic Agents

Property	Sevoflurane	Desflurane	Isoflurane	Nitrous Oxide	Xenon
Boiling point (°C)	59	24	49	−88	−108
Vapor pressure at 20 °C (mm Hg)	157	669	238	38,770	—
Blood:gas partition coefficient	0.65	0.42	1.46	0.46	0.115
Oil:gas partition coefficient	47	19	91	1.4	1.9
Minimum alveolar concentration (MAC)	1.8	6.6	1.17	104	63-71
Metabolized in the body (%)	2-5	0.02	0.2	0	0

volumes of blood and air was exposed to enough isoflurane to produce a 1% concentration of isoflurane in the gas phase (1 mL isoflurane/100 mL of air) and allowed to come to equilibrium (total pressure equal in both air and blood), then 1.46 mL of isoflurane would be dissolved in each 100 mL of blood. The isoflurane would be "partitioned" between the blood and air in a ratio of 1.46:1, so the partition coefficient would be 1.46.

The ***blood:gas*** partition coefficient determines the speed of anesthetic induction, recovery, and change of anesthetic depth. An agent with a relatively high blood:gas partition coefficient (eg, isoflurane = 1.46) will require a longer time for induction (and recovery) compared with an anesthetic with a lower blood:gas partition coefficient (eg, sevoflurane = 0.65). Anesthesia results when the anesthetic is fully dissolved in the blood and an effective partial pressure of the anesthetic is attained in the blood (and brain). It takes longer for induction of anesthesia with an anesthetic with a high blood:gas partition coefficient because more anesthetic is dissolved in blood. And it takes longer for the blood to become "saturated" and the partial pressure exerted by the anesthetic to be high enough to produce a surgical level of anesthesia.

The ***oil:gas*** partition coefficient is a measure of lipid solubility of an inhaled anesthetic. The higher the oil:gas partition coefficient, the more potent the anesthetic and the lower the partial pressure (ie, concentration) required to achieve a surgical plane of anesthesia (see the following section for a discussion of the minimum alveolar concentration).

II. Uptake and Distribution of Inhaled Anesthetic Agents

It is common to discuss the pharmacokinetic behavior of inhaled anesthetics in terms of their uptake and distribution because they are delivered to the patient by inhalation, absorbed or taken up by the blood, and then distributed to organs throughout the body (including the brain!). Furthermore, because it is difficult to measure blood concentrations of inhaled anesthetics, but relatively easy to measure the concentration, or fraction, inspired (F_I), expired (F_E), and in the alveolae (F_A) (which is nearly equivalent to that in the blood and brain), the pharmacokinetics of inhaled anesthetics are typically described in terms of these readily measured values.

A. Alveolar/Inspired Anesthetic Concentration

The speed with which the alveolar anesthetic concentration rises and approaches the inspired concentration determines the speed of onset of action of the anesthetic and correlates with the rapidity of induction of anesthesia. The rise in F_A/F_I is faster with agents that have a low blood:gas partition coefficient (eg, nitrous oxide, sevoflurane, desflurane). If the minute ventilation is high, as with overzealous manual or mechanical ventilation, an increased amount of anesthetic is brought to the alveoli. If cardiac output is low, as from hypovolemia, less anesthetic is carried away from the lungs and the blood becomes "saturated" with anesthetic more rapidly. As a result, the rise in F_A/F_I is faster, induction of anesthesia is more rapid, and unwanted side effects of anesthetics (such as hypotension) can be more profound under these conditions (**Figure 8.1**).

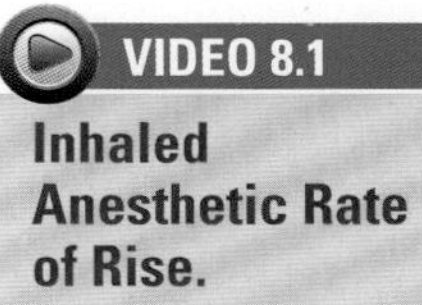

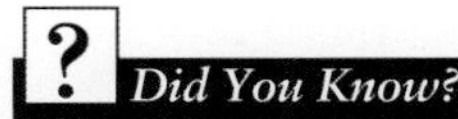

Sevoflurane (alone or in conjunction with nitrous oxide) is the most common agent used for inhalational induction in children.

B. Concentration Effect and Overpressurization

Concentration effect and overpressurization refer to two similar but distinct methods used to speed up the time needed for induction of anesthesia with an

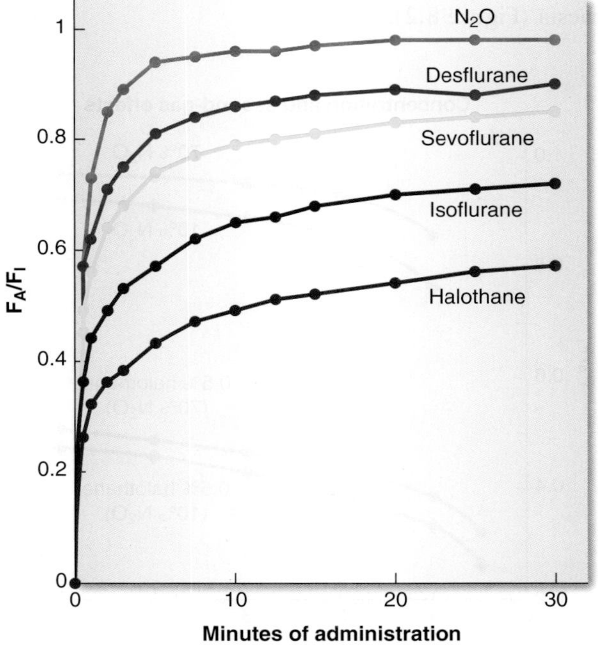

Figure 8.1 The increase in the alveolar anesthetic concentration (F_A) toward the inspired anesthetic concentration (F_I) is most rapid with the least-soluble anesthetics (nitrous oxide, desflurane, and sevoflurane) and intermediate with the more soluble anesthetics (isoflurane and halothane). After 10 to 15 minutes of administration (about three time constants), the slope of the curve decreases, reflecting saturation of vessel-rich group tissues and subsequent decreased uptake of the inhaled anesthetic. (Adapted from Manyam SC, Gupta DK, Johnson KB, et al. Opioid-volatile anesthetic synergy: a response surface model with remifentanil and sevoflurane as prototypes. *Anesthesiology.* 2006;105:267-278 and Inhaled anesthetics. In: Barash PB, Cullen BF, Stoelting RK, et al. *Handbook of Clinical Anesthesia.* 7th ed. Lippincott Williams & Wilkins; 2013:227-251.)

inhaled anesthetic (or an increase in depth of anesthesia during an anesthetic). The ***concentration effect*** refers to the fact that the higher the F_I of an inhaled anesthetic agent, the faster the rise in the F_A/F_I ratio. Uptake of a large volume of anesthetic by the blood causes an increase in alveolar ventilation, which in turn promotes a rapid rise of the F_A/F_I ratio. Although theoretically this applies to all inhaled anesthetics, practically it only has clinical relevance to nitrous oxide and xenon because they are delivered at relatively high concentrations. ***Overpressurization*** refers to the use of a higher F_I than the desired F_A for the patient to achieve a faster rise in the F_A/F_I ratio. Thus, one might use 8% inspired sevoflurane during induction of anesthesia in order to rapidly achieve the 2% alveolar sevoflurane concentration required for surgical anesthesia.

C. Second Gas Effect

The ***second gas effect*** is more of a theoretic than practical phenomenon. It occurs when an anesthetic in high concentration, the "second" gas (eg, nitrous oxide), is acutely added to an already inhaled low concentration, "first" gas (eg, sevoflurane). The initial, rapid uptake of a high volume of nitrous oxide (into the blood) concentrates the sevoflurane in the alveoli and results in a faster rise of the F_A/F_I ratio of sevoflurane. In addition, due to an uptake of large volumes of the nitrous oxide, the resulting replacement of that gas increases inspired ventilation, which also augments the concentration of sevoflurane present in the alveoli. In theory, but probably not clinically obvious, this speeds the induction of anesthesia or more rapidly deepens the level of existing anesthesia (**Figure 8.2**).

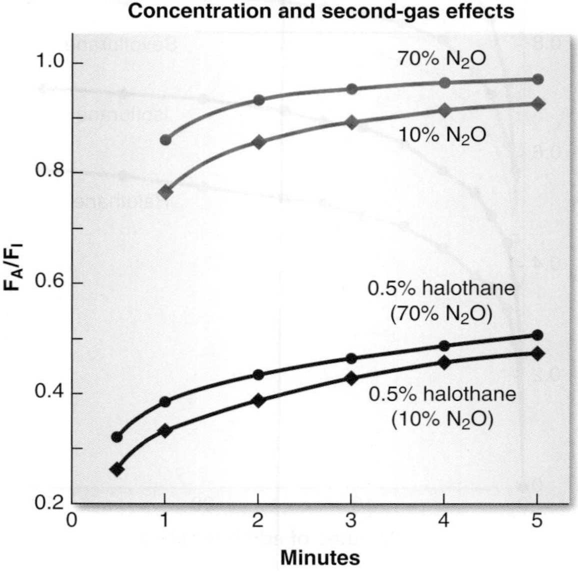

Figure 8.2 The concentration effect is demonstrated in the top half of the graph in which 70% nitrous oxide (N_2O) produces a more rapid increase in the alveolar anesthetic concentration (F_A)/inspired anesthetic concentration (F_I) ratio of N_2O than does administration of 10% N_2O. The second-gas effect is demonstrated in the lower lines in which the F_A/F_I ratio for halothane increases more rapidly when administered with 70% N_2O than with 10% N_2O. (From Inhaled anesthetics. In: Barash PB, Cullen BF, Stoelting RK, et al, eds. *Handbook of Clinical Anesthesia.* 7th ed. Lippincott Williams & Wilkins; 2013:227-251, Figure 17.3.)

Table 8.2 Tissue Groups and Their Perfusion

Group	Body Mass (%)	Cardiac Output (%)	Perfusion (mL/100 g/min)
Vessel rich	10	75	75
Muscle	50	19	3
Fat	20	6	3

D. Distribution

Inhaled anesthetics delivered to the alveoli diffuse into the blood and are distributed to various organs in accordance with the amount of blood flow to those organs (**Table 8.2**). The organs that will be exposed to the most anesthetic early will be in the vessel-rich group, such as the heart, lung, brain, and liver. These organs receive about 75% of the normal cardiac output. The second group of perfused tissues are in the muscle group (including skin) and take longer to become saturated with anesthetic. The least perfused tissues (such as fat) take the longest amount of time to become saturated with anesthetic. But they also take the longest amount of time to be rid of anesthetic when the surgical procedure is terminated. Theoretically, the anesthetic in fat could serve as a depot of anesthetic, which is slowly released back into the circulation and could prolong awakening. In reality, this is not a significant problem with modern anesthetics with low solubility in blood. The dose, duration of anesthetic, and solubility of the agent in various tissues are the primary determinants of the magnitude of this depot or reservoir.

E. Metabolism

Only a small proportion of modern inhaled anesthetics undergo metabolism. Most of the anesthetic is exhaled in an unchanged state (**Table 8.1**). The pharmacokinetic and pharmacodynamic properties of these anesthetics are not significantly affected by their metabolism. Metabolism of halogenated hydrocarbons anesthetics, such as sevoflurane or desflurane, in the liver may be a factor in rare cases of postanesthetic hepatotoxicity.

III. Neuropharmacology of Inhaled Anesthetics

As with other drugs, the clinical effects of inhaled anesthetics are dependent on the administered dose. However, because the concentration of gas in the blood is difficult to measure, the depth of inhaled anesthesia is generally expressed in terms of the more readily measured end-exhalation, or alveolar, concentration. Thus, a 1% alveolar concentration of sevoflurane is equivalent at 1 atmosphere (760 mm Hg) to a partial pressure of 7.6 mm Hg in the blood (and brain).

The concept of ***minimum alveolar concentration (MAC)*** is commonly used to compare the pharmacologic effects of one inhaled anesthetic to another. One MAC is the concentration of an inhaled anesthetic at which 50% of patients do not move in response to a standard surgical stimulation (such as a skin incision). Consequently, if only an inhaled anesthetic is used for a surgical procedure, then more than 1 MAC must be administered to ensure all patients are unresponsive. MAC values are additive. For example, 0.5 MAC of sevoflurane and 0.5 MAC of nitrous oxide is equivalent to 1 MAC. Similarly, concomitant administration of opioids and sedatives reduces MAC. Some of the many factors that may increase or decrease MAC are listed in **Table 8.3**.

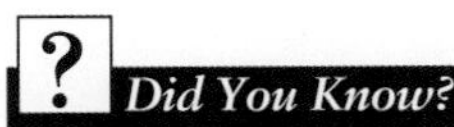

MAC values are more useful to compare potency of different inhaled anesthetic agents. Administering at least 0.7 MAC end-tidal concentration of inhaled anesthetics is needed for prevention of recall and intraoperative awareness.

Table 8.3 Factors That Influence Minimum Alveolar Concentration (MAC) of Inhaled Anesthetics

MAC increases with:
Chronic ethanol use
Hyperthermia
Hypernatremia
Monoamine oxidase inhibitors
Acute dextroamphetamine administration
Cocaine
Ephedrine
Levodopa
MAC decreases with:
Increasing age
Barbiturates
Benzodiazepines
Opioids
Ketamine/verapamil/lithium
Acute ethanol intoxication
Clonidine and dexmedetomidine
Hypothermia/hyponatremia
Pregnancy

All the newer inhaled anesthetics depress cerebral metabolic rate in a similar fashion, resulting in an isoelectric electroencephalogram. They usually produce a loss of consciousness and amnesia at relatively lower inspired concentrations (25%-35% of MAC), although there is considerable variation in sensitivity among individuals. There is controversy whether sevoflurane has any proconvulsant effects, and its use in patients with epilepsy is questioned. All the potent agents cause a dose-dependent increase in cerebral blood flow (**Figure 8.3**). Changes in intracranial pressure parallel the increase in cerebral blood flow at

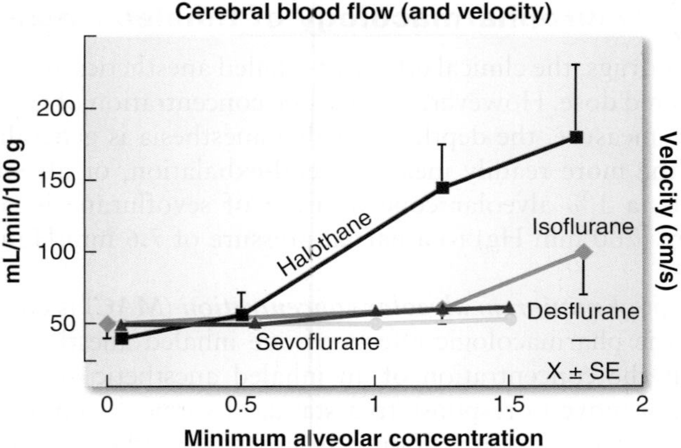

Figure 8.3 Cerebral blood flow (CBF) measured in the presence of normocapnia and in the absence of surgical stimulation in volunteers. At light levels of anesthesia, halothane (but not isoflurane, sevoflurane, or desflurane) increases CBF. Isoflurane increases CBF at 1.6 minimum alveolar concentration. (From Inhaled anesthetics. In: Barash PB, Cullen BF, Stoelting RK, et al, eds. *Handbook of Clinical Anesthesia.* 7th ed. Lippincott Williams & Wilkins; 2013:227-251, Figure 17.5.)

a dose of 1 MAC or above. Inhalation anesthetics offer some degree of cerebral protection from ischemic or hypoxic insults. However, conclusive evidence in humans for sevoflurane and desflurane is lacking. The effects of nitrous oxide on cerebral physiology are not very clear as its effects vary among different species. Nitrous oxide may even have antineuroprotective properties. All the inhaled anesthetics can produce a dose-dependent depression of sensory and motor-evoked potentials. Visual-evoked potentials are the most sensitive to the effects of volatile agents. There is increasing evidence that the inhalation anesthetics may be one of the main contributing factors for the development of short-term cognitive impairment following surgery, particularly in elderly adults.

IV. Cardiovascular Effects

Inhalation anesthetics produce dose-dependent myocardial depression and a decrease in systemic arterial blood pressure. The decrease in blood pressure is mainly due to a reduction of systemic vascular resistance. Heart rate is relatively unchanged by the inhaled anesthetics, although desflurane and to some extent isoflurane can cause sympathetic stimulation, leading to tachycardia and hypertension during induction or when the inspired concentration is abruptly increased (**Figure 8.4**). Nitrous oxide also causes some

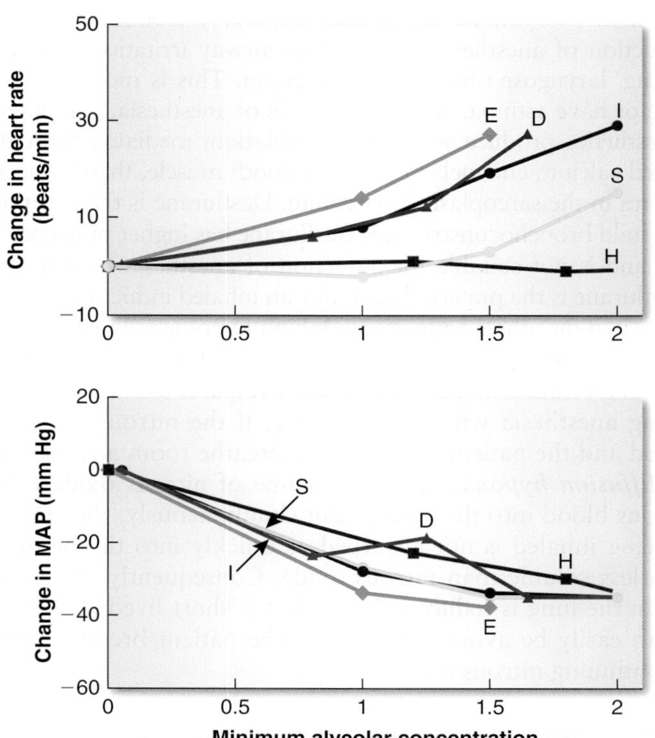

Figure 8.4 Heart rate and systemic blood pressure changes (from awake baseline) in volunteers receiving general anesthesia with a volatile anesthetic. Halothane and sevoflurane produced little change in heart rate at <1.5 minimum alveolar concentration. All anesthetics caused similar decreases in blood pressure. D, desflurane; E, enflurane; H, halothane; I, isoflurane; MAP, mean arterial pressure; S, sevoflurane. (From Inhaled anesthetics. In: Barash PB, Cullen BF, Stoelting RK, et al, eds. *Handbook of Clinical Anesthesia*. 7th ed. Lippincott Williams & Wilkins; 2013:227-251, with permission, Figure 17.6.)

increased sympathetic activity. Its direct cardiac depressive effects are neutralized by this increased sympathetic activity in healthy individuals. Unlike the outdated anesthetic halothane, the newer inhaled anesthetics (isoflurane, sevoflurane, desflurane) do not sensitize the myocardium to circulating catecholamines or predispose patients to dysrhythmias. Inhaled anesthetics are capable of providing myocardial protection against some ischemic and reperfusion injuries that last beyond the elimination of the anesthetic gases. Recent evidence suggests that some inhaled anesthetics, including xenon, also may offer protection against ischemic injury in the kidneys, liver, and brain.

V. Respiratory Effects

Inhaled anesthetics produce dose-dependent respiratory depression with a decrease in tidal volume that is completely compensated for by an increase in respiratory rate. The increase in arterial carbon dioxide partial pressure as a result of respiratory depression is somewhat offset by the stimulation of the attendant surgical procedure. All of the inhaled anesthetics produce a dose-dependent depression of the ventilatory response to hypercarbia and the chemoreceptor response to hypoxia, even at subanesthetic concentrations (as low as 0.1 MAC).

Inhalation of the volatile anesthetics (especially isoflurane and desflurane) during induction of anesthesia can produce airway irritation and may precipitate coughing, laryngospasm, or bronchospasm. This is more likely in patients who smoke or have asthma. At surgical levels of anesthesia, equipotent doses of inhaled anesthetics produce some bronchodilation, mediated through blocking voltage-gated calcium channels in airway smooth muscle, thereby decreasing the calcium stores in the sarcoplasmic reticulum. Desflurane is the exception, in that it produces mild bronchoconstriction. Desflurane has higher pungency than other anesthetics and is not suitable for induction of anesthesia by inhalation of gas alone. Sevoflurane is the preferred agent for an inhaled induction both in children and adults. All of the inhaled anesthetics inhibit hypoxic pulmonary vasoconstriction in animals, producing an intrapulmonary shunt, but their effects in humans during one lung ventilation may be less severe (**Figures 8.5** and **8.6**).

Following anesthesia with nitrous oxide, if the nitrous oxide is abruptly discontinued and the patient is allowed to breathe room air, there is a risk of transient ***diffusion hypoxia.*** A large volume of nitrous oxide diffuses from mixed venous blood into the alveoli. But simultaneously, the large volume of nitrogen being inhaled is not absorbed as quickly into the blood because it is so much less soluble than nitrous oxide. Consequently, the concentration of oxygen in the lung is reduced. This effect is short lived (2-3 minutes), and hypoxia can easily be avoided by having the patient breathe 100% oxygen when discontinuing nitrous oxide.

VI. Effects on Other Organ Systems

Inhaled anesthetics other than nitrous oxide directly relax skeletal muscles; this effect depends on the dose administered. They also potentiate the actions of nondepolarizing neuromuscular blocking drugs. All inhaled anesthetics other than nitrous oxide and xenon can precipitate malignant hyperthermia in susceptible patients.

All volatile inhaled anesthetics directly depress uterine muscle tone in a dose-dependent fashion similar to vascular smooth muscle. This can contribute to

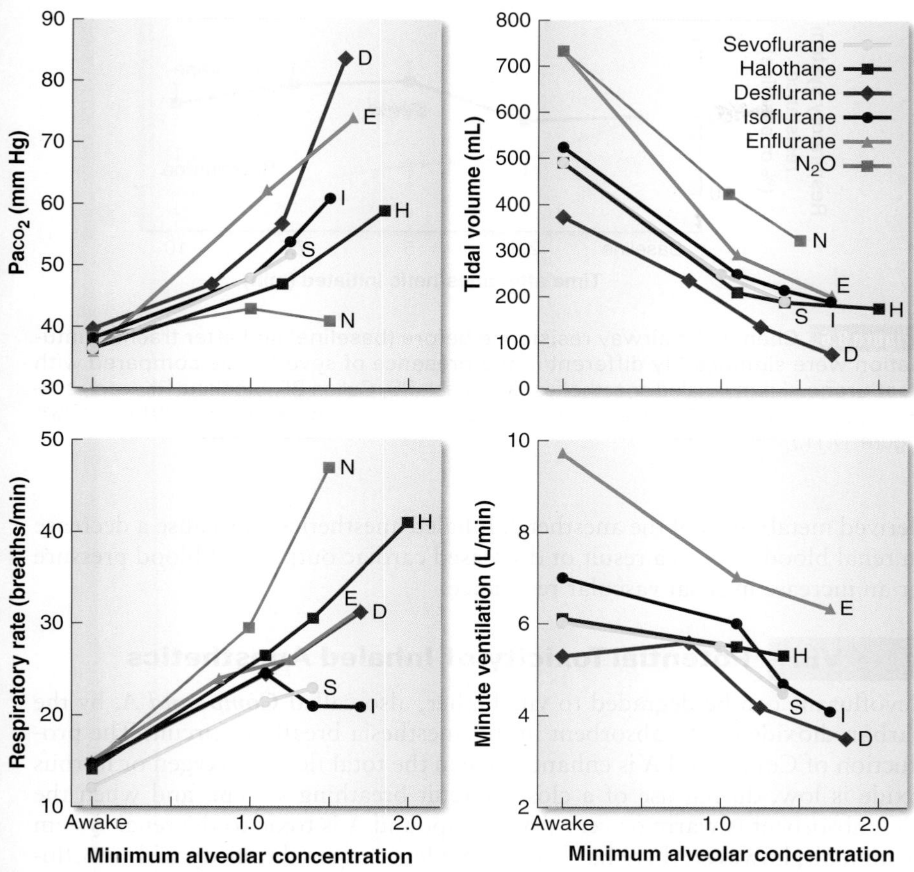

Figure 8.5 **Comparison of mean changes in resting arterial carbon dioxide partial pressure ($Paco_2$), tidal volume, respiratory rate, and minute ventilation in patients receiving an inhaled anesthetic. N_2O, nitrous oxide.** (Adapted from Lockhart SH, Rampil IJ, Yasuda N, et al. Depression of ventilation by desflurane in humans. *Anesthesiology.* 1991;74:484; Doi M, Ikeda K. Respiratory effects of sevoflurane. *Anesth Analg.* 1987;66:241; Fourcade HE, Stevens WC, Larson CP Jr, et al. The ventilatory effects of Forane, a new inhaled anesthetic. *Anesthesiology.* 1971;35:26; and Calverley RK, Smith NT, Jones CW, et al. Ventilatory and cardiovascular effects of enflurane anesthesia during spontaneous ventilation in man. *Anesth Analg.* 1978;57:610; Inhaled anesthetics. In: Barash PB, Cullen BF, Stoelting RK, et al, eds. *Handbook of Clinical Anesthesia.* 7th ed. Lippincott Williams & Wilkins; 2013:227-251.)

excessive uterine bleeding for women undergoing cesarean delivery or a therapeutic abortion, when the concentration of anesthetic exceeds 1 MAC. The anesthetic will also affect the newborn infant in terms of wakefulness, but the effect is short lived. It is common practice to administer lower concentrations of inhaled anesthetics (0.5-0.75 MAC) along with nitrous oxide when general anesthesia is necessary for cesarean delivery. In contrast, the uterine relaxant effects of volatile anesthetics may be desirable in patients with a retained placenta.

Some older inhaled anesthetics are known to decrease liver blood flow. However, the new ether-based anesthetics (isoflurane, desflurane, sevoflurane) maintain or increase hepatic artery blood flow while decreasing or not changing portal vein blood flow. Rarely, patients may develop hepatitis secondary to exposure of an inhaled anesthetic, most notably from halothane (halothane hepatitis), which is an immune-mediated reaction to oxidatively

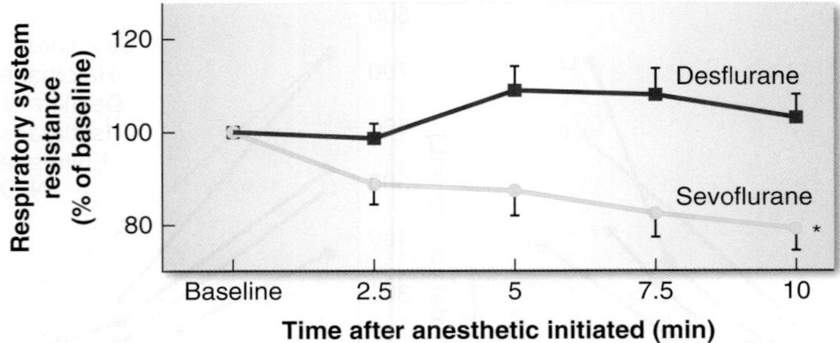

Figure 8.6 **Changes in airway resistance before (baseline) and after tracheal ntubation were significantly different in the presence of sevoflurane compared with desflurane.** (From Inhaled anesthetics. In: Barash PB, Cullen BF, Stoelting RK, et al, eds. *Handbook of Clinical Anesthesia*. 7th ed. Lippincott Williams & Wilkins; 2013:227-251, Figure 17.11.)

derived metabolites of the anesthetic. Inhaled anesthetics may cause a decrease in renal blood flow as a result of decreased cardiac output and blood pressure or an increase in renal vascular resistance.

VII. Potential Toxicity of Inhaled Anesthetics

Sevoflurane can be degraded to vinyl ether, also called ***Compound A***, by the carbon dioxide (CO_2) absorbent in the anesthesia breathing circuit. The production of Compound A is enhanced when the total flow of oxygen or nitrous oxide is low, during use of a closed-circuit breathing system, and when the CO_2 absorbent is warm or very dry. Compound A is toxic to the renal system of animals; however, there has been no evidence of renal toxicity with sevoflurane usage in humans. **Figure 8.7** shows the extent to which Compound A is produced with various CO_2 absorbents.

Desflurane can be degraded to carbon monoxide by CO_2 absorbents. This is most likely when the absorbent is new or dry (water content <5%) and when the absorbent contains barium.

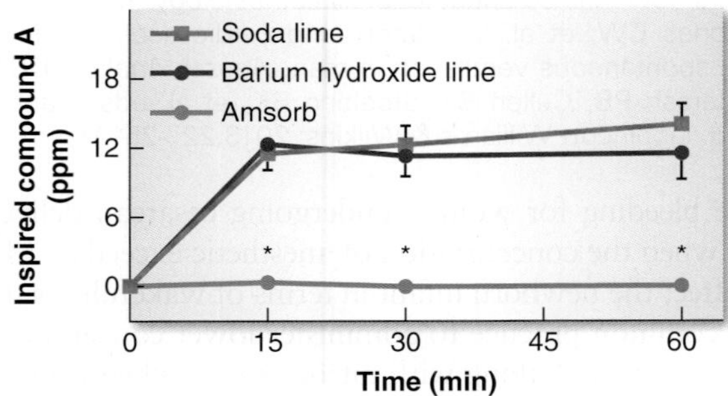

Figure 8.7 **Compound A levels produced from three carbon dioxide absorbents during 1 minimum alveolar concentration sevoflurane anesthesia delivered at a fresh gas flow of 1 L/min (mean ± SE). *Asterisk* indicates $P < .05$ versus soda lime and barium hydroxide lime.** (Adapted from Mchaourab A, Arain SR, Ebert TJ. Lack of degradation of sevoflurane by a new carbon dioxide absorbent in humans. *Anesthesiology*. 2001;94:1007 and Inhaled anesthetics. In: Barash PB, Cullen BF, Stoelting RK, et al, eds. *Handbook of Clinical Anesthesia*. 7th ed. Lippincott Williams & Wilkins; 2013:227-251.)

All the modern volatile anesthetics contain fluoride. This was a problem for older anesthetics, such as methoxyflurane, because metabolism of the drug to a free fluoride ion caused renal toxicity. However, the newer anesthetics undergo limited metabolism, and fluoride-induced renal toxicity has not been demonstrated.

Did You Know?

Inhaled anesthetics and nitrous oxide are greenhouse gases. Nitrous oxide is also destructive to the ozone layer. The global warming potential (GWP) of desflurane is the highest, followed by isoflurane. Sevoflurane has the least GWP. Xenon has none.

VIII. The Nonvolatile Anesthetics

The unique analgesic properties of nitrous oxide and xenon are mediated through inhibition of NMDA receptors. Through the same mechanism, these agents can also produce excitement and euphoria, hence they have a potential for abuse. Given their actions on NMDA receptors, they have been shown to have both neuroprotective as well as neurotoxic effects in animal models.

A. Nitrous Oxide

For many reasons, the clinical use of nitrous oxide is on the decline. First, because it is relatively weak (the MAC is 105%), it cannot be used as the sole anesthetic agent. Second, it can readily diffuse into closed air spaces such as the middle ear, bowel, cranial air sinuses, a pneumoperitoneum (eg, during laparoscopic procedures), a pneumothorax, and gas bubbles inserted during ocular surgery. This can result in either an increase in volume of the space (eg, distension of bowel) or an increase in pressure (eg, in the eye or middle ear). Third, it is associated with a high incidence of PONV when it is used for longer than 1 hour. Fourth, due to its interference with folate metabolism, it has the potential for toxic effects on the developing embryo. Nitrous oxide oxidizes the cobalt atom on vitamin B_{12}, thereby irreversibly inhibiting the B_{12}-dependent enzyme ***methionine synthetase*** and resulting in elevated levels of homocystine. This end product leads to endothelial dysfunction and oxidative stress and destabilizes arterial plaque. Prolonged administration of nitrous oxide, as for sedation in the intensive care unit, is associated with severe anemia. Finally, nitrous oxide, like CO_2, causes ozone depletion in the upper atmosphere. Despite the declining use of nitrous oxide intraoperatively, the administration of a 50:50 mixture of oxygen and nitrous oxide (Entonox) remains useful for brief analgesia in pediatric dentistry, labor analgesia, burn dressing changes, and related procedures.

Did You Know?

All volatile anesthetic agents increase the incidence of postoperative nausea and vomiting (PONV) and the risk increases with the duration of exposure to the anesthetic. They should be avoided in patients at high risk of PONV.

B. Xenon

Xenon is a rare noble gas occurring naturally in air at 0.05 parts per million. Recently, there has been renewed interest in the use of xenon as an anesthetic gas. Xenon has several advantages when compared with not only nitrous oxide but also the potent volatile anesthetics. Xenon has rapid onset and offset of action due to its extremely low blood:gas partition coefficient (**Table 8.1**). Its effects on cardiovascular, neuronal, and respiratory systems are minimal, and it is not a trigger for malignant hyperthermia. Xenon also can be used in low concentrations for analgesia. This action is mediated through inhibition of *N*-methyl-D-aspartate receptors in the central nervous system. The only limitation to routine use of xenon is its cost. The gas exists at very low concentrations in our atmosphere, and there is a high cost associated with its extraction and recycling. New anesthetic systems are being developed that will allow use of xenon in small volumes and will recycle the gas after it is exhaled.

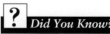

Did You Know?

Shutting off the fresh gas flows (rather than shutting off the vaporizer) during intubation or airway instrumentation is the best approach to prevent operating room pollution with anesthetic gases and reduce wastage.

IX. Clinical Use of Inhaled Anesthetics

Due to a lack of pungency and a low blood:gas partition coefficient, sevoflurane is the agent of choice for an inhaled induction of anesthesia in both children and adults, such as when intravenous access is not possible or desirable. Inhaled anesthetics remain the most popular drugs for maintenance of anesthesia during surgery as they are easy to administer and the dose can be easily titrated in response to highly variable surgical stimuli. Despite their popularity, inhaled anesthetics have some significant drawbacks. These can include profound respiratory depression, hypotension, lack of analgesia at low concentrations, PONV, the potential for triggering malignant hyperthermia in susceptible individuals, and rare toxicity such as hepatitis. The volatile anesthetics also interfere with monitoring of sensory-evoked potentials when administered in doses of more than 0.5 MAC. Nevertheless, despite these drawbacks, when inhaled anesthetics are administered for surgical procedures by appropriately trained specialists, the morbidity and mortality from general anesthesia are remarkably low.

All inhaled anesthetics including nitrous oxide and xenon contribute to postoperative nausea and vomiting (PONV). General anesthesia increases the risk of PONV significantly when compared to regional anesthetic techniques. The incidence of PONV is between 25% to 30% following surgery when general anesthesia is maintained using inhalational agents along with narcotics. However, when propofol is substituted for inhalational agents, the relative risk of PONV is reduced to 19%. Using air as a carrier gas in place of nitrous oxide reduces the relative risk by 12%.

In surgical patients, postoperative immunocompromise is primarily related to the neuroendocrine stress response to surgery, secondary to the activation of the autonomic nervous system and the hypothalamic-pituitary-adrenal axis. The literature concerning the immunomodulatory effects of inhalational anesthetics is somewhat contradictory, but the majority of data suggest that these agents may have immunosuppressive properties. Inhalational anesthetics reduce the production of radical oxygen species (ROS) from neutrophils, which may result in decreased potency in killing bacteria.

For further review and interactivities, please see the associated Interactive Video Lectures and "At a Glance" infographic accessible in the complimentary eBook bundled with this text. Access instructions are located in the inside front cover.

Suggested Readings

1. Becker DE, Rosenberg M. Nitrous oxide and the inhalation anesthetics. *Anesth Prog.* 2008;55(4):124-132. PMID: 19108597.
2. Derwall M, Coburn M, Rex S, et al. Xenon: recent developments and future perspectives. *Minerva Anestesiol.* 2009;75(1-2):37-45. PMID: 18475253.
3. de Vasconcellos K, Sneyd JR. Nitrous oxide: are we still in equipoise? A qualitative review of current controversies. *Br J Anaesth.* 2013;111(6):877-885 PMID: 23801743.
4. Eger II EI. The pharmacology of isoflurane. *Br J Anaesth.* 1984;56(suppl 1):71S-99S. PMID: 6391530.
5. Eger II EI. New inhalational agents—desflurane and sevoflurane. *Can J Anaesth.* 1993;40(5 pt 2):R3-R8. PMID: 8500211.
6. Eger II EI. Age, minimum alveolar anesthetic concentration, and minimum alveolar anesthetic concentration-awake. *Anesth Analg.* 2001;93(4):947-953. PMID: 11574362.
7. Harris PD, Barnes R. The uses of helium and xenon in current clinical practice. *Anaesthesia.* 2008;63(3):284-293. PMID: 18289236.

8. Hirota K. Special cases: ketamine, nitrous oxide and xenon. *Best Pract Res Clin Anaesthesiol.* 2006;20(1):69-79. PMID: 16634415.
9. Jones RM. Desflurane and sevoflurane: inhalation anaesthetics for this decade? *Br J Anaesth.* 1990;65(4):527-536 PMID: 2248821.
10. Kharasch ED. Biotransformation of sevoflurane. *Anesth Analg.* 1995;81(6 suppl):S27-S38. PMID: 7486145.
11. Leighton KM, Koth B. Some aspects of the clinical pharmacology of nitrous oxide. *Can Anaesth Soc J.* 1973;20(1):94-103. PMID: 4571205.
12. Sanders RD, Franks NP, Maze M. Xenon: no stranger to anaesthesia. *Br J Anaesth.* 2003;91(5):709-717. PMID: 14570795.
13. Smith I. Nitrous oxide in ambulatory anaesthesia: does it have a place in day surgical anaesthesia or is it just a threat for personnel and the global environment? *Curr Opin Anaesthesiol.* 2006;19(6):592-596. PMID: 17093360.
14. Smith WD. Pharmacology of nitrous oxide. *Int Anesthesiol Clin.* 1971;9(3):91-123. PMID: 4951009.

Inhaled Anesthetics

AT A GLANCE

Volatile anesthetics are halogenated hydrocarbons. The intended "dose" of these drugs is measured and administered as a percent of inspired gases. As patients inhale them, five factors have significant impact on the speed with which the brain equilibrates to the desired steady state partial pressure of the drug:

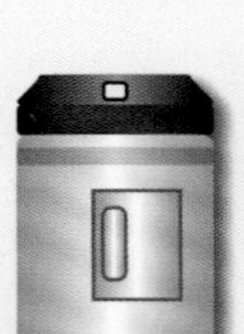

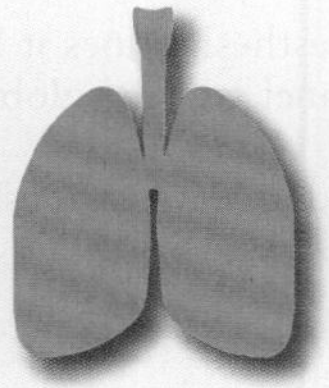

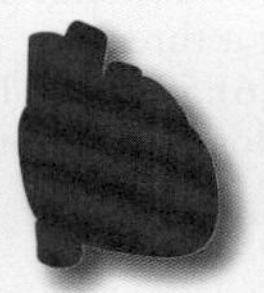

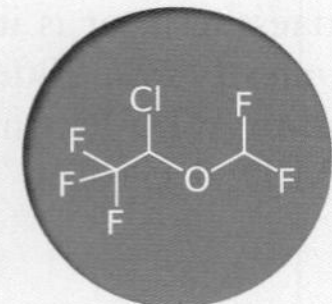

Dialed concentration

The higher the dialed concentration is set on the anesthetic vaporizer, the larger the concentration gradient between the vaporizer and the circuit. This promotes a hastened rise to the desired target dose of inhaled agent.

Fresh gas flow rate

The higher the fresh gas flow rate, the faster the volatile anesthetic equilibrates between the vaporizer and the anesthesia breathing circuit.

Alveolar ventilation

The higher the alveolar ventilation, the faster the patient will equilibrate volatile anesthetic between the anesthesia breathing circuit and the lungs.

Cardiac output

When cardiac output is low, less anesthetic is taken up into circulation which allows the lungs to fully equilibrate with the delivered partial pressure of anesthetic. If the lungs reach steady state, the drug rapidly transfers into circulation and hence the brain.

Physicochemical properties of drug

The less lipid soluble the drug, the less likely it will dissolve into tissues. Thus, it will more rapidly attain a partial pressure equilibrium. For this reason the least lipid soluble drugs like desflurane reach steady state the fastest.

Since young children will not tolerate IV placement, induction of anesthesia is performed by mask inhalation. Sevoflurane is the agent of choice for this since it lacks pungency and is relatively insoluble leading to rapid induction.

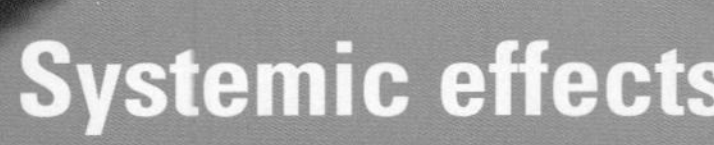

Systemic effects

Central Nervous System

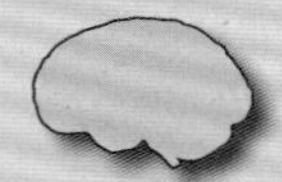

CNS depression

↓ Cerebral O_2 consumption

↑ Cerebral blood flow

↑ Intracranial pressure

Anticonvulsant that can achieve burst suppression on EEG

Cardiovascular System

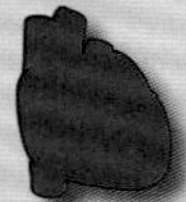

Hypotension results from:

↓ Vascular resistance

↓ Stroke volume

↓ Cardiac output

↓ Baroreceptor response

Heart rate is often unchanged*

*Desflurane may cause tachycardia when its concentration is increased rapidly.

Respiratory System

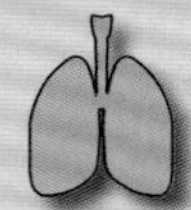

Apnea at higher doses

↓ Tidal volumes

↑ Respiratory rate

↓ Response to hypoxia

↓ Response to hypercarbia

Bronchodilation (sevoflurane)

Bronchoconstriction (desflurane and isoflurane during inhaled induction)

Infographic by: Naveen Nathan MD

Questions

1. **All of the following inhaled anesthetics must be administered using an agent-specific calibrated vaporizer EXCEPT:**

   A. Xenon
   B. Isoflurane
   C. Sevoflurane
   D. Desflurane

2. **Which of the following properties of inhaled anesthetics is the primary determinant of the rapidity with which it can induce anesthesia?**

   A. The vapor pressure at room temperature
   B. The oil:gas partition coefficient
   C. The blood:gas partition coefficient
   D. The minimum alveolar concentration (MAC)

3. **The rate at which the alveolar concentration (F_A) of an inhaled anesthetic approaches that being inspired (F_I) is most rapid under which of the following conditions:**

   A. Increased blood pressure
   B. Increased cardiac output
   C. Increased ventilation
   D. Increased body fat

4. **Which of the following organs or tissue groups has the LEAST effect in determining the rapidity of induction with an inhaled anesthetic?**

   A. Skeletal muscle
   B. Skin
   C. Liver and kidney
   D. Fat

5. **The minimum alveolar concentration (MAC) of an inhaled anesthetic is the concentration necessary to:**

   A. Produce adequate anesthesia for minor surgical procedures (eg, tonsillectomy)
   B. Produce adequate anesthesia for all surgical procedures
   C. Produce analgesia without a loss of consciousness
   D. Prevent movement in response to a skin incision in 50% of patients

6. **All of the following are decreased during general anesthesia with sevoflurane EXCEPT:**

   A. Myocardial contractility
   B. Systemic vascular resistance
   C. Cerebral blood flow
   D. Minute ventilation

7. **A patient with a long history of smoking and asthma requires an inhaled induction of anesthesia. The preferred anesthetic is:**

   A. Nitrous oxide
   B. Sevoflurane
   C. Desflurane
   D. Isoflurane

8. **A spontaneously breathing anesthetized patient becomes accidently disconnected from the anesthetic circuit and breathes room air. A fall in oxygen saturation measured with a pulse oximeter is most likely to occur most rapidly when the anesthetic is:**

   A. 8.0% desflurane
   B. 1.2% isoflurane
   C. 2.5% sevoflurane
   D. 75% nitrous oxide

9. **Anesthesia with isoflurane, as opposed to a combination of nitrous oxide and opioids, is most likely to contribute to excessive bleeding during which of the following procedures:**

   A. Cesarean delivery
   B. Resection of an intracranial meningioma
   C. Transurethral prostatectomy
   D. Repair of a femoral artery laceration

10. **What is the primary reason why xenon is NOT routinely used for general anesthesia?**

    A. It cannot be used as the sole anesthetic (MAC is too high).
    B. It has a high blood:gas partition coefficient.
    C. It has a metabolite that is potentially nephrotoxic.
    D. High cost

Answers

1. A

Xenon is a gas that is stored in a tank and does not require vaporization.

2. C

Inhaled anesthetics that have low solubility in blood can induce anesthesia most rapidly, as well as allow rapid awakening from anesthesia.

3. C

Induction of anesthesia with inhaled anesthetics (rate of rise of F_A relative to F_I) is increased by an increase in alveolar ventilation. It is slower when cardiac output is high. It is relatively unaffected by blood pressure or obesity.

4. A

Because blood flow to fat is a small fraction of total cardiac output, it does not play a significant role in determining the rate of induction with inhaled anesthetics.

5. D

MAC is a tool for comparison of potency of inhaled anesthetics. It is determined in patients by measuring the alveolar concentration of anesthetic required to prevent movement in response to a skin incision in 50% of patients. Patients are unconscious at 1 MAC but not adequately anesthetized for surgery.

6. C

All of the volatile inhaled anesthetics increase cerebral blood flow despite a modest reduction in blood pressure and cardiac output.

7. B

Sevoflurane causes minimal irritation of the upper respiratory tract. Nitrous oxide is not a complete anesthetic. Induction with desflurane and isoflurane is commonly associated with coughing and laryngospasm.

8. D

Abrupt discontinuation of nitrous oxide and inhalation of air can cause diffusion hypoxia. Alveolar oxygen is diluted by an effusion of nitrous oxide into the alveoli from the blood and inhalation of a high concentration of nitrogen.

9. A

All of the volatile anesthetics produce relaxation of uterine muscle. Contraction of the uterus is necessary to control bleeding following delivery of an infant.

10. D

Xenon has many properties of the ideal anesthetic (such as high potency, rapid onset of action, few side effects, no metabolites). However, because it must be extracted from the atmosphere, it is extremely expensive.

9 Intravenous Anesthetics and Sedatives

Jessica R. Black and Sara E. Meitzen

The use of intravenous (IV) anesthetic agents has progressed from the rapid induction of anesthesia to total IV anesthesia (TIVA). TIVA has, in several institutions, it has become the anesthetic of choice for maintenance of anesthesia.

All IV anesthetics are sedative-hypnotics that have the capacity to produce a drug-induced continuum of decreasing consciousness ranging from anxiolysis to general anesthesia. For less invasive procedures, monitored anesthesia care (MAC) is maintained using lower dosages of IV anesthetics. Higher dosages are used to induce general anesthesia and TIVA.

Our current repertoire of IV anesthetics are derived from a variety of pharmacologic drug groups. None are perfect, though each drug combines many of the characteristics of the ideal IV anesthetic: fast-onset, hemodynamic stability, hypnosis, amnesia, analgesia, and rapid recovery. For some IV anesthetics, notable untoward side effects have led to more specific indications (eg, ketamine, etomidate). Today, propofol is by far the most popular and widely used IV anesthetic.

All IV anesthetics are lipophilic and thus have high affinity for lipophilic tissues (brain, spinal cord), which accounts for their rapid onset. As the medication arrives at the effect site and binds to its target receptors (its mechanism of action), the onset of sedation begins. After the drug produces its pharmacodynamic (PD) effect, the body then gets rid of the drug via its pharmacokinetic profile. Regardless of how fast the drug is metabolized, the termination effect of a single induction bolus dose is due to redistribution from highly perfused lipophilic areas into less perfused areas such as skeletal muscle and fat. Consequently, all induction doses of IV anesthetics have a comparable duration of action despite substantial differences in their metabolism.

I. General Pharmacology of IV Anesthetics

A. Mechanism of Action

The most commonly used IV anesthetic agents—the barbiturates, propofol, the benzodiazepines, and etomidate—all act at the site of the gamma aminobutyric acid type A ($GABA_A$) receptor, as shown schematically in **Figure 9.1**. GABA is the main inhibitory neurotransmitter within the central nervous system, and its action at the $GABA_A$ receptor causes increased transport of

> **? *Did You Know?***
>
> GABA is the main inhibitory neurotransmitter within the central nervous system. Its action at the $GABA_A$ receptor causes increased transport of chloride (Cl^-) ions across the membrane, causing it to become hyperpolarized.

chloride (Cl^-) ions across the membrane and into the postsynaptic neuron. The postsynaptic neuron becomes hyperpolarized, which functionally inhibits further propagation of nerve signals. The $GABA_A$ receptor is therefore a ligand-activated ion channel. It is heterogeneously composed of five subunits. IV anesthetics that bind to the $GABA_A$ receptor do not bind at the same location as GABA itself (the orthosteric binding site)—instead, they bind at other locations (allosteric sites) and change the effect of GABA upon the receptor.

These IV anesthetics are therefore positive allosteric modulators of the $GABA_A$ receptor and cause conformational changes in the receptor such that the action of GABA itself is potentiated and sedation occurs. The subunit composition of $GABA_A$ receptors can vary: there are 19 different possible subunits arising from eight different subunit classes (α_{1-6}, β_{1-3}, γ_{1-3}, δ, ε, θ, π, and ρ_{1-3}).

IV anesthetic agents may only be active at receptors expressing certain combinations: the benzodiazepine allosteric binding site occurs only at the interface of α and γ_2 subunits, and etomidate is active primarily at $GABA_A$ receptors that contain β_2 or β_3 subunits.

Unlike the others, ketamine does not interact with GABA receptors. Instead, it principally binds and blockades *N*-methyl-D-aspartate (NMDA) glutamate receptors. The NMDA receptor is an excitatory receptor found throughout the CNS, including areas in the spinal cord, thalamolimbic system, and nucleus tractus solitarius (NTS). Glutamate, the most prominent excitatory neurotransmitter within the CNS, binds to the receptor and (among many other functions) transduces signals for pain, associates sensory signals between the thalamus and cortex, and causes global excitation. Ketamine causes analgesia by blocking the pain signal at the spinal cord and by "disassociating" the communication of pain between the thalamus and limbic system. This state of "dissociative amnesia" causes the patient

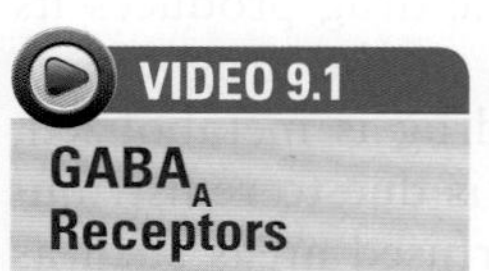

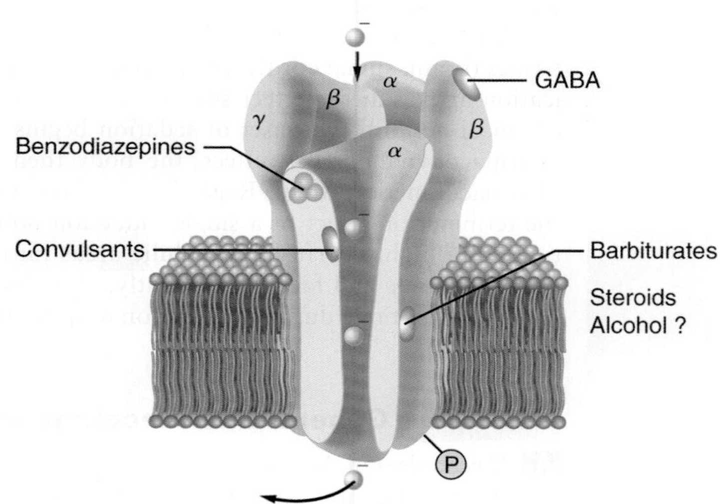

Figure 9.1 Schematic model of the gamma aminobutyric acid type A ($GABA_A$) receptor complex illustrating recognition sites for many of the substances that bind to the receptor (?, secondary to the fact that the actual binding site of alcohol is still questionable.).

to appear conscious (eyes open, staring) but unresponsive to sensory input (pain, questioning).

Ketamine also causes catecholamine release, though the mechanism of action is complex. It is theorized that ketamine blocks the NMDA receptors within the NTS preventing inhibition of the vasomotor center, resulting in a positive release of catecholamines. In isolation, ketamine is a direct myocardial depressant, but secondary to the indirect release of catecholamines, it acts as a cardiac stimulant, causing increased blood pressure, heart rate, and cardiac output. Some caution is required in patients with preexisting sympathetic blockade, such as those with spinal cord lesions, or those with exhaustion of their catecholamine stores, such as patients with shock trauma, for they will not produce these indirect cardiac stimulatory effects. Ketamine also blockades nicotinic, muscarinic, monoaminergic, sodium, calcium, and even kappa opioid receptors. The inhibition of sodium channels provides a modest local anesthetic action, while blockade of calcium channels causes vasodilation.

Dexmedetomidine is an α_2-adrenergic receptor agonist with a high ratio of specificity for the α_2 versus the α_1 receptor at 1600:1. Clonidine, an antihypertensive drug in the same category, exhibits a specificity ratio of 200:1. α_2 receptors are located presynaptically and centrally in the locus ceruleus, an area of the brain responsible for arousal and sympathetic activity. α_2 receptors are inhibitory receptors and, when activated, decrease downstream neurotransmitter release. For sympathetic nerves, this results in less catecholamine release, which causes decreased blood pressure and heart rate. α_2 receptors are also located on axons in the spinal cord involved in pain transmission. When activated, nociceptive transmission is decreased and the perception of pain is attenuated. Activating α_2 receptors in the locus ceruleus cause sedation and decreased sympathetic activity.

B. Pharmacokinetics and Metabolism

Pharmacokinetics, in its simplest terms, can be defined as "what the body does to the drug." Its literal meaning also brings light to its definition "the movement of drug in the body." This movement can be broken into three processes: absorption, distribution, and elimination. All IV anesthetics are lipophilic and, thus when injected, are rapidly absorbed. The prompt sedating effect of IV anesthetics can be attributed to their high lipid profile and the high proportion of cardiac output (20%) that goes to the brain.

The distribution and elimination of IV anesthetic medications within the body can be closely approximated with a simplified three-compartment model of the body. In this model, medications are administered into a first well-mixed central compartment (the brain). Diffusion occurs back and forth between this first compartment and the additional second and third peripheral compartments (muscle, fat). The diffusion constants (shown as k in **Figure 9.2**) are such that one peripheral compartment equilibrates quickly with the central compartment and the other equilibrates more slowly. The drug is not pharmacologically active in these peripheral compartments: instead, they act as reservoirs into which medications are redistributed and sequestered. These peripheral compartments model the way in which the action of the medication may be terminated by redistribution, and also the way in which accumulation of medication within these peripheral compartments can lead to progressively increasing context-sensitive half-times as medication diffuses back into the central compartment. An effect site

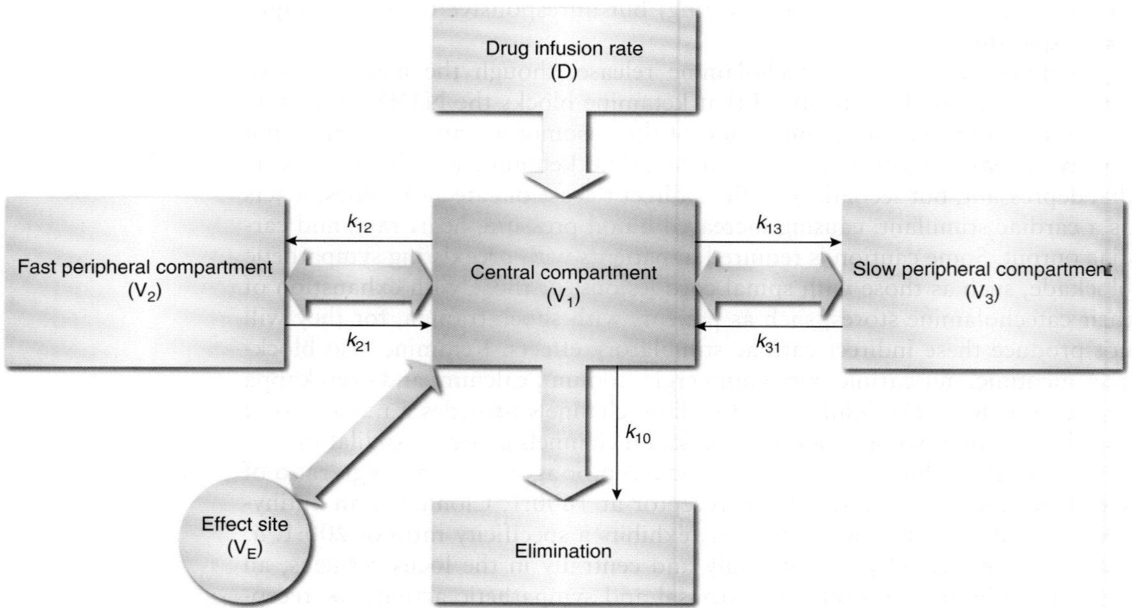

Figure 9.2 Three-compartment model for the pharmacokinetic modeling of intravenous medication administration, redistribution, and elimination. Additionally, an effect site compartment is present. The volume of this compartment is assumed to be sufficiently small that the effect on the quantity of medication in the central compartment is negligible.

compartment models the receptor population at which the medication has its mechanism of action. Diffusion also occurs between the central compartment and the effect site compartment, but because the quantity of drug bound to receptors at any given moment is tiny compared to the total quantity of medication in the body, the effect site compartment is assumed to be sufficiently small that its effect on the mass of medication within the central compartment is negligible.

After distribution, the main form of elimination for IV anesthetics is through hepatic metabolism. IV anesthetics will undergo hepatic enzymatic breakdown via phase I cytochrome P450 (CYP) or phase II glucuronidation. These water-soluble metabolites are then renally excreted. Some metabolites still exhibit pharmacological activity (eg, norketamine).

Although each IV anesthetic travels through similar pathways of absorption, distribution, and elimination, the trajectory is not exact and individual variability exists. Considerations include the amount of protein binding, hepatic function, renal function, preexisting diseases, age, the type of surgery (eg, laparoscopic), body temperature, and drug interactions.

C. Pharmacodynamic Effects

Pharmacodynamics (PD), in its simplest terms, is defined as "what the drug does to the body." Perhaps, a better definition is the relationship between drug concentration in the body and any resulting effects, whether therapeutic or adverse.

Particularly important PD parameters include efficacy (activity) and potency (affinity). Efficacy is defined as the maximum effect that a drug

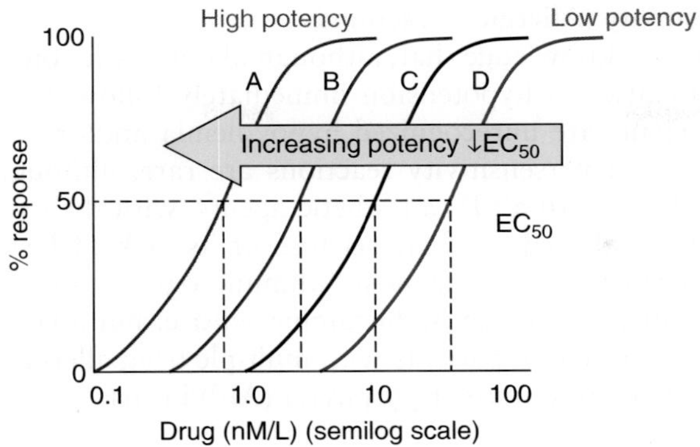

Figure 9.3 Graphical representation of the dose-response curves for a series of drugs (A, B, C, and D) that have the same efficacy but differ in terms of their potency. The most potent drug (drug A) has the lowest EC_{50} value.

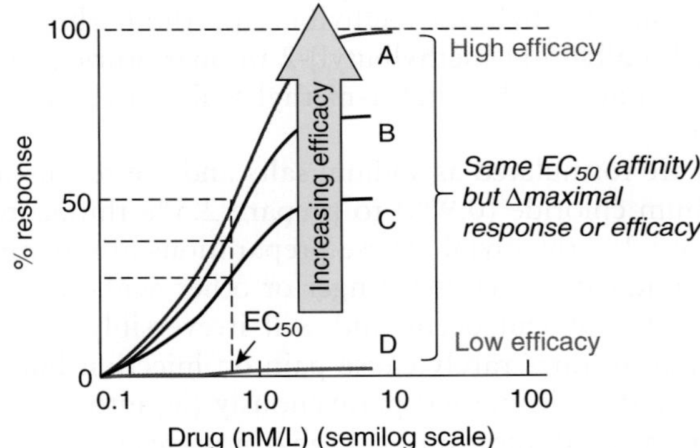

Figure 9.4 Dose-response relationships for four drugs that differ in efficacy. Each drug has essentially the same EC_{50} value (equipotent) but differ in terms of the maximum response they can produce.

can produce regardless of dose, whereas potency is the amount of drug required to produce a given effect. If the drug has low affinity for its receptor, potency will be decreased. A drug may have very high efficacy once bound to its receptor, but if the drug has little affinity, a large dose of medication will be required before maximum efficacy is met. This drug would have little potency despite having high efficacy. On the contrary, a drug may have very little effect once it binds to its receptor but is able to meet its maximum efficacy quickly due to high affinity for its binding site. This drug, although highly potent, would have little efficacy (**Figures 9.3** and **9.4**). The EC_{50} is the concentration or dose of drug that produces 50% of maximum effect. The lower the EC_{50}, the more potent the drug. The EC_{50} can be used to determine the range of target concentrations necessary for effective therapy (ie, the therapeutic window).[1] The therapeutic index is the measurement of the relative safety of a drug. All IV anesthetics have low therapeutic indices—a close margin between the concentration of a drug that is therapeutic versus the concentration that is deadly, and this is why a provider specifically trained in administering these medications is crucial to the safety of the patient.

D. Hypersensitivity (Allergic) Reactions

It is important to acknowledge that, although allergic reactions can occur, the most common causes of hypotension immediately following induction with IV anesthetic agents are unrecognized hypovolemia and/or unexpected drug interactions. True hypersensitivity reactions are rare, although case reports of histamine release with all IV anesthetic agents, with the exception of etomidate, have been alleged. In fact, because of its lack of histamine release, etomidate is considered to be the most "immunologically safe" IV anesthetic. Propofol does not normally cause histamine release, but anaphylactoid reactions have been reported in patients with multiple drug allergies. Barbiturates can precipitate acute intermittent porphyria (AIP) in susceptible patients.

II. Comparative Physiochemical and Clinical Pharmacologic Properties

A. Barbiturates

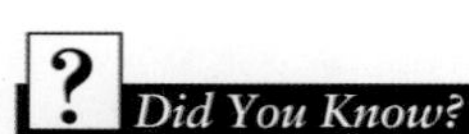

Commonly used intravenous anesthetic agents such as the barbiturates, propofol, benzodiazepines, and etomidate act at the site of the $GABA_A$ receptor.

The most commonly used barbiturates are the thiobarbiturates—thiopental (Pentothal, 5-ethyl-5-[1-methylbutyl]-2-thiobarbituric acid) and thiamylal (Surital, 5-allyl-5-[1-methylbutyl]-2-thiobarbituric acid)—and the oxybarbiturate—methohexital (Brevital, 1-methyl-5-allyl-5-[1-methyl-2-pentanyl] barbituric acid).

Barbiturates are formulated as sodium salts and are reconstituted in water or isotonic sodium chloride (0.9%) to prepare 2.5% thiopental, 1% to 2% methohexital, and 2% thiamylal. These preparations are highly alkaline (pH 9-10), and when added to lactated Ringer or other acidic drug preparations, crystalline precipitation will occur and will irreversibly occlude IV tubing and catheters. Barbiturates rarely cause pain on injection but will cause significant tissue irritation if injected paravenously (ie, into an infiltrated line). Inadvertent intra-arterial injection of thiobarbiturates causes serious complications: crystal formation causing intense vasoconstriction, thrombosis, and tissue necrosis. Immediate treatment includes intra-arterial papaverine and lidocaine or procaine, regional anesthesia–induced sympathectomy (stellate ganglion block, brachial plexus block), and heparinization.

Barbiturates depress the reticular activating system in the brain stem, a center of consciousness control, and are believed to potentiate the action of $GABA_A$ receptors, increasing the duration of an associated chloride ion channel opening. They decrease cerebral metabolic rate of oxygen ($CMRO_2$), cerebral blood flow (CBF), and intracranial pressure (ICP). They can induce an isoelectric electroencephalogram (EEG), maximally decreasing $CMRO_2$.[2]

Thiopental's side effects include decreased respiratory rate, apnea, cardiac arrhythmias, cardiovascular depression, headache, nausea, prolonged awakening, and hangover effects. Methohexital's side effects are similar to thiopental and include respiratory depression, apnea, hiccoughs, cardiovascular depression, and laryngospasm. Of note, a similar concentration of methohexital produces less hypotension than thiopental as the reflex tachycardic response to hypotension is not as acutely blunted compared to thiopental.[3]

The anesthetic action of the barbiturates is primarily terminated by redistribution from the central lipophilic tissues of the brain to peripheral lean muscle compartments. Barbiturates undergo slow terminal elimination via hepatic metabolism, biliary conjugation, and renal excretion leading to a half-life of 10 to 12 hours. Methohexital clearance is more dependent on hepatic blood flow allowing for a shorter elimination half-life of 4 hours.

Care should be taken in patients with porphyrias for barbiturates promote aminolevulinic acid synthetase (barbituric acid is broken down into malonic acid and urea), stimulating porphyrin formation, and can precipitate AIP or variegate porphyria. Acute attacks are usually intermittent and present as severe abdominal pain, peripheral neuropathy, psychiatric symptoms, autonomic dysfunction, and hyponatremia.[3] Barbiturates are strictly contraindicated in patients with a history of AIP.

B. Propofol

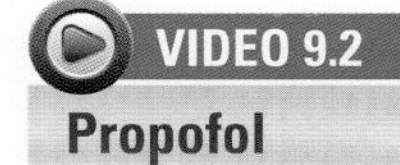

Propofol

Propofol (Diprivan, 2, 6-diisopropylphenol), an oil at room temperature, is insoluble in water. Thus, propofol was introduced as an emulsion: a 1% (10 mg/mL) egg lecithin (egg yolk) formulation consisting of 10% (100 mg/mL) soybean oil, 2.25% (22.5 mg/mL) glycerol, and 1.2% (12.5 mg/mL) egg phosphatide. Each addition to propofol to make the emulsion provides an important role: soybean oil dissolves propofol, glycerol produces isotonicity with blood, and egg lecithin provides stability of the propofol-soybean droplets. These small droplets have large surface areas for rapid diffusion of propofol once injected into the blood stream. The size range of the stable droplets of emulsion refracts light and creates a milky color.[4] To prevent microbial contamination, ethylenediaminetetraacetic acid (0.005%) was added to the solution.

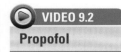

This propofol emulsion often causes venoirritation upon injection into small hand veins. The pain can be minimized by injection into larger veins and by mixing lidocaine with propofol (eg, adding 2 mL 1% lidocaine to 20 mL propofol) or injecting lidocaine alone prior to the propofol injection.

Propofol increases the binding affinity of GABA with the $GABA_A$ receptor. Coupled to a chloride channel, the activation leads to the hyperpolarization of the nerve membrane and is similar to the mechanism of action of the barbiturates. It causes a decrease in arterial blood pressure due to a simultaneous decrease in systemic vascular resistance and a decrease in preload (caused by inhibition of sympathetic tone and direct vascular smooth muscle effect) and negative cardiac inotropy. It also blunts the baroreflex to hypotension, causing a smaller compensatory increase in heart rate than expected for a given drop in blood, thus further exaggerating the hypotension caused. These effects are dose and concentration dependent.

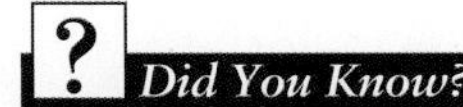

Propofol decreases the arterial blood pressure due to both a decrease in systemic vascular resistance and a decrease in preload (caused by inhibition of sympathetic tone and direct vascular smooth muscle effect). It also causes direct myocardial depression.

Propofol decreases $CMRO_2$, CBF, and ICP. However, in patients with increased cranial pressure, the markedly depressant effect of propofol on systemic arterial pressure will dramatically decrease CPP. It does not affect cerebrovascular regulation or cerebral reactivity to carbon dioxide tension. Its neuroprotective qualities include EEG burst suppression similar to thiopental, anticonvulsive properties, the decrease of intraocular pressure, and free radical scavenging.

Respiratory effects are dose dependent and include a shift of the CO_2 response curve to the right causing hypoventilation, hypercarbia, hypoxemia, and even apnea. Significant interpatient variability exists, and the dose required to induce any of these effects is unique to each patient. Propofol produces bronchodilation and is not an inhibitor of hypoxic pulmonary vasoconstriction.

Propofol has antipruritic and antiemetic properties; while not a first line agent, as little as 10 to 20 mg of propofol may reduce nausea and emesis in the perioperative patient. The same dose may also decrease pruritus associated with spinal opioids. Mechanisms for both are still not entirely understood.

The anesthetic action of propofol is terminated by redistribution from the central lipophilic tissues of the brain to peripheral lean muscle compartments. Terminal metabolism primarily occurs hepatically; the inactive water-soluble metabolites are eliminated renally. However, the presence of even clinically significant hepatic and renal disease does not markedly change propofol pharmacokinetics.[4]

An egg allergy is not necessarily a contraindication to propofol. Most egg allergies involve egg albumin found in egg whites. The egg lecithin in the propofol emulsion is an egg yolk extract. Propofol must be handled with sterile technique as the emulsion can support bacterial growth. Unused propofol should be discarded 6 hours after opening. The use of long-term, high-dose infusion in critically ill children and adults may cause propofol infusion syndrome (PRIS) characterized by cardiac failure, rhabdomyolysis, metabolic acidosis, renal failure, hyperkalemia, hypertriglyceridemia, and hepatomegaly. PRIS is rare, and its pathophysiology is uncertain, but it is often fatal. If suspected, propofol must be immediately discontinued and an alternative sedative employed.

C. Benzodiazepines

Benzodiazepine compounds consist of a benzene ring and a diazepine ring. The most commonly used benzodiazepines in anesthetic practice are midazolam (Versed), lorazepam (Ativan), and diazepam (Valium). Midazolam is water soluble at low pH. Lorazepam and diazepam are insoluble and are formulated with propylene glycol; venoirritation is sometimes seen on administration.

Benzodiazepines bind to the same $GABA_A$ receptors as barbiturates but at a different site on the receptor. The frequency of the associated chloride ion channel opening is increased with binding of GABA to the receptor, causing sedation along the same downstream pathway as propofol and the barbiturates. Benzodiazepines similarly decrease $CMRO_2$, CBF, and ICP. Although benzodiazepines are unable to completely suppress EEG bursts, they are effective in suppressing and controlling grand mal seizures.[5]

Benzodiazepines display minimal cardiorespiratory depression except when large doses are administered or when synergistically administered with opioids. Used alone, they slightly decrease arterial blood pressure, cardiac output, and peripheral vascular resistance. Midazolam can cause vagolysis resulting in changes in heart rate. Other clinically significant adverse effects include paradoxical excitement, which may occur in up to 10% to 15% of patients.

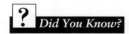

Unlike propofol and the barbiturates, sedation with benzodiazepines can be pharmacologically reversed with flumazenil, a specific competitive antagonist for benzodiazepines.

Unlike propofol and the barbiturates, sedation with benzodiazepines can be pharmacologically reversed. Flumazenil is a specific competitive antagonist for benzodiazepines with a high affinity for the benzodiazepine receptor site. The dosage of flumazenil is 0.5 to 1 mg IV. It is cleared more rapidly than the benzodiazepines, so patients must continue to be monitored as resedation may occur and repeated doses of flumazenil may be required.

Benzodiazepines are hepatically metabolized and are susceptible to hepatic dysfunction and the coadministration of other medications. Being highly protein bound, the free drug fraction is increased in severe liver disease and chronic kidney disease (CKD), with the elimination half-life being either prolonged or shortened, respectively. Hepatic clearance is enhanced if hepatic function is unaffected in the patient with CKD. Primary diazepam metabolites, desmethyldiazepam and 3-hydroxydiazepam, are pharmacologically active and prolong the sedative effects. These metabolites are further conjugated to form inactive water-soluble glucuronidated products. A conjugated midazolam metabolite, α-hydroxymidazolam, may also accumulate in patients with CKD receiving large doses of midazolam.[5]

Although benzodiazepines are not known to be significant teratogens, there is concern that they may cause an increase in the incidence of cleft palate in susceptible patients. Newborns may exhibit withdrawal syndrome from benzodiazepines administered to the mother. Consequently, benzodiazepines are usually avoided during pregnancy.[6]

D. Etomidate

Etomidate (Amidate) is structurally unrelated to other anesthetic agents. It has an imidazole ring that, under physiologic pH, makes it lipid soluble. It is a stereoisomer; only the R(+) isomer possesses clinical anesthetic activity. To allow for an injectable solution, the drug is dissolved in propylene glycol. This solution may cause pain on injection, which may be reduced by pre-IV injection of lidocaine.

Etomidate binds to $GABA_A$ receptors, increasing the receptors affinity for GABA, although etomidate appears to operate preferentially at $GABA_A$ receptors that express only a subset of the possible β subunits.[7] It is thought to cause subcortical disinhibition, explaining the involuntary myoclonic movements and even trismus commonly encountered during induction with this medication. It decreases $CMRO_2$, CBF, and ICP, while maintaining good CPP secondary to hemodynamic stability. It is capable of producing convulsion-like EEG potentials in epileptic patients without creating actual convulsions, helping to localize seizure foci during intraoperative mapping.[7] This property makes it a good second-line agent for those in whom electroconvulsive therapy (ECT) failed with methohexital. Although etomidate may create these potentials, it has anticonvulsant properties and may be used against status epilepticus. Etomidate also increases the amplitude of somatosensory evoked potentials (SSEP) helping in situations where interpretation is needed and SSEP signal quality is poor.

Postoperative nausea and vomiting (PONV) are more common with etomidate than with other IV anesthetics, and it lacks any analgesic properties. Etomidate transiently inhibits 11-β hydroxylase, an enzyme involved in steroidogenesis, which causes adrenocortical suppression. Even after a single induction dose, suppression can be seen for up to 5 to 8 hours. Secondary to this deleterious effect, some practitioners caution against the use of even one dose of etomidate for certain patients (eg, those in septic shock). Additionally, patients with trauma receiving single-dose etomidate for rapid sequence induction (RSI) were found to have an increased risk of adrenal insufficiency and ultimately poorer outcomes compared to a similar group who did not receive etomidate.[8] These concerns have led to the decreased use of etomidate as part of RSI protocols set for patients with trauma at several institutions.

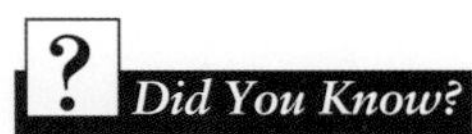

Etomidate transiently inhibits ***11-β-hydroxylase***, an enzyme involved in the production of steroids, even after a single induction dose.

In its favor, however, etomidate lacks histamine release and causes minimal hemodynamic depression and bronchoconstriction even in the presence of cardiovascular and pulmonary disease. It is this hemodynamic stability that underlies the continued use of etomidate in clinical practice. Awakening from etomidate occurs primarily by redistribution to peripheral tissues. Terminal elimination occurs by hepatic biotransformation, where it is broken down by plasma esterases to inactive metabolites that are then renally excreted.

E. Ketamine

Ketamine (Ketalar) is a phencyclidine derivative and is highly lipid soluble. In the United States, intravenous ketamine is sold as a racemic mixture of two enantiomers. Of these two forms, S(+)-ketamine is more potent than the R(−)-stereoisomer and has a greater rate of clearance and faster recovery time.[9] Ketamine has several unique properties to distinguish it from other IV anesthetics: it stimulates the sympathetic nervous system, has minimal respiratory depression, and causes potent bronchodilation. Additionally, it has several routes of administration, making it an excellent choice for uncooperative patients and pediatrics. Although best characterized for its dissociative anesthetic properties, ketamine also exerts analgesic, anti-inflammatory, and antidepressant actions. Its major effects are mediated through its potent antagonism of the NMDA receptor, rather than the action at the $GABA_A$ receptor.

Ketamine is a cerebral vasodilator, causing increased CBF and increased ICP. It also increases $CMRO_2$. It is relatively contraindicated in patients with space occupying lesions within the CNS, especially those with elevated ICP. Research has subsequently shown that normocapnia will blunt the undesirable effects of ketamine on increased CBF, but other induction agents are more appropriate and almost always available. Although ketamine causes myoclonus and increased EEG activity, it is still considered an anticonvulsant and may be used as a last-line agent in status epilepticus.

Secondary to its direct stimulation on the sympathetic nervous system, ketamine can cause an increase in heart rate and an increase in both systemic and pulmonary artery blood pressures. This causes increased cardiac work and myocardial oxygen consumption putting great demand on the heart. Its use is relatively contraindicated in patients with severe coronary artery disease or those with poor right ventricular heart function.

Ketamine has minimal effect on respiratory mechanics and upper airway reflexes. However, patients who are considered full stomachs are still at risk of aspiration and should be intubated during general anesthesia with ketamine. Ketamine causes increased lacrimation and salivation that may lead to laryngospasm. Pretreatment with an antisialagogue such as glycopyrrolate can attenuate this response. Unfortunately, ketamine tends to produce unpleasant emergence reactions, which (controversially) may be minimized with pretreatment of benzodiazepines.[9] Despite its side effect profile, ketamine's unique properties and its multiple documented routes of administration (IV, intramuscular [IM], oral, rectal, and even epidural and intrathecal) give it many adjunct clinical uses. Of note, although the bioavailability of ketamine is 100% following IV or IM injection, it is markedly decreased with oral or rectal administration secondary to first-pass effect, making these modes of drug administration less reliable. Ketamine also appears to be efficacious as a treatment for major depressive disorder with accompanying suicidal ideation, and is available as a nasal spray of S(+)-ketamine (Spravato) for this particular indication.

Termination of the clinical effect of ketamine is primarily due to redistribution from the brain to the peripheral tissues. Ketamine is hepatically metabolized by the CYP450 system into several metabolites of which one, norketamine, retains some anesthetic properties. Its metabolites are then renally excreted. Given its dependence on hepatic metabolism, infusion parameters or repeated doses should be reduced in patients with hepatic dysfunction. It may also have a direct detrimental impact on the interstitial cells of the bladder causing inflammatory cystitis after prolonged use.

Ketamine comes in concentrations of 10 mg/mL (1%), 50 mg/mL (5%), or 100 mg/mL (10%). When drawing up the medication, hypervigilance is critical so as not to confuse the more concentrated solution (ideal for IM injection) with the more dilute solution resulting in a potential overdose with IV injection. With that said, direct deaths caused by ketamine overdose (ie, without physical harm or hypothermia), in the absence of multidrug intoxication, are very rare. In fact, there has been no report involving a lethal dose of ketamine in humans. Most, if not all, side effects of ketamine are dose dependent, transient, and self-resolving.[9]

F. Dexmedetomidine

Dexmedetomidine (Precedex) is the S-enantiomer of medetomidine and is a centrally acting, highly selective α_2 agonist with a relatively long half-life of 2 hours. It produces sedation, anxiolysis, and analgesia without substantial respiratory depression.

Current evidence suggests a dose-dependent reduction of CBF. Mechanisms for such decrease may be due to direct vasoconstriction of the cerebral vasculature and indirectly via effects on the intrinsic neural pathways modulating vascular effects.[10] Decreases in CBF could be secondary to $CMRO_2$ reduction. However, all available evidence suggests that $CMRO_2$ remains unaffected by the use of dexmedetomidine. Unfortunately, no relevant data from human studies exist. Despite the reported neuroprotective effects of dexmedetomidine in models of ischemic brain injury, the possible uncoupling of CBF and $CMRO_2$ raises concerns that decreased CBF with unaltered $CMRO_2$ could prevent adequate cerebral oxygenation of brain tissue at risk for ischemic injury. Lastly, α_2 agonists decrease ICP. This could be due to greater α_2 vasoconstriction on the venous versus the arteriolar side of the cerebral vasculature as the venous compartment comprises most of the cerebral blood volume.[10]

Dexmedetomidine has been associated with serious episodes of bradycardia, hypotension, sinus arrest, and transient hypertension. This hypertension often seen with rapid bolus is secondary to weak α_1 peripheral vasoconstriction.[11] The hypertension is temporary and treatment is usually unnecessary. On the contrary, the more prolonged α_2-mediated hypotension and bradycardia are more likely to necessitate treatment. The preemptive use of anticholinergic agents to prevent bradycardia can be helpful. Unfortunately, even after cessation of the drug, the hypotensive and bradycardic effects can last for several hours. Extreme caution is advised when administering dexmedetomidine to patients with advanced heart block and/or severe ventricular dysfunction.

One of the most frequently cited advantages of dexmedetomidine is its lack of respiratory compromise. Yet, studies comparing dexmedetomidine to midazolam show similar incidences of respiratory complications. On the same note, in a study comparing the effects of dexmedetomidine to propofol, dexmedetomidine proved to have a similar effect to propofol on both hypoxic and hypercapnic regulation of breathing.[12] Lastly, dexmedetomidine can worsen respiratory obstruction in those patients with prior respiratory issues such as sleep apnea.

Dexmedetomidine induces a form of sedation resembling natural sleep from which the patient is easily and quickly aroused. It also reduces shivering, inhibits gastric emptying and gastrointestinal transit times, and reduces intraocular pressure.

The liver rapidly metabolizes dexmedetomidine through mechanisms involving CYP450 and glucuronidation. The drug is rapidly cleared, and metabolites are excreted via bile and urine. Renal or hepatic insufficiency may delay excretion of the metabolites.

III. Clinical Use of IV Anesthetics

A. Use of IV Anesthetics as Induction Agents

Barbiturates

The induction dose of thiopental is 3 to 5 mg/kg in adults, 5 to 6 mg/kg in children, and 6 to 8 mg/kg in infants. The induction of anesthesia occurs in less than 30 seconds, and spontaneous awakening from an induction dose occurs within 20 minutes. Occasionally, barbiturates are associated with a paradoxical reaction of restlessness, excitement, and delirium. Ironically, this effect can be reversed with oral or IV administration of caffeine.[8]

The induction dose of methohexital is 1 to 1.5 mg/kg in adults. At lower doses, methohexital can paradoxically increase or activate cortical EEG seizure discharge. It is with this property that methohexital became the IV anesthetic of choice for ECT as it both decreases seizure threshold and extends seizure duration. The latter is an important quality during ECT, as the duration of seizure has been linked to improved efficacy.[3] It is important to note that although methohexital is the drug of choice for ECT, it is ultimately an anticonvulsant medication and may adversely affect seizure production in patients with high seizure thresholds.

Propofol

The induction dose of propofol in adults is 1 to 2 mg/kg. Propofol causes decreased systemic arterial pressure on induction, due partially to direct action on vascular smooth muscle and blunting of the baroreceptor reflex. Since this effect is related to plasma concentration rather than effect site concentration, it may be possible to blunt the effect by administering the bolus more gradually or in divided doses. Of note, with an induction dose of propofol, some patients may exhibit excitatory motor activity or nonepileptic myoclonus.

Benzodiazepines

The induction dose of midazolam is 0.1 to 0.2 mg/kg IV. However, the prolonged recovery from induction with even short-acting benzodiazepines limits their usefulness as induction agents in routine clinical use.[9]

Etomidate

Etomidate has a very favorable hemodynamic profile on induction, with minimal depression in blood pressure. It is often the drug of choice for anesthetizing patients who have significant cardiovascular disease or for emergent situations in which the need to preserve hemodynamic stability takes precedence over etomidate's other notable drawbacks. Etomidate is only administered intravenously, and the induction dose for adults is 0.2 to 0.3 mg/kg. The onset is extremely rapid, at approximately one arm-to-brain circulation time. The myoclonus and trismus that may follow induction with etomidate can make initial attempts at ventilation and intubation difficult unless the induction is promptly accompanied with a neuromuscular blocker. Etomidate does not inhibit the sympathetic response to laryngoscopy and intubation unless combined with an analgesic.

Ketamine

The induction dose of ketamine in adults is 1 to 2 mg/kg when administered intravenously. However, induction with ketamine via IM administration is frequently used when the patient is unable to tolerate placement of an IV line, such as pediatric patients, uncooperative patients, or patients with cognitive impairments. An IM injection of 4 to 6 mg/kg provides induction of an anesthetic state with maintained spontaneous ventilation, allowing for an IV to be placed and the further management of the patient to proceed. Ketamine's onset is less than 5 minutes when administered via IV or IM routes, with recovery time averaging 45 and 120 minutes. The duration of anesthesia after one induction dose is from 10 to 20 minutes; however, regaining baseline cognitive function may take an additional 60 to 90 minutes.

B. Use of IV Drugs for Maintenance of Anesthesia

Barbiturates

Barbiturates are widely used to improve brain relaxation during neurosurgery and may protect brain tissue from transient episodes of focal ischemia by decreasing $CMRO_2$.[2] However, the dosing required to maintain EEG suppression is associated with prolonged awakening and delayed extubation. In general, the use of barbiturate infusions to maintain anesthesia is not recommended because the capacity of the body to redistribute barbiturates is relatively limited. Continuous administration of barbiturates rapidly causes the concentration of medication in the peripheral compartments to approach the concentration within the central compartment. Termination of the anesthetic effect then depends solely on terminal elimination, leading to a very prolonged context-sensitive half-time.

Propofol

TIVA with propofol is commonly used to maintain a state of general anesthesia. Infusion rates range between 100 and 200 µg/kg/min but variability can exist, and vigilance with such techniques is key. Although a safe and effective technique, questions pertaining to cost-effectiveness have emerged. Schraag et al conducted a systematic review and meta-analysis comparing propofol versus inhalational agents. The study concluded that compared to volatile anesthetics, propofol had a lower risk of PONV, lower pain scores, decreased time in the postanesthesia care unit (PACU), and higher patient satisfaction.[13]

Benzodiazepines

Infusions rates for midazolam for maintaining hypnosis and amnesia are 0.25 to 1.0 µg/kg/min when also combined with an inhalational agent and/or opioid analgesic. Midazolam is the preferred benzodiazepine for continuous infusion due to the long context-sensitive half-lives of diazepam and lorazepam. However, infusions of benzodiazepines for anesthesia are associated with prolonged emergence and are typically used only in patients who are expected to remain intubated.

Etomidate

When etomidate was introduced, its hemodynamic stability appeared to make it an appropriate choice for prolonged sedation—unfortunately, it is now known to be unsafe for this indication. Etomidate potently inhibits steroid synthesis at the 11-β hydroxylase enzyme, and its use results in a significant increase in mortality in sedated ICU patients.[7] Maintenance infusions of etomidate are contraindicated.

Ketamine

Although rarely used as the sole agent for maintenance of anesthesia, ketamine is often used during general anesthesia as an adjunct to provide postoperative analgesia. A subanalgesic infusion (3-5 µg/kg/min) during general anesthesia or a 0.5 mg/kg bolus dose during induction can be used in patients with opioid-resistant chronic pain in whom postoperative pain management is likely to be difficult. There is also evidence for antidepressant responses achieved at doses as low as 0.1 mg/kg with an infusion lasting as little as 5 minutes or given via IM injection. Additionally, the ability of ketamine to reduce proinflammatory cytokine levels may be of clinical relevance, given that elevated interleukin 6 levels have been associated with poor postoperative outcomes and increased trauma-induced hyperalgesia, which could be beneficial regarding chronic postoperative pain.[9] Lastly, like etomidate, ketamine is capable of increasing the amplitude of SSEP, helping in situations where interpretation is needed and SSEP signal quality is poor.

Dexmedetomidine

Like ketamine, dexmedetomidine has been used primarily as an adjunct to general anesthesia for patients who require alternative mechanisms of analgesia, either in the setting of preexisting opioid tolerance in patients with chronic pain or in order to reduce opioid administration in patients at risk of opioid-related postoperative respiratory depression such as in patients with morbid obesity or obstructive sleep apnea. Dexmedetomidine is run intravenously as an infusion, ranging from 0.3 to 0.7 µg/kg/h, and is usually stopped at the onset of closure. Additionally, to reduce the incidence of emergence delirium in pediatrics, 0.5 µg/kg of dexmedetomidine can be given toward the end of the case.

C. Use of IV Anesthetics for Sedation

Barbiturates

Propofol and modern benzodiazepines have largely supplanted the use of barbiturates for sedation. Nevertheless, a small 25 to 50 mg dose of thiopental can be very efficacious if it is necessary to premedicate a patient who is agitated or hostile. There is usually no pain on administration, unlike propofol, and there is usually no sense of the onset of sedation or of disinhibition, unlike midazolam.

Propofol

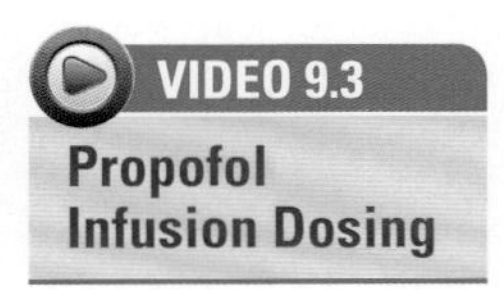

With its relatively quick on-and-off capabilities and favorable side effect profile, propofol is a popular medication for sedation. Propofol infusions, or intermittent bolus doses of comparable quantities of medication, are commonly used for moderate procedural sedation.

Maintenance infusion rates for satisfactory sedation usually range between 25 and 75 µg/kg/min, although higher initial infusion rates may be required to establish a suitable concentration at the effect site if a small bolus (0.25-0.5 mg/kg) is not used prior to the start of infusion. Propofol exhibits respiratory depression in a dose-dependent fashion, a decrease in tidal volumes, and an increased respiratory rate. Inhibition of the hypoxic ventilatory drive and hypercarbic response is observed even at sedating doses of propofol. Nonetheless, with its minimal hangover effects and positive antiemetic properties, propofol is well suited to moderate procedural sedation.

Benzodiazepines

The multiple administration routes of benzodiazepines allow this class to be a key component in sedation. In addition to the IV route of administration, midazolam is routinely given orally to children, although this indication has never been Food and Drug Administration (FDA) approved.

IM, intranasal, transbuccal, and sublingual routes are also possible. IM diazepam should be avoided due to unreliable absorption and pain. When primarily used as premedications and adjuvants, benzodiazepines are dose-dependent anxiolytics, sedatives, anterograde amnestics, anticonvulsants, and muscle relaxants. Midazolam dosing for anesthesia premedication is 0.02 to 0.04 mg/kg IV/IM in adults and 0.4 to 0.8 mg/kg PO in children. Midazolam can be used for procedural sedation with minimal risk of respiratory depression, though in practice a carefully titrated propofol infusion will produce both superior amnesia and a faster recovery. However, the availability of flumazenil to acutely reverse sedation with benzodiazepines can provide a margin of safety that is unavailable when using propofol. Consequently, midazolam may be preferred for sedation in the setting of a jeopardized airway, such as for an awake tracheostomy, because it can be pharmacologically reversed.

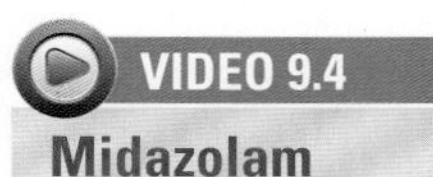

Of note, midazolam has a half-life of roughly 9 minutes. If additional boluses are administered prior to the time to peak effect, over titration may occur leading to hypoventilation, airway obstruction, hypoxia, and hypotension. Although midazolam has a wide margin of safety, repeated doses should only be given with this knowledge in mind to avoid such complications.[12]

Ketamine

In addition to its analgesic properties, ketamine has a relatively high safety profile making it an excellent choice for sedation in certain patient populations. Administration begins with a small dose of 0.25 to 0.5 mg/kg, which is then followed by increments of 10 to 20 mg boluses, titrating to affect. It has an onset of 1 to 2 minutes and approximate duration of 20 to 60 minutes. It produces a dissociative state in which the patient appears conscious (eyes open, staring) but unresponsive to sensory input (pain, questioning). Although airway reflexes are maintained, increased oral secretions increase the risk of laryngospasm and an antisialagogue is often given preemptively. Perhaps the biggest side effect of ketamine is the vivid hallucinations, which (controversially) may be reduced with the use of benzodiazepines. Patient movement may make ketamine less than ideal for procedures requiring a completely motionless patient.

Ketofol

The combination of propofol and ketamine, nicknamed ketofol, is associated with a lower incidence of deleterious side effects than with each medication given alone. Reported advantages of the combination include hemodynamic stability, reduced nausea and vomiting, enhanced procedural conditions, analgesia, and less respiratory compromise. There is no consensus on the exact mixture for ketofol, and ratios of 1:1 to 1:10 of ketamine to propofol can be found in the literature with success. Studies reporting on the use of ketofol, however, should be interpreted and compared with caution as each study may use different ratios of each drug.

Dexmedetomidine

Dexmedetomidine sedation is most commonly administered intravenously as an infusion, ranging from 0.3 to 0.7 µg/kg/h. The rate is titrated based on sedation level and hemodynamic stability and can be preceded by a loading dose of 1 µg/kg given over 10 minutes. Some centers forgo the loading dose as it increases the risk of hemodynamic instability.

Dexmedetomidine induces a form of sedation resembling natural sleep from which the patient is easily and quickly aroused. With this, and the fact that it provides analgesia without causing significant respiratory depression, dexmedetomidine has become a favorable IV sedative. However, when compared with propofol, the target sedation level takes longer to achieve with dexmedetomidine (25 vs 10 minutes), and if loading doses are used, there is an increased risk of hemodynamic instability.

Dexmedetomidine may have completely taken over the IV sedation world had it not been for its prolonged half-life (2 hours) and hemodynamic effects. Hypotension is the most frequently occurring adverse event and can last for several hours after cessation of the infusion. This can delay the release from PACU and ultimately lead to increased cost and patient dissatisfaction.

When used as the sole systemic medication, dexmedetomidine is a good choice of anesthetic for awake fiberoptic intubation (it even causes dry mouth!) or in combination with regional anesthesia. In the ICU, dexmedetomidine can be helpful for weaning intubated patients from the ventilator as it provides sedation with minimal respiratory depression. Compared to benzodiazepines in the ICU, dexmedetomidine is associated with a reduced incidence of delirium and a more physiologic sleep state.[14] Of note, dexmedetomidine has little FDA-approved indications. In fact, regarding sedation with dexmedetomidine of mechanically ventilated adults in the ICU, the FDA has only approved its use up to 24 hours. Additionally, although this medication is often used in the pediatric population, it still does not hold FDA approval for such use. More recently, dexmedetomidine did receive FDA approval for the use of sedation in the operating room.[8]

For further review and interactivities, please see the associated Interactive Video Lectures and "A Closer Look" infographic accessible in the complimentary eBook bundled with this text. Access instructions are located in the inside front cover.

References

1. Felmlee MA, Morris ME, Mager DE. Mechanism-based pharmacodynamic modeling. *Methods Mol Biol.* 2012;929:583-600. doi:10.1007/978-1-62703-050-2_21. PMID: 23007443.
2. Shapiro H. Barbiturates in brain ischaemia. *Br J Anaesth.* 1985;57(1):82-95. doi:10.1093/bja/57.1.82. PMID: 3881116.
3. Qaisar S, Kholi A. *Methohexital.* In: *StatPearls [Internet].* StatPearls Publishing; 2020.
4. Walsh CT. Propofol: milk of amnesia. *Cell.* 2018;175(1):10-13. doi:10.1016/j.cell.2018.08.031. PMID: 30217361.
5. Reves JG, Fragen RJ, Vinik HR, Greenblatt DJ. Midazolam. *Anesthesiology.* 1985; 62(3):310-324. doi:10.1097/00000542-198503000-00017
6. Clinical management guidelines for obstetrician-gynecologists use of psychiatric medications during pregnancy and lactation. *Focus.* 2009;7(3):385-400. doi:10.1176/foc.7.3.foc385
7. Vanlersberghe C, Camu F. Etomidate and other non-barbiturates. *Handb Exp Pharmacol.* 2008;(182):267-282. doi:10.1007/978-3-540-74806-9_13. PMID: 18175096.
8. Tobias J, Leder M. Procedural sedation: a review of sedative agents, monitoring, and management of complications. *Saudi J Anaesth.* 2011;5(4):395-410. doi:10.4103/1658-354x.87270. PMID: 22144928.
9. Zanos P, Moaddel R, Morris PJ, et al. Ketamine and ketamine metabolite pharmacology: insights into therapeutic mechanisms. *Pharmacol Rev.* 2018;70(3):621-660. doi:10.1124/pr.117.015198. PMID: 29945898.
10. Tsaousi G, Bilotta F. Is dexmedetomidine a favorable agent for cerebral hemodynamics? *J Intensive Crit Care.* 2015;01(01):7. doi:10.21767/2471-8505.10007. PMID: 26955209.
11. Keating GM, Hoy SM, Lyseng-Williamson KA. Dexmedetomidine: a guide to its use for sedation in the US. *Clin Drug Invest.* 2012;32(8):561-567. doi:10.1007/bf03261910. PMID: 22741747.
12. Barends CR, Absalom AR, Struys MM. Drug selection for ambulatory procedural sedation. *Curr Opin Anaesthesiol.* 2018;31(6):673-678. doi:10.1097/aco.0000000000000652. PMID: 30124543.
13. Schraag S, Pradelli L, Alsaleh AJO, et al. Propofol vs. inhalational agents to maintain general anaesthesia in ambulatory and in-patient surgery: a systematic review and meta-analysis. *BMC Anesthesiol.* 2018;18(1). doi:10.1186/s12871-018-0632-3. PMID: 30409186.
14. Riker RR. Dexmedetomidine vs midazolam for sedation of critically ill patients: a randomized trial. *J Am Med Assoc.* 2009;301(5):489. doi:10.1001/jama.2009.56. PMID: 19188334.

PROPOFOL

A CLOSER LOOK

Of all the available intravenous anesthetics, propofol is most frequently used. It is commonly employed to induce general anesthesia. Additionally, it is utilized to provide sedation for procedures in the operating room as well as in the intensive care unit.

PROPOFOL
1%
10 mg/mL

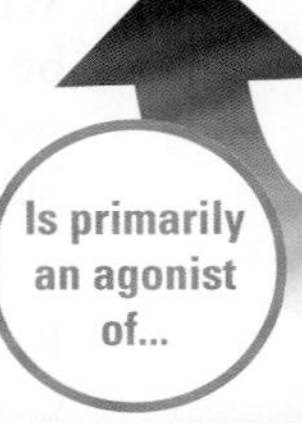

NMDA | Alpha | Acetyl-choline

...but also influences these receptors

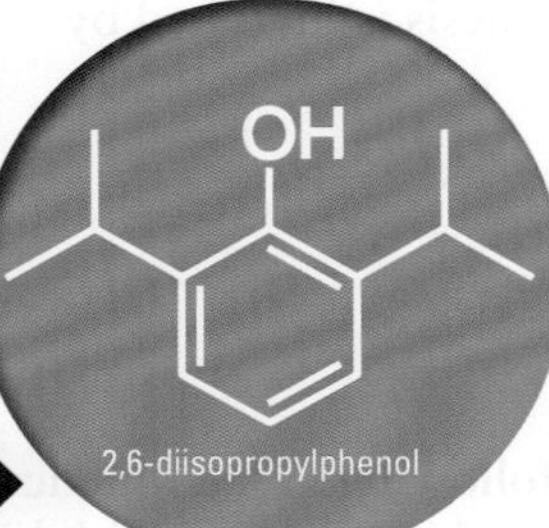

It also contains...

10% soybean oil
2.25% glycerol
1.2% egg phospholipid
EDTA or metabisulfite preservative

Has been used safely in patients with egg allergy

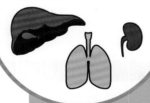

Redistributes rapidly and metabolized by the liver as well as the lung and kidneys

Systemic effects...

Central Nervous System

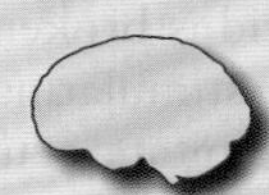

CNS depression
↓ Cerebral O_2 consumption
↓ Cerebral blood flow
↓ Intracranial pressure

Anticonvulsant that can achieve burst suppression on EEG

Cardiovascular System

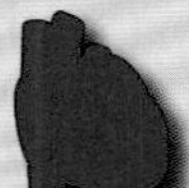

Hypotension results from:
↓ Vascular resistance
↓ Stroke volume
↓ Cardiac output
↓ Baroreceptor response

Heart rate is often unchanged

Respiratory System

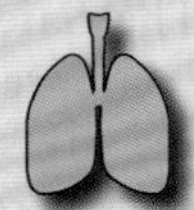

Apnea at higher doses
↓ Tidal volumes
↑ Respiratory rate
↓ Response to hypoxia
↓ Response to hypercarbia

Bronchodilation

Infographic by: Naveen Nathan MD

Questions

1. **When used in the ICU, dexmedetomidine has been associated with a lower risk of delirium when compared to which of the following IV anesthetics?**

   A. Propofol
   B. Etomidate
   C. Barbiturates
   D. Benzodiazepines

2. **Which of the following enzymes involved with steroidogenesis is inhibited by etomidate?**

   A. 17α-hydroxylase
   B. 11β-hydroxylase
   C. 21-Hydroxylase
   D. 18-Oxidase

3. **Which of the following IV anesthetics should be avoided in a patient with history of acute intermittent porphyria?**

   A. Ketamine
   B. Etomidate
   C. Methohexital
   D. Dexmedetomidine

4. **Twenty minutes after starting a sedating infusion for a skin biopsy of the lower extremity, the patient begins complaining of dry mouth. Which of the following IV anesthetics is most likely the culprit?**

   A. Ketamine
   B. Propofol
   C. Midazolam
   D. Dexmedetomidine

5. **Which of the following medications could be given preemptively to prevent increased secretions following the administration of ketamine sedation?**

   A. Glycopyrrolate
   B. Midazolam
   C. Methohexital
   D. Propofol

Answers

1. D

Benzodiazepine use appears to be associated with an increase in delirium when compared to dexmedetomidine. The Safety and Efficacy of Dexmedetomidine Compared With Midazolam (SEDCOM) [Riker et al] study suggests that dexmedetomidine may decrease delirium when compared to benzodiazepines.

2. B

Corticoadrenal suppression is the most significant adverse effect that occurs with the use of etomidate and is the primary limiting factor. Etomidate inhibits function of 11β-hydroxylase (converts 11-deoxycortisol into cortisol), resulting in reversible, dose-dependent inhibition of cortisol and aldosterone synthesis.

3. C

Care should be taken in patients with porphyrias for barbiturates promote aminolevulinic acid synthetase (barbituric acid is broken down into malonic acid and urea), stimulating porphyrin formation, and can precipitate acute intermittent porphyria (AIP) or variegate porphyria. Acute attacks are usually intermittent and present as severe abdominal pain, peripheral neuropathy, psychiatric symptoms, autonomic dysfunction, and hyponatremia. Barbiturates are strictly contraindicated in patients with a history of AIP.

4. D

Dexmedetomidine acts on the presynaptic α_2 receptor to decrease norepinephrine release and hence decrease secretions from the salivary gland, resulting in dry mouth.

5. A

Ketamine causes increased lacrimation and salivation that may lead to laryngospasm. Pretreatment with an antisialagogue such as glycopyrrolate can attenuate this response.

10 Analgesics

Nicole Z. Spence

I. Brief History and Overview

Analgesics are integral to perioperative anesthetic care and postoperative analgesia. As the number of patients consuming chronic opioids has increased in recent years, coupled with a global opioid epidemic, it is important to use a thoughtful and appropriate analgesic regimen for each patient. Resulting from the opioid epidemic, analgesic therapy is now focused on multimodal regimens instead of sole reliance on opioids. This chapter will review both opioid and nonopioid analgesics, including marijuana and tetrahydrocannabinol. Novel analgesics including ketamine, dextromethorphan, esmolol, and dexmedetomidine will also be discussed.

Opioids, derived from natural opiates, have been documented as early as Sumerian times. Opioid formulations were used medicinally in 1500 BC. Opium was then transported across lands and crossed cultural boundaries. Morphine was first isolated in the early 1800s and has been the most studied opioid. With drug use came issues of abuse and addiction, and opioid addiction has flourished today.[1] The United States has a burgeoning national opioid epidemic.

? Did You Know?

Aspirin irreversibly inhibits platelet aggregation for the life of the platelet, while other non-COX-2–specific, NSAIDs reversibly inhibit aggregation in a dose-dependent manner until the drug is cleared from the circulation.

II. Nonopioid Analgesics

A. Acetaminophen

1. Overview

Acetaminophen (paracetamol, para-acetylaminophenol, *N*-acetyl-para-aminophenol) has been used clinically since 1955 and is the most widely used antipyretic in the United States. It is combined with other analgesics, such as opioids, in some formulations. Consequently, the Food and Drug Administration (FDA) has limited the acetaminophen content in those combination formulations to 325 mg per tablet. Acetaminophen remains a leading cause of drug overdose and acute liver failure.[2] ***Centrilobular hepatotoxicity*** occurs with acute overdose and may occur at smaller doses in chronic alcoholics. ***Liver transplantation*** may be offered to patients with acute liver failure.[3]

? Did You Know?

In 2011, the U.S. Food and Drug Administration (FDA) requested that manufacturers of acetaminophen-containing products limit those products to a maximum of 325 mg of acetaminophen per dose to decrease the chance of hepatic toxicity.

2. Mechanism of Action

The exact mechanism of action of acetaminophen is not fully understood. The analgesic effect likely occurs from central sites of action, such as activation of descending inhibitory serotonergic pathways and modulation of cyclooxygenase (COX) pathways. The antipyretic effect results from actions within the hypothalamus.

3. Pharmacokinetics and Pharmacodynamics

See Table 10.1.

4. Metabolism and Excretion

Acetaminophen is metabolized in the liver by ***glucuronidation*** and ***sulfonation***. The nontoxic conjugates that are formed are excreted in the urine and bile. When these pathways become saturated, acetaminophen metabolization occurs via cytochrome P450 (CYP) pathways that produce a toxic metabolite, N-acetyl-p-benzoquinone imine (NAPQI). The NAPQI metabolite interacts with hepatic glutathione to produce a nontoxic compound that is eventually excreted as mercapturic acid and cysteine conjugates. If glutathione levels are depleted, or the system is overwhelmed, oxidative hepatocyte injury and ***hepatocellular centrilobular necrosis*** may ensue because of the NAPQI metabolite. Approximately 2% of ingested acetaminophen is excreted unchanged by the kidneys.

Table 10.1 Common Nonopioid Analgesics[a]

Drug	Formulations Available	Adult Dosing (Max Dose)	Pediatric Dosing (Max Dose)	Pharmacokinetics/ Pharmacodynamics and Special Considerations
Acetaminophen	Oral Rectal Parenteral	325-650 mg q 4-6 h (<4 g/d; depending on factors noted above)	10-15 mg/kg/ dose (75 mg/ kg/d or <4 g/d; do not exceed 5 doses/24 h)	Highly bioavailable after PO dose Onset of action: PO < 1 h Intravenous (IV) 5-10 min Excreted in urine Crosses placenta; present in breast milk
Acetylsalicylic acid (ASA; aspirin)	Oral (can be enteric coated) Rectal	325 mg-1 g q 4-6 h PRN; 81 mg for secondary prevention (usual max dose for antiplatelet effect is 325 mg/d) High doses (4-8 g/d) limited by adverse effects: gastrointestinal, decreased auditory acuity, and tinnitus	Not recommended in children younger than 18 y recovering from viral illness (association of Reye syndrome) Adolescents ≥50 kg: 325-650 mg q 4-6 h PRN (max daily dose 4 g/d)	Extensive first-pass metabolism Bariatric surgery: may alter absorption and efficacy Onset of action: PO < 30 min Food decreases rate of absorption (chewing tablets result in inhibition of platelet aggregation within 20 min) ASA is dialyzable Salicylates cross placenta and enter fetal circulation; salicylic acid found in breast milk

(Continued)

Table 10.1 Common Nonopioid Analgesics[a] (Continued)

Drug	Formulations Available	Adult Dosing (Max Dose)	Pediatric Dosing (Max Dose)	Pharmacokinetics/ Pharmacodynamics and Special Considerations
NSAIDs (ie, ibuprofen, ketorolac)	Oral Topical Parenteral Intramuscular (IM)	For ibuprofen, max dose 3200 mg/d	For ibuprofen, 4-10 mg/kg/dose q 6-8 h, (max dose 40 mg/kg/d or 1200 mg/d)	Negligible first-pass metabolism Highly protein bound to albumin Time to peak effect: 1-2 h (IV ketorolac peak effect within 5 min) Renally excreted; 70%-90% of dose is excreted within 24 h Ibuprofen distributes into cerebrospinal fluid
NMDA receptor antagonists (ie, ketamine)	Oral Parenteral IM	Subanesthetic infusions typically: 2-7 µg/kg/min	Similar to adult but may require higher doses Pharmacokinetics in children similar to adults; children require higher infusion rates and form more norketamine than adults	If given PO, ketamine undergoes extensive first-pass metabolism Bioavailability depends on route of administration: 20% PO, 90% IM, 25% rectal Lipid-soluble, rapidly crosses blood-brain barrier Onset of action: IV or intranasal: 1-2 min; PO: 20-30 min Half-life 2-3 h Termination due to redistribution from the brain and plasma to other tissues
α-2 receptor agonists (ie, dexmedetomidine, clonidine)	IV IM PO Buccal Intranasal	FDA recommends dexmedetomidine use limited to 24 h; if used >24 h, may cause tachyphylaxis and tolerance Typical dexmedetomidine infusion dose 0.2-0.7 µg/kg/h	Typical dexmedetomidine infusion dose 0.2-0.7 µg/kg/h (like adults); consider avoiding boluses in pediatric patients	PO clonidine: nearly 100% bioavailability, peak concentration within 60-90 min; $t_{1/2}$ = 6-23 h $t_{1/2}$ of dexmedetomidine = 6 min-3 h 94% protein bound (mostly albumin)

[a]Notably, acetylsalicylic acid, ibuprofen, and paracetamol are on the World Health Organization (WHO) Model List of Essential Medicines. This WHO list presents the minimum medicine needs for a basic healthcare system and considers the most efficacious, safe, and cost-effective medications.

5. Drug Interactions and Adverse Effects

Patient factors and clinical comorbidities may make patients more prone to liver injury following acetaminophen use. Factors that may increase the risk of acetaminophen toxicity include concomitant use of herbal medications or CYP-inducing drugs such as anticonvulsants and conditions in which glutathione stores are low including malnutrition or alcohol ingestion. ***N-acetylcysteine*** therapy can be provided to patients who have ingested excess acetaminophen to decrease hepatic injury. Administration of N-acetylcysteine requires clinicians to have a high index of suspicion for the nonspecific symptoms of acetaminophen overdose, and treatment should be initiated prior to the onset of liver injury, usually within 8 hours of acute acetaminophen ingestion. Doses of acetaminophen up to 4 g/d are generally safe. Hepatotoxicity has been reported, rarely, at doses less than 4 g/d; therefore, a maximum dose of 3 g/d has been recommended in adults with normal liver function if acetaminophen will be used for more than 7 days. In patients with risk factors, such as malnutrition, advanced age, or heavy alcohol use, a lower maximum dose of 2 g/d may be recommended.[4]

B. Acetylsalicylic Acid

1. Overview

Aspirin, or acetylsalicylic acid (ASA), is one type of nonsteroidal anti-inflammatory drug (NSAID), but it is the only acetylated NSAID. Aspirin was first introduced by ***Bayer*** in 1899. Although NSAIDs decrease inflammation and exhibit analgesic, antipyretic, and antiplatelet properties, aspirin is primarily used for primary and secondary prevention of cardiovascular conditions nowadays.

2. Mechanism of Action

Aspirin ***irreversibly*** inhibits both cyclooxygenase-1 (COX-1) and cyclooxygenase-2 (COX-2), but it is weakly more selective for COX-1. Aspirin's effects vary depending on the dose used. At low doses (ie, 81 mg PO daily), aspirin irreversibly inhibits COX-1 to inhibit platelet generation of thromboxane A_2, which subsequently causes an ***antithrombotic*** effect (**Figure 10.1**). Aspirin acts as an acetylating agent: an acetyl group covalently binds to a serine residue at the active site of the COX enzyme; this interaction is ***irreversible*** and renders the COX enzyme inactive for the duration of the lifetime of the platelet (8-10 days). At intermediate doses (ie, 650-4000 mg/d), both COX-1 and COX-2 are irreversibly inhibited; therefore, prostaglandin production is blocked, resulting in analgesic and antipyretic effects. Higher doses may be used in rheumatologic disorders, but high doses are limited by toxicity and gastrointestinal (GI) irritation. Aspirin may protect cells against oxidative stress.[5]

3. Metabolism and Excretion

Aspirin undergoes extensive first-pass metabolism and has an absorption half-life of 5 to 16 minutes. Aspirin is metabolized to salicylic acid by nonspecific esterases in the liver and less so in the stomach, and salicylic acid excretion is highly variable. Salicylic acid has less metabolic activity, and its serum half-life is dose dependent. Aspirin is highly bound to albumin.[6] Aspirin overdose or toxicity causes an anion gap metabolic acidosis, renal failure, dehydration, tinnitus, or seizures. These patients require ***alkaline diuresis*** to promote salicylate excretion and may require hemodialysis. Patients with aspirin overdose require intensive care.

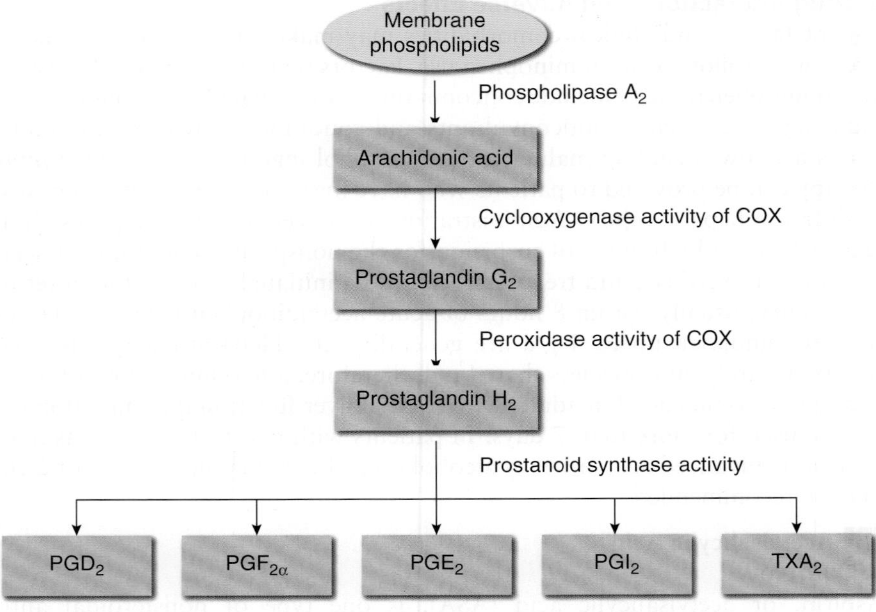

Figure 10.1 Schematic view of prostanoid synthesis. Prostanoids are produced in response to tissue injury and inflammation. These contribute to peripheral pain sensitization, pain perception, and the syndrome of fever, anorexia, and changes in sleep patterns. Arachidonic acid is released from cell membranes during tissue injury and inflammation and generates prostaglandins and thromboxane A_2. COX, cyclooxygenase enzymes; PG, prostaglandin; PGD_2, prostaglandin D_2; PGE_2, prostaglandin E_2; $PGF_{2\alpha}$, prostaglandin $F_{2\alpha}$; PGI_2, prostaglandin I_2; TX, thromboxane; TXA_2, thromboxane A_2.

4. Drug Interactions and Adverse Effects

Aspirin is used as an antithrombotic drug because it irreversibly inactivates COX-1, which then blocks thromboxane A_2 synthesis for the lifetime of the platelet. Therefore, aspirin irreversibly inhibits platelet aggregation and prolongs bleeding time. Once the affected platelets are replaced by normally functioning platelets, bleeding time normalizes. Aspirin, at low doses, is sometimes used in pregnancy for patients at risk for preeclampsia or other hypertensive disorders of pregnancy. Aspirin is rapidly absorbed from the stomach and can ***erode gastric mucosa***. Aspirin causes ***acute tubular necrosis*** secondary to decreased renal blood flow, and patients can exhibit an intolerance to salicylates. An intolerance should be suspected in patients who have ***Samter triad***: asthma or atopy, nasal polyps, and aspirin sensitivity. Aspirin can exacerbate these patients' respiratory disease and ***precipitate bronchospasm***. ***Reye syndrome*** is linked to the use of aspirin in children and young adults who recently had a viral illness; for this reason, it is not recommended to administer aspirin to children younger than 20 years.

C. Other NSAIDs

- Ibuprofen
- Ketorolac
- Indomethacin
- Diclofenac
- Meloxicam
- Celecoxib

1. Overview

Nonselective NSAIDs (nsNSAIDs) are widely used across the world, but NSAIDs are one class of medications that contributes to preventable drug-related hospital admissions. Both COX-1 and COX-2 are inhibited by nsNSAIDs. While many believe nsNSAIDs are safe, their side effect profile includes gastroduodenal ulcers, renal dysfunction, inhibition of platelet aggregation, bronchospasm, and incomplete bone healing. NSAIDs were theorized to reduce bone healing as the inflammatory response is crucial for tissue repair; however, a causal relationship between bone healing following long bone fractures and use of NSAIDs has not been demonstrated. Further, differences in NSAID effects on healing of long bones and spinal bones may exist. COX-2 inhibitors were developed to mitigate the GI and antiplatelet side effects as COX-2 activity has not been found in platelets. Rofecoxib, a COX-2–selective NSAID, was approved by the FDA in 1999 but voluntarily withdrawn from the market in 2004 because patients had an increased risk of cardiovascular events, specifically myocardial infarction and stroke. Valdecoxib was withdrawn from the market a year later. The adverse cardiovascular events are probably due to elevations in blood pressure that occur with all NSAIDs rather than any particular risk associated with COX-2 inhibitors.[7] Prior to the withdrawal of these drugs, studies had shown that older adults prescribed opioids are more likely to die than patients receiving NSAIDs. Celecoxib remains the only COX-2–specific inhibitor that is available in the United States currently. Because celecoxib has no effect on platelet function, it is especially useful in the perioperative period.

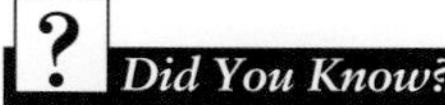

The rate of upper gastrointestinal complications is highest with ketorolac compared with other NSAIDS, and therefore, it should not be used for more than 5 consecutive days.

Ketorolac, an nsNSAID, has similar efficacy to standard doses of morphine and meperidine and is thus ***opioid sparing***. As such, it decreases the common opioid side effects such as postoperative nausea and vomiting, constipation or ileus, and cardiorespiratory depression.

The risk of GI complications exists for all NSAIDs, including COX-2 inhibitors. Ketorolac has one of the ***highest*** relative risks for upper GI complications. Proton pump inhibitors offer protection against peptic ulcers when administered with nsNSAIDs, but COX-2–selective NSAIDs may be more protective of the small intestine. GI prophylaxis is often recommended to patients who are prescribed NSAIDs.

2. Mechanism of Action

The primary mechanism of action of nsNSAIDs is competitive inhibition of the COX enzymes, thereby preventing the creation of prostaglandins, prostacyclin, and thromboxanes from arachidonic acid. COX-1 is expressed ubiquitously, whereas COX-2 is more specifically expressed in the bone, brain, and kidney. Increased expression of COX-2 occurs in states of inflammation and stress. It was hypothesized that inhibiting the COX-2 enzyme would specifically decrease inflammation with minimal effect on the COX-1 functions and limit GI side effects. COX-2–specific inhibitors, like celecoxib, exhibit similar analgesia to nsNSAIDs but have less risk of GI symptoms and inhibition of platelet aggregation and adhesion. These drugs exhibit a 300-fold selectivity for inhibiting COX-2 compared to COX-1. The FDA, however, still markets COX-2–specific inhibitors in the same safety class as nsNSAIDs. COX-2–selective NSAIDs do not precipitate bronchospasm like some nsNAIDs or aspirin. Some NSAIDs are slightly more selective for reversible inhibition of COX-2 than COX-1, including meloxicam and nabumetone. Relative inhibition of COX-2 over COX-1 decreases as the dose of nabumetone increases. The active metabolite of nabumetone equally inhibits both COX isoforms, albeit weakly. Meloxicam and diclofenac also inhibit COX-2 more than COX-1, especially at lower doses. Other anti-inflammatory effects of NSAIDs may exist independent of the COX pathway and include interactions with basic cell functions, neutrophil activity, interference of cell adherence, and inhibition of nitric oxide synthase.[8,9]

3. Metabolism and Excretion

NSAIDs undergo minimal first-pass hepatic metabolism and are highly protein bound to albumin. NSAIDs are metabolized in the liver by ***conjugation*** or ***hydroxylation*** and eliminated ***renally***. Clearance of oral, intravenous, and intramuscular doses is similar.[10]

4. Drug Interactions and Adverse Effects

An acute overdose of NSAIDs presents with nonspecific symptoms, including nausea, vomiting, blurred vision, and drowsiness, but may also can be asymptomatic. Patients may have allergies, or pseudoallergic reactions, to NSAIDs. Concomitant use of NSAIDs with other antithrombotic medications may put patients at higher bleeding risk. Indomethacin can be used as a tocolytic agent in women who present in preterm labor; however, indomethacin (an nsNSAID) is limited to less than 3 days in this patient population given the risk of premature closure of the patent ductus arteriosus. NSAIDs exhibit a risk of adverse cardiovascular events, acute kidney injury, and gastroduodenal ulcers. To mitigate these risks, NSAIDs should be administered at the lowest possible effective dose for the shortest amount of time possible. COX-2–selective NSAIDs, while they may minimize GI side effects, are more likely to cause Stevens-Johnson syndrome than nsNSAIDs. Other adverse effects include anaphylactoid reactions and aseptic meningitis. Topical NSAIDs are absorbed and penetrate locally and may have limited systemic absorption and side effects. Ketorolac is opioid sparing, but the total cumulative dose (either parenteral or parenteral and oral) should be limited to 5 days. NSAIDs are contraindicated in patients with ***renal insufficiency*** because even short courses can produce transient reductions in kidney function.

D. *N*-Methyl-D-Aspartate Receptor Antagonists

- Ketamine
- Methadone
- Dextromethorphan
- Memantine

1. Overview

N-methyl-D-aspartate (NMDA) receptor activation allows the excitatory neurotransmitter, glutamate, to traverse membranes. NMDA receptor activation is associated with noxious stimuli, hyperalgesia, and neuropathic pain, and NMDA receptor overactivation may be responsible for decreased opioid responsiveness. Ketamine is a strong NMDA receptor antagonist, while methadone and dextromethorphan are weaker antagonists; therefore, side effects from NMDA antagonism are more profound with ketamine. The central nervous system (CNS) side effects of ketamine include hallucinations, dissociations, nightmares, and sensory changes. At subanesthetic doses, ketamine can provide analgesia for neuropathic, ischemic, and complex pain syndromes.

At low, subanesthetic doses, ketamine does not alter hemodynamics and many patients tolerate it well with minimal side effects. On the contrary, induction and anesthetic doses (>1 mg/kg) of ketamine may cause hypertension, tachycardia, increased systemic and pulmonary vascular resistances (SVR, PVR). Ketamine should be used cautiously in patients in whom tachycardia, hypertension, or increased SVR and PVR may cause morbidity, such as those with ischemic heart disease or heart failure. As a negative inotrope and direct myocardial depressant, ketamine can cause hemodynamic decompensation. Patients who use or abuse opioids chronically display hyperalgesia; thus, ketamine is especially useful in this patient population. Studies have shown that patients who receive low-dose intravenous ketamine infusions during major surgery have better analgesia and less sedation postoperatively.[11] Methadone has also been used successfully for patients with opioid tolerance and neuropathic pain.

2. Mechanism of Action

The NMDA receptor is found throughout the spinal cord and brain and in many of the same locations as opioid receptors. The NMDA receptor binds glutamate and requires glycine as an endogenous co-agonist. NMDA receptors conduct calcium. Pre- or postsynaptic NMDA receptor activation can potentiate excitatory inputs to dorsal horn neurons and increase synaptic transmission. Together, this may clinically present as hyperalgesia, allodynia, neuropathic, and chronic pain.[12] Ketamine is a noncompetitive NMDA receptor antagonist. NMDA receptor antagonism may block the development of chronic pain states and mitigate the development of tolerance to analgesic effects of opioids.

3. Metabolism and Excretion

Methadone has a long and variable half-life ranging from 6 to 60 hours. Methadone may prolong the QTc of a patient's ECG and interacts with drugs that are metabolized by CYP450 enzymes in the liver, specifically CYP3A4 and CYP2D6. Ketamine undergoes hepatic biotransformation through CYP450 isozymes 3A4, 2B6, and 2C9. CYP3A4 metabolizes ketamine to its active metabolite, ***norketamine*** (**Table 10.1**). Ketamine can be marketed as a racemic mixture, but the *S*-ketamine enantiomer has increased affinity for the NMDA receptor when compared to the *R*-enantiomer. Ketamine is water- and lipid-soluble; thus, ketamine can be administered in multiple routes. Dextromethorphan, commonly found in cough medications, has been investigated for neuropathic pain. It is metabolized by CYP2D6 in the liver to an active metabolite, dextrorphan.

4. Drug Interactions and Adverse Effects

Ketamine and methadone provide analgesia, especially useful for patients who are on chronic opioids or have neuropathic pain. CNS effects of ketamine are limiting and include hallucinations. These ***psychomimetic*** effects may be attenuated by administering a benzodiazepine prior to ketamine. Adverse reactions after ketamine administration, however, are dose related and more likely with anesthetic doses than analgesic doses. Ketamine is a direct myocardial depressant and can lead to hemodynamic decompensation in some patients. Ketamine is also a sialogogue. Weaker NMDA receptor antagonists, such as dextromethorphan and memantine, may possess analgesic benefit but have not been as well studied.

E. α_2-Adrenergic Receptor Agonists: Clonidine and Dexmedetomidine

1. Overview

The α_2-adrenergic receptor is a G-protein–coupled receptor located within the brain and spinal cord and peripherally. Agonists of α_2-receptor are used for sedation and analgesia and decrease agitation and sympathetic tone. Studies support that dexmedetomidine causes a state like non–rapid eye movement physiology without any change in cognitive function. Dexmedetomidine does not inhibit respiratory drive, which makes it a common medication in intensive care units to facilitate extubation. Dexmedetomidine provides effective opioid-sparing analgesia for many patients, including patients who are on high doses of opioids, and may reduce the incidence of opioid-related adverse events. Dexmedetomidine decreases emergence delirium in children.

2. Mechanism of Action

α-Receptor agonists inhibit adenylyl cyclase activity and function ***supraspinally***, where they regulate dopamine, norepinephrine, and other physiologic pathways. Analgesic actions may be related to the effects of α-receptors within the spinal cord, although many of these medications cross the blood-brain barrier. The α_{2A}-receptor subtype is in the spinal cord and brain, including the locus coeruleus and cerebral cortex, where it mediates analgesia and sedation. Dexmedetomidine is a highly selective α_{2A} agonist. Clonidine is a nonselective α_2 agonist. Other receptor subtypes, α_{2B} and α_{2C}, are located within the brain. Medications that have different binding affinities for the α_2-receptor subtypes may have differing indications. For example, α_{2A}-selective agonists, such as guanfacine, are used as antihypertensives. α_2-Receptor antagonists are also used for some psychiatric conditions.

3. Metabolism and Excretion

Clonidine is partially metabolized by the liver into inactive metabolites and excreted unchanged by the kidneys. Dexmedetomidine is metabolized by glucuronidation and oxidation within the liver and excreted in the urine.

4. Drug Interactions and Adverse Effects

α_2-Receptor agonists cause hypotension and bradycardia. Clonidine causes these effects through a reduction in CNS-mediated sympathetic activity. Dexmedetomidine facilitates postoperative recovery and spares opioid usage postoperatively. Research has investigated the addition of α_2 agonists to local anesthetics for administration of peripheral nerve blockade, but there is no widely accepted consensus regarding their use in this specific realm.

III. Novel Nonopioid Analgesics and Future Directions

- Tetrahydrocannabinol
- Esmolol
- Tricyclic antidepressants
- Anticonvulsants

A. Cannabinoids

Cannabis plants have been grown and used throughout the world for thousands of years. Medical cannabis use has increased, and patients and providers cite chronic pain as the most common reason to use cannabis. Cannabis can be inhaled or ingested. Animal models have shed light on the analgesic effects of cannabinoids, which include inhibiting the release of neurotransmitters from presynaptic terminals, modulation of postsynaptic neurons, and activation of descending inhibitory pathways. Cannabinoids may act on multiple native targets including cannabinoid receptor 1 and cannabinoid receptor 2. These are G-protein–coupled receptors and ligand-gated ion channels in the peripheral and central nervous systems. The main component of cannabis is ***delta-9-tetrahydrocannabinol*** (THC), which contributes to the psychoactive effects of cannabis. ***Cannabidiol*** is a nonpsychoactive analogue of THC that possesses analgesic effects. Cannabinoid receptor activation in the CNS causes undesirable side effects including cognitive impairment. Large, longitudinal trials have not been performed; therefore, there is no accepted ideal dose or duration of cannabinoid use.[13] There are two synthetic cannabinoids currently marketed: dronabinol and nabilone. These two medications are FDA approved for the treatment of chemotherapy-induced nausea and vomiting.

B. Esmolol

Esmolol use perioperatively has been studied as a synergistic analgesic. Research has shown that esmolol decreases postoperative pain scores and intraoperative opioid use and mitigates opioid-induced hyperalgesia. The mechanisms have not been elucidated. Theories exist as to how perioperative esmolol may contribute to antinociception; for example, the β-receptor effects may blunt sympathetic arousal transmission.[14] Intraoperative esmolol infusions may contribute to less postoperative pain, but larger studies are needed to further evaluate this correlation and explore esmolol's ability to potentiate analgesia.

C. Antidepressants

Tricyclic antidepressants and serotonin norepinephrine reuptake inhibitors, such as duloxetine, are more efficacious as analgesics than selective serotonin reuptake inhibitors. These medications inhibit neuropathic pain in animal models and are front-line drugs for fibromyalgia. The analgesic effects on chronic pain manifest within a week of use, whereas the effects on depression take 2 to 4 weeks. Norepinephrine reuptake inhibition enhances analgesic effects through α_2-adrenergic receptors in the dorsal horn of the spinal cord. Nortriptyline, a tricyclic antidepressant, is better tolerated than amitriptyline for the treatment of neuropathic pain.

D. Anticonvulsants

Anticonvulsants are commonly used to treat neuropathic pain. They work via voltage- and ligand-gated ion channels in central pain pathways. Gabapentin and pregabalin inhibit voltage-gated calcium channels. Patients who receive anticonvulsants as analgesics or adjuvants for a prolonged period should not have these medications abruptly discontinued as this can precipitate a withdrawal syndrome and seizures. In 2019, the FDA issued a warning regarding respiratory depression with gabapentinoid use and risk of respiratory depression when used in combination with opioids.

IV. Opioid Analgesics

A. Endogenous Opioids

Endogenous opioids are neuropeptides that are produced within the pituitary gland and include endorphins, enkephalins, and dynorphins. Endomorphins have been identified, but their function is still under investigation. These peptides are formed from large protein precursors and act as neurotransmitters.

Endogenous opioids are involved in circuits related to pain modulation, reward, stress response, and autonomic control. Opioids modulate other physiologic processes including endocrine and immune functions, GI transit, ventilation, and mood. β-Endorphins bind to multiple opioid receptors and decrease pain, modulate euphoria, and cause other effects. Enkephalins alter calcium influx and facilitate hyperpolarization of neurons. In the substantia gelatinosa of the spinal cord, enkephalins modulate pain perception. The periaqueductal gray in the brain also contains enkephalins that modulate analgesia and inhibit the release of excitatory neurotransmitters. Overall, β-endorphins and enkephalins have the greatest affinity for the μ- and δ-opioid receptors, whereas dynorphins have a greater affinity for κ-receptors, but all endogenous opioids bind classical opioid receptors. Endogenous opioids and opioid receptors are located throughout the central and peripheral nervous systems.

B. Opioid Receptors

Opioid receptors include the classical μ, δ, κ, and the nonclassical nociceptin-orphanin opioid (or opioid receptor like-1) receptors that are seven transmembrane G-protein–coupled receptors with intra- and extracellular loops and homology among the receptor subtypes. Other receptor subtypes have been suggested but have been dismissed because of lack of naloxone sensitivity. Activation of an opioid receptor facilitates pre- and postsynaptic inhibition that decreases neuronal excitability by inhibition of adenylate cyclase, therefore decreasing cyclic adenosine monophosphate (cAMP) production and calcium influx with increased potassium efflux leading to neuronal hyperpolarization. These mechanisms reduce neuronal excitability with consequential decrease in nerve impulse transmission and inhibition of neurotransmitter release. The differential location and expression of the opioid receptor subtypes provide a range of opioid-induced effects. The main analgesic effects of opioids result from central activation, whereas some of the side effects (reduced GI motility, urinary retention, and pruritus) result from activation of peripherally located opioid receptors. Peripherally acting opioid receptor antagonists, such as methylnaltrexone, treat opioid-induced constipation. Overall, μ- and δ-receptor agonism produces positive reinforcement, whereas κ-receptor agonism provides the more negative effects of opioids (**Figure 10.2**).

The ***μ-opioid receptor*** is located throughout the cerebral cortex, amygdala, basal ganglia, and periaqueductal gray. These receptors are also located presynaptically within the dorsal horn of the spinal cord where they inhibit glutamate release and transmission of nociceptive stimuli from C- and A-delta fibers. Side effects of μ-receptor agonism include inhibition of GI peristalsis and respiratory depression because of a reduction in the sensitivity of chemoreceptors to hypercapnia. μ-Opioid receptor knockout mice exhibit increased sensitivity to thermal pain; these knockout mice also lack the predicted effects and side effects of drugs that act on the μ-opioid receptor.

The ***δ-opioid receptor*** exists in high densities within the cerebral cortex, nucleus accumbens, and putamen. δ-Receptor agonists are involved in analgesia, decreased GI mobility, and respiratory depression. The δ-opioid receptor also modulates mood.

κ-Opioid receptor activation causes sedation and hallucinations, but κ-receptor agonists do not cause respiratory depression. κ-Receptors are located within the nucleus raphe, which are part of the descending inhibitory pathway.

The ***nociceptin-orphanin opioid receptor***, in vitro, exhibits a pronociceptive, anti-analgesic effect supraspinally, but spinal agonism leads to analgesia

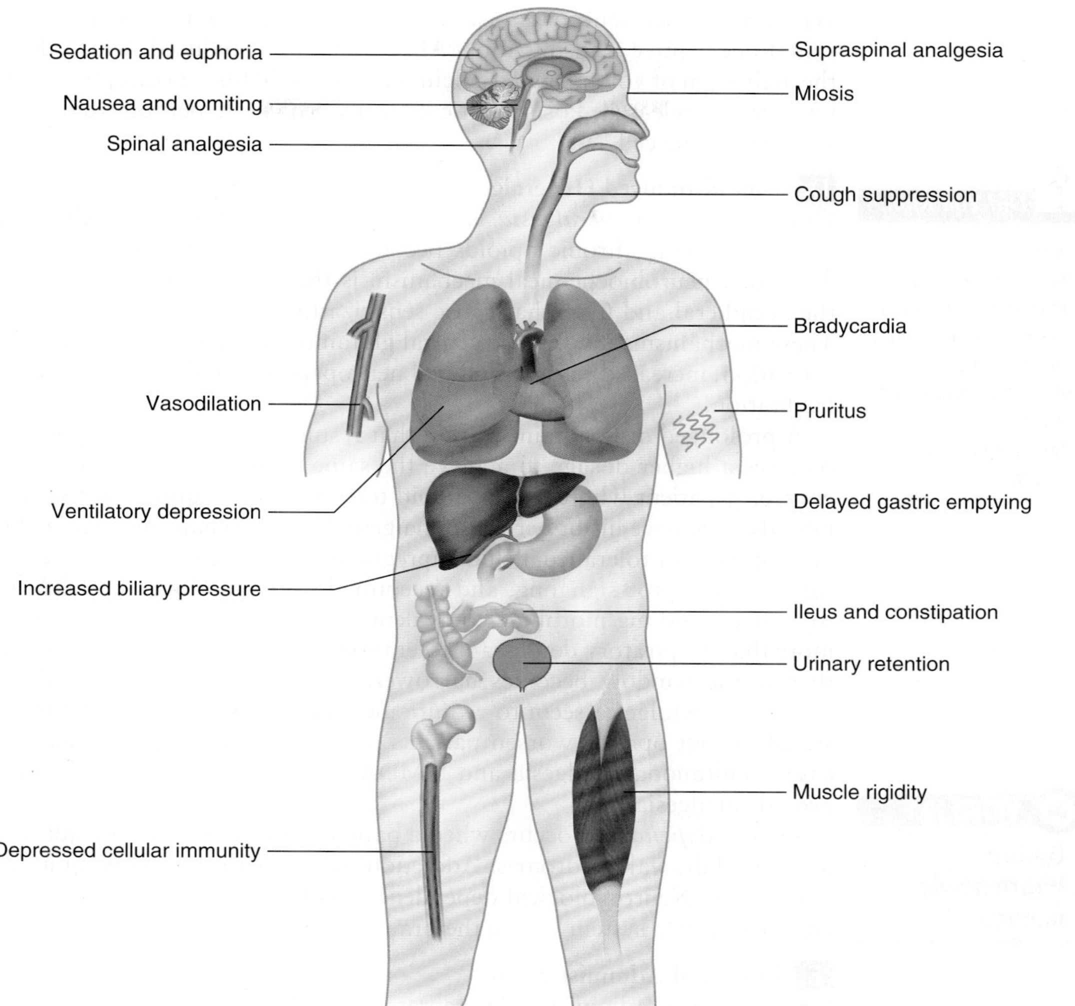

Figure 10.2 Opioid pharmacodynamics. A summary chart of the selected effects of opioids throughout the body.

at high doses balanced with hyperalgesia at low doses. These receptors are also located in the nucleus raphe. Nociceptin-orphanin receptor antagonists produce analgesia. Nociceptin-orphanin receptor knockout mice exhibit loss of tolerance to opioids. Consequently, this receptor may contribute to the development of tolerance observed with chronic opioid use.

C. Mechanism of Opioid Analgesia

Opioid receptors are part of descending inhibitory pathways that modulate the sensation of noxious stimuli. These receptors are localized in subcortical areas of the brain including the thalamus, periaqueductal gray, medulla, and locus coeruleus. Some of these areas are part of the limbic system, which is involved in reward pathways. The dorsal horn of the spinal cord, within lamina I and II, is involved in relaying nociceptive input to the brain. Nociceptive action potentials trigger the release of nociceptive transmitters, including ***substance P, glutamate, calcitonin gene–related peptide***, which relay this information via second-order neurons in ascending pathways. Opioids, therefore, inhibit spinal nociceptive transmission; cAMP signaling is reduced, which decreases the activation of voltage-gated calcium channels. In turn, nociceptive transmitters are not released. Postsynaptic neurons become hyperpolarized as potassium enters the cell.[15,16]

? Did You Know?

With continued use, the tolerance to the analgesic effects of opioids increases more than tolerance to the respiratory depressant effects, thus narrowing the therapeutic window.

D. Opioid-Induced Hyperalgesia, Tolerance, and Dependence

Opioid-induced ***hyperalgesia*** is a paradoxical situation in which a patient who is receiving chronic opioids becomes more sensitive to painful stimuli. The exact neurobiochemical mechanism is thought to arise from changes in the peripheral and CNS that cause sensitization of pronociceptive pathways. These mechanisms involve the central glutaminergic system, NMDA receptor activation, increased release of spinal neuropeptides, and descending pathway facilitation.

A prolonged drug administration that results in a loss of drug potency and requires a higher dosage to achieve the same desired effect is defined as ***tolerance***. A patient who exhibits opioid tolerance will require a higher dose of opioids to achieve his or her prior analgesic level. Mechanisms that lead to the development of tolerance include upregulation of drug metabolism, desensitization of receptor signaling, and receptor downregulation. The FDA defines tolerance as 60 mg morphine equivalents daily. Analgesic tolerance increases more than respiratory depressant tolerance; therefore, as dosages increase, the therapeutic window becomes narrower. Both opioid tolerance and opioid-induced hyperalgesia seem to require increased dosing of opioids for analgesic effect, but opioids worsen patients' opioid-induced hyperalgesia. In both cases, multimodal analgesia and NMDA receptor antagonists are helpful to provide analgesia.

VIDEO 10.1
Opioid Pharmacodynamics

Opioid ***dependence*** occurs when a patient continues to use a medication to avoid withdrawal syndromes. Addiction occurs with drug craving and compulsive use. Neurobiological dependence has been tied to the locus coeruleus and mesolimbic system within the brain.

E. Routes of Administration

Opioids may be administered parenterally, orally, sublingually, transdermally, and intranasally. Most commonly, opioids are administered either via the intravenous or oral route, but some can be administered intrathecally or epidurally, such as fentanyl or preservative-free morphine. Fentanyl and buprenorphine are also marketed as transdermal patches. Fentanyl can be given buccally.

F. Pharmacokinetics and Pharmacodynamics

Plasma and effect site concentrations are important to understand opioid behavior. Medications, like alfentanil, with quick transfer between plasma and effect site, the brain, show that an intravenous dose exerts a quick analgesic response. This example highlights the importance of understanding concepts that define drug kinetics including ***time to peak effect after bolus, time to steady state*** after starting an infusion, and ***context-sensitive half-life***. **Figure 10.3** exhibits common bolus front-end and back-end kinetics of various opioids. When rapid onset analgesia is desired, a rapid onset opioid is most useful, such as remifentanil, alfentanil, or fentanyl. These exert their effects more rapidly than morphine. When using an opioid infusion, it is critical to understand the time to ***steady-state plasma concentration***. Plasma concentrations of opioids, except remifentanil, continue to rise for hours after an infusion is initiated. On the contrary, remifentanil infusions, when started with a bolus

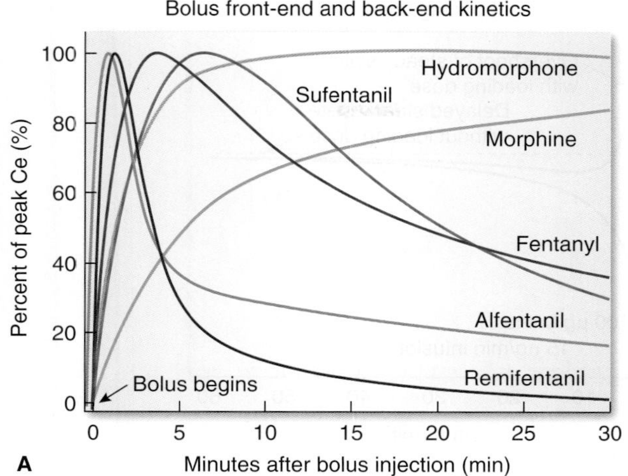

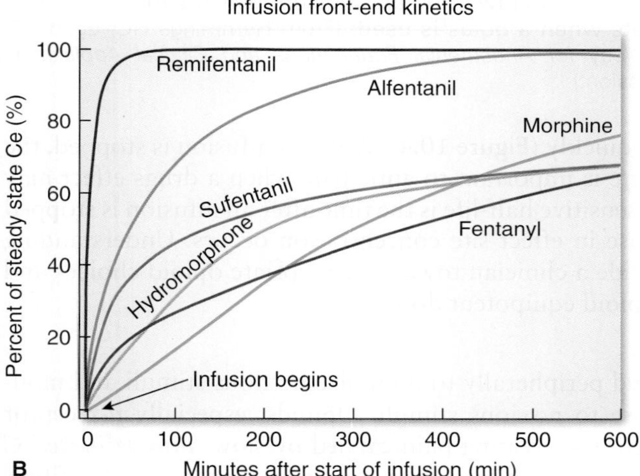

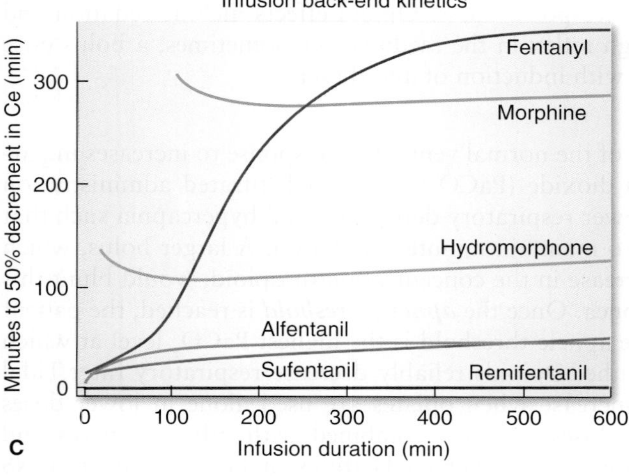

Figure 10.3 Opioid pharmacokinetics. Front-end and back-end pharmacokinetic behavior after administration by bolus injection or continuous infusions for morphine, hydromorphone, fentanyl, alfentanil, sufentanil, and remifentanil. A, Percent of peak effect site concentrations after bolus dosing. B, Percent of steady-state effect site concentrations after beginning an infusion. C, Context-sensitive half-time, or time in minutes to a 50% decrease in effect site concentrations after an infusion is stopped. (From Hemmings HC, Egan TD. *Pharmacology and Physiology for Anesthesia: Foundations and Clinical Application*. Elsevier; 2013, with permission.)

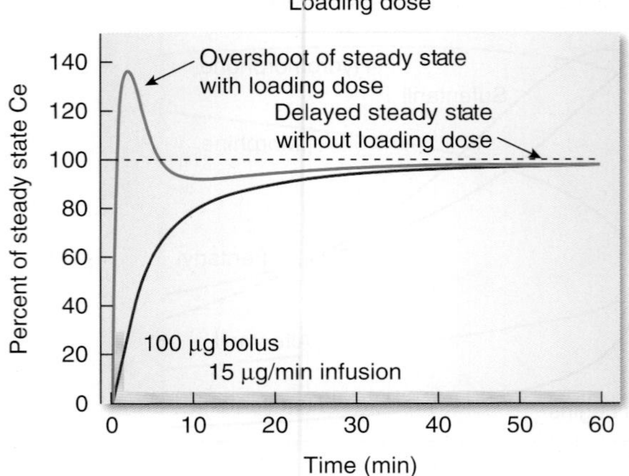

Figure 10.4 Demonstration of plasma concentrations following administration of a bolus dose of remifentanil followed by an infusion, which shows the rapid attainment of steady state when a bolus is used. (From Hemmings HC, Egan TD. *Pharmacology and Physiology for Anesthesia: Foundations and Clinical Application.* Elsevier; 2013, with permission.)

dose, reach steady state quickly (**Figure 10.4**). After an infusion is stopped, the ***context-sensitive half-life*** is important to anticipate when a drugs effect may terminate. The context-sensitive half-life is the time after an infusion is stopped in which a 50% decrease in effect site concentration occurs. Understanding these definitions will guide a clinician toward appropriate opioid choices and uses. **Table 10.2** lists opioid equipotent doses.

G. Therapeutic Effects

Opioids act centrally and peripherally to minimize noxious stimuli and modify the affective response to noxious stimuli. Opioids, especially μ-receptor agonists, are most effective at treating pain carried by slow, ***unmyelinated C fibers***. Neuropathic pain and pain transmitted by fast, myelinated A-δ fibers are not as effectively treated with opioids. The goal of opioid therapy is analgesia, not amnesia or unresponsiveness. Opioid effects include sedation and suppression of the cough reflex in the medulla, but sometimes, a bolus dose may result in coughing with induction of anesthesia.

H. Adverse Effects

Opioids cause blunting of the normal ventilatory response to increases in partial pressure of carbon dioxide ($PaCO_2$). Measured, titrated administration of opioids results in slower respiratory depression and hypercapnia such that the body may be able to maintain minute ventilation. A larger bolus, which could cause a rapid increase in the concentration of opioid, would blunt this response and lead to apnea. Once the ***apneic threshold*** is reached, the patient may breathe again. The apneic threshold is the highest $PaCO_2$ level at which a patient does not breathe. Opioids reliably decrease respiratory rate. Tidal volumes may slightly increase when opiates are used alone in lower doses but decrease at higher doses or when combined with other sedatives and anesthetics. Concomitant use of other medications or factors that are CNS depressants, such as benzodiazepines, large doses of opioids, older age, and hepatic or renal insufficiency, increase the risk of opioid-induced respiratory depression.

> **? *Did You Know?***
>
> The factors that increase the risk of opioid ventilatory depression include high dose, natural sleep, old age, other CNS depressants, and decreased clearance due to hepatic or renal insufficiency.

Table 10.2 Opioid Equipotent Doses[a]

Opioid	Dose
Morphine	1 mg
Hydromorphone	0.2 mg
Fentanyl	50 µg
Alfentanil	150 µg
Sufentanil	5 µg
Remifentanil	50 µg
Meperidine	10 mg
Methadone	1 mg

mg = milligram; µg = microgram.
[a]Note, methadone equivalence is not linear.

Opioids promote parasympathetic over sympathetic activity. When used intraoperatively, this parasympathetic tone manifests as cardiovascular changes; opioids, however, do not have direct cardiovascular depressant effects. Some opioids, such as fentanyl, increase vagal tone and manifest as bradycardia. Chest wall rigidity may be seen following bolus doses of fentanyl or its congeners, which may impair adequate bag mask ventilation.

Opioids may modulate immune function as opioid receptors exist on immune cells. Opioids may be immunosuppressant, but new data suggest they may play a dual role, although the exact mechanism of opioids and their relation to immune function has yet to be elucidated.

I. Metabolism and Active Metabolites

Opioid metabolism generally occurs in the liver by the hepatic cytochrome system. They are highly protein bound and ionized at physiologic pH. Remifentanil is one opioid that is a major exception to this opioid metabolism generalization and is discussed below.

J. Drug Interactions

Sedative drugs, such as benzodiazepines, act ***synergistically*** with opioids to provide greater sedation from their combination rather than from each medication alone. Similarly, gabapentinoids also exhibit synergistic effects of respiratory depression when combined with opioids. In 2019, the FDA issued a new warning regarding respiratory depression with gabapentinoid use and risk of opioid overdose when used in combination with opioids. The synergistic effect of administering an opioid with a benzodiazepine is illustrated in **Figure 10.5**, and a similar effect is seen with propofol (**Figure 10.6**). Opioids, when used at moderate doses intraoperatively, decrease the minimum alveolar concentration (MAC) of volatile anesthetics as much as 75%.

K. Pharmacogenetics and Special Populations

Codeine, a more common outpatient analgesic than inpatient analgesic, may not provide analgesia to patients equally. Codeine is a ***prodrug***; it must be metabolized to morphine to exert an effect. It is metabolized by the CYP450 enzyme, CYP2D6, but in some of the population, this isoform is lacking. The CYP2D6 isoform can be inhibited by other drugs, like fluoxetine or bupropion, rendering a limited response to codeine. Patients exhibit a normal response to morphine even if they may not exhibit a normal cleavage of codeine. Other opioids,

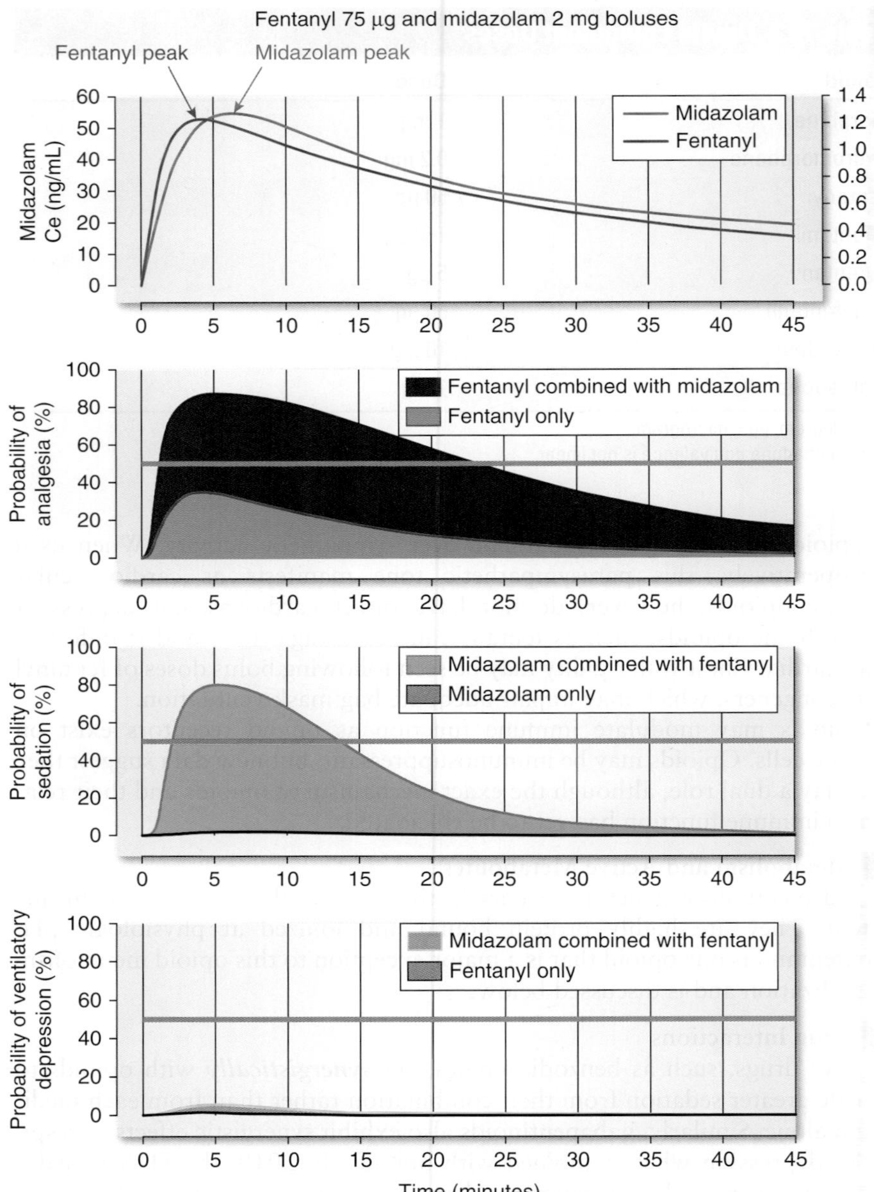

Figure 10.5 Simulation of simultaneous intravenous administration of 75 µg fentanyl and 2 mg midazolam. Top simulation: time to peak plasma concentration of each drug. Middle simulations: synergistic effect of combining opioid with benzodiazepine for the clinical effects of analgesia and sedation. Bottom simulation: low probability of ventilatory depression with this combination, in contrast to the high probability of analgesia and sedation. (Derived from Key Concepts in Safe Sedation. In: Johnson KB. *Clinical Pharmacology for Anesthesiology.* McGraw-Hill Education; 2015 and Safe Sedation Training. https://www.safesedationtraining.com/. Accessed October 6, 2014)

including tramadol, hydrocodone, and oxycodone, are also metabolized by the CYP2D6 isoform. ***Poor metabolizers*** exhibit a decreased analgesic response to these drugs. On the contrary, some patients are ***ultrarapid metabolizers.*** Approximately 1% to 2% of the population falls into this category in which they have duplicated functional genes for CYP2D6. As such, these patients

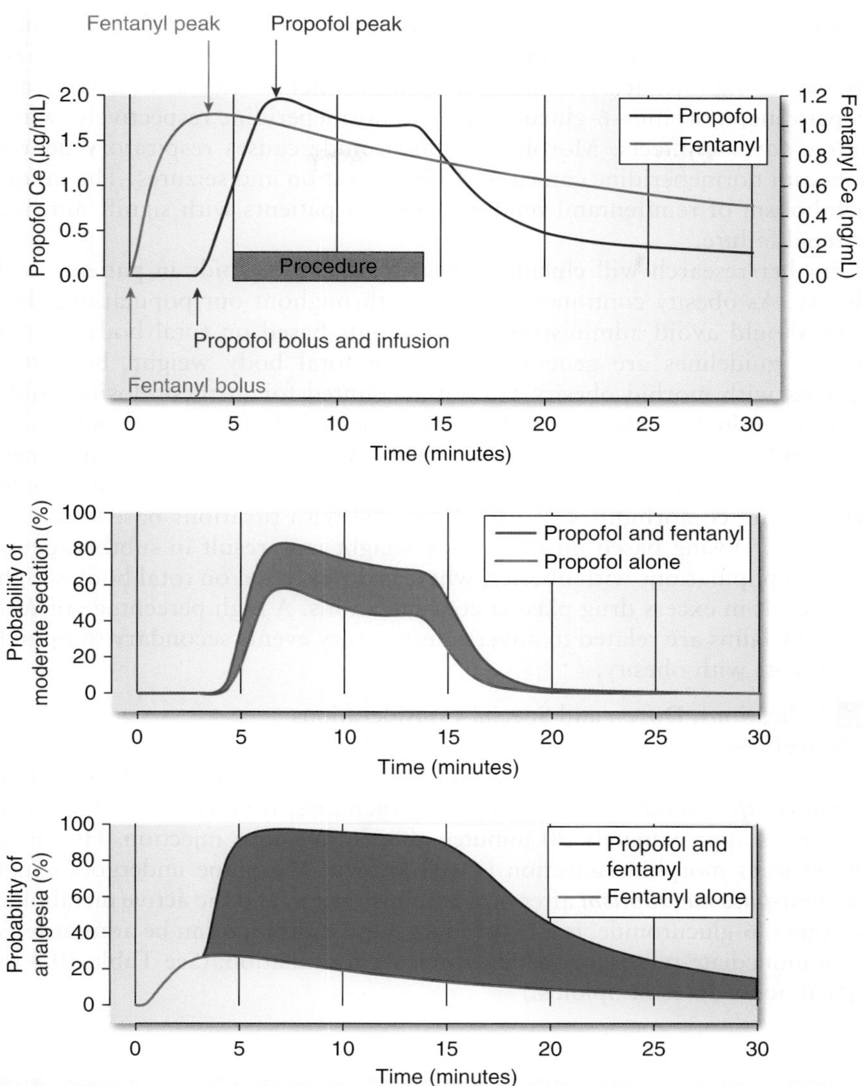

Figure 10.6 Simulation of propofol and fentanyl plasma concentrations. Top simulation: fentanyl is administered as a bolus intravenous dose at time 0. Propofol bolus and infusion is administered 4 minutes later. The middle and bottom simulations represent the probability of moderate sedation and analgesia, respectively, and illustrate the principle of synergism between opioids and propofol. (Derived from Key Concepts in Safe Sedation. In: Johnson KB. *Clinical Pharmacology for Anesthesiology*. McGraw-Hill Education; 2015 and Safe Sedation Training. https://www.safesedationtraining.com/. Accessed October 6, 2014)

metabolize codeine to morphine more rapidly and completely. These patients may then exhibit symptoms of morphine overdose. This clinical effect was seen in pediatric deaths following tonsillectomy, so in 2013, the FDA issued a black box warning against using codeine in pediatric patients undergoing tonsillectomy. Older patients, specifically those older than 65 years, are more sensitive to opioids, and their dosages should be reduced by 50%. Genetic investigations may shed further light on differences in opioid metabolism and responsiveness.

Patients with liver failure or hepatic encephalopathy are particularly sensitive to the sedative effects of opioids. Opioid metabolism is not affected by patients with alterations in their liver function, but the anhepatic phase of orthotopic liver transplantation alters opioid metabolism. Renal failure causes significant accumulation of active metabolites of morphine and meperidine, morphine-6-glucuronide and normeperidine respectively, which causes adverse effects. Morphine-6-glucuronide causes respiratory depression, and normeperidine can cause CNS excitation and seizures. The unique metabolism of remifentanil renders it safe in patients with significant liver or renal failure.

Further research will elucidate the behavior of opioids in patients with obesity. As obesity continues to increase throughout our population, clinicians should avoid administration of opioids based on total body weight. Dosing guidelines are generally based on total body weight, but often, patients with morbid obesity are not accounted for in these dosing guidelines. A limited number of studies have assessed ***dosing scalars*** other than total body weight in patients with obesity. A dosing scalar, or dosing medications based on individual patient characteristics including age, weight, gender, and comorbidities, is useful coupled with titrations based on clinical effect. Dosing based on ideal body weight may result in subtherapeutic doses in populations with obesity, whereas doses based on total body weight may result in excess drug plasma concentrations. A high percentage of ASA Closed Claims are related to adverse respiratory events secondary to opioids in patients with obesity.

L. Indications, Doses, and Special Considerations

1. Morphine

Morphine has been well studied and is the prototypical opioid. Morphine is ***poorly lipid soluble*** and ***hydrophilic***; therefore, it enters the CNS slowly and peaks approximately 90 minutes after intravenous injection. Histamine release after morphine injection is well known. Morphine undergoes extensive ***first-pass metabolism*** after oral administration, and the active metabolite, morphine-6-glucuronide, is a by-product. Oral morphine can be administered as an immediate-release or sustained-release formulation. (See **Table 10.3** for typical bolus doses of opioids.)

Table 10.3 Typical Opioid Bolus Doses and Typical Opioid Oral Doses[a]

Opioid	Typical Bolus Dose	Typical Oral Analgesic Dose
Morphine	1-5 mg IV	15-30 mg PO q 4 h PRN
Hydromorphone	0.2-0.4 mg IV	2-4 mg PO q 4 h PRN
Fentanyl	50-150 µg IV	n/a
Alfentanil	150-300 µg IV	n/a
Remifentanil	25-100 µg IV; continuous infusion: 0.05-0.2 µg/kg/min	n/a
Sufentanil	5-15 µg IV; continuous infusion: 0.1-2 µg/kg/h	30 µg SL (max dose 12 tablets/d up to 72 h; not recommended for outpatient use)
Meperidine	12.5-50 mg IV	n/a

IV = intravenous; kg = kilogram; mg = milligram; SL = sublingual; µg = microgram.
[a]Note, oral to intravenous conversions are not 1:1.

2. Hydromorphone

Hydromorphone is a ***synthetic opioid*** with an onset time similar to morphine but reaches peak effect more quickly, within about 15 minutes. Hydromorphone is more lipophilic than morphine. Oral hydromorphone can be administered as an immediate-release or sustained-release formulation.

3. Meperidine

Meperidine is no longer commonly used as an analgesic today. It is used for anesthetic-related shivering in the postanesthesia care unit. Meperidine is contraindicated in patients receiving monoamine oxidase inhibitors. Meperidine produces an active metabolite, normeperidine, that accumulates in renal failure and causes seizures.

4. Fentanyl

Fentanyl is highly lipophilic; therefore, it crosses the blood-brain barrier rapidly. Fentanyl can be administered intravenously, intranasally, transdermally, and transmucosally. After an intravenous bolus, fentanyl reaches peak effect in 3 to 5 minutes with an analgesic effect that lasts 30 to 45 minutes. Peak respiratory depression occurs between 3 and 5 minutes after an intravenous dose. Fentanyl, however, has a long context-sensitive half-time (**Figure 10.3C**), which may detract from its use as a continuous infusion.

5. Sufentanil

Sufentanil is the most ***potent*** commercially available opioid. It can be administered as a bolus, infusion, or within the intrathecal or epidural spaces. About 5 μg of intravenous sufentanil is the analgesic equivalent to 50 μg of fentanyl.

6. Alfentanil

Alfentanil reaches peak effect rapidly, ~90 seconds after a bolus intravenous dose. The offset is also rapid (**Figure 10.1**). Alfentanil is metabolized by hepatic enzyme CYP3A4, but there is significant interindividual variability; thus the metabolism is less predictable.

7. Remifentanil

Remifentanil is a potent intravenous opioid with a rapid onset (within 90 seconds) and short duration (~3 minutes). Unlike other opioids, it is metabolized by ***ester hydrolysis*** in the plasma and tissues, which accounts for its rapid termination of action. Consequently, it is only used as a continuous infusion, not isolated boluses. Hepatic and renal failure have no impact on the metabolism of remifentanil. Remifentanil is easily titratable but has been implicated in postoperative hyperalgesia.

8. Methadone

Methadone is available for enteral and intravenous use. It is often used as a maintenance therapy for patients with opioid use disorders because of its prolonged pharmacokinetics. Methadone is administered as a racemic mixture, but the dextrorotatory isomer has antagonist activity at the ***NMDA*** receptor, which attenuates the effects of opioid hyperalgesia and tolerance. Methadone prolongs the QT interval.

M. Reversal Agents and Associated Effects

Naloxone is a competitive antagonist at the opioid receptor and is used to reverse opioid intoxication or overdose. It has the greatest affinity for the μ-opioid receptor and lowest affinity for the κ-receptor. Without the presence of opioid, naloxone has no effect. Naloxone can be administered intravenously, intranasally, subcutaneously, or intramuscularly; it can also be administered as a buccal film or tablet in combination with buprenorphine, but naloxone is poorly absorbed after oral administration. Naloxone has a quick onset, but is rapidly metabolized in the liver; thus, naloxone's ***duration of action*** is shorter than the duration of the opioid whose effects it is intended to reverse. As such, patients can renarcotize after naloxone wears off. Naloxone can cause tachycardia, other signs of opioid withdrawal and, rarely, pulmonary edema. Naloxone appears to be safe in pregnancy and crosses the placenta. Naloxone is also on the WHO Model List of Essential Medicines.

> **? *Did You Know?***
>
> Naloxone duration of action is usually substantially shorter than the opioids whose effects it is intended to reverse.

Nalbuphine, like ***butorphanol***, is a mixed opioid agonist-antagonist. It can be administered intravenously or intramuscularly and can be given as an analgesic or to reverse ***opioid-induced pruritus***. Commonly, it is used to attenuate side effects of opioids (ventilatory depression, pruritus) while maintaining some analgesia (partial κ-agonism). Because of its affinity as a μ-receptor antagonist, nalbuphine and butorphanol can precipitate withdrawal in opioid-dependent patients. The analgesic and respiratory effects of these agents reach a ***ceiling effect*** and do not decrease MAC as profoundly as morphine or fentanyl.

Buprenorphine has mixed agonist/antagonist activity at the classical opioid receptors. It has partial agonist activity at the μ- and nociceptin-orphanin opioid receptors. At low and intermediate doses, an analgesic response is created, but at higher doses, the analgesic effects may be decreased, a ***ceiling effect***. Buprenorphine exhibits κ-antagonism. When buprenorphine is administered with full opioid agonists, such as morphine, it can displace the μ-receptor binding of morphine. Buprenorphine is used as an analgesic and in patients with a history of opioid use disorder.

Methylnaltrexone is a peripherally acting μ-opioid receptor antagonist that reverses the side effects of opioids, including constipation, without affecting analgesia or precipitating withdrawal. Methylnaltrexone does not cross the blood-brain barrier because it is a quaternary ammonium cation.

Naltrexone is available as an oral formulation and intramuscular depot and is a competitive opioid antagonist. If administered to a patient who has received opioids, naltrexone will precipitate withdrawal. Naltrexone is metabolized in the liver to an active metabolite. They are both competitive antagonists at the μ-opioid receptor, the κ-opioid receptor to a lesser extent, and the δ-opioid receptor to an even lesser extent. Naltrexone is used in patients who have a history of opioid use disorder and alcohol use disorder.

For further review and interactivities, please see the associated Interactive Video Lectures and "At a Glance" infographic accessible in the complimentary eBook bundled with this text. Access instructions are located in the inside front cover.

References

1. Brownstein MJ. Review: a brief history of opiates, opioid peptides, and opioid receptors. *Proc Natl Acad Sci USA*. 1993;90:5391-5393. PMID: 8390660.
2. Gummin DD, Mowry JB, Spyker DA, Brooks DE, Osterthaler KM, Banner W. 2017 annual report of the American Association of Poison Control Centers' national poison data system (NPDS): 35th annual report. *Clin Toxicol (Phila)*. 2018;56(12):1213-1415. PMID: 30576252.
3. Bunchorntavakul C, Reddy KR. Acetaminophen-related hepatotoxicity. *Clin Liver Dis*. 2013;17(4):587-607. PMID: 24099020.
4. Hayward KL, Powell EE, Irvine KM, Martin JH. Can paracetamol (acetaminophen) be administered to patients with liver impairment? *Br J Clin Pharmacol*. 2016;81(2):210-222. PMID: 26460177.
5. Jian Z, Tang L, Yi X, et al. Aspirin induces Nrf2-mediated transcriptional activation of haem oxygenase-1 in protection of human melanocytes from H_2O_2- induced oxidative stress. *J Cell Mol Med*. 2016;20(7):1307-1318. PMID: 26969214.
6. Needs CJ, Brooks PM. Clinical pharmacokinetics of the salicylates. *Clin Pharmacokinet*. 1985;10(2):164-177. PMID: 3888490.
7. Zhang J, Ding EL, Song Y. Adverse effects of cyclooxygenase-2 inhibitors on renal and arrhythmia events: meta-analysis of randomized trails. *J Am Med Assoc*. 2006;296(13):1619-1632. PMID: 16968832.
8. Silverstein FE, Faich G, Goldstein JL, et al. Gastrointestinal toxicity with celecoxib vs nonsteroidal anti-inflammatory drugs for osteoarthritis and rheumatoid arthritis: the CLASS study. A randomized controlled trial. Celecoxib Long-term Arthritis Safety Study. *J Am Med Assoc*. 2000;284(10):1247. PMID: 10979111.
9. Verbeeck RK, Blackburn JL, Loewen GR. Clinical pharmacokinetics of non-steroidal anti-inflammatory drugs. *Clin Pharmacokinet*. 1983;8(4):297-331. PMID: 6352138.
10. Mroszczak EJ, Jung D, Yee J, Bynum L, Sevelius H, Massey I. Ketorolac tromethamine pharmacokinetics and metabolism after intravenous, intramuscular, and oral administration in humans and animals. *Pharmacotherapy*. 1990;10(6 pt 2):33S-39S. PMID: 2082311.
11. Thompson T, Whiter F, Gallop K, et al. NMDA receptor antagonists and pain relief: a meta-analysis of experimental trials. *Neurology*. 2019;92(14):e1652-e1662. doi:10.1212/WNL.0000000000007238. PMID: 30842296.
12. Miller SL, Yeh HH. *"The NMDA receptor" in chapter 3: neurotransmitters and neurotransmission in the developing and adult nervous system*. In: *Conn's Translational Neuroscience*. Elsevier Academic Press; 2017:49-84.
13. Vučković S, Srebro D, Vujović KS, Vučetić Č, Prostran M. Cannabinoids and pain: new insights from old molecules. *Front Pharmacol*. 2018;9:1259. doi:10.3389/fphar.2018.01259. PMID: 30542280.
14. Gelineau AM, King MR, Ladha KS, Burns SM, Houle T, Anderson TA. Intraoperative esmolol as an adjunct for perioperative opioid and postoperative pain reduction: a systematic review, meta-analysis, and meta-regression. *Anesth Analg*. 2018;126(3):1035-1049. PMID: 29028742.
15. Trang T, Al-Hasani R, Salvemini D, Salter MW, Gutstein H, Cahill CM. Pain and poppies: the good, the bad, and the ugly of opioid analgesics. *J Neurosci*. 2015;35(41):13879-13888. PMID: 26468188.
16. Pasternak GW, Pan YX. Mu opioids and their receptors: evolution of a concept. *Pharmacol Rev*. 2013;65(4):1257-1317. PMID: 24076545.

PERIOPERATIVE MULTIMODAL ANALGESIA

AT A GLANCE

The combination of multiple analgesic drugs targets different nociceptive mechanisms and reduces the side effects of using a single drug class.

NSAIDs

The effect on platelets is **irreversible** for aspirin, **reversible** for other NSAIDs, and **no effect** for celecoxib.

MECHANISM
Inhibition of **cyclooxygenase** 1 and 2 (COX-1, COX-2) leads to ↓ production of inflammatory prostaglandins.
Celecoxib only inhibits COX-2.

Ketorolac when given IV = most rapid onset of NSAIDs, it reaches peak plasma concentration in 5 min.

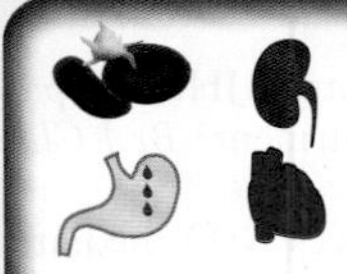

▶NSAIDs (but not COX-2 inhibitors) ↓ platelet function
▶May cause gastric ulceration
▶May cause renal insufficiency
▶COX-2 selective inhibitors may ↑ cardiac events

Opioids

All opioids act **synergystically** with other sedatives, which ↑ the risk of respiratory depression.

MECHANISM
Agonists at μ, κ, δ, and orphanin G-protein receptors leads to ↓ neuronal excitability by way of ↓ Ca^{2+} influx, ↑ K^+ efflux, and ↓ cAMP.

Opioids with ↑ lipophilicity = ↑ **potency** and faster onset. Fentanyl will reach peak effect in 5 min.

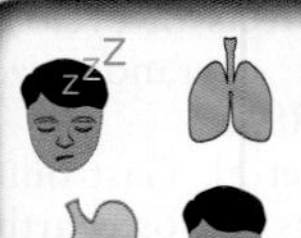

▶Sedation
▶Respiratory depression
▶Bradycardia
▶Nausea and constipation
▶Pruritus
▶Muscle rigidity

Ketamine

MECHANISM
Antagonist at N-methyl-D-aspartate (**NMDA**) receptor leads to ↓ neuronal excitability.

Methadone is an opioid but also antagonizes the NMDA receptor.

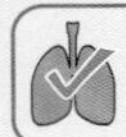

Preserves spontaneous ventilation at lower doses and is also a bronchodilator

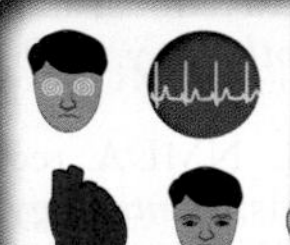

▶May cause hallucinations
▶May cause tachycardia and HTN
▶Is a myocardial depressant
▶Causes salivation
▶May cause ↑ ICP unless other sedatives are used concurrently

Acetaminophen

MECHANISM
Central acting **inhibitor** of **COX** 1, 2, and 3. Also affects opioid, serotonin, and cannabinoid receptors.

Caution if patient is concurrently taking analgesics that are opioid-acetaminophen combination drugs.

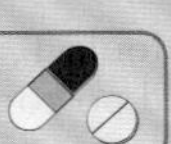

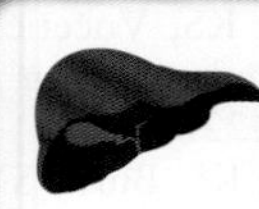

▶An overdose can cause **hepatotoxicity.**
▶The maximum daily dose should be no more than **4 g/d.**

Dexmedetomidine and clonidine

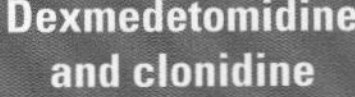

MECHANISM
Agonist at central α_2-receptors and in the posterior horn of the spinal cord.

Dexmedetomidine is also used for sedation in the OR or ICU and as a strategy to ↓ emergence delirium in children.

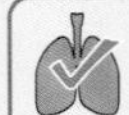

Does not ↓ respiratory drive

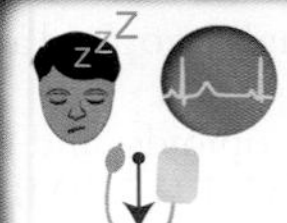

▶Although they can ↓ pain, these drugs cause sedation.
▶They cause bradycardia and hypotension.

Local anesthetics

MECHANISM
Sodium channel antagonists in nerve membranes leads to ↓ neuronal excitability.

Whenever possible, a regional anesthesia technique offers excellent analgesia and reliably reduces or eliminates the need for opioids.

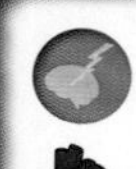

▶Patients must be monitored for the risk of local anesthetic systemic toxicity (LAST) that compromises CNS and cardiac systems.

Infographic by: Naveen Nathan MD

Questions

1. **A patient with a history of opioid use disorder currently receiving a combination of buprenorphine and naloxone is presenting to the operating room. What receptor do you choose to target with your analgesic choices to offer the patient the best multimodal analgesia?**

   A. μ-opioid receptor
   B. κ-opioid receptor
   C. NMDA receptor
   D. δ-opioid receptor
   E. None of the above

2. **A 16-year-old patient presents to the emergency department. The patient's parent believes that the patient ingested multiple acetaminophen tablets. An acute overdose of acetaminophen may cause _____.**

   A. Renal failure
   B. Centrilobular hepatotoxicity
   C. Anion gap metabolic acidosis
   D. Seizures
   E. None of the above

3. **The operation is ending, and your colleague administers an intravenous bolus of hydromorphone. Postoperatively, it is expected that opioids cause all the following effects EXCEPT:**

   A. Sedation
   B. Euphoria
   C. Delayed gastric emptying
   D. Ileus
   E. Miosis
   F. Cough promotion

4. **An intubated and sedated patient in the ICU is receiving dexmedetomidine. He is hemodynamically stable, normotensive, and bradycardic. Dexmedetomidine provides analgesia by:**

   A. Nonselective cyclooxygenase inhibition
   B. Stimulation of the μ-receptor
   C. NMDA receptor antagonism
   D. α_2-receptor simulation
   E. None of the above

5. **A patient is describing significant pain. This patient has an elevated creatine of 2.2 but no other medical problems. It is important to avoid:**

   A. Clonidine administration
   B. Ketorolac administration
   C. Ketamine administration
   D. Hydromorphone administration
   E. None of the above

Answers

1. C

Buprenorphine/naloxone combination medications are used for patients with a history of opioid use disorder. Buprenorphine has a high affinity for the μ-opioid receptor; therefore, giving additional pure opioids, such as morphine, may not provide adequate analgesia. Instead, targeting a different receptor, such as using ketamine, will provide more effective multimodal analgesia. Ketamine is an NMDA receptor antagonist.

2. B

Excess amounts of acetaminophen cause the metabolic pathway of glucuronidation and sulfonation in the liver to become overwhelmed. As such, the toxic metabolite causes hepatocellular injury and contributes to acute liver failure. Acetaminophen overdose is a cause of acute liver failure in the United States. Aspirin overdose causes renal failure, seizures, and anion gap metabolic acidosis and requires treatment in an intensive care unit with alkaline diuresis to promote salicylate excretion.

3. F

Figure 10.2 displays common effects of opioids throughout the body. Sedation, euphoria, delayed gastric emptying and ileus, miosis, and respiratory depression are common side effects after opioid administration.

4. D

Dexmedetomidine, like clonidine, is an α_2-adrenergic receptor agonist. While it may cause hypertension, hypotension, and bradycardia, it can be used in ICUs to provide sedation prior to extubation as it has no effect on respiratory drive. Nonselective cyclooxygenase inhibitors (or nsNSAIDs) include ibuprofen and ketorolac. Opioids are an example of μ-receptor agonists. Ketamine and methadone are examples of NMDA receptor antagonists that provide analgesia.

5. B

Clonidine is an α-agonist and can cause hemodynamic alterations. Ketamine is an NMDA receptor antagonist, and its side effects include hallucinations and excess secretions. Hydromorphone is a potent opioid, like morphine. In patients with renal disease, it is important to avoid NSAIDs as even short courses can produce reductions in renal function.

11 Neuromuscular Blocking Agents

Stephan R. Thilen and Wade A. Weigel

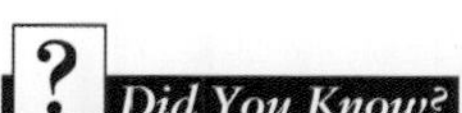

NMBAs are unique, powerful drugs that can inflict serious complications if not used appropriately. It is incumbent on every anesthesia provider to understand how these drugs work and how to safely use them.

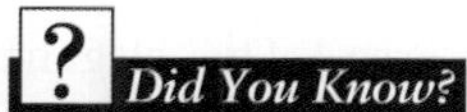

A standardized color code for anesthetic drug labels is used in the United States, Australia, New Zealand, and Canada. In this scheme, only NMBAs are given the color red.

I. History and Introduction

The introduction of neuromuscular blocking agents (NMBAs) into clinical medicine (curare in 1942 and succinylcholine in 1949) has facilitated major advances in anesthesiology. NMBAs are primarily used to facilitate intubation and to improve operating conditions. They may also be used in surgical cases where prevention of any patient movement is critical. NMBAs are also used on specific indication in the intensive care unit, particularly to facilitate mechanical ventilation. Despite their many benefits, NMBAs carry their own set of complications. This class of drugs contributes to the risk of accidental awareness under anesthesia, a rare but serious complication that often leads to devastating posttraumatic stress disorder. A more common complication is a clinically significant lingering effect after emergence from anesthesia. This is referred to as postoperative residual neuromuscular blockade, or residual paralysis; 30% to 40% of patients who receive NMBAs are at risk for this complication. Given that there are over 200 million major surgeries performed every year worldwide, the number of patients exposed to potential complications is significant, and appropriate neuromuscular blockade monitoring is a major patient safety issue. Allergic reactions and anaphylaxis (with an incidence of 1 in 6000-20,000 administrations depending on NMBA), although rare, are also potential problems.

A. Morphology of the Neuromuscular Junction

Muscle contraction occurs when a signal transmitted from the brain via nerve fibers is received by the muscle. A nerve is made up of many axons, and those axons communicate with muscle fibers. The motor unit consists of the motor neuron and the muscle fibers it innervates. Strength of muscle contraction is tied to the number of motor units activated, such that the activation of more motor units leads to a stronger muscle contraction.

The transmission of the nerve signal to the muscle occurs at the neuromuscular junction (**Figure 11.1**). This consists of the end of the motor nerve (presynaptic motor neuron), a gap (synaptic cleft, 50 nm width), and the muscle fiber (motor end plate). Acetylcholine (ACh) is the transmitter utilized to traverse the synaptic cleft, and within the cleft resides the enzyme acetylcholinesterase (AChAse) to keep the process in check. The release of ACh is tightly regulated at the presynaptic nerve. There are folds on the muscle which contain muscle-type nicotinic acetylcholine receptors (nAChRs). More than 90% of all nAChRs in a muscle fiber are located at the synapse, an area that

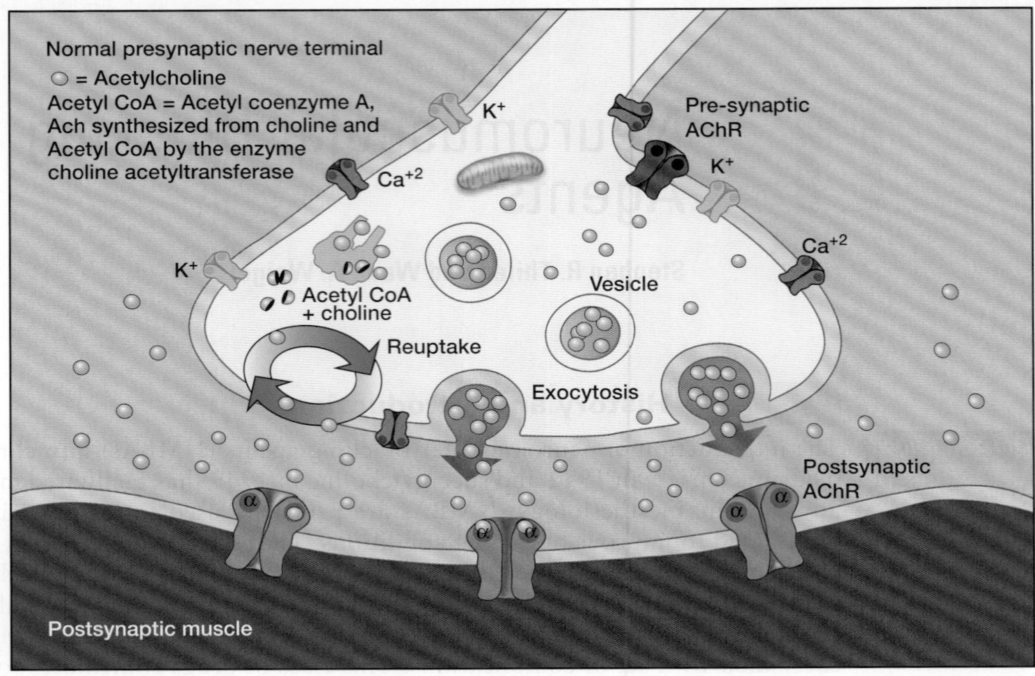

Figure 11.1 Normal neuromuscular transmission across the neuromuscular junction. ACh is synthesized from choline and acetyl CoA by the enzyme choline acetyltransferase. acetyl CoA, acetyl coenzyme A; Ach, acetylcholine.

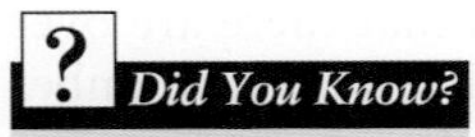

The ACh vesicle transport system cannot keep up when exogenous electrical signals are sent to a nerve at very high frequencies (typically above 70 Hz). When 100 Hz stimulation is applied over 5 seconds, muscle contraction often cannot be sustained. This is known as physiologic fade.

represents <0.1% of the total muscle membrane surface area.[1] This elegant process strings together electrical (motor nerve end), chemical (ACh release), and mechanical (muscle contractions) events.

B. Presynaptic Events: Mobilization and Release of Acetylcholine

An electrical signal reaching the presynaptic motor neuron ending, the nerve terminal, activates voltage-gated calcium (Ca^{2+}) channels allowing the influx of calcium. ACh is synthesized in the presynaptic nerve terminal from choline and acetyl coenzyme A (acetyl CoA) by the enzyme choline acetyltransferase. The calcium influx mobilizes small vesicles containing ACh to migrate toward the synaptic cleft, fuse with the nerve membrane, and release quanta (50,000-100,000 molecules) of ACh into the synaptic cleft. Some ACh-containing vesicles reside in the active zone very near the membrane, where they are immediately available for fusion. A much larger number or ACh vesicles reside away from the active zone in a reserve pool. Proteins present in the nerve terminal facilitate vesicle movement from the reserve pool to the active zone. Release of ACh from vesicles also occur spontaneously and randomly, leading to miniature end plate potentials (MEPPs) which represent release of hundreds of ACh molecules. In contrast, an action potential initiates a coordinated fusion of thousands of ACh vesicles releasing millions of ACh into the synaptic cleft.

ACh vesicle migration and fusion are hindered if there is insufficient calcium available (hypocalcemia). In high concentrations, magnesium can bind and block the calcium channel, limiting calcium influx and ACh vesicle release leading to weakness. This is seen in women receiving magnesium infusions to slow the progress of labor. In Eaton-Lambert syndrome, antibodies target the calcium channels, again hindering calcium influx and resulting in weakness.

C. Postsynaptic Events

ACh traverses the synaptic cleft to the motor end plate of the muscle where it binds to postsynaptic nicotinic acetylcholine receptors (muscle-type nAChR) which are made up of five subunits. If sufficient ACh is released, depolarization of the muscle membrane occurs, resulting in actin-myosin–mediated muscle contraction. Two types of nAChR exist, mature and immature, which have four subunits in common (alpha, alpha, beta, delta). Mature nAChR, which only reside at the muscle endplate, contains an epsilon subunit (think "ε" as an E in elderly). The immature nAChR is predominately extrajunctional and contains gamma as the fifth subunit. ACh must bind to both α subunits (think two "launch keys" are required) of the nAChRs to induce a conformational change of the receptor that results in the formation of a central channel (pore). The central channel allows sodium ion (Na^+) influx and potassium (K^+) efflux, resulting in muscle cell membrane depolarization (resting −90 mV to positive). Voltage-gated Na^+ channels on the muscle membrane propagate the action potential across the membrane, leading to the development of muscle tension (excitation-contraction coupling). Upon release from the receptor, ACh undergoes rapid and efficient hydrolysis by AChAse into choline and acetic acid. Choline is then reabsorbed into the presynaptic nerve terminal. ACh can also bind to presynaptic neuronal nAChRs, which facilitates ACh movement from the reserve pool to the active zone, thus providing positive feedback allowing for an adequate concentration of ACh in the active zone also for repetitive muscle activity.

> **? Did You Know?**
>
> The migration of ACh vesicles is accomplished by a group of proteins that are digested by botulinum toxin, impairing release of ACh and leading to weakness.

D. Receptor Up- and Downregulation

Upper or lower motor neuron disruption, severe burns, immobilization, sepsis, prolonged use of NMBAs in the intensive care unit, or cerebrovascular accidents, all decrease the frequency of motor nerve stimulations. When these conditions persist over days, the number of immature nAChRs increases (upregulation). The immature nAChRs have increased sensitivity to agonists (ACh and succinylcholine [SCh]) and decreased sensitivity to nondepolarizing NMBAs. The channel opening time of the immature nAChRs is up to tenfold longer and may allow systemic release of lethal doses of intracellular K^+ in response to administration of SCh. Downregulation of mature nAChRs occurs during periods of sustained agonist stimulation, for instance, chronic neostigmine use (in patients with myasthenia gravis), or organophosphorus poisoning. This leads to SCh resistance and extreme sensitivity to nondepolarizing NMBAs.

II. Neuromuscular Blocking Agents

A. Pharmacologic Characteristics of Neuromuscular Blocking Agents

Potency of a drug is determined by the dose required to produce a certain effect and is typically expressed in a dose versus response curve. Commonly, drug potency is expressed as the effective dose for a percentage of patients. As such, ED_{95} represents the effective dose for 95% of patients. The expression of NMBA potency does not follow this convention. Most NMBA potencies are described as the dose required in half the population for 95% depression of maximal muscle contraction after nerve stimulation. This is more accurately captured by the notation $ED_{50}95\%$ (in 50% of patients there is a 95% twitch reduction). ED_{95} will be used in this chapter to indicate $ED_{50}95\%$. Onset of action (onset time) for all NMBAs is defined as the time from its administration (usually intravenous) until maximal neuromuscular block (disappearance

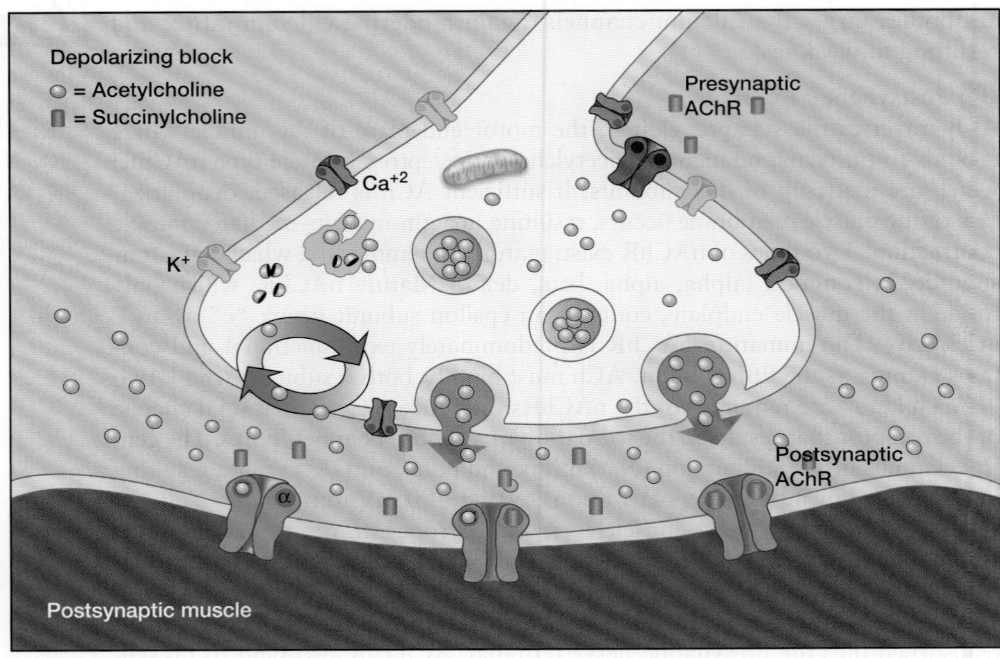

Figure 11.2 The effects of a depolarizing neuromuscular block at the neuromuscular junction.

of the single twitch, ST). Conventionally, two or three times the ED_{95} is used for initiating paralysis. Onset time is inversely related to dose and can be affected by rate of delivery to the action site (blood flow, speed of injection, use of saline flush etc.), receptor affinity, mechanism of action (depolarizing vs competitive nondepolarizing), and plasma clearance (metabolism, redistribution). Duration of action until recovery to 25% (DUR 25%) is defined as the time from drug administration until recovery of ST to 25% of baseline (normal) strength. Significant paralysis persists at DUR 25% and it does not reflect return of adequate strength for extubation. A clinically more meaningful metric is the total duration of action defined as the time from drug administration until recovery of train-of-four ratio (TOFR) to 0.90 (DUR 0.90). Duration of action is directly related to the dose of NMBA administered.

NMBAs can be classified based on their mode of action: depolarizing NMBAs (eg, SCh) produce muscle relaxation by directly depolarizing the nAChRs (**Figure 11.2**). This occurs because SCh (made up of two ACh molecules joined end to end) acts as a "false transmitter," mimicking ACh (**Figure 11.3**). Nondepolarizing NMBAs compete with ACh for the two α subunit recognition sites, preventing normal nAChR function. Nondepolarizing agents can be classified according to their chemical structure (benzylisoquinolinium or aminosteroid) or to their duration of action (short, intermediate, or long duration).

III. Depolarizing Neuromuscular Blocking Drugs: Succinylcholine

VIDEO 11.1
Fasciculations After Succinylcholine

A. Neuromuscular Effects

Succinylcholine is the only depolarizing NMBA clinically available (**Table 11.1; Figure 11.3**). Because of its molecular similarity to ACh, SCh depolarizes both postsynaptic and extrajunctional receptors, although not prejunctional

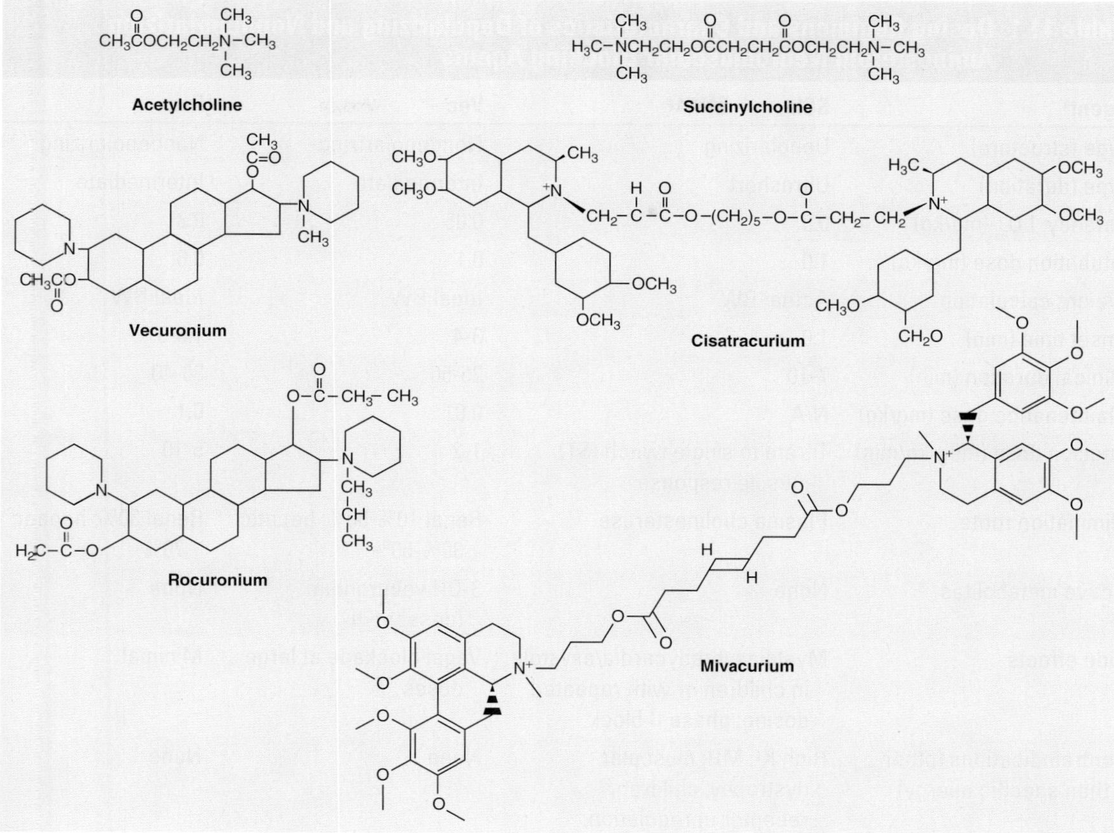

Acetylcholine

Succinylcholine

Vecuronium

Cisatracurium

Rocuronium

Mivacurium

Figure 11.3 Chemical structures of common neuromuscular blocking drugs.

neuronal nAChRs. The mechanism of paralysis is related to prolonged attachment to the AChR, inactivation of muscle membrane Na^+ channels, and lack of metabolism by acetylcholinesterase. Initial receptor activation manifests clinically as muscle "fasciculations"; thereafter, muscle membrane polarization cannot be reestablished, and flaccid paralysis persists.

B. Characteristics of Depolarizing Blockade

As with all NMBAs, increasing the dose of SCh leads to a progressive decrease in force of muscle contraction. However, the response to repetitive stimulation (train-of-four, TOF, and tetanus patterns, see Monitoring Modalities) is maintained (no fade) because SCh has no affinity for the presynaptic neuronal nAChRs, allowing ACh to continue to signal ACh vesicles to move to the active zone. Additionally, after a brief period of high-frequency stimulation (tetanus), there is no increase or amplification in the force of subsequent muscle contractions (no posttetanic potentiation). Large doses (7-10 mg/kg), prolonged (>30 minutes) exposure to SCh, presence of atypical pseudocholinesterase, or plasma cholinesterase deficiency may lead to phase II block. This is characterized by fade of responses to repetitive stimulation and amplification of muscle responses after high-frequency stimulation (posttetanic potentiation), similar to a nondepolarizing block.

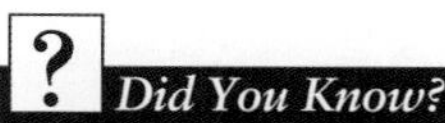

There are also nAChRs on the nerve terminal that signal the migration of ACh vesicles to the active zone. Nondepolarizing muscle relaxants bind and inactivate these receptors leading to fade with successive nerve stimulations. Succinylcholine does not bind these presynaptic nAChR receptors, so there is no fade with successive nerve stimulations.

Table 11.1 Dosing Regimens and Characteristics of Depolarizing and Nondepolarizing Aminosteroid Neuromuscular Blocking Agents

Agent[a]	SCh	Vec	Roc
Type (structure)	Depolarizing	Nondepolarizing	Nondepolarizing
Type (duration)	Ultrashort	Intermediate	Intermediate
Potency: ED_{95} (mg/kg)	0.3	0.05	0.3
Intubation dose (mg/kg)	1.0	0.1	0.6
Weight calculation	Actual BW	Ideal BW	Ideal BW
Onset time (min)	1.0	3-4	1.5-3
Clinical duration (min)	7-10	25-50	30-40
Maintenance dose (mg/kg)	N/A	0.01	0.1
Infusion dose (mcg/kg/min)	Titrate to single twitch (ST) muscle response	1-2	5-10
Elimination route	Plasma cholinesterase	Renal 10%-50%; hepatic 30%-50%	Renal 30%; hepatic 70%
Active metabolites	None	3-OH vecuronium (desacetyl)	None
Side effects	Myalgias; bradycardia/asystole in children or with repeated dosing; phase II block	Vagal blockade at large doses	Minimal
Contraindications (other than specific allergy)	High K^+; MH; muscular dystrophy, children, receptor upregulation, pseudocholinesterase deficiency	None	None
Comments	Fastest onset	Not for prolonged intensive care administration (myopathy); reversible by sugammadex	Pain on injection; easily reversible by sugammadex

BW, body weight; ED_{95}, the dose required in half the population for 95% depression of a single twitch; K^+, potassium; MH, malignant hyperthermia; Roc, rocuronium; SCh, succinylcholine; Vec, vecuronium.

[a]Agents in current clinical use in the United States. The data are averages obtained from published literature, assuming there is no potentiation from other coadministered drugs (such as volatile inhalational anesthetics) and the effects are measured at the adductor pollicis muscle. Other factors, such as muscle temperature, mode of evoked response monitoring, type or site of muscle monitoring, will affect the data.

C. Pharmacology of Succinylcholine

The onset of SCh at peripheral muscles (such as adductor pollicis muscle) is the fastest of any NMBA (1-2 minutes). Its ED_{95} is approximately 0.30 mg/kg, and at doses of 1 to 1.5 mg/kg (3-5 × ED_{95}), the DUR 25% of SCh is 10 to 12 minutes. In large doses, the DUR 25% is prolonged beyond 15 minutes. The recovery from SCh is slower than from rocuronium when sugammadex is administered for reversal (**Figure 11.4**). SCh is most commonly administered intravenously (IV), but intraosseous, intralingual, and intramuscular routes

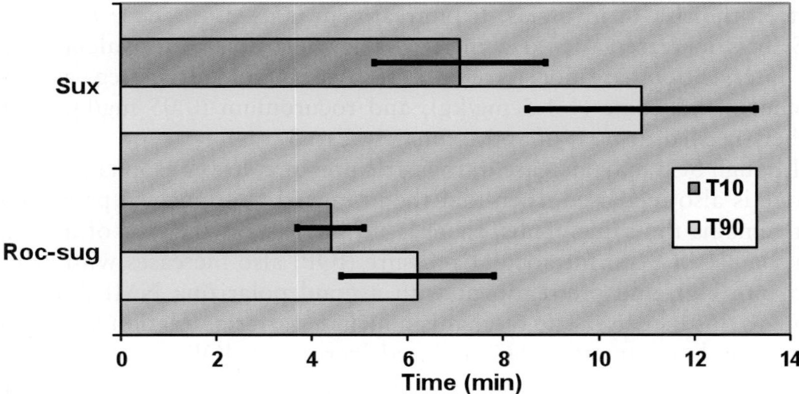

Figure 11.4 **Comparison of time to recovery after administration of succinylcholine (Sux) versus the combination of rocuronium and then sugammadex administered 3 minutes later. Bars indicate standard deviation. T10, time to 10% single twitch; T90, time to 90% single twitch recovery.** (Data from Lee C, Jahr JS, Candiotti KA, Warriner B, Zornow MH, Naguib M. Reversal of profound neuromuscular block by sugammadex administered 3 minutes after rocuronium. *Anesthesiology.* 2009;110:1020-1025. Originally published in Brull SJ. Neuromuscular blocking agents. In: Barash PG, Cahalan MK, Cullen BF, et al, eds. *Clinical Anesthesia.* 8th ed. Wolters Kluwer; 2018:527-563, Figure 21.16.)

have been successfully reported if an IV cannot be established. Onset is delayed with these alternative routes, particularly with intramuscular administration.

Hydrolysis of SCh by plasma cholinesterase (also known as pseudocholinesterase or butyrylcholinesterase) occurs away from the neuromuscular junction in the plasma. Plasma cholinesterase activity may be reduced in liver disease, pregnancy, acute infection, uremia, burns, with oral contraceptive use, and in some forms of cancer. A variant of plasma cholinesterase, atypical pseudocholinesterase, does not metabolize SCh efficiently. Heterozygous atypical pseudocholinesterase occurs in approximately 1:250 patients and leads to prolonged SCh effect of approximately 30 minutes. Homozygous atypical pseudocholinesterase is uncommon (1:3000) and leads to up to 8 hours of paralysis after SCh administration. Dibucaine is a local anesthetic that very effectively inactivates normal plasma cholinesterase, reducing activity by 80% to 100%. It inactivates atypical pseudocholinesterase less well—40% to 60% with heterozygous atypical pseudocholinesterase and 20% with homozygous atypical pseudocholinesterase. The dibucaine number reflects the degree of enzyme inhibition and can be used clinically to elucidate the cause of prolonged paralysis after succinylcholine administration.

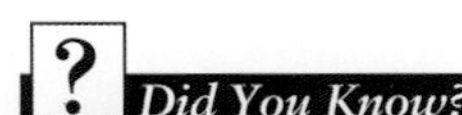

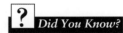

Almost 90% of the intravenous dose of SCh is hydrolyzed in the plasma before reaching the neuromuscular junction.

D. Side Effects

SCh can induce significant bradycardia or even asystole, particularly in children, and after redosing. Premature ventricular escape beats are also common. Cardiac effects can be attenuated by pretreatment with anticholinergics. Disorganized muscle contractions (fasciculations) after SCh administration are very common (80%-90% of patients). Myalgias are also very common 1 to 2 days postoperatively (50%-60% of patients). The relationship between fasciculations and myalgias is unclear; a "defasciculating" pretreatment with a small dose of nondepolarizing NMBA (10% ED_{95}) appears to have limited effect on the risk of myalgias. If pretreatment is used, the dose requirement for SCh is increased (up to 2 mg/kg). The most effective myalgia prophylaxis interventions are nonsteroidal anti-inflammatory drugs (eg, aspirin or diclofenac), lidocaine (1-1.5 mg/kg), and rocuronium (0.05 mg/kg), with a numbers-needed-to-treat of approximately 2 to 3.[2]

Although SCh may increase intragastric pressure, lower esophageal sphincter tone is also increased, such that the intragastric-esophageal pressure gradient remains the same. Thus, there is no increase in the risk of aspiration from the use of SCh. Intraocular pressure (IOP) also increases with SCh (up to 15 mm Hg), and pretreatment with a nondepolarizing NMDA does not attenuate this increase. The mechanism includes arterial dilation and perhaps ocular muscle contraction. SCh-induced increase in IOP is unlikely to lead to clinically impactful extrusion of ocular contents in patients with an open-globe injury, so SCh does not need to be avoided in this situation. Elevation in intracranial pressure from SCh may occur, though there is evidence to the contrary.[3] More importantly, inadequate levels of anesthesia during laryngoscopy and tracheal intubation increase intracranial pressure. Although SCh administration induces an elevation in the plasma level of potassium of 0.5 mEq/L, severe hyperkalemia with attendant cardiac arrest has only been reported in cases in which there is a proliferation of immature nAChRs (see "Receptor Up- and Downregulation"). Particularly important is the association between pediatric myotonia and muscle dystrophies and SCh administration, leading to fatal hyperkalemia and rhabdomyolysis. For this reason, the U.S. Food and Drug Administration has a black box warning on the use of SCh, and clinicians should avoid its use in children. SCh may also trigger lethal malignant hyperthermia (MH), especially in patients anesthetized with volatile anesthetics.[4] Some patients (both adults and children) may exhibit masseter muscle spasm after SCh administration, making intubating conditions difficult. SCh can produce allergic reactions (anaphylaxis) in about 1 of 10,000 administrations.

E. Clinical Uses

SCh is indicated for rapid attainment of optimal intubating conditions and prevention of regurgitation and pulmonary aspiration of gastric contents in patients at risk (those unfasted, with gastroparesis or gastrointestinal obstruction) in the rapid sequence induction and intubation (RSII) scenario. SCh has the shortest onset time (1 minute at 1.5 mg/kg) and a short clinical duration (5-10 minutes at 1 mg/kg dose). The short onset of action may be offset by a faster time to desaturation in patients given succinylcholine compared to those given rocuronium.[5] In obese individuals who need RSII, the dose of SCh should be calculated on the basis of actual body weight, rather than ideal body weight. Children are more resistant than adults to the actions of SCh, and the usual dose (see "Side Effects") is 1.5 to 2.0 mg/kg (up to 3 mg/kg in infants).

F. Contraindications to Use of Succinylcholine

Use of SCh is contraindicated in patients (and their relatives) with a history of MH. Other settings in which SCh is contraindicated include states of receptor upregulation such as critical care patients or those immobilized for prolonged periods (eg, weeks) due to the potential for lethal hyperkalemia. Due to upregulation of immature nAChR, succinylcholine should be avoided 48 hour after a burn or denervation process. This danger persists for the duration of the disease process.[6] In patients with renal failure, SCh may be administered if the plasma K^+ is not elevated. Lethal hyperkalemia following administration of SCh has been reported in severely acidotic and hypovolemic patients. Finally, SCh should be avoided in patients with pseudocholinesterase deficiency or atypical pseudocholinesterase.

IV. Nondepolarizing Neuromuscular Blocking Agents

A. Characteristics of Nondepolarizing Blockade

Nondepolarizing NMBAs compete with ACh for binding to one or both of the α subunits of the muscular nAChRs, inhibiting activation (**Figure 11.5**). They also bind and inactivate neuronal presynaptic nAChRs which explains why repetitive stimulation (0.1-2 Hz) during partial block leads to muscle contraction fade. The degree of fade can be determined by a sequence of four stimuli delivered at 2 Hz by calculating the ratio of the amplitude of the fourth response (T4) to the amplitude of the first response (T1). This is the train-of-four ratio (TOFR or T4/T1). Another characteristic of nondepolarizing block is the transient amplification of responses that follows a 5-second period of tetanic stimulation (posttetanic potentiation) that lasts up to 3 minutes following tetanic stimulation. Unlike depolarizing blockade, which is potentiated by the administration of anticholinesterases, the nondepolarizing block can be antagonized by anticholinesterases if the level of block is sufficiently shallow (see "Reversal of Neuromuscular Blockade").

B. Pharmacology of Nondepolarizing Neuromuscular Blocking Drugs

Nondepolarizing NMBAs can be classified as long, intermediate, and short acting, and their duration of action depends on metabolism, redistribution, and elimination (**Tables 11.1 and 11.2; Figures 11.3** and **11.5**). They also can be classified based on their chemical structure as benzylisoquinolinium (cisatracurium, mivacurium) or aminosteroid (rocuronium, vecuronium) compounds. Nondepolarizing NMBAs are almost always administered intravenously. Intramuscular delivery leads to very slow and variable onset of action. Since they are positively charged, nondepolarizing NMBAs are distributed mostly in the extracellular fluid (ECF). Thus, in patients with renal or hepatic failure (who have increased ECF), larger initial doses may be required.

C. Onset and Duration of Action

Onset of nondepolarizing NMBAs generally depends on potency; less potent agents such as rocuronium (ED_{95} of 0.3 mg/kg) have more molecules per equivalent dose than a potent NMBA such as vecuronium (ED_{95} of 0.05 mg/kg), resulting in faster onset. Thus, an ED_{95} dose of rocuronium will have six times more molecules than an equipotent dose of vecuronium, and the plasma concentration of rocuronium will be greater than that of vecuronium. This greater concentration difference between plasma and the synaptic cleft partly explains the more rapid onset of rocuronium. A similar plasma to synaptic cleft concentration gradient might be achieved by administering six times the ED_{95} of vecuronium. Although this will speed up the onset of action, the much larger dose will also markedly prolong the total duration of action. Typically, a dose of 2 to 3 × ED_{95} of a nondepolarizing NMBA is used to facilitate tracheal intubation.

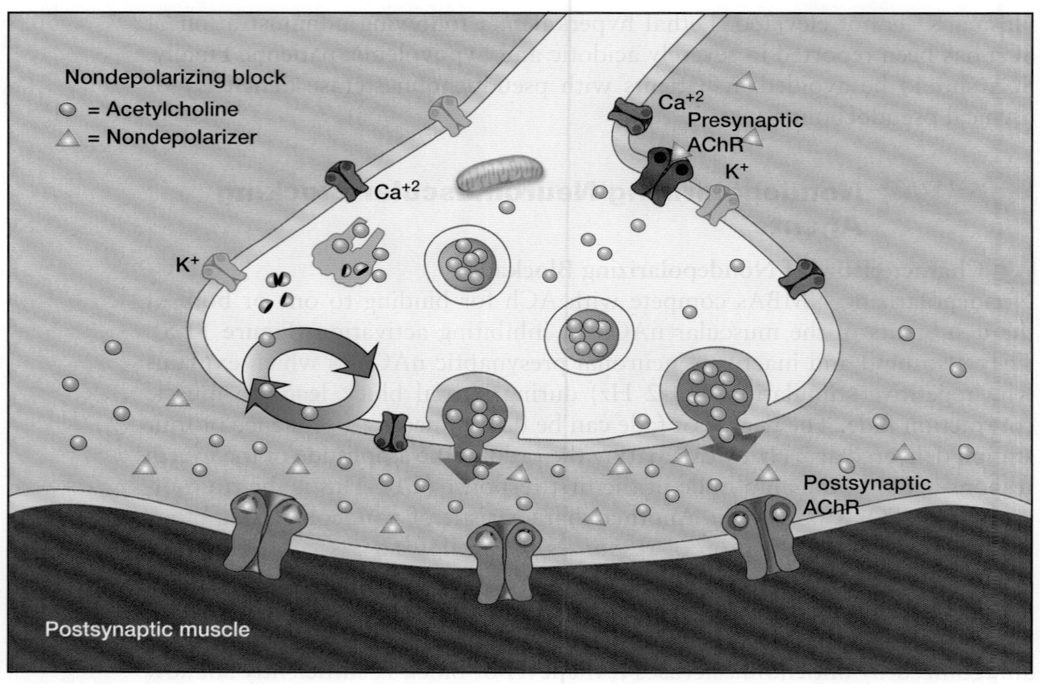

Figure 11.5 The effects of a nondepolarizing (competitive) block at the neuromuscular junction.

D. Nondepolarizing Agents

Vecuronium is an intermediate-duration NMBA that is devoid of cardiovascular effects; because it is more potent than rocuronium, its onset of action is slower (**Table 11.1**). Vecuronium can precipitate in the intravenous tubing if administered immediately after thiopental (but not propofol) administration. Since the introduction of rocuronium, vecuronium is no longer recommended for RSII.

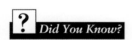

> **Did You Know?**
>
> The vecuronium metabolite (3-desacetyl) has 60% of the parent compound potency. It accumulates with large or repeated doses in intensive care patients and likely contributes to the condition of persistent paralysis in the critically ill.

Rocuronium is structurally similar to vecuronium (**Table 11.1**). Because of its low potency, the high plasma concentration achieved after bolus administration decreases rapidly, so that its duration of action in patients with normal renal and hepatic function is determined mostly by its redistribution, not its elimination. Unlike vecuronium, rocuronium metabolites (17-OH rocuronium) have very low neuromuscular blocking activity. Rocuronium can be used in high doses (1-1.2 mg/kg) in the RSII setting, particularly in those patients in whom the use of SCh is contraindicated. The mean onset time at this dose rivals that of SCh, with similar intubation conditions.[3] After large doses, the DUR 25% is significantly prolonged (>60 minutes), and if rapid reversal is considered in the "cannot-intubate, cannot-ventilate" scenario, a large dose (16 mg/kg) of sugammadex is necessary. Similar to vecuronium, rocuronium has no effect on hemodynamics and does not release histamine. However, allergic reactions have been documented. Reports from around the world suggest that the incidence of anaphylaxis following rocuronium may be higher than with other NMBAs. This has been ascribed to sensitization to an antitussive medication, pholcodine, available in some countries. Potency appears to be greater in

Table 11.2 Dosing Regimens and Characteristics of Benzylisoquinolinium Nondepolarizing Neuromuscular Blocking Agents

Agent[a]	Cisatracurium	Mivacurium
Type (duration)	Intermediate	Short
Potency: ED_{95} (mg/kg)	0.05	0.08
Intubation dose (mg/kg)	0.15	0.2-0.25
Weight-based dosing	Actual BW	Actual BW
Onset time (min)	5-7	3-4
Clinical duration (min)	35-50	15-20
Maintenance dose (mg/kg)	0.01	0.25
Infusion dose (mg/kg/min)	1-3	5-7
Elimination route	Hofmann 30%; ester hydrolysis 60%	Plasma cholinesterase
Active metabolites	None	None
Side effects	Rare; histamine release at high doses	Histamine release, flushing and erythema at doses >0.2 mg/kg
Contraindications (other than specific allergy)	None	Reactive airway disease, atypical pseudocholinesterase, plasma cholinesterase deficiency
Comments	Results in trivial histamine, laudanosine and acrylate levels	Slow onset and short duration limit clinical usefulness

BW, body weight; ED_{95}, the dose required in half the population for 95% depression of a single twitch; SCh, succinylcholine. Actual BW for cisatracurium is based on conflicting data for atracurium; there are limited data on cisatracurium. Actual BW is presumed for mivacurium based on similarities with SCh pharmacodynamics.

[a]The information is estimated based on data from published literature, assuming there is no potentiation from other coadministered drugs (such as volatile inhalational anesthetics), and with effects measured at the adductor pollicis muscle. Other factors, such as muscle temperature, mode of evoked response monitoring, type or site of muscle monitoring, will affect the data.

women than in men, and the dose should be reduced 20% in women. In the pediatric population, onset and duration of action are shorter, and dose requirements are slightly increased.

Cisatracurium is a benzylisoquinolinium compound of the curare family. It is the more contemporary version of atracurium, which is composed of a mixture of 10 optical isomers (**Table 11.2**) that has a propensity to release histamine. Cisatracurium is composed of the cis-cis isomer, which is more potent than atracurium and does not release histamine. It has a unique, dual metabolic pathway: a nonenzymatic degradation that is directly proportional with temperature and pH (Hofmann degradation) and a secondary pathway that involves hydrolysis by nonspecific plasma esterases. As seen with more potent NMBAs, cisatracurium has a slower onset of action. Even at 3 times ED_{95}, onset is 5 to 7 minutes, which may be shortened by increasing the dose. DUR 25% is intermediate (30-45 minutes) but is slightly more predictable than other intermediate-duration agents, likely because of the dual metabolic pathway. Potency is similar for both men and women and is not affected appreciably by age or organ failure. Allergic reactions have been reported at a low frequency.

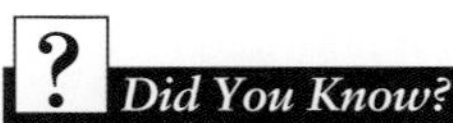

Rocuronium dose should be reduced 20% for females. Elderly women are at particularly high risk of prolonged paralysis from rocuronium with standard doses.

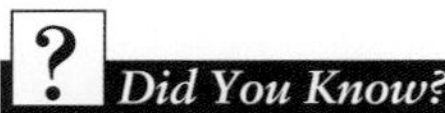

Cisatracurium is metabolized by the same enzyme that degrades esmolol and remifentanil.

Mivacurium is a benzylisoquinolinium and the only nondepolarizing NMBA with a short duration of action (**Table 11.2**). Potency is intermediate (ED_{95} is 0.08-0.15 mg/kg) partially explaining the slow onset of action (3-4 minutes). Slow onset is also due to rapid metabolism of mivacurium en route to the neuromuscular junction. Metabolism occurs by plasma cholinesterase, similar to succinylcholine, and there are no active metabolites. Histamine release occurs at doses >0.2 mg/kg, which may manifest as cutaneous flushing, erythema, and hypotension. Reversal of this drug is unique in that a buildup of ACh in the synapse by acetylcholinesterase inhibition is desired to overcome the competitive nondepolarizing block; however, inhibition of plasma cholinesterase also slows metabolism of mivacurium. Neostigmine blocks both plasma cholinesterase and acetylcholinesterase, making the preferred reversal agent for mivacurium one that only acts on acetylcholinesterase, such as edrophonium.

V. Drug Interactions

A. Additive and Synergistic Effects

Nondepolarizing NMBAs can have either additive or synergistic effects when combined. Usually, combining two chemically similar drugs with similar duration of action (eg, rocuronium and vecuronium) results in an additive potency and no effect on total duration. When drugs of different classes are combined (eg, cisatracurium and rocuronium), the effect in terms of total dose are synergistic and both potency and total duration are increased.

B. Antagonism

Adding depolarizing and nondepolarizing NMBAs results in mutual antagonism. For instance, defasciculating doses of a nondepolarizing NMBA prior to administration of SCh will increase the SCh dose requirement and shorten the SCh duration of action.

C. Potentiation

Inhalational anesthetic agents potentiate neuromuscular block (desflurane > sevoflurane > isoflurane > nitrous oxide), likely by direct effects at the postjunctional receptors. Higher concentration (minimum alveolar concentration) and longer agent exposure will potentiate the neuromuscular block to a greater extent. The intravenous agent propofol has no effect on neuromuscular transmission. Local anesthetics potentiate the effects of both depolarizing and nondepolarizing NMBAs; the onset time is not significantly affected, but duration of action is prolonged.

The common antibiotics penicillin, cephalosporin, tetracycline, and erythromycin do not appreciably prolong the effects of NMBAs. Clindamycin and lincomycin do have pre- and postsynaptic effects, but at typical doses, they have no clinically noticeable effect on muscle blockade. Older antibiotics, such as streptomycin and neomycin, which are known to depress neuromuscular function, have more prominent but still limited effects. Hypercarbia, acidosis, and hypothermia, however, may potentiate the depressant effects of antibiotics in the critically ill. In patients receiving acute administration of anticonvulsants (phenytoin, carbamazepine), neuromuscular block is potentiated. Chronic administration significantly decreases the duration of action of aminosteroid but not benzylisoquinolinium compounds. Beta-receptor and calcium channel antagonists have insignificant effects on NMBAs, but ephedrine has been shown to speed the onset of rocuronium, likely as a result of its impact on cardiac output.

Corticosteroids administered in conjunction with neuromuscular blockade, particularly in critically ill patients and for prolonged periods, markedly increase the risk of myopathy (up to 50% of mechanically ventilated patients who receive both drugs).

VI. Altered Responses to Neuromuscular Blocking Agents

Multiple factors affect the pharmacokinetics of all drugs, including NMBAs. Intraoperative hypothermia prolongs the duration of NMBAs by decreasing receptor sensitivity and ACh mobilization, decreasing the force of muscle contraction, and reducing renal and hepatic metabolism as well as the Hofmann degradation pathway.

Aging results in a decrease in total body water and serum albumin concentration, which reduces the volume of distribution of NMBAs. Decreased cardiac function, glomerular filtration rate, and liver blood flow all contribute to a reduced rate of NMBA elimination (especially the aminosteroid compounds).

Acid-base and electrolyte imbalance affect the duration of action of NMBAs, including their metabolism and elimination. Hypokalemia potentiates nondepolarizing block and decreases the effectiveness of anticholinesterases (neostigmine) in antagonizing nondepolarizing block. Hypermagnesemia prolongs the duration of action of NMBAs by inhibiting pre- and postsynaptic Ca^{2+} channels. Acidosis interferes with the ability of anticholinesterases to reverse a nondepolarizing block. Hypercarbia also leads to acidosis, impairing NMBA antagonism.

The duration of action of aminosteroid NMBAs is prolonged by liver and kidney dysfunction. For this reason, benzylisoquinolinium-class NMBAs are preferred in patients with organ dysfunction (such as critically ill patients in the intensive care unit), because they are metabolized by organ-independent, nonenzymatic pathways.

VII. Monitoring Neuromuscular Blockade

A. Subjective Evaluation and Quantitative Monitoring

Monitoring involves the stimulation of a peripheral nerve and evaluating the response (contraction or twitch) of the innervated muscle. Peripheral nerve stimulators (PNS) are generally battery-operated, stand-alone units that provide the stimulus via wires connected to surface (skin) electrodes. When a PNS is used, the response is evaluated subjectively either visually or manually (tactile assessment). Subjective evaluation has consequential limitations stemming from the inability of humans to detect subtle variations in movement. Quantitative monitors objectively measure the evoked muscle response. Importantly, these monitors provide real-time accurate measurements of the TOFR (see "Pharmacologic Characteristics of Neuromuscular Blocking Agents for definition"); there is expert consensus that best practice includes the routine use of quantitative monitoring of neuromuscular blockade.[7] PNS and quantitative monitors both stimulate a nerve (the ulnar nerve and the evoked response of the adductor pollicis muscle is the gold standard) in the same manner; the difference is in the assessment of the response. They deliver a range of currents up to 80 mA. The current should be constant (square wave) over the duration of the impulse. The most commonly used duration is 200 μs; it should not exceed 300 μs to avoid exceeding the nerve refractory period.

The current is delivered via surface (skin) stimulating electrodes that have a silver-silver chloride interface with the skin, reducing its resistance. Standard electrocardiogram (ECG) electrodes are acceptable, but specialized electrodes are also used. Skin can have very high resistance, and preparing the skin by cleaning with alcohol and abrading with a gauze is useful to improve delivery of the electrical stimulus.

B. Monitoring Modalities

The first nerve stimulators delivered single repetitive stimuli at frequencies between 0.1 and 10 Hz. The muscle response was a single twitch (ST) to each stimulus (**Figure 11.6**). If the frequency of stimulation exceeds 0.1 Hz (1 stimulus every 10 seconds) some degree of muscle fatigue may occur. To measure the extent of neuromuscular block, the current intensity is increased progressively (prior to NMBA administration) from 0 mA in 5 to 10 mA steps. The amplitude of the evoked muscle response is plotted over time and has a sigmoidal shape. Once the amplitude of the muscle response no longer increases despite increasing current intensity, the response is maximal, and the current required is called maximal current. Increasing the current value by 20% above maximal ensures that all fibers in the innervated muscle will consistently depolarize, despite skin resistance changes over time. This is termed supramaximal current. If a baseline control force is measured and recorded before NMBA administration, the force of subsequent contractions can be compared and expressed as twitch height (% of control). This modality (ST) is useful clinically to determine onset of neuromuscular block. Because the onset of neuromuscular block at the laryngeal muscles precedes the block at the adductor pollicis due to preferential blood flow to central musculature, satisfactory intubation conditions are often achieved before complete depression of the ST response at the adductor pollicis. The ST mode is not useful for monitoring of recovery from nondepolarizing block.

TOF stimulation was introduced clinically in 1971 and consists of four sequential ST stimuli (named T1, T2, T3, and T4) delivered at a frequency of 2 Hz (**Figure 11.7A** and **B**). Each train can be delivered every 15 to 20 seconds.

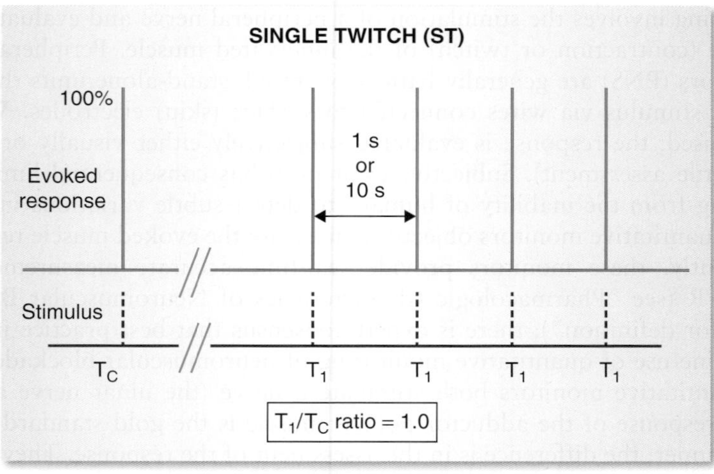

Figure 11.6 Single twitch nerve stimulation. If single twitches occur less than 2 seconds apart, there is some risk of physiologic fade with >4 subsequent twitches.

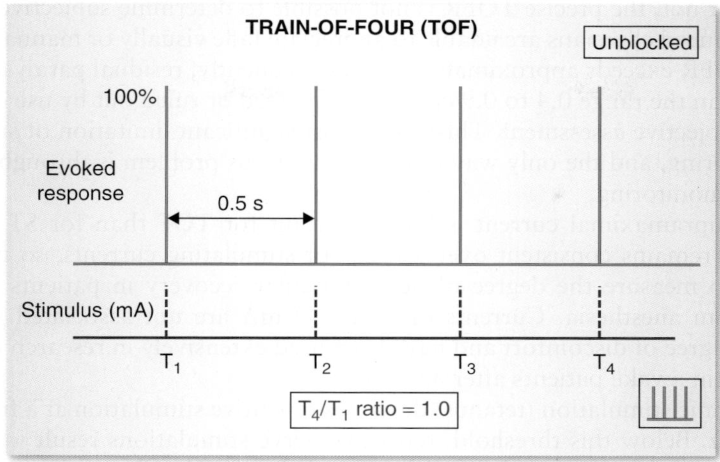

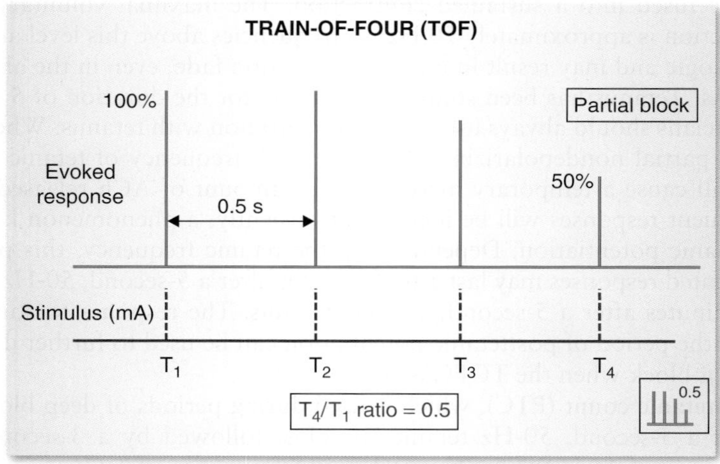

Figure 11.7 A, Following train-of-four (TOF) stimulation, TOF baseline ratio (T4/T1 = 1.0) is observed. B, Following TOF stimulation, depression of response to TOF (T4/T1 = 0.5) is noted following administration of a nondepolarizing neuromuscular blocking agent.

The TOFR is calculated by dividing the T4 amplitude by the T1 amplitude. The control TOF response (before administration of NMBA) is four twitches of equal amplitude and the TOFR is 1.0 (100%). During a partial nondepolarizing block, the ratio decreases (ie, there is increasing fade) as the degree of block increases. A TOFR of 0.9 is considered acceptable clinical recovery, and residual paralysis is defined as a TOFR <0.9 at the adductor pollicis. TOFR does not require a baseline measurement—all subsequent responses are measured as a fraction of T1. By eliciting four responses, the clinician sometimes is able to assess the degree of fade subjectively by visual or tactile means or, more reliably, by counting the number of evoked responses (twitches) known as the train-of-four count (TOFC). When subjectively assessed, the TOFC has six possible classifications, namely 0, 1, 2, 3, 4 with fade, and 4 without fade. The term "four out of four" should be avoided as it conflates two distinct classifications. While it is possible to subjectively determine whether there is fade, or not, the precise TOFR is not possible to determine subjectively. Even experienced clinicians are unable to appreciate fade visually or manually when the TOFR exceeds approximately 0.4. Consequently, residual paralysis with a TOFR in the range 0.4 to 0.9 cannot be detected or ruled out by use of a PNS and subjective assessment. This is the most significant limitation of subjective monitoring, and the only way of overcoming this problem is through quantitative monitoring.

A supramaximal current is less important for TOF than for ST and the TOFR remains consistent over a range of stimulating currents, so it can be used to measure the degree of neuromuscular recovery in patients recovering from anesthesia. Currents of 30 to 40 mA are not associated with the high degree of discomfort and have been used extensively in research to assess TOFR in awake patients after anesthesia.

Tetanic stimulation (tetanus) describes repetitive stimulation at a frequency >30 Hz. Below this threshold, repetitive nerve stimulations result in individual, rapid contractions. At frequencies above 30 Hz, the muscle responses become fused into a sustained contraction. The maximal voluntary muscle contraction is approximately 70 Hz, so frequencies above this level are supraphysiologic and may result in muscle contraction fade, even in the absence of NMBAs. Tetanus has been studied extensively for the duration of 5 seconds, so clinicians should always use a 5-second duration with tetanus. When tested during partial nondepolarizing block, the high frequency of tetanic stimulation will cause a temporary increase in the amount of ACh released so that subsequent responses will be increased transiently, a phenomenon known as posttetanic potentiation. Depending on the tetanic frequency, this period of potentiated responses may last 1 to 2 minutes after a 5-second, 50-Hz tetanus, or 3 minutes after a 5-second, 100-Hz tetanus. The response to stimulation during the period of posttetanic potentiation can be used to further define the depth of block when the TOFC is zero.

? *Did You Know?*

Both visual and tactile (subjective) evaluation of fade to TOF stimulation fail to recognize significant degrees of residual block.

Posttetanic count (PTC), which is used during periods of deep block, consists of a 5-second, 50-Hz tetanic stimulus, followed by a 3-second pause and a series of 15 to 20 single twitches at a frequency of 1 Hz (**Figure 11.8**).

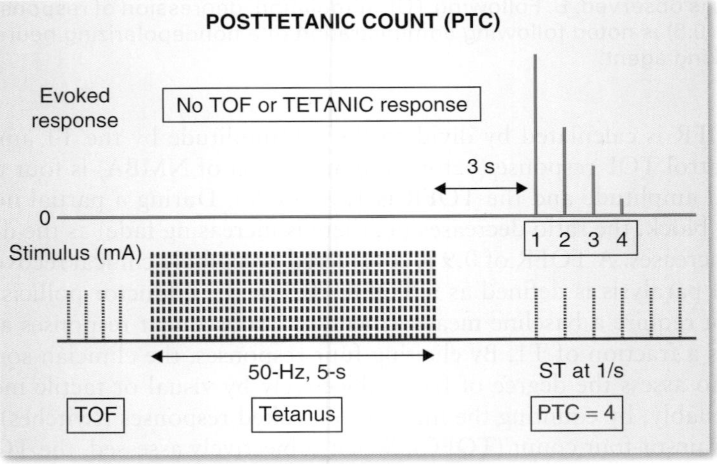

Figure 11.8 Posttetanic count (PTC). The number of posttetanic twitches is inversely related to the degree of neuromuscular block.

The number of posttetanic twitches is inversely proportional to the depth of block: the fewer the number of posttetanic twitches, the deeper the block. With a PTC of 1, the time until recovery to a TOFC of 1 is about 20 to 30 minutes; however, recovery time may be significantly longer in some patients.

Double burst stimulation was developed to increase the sensitivity when attempting to assess residual paralysis subjectively. By delivering two (instead of four) intense stimuli (minitetanic bursts) separated by 0.75 second, two fused responses can be evaluated directly instead of comparing the fourth response of the TOF to the first. This modality is termed double burst stimulation ($DBS_{3,3}$) (**Figure 11.9**). The numbers 3,3 signify that each burst contains three stimuli at a frequency of 50 Hz. Because the two individual bursts are tetanic in frequency, a longer recovery period between successive DBS stimulations is necessary (20 seconds). Using DBS subjectively, clinicians are able to detect fade when the TOFR is <0.60, an improvement over subjectively detected TOF fade. The inability to appreciate residual paralysis with TOFR in the range 0.6 to 0.9 is a significant shortcoming of DBS.

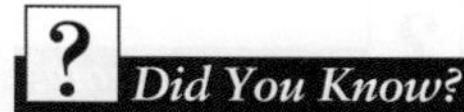

Even the often-used test of 5-second head lift has the same poor predictive value as other clinical tests (PPV ≤ 0.5). A majority of volunteers were able to maintain head lift for >5 seconds at a TOFR of 0.5.

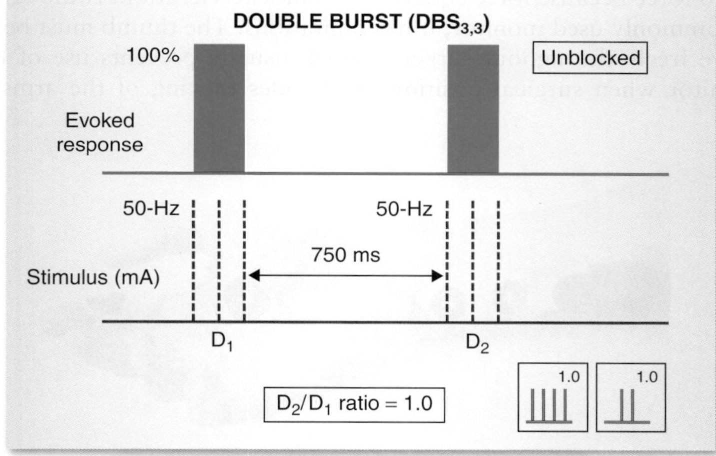

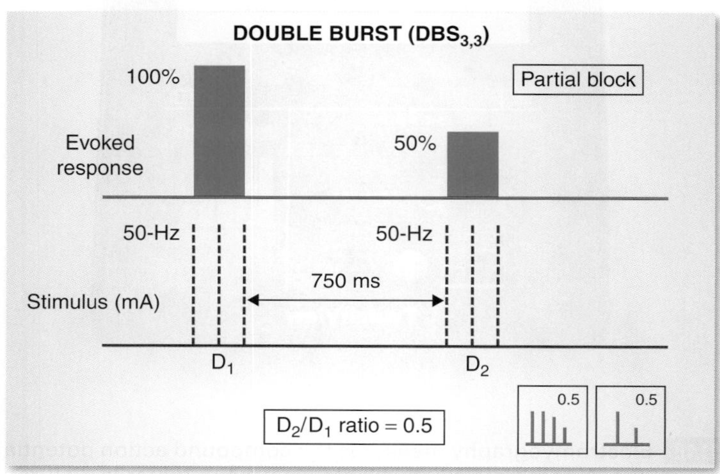

Figure 11.9 A, Double burst stimulation ($DBS_{3,3}$). B, Double burst stimulation ($DBS_{3,3}$) ratio = 0.5.

? *Did You Know?*

It is estimated that postoperative mortality is increased 90-fold if patients have residual paralysis that requires unplanned tracheal reintubation and intensive care postoperatively.

C. Quantitative Monitoring

There are different technologies for precise measurement of the evoked response. Mechanomyography (MMG) is considered the gold standard. It is an isometric measurement of the force of the thumb contraction. The equipment is cumbersome and not used in clinical practice.

Electromyography (EMG) is one of the oldest methods of measuring neuromuscular transmission which yields measurements that do not differ significantly from MMG (**Figure 11.10**). For EMG monitoring, a peripheral nerve (usually the ulnar nerve) is stimulated via surface electrodes, and the action potential generated at the innervated muscle (adductor pollicis) is measured. Measurement of the evoked response involves either area under the curve of the compound muscle action potential, the peak-to-baseline, or the peak-to-peak amplitude of the signal.

Acceleromyography (AMG) has been the most commonly used clinical method of measuring muscle function in the past 3 decades (**Figure 11.11**). AMG consists of an accelerometer attached to a moving body part (usually the thumb) that measures the acceleration in response to nerve stimulation (the ulnar nerve and muscle contraction). Acceleration is directly proportional to force because force equals mass times acceleration. Although it is the most commonly used monitor, it has limitations. The thumb must be allowed to move freely throughout surgery, which usually prevents use of this type of monitor when surgical positioning includes tucking of the arms. Newer

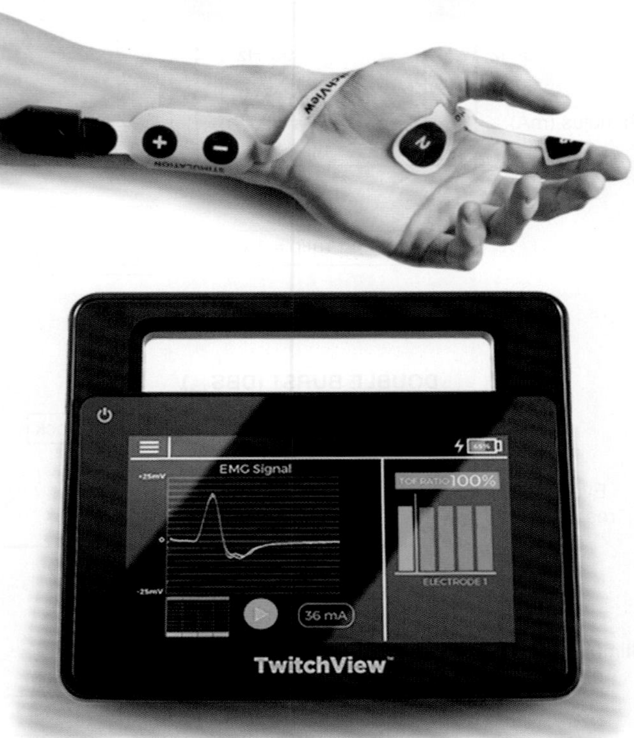

Figure 11.10 Electromyography measures the compound action potential from an applied stimulus. A commercially available electromyometer is pictured. (© 2021 Blink Device Company All rights reserved.)

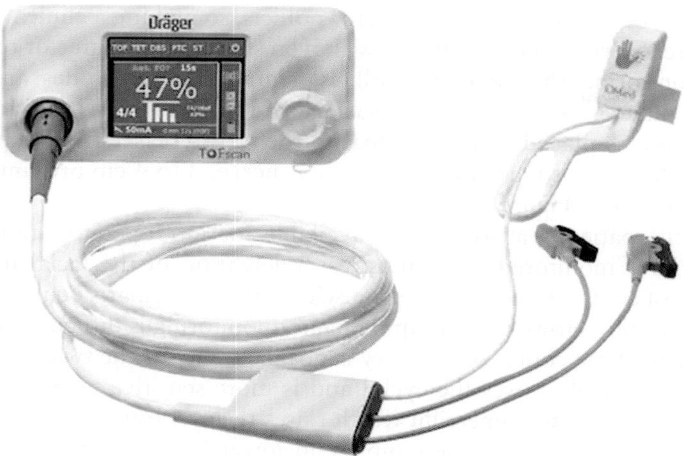

Figure 11.11 An accelerometer measures the acceleration of the thumb with each applied stimulus. Force is directly proportional to acceleration by F = mA (F, force; m, mass; A, acceleration). A commercially available accelerometer is pictured. (© Drägerwerk AG & Co. KGaA, Lubeck,. All rights reserved.)

models employ triaxial vectoring, but keeping the arm and hand in a consistent position remains important for ideal monitor performance. Compared to MMG and EMG, AMG gives inflated values for TOFR; the baseline value before NMDA administration is often 1.1 to 1.15 but can be higher. The measurements provided by the AMG monitor are referred to as the raw values and there are two approaches to compensating for the inflated raw TOFR values. One can determine the individual baseline value before paralysis and divide all subsequent measurements by this value. This is called normalization to baseline value. As an example, if the baseline value is 1.12 and the postoperative TOFR is 0.94, the normalized TOFR will be 0.94/1.12 = 0.84. The alternative approach is to adjust the threshold for acceptable recovery to a raw value of 1.0. In this example, both approaches would lead to the raw value of TOFR = 0.94 being classified as residual paralysis.

D. Differential Muscle Sensitivity

It has long been known that NMBAs do not affect all muscles at the same time nor do they produce the same depth of relaxation. It is also important to note that NMBAs are administered to produce good intubating conditions, vocal cord paralysis, abdominal muscle relaxation, or diaphragmatic immobility. Yet, laryngeal muscles, abdominal muscles, and the diaphragm are not monitored. Understanding the relation between the response of the different muscles to the effects or NMBAs is therefore clinically important.

The adductor pollicis is most commonly monitored (subjectively or objectively). Being a peripheral muscle, the onset time at the adductor pollicis is longer than in centrally located muscles, where blood flow (and thus drug delivery) is greater. At the same time, the adductor pollicis is more sensitive to nondepolarizing NMBAs, so recovery is delayed compared to central muscles (diaphragm, laryngeal muscles). Even monitoring of similar but different peripheral muscles innervated by a common nerve can induce error: stimulation of the ulnar nerve produces flexion of the fifth finger as well as adductor pollicis contraction. However, the recovery of the fifth finger contraction occurs more rapidly than at the adductor pollicis, so making a clinical decision based on recovery of the fifth finger will overestimate the degree of recovery.

For monitoring the adductor pollicis, stimulating electrodes are placed along the ulnar nerve on the volar surface of the forearm. The distal (negative) electrode is placed 2 cm proximal to the wrist crease, and the proximal (positive) electrode is placed along the ulnar nerve, 3 to 4 cm proximal to the negative electrode (**Figure 11.12**).

When the patient's arms are not available for intraoperative monitoring, clinicians have monitored facial muscles: innervation of the facial nerve and evaluation of contractions of the eye muscles, either orbicularis oculi or the corrugator supercilii. However, this approach to monitoring is difficult and unreliable. First, the time course of recovery is not the same for the two eye muscles: the orbicularis oculi moves the eyelid and is more sensitive to NMDAs compared to the corrugator supercillii which raises the eyebrow. Second, improper placement of electrodes on the temple and lower jaw leads to direct muscle stimulation and false assessment of neuromuscular recovery. Gätke, in her detailed report on technical aspects of acceleromyographic monitoring of the orbicularis oculi, concluded: "when monitoring in the face, with its many small nerves and muscles, it is difficult to ensure that only one single nerve is being stimulated and accordingly that only one muscle is contracting."[8] Therefore, it may be quite difficult for anesthesia providers to distinguish between twitches of different muscles surrounding the eye. Third, although frequently used, the effectiveness of this approach to monitoring has not been validated. Fourth, current clinical practice of monitoring eye muscles has been shown to result in a fivefold increased risk of residual paralysis.[9] When the wrists and thumbs are unavailable for monitoring of the adductor pollicis, the great toe offers a better alternative. Stimulation of the posterior tibial nerve along the medial malleolus produces flexion of the great toe and has a time course that is comparable to the adductor pollicis. Importantly, if facial nerve stimulation is used during surgery because it is the only available site, it is prudent to switch from facial to ulnar nerve stimulation before pharmacological reversal at the end of the surgical procedure. An appropriate choice of reversal drug and dose requires a valid assessment of the level of neuromuscular blockade obtained at the gold standard site which is the ulnar nerve and adductor pollicis.

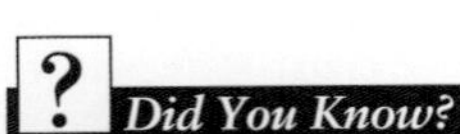

The twitch response of the great toe with stimulation of the posterior tibial nerve is preferred over evaluation of eye muscles with stimulation of the facial nerve when monitoring at the adductor pollicis is not available.

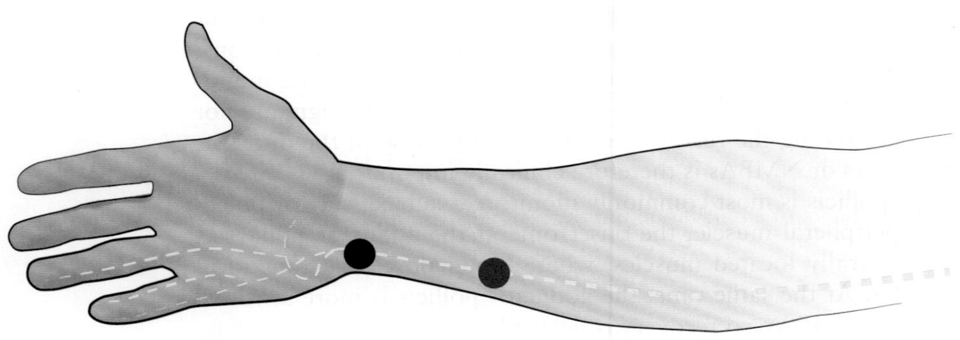

Figure 11.12 Proper electrode placement on the volar surface of the arm. The black electrode is near the wrist, the red electrode is more proximal ("red near the head").

E. Clinical Applications

Neuromuscular monitoring should routinely commence immediately after induction of anesthesia, before NMBA administration. This has important advantages; it allows for confirmation that the monitor works, and it gives the clinician a good indication of the baseline response to stimulation. Restoration of normal neuromuscular function before extubation should yield the same response as at baseline. Moreover, modern monitors can automatically determine the appropriate supramaximal current and perform better when they are calibrated prior to NMBA administration. Knowledge of the time course for onset, duration, and recovery of neuromuscular block of NMBAs allows optimal care (**Figure 11.13**). Satisfactory intubating conditions are usually present before complete depression of the adductor pollicis twitch response.

Most surgical procedures can be performed under moderate block (TOFC 1-3). Deep block is defined as a level with TOFC = 0 and PTC of at least 1. The role for deep block remains controversial; however, it is rarely required for lower abdominal surgery. If a level of block that prevents diaphragmatic movement is required, a PTC of 1 or 2 is usually sufficient.

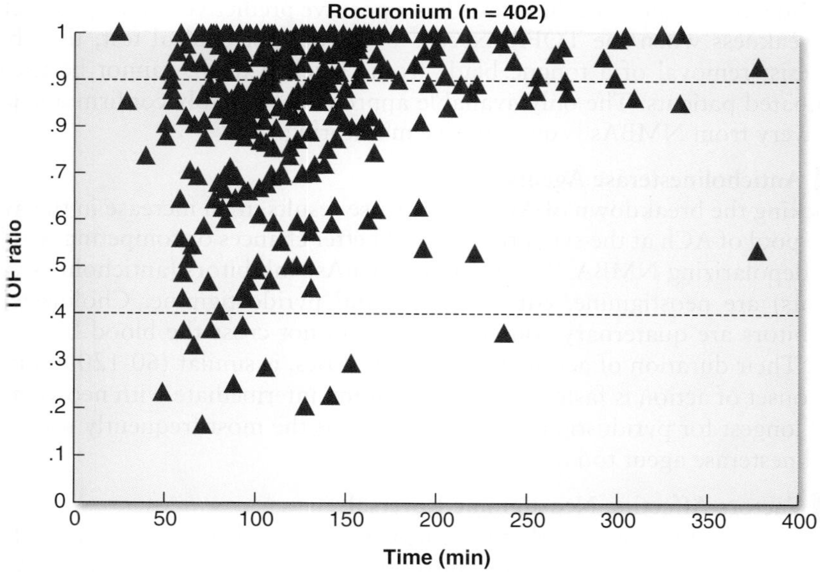

Figure 11.13 The plot shows train-of-four (TOF) ratios for 402 patients on arrival to the postanesthesia care unit. Each patient received only one dose of rocuronium 0.6 mg/kg and did not receive pharmacological reversal. There is substantial interpatient variation in duration of rocuronium, and the duration cannot be predicted in an individual patient. The dotted lines correspond to TOF ratio 0.4 and 0.9, respectively. With use of a peripheral nerve stimulator and subjective assessment, the majority of patients with TOF ratio >0.4 would be expected to have a TOF count of 4 without appreciable fade. Quantitative monitoring is necessary to be able to determine the TOF ratio for these patients. Quantitative monitoring would also identify the 55% of patients who have spontaneously recovered to TOF ratio ≥0.9 and therefore should not be exposed to pharmacological reversal drugs and their associated costs and potential side effects. (Redrawn from Debaene B, Plaud B, Dilly MP, Donati F. Residual paralysis in the PACU after a single intubating dose of nondepolarizing muscle relaxant with an intermediate duration of action. *Anesthesiology*. 2003;98:1042-1048, Figure 1).

VIII. Reversal of Neuromuscular Blockade

A. Residual Neuromuscular Blockade

For decades, investigators have shown that regardless of the NMBA used, over 40% of patients managed intraoperatively by clinical criteria or subjective evaluation had residual paralysis (TOFR < 0.90) when tested objectively in the postanesthesia care unit.[10,11] Residual paralysis is associated with adverse clinical consequences, especially pertaining to the respiratory system. These include impaired pharyngeal function with increased risk of aspiration, airway obstruction, hypoxemia, respiratory failure, reintubation, and postoperative atelectasis and pneumonia. Residual paralysis is an iatrogenic complication; it can and should be prevented. First, when paralysis is no longer required, a valid prereversal assessment should be obtained from the adductor pollicis muscle. Second, unless the block has recovered spontaneously to at least TOFR = 0.9, an effective pharmacological reversal should be administered. Third, adequacy of neuromuscular function should be confirmed by quantitative monitoring before the final stage of emergence from anesthesia and tracheal extubation.

Clinical testing has been advocated for decades; tests such as grip strength, vital capacity, tidal volume, or leg lift are notoriously poor at detecting residual fade. In fact, none of these tests has a positive predictive value for detection of weakness when the TOFR exceeds 0.5. The best clinical test, the ability to resist removal of a tongue blade from clenched teeth, cannot be used in intubated patients. The only available approach to reliably confirm adequate recovery from NMBAs is quantitative monitoring.

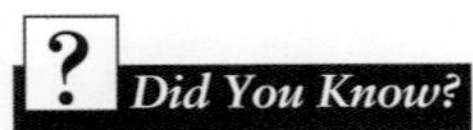

Neostigmine is most effective for reversal of minimal block (TOFR between 0.4 and 0.9). Its use is acceptable for shallow block (TOFR < 0.4) only if quantitative monitoring is used.

B. Anticholinesterase Agents

Blocking the breakdown of ACh by AChAse results in an increase in the available pool of ACh at the synaptic cleft and better chances of competing with the nondepolarizing NMBA. The available AChAse inhibitors (anticholinesterase agents) are neostigmine, edrophonium, and pyridostigmine. Cholinesterase inhibitors are quaternary compounds and do not cross the blood-brain barrier. Their duration of action at equivalent doses, is similar (60-120 minutes), but onset of action is fastest for edrophonium, intermediate with neostigmine, and longest for pyridostigmine. Neostigmine is the most frequently used anticholinesterase agent today.

C. Factors Affecting Neostigmine Reversal

It is important to consider that once neostigmine has been administered, there are two parallel processes that contribute to recovery. One is the inhibition of acetylcholinesterase which leads to an increased concentration of Ach; the other is the continued metabolism and elimination of NMBA. A major determinant of the effectiveness of neostigmine is the level of neuromuscular block. Traditionally, neostigmine reversal has been attempted for moderate block (TOFC 1-3). This is no longer recommended as its effectiveness is unreliable.[12] Even when the block is shallow, that is TOFC of 4 with subjective fade, there is no dose of neostigmine that can guarantee complete reversal to TOFR 0.9 within 10 minutes in 95% of patients.[13,14] Only when the block is minimal (TOFC of 4 without fade or TOFR ≥ 0.4) is neostigmine highly effective. Administration of neostigmine earlier than 10 to 15 minutes before anticipated extubation is not optimal because neostigmine has peak effect at approximately 10 minutes.[15,16] Therefore, if full recovery to TOFR ≥0.9 is not accomplished by 10 minutes after neostigmine administration, the most likely explanation is that the block was too deep for reversal with neostigmine. In this case, spontaneous recovery will continue (while neostigmine's effect somewhat diminishes after its peak), and the patient will eventually reach full recovery. When monitoring is performed by PNS and subjective evaluation, early administration of neostigmine for a block deeper than minimal has a significant disadvantage, namely that a longer and unpredictable period of time will be spent in the TOFR range 0.4 to 0.9.[17] This range has been referred to as the zone of blind paralysis and it is not possible to subjectively determine when the patient is fully recovered.[18] Neostigmine is relatively inexpensive and if quantitative monitoring is used, it is acceptable to attempt neostigmine reversal for a block with TOFC of 4 with fade, because a minority of patients will be successfully reversed. This approach is more likely to be successful in the context of total intravenous anesthesia and less likely to succeed with volatile anesthetics. For reversal of a block with TOFC of 4 with fade (and quantitative monitoring), an appropriate dose of neostigmine is 50 μg/kg. Higher doses than 50 μg/kg have not been shown to increase effectiveness. For neostigmine reversal of minimal block (TOFC 4 without fade or TOFR ≥ 0.4), a dose of 20 to 30 μg is recommended. There is no significant difference in the speed of recovery induced by neostigmine among the intermediate-acting nondepolarizing NMBAs. Age affects neostigmine-induced speed of reversal, being faster in children than in adults and slower in the elderly. Finally, drugs and conditions that potentiate the effect of nondepolarizing NMBAs will also prolong neostigmine-induced recovery time: volatile anesthetics, magnesium, and hypothermia.

D. Neostigmine: Other Effects

Neostigmine and edrophonium inhibit acetylcholinesterase at all cholinergic sites, including muscarinic receptors and therefore induce vagal stimulation. Therefore, anticholinergic agents such as atropine or glycopyrrolate are coadministered with anticholinesterase agents. Atropine is faster in onset than glycopyrrolate, produces more tachycardia, and crosses the blood-brain barrier. For these reasons, glycopyrrolate is preferred. Other side effects of neostigmine include increased salivation and bowel motility. Although anticholinergic agents are effective in preventing salivation, their effects on bowel motility are limited. A meta-analysis of the effects of neostigmine on postoperative nausea and vomiting (PONV) have not supported a connection and the current guideline for management of PONV advises only against high dose neostigmine.[19]

E. Selective Relaxant Binding Agents: Sugammadex

Sugammadex is a γ-cyclodextrin with a central cavity that encapsulates the steroid nucleus of rocuronium and vecuronium. It has no affinity for any of the other depolarizing or nondepolarizing NMBAs. Binding to rocuronium is extremely tight, with no clinically relevant dissociation. Binding to vecuronium is one-third as tight, and the dose requirement for reversal of vecuronium is higher. Binding occurs in plasma and creates a rapid decrease in the plasma concentrations of NMBA. Free NMBA molecules at the neuromuscular junction move with the concentration gradient to the plasma compartment. As long as a sufficient dose of sugammadex is administered, the result is a highly effective reversal within a few minutes. The recommended dose is 2 mg/kg when the level of block has recovered to TOFC of 2, and 4 mg/kg for deeper blocks as long as the PTC is at least 1 (**Table 11.3**). These dose recommendations are adequate for reversal of both vecuronium- and rocuronium-induced

Table 11.3 Reversal of Rocuronium-Induced Neuromuscular Blockade

Level of Block	Type of Monitoring		Reversal Agent	
	PNS + Subjective Evaluation	Quantitative Monitoring	Neostigmine	Sugammadex
Complete (intense)	No twitch PTC 0	PTC 0	Wait	Wait
Deep	TOFC 0 PTC ≥ 1	TOFC 0 PTC ≥ 1	Wait	4 mg/kg
Moderate	TOFC 1-3	TOFC 1-3	Wait	2 mg/kg
Shallow	TOFC 4 with fade	TOFR <0.4	Wait[a]	2 mg/kg
Minimal	TOFC 4 without fade	TOFR 0.4-0.9	15-30 µg/kg	2 mg/kg
Acceptable recovery	Unable to assess	TOFR ≥ 0.9	None	None

PNS, peripheral nerve stimulator; PTC, posttetanic count; TOFC, train-of-four count; TOFR, train-of-four ratio.
[a]With quantitative monitoring, neostigmine reversal with 40 µg/kg can be attempted, as some patients can be successfully reversed from this level of block.

neuromuscular block; however, reversal of rocuronium will be more rapid. Underdosing of sugammadex can lead to an incomplete reversal or to an initial reversal with reparalysis 15 to 30 minutes later. Therefore, it is critical that a valid prereversal assessment of neuromuscular blockade from the adductor pollicis is obtained and that dose recommendations are followed. Importantly, if no neuromuscular monitor is used, there is a risk of significant residual weakness, even with administration of sugammadex 2 to 4 mg/kg.[20] The dose recommendations above are not applicable if reversal is guided by assessment of the corrugator supercilii muscle.[21] As mentioned above, 16 mg/kg can effectively reverse rocuronium 1.2 mg/kg in an emergency situation, however, a number of other factors influence whether spontaneous ventilation will be restored. Unlike with anticholinesterase reversal, the type of anesthesia (intravenous or volatile) does not influence the ability of sugammadex to reverse rocuronium. The sugammadex-rocuronium complexes are excreted via the kidneys, with an elimination half-life of 100 minutes. It is not FDA-approved for use in patients with renal failure (CrCl < 30 mL/min), although reports of successful use have been published.[22]

1. Clinical Use, Side Effects, and Safety

Sugammadex is an important addition to the anesthesiologist's armamentarium. The leading safety concern is the potential for hypersensitivity reactions, including anaphylactic shock. The perioperative prevalence of anaphylactic reactions is estimated to be between 1:3500 and 1:20,000 cases, with an associated mortality of up to 9%.[23] The risk of hypersensitivity reactions is significantly greater with sugammadex than with neostigmine, and the risk has been reported to increase when higher doses are administered.[24] There has been concern that the risk of hypersensitivity reactions will increase with more widespread use.

Sugammadex has been associated with cardiac arrhythmias, including marked bradycardia and asystole. ECG monitoring should be routine when sugammadex is administered.[25]

Sugammadex can bind also hormonal contraceptives and therefore inhibit their effectiveness. Women of childbearing age should be advised to use alternative nonhormonal means of birth control for 1 week after exposure.

IX. Conclusion

Neuromuscular blockade has facilitated many advances in anesthesia but also carries considerable risk. Understanding the physiology of the neuromuscular junction yields an appreciation for the effects of NMBAs and the need to follow patient response to these agents. Proper monitoring during maintenance paralysis allows selection of an effective reversal strategy to minimize the risk of complications associated with residual weakness.

For further review and interactivities, please see the associated Interactive Video Lectures and "A Closer Look" infographic accessible in the complimentary eBook bundled with this text. Access instructions are located in the inside front cover.

References

1. Scholz A. Mechanisms of (local) anaesthetics on voltage-gated sodium and other ion channels. *Br J Anaesth*. 2002;89(1):52-61. PMID: 12173241.
2. Schreiber JU, Lysakowski C, Fuchs-Buder T, Tramèr MR. Prevention of succinylcholine-induced fasciculation and myalgia: a meta-analysis of randomized trials. *Anesthesiology*. 2005;103(4):877-884. PMID: 16192781.
3. Kovarik WD, Mayberg TS, Lam AM, Mathisen TL, Winn HR. Succinylcholine does not change intracranial pressure, cerebral blood flow velocity, or the electroencephalogram in patients with neurologic injury. *Anesth Analg*. 1994;78(3):469-473. PMID: 8109761.
4. Dexter F, Epstein RH, Wachtel RE, Rosenberg H. Estimate of the relative risk of succinylcholine for triggering malignant hyperthermia. *Anesth Analg*. 2013;116(1):118-122. PMID: 23223104.
5. Tang L, Li S, Huang S, Ma H, Wang Z. Desaturation following rapid sequence induction using succinylcholine vs. rocuronium in overweight patients. *Acta Anaesthesiol Scand*. 2011;55(2):203-208. PMID: 21226862.
6. Martyn JA, Richtsfeld M. Succinylcholine-induced hyperkalemia in acquired pathologic states: etiologic factors and molecular mechanisms. *Anesthesiology*. 2006;104(1):158-169. PMID: 16394702.
7. Naguib M, Brull SJ, Kopman AF, et al. Consensus statement on perioperative use of neuromuscular monitoring. *Anesth Analg*. 07 2018;127(1):71-80. PMID: 29200077.
8. Gätke MR, Larsen PB, Engbaek J, Fredensborg BB, Berg H, Viby-Mogensen J. Acceleromyography of the orbicularis oculi muscle I: significance of the electrode position. *Acta Anaesthesiol Scand*. 2002;46(9):1124-1130. PMID: 12366508.
9. Thilen SR, Hansen BE, Ramaiah R, Kent CD, Treggiari MM, Bhananker SM. Intraoperative neuromuscular monitoring site and residual paralysis. *Anesthesiology*. 2012;117(5):964-972. PMID: 16394702.
10. Viby-Mogensen J, Jørgensen BC, Ording H. Residual curarization in the recovery room. *Anesthesiology*. 1979;50(6):539-541. PMID: 156513.
11. Fortier LP, McKeen D, Turner K, et al. The RECITE study: a Canadian prospective, multicenter study of the incidence and severity of residual neuromuscular blockade. *Anesth Analg*. 2015;121(2):366-372. PMID: 25902322.
12. Kirkegaard H, Heier T, Caldwell J. Efficacy of tactile-guided reversal from cisatracurium-induced neuromuscular block. *Anesthesiology*. 2002;96(1):45-50. PMID: 11753000.
13. Kopman A, Naguib M. Neostigmine-induced weakness after sugammadex – A reply. *Anaesthesia*. 2019;74(2):254. PMID: 30656654.
14. Kaufhold N, Schaller SJ, Stäuble CG, et al. Sugammadex and neostigmine dose-finding study for reversal of residual neuromuscular block at a train-of-four ratio of 0.2 (SUNDRO20)†. *Br J Anaesth*. 2016;116(2):233-240. PMID: 26787792.
15. Miller R, Van Nyhuis L, Eger E., Vitez T, Way W. Comparative times to peak effect and durations of action of neostigmine and pyridostigmine. *Anesthesiology*. 1974;41(1):27-33. PMID: 4834375.
16. Kirkegaard-Nielsen H, Helbo-Hansen HS, Lindholm P, Severinsen IK, Bülow K. Time to peak effect of neostigmine at antagonism of atracurium- or vecuronium-induced neuromuscular block. *J Clin Anesth*. 1995;7(8):635-639. PMID: 8747561.

17. Donati F. Residual paralysis: a real problem or did we invent a new disease? *Can J Anaesth*. 2013;60(7):714-729. PMID: 23625545.
18. Plaud B, Debaene B, Donati F, Marty J. Residual paralysis after emergence from anesthesia. *Anesthesiology*. 2010;112(4):1013-1022. PMID: 20234315.
19. Gan TJ, Belani KG, Bergese S, et al. Fourth consensus guidelines for the management of postoperative nausea and vomiting. *Anesth Analg*. 2020;131(2):411-448. PMID: 32467512.
20. Kotake Y, Ochiai R, Suzuki T, et al. Reversal with sugammadex in the absence of monitoring did not preclude residual neuromuscular block. *Anesth Analg*. 2013;117(2):345-351. PMID: 23757472.
21. Yamamoto S, Yamamoto Y, Kitajima O, Maeda T, Suzuki T. Reversal of neuromuscular block with sugammadex: a comparison of the corrugator supercilii and adductor pollicis muscles in a randomized dose-response study. *Acta Anaesthesiol Scand*. 2015;59(7):892-901. PMID: 25962400.
22. de Souza CM, Tardelli MA, Tedesco H, et al. Efficacy and safety of sugammadex in the reversal of deep neuromuscular blockade induced by rocuronium in patients with end-stage renal disease: a comparative prospective clinical trial. *Eur J Anaesthesiol*. 2015;32(10):681-686. PMID: 25829395.
23. Galvão VR, Giavina-Bianchi P, Castells M. Perioperative anaphylaxis. *Curr Allergy Asthma Rep*. 2014;14(8):452. PMID: 24951238.
24. Orihara M, Takazawa T, Horiuchi T, et al. Comparison of incidence of anaphylaxis between sugammadex and neostigmine: a retrospective multicentre observational study. *Br J Anaesth*. 2020;124(2):154-163. PMID: 31791621.
25. Savic L, Savic S, Hopkins PM. Anaphylaxis to sugammadex: should we be concerned by the Japanese experience? *Br J Anaesth*. 2020;124(4):P370-P372. PMID: 31982112.

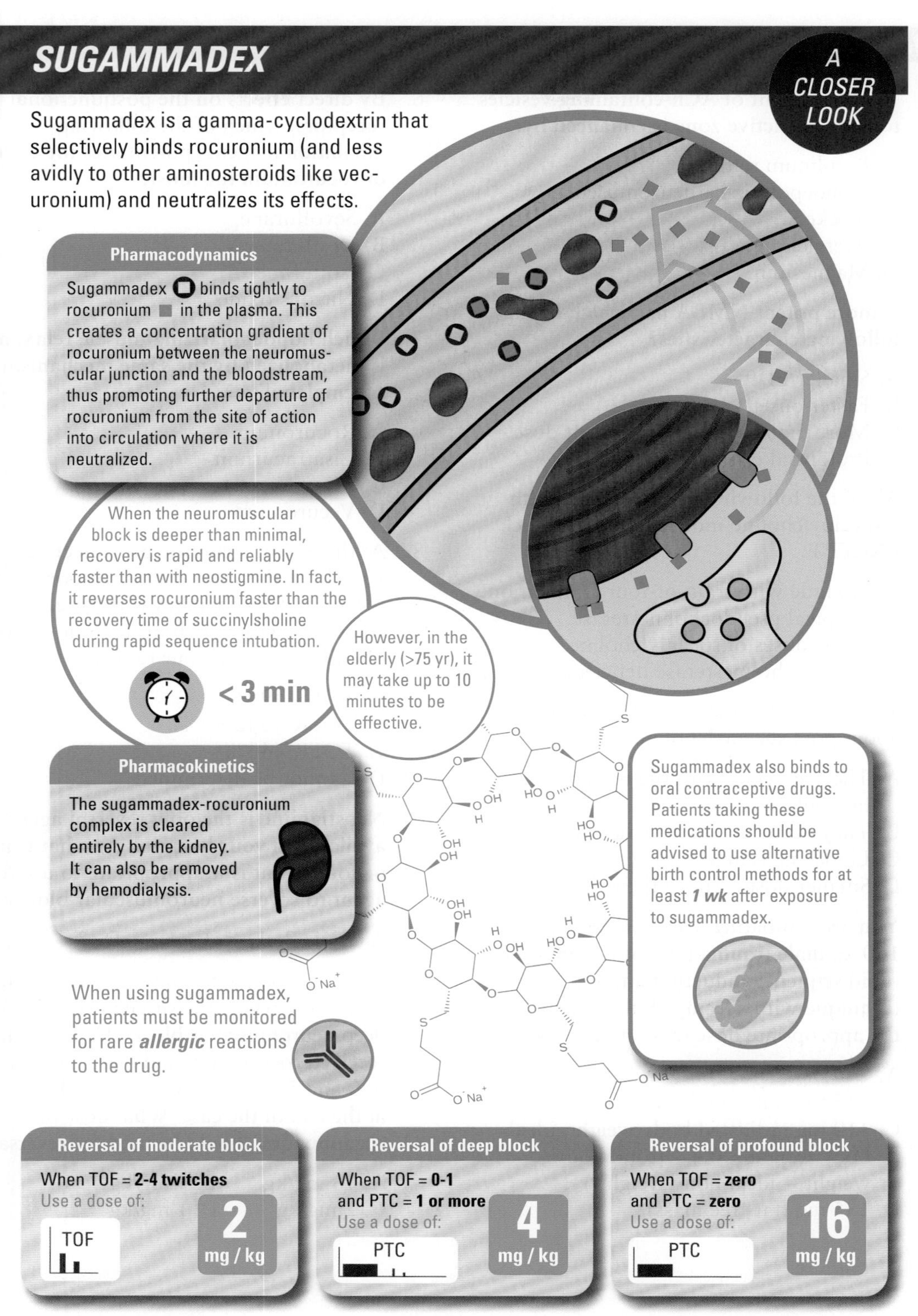

SUGAMMADEX
A CLOSER LOOK
Sugammadex is a gamma-cyclodextrin that selectively binds rocuronium (and less avidly to other aminosteroids like vecuronium) and neutralizes its effects.
Pharmacodynamics
Sugammadex binds tightly to rocuronium in the plasma. This creates a concentration gradient of rocuronium between the neuromuscular junction and the bloodstream, thus promoting further departure of rocuronium from the site of action into circulation where it is neutralized.
When the neuromuscular block is deeper than minimal, recovery is rapid and reliably faster than with neostigmine. In fact, it reverses rocuronium faster than the recovery time of succinylsholine during rapid sequence intubation.
< 3 min
However, in the elderly (>75 yr), it may take up to 10 minutes to be effective.
Pharmacokinetics
The sugammadex-rocuronium complex is cleared entirely by the kidney. It can also be removed by hemodialysis.
Sugammadex also binds to oral contraceptive drugs. Patients taking these medications should be advised to use alternative birth control methods for at least 1 wk after exposure to sugammadex.
When using sugammadex, patients must be monitored for rare allergic reactions to the drug.
Reversal of moderate block
When TOF = 2-4 twitches
Use a dose of:
TOF
2 mg / kg
Reversal of deep block
When TOF = 0-1 and PTC = 1 or more
Use a dose of:
PTC
4 mg / kg
Reversal of profound block
When TOF = zero and PTC = zero
Use a dose of:
PTC
16 mg / kg

Sugammadex **should not be used without monitoring** and proper dosing should always be guided by obtaining a **prereversal assessment** from the adductor pollicis.

Infographic by: Naveen Nathan MD

Questions

1. **The movement of ACh-containing vesicles toward the active zone is enhanced by:**

   A. Botulinum toxin.
   B. Nondepolarizing neuromuscular blockers.
   C. Acetylcholine.
   D. Magnesium.

2. **A more potent NMBA has which of the following characteristics?**

   A. Smaller ED95
   B. Faster onset
   C. More molecules per equivalent dose
   D. Prolonged duration

3. **All of the following are associated with a succinylcholine-induced phase II block EXCEPT:**

   A. No fade with train-of-four stimulation.
   B. Atypical pseudocholinesterase.
   C. Large doses of succinylcholine.
   D. Plasma cholinesterase deficiency.

4. **Which of following is most likely true about post-succinylcholine myalgias?**

   A. They correlate with the presence of fasciculations.
   B. They occur in 1% of patients.
   C. Lidocaine is an effective prophylaxis.
   D. Smaller doses reduce the risk.

5. **You are intubating a 183 cm (6 ft), 160 kg male trauma patient utilizing the rapid sequence induction and intubation technique with succinylcholine. Which is the appropriate dose (assume 1.5 mg/kg)?**

   A. 240 mg (actual body weight)
   B. 115 mg (ideal body weight)
   C. 110 mg (adjusted body weight, ideal body weight + 0.4 × [total body weight – ideal body weight])
   D. 135 mg (fat-free mass)

6. **By direct effects on the postjunctional receptors, which of the following inhalational agents potentiates the effects of rocuronium the most?**

   A. Sevoflurane
   B. Desflurane
   C. Isoflurane
   D. Nitrous oxide

7. **Which nondepolarizing muscle relaxant is metabolized by the same mechanism as succinylcholine?**

   A. Rocuronium
   B. Cisatracurium
   C. Mivacurium
   D. Vecuronium

8. **At the end of a robotic prostatectomy you check the train-of-four response and recognize four twitches with fade. This correlates with which of the following? (TOFR = train-of-four ratio.)**

   A. TOFR ≥90%
   B. TOFR 40 to 90%
   C. TOFR <40%
   D. Cannot be determined

9. **Neostigmine is the only reversal agent available in your hospital. At what train-of-four count is it appropriate to use this agent to reverse neuromuscular blockade?**

   A. 2 B. 1 C. 4 D. 3

10. **A 65 kg woman has undergone a left upper lobectomy where the surgeon requested deep neuromuscular blockade. The patient received rocuronium and has a TOF count of 0 and 5 post-tetanic twitches (PTC = 5) at the end of the case. What dose of sugammadex should be used for reversal?**

    A. 16 mg/kg B. 4 mg/kg
    C. 2 mg/kg D. 1 mg/kg

Answers

1. C

Acetylcholine binds to presynaptic neuronal nAChRs in a positive feedback loop, causing migration of Ach vesicles to the active zone. Nondepolarizing NMBs bind presynaptic neuronal nAChRs impeding this process, leading to TOF fade. Botulinum toxin degrades the proteins that facilitate Ach vesicle movement to the active zone causing weakness. Calcium influx cause Ach vesicles in the active zone to fuse with the nerve membrane resulting in release of Ach into the cleft. Magnesium acts as a false transmitter for calcium, slowing calcium influx and hindering ACh release from vesicles.

2. A

Fewer molecules are required for effect with more potent NMBs; thus, the effective dose for 95% twitch reduction in half the patients (ED_{95}) is smaller. Potency is inversely related to speed of onset; thus, more potent NMBs have slower onset. Potency does not affect duration.

3. A

Phase II block occurs with relatively large doses of succinylcholine and shares characteristics with a nondepolarizing block, such as fade with train-of-four stimulation. Lack of efficient metabolism of succinylcholine, which occurs with atypical pseudocholinesterase or a deficiency of normal pseudocholinesterase, leads to build up of succinylcholine even when normal doses are administered; this can result in a phase II block.

4. C

Myalgias are reported in up to half the patients who receive succinylcholine. There is no correlation between fasciculations and the development of myalgias. Lidocaine and nonsteroidal anti-inflammatory drugs are effective pharmacologic prophylactic options. Interestingly, patients receiving larger doses of succinylcholine are less likely to experience myalgias.

5. A

Succinylcholine is dosed based on actual body weight, as are the benzylisoquinoline neuromuscular blockers (cisatracurium and mivacurium). The aminosteroidal neuromuscular blockers (rocuronium and vecuronium) are dosed based on ideal body weight.

6. B

Desflurane potentiates neuromuscular blockade more than sevoflurane and isoflurane. Nitrous oxide potentiates neuromuscular blockade the least of the listed agents.

7. C

Mivacurium and succinylcholine are metabolized by pseudocholinesterase. Rocuronium and vecuronium are eliminated via a combination of hepatic and renal routes. Cisatracurium is eliminated via Hoffman degradation and nonspecific ester hydrolysis.

8. C

TOFR cannot be determined by objective assessment. However, human detection of a reduction in the fourth twitch (TOF with fade) correlates with a measured TOFR less than 40%. If there is no fade, then all that can be determined is that the TOFR is greater than 40%. Based solely on this objective assessment, it cannot be determined if the TOFR is acceptable for extubation (TOFR ≥ 90%). Quantitative monitoring is required to determine if the TOFR is above 90%.

9. C

The practice of reversing deep levels of neuromuscular block with neostigmine is very likely the main contributing factor in the ongoing problem of postoperative residual paralysis. To combat this disturbing trend, experts recommend waiting until the fourth twitch has returned before reversing with neostigmine. If neostigmine is used to reverse at deeper levels of block, then quantitative monitoring should be used to verify that a TOFR ≥ 90% has been attained before extubation.

10. B

The manufacturer-recommended dose is 16 mg/kg for profound block (zero posttetanic twitches, PTC = 0). When at least one twitch can be elicited after tetany (PTC ≥ 1) up to a TOF count of 1, the recommended dose is 4 mg/kg. After the second twitch has returned (TOFC ≥ 2), then only 2 mg/kg is needed.

12 Local Anesthetics

Andrew M. Walters and Francis V. Salinas

Introduction

Local anesthetics are a class of drugs that transiently and reversibly inhibit the conduction of sensory, motor, and autonomic neural impulses. Clinically, local anesthetics are primarily used to provide perioperative anesthesia or analgesia. This chapter presents the mechanism of action of local anesthetics, the physiochemical properties that determine their clinical pharmacology, clinical applications, and potential for toxicity. Relevant peripheral nerve anatomy and physiology are briefly reviewed here, with more detailed information presented in Chapter 4. Chapters 21 and 31 will present common clinical applications for local anesthetics.

I. Mechanism of Action of Local Anesthetics

A. Anatomy of Nerves

The neuron is the basic functional unit responsible for the conduction of neural impulses. It consists of a spherical cell body (soma) that contains the nucleus. The cell body is connected to several branching processes (dendrites), which transmit neural impulses to the neuron, and a single axon, which transmits neural impulses away from the cell body to other neurons (**Figure 12.1A**). Axons are cylinders of axoplasm encased within a lipid bilayer cell membrane that is embedded with various proteins, including voltage-gated sodium (Na^+; VG_{Na}) channels. Glial cells (oligodendrocytes in the ***central nervous system*** [CNS] and Schwann cells in the ***peripheral nervous system***) are closely associated with neurons and function to support, insulate, and nourish axons. A nerve fiber is composed of an axon, its associated glial cell, and the surrounding endoneural connective tissue.

Peripheral nerve fibers are organized within three layers of connective tissue (**Figure 12.1B**). Individual nerve fibers are immediately surrounded by ***endoneurium***, consisting of delicate connective tissue that consists of Schwann cells and fibroblasts along with capillaries. A dense layer of collagenous connective tissue, the ***perineurium***, encloses bundles of nerve fibers into a fascicle. It functionally provides an effective barrier against penetration of the nerve fibers by foreign substances. The ***epineurium*** is also a dense connective tissue layer that surrounds and encases bundles of fascicles together into a cylindrical sheath structurally similar to a coaxial cable. It is looser in between fascicles, but denser and fibrous externally, where it forms the outer boundary of the

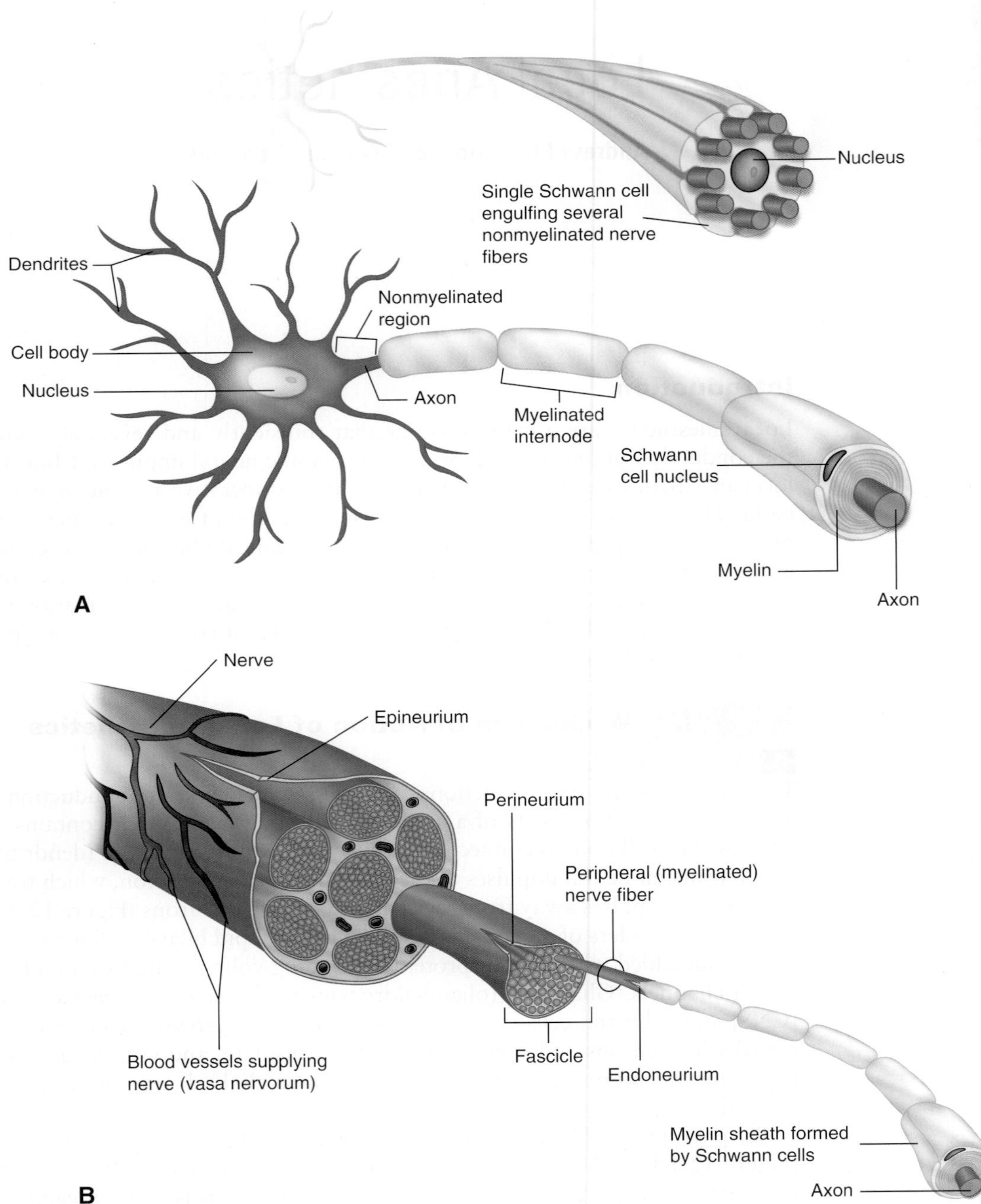

Figure 12.1 A, Representative neuron and myelinated and nonmyelinated axon. The neuron consists of a cell body (soma), dendrites, and an axon. Myelinated nerve fibers have a sheath composed of a continuous series of neurolemma (derived from Schwann cells) that surround the axon and form a series of myelin segments. Multiple nonmyelinated nerve fibers are individually encased within a single neurolemma that does not produce myelin. B, Arrangement of perineural connective tissue layers in a representative nerve. Peripheral nerves consist of bundles of nerve fibers, the layers of the connective tissues (endoneurium, perineurium, and epineurium) that serve to bind them, and associated blood vessels (vasa nervorum) that supply them. All but the smallest peripheral nerves are arranged in bundles called fascicles.

Table 12.1 Classification of Peripheral Nerve Fibers

Fiber Classification	Diameter (mm)	Myelination	Conduction Velocity (m/s)	Anatomical Location	Function	Local Anesthetic Susceptibility
Aa	6-22	Yes	30-120	Efferent to muscles	Motor	++
Ab	6-22	Yes	30-120	Afferent from skin and joints	Touch and proprioception	++
Ag	3-6	Yes	15-35	Efferent to muscle spindles	Muscle tone	++++
Ad	1-4	Yes	5-25	Afferent sensory	Distinct, well-localized (fast) pain, cold temperature, touch	+++
B	<3	Yes	3-15	Preganglionic sympathetic	Autonomic	++
C	0.3-1.3	No	0.7-1.3	Afferent sensory, postganglionic sympathetic	Autonomic, warm temperature, touch, and diffuse (slow) pain	+

+ (least susceptible), ++, +++, ++++ (most susceptible) to conduction blockade.

nerve. An additional connective tissue layer that forms a ***paraneural*** sheath further encases peripheral nerves. Together, these tissue layers offer protection to peripheral nerves but also present a significant barrier to passive diffusion of local anesthetics toward the axonal cell membrane.

Peripheral nerves are mixed nerves containing both afferent and efferent nerve fibers that are either myelinated or nonmyelinated (**Figure 12.1A**). Myelinated nerve fibers contain axons, which are concentrically wrapped multiple times by the cell membrane (neurolemma) of Schwann cells. These layers of neurolemma form a myelin sheath, which provide insulation around the nerve allowing electrical signals to travel the distance of the sheath with minimal attenuation. Voltage-gated sodium channels (VG_{Na}) cluster on the axonal cell membrane in gaps between each Schwann cell, referred to as nodes of Ranvier. Nonmyelinated nerve fibers consist of multiple axons that are simultaneously encased by the neurolemma of a single Schwann cell. Voltage-gated sodium channels (VG_{Na}) are uniformly distributed along the entire axon of nonmyelinated nerve fibers (**Table 12.1**).

B. Electrophysiology of Neural Conduction and Voltage-Gated Sodium Channels

Neural impulses are conducted along axons as action potentials, which are transient membrane depolarizations initiated by various mechanical, chemical, or thermal stimuli. Depolarization of the cell membrane is mediated primarily via rapid intracellular influx of Na^+ ions flowing down its electrochemical gradient through VG_{Na}. As one area of the cell membrane is depolarized, the change in polarization is sensed by adjacent VG_{Na}, which subsequently open and cause further depolarization. In nonmyelinated nerve fibers, this wave of depolarization propagates along the axon as sequential VG_{Na} open. In myelinated nerve fibers, action potentials propagate by hopping between VG_{Na} clustered in the nodes of Ranvier in a process known as ***saltatory conduction***, which enhances the speed of signal transmission along the axon.

The potential energy utilized to facilitate electrical conduction down the axon is provided by an electrochemical concentration gradient across the cell membrane. Transmembrane Na^+-K^+ (potassium) pumps establish this gradient actively cotransporting three Na^+ ions out of the cell for every two K^+ ions into the cell. The resulting chemical concentration gradient favors the movement of Na^+ ions into the cell and K^+ ions out of the cell. At rest, the cell membrane is relatively more permeable to K^+ ions, preventing an influx of Na^+ ions while allowing for a passive efflux of K^+ ions down their concentration gradient and out of the cell. This creates a relative net excess of negatively charged ions (polarized) within the axoplasm. The difference in charge across the cell membrane is referred to as the resting membrane potential, which measures approximately −60 to −70 mV in the neuron.

The VG_{Na} spans the axonal membrane and consists of an α-subunit and one or two varying auxiliary β-subunits. The α-subunit forms the ion-conducting pore of the VG_{Na} and it comprises four homologous domains (I to IV), each with six α-helical transmembrane segments. The loops that link the S5 and S6 segments of the α-helices of each of the four domains are located extracellular, extending inward to form the narrowest section of the channel pore. They are believed to provide its ion selectivity.

At the resting membrane potential, the channel pore is in a resting (closed) conformation. Upon an initial depolarization, movement of the S1-S4 voltage-sensing segments leads to rearrangement of the S6 segment. This results in activation (opening) of the channel pore, inducing a sudden increase in Na^+ ion permeability. The resultant rapid inward Na^+ current activates and opens additional VG_{Na}. This further accelerates depolarization until a threshold membrane potential is reached, triggering an action potential. During the depolarization phase, the inward Na^+ current flows into the axoplasm and spreads to the adjacent (inactive) cell membrane, resulting in a wave of sequential depolarization (and the action potential) propagating along the axon. Although the wave of depolarization spreads from the initial area of excitation in both directions, the just activated membrane behind the impulse is temporarily refractory to subsequent depolarization. Thus, the propagation of the impulse is unidirectional. The activated VG_{Na} is inactivated within milliseconds by an additional conformational change. This leads to binding of the cytoplasmic loop located between domains III and IV to the cytoplasmic opening of the VG_{Na} to form the rapid inactivation gate. The rapid inactivation gate functions as an intracellular blocking particle that folds into and blocks the channel pore. This rapid inactivation process is required for repetitive firing of action potentials in neural circuits and for control of excitability in neurons. Repolarization occurs due to a combination of a progressive decrease in the driving force for the inward Na^+ current and inactivation of VG_{Na}. In addition, membrane depolarization simultaneously activates voltage-gated K^+ channels. This leads to an outward positive current of K^+ ions, which in conjunction with VG_{Na} inactivation eventually returns the axonal membrane to or just beyond (hyperpolarization) its resting membrane potential. In summary, inward positive currents, mediated by Na^+ ions, depolarize the membrane, and in contrast, outward positive currents, mediated by K^+ ions, repolarize the membrane.

C. Voltage-Gated Sodium Channels and Interactions With Local Anesthetics

Local anesthetics act at the axonal membrane by binding to a specific region within the α-subunit. This prevents VG_{Na} activation, thus inhibiting the inward Na^+ current that mediates membrane depolarization. The binding site for local anesthetics is located within the channel pore and is formed from amino acid residues in the S6 segments of domains I, III, and IV. The binding site may be approached from two pathways: from the intracellular aspect of the channel pore (hydrophilic pathway) or laterally from within the lipid membrane (hydrophobic pathway). As the amount of administered local anesthetic increases, an increasing percentage of VG_{Na} bind to local anesthetics, further inhibiting the inward Na^+ current. Subsequently, the rate of depolarization (in response to stimulation) is attenuated, inhibiting the achievement of the threshold membrane potential. Consequently, achievement of an action potential becomes increasingly difficult. With a sufficient number of local anesthetic-bound VG_{Na}, an action potential can no longer be generated, and impulse propagation is blocked. Local anesthetic binding to VG_{Na} does not alter the resting membrane potential nor does it alter the threshold potential.

Local anesthetics bind more avidly to VG_{Na} in the activated (open) and inactivated (channel pore is ***open*** but closed by movement of the inactivation gate) conformations. The difference in binding affinity is attributable to the difference in the availability of the two pathways for local anesthetic to reach the binding site. Local anesthetics produce a concentration-dependent decrease in inward Na^+ current characterized as ***tonic blockade***, representing a decrease in the number of open confirmation VG_{Na}.[1] When undergoing repeated depolarization, a greater number of VG_{Na} are in either the activated or inactivated conformations with high binding affinity for local anesthetics. Thus, repeated stimulation results in accumulation of local anesthetic-bound VG_{Na} characterized as ***frequency (or use)-dependent blockade.***

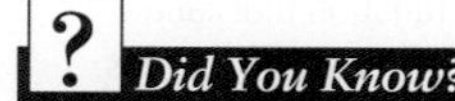

Not only do local anesthetics prevent nerve impulse propagation by adhering to binding sites on voltage-gated sodium channels in the cell membrane (tonic blockade), they also bind more readily to nerves undergoing repeated stimulation (frequency [or use]-dependent blockade).

D. Mechanisms of Nerve Block

In order for local anesthetics to bind VG_{Na}, they must reach the neural membrane. Thus, local anesthetics must penetrate through variable amounts of perineural tissue and still maintain a sufficient concentration gradient to diffuse through the lipid bilayer. Only a small fraction (1%-2%) of local anesthetic reaches the neural membrane even when deposited in close proximity to peripheral nerves. Peripheral nerves that have been desheathed in vitro require about a 100-fold lower local anesthetic concentration than peripheral nerves in vivo. In contrast, central neuraxial nerves are encased in three layers of meninges: the pia mater, arachnoid membrane, and dura mater. The pia mater is adherent to the nerves themselves and is separated from the arachnoid membrane by cerebrospinal fluid that fills the space between these two layers. The ***subarachnoid*** space, where the spinal nerves are only covered by the pia mater, is the target location for spinal anesthesia. The dura mater further encases the arachnoid membrane, forming the dural sac, a tough covering around the central neuraxis. The epidural space consists of everything located within the vertebral canal but outside the dural sac. The presence of the arachnoid membrane and dura mater result in 10-fold higher local anesthetic dose requirements to produce complete epidural blockade compared with that required in the subarachnoid space.

The quality of nerve block is determined not only by the intrinsic potency of the chosen local anesthetic but also by the concentration and volume of the administered local anesthetic. The potency of a local anesthetic can be expressed as the minimum effective concentration required to establish complete nerve blockade. The volume of local anesthetic is also important, as a sufficient length of axon or adjacent nodes of Ranvier must be blocked in order to inhibit regeneration of the neural impulse. This is due to the phenomenon of ***decremental conduction***. Membrane depolarization passively decays with distance away from the front of the action potential to the point that impulse propagation stops when depolarization falls below the threshold for VG_{Na} activation. If less than a critical length of axon is blocked, the action potential may still be regenerated in the proximal neural membrane segment or node of Ranvier when the decaying depolarization is still above the threshold potential for Na^+ channel activation.

? *Did You Know?*

Differential blockade refers to the predictable progression of sensory and motor function blockade by local anesthetics, starting with loss of temperature sensation and followed by impaired proprioception, motor function, sharp pain, and lastly light touch.

Different types of nerve fibers demonstrate varying minimal blocking concentrations and local anesthetic susceptibilities (**Table 12.1**). Clinically, there is a predictable progression of sensory and motor function blockade, starting first with loss of temperature sensation, followed by proprioception, motor function, sharp pain, and lastly light touch. Termed ***differential block***, this progression was initially attributed to differences in axon diameter, with smaller fibers inherently more susceptible to conduction blockade compared with that of larger fibers. However, small myelinated fibers (Aγ and Aδ) are the most susceptible to conduction blockade. Next in order of block susceptibility are large myelinated fibers (Aα and Aβ), and the least susceptible are small, nonmyelinated C fibers.

Within peripheral nerves, longitudinal and radial diffusion of local anesthetic will produce varying drug concentrations along and within the nerve during the onset and recovery from clinical block. When local anesthetics are deposited around a peripheral nerve, diffusion progresses from the outer surface (mantle) toward the center (core) along a concentration gradient. Consequently, nerve fibers arranged in the mantle of mixed peripheral nerves are blocked initially. These outer nerve fibers are typically distributed to more proximal anatomic structures, whereas core fibers innervate more distal structures. This topographical arrangement explains the initial development of proximal, followed by distal anesthesia, as local anesthetic diffuses to the more centrally located core nerve fibers. In summary, the sequence of onset and recovery from peripheral nerve block depends on a combination of the topographical arrangement of the nerve fibers within a mixed peripheral nerve and their inherent susceptibility to local anesthetic blockade.

? *Did You Know?*

Although the linkage between a local anesthetic's hydrophobic aromatic ring and its hydrophilic amine group determines the molecule's class (aminoamide or aminoester) and metabolic pathway, it is the chemical substitutions on the aromatic ring or amine group that determine the drug's potency, onset, and duration of action.

II. Local Anesthetic Pharmacodynamics

A. Physiochemical Properties and Relationship to Activity and Potency

Local anesthetics in solution are weak bases that typically carry a positive charge at the amine group at physiologic pH. The prototypical local anesthetic structure consists of a hydrophobic group (typically a lipid-soluble aromatic ring) connected to a hydrophilic group (charged amine) by either an amide or ester linkage (**Figure 12.2**). The nature of the chemical bond is the basis for classification of local anesthetics as either an aminoamide or aminoester (**Table 12.2**). Although the nature of the linkage determines the basis for metabolism (aminoamides are metabolized in the liver, whereas aminoesters are metabolized by plasma cholinesterase), the physiochemical properties are largely determined by the nature of the alkyl substitutions on either the aromatic ring or the amine group, the charge of the amine group, or the stereochemistry of the related isomers (**Table 12.2**). These physiochemical properties largely determine the potency, onset and duration of action, and tendency for differential nerve block.

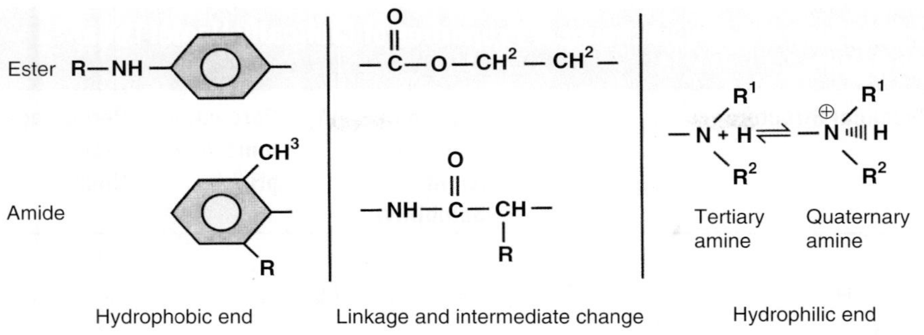

Ester R—NH—⟨ring⟩— | —C(=O)—O—CH² — CH²— | Tertiary amine ⇌ Quaternary amine

Amide ⟨ring with CH³ and R⟩— | —NH—C(=O)—CH(R)— |

Hydrophobic end | Linkage and intermediate change | Hydrophilic end

Figure 12.2 **The prototypical structures of aminoester and aminoamide local anesthetics.** (From Mulroy F, Bernards CM, McDonald SB, Salinas FV. *A Practical Approach to Regional Anesthesia*. 4th ed. Wolters Kluwer; 2009:2.)

The potency and, to a lesser extent, the duration of action of local anesthetics correlates with lipid solubility. Lipid solubility is determined by the degree of alkyl substitutions on either the aromatic ring or the amine group, and it is typically expressed by the partition coefficient in a hydrophobic solvent (typically octanol). Compounds with increased octanol solubility are more lipid soluble (**Table 12.2**). Increased lipid solubility enhances the ability to penetrate the lipid membrane and deliver local anesthetic in closer proximity to the membrane-bound VG_{Na}. Although lipid solubility correlates with octanol solubility (and inherent potency in vitro), the minimum in vivo local anesthetic concentration that will block impulse conduction may be affected by numerous factors such as fiber size, type, and myelination; tissue pH (see below); local tissue redistribution and sequestration into lipid-rich perineural compartments; and inherent vasoactive properties of the specific local anesthetic.

The time to onset of action of local anesthetics correlates with the dissociation constant (pK_a). At physiological pH, local anesthetics are weak bases that exist in equilibrium between either the lipid-soluble base form or the water-soluble ionized form. The relative percentage of each form is determined by the pK_a and surrounding tissue pH. The pK_a is the pH at which the percentage of each form is equal (**Table 12.2**), which is defined by the Henderson-Hasselbalch equation:

$$pK_a = pH + \log\left[BH^+\right]/[B]$$

where $[BH^+]$ is the concentration of the charged, lipid-insoluble form of the local anesthetic, and [B] is the concentration of the uncharged lipid-soluble form of local anesthetic.

The lower the pK_a for a given local anesthetic, the higher the percentage of the lipid-soluble base form that exists to more readily penetrate the lipid cell membrane, thus speeding the onset of action. After penetration through the cell membrane into the axoplasm, equilibrium between the base form and the charged form is reestablished. It is the charged form within the axoplasm that more avidly binds to local anesthetic binding sites within the channel pore of the VG_{Na}.

The duration of action of local anesthetics correlates with protein binding affinity. Freely circulating local anesthetic molecules bind predominantly to α_1-acid glycoprotein and albumin in plasma. Molecules with high binding affinity have a relatively longer duration of action, which is theorized to be due to a similar increased affinity for binding sites on the VG_{Na}. Duration of action is also influenced by rate of vascular absorption of local anesthetic from

Table 12.2 Chemical Structure and Physiochemical Properties of Clinically Useful Local Anesthetic Agents

Local Anesthetic	Chemical Structure	Partition Coefficient (Lipid Solubility)	pK_a	Percentage Ionized at pH 7.4	Percentage Protein Bound
Aminoamides					
Lidocaine	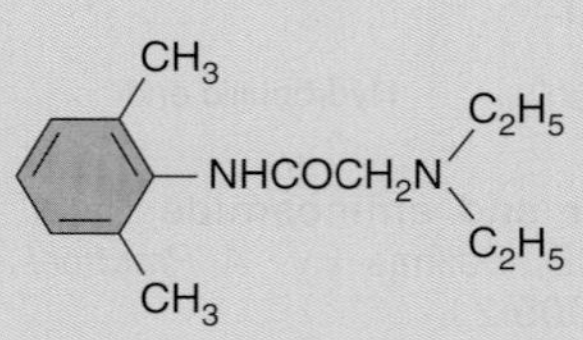 CH_3; C_2H_5; $NHCOCH_2N$; C_2H_5; CH_3	366	7.9	76	65
Prilocaine	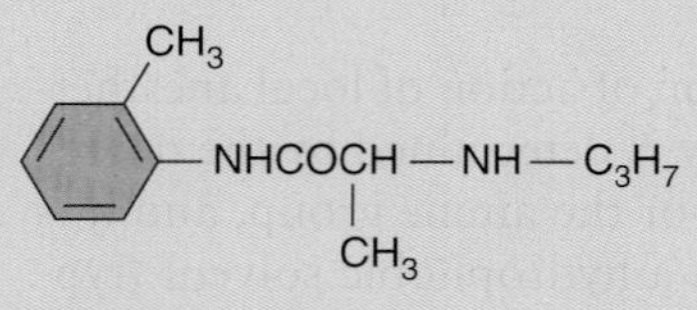 CH_3; $NHCOCH—NH—C_3H_7$; CH_3	129	7.9	76	55
Mepivacaine	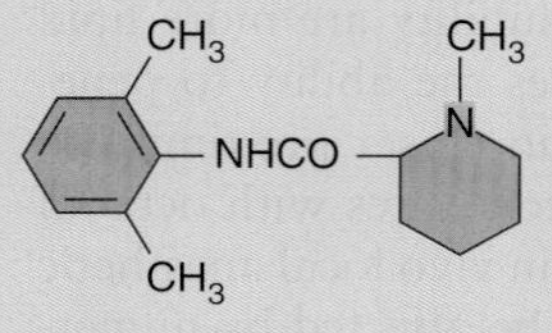 CH_3; CH_3; N; NHCO; CH_3	130	7.6	61	78
Bupivacaine	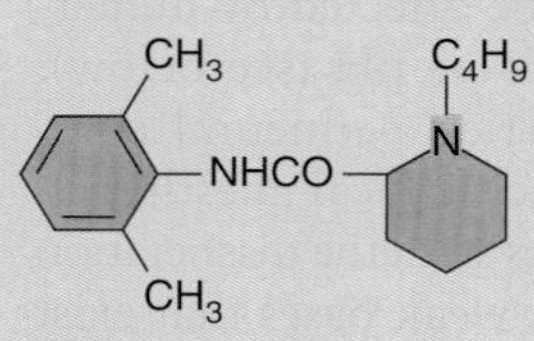 CH_3; C_4H_9; N; NHCO; CH_3	3420	8.1	83	96
Ropivacaine	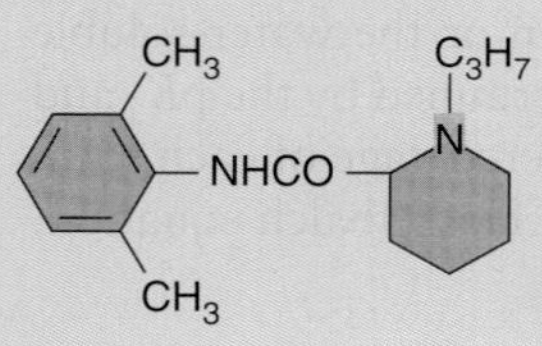 CH_3; C_3H_7; N; NHCO; CH_3	775	8.1	83	94
Aminoesters					
Procaine	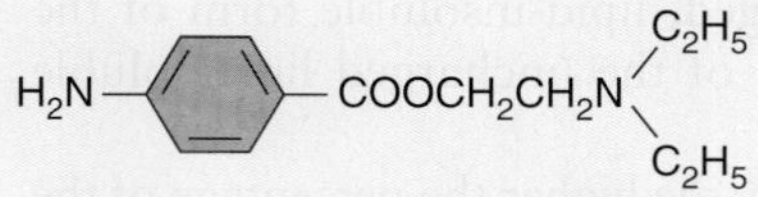 C_2H_5; H_2N—; —$COOCH_2CH_2N$; C_2H_5	100	8.9	97	6
2-Chloroprocaine	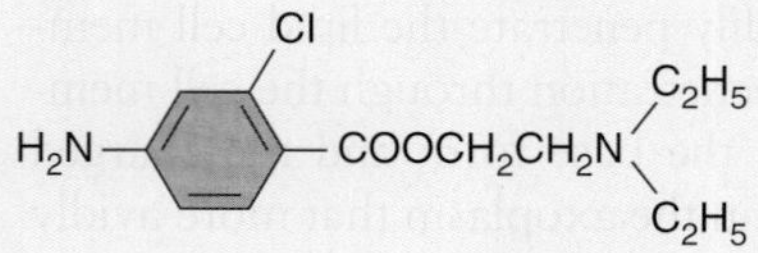 Cl; C_2H_5; H_2N—; —$COOCH_2CH_2N$; C_2H_5	810	8.7	95	N/A
Tetracaine	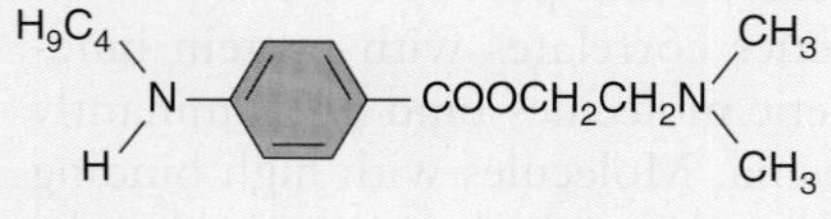 H_9C_4; N—; H; CH_3; —$COOCH_2CH_2N$; CH_3	5822	8.5	93	76

the injection site. Thus, administration of local anesthetics at a highly vascular site is associated with a higher rate of vascular absorption. Vasoconstrictors decrease the rate of vascular absorption and thus, prolong the duration of action (see the section that follows).

The majority of clinically useful local anesthetics are formulated as racemic compounds. These are one-to-one mixtures of enantiomeric stereoisomers bearing identical chemical composition, but with a different three-dimensional spatial orientation around an asymmetric carbon atom. Although enantiomers of local anesthetics have identical physiochemical properties, they exhibit different clinical pharmacodynamics (potency) due to subtle differences in interaction and binding of VG_{Na}. For example, levobupivacaine (the *S*-enantiomer of bupivacaine) and ropivacaine (the *S*-enantiomer of the bupivacaine, but with a propyl alkyl group rather than the butyl group found in bupivacaine) appear to have equipotent clinical efficacy for neuronal conduction block. However, they have a lower potential for cardiac systemic toxicity than either the *R*-enantiomer or the racemic mixtures.

B. Additives to Augment Local Anesthetic Activity

Local anesthetics are formulated as hydrochloride salts to increase their solubility and stability. The pH of commercially prepared local anesthetic solutions ranges from 3.9 to 6.47 and is especially acidic when prepackaged with epinephrine (see the section that follows). Given that the pK_a of the most commonly used local anesthetics ranges from 7.6 to 8.9 (**Table 12.2**), <3% of the local anesthetic solution is in the lipid-soluble neutral form at physiologic pH. This slows penetration through the cell membrane and delays the onset of conduction block. An even lower lipid-soluble fraction may be encountered clinically when local anesthetics are injected into infected tissues that have a more acidic pH. Thus, alkalinization of local anesthetic solutions by the addition of sodium bicarbonate may potentially increase the onset and the quality of conduction block by increasing the percentage of lipid-soluble base form. Clinical experience demonstrates that the addition of sodium bicarbonate may speed the onset of intermediate-acting local anesthetics (lidocaine and mepivacaine). In addition, decreasing the acidity of the local anesthetic solution reduces the burning sensation that occurs with subcutaneous injection. However, this modification has minimal effect with the longer acting, more potent amide local anesthetics (bupivacaine or ropivacaine).[2]

Epinephrine is commonly added to local anesthetic solutions to induce vasoconstriction at the site of injection. The α_1-adrenoreceptor–mediated vasoconstrictive effect of epinephrine augments local anesthetic activity by antagonizing the inherent vasodilating effect of most local anesthetics. Consequently, decreased vascular absorption maintains an increased concentration of anesthetics at the site of action. The reported clinical benefits include enhancement of the quality of conduction block and prolongation of the duration of action. It also decreases the peak systemic local anesthetics levels, potentially limiting toxic effects.[3] The extent to which epinephrine prolongs the duration of conduction block largely depends on the physiochemical properties of the local anesthetic as well as the site of injection. For example, the addition of epinephrine to lidocaine typically extends the conduction block by at least 50%, but the addition of epinephrine to bupivacaine has little or no clinically relevant effect on the duration of blockade. Additional analgesic effects due to epinephrine (and clonidine) may also occur through interaction with α_2-adrenoreceptors in the CNS, directly activating endogenous analgesic mechanisms.

Dexamethasone may be administered to prolong the duration of peripheral nerve blocks by 40% to 70%. The exact mechanism explaining this action is unclear. Motor and sensory block is prolonged after either perineural or intravenous administration, with perineural administration appearing to have slightly increased efficacy compared to systemic administration. Side effects are minimal, although publications of neurotoxicity in animal models exist. Future research should focus identifying the effects (if any) on axonal transmission and neural blood flow (in the presence and absence of local anesthetic).[4]

Clonidine is a direct-acting α_2-agonist, but it also possesses direct inhibitory effects on neural conduction (A and C peripheral nerve fibers).[5] In contrast to epinephrine, clonidine will improve the duration of conduction block, regardless of whether lidocaine or bupivacaine is used. However, potential clonidine-associated side effects of bradycardia and orthostatic hypotension have limited its more widespread clinical use.

Dexmedetomidine is another direct-acting α_2-agonist which, compared to clonidine, is seven times more specific for the α_2 receptor. Perineural administration of 0.5 to 1.0 μg/kg during peripheral nerve blocks can increase block duration by up to 50% and speed the onset of longer acting local anesthetics. Side effects include sedation, bradycardia, and hypotension requiring close postprocedural monitoring.[6]

III. Local Anesthetic Pharmacokinetics

Local anesthetics are most commonly delivered to extravascular tissue in close proximity to the intended target site. The resulting plasma concentration is influenced by the total dose of administered local anesthetic, the extent of systemic absorption, tissue redistribution, and the rate of elimination. Patient-specific factors such as age, cardiovascular and hepatic function, and plasma protein binding also influence subsequent plasma levels. An understanding of these factors should maximize the clinical application of local anesthetics, while minimizing potential complications associated with toxic systemic drug levels.

A. Systemic Absorption

In general, decreased systemic local anesthetic absorption provides a greater margin of safety in clinical practice. The rate and extent of systemic absorption are influenced by a number of factors, including total local anesthetic dose, site of administration, physiochemical properties of individual local anesthetics, and addition of vasoconstrictors (epinephrine). For any given site of administration, the greater the total dose of local anesthetic, the greater the extent of systemic absorption and peak plasma levels (C_{max}). Furthermore, an increased rate of absorption will also decrease the time to peak plasma levels (T_{max}). Within the clinical range of commonly used doses, the dose-response relationship is nearly linear and is relatively unaffected by anesthetic concentration or speed of injection. The extent of perineural tissue perfusion significantly influences systemic absorption, so that local anesthetic administration in highly perfused perineural tissues results in higher C_{max} and shorter T_{max}. Thus, the rate of systemic absorption from highest to lower is intrapleural > intercostal > caudal > epidural > brachial plexus > sciatic/femoral > and subcutaneous tissue. The rate of systemic absorption is also influenced by the physiochemical properties of the individual local anesthetic agents. In general, the more potent, lipid-soluble local anesthetics will result in decreased systemic absorption. The greater the lipid solubility, the more likely it will be

? *Did You Know?*

The rate and extent of systemic local anesthetic absorption and, hence, the risk of local anesthetic systemic toxicity, are determined by the total anesthetic dose, the site of administration, physiochemical properties of the specific drug (eg, lipid solubility), and the addition of vasoconstrictors.

sequestered in the lipid-rich compartments of both the axonal membrane and perineural tissues. The effects of epinephrine have been previously discussed and counteract the inherent vasodilator characteristics of most local anesthetics. The reduction in C_{max} associated with epinephrine is more pronounced for the less lipid-soluble local anesthetics, while increased neural and perineural tissue binding may be a greater determinant of systemic absorption with increased lipid solubility.

B. Distribution

After systemic absorption, local anesthetics are rapidly distributed throughout all body tissues and can be described by a two-compartment model (see Chapter 7). The pattern of distribution (and relative tissue concentration) is influenced by the perfusion, partition coefficient, and mass of specific tissue compartments. The highly perfused organs (brain, lung, heart, liver, and kidneys) are responsible for the initial rapid uptake (α-phase), which is followed by a slower redistribution (β-phase) to less perfused tissues (muscle and gut). In particular, the lung extracts significant amounts of local anesthetic. Consequently, C_{max} and the threshold for systemic toxic effects require much lower doses of local anesthetics following arterial injections compared with that for venous injections.

> **? *Did You Know?***
>
> Allergic reactions to local anesthetics are rare but typically associated with either the breakdown product of aminoester metabolism (para-aminobenzoic acid) or the related compound methylparaben used as a preservative in some formulations of aminoamide local anesthetics.

C. Elimination

The chemical linkage determines the biotransformation and elimination of local anesthetics (see **Figure 12.2**). Aminoamides are metabolized in the liver by cytochrome P-450 enzymes via *N*-dealkylation and hydroxylation. Aminoamide metabolism is highly dependent on hepatic perfusion, hepatic extraction, and enzyme function. Therefore, local anesthetic clearance is decreased by conditions such as cirrhosis and congestive heart failure. Excretion of the aminoamide metabolites occurs by renal excretion, with <5% of unmetabolized local anesthetic excreted by the kidney. Prilocaine is the only aminoamide local anesthetic that is hydrolyzed to o-toluidine, which can oxidize hemoglobin to methemoglobin in a dose-dependent fashion. Prilocaine doses as low as 8 mg/kg may be expected to produce sufficient methemoglobin levels to cause cyanosis (methemoglobinemia).

Aminoester local anesthetics are rapidly metabolized by plasma cholinesterase. Procaine and benzocaine are metabolized to ***para-aminobenzoic acid*** (PABA), which has been associated with rare anaphylactic reactions with the use of these local anesthetics. Patients with genetically abnormal plasma cholinesterase or those who are taking cholinesterase inhibitors have decreased aminoester metabolism. They would theoretically be at increased risk for systemic toxic effects, but clinical evidence is lacking.

D. Clinical Pharmacokinetics

The metabolism of local anesthetics is of significant clinical relevance as systemic toxicity (determined principally by C_{max}) depends on the balance between systemic absorption and elimination. Local anesthetics are largely bound to tissue and plasma proteins, yet systemic toxicity is related to the free (unbound) plasma concentration. Thus, plasma protein binding of local anesthetics reduces the free concentration in the systemic circulation and also reduces the risk of systemic toxicity. The extent of plasma protein binding is primarily dependent on the level of α_1-acid glycoprotein and albumin, and it is also influenced by the pH of the plasma. Clinical conditions that decrease plasma proteins (cirrhosis, pregnancy, newborn status) decrease binding capacity and increase the risk of systemic toxicity. Furthermore, the percentage of protein binding decreases as the pH decreases. Thus, in the presence of acidosis (seizures, cardiac arrest, renal failure), the amount of unbound drug increases. Altered hepatic clearance may also influence the elimination of local anesthetics. For example, neonates have immature hepatic microsomal enzymes, leading to decreased elimination of aminoamide local anesthetics. Some medications such as beta-blockers, H_2 receptors, and fluvoxamine inhibit specific hepatic microsomal enzymes and may also contribute to decreased aminoamide local anesthetic metabolism. All of the previously described factors that influence systemic absorption, distribution, and patient-specific factors should be taken into account to minimize the risk for systemic toxicity. These factors form the basis for current recommendations of "maximal doses" of local anesthetics.[7]

IV. Toxicity of Local Anesthetics

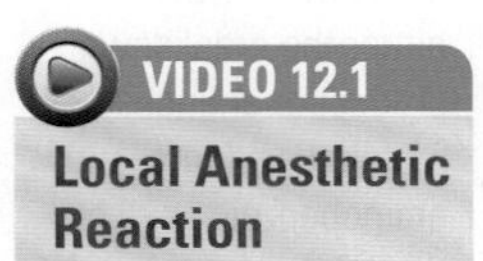

Clinically significant adverse effects of local anesthetics include ***local anesthetic systemic toxicity*** (LAST), local tissue toxicity, allergic reactions, and local anesthetic-specific effects. LAST results from excessive plasma concentrations of local anesthetic, either due to unintentional direct intravascular injection or from systemic absorption of larger doses of local anesthetics performed during peripheral nerve blocks, epidural anesthesia, or even large-volume infiltration (***tumescent***) anesthesia. As previously discussed, plasma concentration is determined by the balance between systemic absorption and elimination. Clinically significant symptoms of LAST manifest primarily in the CNS and cardiovascular system (CVS).

Risk factors for LAST include extremes of age, low muscle mass, female sex, pregnancy, or preexisting cardiac, neurologic, hepatic disease. The use of ultrasound guidance to direct local anesthetic administration during regional anesthesia has been shown to decrease the risk of LAST.

A. Central Nervous System Toxicity

Local anesthetics readily cross the blood-brain barrier and produce dose-dependent signs and symptoms of CNS toxicity. Initial symptoms may include drowsiness, circumoral numbness, facial tingling, restlessness, tinnitus, or auditory hallucinations. Objective signs of progressive CNS excitation may manifest as tremors or muscle twitching and can progress to generalized tonic-clonic convulsions.[8] If local anesthetic plasma levels are sufficiently elevated or the rate of rise is rapid, CNS excitation may progress to generalized CNS depression, leading to coma or respiratory or even cardiac arrest. The apparent biphasic pattern of CNS toxicity reflects neuronal depression by local anesthetics. At lower plasma concentrations, selective depression of cortical inhibitory neurons permits relatively unopposed actions of excitatory neurons, manifesting as CNS excitation. In contrast, markedly elevated plasma levels reflect the added inhibition of excitatory neurons and present clinically as profound CNS depression. The potential for CNS toxicity directly parallels the intrinsic potency of local anesthetics and can be augmented by various clinical factors. Untreated convulsions, for example, can rapidly cause both respiratory and metabolic acidosis, increasing the risk for CNS toxicity by decreasing plasma protein binding, increasing cerebral perfusion, and favoring intracellular trapping of the uncharged form of the local anesthetic.

B. Cardiovascular System Toxicity

Local anesthetic–induced cardiovascular system (CVS) toxicity can lead to hemodynamic instability due to a combination of direct myocardial depression, direct arteriolar vasodilation, the potential to cause significant dysrhythmias, and impaired autonomic regulation of the CVS system. Classically, LAST was taught as a progression from CNS to CVS symptoms when significantly larger doses of local anesthetic were administered. However, recent case series and registries show frequent presentations of CVS toxicity without the presence of CNS toxicity; therefore, LAST should always be considered in any case of cardiovascular collapse in patients who have received local anesthetics.

Similar to CNS toxicity, the more potent lipid-soluble local anesthetics appear to have greater inherent CVS toxicity compared with the less potent local anesthetics. For example, the ratio of the dose required for irreversible CVS collapse relative to that required for CNS toxicity is much lower for bupivacaine than for lidocaine. Additionally, the more potent lipid soluble agents (eg, bupivacaine) produce a different pattern of CVS toxicity compared with the less potent agents. At progressively increasing plasma concentrations, all local anesthetics can cause hypotension, myocardial depression, and dysrhythmias. However, toxic levels of bupivacaine can result in sudden cardiovascular collapse caused by malignant ventricular dysrhythmias that are often resistant to traditional resuscitation protocols.

> **? Did You Know?**
>
> Lipid-soluble local anesthetics (eg, bupivacaine) cause cardiovascular system toxicity by blocking cardiac voltage-gated sodium channels, resulting in cardiac conduction system abnormalities, including prolongation of the PR and QRS intervals, as well as more ominous ventricular dysrhythmias.

The more potent lipid-soluble local anesthetics display greater potential for direct electrophysiologic toxicity (prolongation of the PR and QRS intervals). Although all local anesthetics block the conduction system through a dose-dependent block of cardiac VG_{Na}, several features of bupivacaine's Na^+ channel blocking abilities may enhance its CVS toxicity. First, bupivacaine exhibits a much stronger binding affinity to resting and inactivated cardiac VG_{Na} compared with that for lidocaine. Second, although all local anesthetics bind to VG_{Na} during systole and subsequently dissociate during diastole, bupivacaine dissociates much slowly compared with lidocaine. Bupivacaine dissociates slowly enough that there is inadequate time during diastole for complete recovery of VG_{Na}, and conduction block accumulates with successive cardiac cycles.[9] In contrast, lidocaine completely dissociates with each cardiac cycle, and minimal accumulation of conduction block occurs. Lastly, bupivacaine displays a greater degree of direct myocardial depression compared with that for lidocaine or ropivacaine. Ropivacaine's safer CVS toxicity profile compared with that for bupivacaine stems from a combination of its slightly decreased potency due to its chemical structure (propyl alkyl substitution compared to butyl alkyl substitution on bupivacaine) as well as its formulation as the less cardiotoxic single *S*-enantiomer.

C. Treatment of Local Anesthetic Systemic Toxicity

LAST is best managed by preventing the occurrence of toxic plasma levels of local anesthetics by using the minimum effective dose required for a specific regional anesthetic technique, vigilance for inadvertent direct intravascular injection, and awareness of the early signs and symptoms of LAST. The basic treatment needed for CNS toxicity is initially supportive. Maintenance of adequate oxygenation and ventilation is mandatory, and if needed, the airway may be secured. Generalized tonic-clonic convulsions rapidly lead to metabolic acidosis, and their associated hypoventilation leads to hypoxemia and hypercapnea, all of which can potentiate LAST and exacerbate CNS toxicity. Convulsions that persist despite adequate oxygenation and ventilation should be promptly treated with titrated doses of the most readily available sedative hypnotic agent (such as midazolam [0.05-0.1 mg/kg] or propofol [0.5-1.5 mg/kg]).[10] Caution should be used when administering propofol due to its cardiac depressant effects, and it should be avoided if there is concern for CVS toxicity. If convulsions are not readily terminated with appropriate doses of sedative hypnotic agents, a neuromuscular blocker (typically succinylcholine) should be administered to terminate the intense muscular activity and attenuate worsening metabolic acidosis. It should be noted that neuromuscular blockade, however, does not decrease CNS excitation associated with CNS toxicity.

In the event of CVS toxicity, prompt attention should be turned to maintaining adequate oxygenation and, more important, coronary perfusion pressure. Local anesthetics themselves do not irreversibly damage cardiac myocytes. Experimental evidence demonstrates that with adequate coronary perfusion, bupivacaine promptly leaves cardiac tissue with a simultaneous return of normal cardiac function.

Intravenous lipid emulsion (ILE) can significantly attenuate bupivacaine-induced CVS toxicity as demonstrated by numerous case reports of successful rapid resuscitation with ILE administration in cases of severe CVS toxicity from both bupivacaine and ropivacaine.[11] Recent guidelines recommend administration of ILE early in the presentation or suspicion of a severe LAST event. The mechanism of action of intralipid is not completely elucidated but is thought to be mediated by (1) shuttling of local anesthetics from the heart and brain to muscle for temporary storage and the liver for detoxification, (2) cardiotonic effects including increased inotropy and peripheral vascular resistance, and (3) cardiac ischemic postconditioning. Dosing guidelines for ILE are shown in **Table 12.3**.

In the event of cardiac arrest due to LAST, standard advanced cardiac life support measures should be instituted with the following modifications: vasopressin is not recommended, smaller initial epinephrine dosing (≤1 μg/kg) is preferred, and if ventricular dysrhythmias develop, amiodarone is preferred instead of lidocaine. Cardiac bypass may be required in refractory cases to support perfusion until systemic levels of local anesthetic are reduced. Current recommendations call for monitoring patients for at least 2 hours after a limited CNS event or at least 4 to 6 hours after a significant CVS event.[12]

Table 12.3 Treatment of LAST With Lipid Emulsion

Lipid Emulsion 20%	
Greater than 70 kg patient • Bolus 100 mL rapidly over 2-3 min • Start infusion of 200-250 mL over 15-20 min	Less than 70 kg patient • Bolus 1.5 mL/kg rapidly over 2-3 min • Start infusion of approximately 0.25 mL/kg/min (ideal body weight)
If patient remains unstable • Re-bolus once or twice at the same dose and double infusion rate; be aware of dosing limit (12 mL/kg) • Total volume of lipid emulsion can approach 1 L in a prolonged resuscitation	

From Neal JM. The Third American Society of Regional Anesthesia and Pain Medicine Practice Advisory on local anesthetic systemic toxicity: executive summary 2017. *Reg Anesth Pain Med.* 2018;43:113-123.

D. Neural Toxicity and Myotoxicity

Direct neural toxicity has been described with clinical application of multiple local anesthetic agents.[13] Case reports of cauda equina syndrome associated with the administration of high concentrations of lidocaine through spinal microcatheters began to appear in the late 1980s. Subsequent in vitro and in vivo investigations suggested that a combination of maldistribution (pooling) and high doses of local anesthetics led to neurotoxic concentrations localized to the lumbosacral subarachnoid space. Similarly, 2-chloroprocaine was associated with cauda equina syndrome in the 1980s, with the mechanism linked to the preservative used at that time (sodium metabisulfite) when large doses were accidentally administered into the subarachnoid space during attempted epidural administration. Subsequently, 2-chloroprocaine was reformulated as a preservative-free solution.

Transient neurologic symptoms (TNS) are associated with the subarachnoid administration of local anesthetics (most notably lidocaine) and characterized by transient pain or sensory abnormalities in the lower back radiating to the lower extremities and buttocks.[13] Additional risk factors for TNS include surgical lithotomy position and ambulatory surgical procedures. Overall, there appears to be a paucity of electrophysiologic evidence to support a direct neurotoxic mechanism for TNS. Furthermore, effective treatment modalities, such as nonsteroidal anti-inflammatory drugs or trigger point injections, indicate a myofascial rather than a neuropathic mechanism for TNS.

Local anesthetics have also been shown to cause direct toxic effects to muscle tissue, leading to destruction of myocytes.[14] Despite the predictable nature of muscle damage, local anesthetic myotoxicity is only rarely a clinical problem, as complete muscle regeneration typically occurs within 3 to 4 weeks. Risk factors include potency of the individual local anesthetic agent, direct intramuscular injection, and dose, which is exacerbated with serial or continuous administration. A notable exception to the generally low clinical consequence of local anesthetic myotoxicity is extraocular muscle damage, where there is a reported 0.25% incidence of prolonged extraocular muscle dysfunction (diplopia) after regional anesthesia for ocular surgery.

E. Allergic Reactions

True immune-mediated allergic reactions to local anesthetics are rare. A careful history should be elucidated from patients with local anesthetic allergies as many reactions are secondary effects of epinephrine coadministered during dental or other procedures. When true allergies do occur, the vast majority are associated with aminoester local anesthetics, most likely due to their metabolism to the pure allergen PABA. Some preparations of aminoamide local anesthetics also contain methylparaben, which has a similar chemical structure to PABA and is the most likely cause of allergic reactions to aminoamide local anesthetics.

V. Local Anesthetic Agents and Their Common Clinical Applications

A. Aminoamide Local Anesthetics

1. Lidocaine

Lidocaine was the first widely used local anesthetic and remains the most commonly used local anesthetic. It may be used for infiltration, intravenous regional anesthesia (Bier block), peripheral nerve block, and central neuraxial (subarachnoid and epidural) anesthesia. It is characterized by a rapid to intermediate onset of action and intermediate duration of action for peripheral nerve blocks and epidural anesthesia. Although concerns over TNS have led to decreased use for subarachnoid anesthesia, it remains popular for epidural anesthesia. Lidocaine may be applied topically as a jelly, an ointment, a patch, or in aerosol form to anesthetize the upper airway. Intravenous injections targeting relatively low plasma levels (<5 μg/mL) produce systemic analgesia and have been used as an adjunct to blunt the sympathetic response to laryngoscopy and intubation. One of its most common uses involves intravenous injection to decrease the discomfort associated with intravenous administration of propofol. Lidocaine infusions have been administered to treat chronic neuropathic pain as well as acute postoperative pain. More recently, lidocaine (5% patch) was U.S. Food and Drug Administration (FDA)-approved for the treatment of chronic pain associated with neuropathic postherpetic neuralgia. The patch is a topical delivery system designed to deliver low doses of lidocaine to superficially involved nociceptors in an amount that produces analgesia devoid of sensorimotor block.

2. Mepivacaine

Mepivacaine has a chemical structure combining the piperidine ring of cocaine with the xylidine ring of lidocaine. It shares a similar clinical profile to lidocaine but with a slightly longer duration of action because it results in less vasodilation and has a higher protein binding affinity. It is relatively ineffective when applied topically. As a spinal anesthetic agent, it appears to have a lower, although not clinically insignificant, incidence of TNS compared with that of lidocaine. Metabolism in the fetus and neonate is prolonged and, therefore, it is not used for obstetric analgesia.

3. Prilocaine

Prilocaine also has a similar clinical profile to lidocaine and is used for infiltration, peripheral nerve blocks, and spinal and epidural anesthesia. Due to its high clearance, it demonstrates the least systemic toxicity of all the amide local anesthetics and is therefore potentially useful for intravenous regional anesthesia. However, administration of higher doses (>500-600 mg) may result in methemoglobinemia. Clinically significant methemoglobinemia may be effectively treated with intravenous administration of methylene blue (1-2 mg/kg). Nonetheless, concerns over methemoglobinemia and lack of FDA approval have limited more widespread clinical use.

4. Bupivacaine

Bupivacaine is a more lipid-soluble, structural homologue of mepivacaine due to a butyl group, rather than a methyl group, on its piperidine ring. Thus, it is characterized by a relatively slower onset compared with that of lidocaine, but it has an extended duration of action. It provides prolonged sensory anesthesia and analgesia that typically outlasts the duration and intensity of its motor block, especially with the use of lower concentrations in continuous infusions. This characteristic has established bupivacaine as the most widely used local anesthetic for labor epidural analgesia and for acute postoperative pain management. Single injections for peripheral nerve block applications may provide surgical anesthesia for up to 12 hours and sensory analgesia lasting as long as 24 hours. It is widely used for subarachnoid anesthesia, typically with duration of action of 2 to 3 hours and, in contrast to lidocaine or mepivacaine, it has rarely been associated with TNS.

5. Ropivacaine

Ropivacaine is another structural homologue of mepivacaine and bupivacaine, but with a propyl group on its piperidine ring, and it is also formulated as an *S*-enantiomer. Together, these two characteristics result in clinically equivalent potency for neural blockade, but with a less cardiotoxic profile compared with that for bupivacaine. It has an inherent vasoconstricting effect, which may contribute to its reduced cardiotoxic profile and possibly augment its duration of action (notably, the addition of epinephrine does not further prolong block duration). Although there is some evidence to suggest that ropivacaine may produce a more favorable sensorimotor differential block compared with bupivacaine, the lack of equivalent potency hinders true comparisons. Overall, the clinical profile is similar to that of bupivacaine, taking into account its decreased potency compared with that of bupivacaine.

B. Aminoester Local Anesthetics

1. Procaine

Procaine was used primarily for infiltration and spinal anesthesia during the first half of the 20th century. Its low potency, relatively slow onset of action (likely due to its high pK_a), and short duration of action limit the widespread use of procaine. Concerns regarding TNS with lidocaine prompted a renewed interest in the use of procaine for intermediate duration subarachnoid anesthesia. Despite its lower incidence of TNS compared with that of lidocaine, the increased risk of block failure and associated nausea have limited its clinical utility.

2. 2-Chloroprocaine

Due to its relative low potency and extremely rapid metabolism by plasma cholinesterases, 2-chloroprocaine may be used in relatively higher concentrations (2%-3%), yet with the lowest potential for systemic toxicity of all the clinically useful local anesthetic agents. Despite its relatively high pK_a, chloroprocaine is administered at relatively higher concentrations, resulting in rapid onset of anesthesia. This characteristic, along with virtually no transmission to the fetus, makes it particularly useful when a rapid onset of surgical epidural anesthesia (ie, urgent or emergent cesarean delivery) is required. The preservative-free solution of 2-chloroprocaine has gained increased popularity for ambulatory subarachnoid anesthesia, where a rapid onset of action along with a predictably short duration of action is desired. Furthermore, the use of 2-chloroprocaine has been associated with very low incidence of TNS. Isobaric 1% 2-chloroprocaine received FDA approval for spinal anesthesia in 2019.

3. Tetracaine

Tetracaine is a potent aminoester local anesthetic, characterized by a slow onset and long duration of action. In contrast to bupivacaine, the duration of action of tetracaine is significantly prolonged with the addition of a vasoconstrictor. Due to its slow onset of action and lack of sensorimotor dissociation (resulting in significant motor blockade), it is rarely indicated for epidural anesthesia or peripheral nerve block, and its primary clinical application is for extended duration subarachnoid anesthesia.

4. Cocaine

Cocaine is the only naturally occurring local anesthetic agent. Current clinical applications for cocaine are largely restricted to topical anesthesia for ear, nose, and throat procedures, where its intense vasoconstriction is clinically useful to reduce bleeding when instrumenting the nasopharynx. Cocaine inhibits the neuronal reuptake of norepinephrine, mediating its neurogenic vasoconstrictive effects. But it can also result in significant cardiovascular side effects, such as hypertension, tachycardia, and dysrhythmias. Concerns regarding its potential for cardiovascular toxicity, along with its potential for diversion and abuse, have markedly limited its clinical use.

5. Eutectic Mixture of Local Anesthetics

A eutectic mixture of lidocaine and prilocaine, each at a 2.5% concentration, is formulated as viscous liquid (eutectic mixture of local anesthetics [EMLA] cream). This mixture has a lower melting point than either individual local anesthetic, allowing it to exist as oil at room temperature, facilitating its penetration and absorption through dermis. EMLA cream is primarily used to provide dermal analgesia, and it is particularly useful in decreasing the pain associated with venipuncture or placement of a peripheral intravascular catheter. EMLA cream should only be applied to intact skin surfaces as application to breached skin may lead to unpredictably rapid systemic absorption.

6. Controlled Release Local Anesthetics

Multiple formulations for controlled release of local anesthetics have been developed in an attempt to extend the duration of neuronal blockade, and specifically postoperative analgesia. Liposomal bupivacaine, the only delivery system to have received FDA approval, controls the release of bupivacaine by encapsulating molecules in liposomes. These liposomes are multivesicular, spherical structures composed of lipidlike particles arranged in bilayers. As liposomes degrade, bupivacaine is slowly released, with plasma levels persisting for up to 96 hours. Pain control may last for up to 24 hours. Due to concerns for uncontrolled lysis of liposomes causing rapid release of bupivacaine, other local anesthetics should not be administered with liposomal bupivacaine and be avoided for 96 hours after use. Other delivery systems, including bupivacaine encapsulated in a biodegradable sucrose acetate isobutyrate biolayer, a bioerodible polymer consisting of bupivacaine and low-dose meloxicam (HTX-011), and a bupivacaine-collagen bioresorbable implant, are in development and undergoing phase III clinical trials.

For further review and interactivities, please see the associated Interactive Video Lectures and "At a Glance" infographic accessible in the complimentary eBook bundled with this text. Access instructions are located in the inside front cover.

References

1. Scholz A. Mechanisms of (local) anaesthetics on voltage-gated sodium and other ion channels. *Br J Anaesth*. 2002;89:52-61. PMID: 12173241.
2. Lambert DH. Clinical value of adding sodium bicarbonate to local anesthetics. *Reg Anesth Pain Med*. 2002;27:328-329. PMID: 12016613.
3. Neal JM. Effects of epinephrine in local anesthetics on the central and peripheral nervous system. *Reg Anesth Pain Med*. 2003;28:124-134. PMID: 12677623.
4. Pehora C, Pearson AME, Kaushal A, Crawford MW, Johnston B. Dexamethasone as an adjuvant to peripheral nerve block. *Cochrane Database Syst Rev*. 2017;11:CD011770. PMID: 29121400.
5. Brummett CM, Williams BA. Additives to local anesthetics for peripheral nerve block. *Int Anesthesiol Clin*. 2011;49:104-116. PMID: 21956081.

6. Vorobeichik L, Brull R, Abdallah FW. Evidence basis for using perineural dexmedetomidine to enhance the quality of brachial plexus nerve blocks: a systematic review and meta-analysis of randomized controlled trials. *Br J Anaesth*. 2017;118:167-181. PMID: 28100520.
7. Rosenberg PH, Veering BT, Urmey WF. Maximum recommended doses of local anesthetics: a multifactorial concept. *Reg Anesth Pain Med*. 2004;29:564-575. PMID: 15635516.
8. Di Gregorio G, Neal JM, Rosenquist RW, et al. Clinical presentation of local anesthetic systemic toxicity: a review of published cases, 1979 to 2009. *Reg Anesth Pain Med*. 2010;35:181-187. PMID: 20301824.
9. Clarkson CW, Hondeghem LM. Mechanisms for bupivacaine depression of cardiac conduction: fast block of sodium channels during the action potential with slow recovery from block during diastole. *Anesthesiology*. 1985;62:396-405. PMID: 2580463.
10. Weinberg GL. Treatment of local anesthetic systemic toxicity. *Reg Anesth Pain Med*. 2010;35:188-193. PMID: 20216036.
11. Weinberg GL. Lipid emulsion infusion: resuscitation for local anesthetic and other drugs. *Anesthesiology*. 2012;117:180-187. PMID: 22627464.
12. Neal JM. The Third American Society of Regional Anesthesia and Pain Medicine Practice Advisory on local anesthetic systemic toxicity: executive summary 2017. *Reg Anesth Pain Med*. 2018;43:113-123.PMID: 29356773.
13. Pollock JE. Neurotoxicity of intrathecal local anaesthetics and transient neurological symptoms. *Best Pract Res Clin Anaesthesiol*. 2003;17:471-484. PMID: 14529015.
14. Hussain N, McCartney CJL, Neal JM, et al. Local anaesthetic-induced myotoxicity in regional anaesthesia: a systematic review and empirical analysis. *Br J Anaesth*. 2018;121:822-841. PMID: 30236244.

LOCAL ANESTHETIC TOXICITY

AT A GLANCE

Excessive plasma levels of local anesthetic drugs may result in both central nervous system and cardiovascular toxicity. This may result from administration of local anesthetics in excess of the recommended maximum dose or inadvertent intravascular injection.

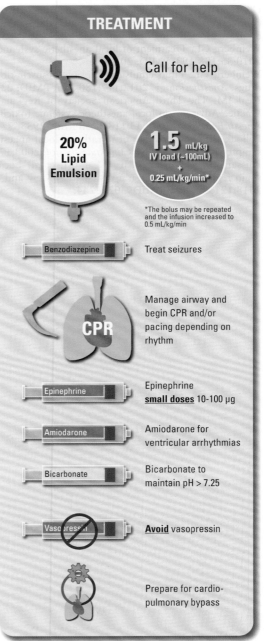

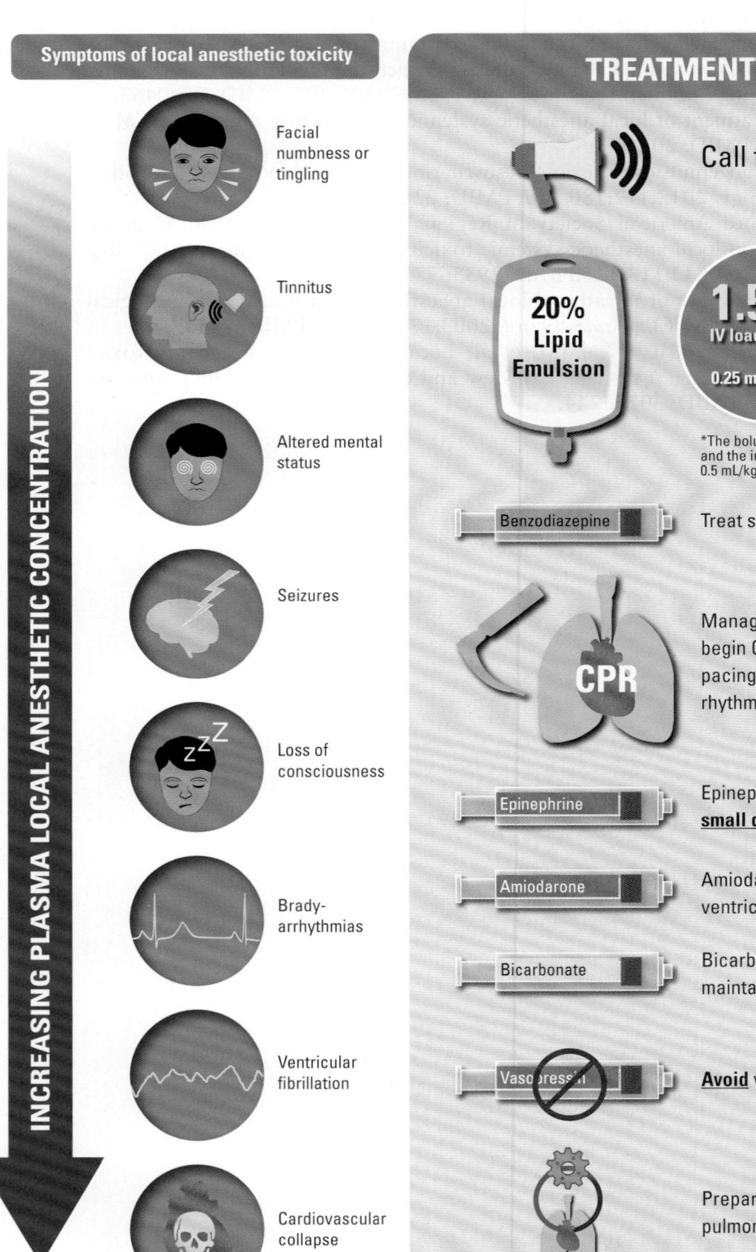

Symptoms of local anesthetic toxicity
Facial numbness or tingling
Tinnitus
Altered mental status
Seizures
Loss of consciousness
Brady-arrhythmias
Ventricular fibrillation
Cardiovascular collapse
INCREASING PLASMA LOCAL ANESTHETIC CONCENTRATION
TREATMENT
Call for help
20% Lipid Emulsion
1.5 mL/kg IV load (~100mL) + 0.25 mL/kg/min*
*The bolus may be repeated and the infusion increased to 0.5 mL/kg/min
Benzodiazepine
Treat seizures
CPR
Manage airway and begin CPR and/or pacing depending on rhythm
Epinephrine
Epinephrine small doses 10-100 μg
Amiodarone
Amiodarone for ventricular arrhythmias
Bicarbonate
Bicarbonate to maintain pH > 7.25
Avoid vasopressin
Prepare for cardio-pulmonary bypass

Infographic by: Naveen Nathan MD

Questions

1. **A patient with which preexisting condition is MOST likely to tolerate standard maximum doses of local anesthetics?**

   A. COPD
   B. Elderly
   C. Pregnancy
   D. Liver failure

2. **Addition of epinephrine to which local anesthetic would have the LEAST impact on duration of nerve block?**

   A. Lidocaine
   B. Mepivacaine
   C. Ropivacaine
   D. Bupivacaine

3. **A 66-year-old 80 kg man with ischemic cardiomyopathy presents after a mechanical fall for operative fixation of a distal radius fracture under regional anesthesia. After placement of an infraclavicular catheter, the patient becomes hypotensive and a pulse is no longer palpable. Which medication would be the MOST appropriate?**

   A. 1 mg epinephrine
   B. 50 mg propofol
   C. 100 mL lipid emulsion 20%
   D. 40 units vasopressin

4. **An otherwise healthy 26-year-old woman presents for knee arthroscopy. The procedure is expected to last 30 minutes. Which would be the MOST appropriate spinal anesthetic to facilitate rapid discharge?**

   A. 40 mg 2-chloroprocaine
   B. 7.5 mg bupivacaine
   C. 40 mg mepivacaine
   D. 40 mg lidocaine

5. **A 43-year-old woman undergoes hysteroscopy and myomectomy under spinal anesthesia in the lithotomy position. The following day she calls to report bilateral pain in the back of her legs and buttocks with no motor weakness or change in bowel or bladder function. Which statement is MOST likely to be true?**

   A. MRI will likely show a gadolinium enhancing lesion.
   B. These symptoms may indicate the need for emergent surgery.
   C. If symptoms do not improve, a blood patch may bring relief.
   D. Pain should self-resolve in about 72 hours.

Answers

1. A

All of the other preexisting conditions are known to increase the risk of local anesthetic systemic toxicity

2. C

Lidocaine and mepivacaine are both significantly prolonged by addition of epinephrine. Bupivacaine is also prolonged, however not at the same magnitude of lidocaine or mepivacaine. Ropivacaine is not prolonged likely due to its inherent vasoconstrictive properties and its long duration of action.

3. C

During a LAST event, vasopressin should be avoided and epinephrine should be dosed at ≤1 μg/kg. Propofol would be contraindicated with cardiac toxicity due to its cardiac depressant effects and should be used cautiously in patients with only neurologic symptoms.

4. A

Chloroprocaine is rapid acting and demonstrates for rapid recovery after ambulatory surgery. Mepivacaine and lidocaine have longer durations of action. Although 7.5 mg of bupivacaine is a low dose, there is a significant amount of variability to low-dose bupivacaine blocks, and ambulation is still likely to be delayed.

5. D

These symptoms most likely represent transient neurologic symptoms (TNS), which can be present after spinal anesthesia, especially in the lithotomy position. As the name implies, these symptoms are transient and usually resolve within 72 hours. Gadolinium enhancing lesions are seen in disorders such as transverse myelitis, which would be uncommon. Surgery may be indicated for cauda equina or epidural abscess/hematoma, but these are rare and would likely also present with motor, bowel, or bladder dysfunction. A blood patch would improve headache for patients with postdural puncture headache (PDPH); however, PDPH presents as headache that improves with lying flat.

13 Cardiovascular Pharmacology

Paul S. Pagel, Justin N. Tawil, Brent T. Boettcher, and Julie K. Freed

This chapter reviews the cardiovascular pharmacology of medications used to alter hemodynamics during surgery and in the intensive care unit, including endogenous and synthetic catecholamines, sympathomimetics, milrinone, vasopressin, and antihypertensive medications.

I. Catecholamines

Did You Know?

Catecholamines activate β_1-adrenoceptors, which in turn accelerate the formation of the second messenger, cyclic adenosine monophosphate.

The α, β, and dopamine adrenergic receptor subtypes are responsible for mediating the cardiovascular effects of endogenous (epinephrine, norepinephrine, dopamine) and synthetic (dobutamine, isoproterenol) catecholamines. These drugs activate β_1-adrenoceptors located on the sarcolemmal membrane of atrial and ventricular myocytes to varying degrees. This β_1-adrenoceptor stimulation causes positive chronotropic (heart rate), dromotropic (conduction velocity), inotropic (contractility), and lusitropic (relaxation) effects. The β_1-adrenoceptor is coupled to a stimulatory guanine nucleotide–binding (G_s) protein that activates the key intracellular enzyme adenylyl cyclase, thereby accelerating formation of the second messenger cyclic adenosine monophosphate (cAMP) from adenosine triphosphate (ATP; **Figure 13.1**). Three major consequences result from activation of this signaling cascade: (1) more calcium (Ca^{2+}) is available for contractile activation; (2) the efficacy of activator Ca^{2+} at troponin C (TnC) of the contractile apparatus is enhanced; and (3) removal of Ca^{2+} from the contractile apparatus and the sarcoplasm after contraction is accelerated. The first two of these actions produce a direct increase in contractility, whereas the third results in more rapid myocardial relaxation during early diastole. Treatment of acute or chronic left ventricular (LV) systolic dysfunction is the primary reason for the perioperative use of catecholamines. It is noteworthy that the efficacy of catecholamines under these clinical conditions is affected by the relative density and functional integrity of the β_1-adrenoceptor and its signaling cascade because receptor downregulation and abnormal intracellular Ca^{2+} homeostasis are characteristic features of heart failure.

The vasoactive effects of catecholamines in other perfusion territories are dependent on the tissue-specific distribution of α- and β-adrenoceptor subtypes. Differences in each catecholamine's chemical structure and its relative selectivity for adrenoceptors also influence the peripheral vascular actions of these medications. This selectivity is often dose related; dopamine provides a useful

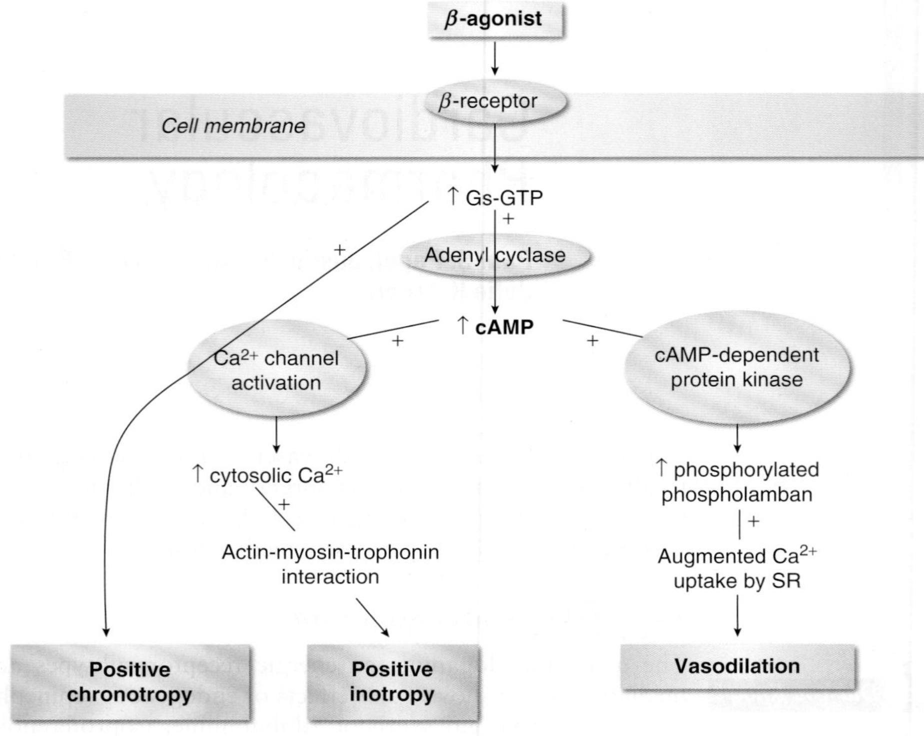

Figure 13.1 Schematic illustration of β-adrenoceptor agonist mechanism of action. cAMP, cyclic adenosine monophosphate; SR, sarcoplasmic reticulum. (From Gillies M, Bellomo R, Doolan L, et al. Bench-to-bedside review: inotropic drug therapy after adult cardiac surgery—A systematic literature review. *Crit Care*. 2005;9:266-279, with permission.)

pedagogical illustration of this principle. Low doses of this catecholamine predominantly stimulate dopamine subtype 1 and 2 (DA_1 and DA_2, respectively) receptors, causing arterial vasodilation, but progressively larger doses sequentially activate β_1- and α_1-adrenoceptors, augmenting contractility and causing arterial vasoconstriction, respectively. The α_1-adrenoceptors are major regulators of vasomotor tone as a result of their location in arteries, arterioles, and veins. Thus, catecholamines that exert substantial α_1-adrenoceptor agonist activity (eg, norepinephrine) increase systemic vascular resistance and reduce venous capacitance through arterial and venous vasoconstriction, respectively. This α_1-adrenoceptor–mediated vasoconstriction occurs through phospholipase C-inositol 1,4,5-triphosphate signaling through an inhibitory guanine nucleotide-binding (G_i) protein (**Figure 13.2**). This cascade opens Ca^{2+} channels, releases Ca^{2+} from intracellular stores (sarcoplasmic reticulum and calmodulin), and activates several Ca^{2+}-dependent protein kinases. Collectively, these actions increase intracellular Ca^{2+} concentration and cause contraction of vascular smooth muscle cell. α_1-adrenoceptors are the major target for catecholamines in cutaneous blood vessels, whereas β_2-adrenoceptors predominate in skeletal muscle. Stimulation of the β_2-adrenoceptor subtype produces arteriolar vasodilation via adenylyl cyclase–mediated signaling, thereby increasing blood flow to skeletal muscle.

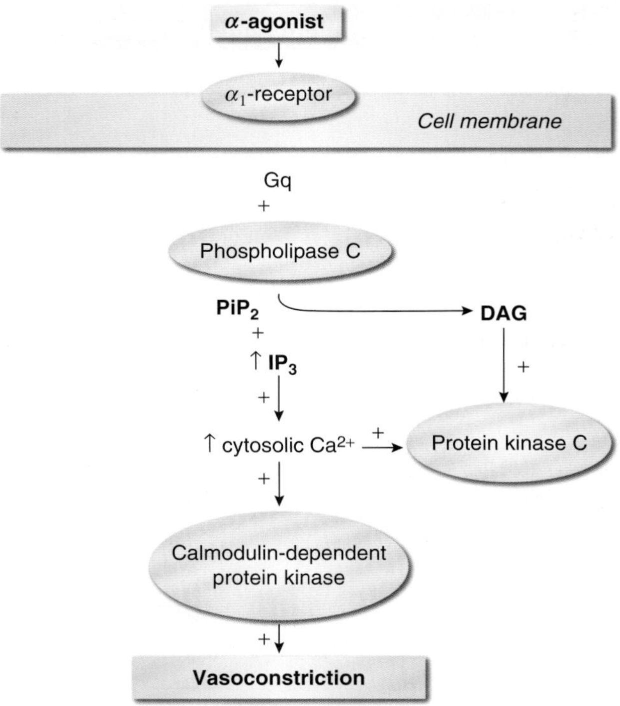

Figure 13.2 Schematic illustration of β-adrenoceptor agonist mechanism of action. DAG, diacylglycerol; IP_3, inositol 1,4,5-triphosphate; PIP_2, inositol 4,5-bisphosphate. (From Gillies M, Bellomo R, Doolan L, et al. Bench-to-bedside review: inotropic drug therapy after adult cardiac surgery—A systematic literature review. *Crit Care*. 2005;9:266-279, with permission.)

The actions of each specific catecholamine on heart rate, myocardial contractility, and LV preload and afterload combine to determine its overall effect on arterial pressure (**Table 13.1**). For example, if a catecholamine acts primarily through the α_1-adrenoceptor (eg, norepinephrine), an increase in arterial pressure will most likely be observed because enhanced arterial and venous vasomotor tone increases systemic vascular resistance (greater afterload) and augments venous return to the heart (increased preload), respectively. In contrast, a catecholamine with β_1- and β_2-adrenoceptor activity and little or no effect on the α_1-adrenoceptor (eg, isoproterenol) would be expected to modestly decrease arterial pressure because reductions in systemic vascular resistance offset increases in cardiac output caused by tachycardia and enhanced myocardial contractility. All catecholamines have the potential to cause detrimental increases in myocardial oxygen consumption in patients with flow-limiting coronary artery stenoses and may contribute to the development of acute myocardial ischemia. As a result, the use of catecholamines to support LV function in patients with coronary artery disease complicated by congestive heart failure should be approached with caution. Thus, it should come as no surprise that a drug that reduces LV afterload, and not one that causes a positive inotropic effect, is usually chosen first to improve cardiac output in a patient with coronary artery disease and LV systolic dysfunction.

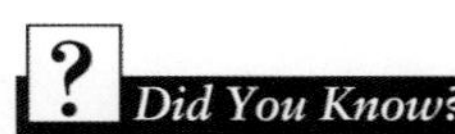

The α_1-adrenoreceptors are major regulators of vasomotor tone, including systemic vascular resistance and venous capacitance.

Table 13.1 Comparative Effects of Endogenous and Synthetic Catecholamines

Name	Chemical Structure	β_1	β_2
Epinephrine	HO; HO–(benzene ring)–CH(HO)–CH_2–NH–CH_3	++++	+++
Norepinephrine	HO; HO–(benzene ring)–CH(HO)–CH_2–NH_2	+++	+
Dopamine	HO; HO–(benzene ring)–CH_2–CH_2–NH_2	++++	++
Dobutamine	HO; HO–(benzene ring)–CH_2–CH_2–NH–CH(CH_3)–CH_2–CH_2–(benzene ring)–HO	+++++	+++
Isoproterenol	HO; HO–(benzene ring)–CH(HO)–CH_2–NH–CH(CH_3)(CH_3)	+++++	+++++
Phenylephrine	HO; OH; H; N	0	0

From Pagel PS, Grecu L. Cardiovascular Pharmacology. In: Barash PG, Cahalan MK, Cullen BF, et al, eds. *Clinical Anesthesia.* 8th ed. Wolters Kluwer; 2018:301-332, Table 13.5.

A. Epinephrine

Epinephrine is an endogenous catecholamine that exerts its cardiovascular effects by activating α_1-, β_1-, and β_2-adrenoceptors. Epinephrine stimulates β_1-adrenoceptors located on the cell membranes of sinoatrial node cells and cardiac myocytes to produce positive chronotropic and inotropic effects, respectively. Epinephrine-induced activation of β_1-adrenoceptors also enhances the rate and extent of myocardial relaxation, thereby facilitating greater LV filling during early diastole. The combination of these actions on heart rate and LV systolic and diastolic function causes dramatic increases in cardiac output. The increase in heart rate initially observed during an infusion of epinephrine may subsequently be attenuated to some extent as baroreceptor-mediated reflexes are activated. As a result, epinephrine is especially useful for the treatment of acute LV failure during cardiac surgery because it predictably increases cardiac output. Epinephrine also enhances cardiac output and oxygen delivery without causing deleterious increases in heart rate in septic, hypotensive patients. However, epinephrine's efficacy as a positive inotropic medication may be limited because the catecholamine stimulates the development of atrial or ventricular arrhythmias. Epinephrine increases conduction velocity and reduces refractory period in the atrioventricular (AV) node, His bundle, Purkinje fibers, and ventricular muscle. The positive dromotropic effect of epinephrine on AV nodal conduction may produce supraventricular tachyarrhythmias or cause marked increases in ventricular rate in the presence of atrial flutter or fibrillation. These adverse consequences may inadvertently result in hypotension because profound tachycardia reduces LV filling time and compromises coronary perfusion. Irritability in other parts of the conduction system may also precipitate ventricular arrhythmias including premature ventricular contractions, ventricular tachycardia, and ventricular fibrillation, especially in the presence of a preexisting arrhythmogenic substrate (eg, myocardial ischemia, cardiomyopathy).

Epinephrine causes vasoconstriction in the cutaneous, splanchnic, and renal perfusion territories through its effects at the α_1-adrenoceptor, but the catecholamine also simultaneously produces vasodilation in the skeletal muscle circulation as a result of β_2-adrenoceptor activation. Thus, epinephrine's overall effect on blood flow is dependent on the organ-specific distribution of α_1- and β_2-adrenoceptors. These actions are also dose dependent: lower doses of epinephrine stimulate β_2-adrenoceptors to cause peripheral vasodilation and modestly reduce arterial pressure, whereas higher doses activate α_1-adrenoceptors to increase systemic vascular resistance and arterial pressure. A high density of α_1-adrenoceptors is also present in the venous circulation, and as a result, epinephrine produces venoconstriction and augments venous return. Epinephrine also causes vasoconstriction of the pulmonary arterial tree and increases pulmonary arterial pressures through α_1-adrenoceptor activation. The α_1- and β_2-adrenoceptors are present in the coronary circulation, but selective activation of either of these receptor subtypes does not play a major role in determining coronary blood flow during administration of epinephrine. Instead, epinephrine-induced increases in coronary perfusion occur almost exclusively because of metabolic autoregulation: increases in myocardial oxygen demand resulting from increases in heart rate, contractility, preload, and afterload are responsible for coronary vasodilation. Nevertheless, epinephrine may cause epicardial coronary vasoconstriction and reduce coronary blood flow in situations where maximal coronary vasodilation is present (eg, acute myocardial ischemia distal to a severe coronary stenosis) via direct stimulation of α_1-adrenoceptors. The vasoconstrictor properties of epinephrine make it useful for a number of other clinical applications. Subcutaneous infiltration of epinephrine is used to substantially reduce bleeding during dental, otolaryngology, and plastic surgery procedures. The mixture of a local anesthetic (eg, lidocaine) with a dilute concentration of epinephrine reduces blood loss during tumescent anesthesia for liposuction. Anesthesiologists often use epinephrine as a vasoconstrictor to delay the absorption of local anesthetics to prolong the duration of neuraxial anesthesia or peripheral nerve blocks. This effect also decreases serum local anesthetic concentration and reduces the risk of systemic toxicity. Mucosal vasoconstriction resulting from inhalation of aerosolized racemic epinephrine is frequently used to treat airway edema associated with prolonged endotracheal intubation, airway trauma, or croup.

Prior administration of α- or β-adrenoceptor antagonists influences the cardiovascular effects of epinephrine. For example, epinephrine causes greater increases in systemic vascular resistance and arterial pressure when administered after the nonselective β-blocker propranolol because β_2-adrenoceptor–mediated arterial vasodilation no longer opposes α_1-adrenoceptor–induced vasoconstriction. Established β-blockade also competitively inhibits β_1-adrenoceptor activation by epinephrine, thereby attenuating the positive chronotropic and inotropic effects of the catecholamine. Such a competitive blockade may only be overcome by larger doses of epinephrine. Indeed, the hemodynamic effects of epinephrine may be similar to those of the pure α_1-adrenoceptor agonist phenylephrine (see section that follows) in the presence of complete β_1- and β_2-adrenoceptor blockade. Conversely, epinephrine's β_2-adrenoceptor–meditated vasodilation is unmasked in the presence of α_1-adrenoceptor blockade, which may cause hypotension when the catecholamine is administered under these conditions.

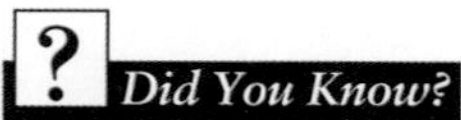

In patients with complete β_1- and β_2-blockade, epinephrine produces hemodynamic effects similar to a pure α_1-adrenoceptor agonist like phenylephrine.

B. Norepinephrine

Norepinephrine is the neurotransmitter that is released from postganglionic neurons of the sympathetic nervous system. This catecholamine activates α_1-, α_2-, and β_1-adrenoceptors similar to epinephrine, but norepinephrine exerts few if any effects on the β_2-adrenoceptor. As a result, norepinephrine enhances myocardial contractility and causes intense arterial vasoconstriction. These actions dramatically increase arterial pressure, but cardiac output remains largely unchanged. In contrast, a pure α_1-adrenoceptor agonist (eg, phenylephrine) causes predictable, dose-related decreases in cardiac output because simultaneous increases in contractility mediated through the β_1-adrenoceptor do not occur. Unlike epinephrine, norepinephrine usually does not produce tachycardia because elevated arterial pressure activates baroreceptor-mediated reflexes and, in so doing, mitigates the direct positive chronotropic actions of β_1-adrenoceptor stimulation. In general, greater increases in systemic vascular resistance and diastolic arterial pressure are observed during administration of norepinephrine compared with similar doses of epinephrine. Norepinephrine also causes constriction of venous capacitance vessels through α_1-adrenoceptor stimulation, thereby increasing venous return and augmenting stroke volume.

Norepinephrine is especially useful for treatment of refractory hypotension resulting from pronounced vasodilation. For example, norepinephrine increases arterial pressure, cardiac index, and urine output in patients with sepsis. Norepinephrine is also useful for the treatment of vasoplegic syndrome, a hypotensive state characterized by low systemic vascular resistance that sometimes occurs during prolonged cardiopulmonary bypass in patients undergoing cardiac surgery. Norepinephrine increases coronary perfusion pressure in patients with severe coronary artery disease, but the drug increases myocardial oxygen demand and may cause spasm of internal mammary or radial artery grafts used during coronary artery bypass graft (CABG) surgery through α_1-adrenoceptor activation. Either of these adverse effects may contribute to the development of acute myocardial ischemia. Administration of norepinephrine is associated with ventricular and supraventricular arrhythmias, but arrhythmogenic effects of this catecholamine are less than those of epinephrine. As a result, it may be appropriate to substitute norepinephrine for epinephrine when treating cardiogenic shock in the presence of hemodynamically significant atrial or ventricular arrhythmias. Norepinephrine stimulates pulmonary arterial α_1-adrenoceptors and produces dose-related increases in pulmonary arterial pressures that may precipitate right ventricular (RV) dysfunction because the relatively thin-walled RV is less able to tolerate acute elevations in afterload than the thicker, more muscular LV. Addition of a selective inhaled pulmonary vasodilator (eg, nitric oxide, epoprostenol) may be useful to attenuate norepinephrine's actions as a direct pulmonary vasoconstrictor when the drug is used to treat LV dysfunction in patients with pulmonary hypertension. Dose-dependent decreases in hepatic, skeletal muscle, splanchnic, and renal blood flow occur during administration of norepinephrine via α_1-adrenoceptor activation when blood pressure is normal or modestly reduced, but in the presence of profound hypotension (eg, sepsis), norepinephrine increases perfusion pressure and blood flow to these vascular beds. Nevertheless, sustained reductions in renal and splanchnic blood flow represent a major limitation of prolonged use of norepinephrine. The endogenous catecholamine should be administered through a central venous catheter to avoid the possibility of tissue necrosis in the event that peripheral extravasation occurs.

C. Dopamine

Dopamine is the biochemical precursor of norepinephrine and differentially activates several adrenergic and dopaminergic receptor subtypes in a dose-related manner. Low doses (typically below 3 µg/kg/min) of dopamine selectively increase renal and splanchnic blood flow via activation of DA_1 receptors and also reduce norepinephrine release from autonomic nervous system ganglia and adrenergic neurons through a DA_2 receptor–mediated mechanism. These combined effects produce a modest decline in arterial pressure. Moderate doses (3-8 µg/kg/min) of dopamine activate both α_1- and β_1-adrenoceptors, whereas high doses (in excess of 10 µg/kg/min) almost exclusively act on α_1-adrenoceptors to increase arterial pressure through arteriolar vasoconstriction. Although easily understood, this simplistic dose-response description of dopamine pharmacodynamics is strictly incorrect because differences in receptor density and regulation, drug interactions, and patient variability cause a broad range of clinical responses to the catecholamine. For example, low doses of dopamine were once thought to provide renal protection through DA_1 receptor–mediated increases in renal blood flow alone, but it is now clear that even low doses of dopamine also stimulate α_1- and β_1-adrenoceptors that may attenuate the catecholamine's intended dopaminergic effect. Conversely, renal blood flow and urine output may be maintained (and not decreased) during administration of higher doses of dopamine because DA_1 receptors continue to be activated despite a predominant α_1-adrenoceptor agonist effect. Such varied responses may explain, at least in part, why dopamine fails to consistently provide renal protective effects despite causing modest increases in renal perfusion and urine output.

Dopamine continues to be used for inotropic support in patients with acute LV dysfunction, although we prefer to use more potent catecholamines with more predictable pharmacodynamic characteristics in our practice. Activation of β_1-adrenoceptors is responsible for increases in myocardial contractility produced by the drug. Dopamine also stimulates arterial and venous α_1-adrenoceptors, thereby increasing LV afterload and enhancing venous return, respectively. These actions augment arterial pressure. The use of dopamine for the treatment of hypotension associated with depressed contractile function may be limited to some degree in patients with preexisting pulmonary hypertension or elevated preload because dopamine increases right atrial, mean pulmonary arterial, and pulmonary capillary occlusion pressures. Infusion of an arterial vasodilator (eg, sodium nitroprusside) may be used to mitigate the increases in LV afterload associated with administration of dopamine and, in so doing, may further augment cardiac output. However, administration of an inotrope-vasodilator ("inodilator") such as milrinone has largely replaced this "dopamine plus nitroprusside" approach. Like epinephrine and norepinephrine, dopamine increases myocardial oxygen consumption and may worsen myocardial ischemia in the presence of hemodynamically significant coronary stenoses.

D. Dobutamine

Dobutamine is a synthetic catecholamine composed of two stereoisomers (– and +), both of which stimulate β-adrenoceptors, whereas these stereoisomers produce opposing agonist and antagonist effects on α_1-adrenoceptors. As a result, dobutamine causes potent β-adrenoceptor stimulation but exerts little or no effect on α_1-adrenoceptors when administered at infusion rates less than 5 µg/kg/min. This unique pharmacology allows dobutamine to enhance myocardial contractility and simultaneously reduce arterial vasomotor tone through activation of β_1- and β_2-adrenoceptors, respectively. These properties combine to substantially increase cardiac output in normal and failing hearts. Notably, the isomer of dobutamine begins to stimulate the α_1-adrenoceptor at infusion rates greater than 5 µg/kg/min, an action that limits the magnitude of β_2-adrenoceptor–mediated vasodilation. This effect preserves LV preload, afterload, and arterial pressure; sustains increases in cardiac output; and may serve to attenuate profound baroreceptor reflex–mediated tachycardia that might otherwise occur. Despite this latter effect, dobutamine often markedly increases heart rate by direct chronotropic effects resulting from β_1-adrenoceptor stimulation. Indeed, dobutamine causes significantly higher heart rates than epinephrine at equivalent values of cardiac index in patients after coronary artery surgery. Dobutamine-induced tachycardia and enhanced contractility directly increase myocardial oxygen consumption and may cause "demand" myocardial ischemia in patients with flow limiting coronary stenoses. The propensity for dobutamine to produce demand myocardial ischemia under these circumstances is the underlying principle behind dobutamine stress echocardiography as a diagnostic tool for the detection of coronary artery disease because regional wall motion abnormalities in the affected coronary perfusion territories occur in response to the transient myocardial oxygen supply-demand mismatch. Conversely, dobutamine may reduce heart rate in patients with decompensated heart failure because increases in cardiac output and systemic oxygen delivery resulting from administration of the drug are capable of decreasing the chronically elevated sympathetic nervous system tone that occurs in heart failure. Dobutamine may also favorably reduce myocardial oxygen consumption in the failing heart because β_2-adrenoceptor activation decreases LV preload and afterload and, consequently, LV end-diastolic and end-systolic wall stress, respectively.

Declines in pulmonary arterial pressures and pulmonary vascular resistance mediated through β_2-adrenoceptor activation occur during administration of dobutamine. This property makes dobutamine a useful inotropic drug to enhance cardiac output in patients undergoing cardiac surgery with preexisting pulmonary hypertension. In contrast to dobutamine, dopamine activates α_1-adrenoceptors in the pulmonary circulation and venous capacitance vessels, thereby increasing pulmonary arterial pressures and LV preload, respectively. Thus, dobutamine may offer a distinct advantage over dopamine in patients with heart failure accompanied by increased pulmonary vascular resistance and elevated LV filling pressures. Nevertheless, dobutamine-induced pulmonary vasodilation has the potential to increase transpulmonary shunt and cause relative hypoxemia. Dobutamine does not activate dopaminergic receptors, but the drug may improve renal perfusion as a result of increases in cardiac output. Despite the aforementioned theoretical beneficial cardiovascular effects of the drug, several clinical trials showed that use of dobutamine is linked to an increased incidence of major adverse cardiac events including mortality in patients with heart failure. We no longer recommend the use of dobutamine for inotropic support in this setting as a result.

E. Isoproterenol

Isoproterenol is a nonselective β-adrenoceptor agonist synthetic catecholamine that exerts almost no activity at α-adrenoceptors. Historically, isoproterenol was used for "pharmacological pacing" because it increases heart rate in patients with symptomatic bradyarrhythmias or AV conduction block (eg, Mobitz type II second degree block, third degree block). Isoproterenol was also used during cardiac transplantation to increase heart rate and augment myocardial contractility in the denervated donor heart. However, use of the catecholamine for these indications has been largely supplanted by transcutaneous or transvenous pacing, especially in view of the drug's propensity to cause untoward supraventricular and ventricular tachyarrhythmias. Isoproterenol was previously used to treat RV dysfunction associated with severe pulmonary hypertension because the drug reduces pulmonary vascular resistance, but selective inhaled pulmonary vasodilators are more efficacious and cause fewer adverse effects in this setting as well. The clinical utility of isoproterenol is quite limited at present, but the drug's unique pharmacology compared with that of other catecholamines continues to make it worthy of discussion.

Isoproterenol causes β_2-adrenoceptor–mediated arteriolar vasodilation in skeletal muscle and also dilates the renal and splanchnic circulations, thereby reducing systemic vascular resistance. As a result of these peripheral vascular effects, the drug selectively decreases diastolic and mean arterial pressures while systolic arterial pressure is usually maintained. Isoproterenol causes direct positive chronotropic and dromotropic effects through activation of β_1-adrenoceptors, but heart rate also increases because baroreceptor reflexes are stimulated in response to declines in arterial pressure. Isoproterenol is a positive inotrope, but cardiac output may not be reliably increased during the drug's administration because pronounced tachycardia prevents optimal LV filling, and β_2-adrenoceptor–mediated venodilation decreases venous return. Dose-related increases in myocardial oxygen consumption occur with isoproterenol accompanied by simultaneous decreases in coronary perfusion pressure and diastolic filling time. These actions may contribute to acute myocardial ischemia or subendocardial necrosis, especially in the presence of coronary artery disease.

II. Sympathomimetics

A. Ephedrine

Ephedrine is a sympathomimetic drug that exerts direct and indirect actions on adrenoceptors. Transport of ephedrine into α_1- and β_1-adrenoceptor presynaptic terminals displaces norepinephrine from the synaptic vesicles, the latter of which is then released to activate the corresponding postsynaptic receptors to cause arterial and venous vasoconstriction and increased myocardial contractility, respectively. This indirect effect is the ephedrine's predominant pharmacological effect, but the drug also directly stimulates β_2-adrenoceptors, thereby limiting increases in arterial pressure resulting from α_1-adrenoceptor activation. In this regard, ephedrine's initial cardiovascular effects resemble those of epinephrine because dose-related increases in heart rate, cardiac output, and systemic vascular resistance are observed. However, tachyphylaxis to the hemodynamic effects of ephedrine occurs with repetitive administration of the drug because presynaptic stores of norepinephrine are rapidly depleted. This tachyphylaxis is not observed with epinephrine because the catecholamine acts directly on α1- and β-adrenoceptors independent of indirect stimulation of norepinephrine release. Notably, drugs that block the ephedrine uptake into adrenergic nerves (eg, cocaine) and those that deplete norepinephrine reserves (eg, reserpine) predictably attenuate ephedrine's cardiovascular effects. Ephedrine is most often used as an intravenous bolus to treat acute hypotension accompanied by decreases in heart rate.

B. Phenylephrine

The chemical structure of phenylephrine is very similar to epinephrine, but the sympathomimetic drug lacks the hydroxyl moiety that is present on the phenyl ring of the endogenous catecholamine. As a result of this minor modification, phenylephrine almost exclusively stimulates α_1-adrenoceptors to produce vasoconstriction while exerting little or no effect on β-adrenoceptors except when large doses are administered. Unlike ephedrine, phenylephrine is not dependent on presynaptic norepinephrine displacement and, instead, acts directly on the α_1-adrenoceptor to produce its cardiovascular effects. Phenylephrine constricts venous capacitance vessels and causes cutaneous, skeletal muscle, splanchnic, and renal vasoconstriction to increase preload and afterload, respectively. These actions produce dose-related increases in arterial pressure. Decreases in heart rate mediated by baroreceptor reflex activation also occur. Cardiac output remains relatively constant when normal LV systolic and diastolic functions are present, but cardiac output may fall when LV function is compromised because failing myocardium is more sensitive to increases in afterload. Phenylephrine causes pulmonary arterial vasoconstriction and increases pulmonary artery pressures. Intravenous boluses or infusions of phenylephrine are most often used intraoperatively for short-term treatment of hypotension resulting from vasodilation. Unlike catecholamines, phenylephrine is not arrhythmogenic.

> **? *Did You Know?***
>
> Phenylephrine stimulates α_1-adrenoreceptors almost exclusively and has little or no effect on β-adrenoreceptors.

III. Milrinone

Phosphodiesterases (PDEs) are enzymes that hydrolyze and terminate the intracellular actions of cyclic monophosphate second messengers including cAMP in a variety of tissues. Of most relevance to this chapter, human myocardium contains the type III PDE isoenzyme that is bound to the sarcoplasmic reticulum and cleaves active cAMP to its inactive metabolite adenosine monophosphate. Milrinone is a relatively selective bipyridine inhibitor of this cardiac type III PDE that preserves intracellular cAMP concentration by preventing the second messenger's degradation (**Table 13.2**). This action increases systolic Ca^{2+} availability by enhancing transsarcolemmal Ca^{2+} influx and Ca^{2+}-induced Ca^{2+} release from the sarcoplasmic reticulum to produce a positive inotropic effect independent of the β_1-adrenoceptor. The inhibition of cAMP metabolism by milrinone simultaneously facilitates diastolic Ca^{2+}

Table 13.2 Comparative Effects of Milrinone, Levosimendan, and Vasopressin

Name	Chemical Structure	Mechanism of Action	Dose Range	Clinical Indications	Major Side Effects
Milrinone	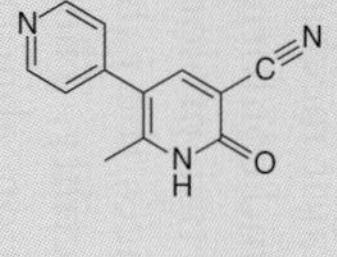	PDE III inhibition	Load: 25-50 μg/kg; IV: 0.375-0.75 μg/kg/min	Acute LV dysfunction	Arrhythmias Myocardial ischemia Sudden cardiac death Hypertension Stroke
Levosimendan	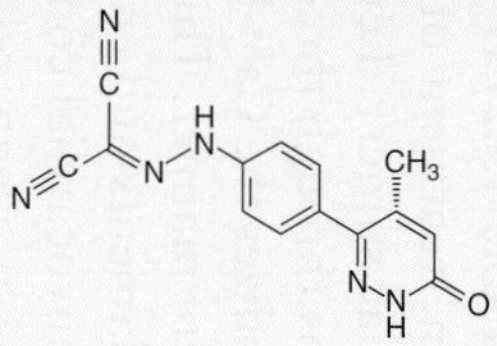	Myofilament Ca^{2+} sensitization PDE III Inhibition K_{ATP} channel opener	Load: 12-24 μg/kg; IV: 0.05-0.2 μg/kg/min	Acute LV dysfunction Heart failure	Tachycardia Hypotension
Vasopressin	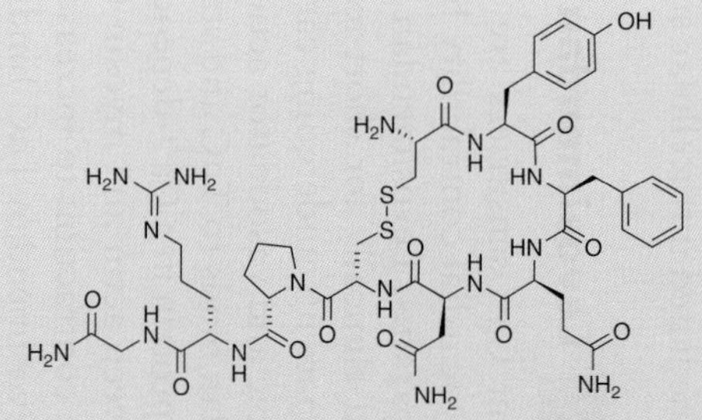	V_1 (vascular smooth muscle) and V_2 (renal collecting tubules) agonist	IV: 0.01-0.1 U/min	Shock (vasodilatory, cardiogenic) Cardiac arrest	Arrhythmias Hypertension Myocardial ischemia Reduced cardiac output Peripheral ischemia Splanchnic vasoconstriction

Ca^{2+}, calcium; IV, intravenous; K_{APT}, adenosine triphosphate–sensitive potassium channel; LV, left ventricular; PDE, phosphodiesterase.

From Pagel PS, Grecu L. Cardiovascular Pharmacology. In: Barash PG, Cahalan MK, Cullen BF, et al, eds. *Clinical Anesthesia*. 8th ed. Wolters Kluwer; 2018:301-332, Table 13.7.

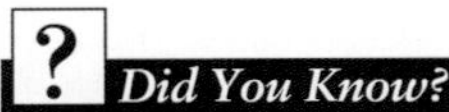

Milrinone increases cardiac contractility by inhibiting cardiac type III PDE, the enzyme responsible for the breakdown of cyclic adenosine monophosphate.

removal from the sarcoplasm to enhance the rate and extent of myocardial relaxation. This positive lusitropic effect of milrinone may improve diastolic function in patients with heart failure. Milrinone causes potent systemic and pulmonary arterial vasodilation by attenuating cyclic guanosine monophosphate (cGMP) degradation in vascular smooth muscle. Indeed, milrinone produces greater vasodilation than catecholamines including dobutamine and isoproterenol. The combination of positive inotropic effects and arterial vasodilation ("inodilator") increases cardiac output in a dose-related manner despite declines in preload resulting from dilation of venous capacitance vessels. Mean arterial pressure may be modestly reduced during infusion of the drug unless additional preload is administered.

Milrinone decreases pulmonary vascular resistance, and this action may be especially beneficial in patients with pulmonary hypertension who are undergoing cardiac surgery. However, the pulmonary vasodilating properties of milrinone have the potential to increase intrapulmonary shunt and cause arterial hypoxemia. Milrinone causes less pronounced increases in heart rate than catecholamines such as dobutamine, but the PDE inhibitor is arrhythmogenic because of its actions on intracellular Ca^{2+} homeostasis. Milrinone also inhibits platelet aggregation without producing thrombocytopenia, blunts the inflammatory cytokine response to cardiopulmonary bypass, and dilates native epicardial coronary arteries and arterial graft conduits. These actions are potentially anti-ischemic in patients with coronary artery disease undergoing coronary artery surgery. The relative utility of milrinone as a positive inotrope may be partially attenuated in the failing heart, but not to the degree that is commonly seen with β_1-adrenoceptor agonists. As a result, the PDE inhibitor continues to effectively enhance myocardial contractility in decompensated heart failure despite the presence of β_1-adrenoceptor downregulation. Indeed, the combination of milrinone and a β_1-adrenoceptor agonist is frequently used to assist weaning from cardiopulmonary bypass in patients with substantially depressed LV systolic function because of the synergistic actions of these drugs on cAMP-mediated intracellular signaling.

IV. Levosimendan

Myofilament Ca^{2+} sensitizers are positive inotropic, vasodilating drugs that enhance myocardial contractility by increasing the Ca^{2+} sensitivity of the contractile apparatus. Levosimendan (**Table 13.2**) is the only drug in this class that is used clinically for short-term treatment of heart failure or inotropic support in patients undergoing cardiac surgery. Levosimendan exerts its positive inotropic and vasodilator actions through three major mechanisms. First, levosimendan binds to TnC and stabilizes the Ca^{2+}-bound conformation of the regulatory protein in a Ca^{2+}-dependent manner. This action prolongs the interaction between actin and myosin filaments and enhances the rate and extent of myocyte contraction to increase myocardial contractility. The Ca^{2+} dependence of levosimendan-TnC binding prevents relaxation abnormalities that would otherwise be expected to occur. Second, levosimendan is a potent PDE III inhibitor that produces positive inotropic and lusitropic effects and causes systemic, pulmonary, and coronary vasodilation. Finally, levosimendan opens ATP-dependent K^+ (K_{ATP}) channels, which contribute to the drug's vasodilator properties and may also produce the additional benefit of myocardial protection against ischemic injury. Levosimendan decreases LV filling pressures, mean arterial pressure, and pulmonary and systemic vascular resistances and increases cardiac output in patients with heart failure. The modest reductions in arterial pressure observed with levosimendan are similar to those produced by milrinone and usually respond to volume administration. Levosimendan causes only minimal increases in heart rate and myocardial oxygen consumption in patients with heart failure. The drug also improves cardiac performance concomitant with reductions in pulmonary capillary occlusion pressure and systemic vascular resistance in patients with normal and depressed LV systolic function undergoing cardiac surgery. Levosimendan has a biologically active metabolite that contributes to the parent drug's more prolonged hemodynamic effects compared with catecholamines or milrinone. Use of levosimendan is more common in Europe than in the United States.

V. Vasopressin

Vasopressin (antidiuretic hormone; **Table 13.2**) is a peptide hormone released from the posterior pituitary that regulates water reabsorption in the kidney and exerts potent hemodynamic effects independent of adrenergic receptors. Vasopressin receptors consist of three subtypes (V_1, V_2, and V_3), all of which are five-subunit helical membrane proteins coupled to G-proteins. Vasopressin's cardiovascular effects are predominately mediated through V_1 receptors, which are located in the cell membrane of vascular smooth muscle. Activation of the V_1 receptor subtype stimulates phospholipase C and triggers hydrolysis of inositol 4,5-bisphosphate (PIP_2) to inositol 1,4,5-triphosphate (IP_3) and diacylglycerol. These second messengers increase intracellular Ca^{2+} concentration and produce contraction of the vascular smooth muscle cell. V_2 receptors are present on renal collecting duct cells and, when activated, increase reabsorption of free water, whereas the V_3 receptors are located in the pituitary gland and act as autacoid modulators.

Along with the sympathetic nervous system and renin-angiotensin-aldosterone axis, endogenous vasopressin plays a crucial role in the maintenance of arterial pressure. Exogenous administration of vasopressin does not substantially affect arterial pressure in conscious, healthy patients because activation of central V_1 receptors in the area postrema increases baroreceptor reflex–mediated inhibition of efferent sympathetic nervous outflow that counterbalances the elevated system vascular resistance resulting from V_1-induced arterial vasoconstriction. In contrast, vasopressinergic mechanisms are essential for maintaining arterial pressure under conditions in which sympathetic nervous system or renin-angiotensin-aldosterone axis dysfunction is present. Indeed, exogenous administration of vasopressin has been shown to effectively support arterial pressure when there is a relative vasopressin deficiency (eg, catecholamine-refractory hypotension, vasodilatory shock, sepsis, cardiac arrest). Angiotensin-converting enzyme inhibitors and angiotensin II receptor blockers used to treat hypertension also affect autonomic nervous system and renin-angiotensin-aldosterone axis function. Intraoperative hypotension that is relatively refractory to administration of catecholamines or sympathomimetics has been repeatedly described in patients who are treated with these medications. General or neuraxial anesthesia also reduces sympathetic nervous system tone, resulting in decreased plasma stress hormone concentrations including vasopressin. Under these circumstances, administration of vasopressin activates V_1 vascular smooth muscle receptors and rapidly increases arterial pressure during anesthesia by causing arterial vasoconstriction. Vasopressin therapy has been shown to reduce mortality associated with acute vasodilatory states such as anaphylaxis. In addition, infusion of vasopressin is indicated for the treatment of severe hypotension after prolonged cardiopulmonary bypass in patients who are otherwise unresponsive to phenylephrine or norepinephrine (vasoplegia).

Vasopressin is a useful drug for the treatment of sepsis. Vasodilation that is refractory to fluid resuscitation combined with a relative deficiency of endogenous vasopressin is a characteristic feature of sepsis. Inadequate sympathetic nervous system and renin-angiotensin-aldosterone axis responses to hypotension are also present in sepsis. Administration of vasopressin in the absence or presence of other vasoactive medications often improves hemodynamics and facilitates survival in patients with sepsis. The combined use of vasopressin with other vasoactive medications often reduces the overall dose of vasopressin required to maintain arterial pressure, thereby limiting the adverse effects of vasopressin on organ perfusion. In fact, sustained administration of higher doses of vasopressin may produce mesenteric ischemia, peripheral vascular insufficiency, and cardiac arrest because the drug causes pronounced vasoconstriction of cutaneous, skeletal muscle, splanchnic, and coronary vascular beds concomitant with reduced perfusion of and oxygen delivery to these tissues.

VI. Antihypertensive Medications

A. β-Blockers

Many of the cardiovascular actions of β-adrenoceptor antagonists ("β-blockers") may be anticipated based on the previous discussion of catecholamines (**Table 13.3**). β-blockers produce important anti-ischemic effects and are considered a first-line therapy for treatment of patients with ST segment elevation myocardial infarction in the absence of cardiogenic shock, hemodynamically significant bradyarrhythmias, or reactive airway disease. Indeed, β-blockers have been repeatedly shown to reduce mortality and morbidity associated with myocardial infarction in a number of large clinical trials. The American College of Cardiology/American Heart Association guidelines recommend continuation of β-blockers in patients who are receiving them chronically for established cardiac indications. β-blockers should be considered for patients undergoing vascular surgery and those at high risk of myocardial ischemia who are schedule to undergo intermediate- or high-risk noncardiac surgery. Perioperative β-blocker therapy should be initiated well before anticipated elective surgery to mitigate the elevated risk of severe stroke and death that was reported when a large dose of one of these drugs (metoprolol) was first administered on the day of surgery. β-blockers are effective for the treatment of essential hypertension and also exert useful antiarrhythmic effects, especially in the presence of increased sympathetic nervous system tone associated with surgery or during conditions characterized by elevated levels of circulating catecholamines (eg, pheochromocytoma, hyperthyroidism). β-blockers reduce heart rate, myocardial contractility, and arterial pressure by binding to β_1-adrenoceptors and inhibiting the actions of circulating catecholamines and norepinephrine released from postganglionic sympathetic nerves. The decrease in heart rate produced by β-blockers prolongs diastole, increases coronary blood flow to the LV, enhances coronary collateral perfusion to ischemic myocardium, and improves oxygen delivery to the coronary microcirculation.

Table 13.3 Comparative Effects of β-blockers

Name	Chemical Structure	Selectivity β_1	β_2	α_1	Plasma Half-Life (hrs)	Intrinsic Sympathomimetic Activity	Membrane Stabilizing Activity	Lipid Solubility	Metabolism
Propranolol	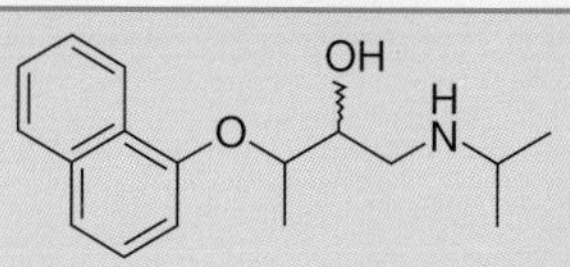	+	+	0	3-4	0	+	+++	Liver
Metoprolol	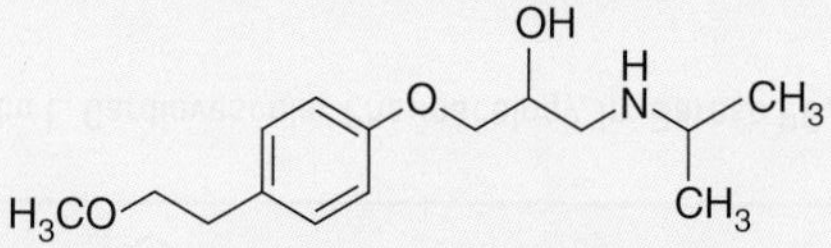	+	0	0	3-4	0	0	++	Liver
Atenolol	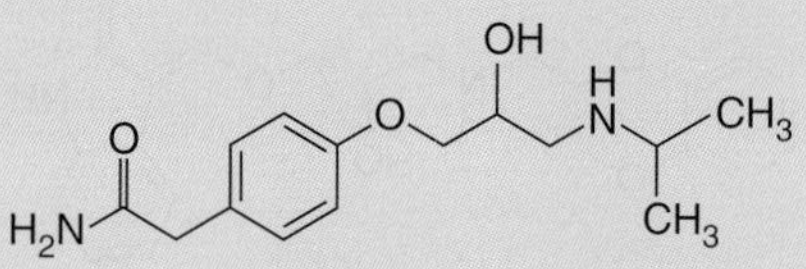	+	0	0	6-9	0	0	+	Renal
Esmolol	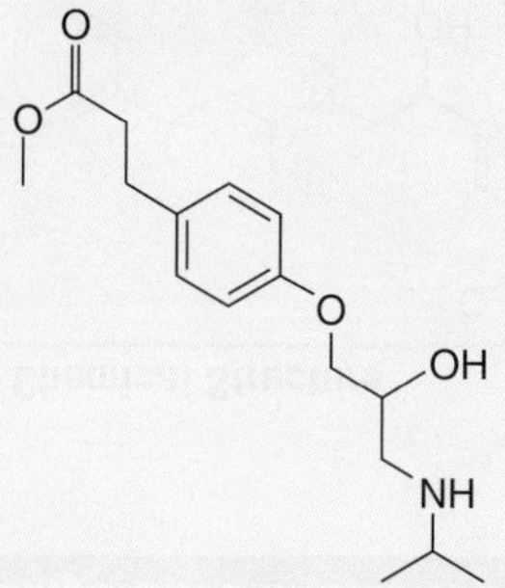	+	0	0	0.15	0	0	+	RBC esterase

(Continued)

Table 13.3 Comparative Effects of β-blockers (Continued)

Name	Chemical Structure	Selectivity β_1	β_2	α_1	Plasma Half-Life (hrs)	Intrinsic Sympathomimetic Activity	Membrane Stabilizing Activity	Lipid Solubility	Metabolism
Labetalol	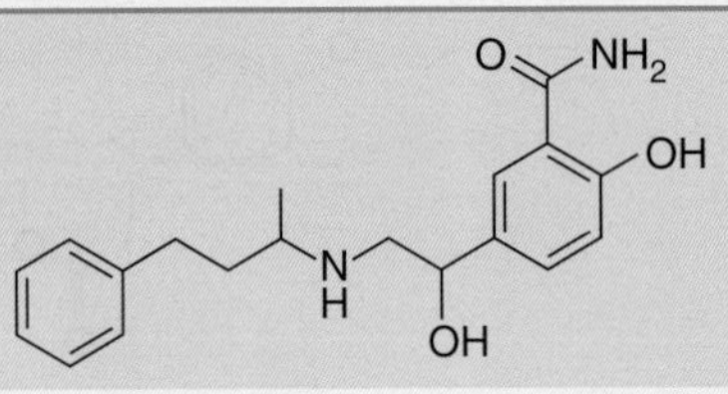	+	+	+	6	+	0	+	Liver
Carvedilol	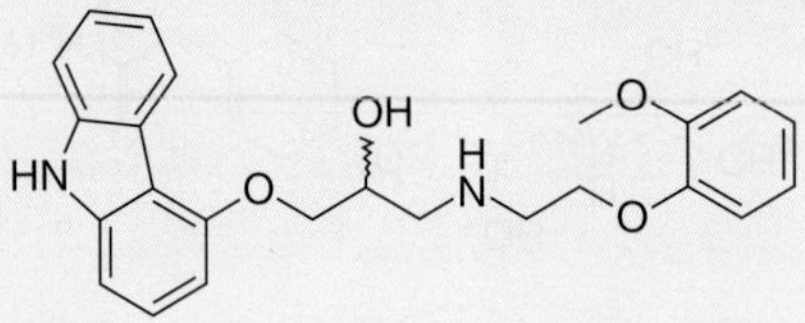	+	+	+	2-8	0	+	+++	Liver

RBC, red blood cell.

From Pagel PS, Grecu L. Cardiovascular Pharmacology. In: Barash PG, Cahalan MK, Cullen BF, et al, eds. *Clinical Anesthesia*. 8th ed. Wolters Kluwer; 2018:301-332, Table 13.6.

These combined effects serve to reduce myocardial oxygen demand while simultaneously increasing supply. β-blockers have also been shown to inhibit platelet aggregation. This latter action is particularly important during acute myocardial ischemia or evolving myocardial infarction because platelet aggregation at the site of an atherosclerotic plaque may worsen a coronary stenosis or produce acute occlusion of the vessel. β-blockers vary in their affinity for and relative selectivity at the β_1-adrenoceptor, while some of these drugs exert "intrinsic sympathetic activity" by acting as partial β-adrenoceptor agonists. Nevertheless, all β-blockers effectively reduce arterial pressure.

Esmolol

Esmolol is a relatively selective β_1-adrenoceptor blocker. The chemical structure of esmolol is very similar to that of propranolol and metoprolol, but esmolol contains an additional methylester group that facilitates the drug's rapid metabolism via hydrolysis by red blood cell esterases, resulting in an elimination half-life of approximately 9 minutes. The rapid onset and metabolism of esmolol makes the drug very useful for the treatment of acute tachycardia and hypertension during surgery. Esmolol is most often administered as an intravenous bolus, which causes almost immediate dose-related decreases in heart rate and myocardial contractility; arterial pressure declines as a result of these direct negative chronotropic and inotropic effects. Esmolol is often used to attenuate the sympathetic nervous system response to laryngoscopy, endotracheal intubation, or surgical stimulation, particularly in patients with known or suspected coronary artery disease who may be at risk of myocardial ischemia. Esmolol is also useful for rapid control of heart rate in patients with supraventricular tachyarrhythmias (eg, atrial fibrillation, atrial flutter). Esmolol effectively blunts the sympathetically mediated tachycardia and hypertension that occur shortly after the onset of seizure activity during electroconvulsive therapy. Because esmolol does not appreciably block β_2-adrenoceptors due to its relative β_1-selectivity, hypotension is more commonly observed after administration of this drug compared with other nonselective β-blockers.

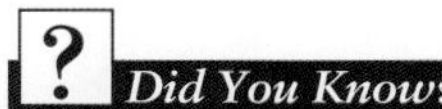

Esmolol has an elimination half-life of approximately 9 minutes because it is hydrolyzed by red cell esterases.

Labetalol

Labetalol is composed of four stereoisomers that inhibit α- and β-adrenoceptors to varying degrees. One of the four stereoisomers is an α_1-adrenoceptor antagonist, another is a nonselective β-adrenoceptor blocker, and the remaining two do not appreciably affect adrenergic receptors. The net effect of this mixture is a drug that selectively inhibits α_1-adrenoceptors while simultaneously blocking β_1- and β_2-adrenoceptors in a nonselective manner. The intravenous formulation of labetalol contains a ratio of α_1- to β-adrenoceptor blockade of approximately 1:7. Blockade of the α_1-adrenoceptor causes arteriolar vasodilation and decreases arterial pressure through a reduction in systemic vascular resistance. This property makes the drug very useful for the treatment of perioperative hypertension. Despite its nonselective β-blocking properties, labetalol is also a partial β_2-adrenoceptor agonist; this latter characteristic also contributes to vasodilation. Labetalol-induced inhibition of β_1-adrenoceptors decreases heart rate and myocardial contractility. Stroke volume and cardiac output are essentially unchanged as a result of the combined actions of labetalol on α_1- and β-adrenoceptors. Unlike other vasodilators, labetalol produces vasodilation without triggering baroreceptor reflex tachycardia because the drug blocks expected increases in heart rate mediated through β_1-adrenoceptors. This latter action may be especially beneficial for the treatment of hypertension in the setting of acute myocardial ischemia. Labetalol is most commonly used for the treatment of perioperative hypertension. Labetalol may also be useful for controlling arterial pressure without producing tachycardia in patients with hypertensive emergencies and those with acute type A aortic dissection. Labetalol has been shown to attenuate the sympathetic nervous system response to laryngoscopy and endotracheal intubation, although the drug's relatively long elimination half-life (approximately 6 hours) limits its utility in this setting.

B. Nitrovasodilators

Nitrovasodilators include organic nitrates (eg, nitroglycerin) and nitric oxide (NO) donors (eg, sodium nitroprusside) that release NO through enzymatic sulfhydryl group reduction or through a spontaneous mechanism that occurs independent of metabolism, respectively. Like endogenous NO produced by vascular endothelium, exogenous NO stimulates guanylate cyclase within the vascular smooth muscle cell to convert guanosine triphosphate to cGMP. The second messenger activates a cGMP-dependent protein kinase (protein kinase G) that dephosphorylates myosin light chains and contributes to relaxation of vascular smooth muscle. NO stimulates Ca^{2+} reuptake into the sarcoplasmic reticulum by activating the sarcoplasmic reticulum Ca^{2+} ATPase through a cGMP-independent mechanism, thereby reducing intracellular Ca^{2+} concentrations and causing relaxation. NO also stimulates potassium (K^+) efflux from the cell by activating the K^+ channel. The net effect of this shift in K^+ balance is cellular hyperpolarization, which closes the sarcolemmal voltage-gated Ca^{2+} channel and also facilitates relaxation.

Nitrovasodilators are often used to improve hemodynamics and myocardial oxygen supply–demand relations in patients with heart failure. Vasodilation reduces venous return, contributing to declines in LV and RV end-diastolic volume, pressure, and wall stress, and also reduces systemic and pulmonary arterial pressures, which decreases LV and RV end-systolic wall stress, respectively. These actions combine to decrease myocardial oxygen consumption. Simultaneously, nitrovasodilators increase myocardial oxygen supply through direct dilation of epicardial coronary arteries in the absence and presence of flow-limiting stenoses. The reduction in LV end-diastolic pressure observed during administration of nitrovasodilators coupled with coronary vasodilation substantially enhances subendocardial perfusion. The clinical efficacy of nitrovasodilators may display some initial variability between patients, but the cardiovascular effects of these drugs inevitably diminish with prolonged use. Some patients may be relatively resistant to the effects of organic nitrates in the presence of oxidative stress because superoxide anions scavenge NO, cause reversible oxidation of guanylate cyclase, and inhibit aldehyde dehydrogenase. The latter action prevents the release of NO from organic nitrates. A progressive attenuation of hemodynamic responses to nitrovasodilators may develop in other patients as a result of sympathetic nervous system and renin-angiotensin-aldosterone axis activation; this phenomenon ("pseudotolerance") accounts for the rebound hypertension that may be observed after abrupt discontinuation of nitrovasodilator therapy. Inhibition of guanylate cyclase activity is most likely responsible for true tolerance to organic nitrates. A "drug holiday" is a useful strategy for reversing this effect in patients requiring prolonged treatment in the intensive care unit. Administration of *N*-acetylcysteine, a sulfhydryl donor, may also be effective for reversing true tolerance. Notably, prolonged use of organic nitrates may also cause methemoglobinemia, interfere with platelet aggregation, and produce heparin resistance. It is also important to recognize that organic nitrates should also be used with caution in patients receiving phosphodiesterase type V inhibitors (eg, sildenafil) because NO-induced vasodilation is enhanced and profound hypotension, myocardial ischemia or infarction, and death may result.

Nitroglycerin

Nitroglycerin dilates venules to a greater degree than arterioles. At lower doses, the organic nitrate produces venodilation without causing a significant decrease in systemic vascular resistance. Arterial pressure and cardiac output fall in response to the reduction in preload despite a modest baroreceptor reflex–mediated increase in heart rate. Nitroglycerin also decreases pulmonary arterial pressures and vascular resistance. At higher doses, nitroglycerin dilates arterioles, reducing LV afterload, causing more pronounced decreases in arterial pressure, and stimulating greater reflex tachycardia. Overshoot hypotension and tachycardia is particularly common setting of hypovolemia, such as is often observed in patients with poorly controlled essential hypertension and parturients with pregnancy-induced hypertension.

Nitroglycerin improves the balance of myocardial oxygen supply to demand through its actions as a direct coronary vasodilator (which increase supply) and its systemic hemodynamic effects (which reduce demand). Nitroglycerin dilates both normal and poststenotic epicardial coronary arteries, enhances blood flow through coronary collateral vessels, and preferentially improves subendocardial perfusion. The drug also inhibits coronary vasospasm and dilates arterial conduits used during CABG surgery. Nitroglycerin decreases myocardial oxygen demand by reducing LV preload, and to a lesser extent afterload, thereby producing corresponding reductions in LV end-diastolic and end-systolic wall stress. These effects are particularly important in patients with acutely decompensated heart failure resulting from myocardial ischemia. Thus, nitroglycerin is a very effective first-line drug for the treatment of myocardial ischemia, but caution should be exercised when using nitroglycerin in patients with ischemia who are also hypovolemic. Under these circumstances, administration of nitroglycerin may precipitate life-threatening hypotension by compromising coronary perfusion pressure, reducing coronary blood flow despite epicardial vasodilation, and worsening ischemia.

Sodium Nitroprusside

Sodium nitroprusside is an ultrashort-acting direct NO donor. It is a potent venous and arterial vasodilator devoid of inotropic effects that rapidly reduces arterial pressure by decreasing LV preload and afterload. These characteristics make sodium nitroprusside a first-line drug for the treatment of hypertensive emergencies. Sodium nitroprusside is also useful for the treatment of cardiogenic shock because arterial vasodilation improves forward flow by reducing impedance to LV ejection, while venodilation decreases LV filling pressures. Unlike nitroglycerin, sodium nitroprusside is relatively contraindicated in patients with acute myocardial ischemia because the drug causes abnormal redistribution of coronary blood flow away from ischemic myocardium ("coronary steal") by producing greater coronary vasodilation in vessels that perfuse normal myocardium compared with those that supply the ischemic territory. Baroreceptor reflex–mediated tachycardia is also more pronounced during administration of sodium nitroprusside compared with nitroglycerin because the direct NO donor is a more potent arteriolar vasodilator than the organic nitrate. This reflex tachycardia dramatically increases heart rate and myocardial oxygen demand, thereby exacerbating acute myocardial ischemia. Sodium nitroprusside is often combined with a β_1-adrenoceptor antagonist such as esmolol to decrease arterial pressure, depress myocardial contractility, and reduce ascending aortic wall stress in patients with acute type A aortic dissection until direct surgical control of the injury can be achieved. Clinical use of sodium nitroprusside is limited by its toxic metabolites, which predictably accumulate when administration is prolonged or relatively high doses are used. Metabolism of sodium nitroprusside produces cyanide, which binds with cytochrome C to inhibit aerobic metabolism and cause lactic acidosis. Cyanide derived from sodium nitroprusside metabolism also binds with hemoglobin to form methemoglobin and with sulfur to form thiocyanate. The latter metabolite may accumulate in patients with renal insufficiency and produce neurological complications including delirium and seizures.

C. Hydralazine

Hydralazine is a direct vasodilator that reduces intracellular Ca^{2+} concentration in vascular smooth muscle, at least in part, by activating ATP-sensitive potassium (K_{ATP}) channels. This action produces direct relaxation of small arteries and arterioles in coronary, cerebral, splanchnic, and renal vascular beds, declines in systemic vascular resistance, and decreases in arterial pressure. LV preload is relatively preserved because hydralazine does not dilate venous capacitance vessels. The primary reduction in afterload stimulates baroreceptor reflex–mediated tachycardia and increases cardiac output. The magnitude of tachycardia observed with administration of hydralazine is often greater than expected based solely on baroreceptor reflexes alone and may instead reflect a direct effect of the drug on other centrally mediated cardiovascular regulatory mechanisms. The pronounced tachycardia associated with administration of hydralazine may produce acute myocardial ischemia in patients with critical coronary stenoses based on increases in myocardial oxygen demand and reductions in coronary perfusion pressure. Hydralazine-induced tachycardia responds appropriately to β_1-adrenoceptor antagonists, but caution should be exercised because further declines in arterial pressure may also occur. Hydralazine is commonly used for management of sustained postoperative hypertension in the absence of tachycardia.

D. Calcium Channel Antagonists

Calcium channels are asymmetric biochemical pores consisting of at least four subunits (α_1, α_2/δ, and β with or without γ) that traverse many biological membranes. Under quiescent conditions, Ca^{2+} channels are closed, but they may open through a voltage-dependent (requiring cell depolarization) or receptor-operated (activation) mechanism to allow Ca^{2+} entry into the cell or an organelle (eg, mitochondria, sarcoplasmic reticulum), most often down an electrochemical gradient. Myocardial and vascular smooth muscle cell membranes contain two distinct types of voltage-dependent Ca^{2+} channels that are denoted based on the relative duration of pore opening: T (transient) and L (long). The L-type Ca^{2+} channel is the predominant target of all Ca^{2+} channel antagonists in current clinical use (these drugs do not block the T-type Ca^{2+} channel). There are four major classes of chemically distinct Ca^{2+} channel antagonists (**Table 13.4**): (1) 1,4-dihydropyridines (eg, nifedipine, nicardipine, clevidipine), (2) benzothiazepines (diltiazem), (3) phenylalkylamines (verapamil), and (4) diarylaminopropylamine ethers (bepridil). In general, Ca^{2+}

Table 13.4 Comparative Effects of Ca^{2+} Channel Blockers

Name	Chemical Structure	Myocardial Depression	Coronary Blood Flow	Suppression of SA Node (Automaticity)	Suppression of AV Node (Conduction)
Nifedipine	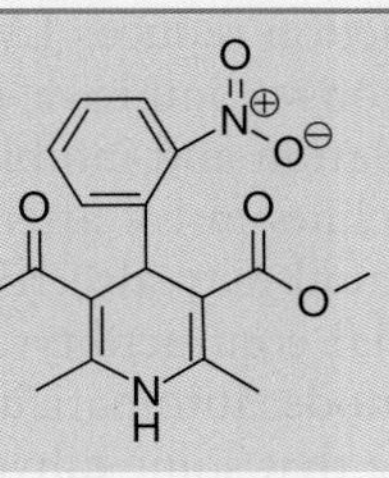	+	+++++	+	0
Nicardipine	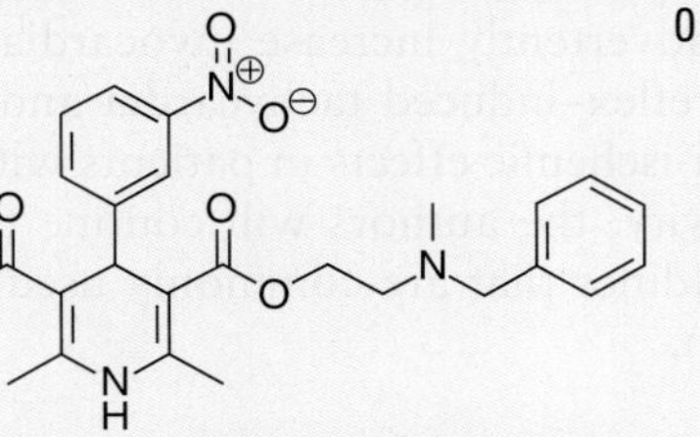	0	+++++	+	0
Clevidipine	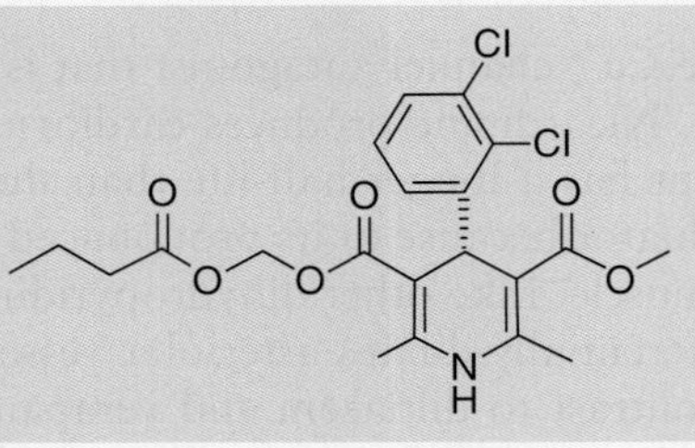	+	+++++	+	0
Nimodipine	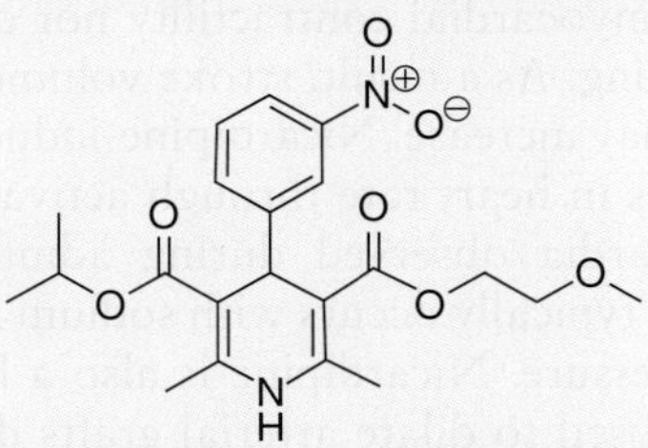	+	++++	+	0
Diltiazem	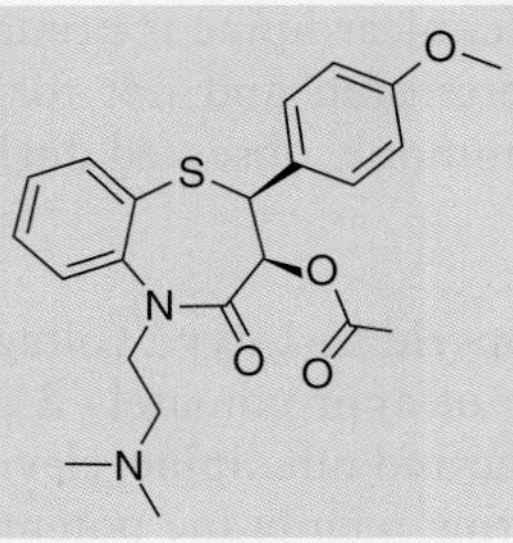	++	+++	+++++	++++
Verapamil	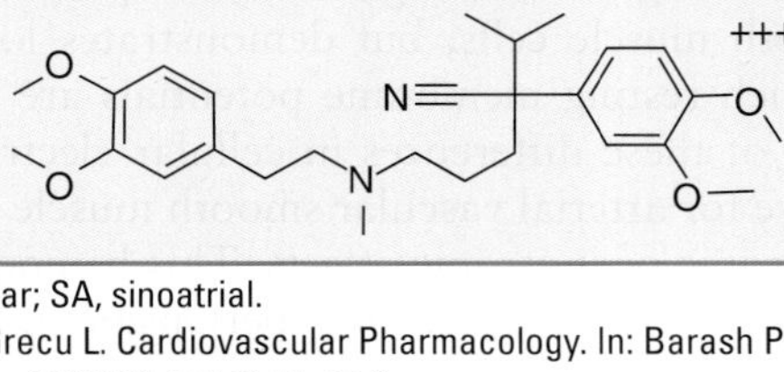	++++	++++	+++++	++++

AV, atrioventricular; SA, sinoatrial.

From Pagel PS, Grecu L. Cardiovascular Pharmacology. In: Barash PG, Cahalan MK, Cullen BF, et al, eds. *Clinical Anesthesia*. 8th ed. Wolters Kluwer; 2018:301-332. Table 13.8.

channel antagonists produce vasodilation, direct negative chronotropic, dromotropic, and inotropic effects and baroreceptor reflex–mediated increases in heart rate to varying degrees depending on each drug's relative selectivity for voltage-gated Ca^{2+} channels in myocardium and vascular smooth muscle. All Ca^{2+} channel antagonists cause greater relaxation of arterial compared with venous vascular smooth muscle. This action reduces LV afterload while preserving preload. Calcium channel antagonists improve myocardial oxygen supply through coronary arterial vasodilation and inhibition of coronary artery vasospasm. In addition to eliciting declines in LV afterload, Ca^{2+} channel antagonists such as diltiazem and verapamil may also reduce myocardial oxygen demand via depression of myocardial contractility and decreases in heart rate mediated by reduced sinoatrial node automaticity and AV node conduction. However, it is important to note that some dihydropyridine Ca^{2+} channel antagonists may inadvertently increase myocardial oxygen demand as a result of baroreceptor reflex–induced tachycardia and, as a result, may not consistently produce anti-ischemic effects in patients with coronary artery disease. For the sake of brevity, the authors will confine their discussion to two intravenous dihydropyridines that are commonly used for the treatment of perioperative hypertension.

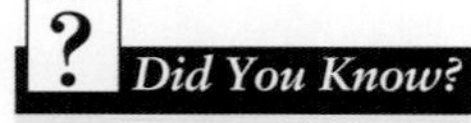

All Ca^{2+} channel blockers produce greater relaxation of arterial than venous vascular smooth muscle.

Nicardipine

Nicardipine is a dihydropyridine Ca^{2+} channel antagonist that is highly selective for vascular smooth muscle. Nicardipine produces cardiovascular effects that are similar to nifedipine, but has a longer half-life than the latter drug. Nicardipine is a profound vasodilator because of its pronounced inhibition of Ca^{2+} influx in vascular smooth muscle. Like other dihydropyridine Ca^{2+} channel antagonists, nicardipine preferentially dilates arteriolar vessels; this effect decreases arterial pressure. In contrast to diltiazem and verapamil, nicardipine does not substantially depress myocardial contractility nor does the drug affect the rate of sinoatrial node firing. As a result, stroke volume and cardiac output are relatively preserved or may increase. Nicardipine-induced decreases in arterial pressure trigger increases in heart rate through activation of baroreceptor reflexes, but the tachycardia observed during administration of nicardipine is less pronounced than typically occurs with sodium nitroprusside at comparable levels of arterial pressure. Nicardipine is also a highly potent coronary vasodilator and is often used to dilate arterial grafts during CABG surgery. Because of its relative long half-life, nicardipine is primarily used for treatment of sustained perioperative hypertension and not for acute, often transient hypertensive episodes that are commonly observed during surgery.

Clevidipine

Clevidipine is an ultrashort-acting dihydropyridine L-type voltage-gated Ca^{2+} channel antagonist with a plasma half-life of approximately 2 minutes after intravenous administration. Like nicardipine and nifedipine, clevidipine exerts pronounced effects at the less negative resting membrane potentials typically observed in vascular smooth muscle cells, but demonstrates lower potency in cardiac myocytes in which resting membrane potentials are substantially more negative. As a result of these differences in cellular electrophysiology, clevidipine is highly selective for arterial vascular smooth muscle and is nearly devoid of negative chronotropic or inotropic effects. This hemodynamic profile may be especially useful for the treatment of hypertension in patients with compromised LV function. Clevidipine causes dose-related arteriolar vasodilation while sparing venous vasomotor tone, thereby reducing systemic vascular resistance and arterial pressure without affecting LV preload. These actions may combine to augment cardiac output. Modest increases in heart rate may also occur during administration of clevidipine as a result of baroreceptor reflex activation. Unlike other short-acting antihypertensive drugs, administration of clevidipine is not associated with the development of tachyphylaxis, and abrupt discontinuation of the drug does not appear to cause rebound hypertension. Because tissue and plasma esterases are responsible for clevidipine metabolism, little to no accumulation of the drug occurs even in the setting of hepatic or kidney dysfunction.

For further review, please see the associated Interactive Video Lectures accessible in complimentary eBook bundled with this text. Access instructions are located on the inside front cover.

Suggested Readings

1. Benham-Hermetz J, Lambert M, Stephens RC. Cardiovascular failure, inotropes and vasopressors. *Br J Hosp Med (Lond)*. 2012;73:C74-C77.
2. Bozkurt B. What is new in heart failure management in 2017? Update on AHA/ACC heart failure guidelines. *Curr Cardiol Rep*. 2018;20:39.
3. Fleisher LA, Fleischmann KE, Auerbach AD, et al. 2014 ACC/AHA guideline on perioperative cardiovascular evaluation and management of patients undergoing noncardiac surgery: a report of the American College of Cardiology/American Heart Association Task Force on practice guidelines. *J Am Coll Cardiol*. 2014;64:e77-e137.
4. Friederich JA, Butterworth JF. Sodium nitroprusside: twenty years and counting. *Anesth Analg*. 1995;81:152-162.
5. Iachini Bellisarii F, Radico F, Muscente F, Horowitz J, De Caterina RD. Nitrates and other nitric oxide donors in cardiology: current positioning and perspectives. *Cardiovasc Drugs Ther*. 2012;26:55-69.
6. MacCarthy EP, Bloomfield SS. Labetalol: a review of its pharmacology, pharmacokinetics, clinical uses and adverse effects. *Pharmacotherapy*. 1983;3:193-219.
7. Overgaard CB, Dzavik V. Inotropes and vasopressors: review of physiology and clinical use in cardiovascular disease. *Circulation*. 2008;118:1047-1056.
8. Pagel PS, Warltier DC. Positive inotropic drugs, In: Evers AS, Maze M, Kharasch E, eds. *Anesthetic Pharmacology: Physiologic Principles and Clinical Practice*. 2nd ed. Cambridge University Press; 2011:706-723.
9. Prlesi L, Cheng-Lai A. Clevidipine: a novel ultra-short-acting calcium antagonist. *Cardiol Rev*. 2009;17:147-152.
10. Putzu A, Clivio S, Belletti A, Cassini T. Perioperative levosimendan in cardiac surgery: a systematic review with meta-analysis and trial sequential analysis. *Int J Cardiol*. 2018;251:22-31.
11. Treschan TA, Peters J. The vasopressin system: physiology and clinical strategies. *Anesthesiology*. 2006;105:599-612.
12. van Diepen S, Katz JN, Albert NM, et al. Contemporary management of cardiogenic shock: a scientific statement from the American Heart Association. *Circulation*. 2017;136:e232-e268.

Questions

1. A 56-year-old woman with aortic valve endocarditis and septic shock is hypotensive (mean arterial pressure of 45 mm Hg) despite receiving an intravenous infusion of norepinephrine (0.15 μg/kg/min). The central venous pressure is 12 mm Hg and the cardiac index is 4.5 L/min/m². Administration of which of the following medications is MOST likely to be indicated?

   A. Phenylephrine
   B. Dobutamine
   C. Epinephrine
   D. Vasopressin

2. Which of the following medications is MOST likely to be indicated for treatment of right ventricular dysfunction associated with acute pulmonary hypertension?

   A. Ephedrine
   B. Phenylephrine
   C. Milrinone
   D. Dopamine

3. A 72-year-old man undergoing coronary artery bypass graft surgery separates from cardiopulmonary bypass while receiving intravenous infusions of milrinone (0.5 μg/kg/min) and norepinephrine (0.1 μg/kg/min). The mean arterial pressure is 50 mm Hg and the cardiac index is 1.6 L/min/m². Transesophageal echocardiography demonstrates global left ventricular hypokinesis. Administration of which of the following medications is the MOST appropriate next step?

   A. Epinephrine
   B. Vasopressin
   C. Dopamine
   D. Phenylephrine

4. Administration of which of the following medications is MOST likely to attenuate the sympathetic nervous system responses to direct laryngoscopy and endotracheal intubation?

   A. Lidocaine
   B. Fentanyl
   C. Esmolol
   D. Verapamil

5. Administration of which of the following vasodilators is MOST likely to be associated with the development of lactic acidosis?

   A. Clevidipine
   B. Milrinone
   C. Nitroglycerin
   D. Sodium nitroprusside

Answers

1. D

The patient requires an additional vasopressor to increase mean arterial pressure. Norepinephrine and vasopressin are potent vasoconstrictors and are indicated for treatment of hypotension associated with septic shock.

2. C

Milrinone enhances myocardial contractility and is a pulmonary vasodilator.

3. A

Epinephrine is the treatment of choice for management of acute cardiogenic shock if other inotropic medications are insufficient.

4. C

The short-acting β-blocker esmolol effectively blunts the sympathetic nervous system–mediated tachycardia and hypertension associated with direct laryngoscopy and endotracheal intubation.

5. D

Higher doses of sodium nitroprusside cause cyanide toxicity, interfering with cellular metabolism and resulting in progressive lactic acidosis.

PART C
Technology

14 The Anesthesia Workstation

Naveen Nathan

? Did You Know?

The modern anesthesia workstation is a sophisticated device that contributes to patient safety, but like many modern devices, it is complex and may fail. A simple self-inflating bag and mask must always be immediately available.

It is common for students, nurses, and physicians in the earliest phases of their anesthesiology training to be intimidated when confronted by the anesthesia workstation. The sheer number of cables, hoses, knobs, digital displays, and alarms may seem formidable. This chapter aims to deconstruct the anatomy and functionality of the conventional anesthesia workstation and characterize the principles underlying its use.

As a salient and indispensable component of the operating room, the anesthesia workstation serves to achieve four goals: (1) provide a reliable mechanism to continually ventilate the anesthetized patient, (2) serve as a source for supplemental O_2, (3) provide a mechanism for the delivery of volatile anesthetic agents, and (4) serve as a monitor and early warning system for several potential hazards encountered in clinical anesthetic care. Note that a variety of simple tools exist to achieve each of these goals individually (eg, a bag valve mask device [Ambu bag] may be used to ventilate a patient's lungs, and a simple E-cylinder filled with pressurized oxygen may be used to increase the fraction of inspired oxygen [FiO_2]). The anesthesia workstation, however, incorporates and consolidates all of the above goals in a manner that is convenient and allows the anesthesiologist to be more vigilant in performing other equally important facets of anesthetic care. It cannot be overemphasized that this convenience comes at the price of complexity. Many intraoperative crises can be avoided by appreciating the design, functionality, and limitations of modern anesthesia workstations.

I. Functional Anatomy of the Anesthesia Workstation

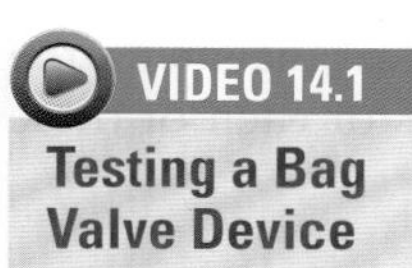

In its entirety, the anesthesia workstation encompasses a broad range of equipment, including the anesthesia machine, physiologic monitors, and accessories such as active suction equipment and adjunctive bag valve mask device. Patient monitoring and airway management are discussed elsewhere. The remainder of this chapter directs attention specifically to the anesthesia machine. The basic construct of the anesthesia machine is defined by three concepts (**Figure 14.1**). The first is a system that originates with a *gas*; typically, this is pressurized oxygen/air delivered from a central hospital source, directly into the operating room. A series of ***pressure-reducing systems*** follows, after which

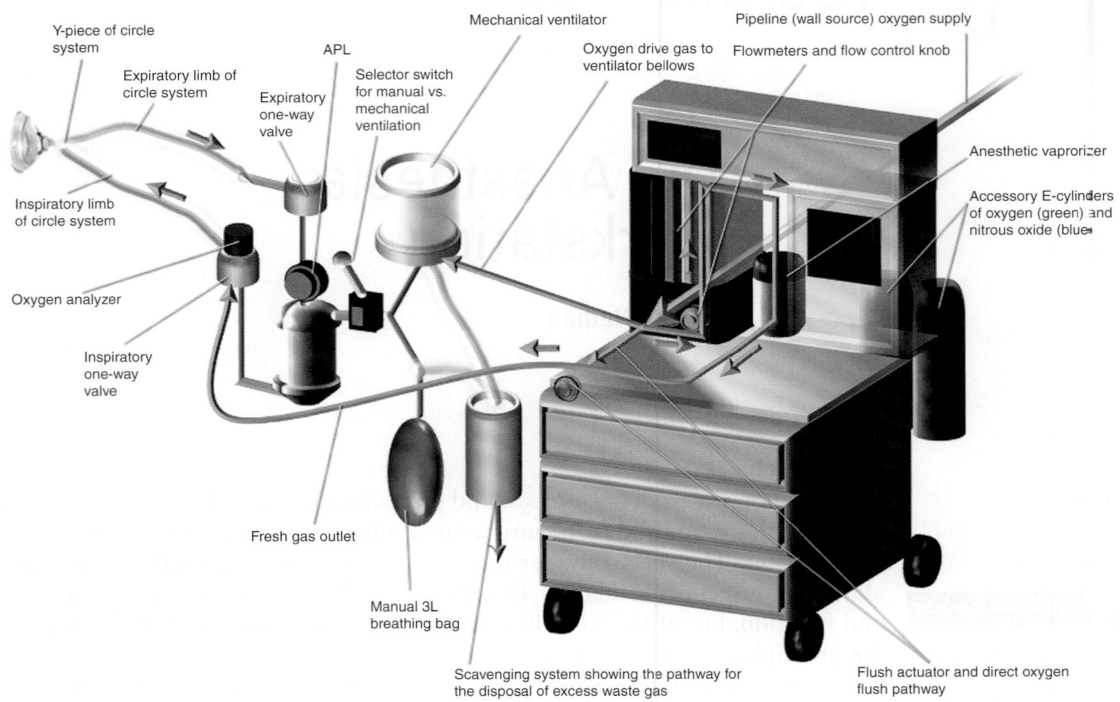

Figure 14.1 Representation of a typical anesthesia workstation. Arrows indicate direction of oxygen flow. Pipeline sources of air and nitrous oxide are not shown. APL, adjustable pressure-limiting valve.

the anesthesiologist directly controls the flow of these gases to achieve the desired flow rate and oxygen concentration that is delivered to the second system. Integrated into this gas delivery design is the anesthetic ***vaporizer***, which allows for the administration of volatile anesthetic to the patient.

The system described above converges on the ***fresh gas outlet***, which delivers the desired concentrations of gases and volatile anesthetics into the next conceptual framework (system) of the anesthesia machine: the ***anesthesia breathing apparatus***. Patient ventilation is achieved using either the automated controlled mechanical ventilator or manually through the breathing bag, both of which are incorporated into a system of corrugated tubes and unidirectional valves known as the ***circle system***. This design enables reciprocal inflation and deflation of the patient's lungs with the ventilator or breathing bag. It also incorporates an absorbent compound to neutralize expired carbon dioxide.

Lastly, there must be a mechanism to remove excess gas or pressure from the system. This is accomplished through another structural arrangement, the ***scavenging system***. The mechanics, safeguards, and hazards of each of these three systems will be discussed below.

II. Delivery of Gases: High-, Intermediate-, and Low-Pressure Systems

Most anesthesia workstations receive a dual supply of medical-grade gases. Oxygen is delivered at high pressure from the central hospital supply source (liquid oxygen tanks) into the operating room through readily

Table 14.1 Pressure Readings Encountered in an Anesthesia Workstation

	Psi	mm Hg	cm H_2O
Anesthesia workstation: High-pressure oxygen or air source (a full E-cylinder containing 625 L of gas)	**2,200**	113,773	154,675
Anesthesia workstation: High-pressure nitrous oxide source (a full E-cylinder containing 1590 L of gas)	**745**	38,528	52,379
Anesthesia workstation: Intermediate pressure oxygen, air, or nitrous oxide (in-line working pressure within the machine)	**50-55**	2586	3515
Typical peak airway pressure during mechanical ventilation of a healthy patient at 6 mL/kg tidal volume and respiratory rate of 10 breaths/min	0.2-0.3	11-18	**15-25**

The most commonly used unit of measurement is indicated in bold text.

visible green hoses or, alternatively, can be delivered from a cylinder (size E) of oxygen attached to the anesthesia machine. Air is color coded in yellow. Note that these color designations apply to medical centers located in the United States and vary internationally. A third supply line of nitrous oxide at high pressure, coded in blue, or a backup supply of nitrous oxide stored in an E-cylinder attached to the anesthesia machine may also be present.[1] The delivery of these gases through the anesthesia machine and ultimately to the patient is marked by a progressive, regulated decrement in pressure. Wall source gases are delivered to the anesthesia machine at a pressure of 50 pounds per square inch (psi). E-cylinders contain considerably higher pressures but are regulated to 45 psi prior to their interface with the anesthesia machine.[1,2] The user further regulates and fine-tunes the low-pressure flow of gases to the patient using flow control knobs specific to each gas. **Table 14.1** lists pressure readings encountered in the anesthesia workstation.

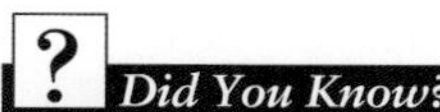

Most operating rooms have a reliable wall source of oxygen. However, if this should fail, a low-pressure alarm will be triggered. The green oxygen hose attached to the back of the anesthesia machine should be disconnected and the auxiliary oxygen E-cylinder turned on.

Pressure gauges reflective of both wall and cylinder sources of medical gases are displayed on the anesthesia machine. The gauges for the central hospital gas sources measure the ***intermediate*** in-line working pressure and typically read approximately 50 to 55 psi. The most common reason why this pressure reading would decrease is that the hose from the wall source has been disconnected from the anesthesia machine, but it could also result from a complete or partial failure of the central hospital gas source. This pressure gauge reading remains constant through the routine and continuous use of wall source gases even when used at high flow rates. In contrast, the gauges for medical gas cylinders reflect the ***high*** internal pressure of the cylinders themselves. A full E-cylinder of oxygen or air will contain roughly 625 L of gas at a pressure of 2200 psi. The pressure will drop proportionately as these gases are used.[1-4] If a tank is used to oxygenate the patient at 10 L/min, then it will only last approximately 60 minutes.[5] A full tank of nitrous oxide contains 1590 L of gas at a pressure of 745 psi. Nitrous oxide, in contrast to oxygen and air, exists as a combination of liquid and gas inside its compressed cylinder due to its physicochemical properties and critical temperature. As a result, continuous use of a nitrous oxide cylinder will ***not*** result in a pressure drop at the gauge until nearly 75% (1200 L) of the nitrous oxide in the cylinder has

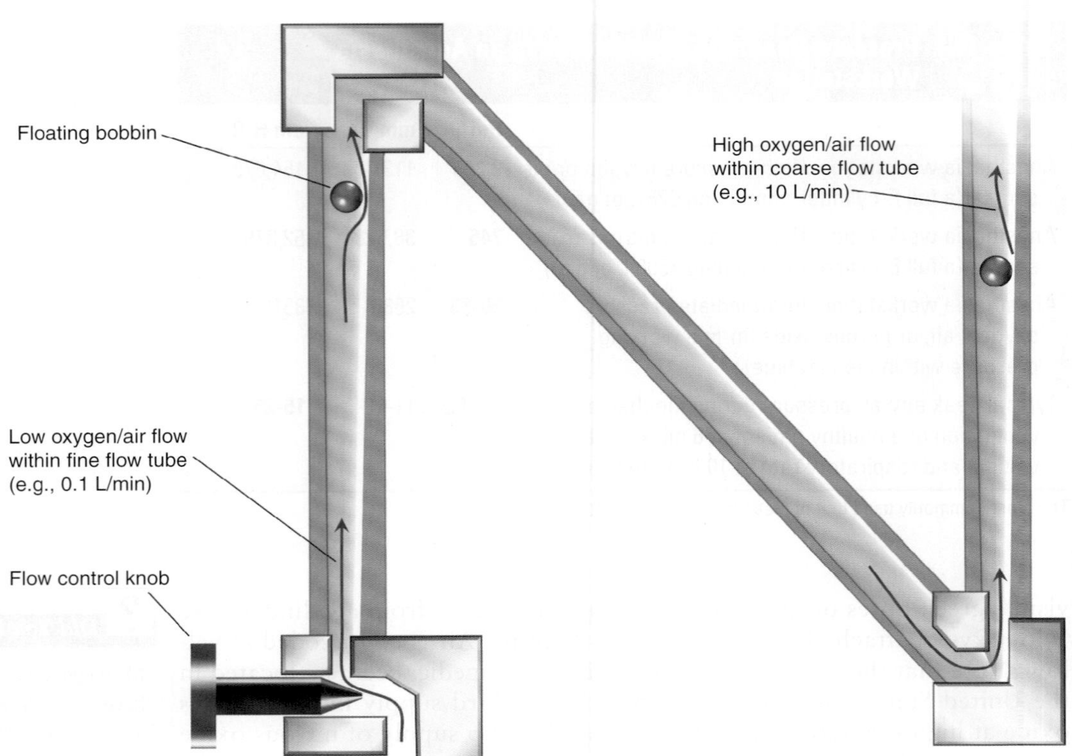

Figure 14.2 A flowmeter assembly and Thorpe tube. The black circle represents the floating bobbin, which indicates the current flow rate being used. Low flows at the narrow end of the tapered glass tube (eg, 100 mL/min) are characterized as laminar and viscosity dependent. In contrast, high flows at the large diameter end of the tube (eg, 10 L/min) are turbulent and density dependent.

been used. During the routine use of the anesthesia machine, the E-cylinder sources are kept in the off position as these are intended for use only during central pipeline failure. If such an event occurs, two actions are to be undertaken. First, the central pipeline gas source is disconnected from the anesthesia machine. Second, the E-cylinder is turned to the on position so that continued oxygenation and ventilation of the patient may proceed.[1-4]

A. Flowmeters

From the flowmeter assembly onward, the anesthesia machine is considered a ***low***-pressure system. The anesthesiologist may individually manipulate the flow of air, oxygen, and nitrous oxide to achieve flow rates of 0.2 L/min to more than 10 L/min for each gas. The fine control over the flow of these gases is achieved as they pass through specialized, variable orifice glass tubes known as Thorpe tubes. The height of a floating bobbin within the tapered lumen (increasing internal diameter) of these tubes indicates the current flow rate being used (**Figure 14.2**). At very low flow rates (0.1-0.3 L/min), the passage of gas molecules through the smaller diameter section of these tubes is laminar. Concentric telescoping tubes of gas molecules moving parallel to one another in this fashion are influenced by gas ***viscosity*** or, in other words, the frictional properties between the inner surface of an outer layer of gas flow and the outer surface of the inner layer adjacent to it. In contrast, at high flow rates in the large diameter section of the Thorpe tube (5-10 L/min), gas flow is turbulent, which is characterized by the random trajectory of gas molecules, although en masse, there is bulk movement of air in the antegrade direction. In this scenario, flow is significantly affected by gas ***density***. Larger gas molecules will result in greater intermolecular collisions and hence greater impedance to gas flow.[1,2]

B. Flush Actuator and One-Way Check Valve

Thus far, the discussion of gas delivery from its source to the patient has followed a single path that begins with very high pressures. However, it is ultimately received by the patient's lungs under low pressure conditions within agreeable physiologic limits. Anesthesia machines are equipped with an alternate pathway for oxygen that may expose the patient to the intermediate pressure system. The ***flush actuator*** permits the application of oxygen flow from the in-line working pressure of 55 psi through the common gas outlet to the patient. Flow rates of oxygen through this alternate pathway that bypass the flowmeters can range from 35 to 75 L/min. As a matter of perspective, using the flush valve to inflate a patient's lungs exposes the patient to roughly 200 times the typical inflation pressures used during routine mechanical ventilation. One may wonder why this pathway exists at all. Should the patient somehow become disconnected from the anesthesia breathing apparatus during controlled ventilation, the ventilator bellows (or the breathing bag) will immediately deflate as the volume of gas within will be drained into the operating room environment. The flush actuator could be used to rapidly increase the volume of gas in the system, so that normal tidal volumes may resume. This should be undertaken with care and advisably only during the ***expiratory*** phase of respiration when any excess gas or pressure resulting from the use of the flush valve can be scavenged away from the system (see "Scavenging Systems" later in this chapter). Additionally, the flush valve may be used for more complex ventilation strategies such as high-frequency jet ventilation.[1,2]

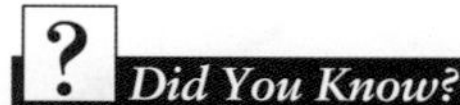

The oxygen flush actuator ("flush valve") delivers oxygen at high pressure and flow directly to the common gas outlet. Its primary purpose is to enable rapid filling of a deflated rebreathing bag or ventilator bellows.

A further consideration involves the potential presence of a one-way check valve just ***upstream*** of where the flush actuator joins the fresh gas outlet to the patient. This valve is present on many models of Datex-Ohmeda (GE Healthcare Company) brand workstations and allows for the unidirectional flow of gas only in the antegrade route. As a consequence, using the flush valve exposes the patient to ***all*** of the oxygen flow from the intermediate pressure system. In the absence of this one-way check valve, as is the case in Dräger workstations (Dräger Medical Inc), some of the oxygen flow from flushing the system may course in a retrograde fashion (**Figure 14.3**).[1]

C. Safeguards in the Delivery of Medical Gases

It is imperative that the anesthesiologist verifies the presence of adequate gas supply pressures for both the wall source and the auxiliary E-cylinder(s) during the preuse check of the workstation (see "Anesthesia Workstation Preuse Checkout" later in this chapter). Acceptable gas pressure readings, however, still do not guarantee that the ***correct*** gas is in fact being delivered to the patient. Misconnecting a nitrous oxide wall hose or nitrous cylinder to the noncorresponding interface for oxygen could result in the delivery of a hypoxic gas mixture. Thankfully, modern anesthesia systems help prevent such catastrophic occurrences. Wall source hoses are connected to the back of the anesthesia machine through noninterchangeable fittings, each with a diameter specific to its respective gas (the ***diameter index safety system***). Additionally, E-cylinders for oxygen, air, and nitrous oxide each have a specific arrangement of two holes that mate with their corresponding pins on the yoke of the anesthesia machine (the Pin Index Safety System) (**Figure 14.4**).[1,2]

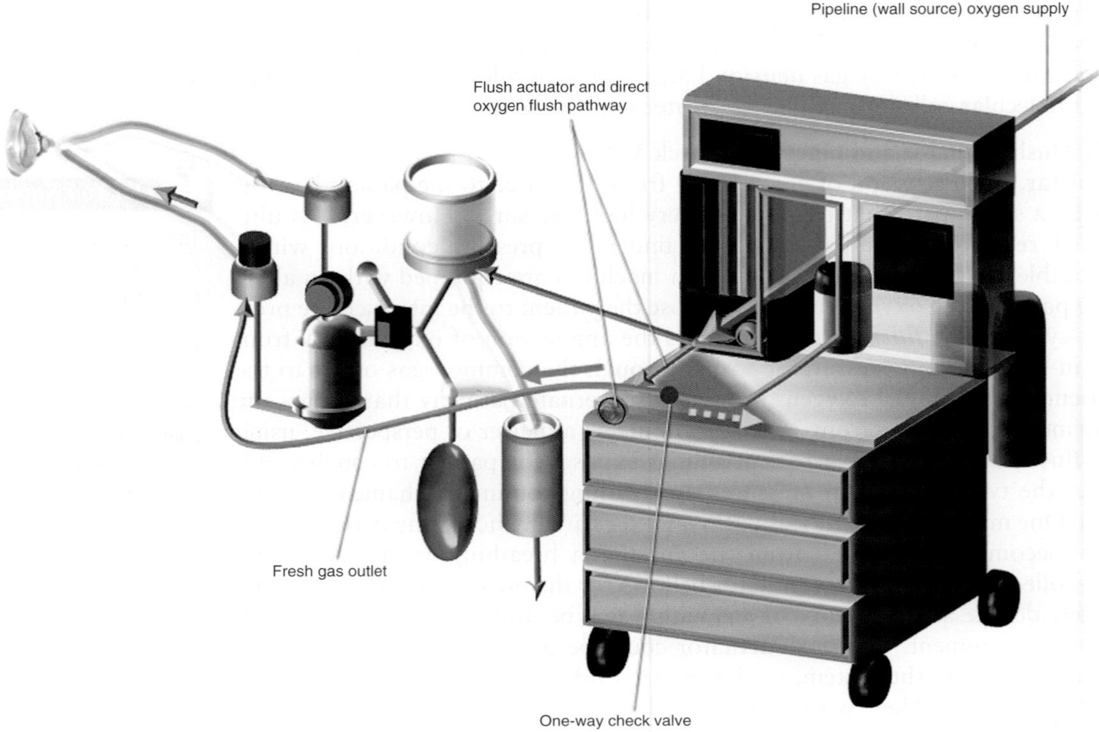

Figure 14.3 Oxygen flush actuator showing how the high pressure (50 psi) of oxygen can bypass the flowmeters and be directly administered to the patient. The presence of a one-way check valve (*red dot*) forces all of the high-flow oxygen to course antegrade into the fresh gas outlet (*solid green arrow*). In the absence of such a check valve, some of the oxygen will flow retrograde into the anesthesia machine (*dotted yellow arrow*).

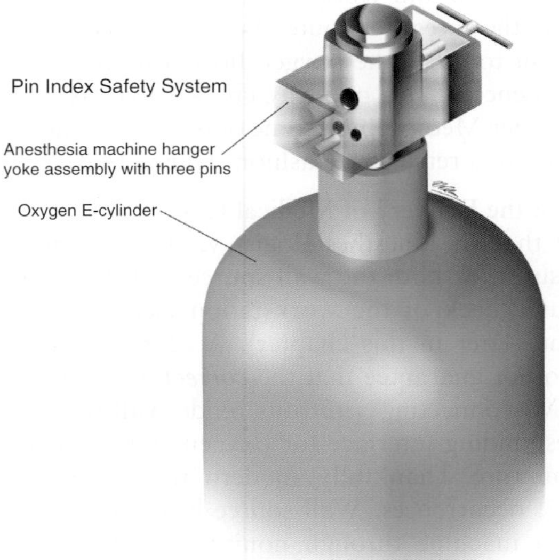

Figure 14.4 Pin Index Safety System for medical gas cylinders.

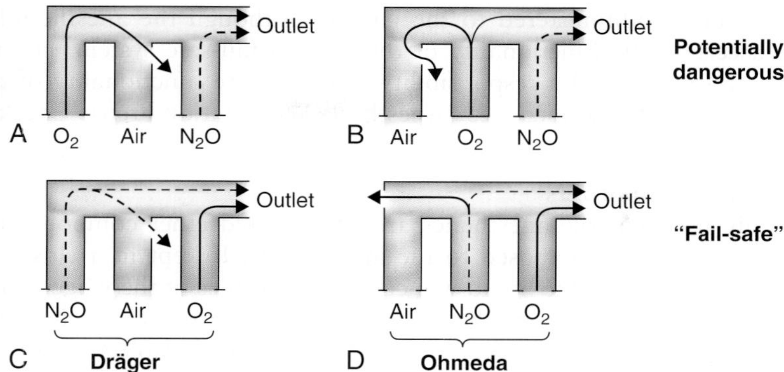

Figure 14.5 Flowmeter sequence—a potential cause of hypoxia. In the event of a flowmeter leak, a potentially dangerous arrangement exists when nitrous oxide is located in the downstream position (**A** and **B**). The safest configuration exists when oxygen is located in the downstream position (**C** and **D**). O_2, oxygen; N_2O, nitrous oxide. (Adapted from Eger II EI, Hylton RR, Irwin RH, et al. Anesthetic flowmeter sequence—a cause for hypoxia. *Anesthesiology.* 1963;24:396 and from Riutort KT, Eisenkraft JB. The anesthesia workstation and delivery systems for inhaled anesthetics. In: Barash PG, Cahalan MK, Cullen BF, et al, eds. *Clinical Anesthesia.* 8th ed. Wolters Kluwer; 2018:644-705, Figure 25.21.)

Additional measures exist to ensure appropriate oxygenation of the patient. Consider the scenario in which a fresh gas mixture of 50% oxygen and 50% nitrous oxide is being used and an isolated drop in oxygen pipeline pressure occurs. The sequence in which these two gases enter the fresh gas main line impacts the resulting gas mixture delivered to the patient. Oxygen is always the last gas to sequentially enter the fresh gas mixture to minimize (but not eliminate) the alteration in inspired oxygen (**Figure 14.5**).

Although inspection of the oxygen pipeline pressure gauge, a low O_2 pressure alarm, and low fraction of inspired oxygen (FiO_2) concentration alarm would alert the user to the hazardous event described above, a mechanism known as the oxygen ***fail-safe system*** exists to minimize the decrement in FiO_2. The fail-safe system proportionally decreases the flow of all other gases in use or halts their administration completely when a decline in oxygen pressure occurs. This prevents a disproportionate increase in the relative contribution of fresh gases that do not contribute to the oxygenation of the patient.[1-4]

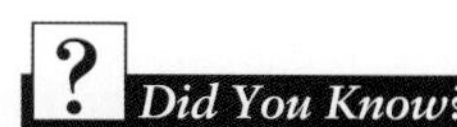

A properly functioning and calibrated oxygen analyzer is a mandatory part of the anesthesia workstation. There are several safeguards in modern machines to prevent delivery of a hypoxic gas mixture to the patient, but the oxygen analyzer is last in line and is the only device that actually measures the concentration.

Even under conditions in which the integrity of the oxygen pipeline source is maintained, it would still be possible to deliver a hypoxic fresh gas mixture to a patient. Imagine that oxygen flow is set to 1 L/min and nitrous oxide is delivered concurrently at 4 L/min. In this situation, the consequent FiO_2 would be 20%, less than that of room air. ***Proportioning systems*** within the flowmeter assembly prevent exactly this type of problem from occurring. One possible design is the use of chain-linked sprockets that unite the control knobs for nitrous oxide and oxygen to each other. The effect imposes limits such that the ratio of nitrous oxide flow to oxygen flow never exceeds 3:1 (an FiO_2 of 25%). Other types of proportioning mechanisms actively reduce nitrous oxide flows when oxygen flows are decreased by the user.[1]

Lastly, an ***oxygen analyzer*** oversees the delivered concentration of oxygen just beyond the fresh gas outlet. Although not a constituent of the anesthesia machine per se, it is a final check on what concentration of oxygen is in fact ultimately being administered to the patient. Although the anesthesiologist cannot ascertain the functionality of the oxygen fail-safe system, he or she has an opportunity and a responsibility to certify the functionality of *all* of the safeguards just described (see "Anesthesia Workstation Preuse Checkout" later in this chapter).

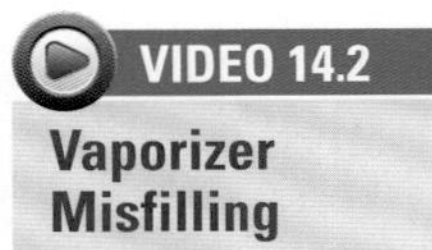

D. Anesthetic Vaporizers

Commonly used volatile anesthetics are halogenated ether compounds that readily vaporize when exposed to the atmosphere. If kept in a closed container, the space above the liquid will contain molecules of these agents in the vapor state, equilibrating with the liquid surface. The pressure exerted against the walls of the container in this space by the gas-phase molecules is known as ***vapor pressure***. At standard temperature and pressure, the measured vapor pressure for volatile anesthetics reflects the unique physicochemical characteristics of these drugs. Vapor pressure, however, is not a static value and will increase if the ambient temperature rises. The temperature at which the kinetic energy of these molecules is sufficient to counterbalance the pressure of the atmosphere (760 mm Hg at sea level) is known as the agent's ***boiling point***. At this temperature and beyond, ***all*** of the liquid agent will readily vaporize into gas.[1,2]

Figure 14.6 illustrates how the concept of saturated vapor pressure is exploited to allow the safe use of volatile anesthetics in clinical anesthesia. ***Variable bypass vaporizers*** are typically installed on most anesthesia machines. They contain an internal reservoir of liquid anesthetic agent that saturates a large wick. Molecules of anesthetic in the gaseous state emanate from this wick to create a saturated vapor pressure within the vaporizing chamber. These vaporizers are referred to as ***variable bypass*** because when they are not in use, the fresh gas flow of oxygen/air/nitrous oxide "bypasses" these vaporizers and continues onward to the patient. When the control dial of the anesthetic vaporizer is rotated in the counterclockwise direction, it diverts a portion of the carrier gas to the internal vaporizing chamber, where it will incorporate a certain amount of anesthetic gas and then return to join the fresh gas flow where the mixture of anesthetic and oxygen will be delivered to the common gas outlet. The more the dial is turned, the greater the amount of anesthetic vapor incorporated and administered to the patient.

The transformation of a substance from the liquid state into the gas phase is an endothermic process. It requires energy to make this transition. Yet, most variable bypass vaporizers are not actively heated. Therefore, the energy required to continually vaporize liquid anesthetic into gas comes from the environment: the existing thermal energy of the operating room and the walls of the vaporizer itself. If the operating room is unusually cold or high fresh gas flow is being used, which requires vaporization of a large volume of anesthetic, the temperature in the vaporizing chamber may drop. Consequently, there will be a predictable and proportional decrease in the vapor pressure of the agent, and less anesthetic will be available in the gas state to be delivered to the patient. To allow for changing temperatures in the vaporizing chamber, a bimetallic switch is placed at the interface where fresh gas flow enters the vaporizing chamber. When two metals of differing thermal conductivities are joined together, one will expand or shrink at a rate much different from the other when the local temperature increases or decreases, respectively. The result will create shearing of one metal against another. When the internal

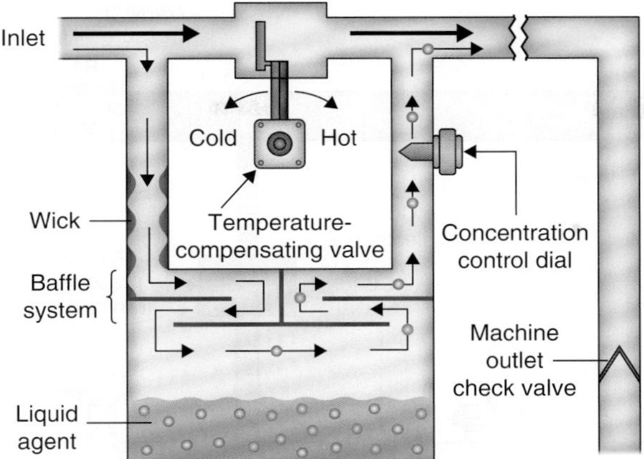

Figure 14.6 Simplified schematic of the GE Datex-Ohmeda Tec-type vaporizer. Note bimetallic strip temperature-compensating mechanism in the bypass chamber. (From Riutort KT, Eisenkraft JB. The anesthesia workstation and delivery systems for inhaled anesthetics. In: Barash PG, Cahalan MK, Cullen BF, et al, eds. *Clinical Anesthesia*. 8th ed. Wolters Kluwer; 2018:644-705, Figure 25.31.)

temperature or vapor pressure falls, the bimetallic strip bends and allows more fresh gas flow to enter the vaporizing chamber to compensate (**Figure 14.6**).[1,2]

E. Desflurane and the Tec 6 Vaporizer

Each variable bypass vaporizer described above is constructed to be agent specific and calibrated to accommodate an individual drug's unique vapor pressure and potency. Currently, these vaporizers are used to deliver isoflurane and sevoflurane.

Desflurane, however, is a newer volatile anesthetic, which, unlike its predecessors, has a boiling point close to that of room temperature. This prohibits its use in a conventional variable bypass vaporizer. Whereas a conventional variable bypass vaporizer is characterized by two parallel circuits (a bypass pathway and a vaporizing pathway), the Tec 6 vaporizer (GE Healthcare, Little Chalfont, UK) is more appropriately described as a ***single circuit gas-vapor blender*** (**Figure 14.7**).[4,6] The Tec 6 vaporizer is uniquely designed to overcome the challenges posed by desflurane's low boiling point. In this system, a reservoir of liquid desflurane is actively heated to twice its boiling point, generating pure desflurane gas. This gas is then "fuel injected" directly into the fresh gas flow line based on how far the control dial setting is opened. Truthfully, with progress in medical technology, modern anesthesia machines have now incorporated the advanced pressure, temperature, and flow sensors developed in the Tec 6 into current models of variable bypass vaporizers. With the addition of advanced microprocessors, the result is a wide variety of proprietary vaporizer technology.

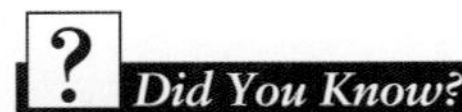

Anesthetic vaporizers must be filled with the correct agent. Failure to do so could have disastrous consequences. This is particularly true for desflurane, which requires a specially designed heated vaporizer.

III. Anesthesia Breathing Systems

Thus far, this chapter has characterized the confluence of oxygen/air/nitrous oxide and volatile anesthetics on the common fresh gas flow outlet. This section will explain what happens to this fresh gas as it enters the anesthesia breathing system. The ***circle system*** is the most commonly used design. In this system, a breathing bag (or ventilator bellows) contracts and delivers a tidal

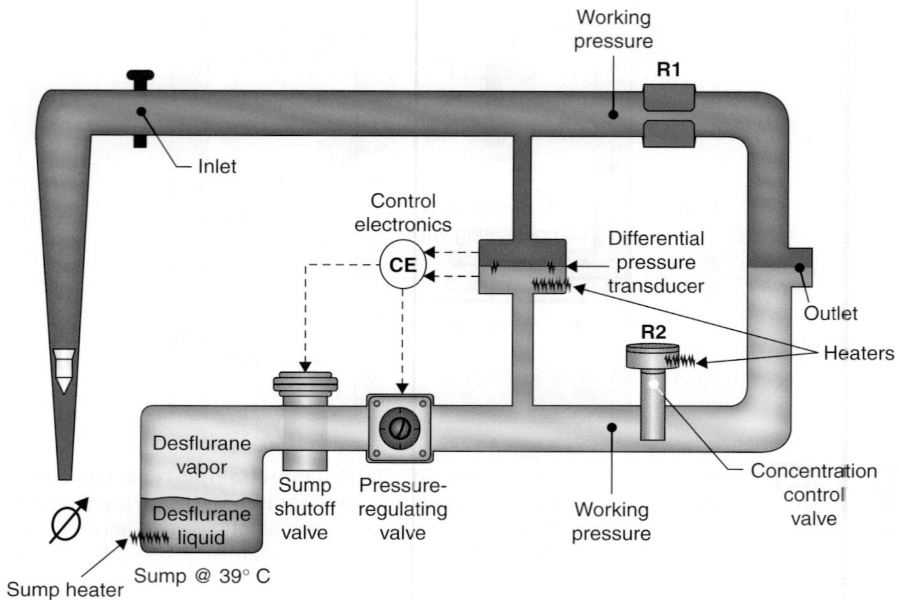

Figure 14.7 **Simplified schematic of the Tec 6 desflurane vaporizer.** (Adapted from Andrews JJ. *Operating Principles of the Ohmeda Tec 6 Desflurane Vaporizer: A Collection of Twelve Color Illustrations*. Library of Congress; 1996 and Riutort KT, Eisenkraft JB. The anesthesia workstation and delivery systems for inhaled anesthetics. In: Barash PB, Cullen BF, Stoelting RK, et al, eds. *Clinical Anesthesia*. 7th ed. Lippincott Williams & Wilkins; 2013:641-696.)

> **? Did You Know?**
>
> It is routine to administer 3 to 5 L/min of oxygen at the beginning of an anesthetic. This far exceeds the oxygen consumed by the patient. The waste gas must be vented. During manual ventilation, the APL (or "pop-off" valve) opens when pressure in the circle system exceeds the set limit. During mechanical ventilation, waste gas is vented during the expiratory phase at zero (or very low) pressure.

volume of gas into a patient's lungs. The patient exhales back into the breathing bag (or ventilator). This to-and-fro reciprocal exchange of gas between the breathing bag/ventilator and the patient's lungs allows for ***rebreathing*** of exhaled gases (**Figure 14.8**). The components of this system are as follows. First, just past the point where the fresh gas flow enters the circle system exists the ***one-way inspiratory valve***. This allows for both the delivered tidal volume and fresh gas flow to travel only in the antegrade direction to the patient through a section of corrugated tubing known as the ***inspiratory limb***. The inspiratory limb attaches to a ***Y-piece*** connector that, in turn, is connected to the patient via a mask, laryngeal mask, or endotracheal tube.

Second, during expiration, the exhaled tidal volume courses out through the Y-piece and through the ***expiratory limb*** of corrugated tubing past the ***expiratory one-way valve***. Again, this valve allows for unidirectional flow of expired gases. Between the inspiratory and expiratory valves, flow is unidirectional, as seen in **Figure 14.8**.

Third, the expired tidal volume may enter two different paths. During manual or spontaneous ventilation, some of the expired volume will pass through the ***adjustable pressure-limiting (APL) valve*** (commonly referred to as the pop-off valve) and enter the scavenging system or instead go on to reinflate the breathing bag. What fraction of the tidal volume enters scavenging versus reinflates the breathing bag is largely determined by how open or closed the APL valve position might be and the fresh gas flow rate entering the system. Additionally, a positive pressure is needed to exit through the APL valve. Hence, this typically only happens during manual, positive-pressure inspiration or at end exhalation when the breathing bag is full. Analogously,

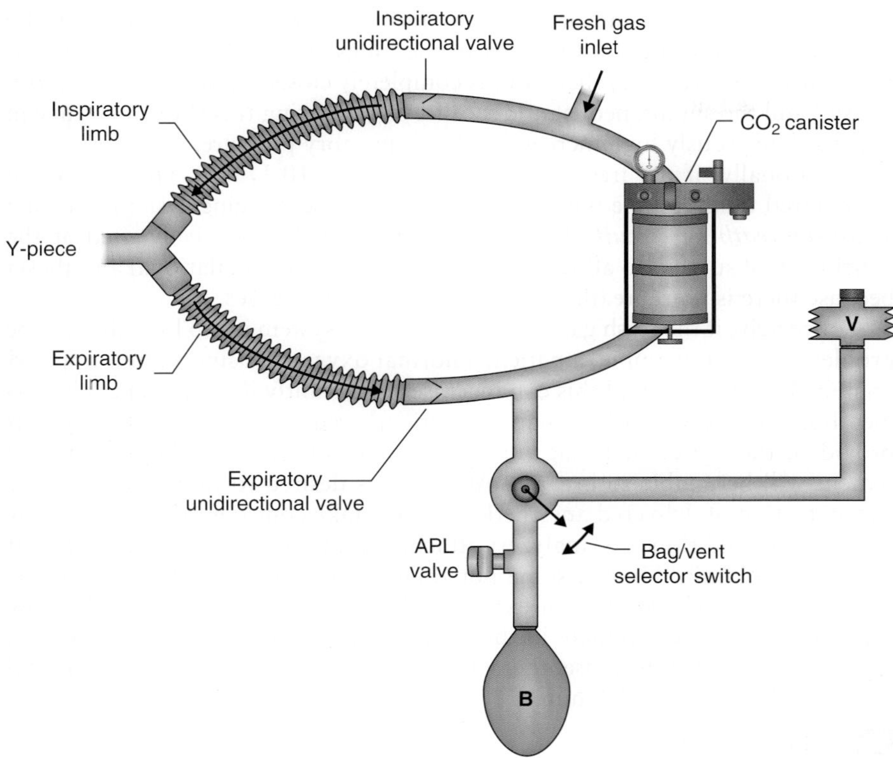

Figure 14.8 Components of the circle breathing system. APL, adjustable pressure-limiting (pop-off) valve; B, reservoir bag; CO_2, carbon dioxide; V, ventilator. (Adapted from Brockwell RC. Inhaled anesthetic delivery systems. In: Miller RD, ed. *Anesthesia*. 6th ed. Churchill Livingstone; 2004:295 and from Riutort KT, Eisenkraft JB. The anesthesia workstation and delivery systems for inhaled anesthetics. In: Barash PG, Cahalan MK, Cullen BF, et al, eds. *Clinical Anesthesia*. 8th ed. Wolters Kluwer; 2018:644-705, Figure 25.9.)

during mechanical ventilation, expired gases will act to reinflate the ventilator bellows. The ventilator contains its own pressure-relief valve, which allows expired gases to enter the scavenging system (discussed later).

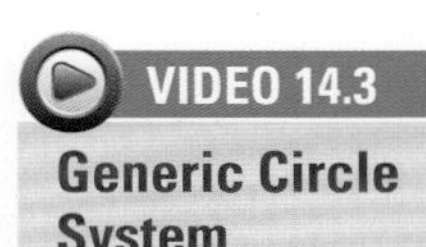

Fourth, upon the next inspiratory cycle, another tidal volume enters the inspiratory limb. Prior to doing so, however, this volume of gas must first pass through a canister filled with absorbent material aimed at neutralizing any carbon dioxide. Recall that this is a ***circle*** system that allows for ***rebreathing.*** Were it not for the presence of this carbon dioxide absorbent, the patient would ultimately sustain increasing carbon dioxide tension and hypercapnia. The circle system is intrinsically complex. Disadvantages naturally arise from multiple connections and constituent components that may malfunction or be misconnected. Adding to the intricacy is the fact that some components are disposable and others are permanent. However, this design is a popular one owing to its allowance for very low fresh gas flows and conservation of anesthetic gases, heat, and humidity.[1-4] Several interesting considerations related to the use of the circle breathing system are illustrated in the section that follows.

A. Impact of Fresh Gas Flow

Proper function of the circle system depends significantly on the fresh gas flow rate being delivered from the common gas outlet. If a very high flow (eg, >10 L/min) enters the circle system and the patient is being mechanically ventilated, there is a risk of trauma to the lungs. This is because the ventilator's automatic pressure relief valve is completely closed during the inspiratory phase,[2] and the simultaneous inflow of fresh gas during this short interval can cause a dangerously high increase in the inspiratory pressure.

Additionally, if the fresh gas flow is high (eg, 10 L/min), virtually ***all*** of the expired tidal volume will escape through the scavenging system, creating a ***non-rebreathing circuit***. This phenomenon can be effectively used at the conclusion of surgery to allow patients to emerge from inhalational anesthesia because there is no rebreathing of exhaled anesthetic gases.

Conversely, if the fresh gas flow into the circle system is too low, this can be problematic. For example, a patient's normal oxygen consumption is approximately 300 mL/min, and this can increase significantly if the patient is hypermetabolic (eg, fever). If less than the patient's required volume of oxygen is provided, the rebreathing bag (or ventilator bellows) will collapse, and the patient will be unable to breathe. Also, if it is desired to rapidly change the concentration of delivered anesthetic, this will take considerable time at a low flow rate. In addition, gas analyzers attached to the circle system can draw off up to 150 mL/min. Finally, some potentially harmful metabolites of volatile anesthetics are exhaled. Use of extremely low fresh gas flow rates will allow these products to accumulate in the circle system. Under most circumstances when a circle system is in use, there are only rare indications for use of a total fresh gas flow rate of <1 L/min.

B. Unidirectional Valves

As mentioned earlier, the presence of one-way valves ensures that a delivered tidal volume enters a patient's lungs during inspiration and exits the system during expiration. Incompetent seating of either of these valves results in ***bidirectional*** flow, which allows expired gases, particularly carbon dioxide, to contaminate the inspiratory gas. This carbon dioxide oscillates between the inspiratory and expiratory limb and is therefore immune to the presence of the carbon dioxide absorbent.[1]

C. Adjustable Pressure-Limiting Valve

During manual (bag) ventilation, the APL valve is carefully adjusted. It is partially closed off just enough to allow a sufficient tension in the breathing bag to develop. This permits the user to squeeze the bag and reliably insufflate the patient's lungs with an appropriate tidal volume. With practice, one quickly appreciates that if the APL valve is too constricted, pressure will build in the system as evidenced by high pulmonary pressures and a swelling breathing bag. Conversely, an APL valve left completely open will not enable any tension in the circuit to occur. Therefore, the anesthesiologist will not be able to manually deliver a tidal volume to the patient.

When a patient is breathing spontaneously through the circle system, the breathing bag does not require any manual compression by the anesthesiologist. Therefore, the APL valve may remain in the open position to discourage any accumulation of gas and pressure within the system. In some circumstances, such as with a patient who is developing atelectasis, the APL can be adjusted to enable a small amount of continuous positive pressure to develop in the system and expand collapsed alveoli.

D. The Breathing Bag

During the anesthetic management of adult patients, a 3-L breathing bag is typically affixed to the circle system. Smaller volume bags are available for pediatric and neonatal use. Breathing bags are considered high-volume, low-pressure systems. Beyond 3 L, the pressure within a breathing bag will rise steeply with increasing volume. However, these bags are designed so that their compliance will actually change at extremes of capacity. This limits the rise in internal pressure that can be attained.[1,2]

E. Carbon Dioxide Absorbents

Carbon dioxide absorbents consist of fine, solid-phase granules that participate in an acid-base reaction with carbon dioxide. Smaller-sized granules result in greater absorptive capacity; however, this also creates increased resistance to gas flow through the absorbent. The primary purpose of these absorbents is to ultimately convert carbon dioxide into an inert salt, calcium carbonate. Classically, older absorbents such as soda lime consisted of water, calcium hydroxide $Ca(OH)_2$, and a more potent base, sodium hydroxide (NaOH). The reaction between soda lime and carbon dioxide proceeded as follows:

1. $CO_2 + H_2O \rightarrow H_2CO_3$ (carbonic acid)
2. $H_2CO_3 + 2NaOH \rightarrow Na_2CO_3$ (sodium carbonate) + $2H_2O$
3. $Na_2CO_3 + Ca(OH)_2 \rightarrow 2NaOH + CaCO_3$ (calcium carbonate)

Of note, soda lime also contained small amounts of another reactive base, potassium hydroxide (KOH), which also participated in the above reaction in a manner entirely analogous to sodium hydroxide. Although carbon dioxide absorbents are highly effective at mitigating the risks of hypercapnia in the circle system, they impose their own brand of hazards. Strong bases such as NaOH and KOH are highly reactive, so much so that they react not only with carbon dioxide but also with the volatile anesthetics that must pass through the absorbent. Specifically, the use of sevoflurane with older absorbents has been noted to generate an intense amount of thermal energy, to the point of inciting absorbent canister fires. By-products of anesthetic degradation have also been problematic. Sevoflurane may react with carbon dioxide absorbents to form Compound A, a vinyl ether that could theoretically be nephrotoxic. Desflurane, more than any other anesthetic, is also notable for its degradation to carbon monoxide in the presence of desiccated absorbent. All of these untoward effects of anesthetic reactions with carbon dioxide absorbents are augmented when older, dry absorbent is used for prolonged periods under low fresh gas flow conditions.[1-4] Modern carbon dioxide absorbents (ie, Amsorb, Armstrong Medical, Coleraine, Northern Ireland; Drägersorb, Dräger, East Tamaki, New Zealand) have addressed the potential toxicities listed above by completely eliminating the presence of highly reactive bases such as sodium hydroxide. They consist solely of calcium hydroxide and water.[7] This results in a somewhat diminished capacity to absorb carbon dioxide. Alternatively, absorbents with a new chemical composition using lithium (Litholyme, Allied Health Care Products, St Louis, Missouri) are characterized by different chemical reactions with carbon dioxide and greater absorbent capacity.

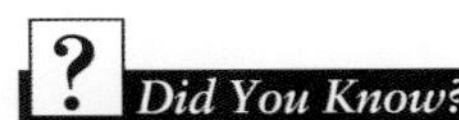

Evidence of exhausted carbon dioxide absorbent includes a change to violet color, attempts by the patient to hyperventilate, and elevated inspired carbon dioxide with capnography.

Continued use of absorbent will eventually extinguish its capacity to absorb any further carbon dioxide. Carbon dioxide absorbents are typically impregnated with an indicator dye that responds to decreasing pH when the absorbent is exhausted. Ethyl violet is most commonly used. This dye imparts a violet hue to the absorbent when it is exhausted.

F. End-Tidal Gas Monitoring, Oxygen Analyzer, and Spirometry

Measurements of respiratory gases and pulmonary volumes are not required components for a functional circle system, but they provide valuable added safety. The ***oxygen analyzer*** sits atop the inspiratory one-way valve. This location for the analyzer is particularly suitable as it will gauge the FiO_2 immediately downstream of the fresh gas flow inlet. The most commonly used analyzers use galvanic cell analysis to measure oxygen. These analyzers measure the current produced as oxygen diffuses across a membrane within, ultimately being reduced to hydroxide at the anode of an electrical circuit. The amount of current produced is proportional to the partial pressure of oxygen present.[2]

Whereas inspiratory gas analysis focuses on the fraction of inspired oxygen, ***expiratory gas analysis*** measures and displays the tensions of carbon dioxide and volatile anesthetics. Most often, a Luer-lock port at the Y-piece connector draws away expired gas at a rate of 50 to 150 mL/min to an independent infrared absorbance analyzer. This device is capable of identifying the presence and concentrations of carbon dioxide, nitrous oxide, and volatile anesthetics.[2]

Lastly, the patient's ***expired tidal volumes*** are typically measured in the expiratory limb just upstream of the expiratory one-way valve. Spirometers use a rotating vane, ultrasound, or a heated wire to measure gas flow and display the values electronically.

G. Mechanical Ventilators

Frequently, a mechanical ventilator is employed to ventilate the patient during anesthesia. This can be done to permit the anesthesiologist to have a "hands-free" method for delivering a reliable volume of ventilation, or it can be a necessity when the patient is paralyzed or has significant lung disease.

Ventilators associated with the anesthesia workstation often use a dual-circuit, gas-driven design (**Figure 14.9**). A compressible bellows assembly delivers a volume of gas to the patient. These bellows are compressed through the action of a "drive" gas, which is external to the bellows. Thus, there are ***two circuits of gas***: one for the patient's lungs, the other to drive the bellows. The drive gas may either be compressed air, oxygen, or a mixture of the two. If oxygen is used as the drive gas, then any disruption of the central supply of oxygen to the workstation will not only compromise delivery of carrier gas to the fresh gas outlet but will also render the mechanical ventilator incapable of delivering a tidal volume. Newer anesthesia machines may use a ventilator that incorporates a single-circuit, ***piston-driven*** design. In such cases, an electrically powered piston delivers a tidal volume to the patient. This of course means that failure of electrical power will incapacitate the ventilator. The latest design for delivery of controlled tidal volumes has been the inclusion of an electrically driven compressor turbine within the inspiratory limb of the circle system.[1-4]

Regardless of the mechanism through which the ventilator delivers the proposed tidal volume, there must be a route for the escape of excess gas during expiration. Similar to how the APL valve interfaces with the scavenging system during spontaneous or manual bag ventilation, a dedicated ***spill valve*** directs excess expiratory gas through this evacuation route during mechanical ventilation.[1]

Characterizing the settings of a mechanical ventilator requires defining how each breath is ***cycled*** and by what measure it is ***limited.*** Most often, mechanical ventilation is ***time cycled***, that is, the selected respiratory rate will define how often the ventilator delivers a breath. Very commonly,

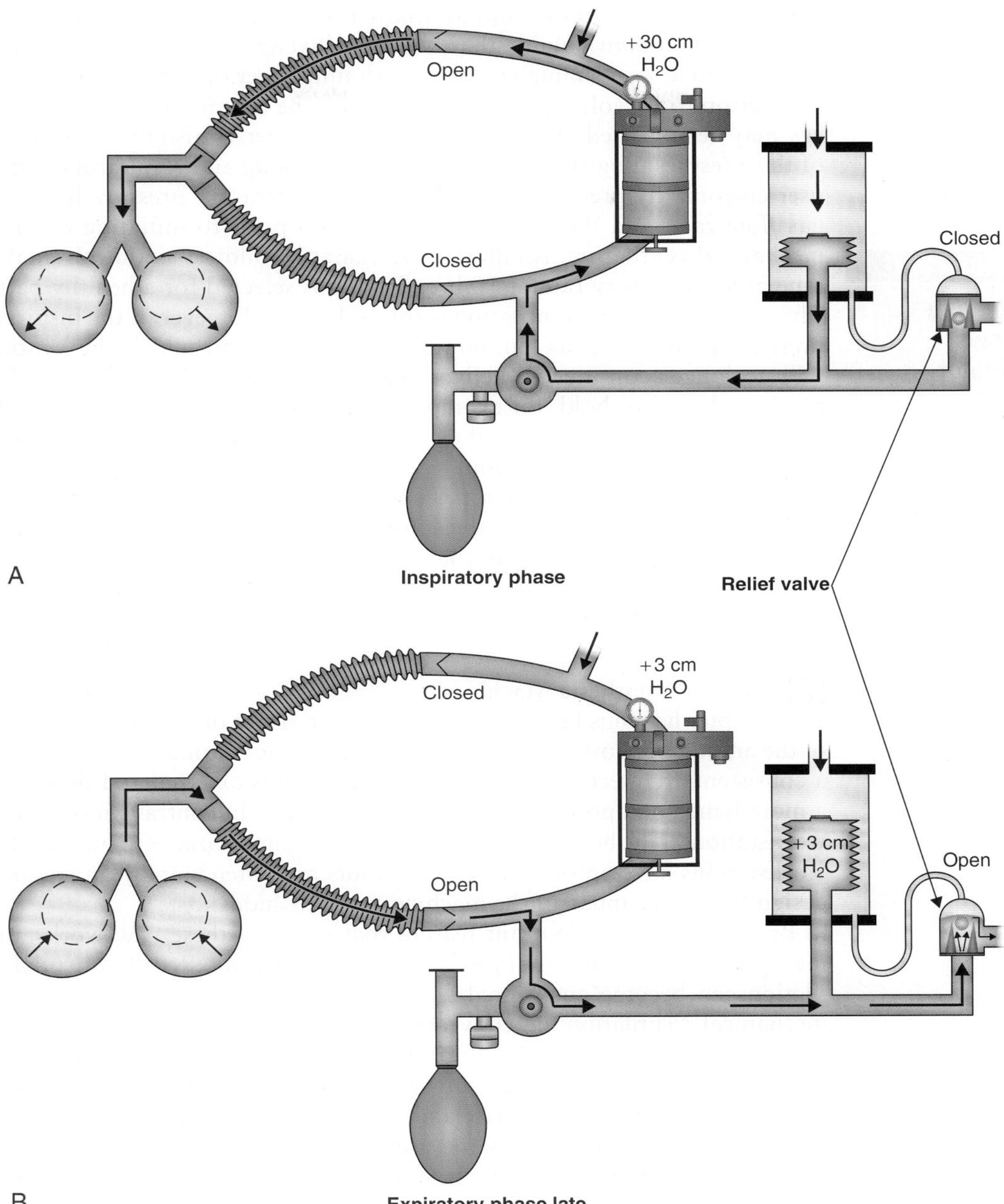

Figure 14.9 Inspiratory (**A**) and expiratory (**B**) phases of gas flow in a traditional circle system with an ascending bellows ventilator. The bellows physically separates the driving gas circuit from the patient gas circuit. The driving gas circuit is located outside the bellows, and the patient gas circuit is inside the bellows. During inspiratory phase (**A**), the driving gas enters the bellows chamber, causing the pressure within it to increase. This causes the ventilator relief valve to close, preventing anesthetic gas from escaping into the scavenging system, and the bellows to compress, delivering anesthetic gas within the bellows to the patient's lungs. During expiratory phase (**B**), pressure within the bellows chamber and the pilot line decreases to zero, causing the mushroom portion of the ventilator relief valve to open. Gas exhaled by the patient refills the bellows before any scavenging occurs because a weighted ball is incorporated into the base of the ventilator relief valve. Scavenging occurs only during the expiratory phase because the ventilator relief valve is only open during expiration. (Adapted from Andrews JJ. *The Circle System. A Collection of 30 Color Illustrations*. Library of Congress; 1998 and Riutort KT, Eisenkraft JB. The anesthesia workstation and delivery systems for inhaled anesthetics. In: Barash PG, Cahalan MK, Cullen BF, et al, eds. *Clinical Anesthesia*. 8th ed. Wolters Kluwer; 2018:644-705.)

mechanical ventilation is ***volume limited***, that is, the set tidal volume predicts the maximum volume that will be delivered to the patient. Although defining these two simple parameters should generate a predictable minute ventilation (tidal volume × respiratory rate), the true limitation of this strategy may be governed by a variety of other parameters also under the control of the anesthesiologist. In addition to ***tidal volume*** and respiratory ***rate***, the user customarily predefines the settings for inspiratory ***pressure*** limit, drive gas ***flow*** rate, and the ***inhale-to-exhale ratio*** prior to initiating controlled mechanical ventilation. An illustrative example follows: a 600-mL tidal volume at a respiratory rate of 10 breaths/min is selected for a healthy patient. The predicted minute ventilation is thus 6 L/min. However, if the inspiratory pressure limit (the peak pulmonary pressure beyond which the ventilator will no longer continue to deliver any further volume) is inadvertently set to a very low threshold, for example, 10 cm H_2O, only a small tidal volume will be delivered. In this case, the inspiratory pressure limit serves as the true limitation to minute ventilation.

VIDEO 14.4
Ascending Bellows Ventilator

Additionally, depending on the surgical procedure and the patient's underlying illnesses, the anesthesiologist may select from a variety of profiles that define how the mechanical breath is delivered. These include volume-controlled ventilation, pressure-controlled ventilation, and pressure-support ventilation with or without the inclusion of positive end-expiratory pressure.

H. Modern Anesthesia Machines

This chapter has thus far described the characteristics of a conventional model of the anesthesia workstation. Such classic machines of older generations have a consistent architecture; much of the machinery is external and they require a more hands-on approach to checkout and usage. In contrast, more modern workstations rely heavily on sophisticated, computerized processing. These workstations have automated self-checkouts and often employ an ergonomic design that keeps much of the machine anatomy hidden.[8]

By far, the most important feature that many of these new workstations incorporate is the concept of ***fresh gas flow decoupling***. Recall how tidal ventilation can become augmented when high fresh gas flows are used during mechanical ventilation in conventional anesthesia machines. This occurs because the fresh gas flow is "coupled" to the circle system during inspiration. Many new workstation designs divorce the fresh gas flow from the circle system during the inspiratory phase and, as a result, the patient only receives the prescribed tidal volume set by the user. A decoupling valve diverts fresh gas flow typically into the breathing bag during the inspiratory phase. Once exhalation commences, fresh gas flow is coupled and the gas within the breathing bag deploys into the circuit, refilling the ventilator bellows. This remarkably different design in the anesthesia workstation virtually eliminates the risk of fresh gas flow–induced volutrauma or barotrauma. The major disadvantage to fresh gas decoupled machines is the reliance imposed on the breathing bag as a fresh gas reservoir. Should the breathing bag become partially or fully disconnected, two problems arise. First, anesthetic gas will pollute the operating room. Second, room air will be entrained into the circuit, which will dilute the intended fraction of oxygen and anesthetic desired for the patient.[8]

In addition to the fundamental changes in gas delivery described above, modern anesthesia workstations are asked to accomplish far more than merely ventilate a patient's lungs. They are frequently integrated with computing systems to serve as a data processing station. In the current era of healthcare delivery in the developed world, patient data are almost exclusively tracked and logged in an electronic health record (EHR). In contrast to other fields of medicine, anesthesiology is characterized by the simultaneous acute management of the patient alongside real-time record keeping. As the latter may be construed as a distraction while performing intense cognitive and physical tasks, automated data recording systems have emerged. Anesthesia care providers may now focus primarily on clinically managing a patient, while computer systems automatically populate the EHR with ongoing vital signs, ventilatory parameters, and respiratory gas concentrations. This convenience has its own drawbacks. Each patient monitor must interface with a data hub that then transposes the information to the computing system running the EHR. The entire system is within the domain of an encrypted, hospital-based data network. For this to function properly, it requires the integrity of an enormous amount of hardware and software to be maintained. It is strongly advised that anesthesia providers become proficient in using the EHR and familiarize themselves with the basic hardware connectivity of their workspace. As one can imagine, the dysfunction of any single component of hardware or software that cannot be readily diagnosed and rectified can lead to a tremendous diversion of attention from patient care.

IV. Scavenging Systems

The primary determinant of the amount of waste gas scavenged is the fresh gas flow out of the common gas outlet. At very low flow rates, a relatively unchanging volume of gas will constantly oscillate between the patient's lungs and the breathing bag or ventilator, and very little gas will escape through the waste gas scavenging system. At high fresh gas flow rates, excess gas will vent through the scavenging system to prevent a buildup of volume and pressure. Both the mechanical ventilator and the breathing bag are connected to the scavenging terminal through 19-mm hose connectors. During manual or spontaneous ventilation, waste gas is vented through the APL. When the ventilator is in use, waste gas is vented during expiration. During that interval in the respiratory cycle, after a certain pressure threshold has been reached, typically 2 cm H_2O, the spill valve will open and vent the excess gas into the scavenging hose. From the scavenging terminal, a third hose directs the waste gas out of the operating room and ultimately out of the hospital (**Figure 14.10**).

Once waste gas exits the anesthesia workstation, a variety of systems exist to dispose of them. A defining characteristic of scavenging systems relates to the dynamics of gas flow, which may be either ***active*** or ***passive***. In active systems, negative pressure is applied through the hospital vacuum to facilitate the removal of waste gas. Passive systems rely simply on the small amount of positive pressure generated during exhalation to promote waste gas disposal. Scavenging systems may additionally be defined according to their anatomic design, either open or closed. Closed systems are self-explanatory: a system of hoses evacuates exhaled gas in a contained manner that prohibits the waste gas from entering the operating room. Open systems contain vents in the scavenging reservoir that ***do*** allow waste gas to ***potentially*** enter the operating room. At first glance, one may question the merit of an open system, a design that decidedly allows waste gas to contaminate the operating room environment. The following two examples serve to justify how open systems may be intrinsically safer than closed systems.

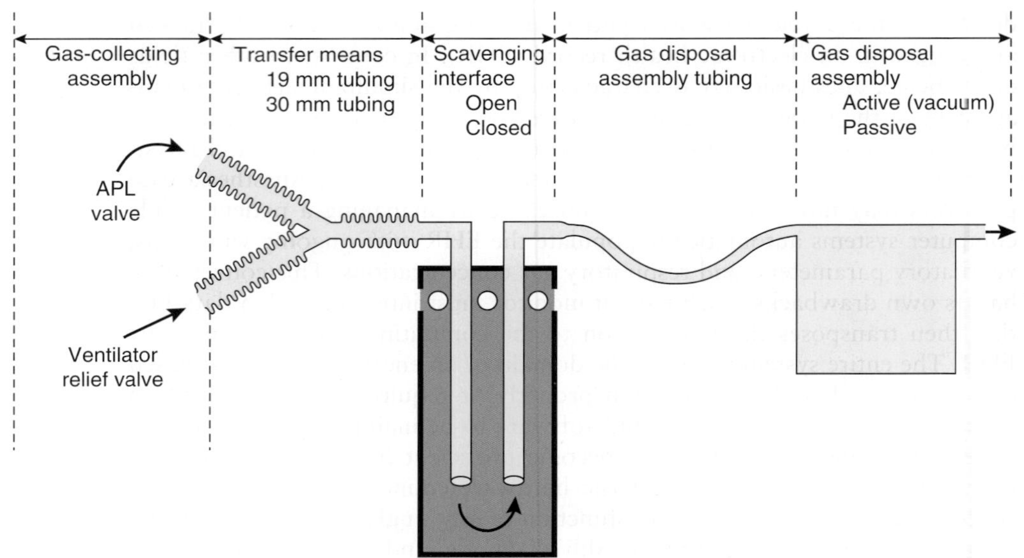

Figure 14.10 **Components of a scavenging system. APL, adjustable pressure-limiting valve.** (Riutort KT, Eisenkraft JB. The anesthesia workstation and delivery systems for inhaled anesthetics. In: Barash PG, Cahalan MK, Cullen BF, et al, eds. *Clinical Anesthesia*. 8th ed. Wolters Kluwer; 2018:644-705, Figure 25.49.)

Think about what might happen if the hose that sends waste gases out of the room becomes occluded. In a closed system, waste gas would accumulate, generating positive pressure that could theoretically be conveyed to the patient. The presence of vents in the scavenging reservoir in an open system, however, would allow this excess pressure to dissipate into the operating room. Consider the opposite problem as well. Perhaps an excessive amount of negative pressure is applied to evacuate waste gas. In such a scenario, too ***much*** gas is being relieved from the circle system in closed designs. The very same vents described earlier in open systems would entrain room air to accommodate this excessive negative pressure. Closed systems are acceptable for use, but they must retain mechanisms that mitigate the problems illustrated by the above examples. Closed systems harbor positive-pressure and negative-pressure relief valves. The former bleeds open into the operating room when excessive pressure accumulates within the scavenging system. Negative-pressure relief valves, however, respond to excessive negative pressure and entrain room air to compensate.[1-4]

? *Did You Know?*

Like competent pilots before they fly, it is highly recommended that the anesthesiologist performs a thorough check of the anesthesia workstation before use and, for quality control purposes, documents that it was done.

V. Anesthesia Workstation Preuse Checkout

The American Society of Anesthesiologists (ASA) has published, and regularly revises, recommendations for a preuse checkout of the anesthesia workstation. A basic summary of the 15-point checklist is provided in **Table 14.2**. However, the full, comprehensive elaboration of the checklist can be found at the ASA website.[9] Anesthesiologists are advised to follow these recommendations. Additionally, they are encouraged to become familiar with the manufacturer's operations manual for the specific workstation(s) they intend to use.

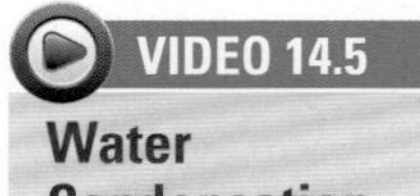

VIDEO 14.5

Water Condensation in Breathing Circuit

Table 14.2 Summary of the American Society of Anesthesiologists Preanesthesia Checkout Recommendations

ITEMS TO BE COMPLETED (*, daily; +, before each procedure):
Item 1*: Verify auxiliary oxygen cylinder and self-inflating manual ventilation device are available and functioning.
Item 2*+: Verify patient suction is adequate to clear the airway.
Item 3*: Turn on anesthesia delivery system and confirm that AC power is available.
Item 4*+: Verify availability of required monitors and check alarms.
Item 5*: Verify that pressure is adequate on the spare oxygen cylinder mounted on the anesthesia machine.
Item 6*: Verify that piped gas pressures are ≥50 psi gauge.
Item 7*+: Verify that vaporizers are adequately filled and, if applicable, that the filler ports are tightly closed.
Item 8*: Verify that there are no leaks in the gas supply lines between the flowmeters and the common gas outlet.
Item 9*: Test scavenging system function.
Item 10*: Calibrate, or verify calibration of, the oxygen monitor and check the low oxygen alarm. Verify the function of the carbon dioxide analyzer.
Item 11*+: Verify carbon dioxide absorbent is not exhausted.
Item 12*+: Breathing system pressure and leak testing.
Item 13*+: Verify that gas flows properly through the breathing circuit during both inspiration and exhalation. Check function of one-way valves.
Item 14*+: Document completion of checkout procedures.
Item 15*+: Confirm ventilator settings and evaluate readiness to deliver anesthesia care.

From The American Society of Anesthesiologists. *2008 Recommendations for Preanesthesia Checkout.* 2008. www.asahq.org/For-Members/Clinical-Information/2008-ASA-Recommendations-for-PreAnesthesia-Checkout.aspx

For further review and interactivities, please see the associated Interactive Video Lectures and "A Closer Look" infographic accessible in the complimentary eBook bundled with this text. Access instructions are located in the inside front cover.

References

1. Dorsch JA, Dorsch SE. *A Practical Approach to Anesthesia Equipment.* Lippincott Williams & Wilkins; 2011.
2. Davey AJ, Ali D.. *Ward's Anaesthetic Equipment.* 6th ed. Elsevier; 2012.
3. Baha A. *Essentials of Equipment in Anaesthesia, Critical Care and Peri-Operative Medicine.* 5th ed. Elsevier; 2019.
4. Ehrenwerth J. *Anesthesia Equipment: Principles and Applications.* 2nd ed. Saunders; 2013.
5. Atlas G. A method to quickly estimate remaining time for an oxygen E-cylinder. *Anesth Analg.* 2004;98:1190.
6. Andrews JJ, Johnston RV Jr, Kramer GC. Consequences of misfilling contemporary vaporizers with desflurane. *Can J Anaesth.* 1993;40:71.
7. Versichelen LF, Bouche MP, Rolly G, et al. Only carbon dioxide absorbents free of both NaOH and KOH do not generate compound-A during in vitro closed system sevoflurane. *Anesthesiology.* 2001;95:750.
8. Olympio MA. *Modern Anesthesia Machines Offer New Safety Features. Anesthesia Patient Safety Foundation Newsletter.* 2003. https://www.apsf.org/article/modern-anesthesia-machines-offer-new-safety-features/
9. The American Society of Anesthesiologists. *2008 Recommendations for Preanesthesia Checkout.* 2008. https://www.asahq.org/standards-and-guidelines/2008-asa-recommendations-for-pre-anesthesia-checkout

ASA PREANESTHESIA CHECKOUT

A CLOSER LOOK

Illustrated below is a visual checklist of mandatory items that must be verified before providing anesthetic care according to the ASA preanesthesia checkout.

These items must be completed daily.

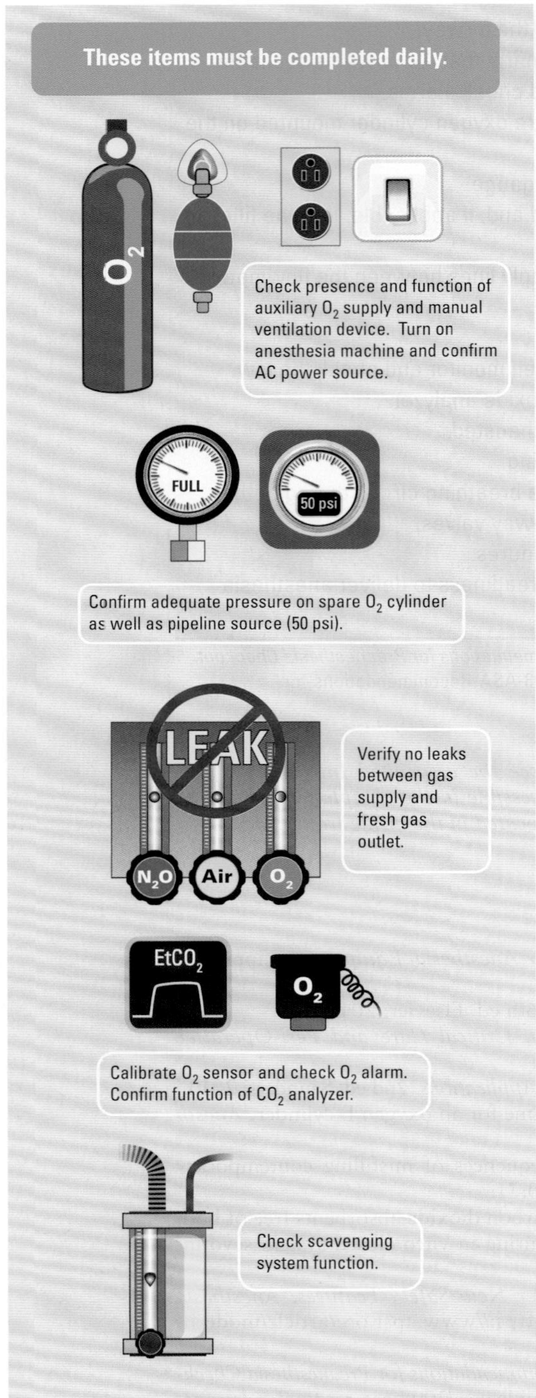

O_2
Check presence and function of auxiliary O_2 supply and manual ventilation device. Turn on anesthesia machine and confirm AC power source.
FULL
50 psi
Confirm adequate pressure on spare O_2 cylinder as well as pipeline source (50 psi).
LEAK
N_2O
Air
O_2
Verify no leaks between gas supply and fresh gas outlet.
$EtCO_2$
O_2
Calibrate O_2 sensor and check O_2 alarm. Confirm function of CO_2 analyzer.
Check scavenging system function.

These items must be completed before *each procedure.*

Check that suction is set up and operational.

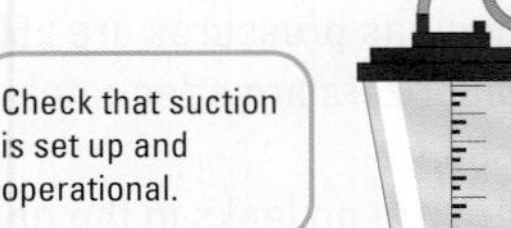

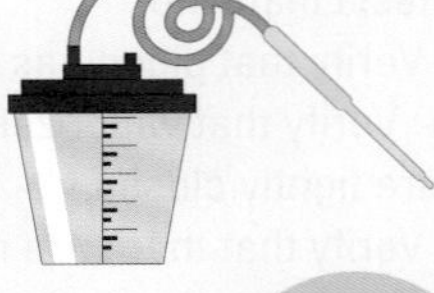

Confirm presence of all monitors and alarms.

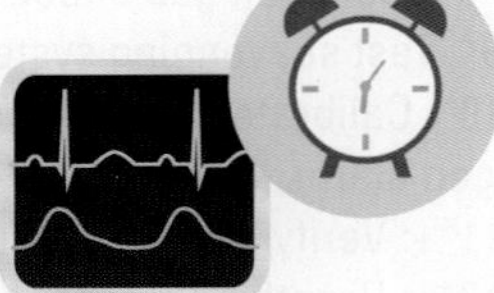

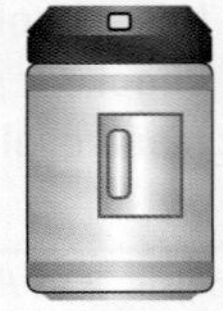

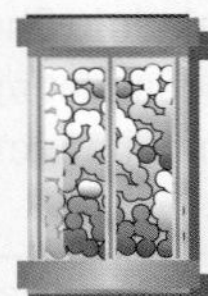

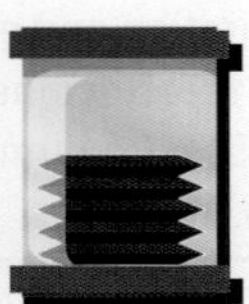

Check vaporizer level and confirm filler ports are tightly closed. Verify CO_2 absorbent is not exhausted. Confirm ventilator settings.

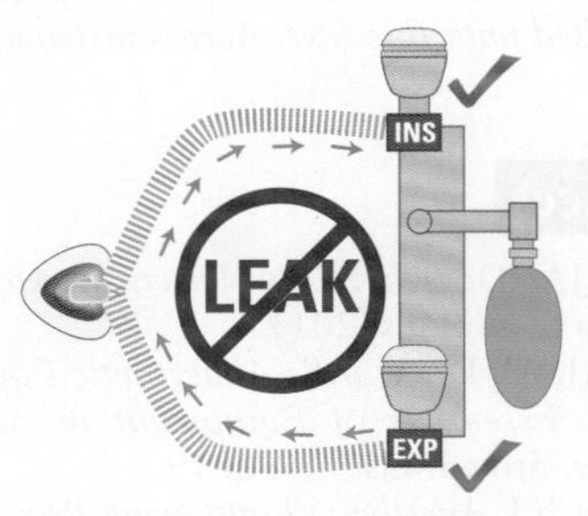

Confirm that the circle system can hold positive pressure and also pass the leak test. Verify proper gas flow through breathing circuit and integrity of one-way valves.

Document completion of checkout procedures.

Infographic by: Naveen Nathan MD

Questions

1. **Your department has purchased brand new anesthesia machines and you are using one for the first time. As compared to older, conventional anesthesia machines, the main hazard to be mindful of with new machines is which of the following?**

   A. Volutraumatic lung injury when using high fresh gas flows during mechanical ventilation
   B. Patient awareness during mechanical ventilation if the breathing bag becomes disconnected
   C. Consumption of oxygen for use as a drive gas for the ventilator bellows
   D. Greater chance of malfunction of inspiratory and/or expiratory one-way valves

2. **Modern carbon dioxide absorbents are considered safer with respect to potential toxic by-products when exposed to volatile anesthetics. The main component in older absorbents that imposed this risk was which of the following?**

   A. Lithium salts
   B. Calcium carbonate
   C. Calcium hydroxide
   D. Sodium hydroxide

3. **Variable bypass vaporizers are calibrated to exploit which property of volatile anesthetics to deliver these drugs into the fresh gas flow path of the anesthesia machine?**

   A. Boiling point
   B. Lipid solubility
   C. Vapor pressure
   D. Thermal conductivity

4. **Which of the following mechanisms helps ensure that a medical gas supply line like nitrous oxide will not be inadvertently connected to the wrong coupling interface on the back of an anesthesia machine?**

   A. Fail-safe system
   B. Diameter index system
   C. Proportioning system
   D. Pin index system

5. **A healthy 3-year-old boy requires general anesthesia. An inhalational induction with sevoflurane is performed using 100% oxygen at 10 L/min fresh gas flow. Gas flow at this rate is characterized by which of the following properties?**

   A. Dependence on gas density
   B. Laminar flow dynamics
   C. Lower risk of depletion of volatile anesthetic
   D. Flow through a smaller diameter Thorpe tube

Answers

1. B

New machines use fresh gas flow decoupling in which the fresh gas flow is diverted into the breathing bag during mechanical inspiration. Thus, the breathing bag is directly involved even during mechanical ventilation. If the breathing bag becomes disconnected, volatile anesthetic will spill into the operating room contaminating it and the patient will not receive sufficient anesthesia as the leak entrains room air into the circuit.

2. D

Sodium hydroxide is a very reactive base that leads to potentially toxic by-products when it encounters volatile agents in the absorbent.

3. C

Vaporizers are calibrated to the saturated vapor pressure of an inhalational anesthetic, which determines the vapor tension inside the vaporizer during use.

4. B

The diameter index safety system ensures hospital supply gases are interfaced to the correct coupling on the anesthesia machine. A given gas hose has a unique diameter that will not fit on an incorrect gas coupling.

5. A

The question describes high gas flows that are turbulent. Turbulent gas flow is dependent on gas density.

15 Standard Anesthesia Monitoring Techniques and Instruments

Grace C. McCarthy and Jonathan B. Mark

Monitoring of patients during anesthesia begins with a ***vigilant anesthesia provider***—visual inspection of chest rise and patient color for ventilation and oxygenation and palpation of the pulse for heart rate and blood pressure estimation. Although technology has enhanced the anesthesia provider's ability to monitor and treat patients during anesthesia and surgery, a vigilant anesthesia provider with good clinical decision-making skills is still required. Standards for basic anesthetic monitoring published by the American Society of Anesthesiologists emphasize the need for a qualified anesthesia provider to be in the room for all anesthetics and monitored anesthesia care (**Table 15.1**).

I. Basic Anesthesia Monitoring

The "Standards for Basic Anesthetic Monitoring" were first published in 1986 and updated in 2015 (**Table 15.1**).[1] These standards lay the foundation for the minimal monitoring needed during all anesthesia care, and they begin with the continual presence of a qualified anesthesia provider. Depending on the clinical judgment of this provider, more intensive monitoring may be needed in some cases.

A. Oxygenation

Proper ***oxygenation*** of the patient is ensured in two ways. During general anesthesia using an anesthesia machine, the provider needs to confirm that there is a sufficient concentration of oxygen being delivered. Most anesthesia machines use a galvanic cell analyzer located in the inspired limb of the anesthesia circuit and are equipped with a low oxygen concentration alarm that will alert the provider to a dangerous hypoxic gas mixture. The oxygen analyzer may require daily calibration and intermittent replacement. If a patient is receiving supplemental oxygen by nasal cannula or facemask during regional anesthesia or monitored anesthesia care, the provider must ensure the proper flow of oxygen from the wall oxygen supply or gas cylinder.

After ensuring sufficient oxygen delivery to the patient or the breathing circuit, oxygenation of the patient's blood must be monitored qualitatively, most often via the patient's skin or mucous membrane color, and quantitatively with a ***pulse oximeter***. This device has become ubiquitous both inside and outside the operating room because it provides a continuous, noninvasive, and accurate measurement of arterial hemoglobin oxygen saturation.

Table 15.1 Summary of the American Society of Anesthesiologists "Standards for Basic Anesthetic Monitoring"

Standard 1
Qualified anesthesia personnel shall be present in the room throughout the conduct of all general anesthetics, regional anesthetics, and monitored anesthesia care.
Standard 2
During all anesthetics, the patient's oxygenation, ventilation, circulation, and temperature shall be continually evaluated.
Oxygenation
Oxygen concentration of the inspired gas
Observation of the patient's skin and mucous membrane color
Pulse oximetry
Ventilation
Observation of the patient and reservoir bag
Mechanical ventilation circuit disconnection alarms
Auscultation of breath sounds
Continuous end-tidal carbon dioxide measurement
Circulation
Continuous ECG display
Heart rate and blood pressure measured at least every 5 minutes
Evaluation of the circulation: auscultation of heart sounds, palpation of pulse, pulse plethysmography, pulse oximetry, intra-arterial pressure tracing
Temperature
Continual temperature monitoring, when significant changes are anticipated or suspected

ECG, electrocardiogram.
From American Society of Anesthesiologists. Standards for Basic Anesthetic Monitoring. https://www.asahq.org/standards-and-guidelines/standards-for-basic-anesthetic-monitoring

? *Did You Know?*

The pulse oximeter has a significant delay (15-30 seconds) in the detection of changes in arterial oxygen saturation.

The pulse oximeter emits two wavelengths of light (red and near-infrared) and uses a photo detector to measure the absorbance of oxygenated and deoxygenated hemoglobin in the blood. The oximeter then uses an algorithm to calculate the percentage of the total hemoglobin that exists as oxyhemoglobin, and displays this as the hemoglobin saturation (SpO_2). This monitor must also differentiate the ***pulsatile arterial signal*** (and thus the ***arterial*** hemoglobin oxygen saturation) from the nonpulsatile venous (and other tissue) saturation. Although a pulse oximeter is considered to be a continuous monitor, there can still be a significant delay (of up to 15-30 seconds) before it alarms to note a decrease in the SpO_2.

The pulse oximeter has a variable-pitch tone to signal changes in SpO_2, and an abnormally low or suddenly decreasing SpO_2 (<90%) triggers the monitor to provide an audible warning alert of impending patient deterioration. However, like any monitor, the pulse oximeter is subject to artifacts and inaccurate readings (**Table 15.2**). A vigilant anesthesia provider is necessary to determine whether a low SpO_2 on the monitor is artifactual or a real event that necessitates intervention.

Beyond measurement of SpO_2, the pulse oximeter has other features that are useful during anesthesia. The pulse oximeter ***plethysmographic waveform*** provides a measurement of heart rate (pulse rate) and a crude estimation of

Table 15.2 Limitations of the Pulse Oximeter

Low Blood Flow Conditions (or decrease in arterial pulsatility)
• Hypotension
• Hypothermia causing peripheral vasoconstriction
• High-dose vasopressors
• Cardiopulmonary bypass
Movement Artifacts
• Light anesthesia/no paralysis
• Surgical interference
• Neuromuscular twitch monitor causing motion artifact
• Shivering
Varying Light Absorbance
• Methemoglobinemia
• Carboxyhemoglobinemia
• Methylene blue/indigo carmine
• Nail polish
• Ambient light

blood pressure, because the waveform will appear dampened or disappear altogether when there is severe hypotension. Newer generations of pulse oximeters are less influenced by patient motion and other sources of artifact. Some devices measure the concentration of other forms of hemoglobin (ie, carboxyhemoglobin and methemoglobin) and even measure the total hemoglobin concentration. Pulse oximeter waveform analysis may also be used to estimate intravascular volume status and volume responsiveness through analysis of the changes in pulse wave contour during the respiratory cycle.[2] Although the pulse oximeter is mostly used with a finger probe, other probes can be used on the ear, nares, cheek, or forehead. Pulse oximeters will not work when there are no arterial pulsations (eg, on cardiopulmonary bypass), and other techniques must be used, such as reflectance oximetry, which does not depend on arterial pulsations.

B. Ventilation

Ventilation, or the movement of gases between the environment and the alveoli, is another important aspect of a patient's physiology to monitor during anesthesia (**Table 15.1**). This can be accomplished by visual inspection of chest rise and fall, condensation of airway water vapor in the endotracheal tube or facemask during expiration, or the cyclic filling and emptying of the reservoir bag or ventilator bellows. The anesthesia machine measures tidal volume and respiratory rate and can alarm if these ventilator parameters fall outside a predetermined range.

During general anesthesia, the best monitor for determining adequacy of ventilation is the measurement of ***exhaled carbon dioxide*** (***CO_2***) and its end-tidal or end-expiratory value. A small sample of respiratory circuit gas is continually removed from the anesthesia breathing circuit for measurement of CO_2 and other gases using an infrared absorption spectrophotometer. The CO_2 concentration is continually displayed as a time-dependent waveform, called a ***capnogram*** (**Figure 15.1**), and is usually reported in millimeters of mercury (mm Hg).

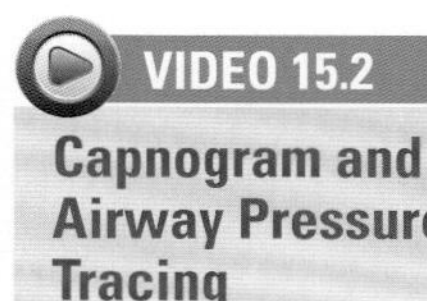

At the beginning of a general anesthetic, a normal-appearing capnogram confirms correct placement of the endotracheal tube in the trachea rather than

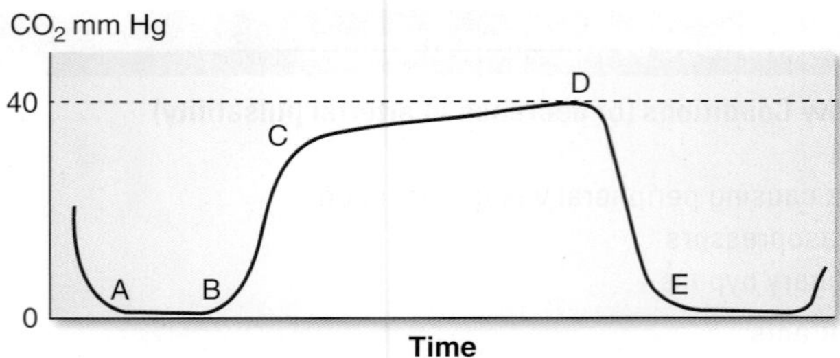

A-B: Initial expiration, mostly dead space with no CO_2
B-C: Exhaled CO_2 begins to reach the analyzer
C-D: Expiratory plateau, alveolar CO_2 being measured
Point D: End-tidal CO_2 measurement taken here
D-E: Inspiration

Figure 15.1 **Normal capnogram and phases of the respiratory cycle.** (From Connor CW, Conley CM. Commonly used monitoring techniques. In: Barash PG, Cahalan MK, Cullen BF, et al, eds. *Clinical Anesthesia*. 8th ed. Wolters Kluwer; 2018:706-730. Figure 26.3.)

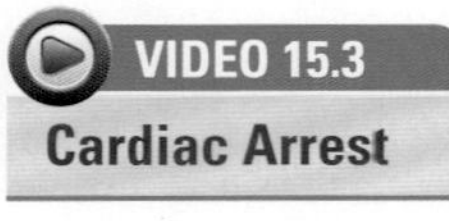

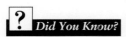

? Did You Know?

The shape of the capnograph provides important information including the presence of bronchospasm.

the esophagus. Both the CO_2 value and the shape of the capnogram provide important diagnostic clues about metabolic, respiratory, circulatory, or technical problems with the patient or anesthesia machine (**Figure 15.2; Table 15.3**). For example, a decrease in the end-expiratory or end-tidal CO_2 ($ETCO_2$) indicates a potentially serious problem that must be addressed. Although the most common cause of low $ETCO_2$ is hyperventilation or increased dead space ventilation, a sudden and large decrease may be a sign of a misplaced endotracheal tube or a reduction in lung perfusion resulting from pulmonary embolism, anaphylaxis, or cardiac arrest. Capnography is also an important monitor during regional anesthesia or monitored anesthesia care. Although the CO_2 value measured from a nasal cannula or facemask will likely underestimate the true $ETCO_2$, owing to dilution with room air, a marked change

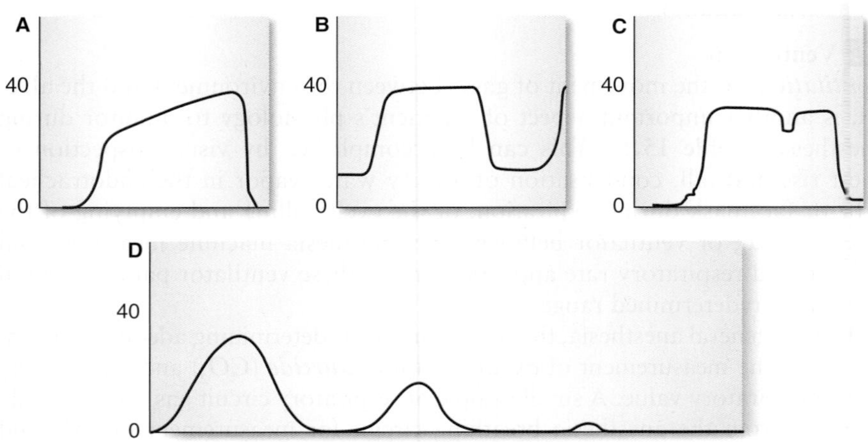

Figure 15.2 Abnormal capnograms. A, Steep, prolonged upslope indicating bronchospasm or expiratory airway obstruction. B, Increase in the baseline due to rebreathing carbon dioxide (CO_2), such as with an exhausted CO_2 absorbent. C, "Curare cleft," which may indicate a patient's attempt at spontaneous ventilation during positive pressure mechanical ventilation. D, Esophageal intubation.

Table 15.3 Factors That May Change the End-Tidal CO_2 Measurement or Waveform During Anesthesia

Increases in $ETCO_2$	Decreases in $ETCO_2$
Changes in CO_2 Production	
Increases in metabolic rate:	Decreases in metabolic rate:
• Hyperthermia • Sepsis • Malignant hyperthermia • Shivering • Hyperthyroidism	• Hypothermia • Hypothyroidism
Changes in CO_2 Elimination	
• Hypoventilation • Rebreathing	• Hyperventilation • Hypoperfusion • Pulmonary embolism

CO_2, carbon dioxide; $ETCO_2$, end-tidal carbon dioxide.
Adapted from Connor CE. Commonly used monitoring techniques. In: Barash P, Cullen B, Stoelting R, et al, eds. *Clinical Anesthesia*. 7th ed. Wolters Kluwer/Lippincott Williams & Wilkins; 2013:263-285, with permission.

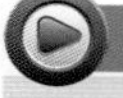
VIDEO 15.4
Hypocarbia Differential Diagnosis

in the capnogram or loss of the waveform entirely provides a prompt alert that there may be severe hypoventilation, apnea, or obstruction of the airway. Particularly in patients who are breathing supplemental oxygen, the capnogram is an early warning that occurs before a low SpO_2 is detected by the pulse oximeter.

C. Circulation

A patient's ***circulation*** is monitored in multiple different ways during anesthesia. ***Continuous electrocardiogram (ECG) monitoring*** is standard of care in anesthesia and provides important information (**Table 15.4**), including cardiac rate and rhythm. A wide range of rhythm disturbances may occur during anesthesia, and most all can be detected and diagnosed with a simple three-lead ECG system using the standard bipolar limb leads I, II, and III (**Figure 15.3**). However, cardiac ischemia is best detected by monitoring a five-lead ECG and displaying both leads II and V_5, a technique that can have a sensitivity of up to 80%. V_5 is often used instead of the potentially more sensitive medial precordial leads (**Figure 15.4**), because the latter often interfere with the sterile surgical field.[3] ST-segment depression, or ***subendocardial ischemia*** (**Figure 15.5**), is probably the most common form of perioperative cardiac ischemia, reflecting an oxygen supply-demand mismatch, or ***demand ischemia***. However, transmural or ***supply ischemia*** reflected by ECG ST elevations can also be seen in the perioperative setting (**Figure 15.6**).

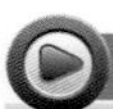
VIDEO 15.5
Electrocardiogram Principles

VIDEO 15.6
Heart Electrical Conduction System

Table 15.4 Goals of Intraoperative Electrocardiogram Monitoring

- Heart rate monitoring
- Detection of arrhythmias and conduction abnormalities
- Detection of myocardial ischemia
- Monitoring pacemaker function or malfunction
- Identification of electrolyte abnormalities

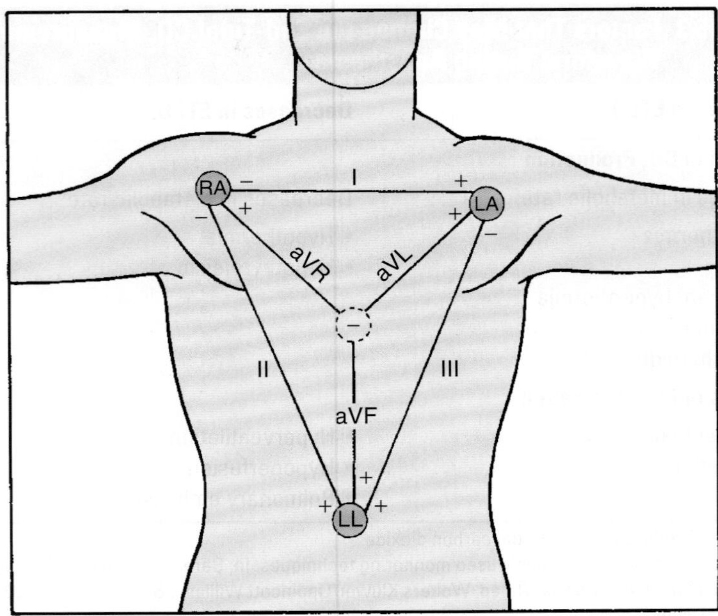

Figure 15.3 Three-lead ECG bipolar limb leads.

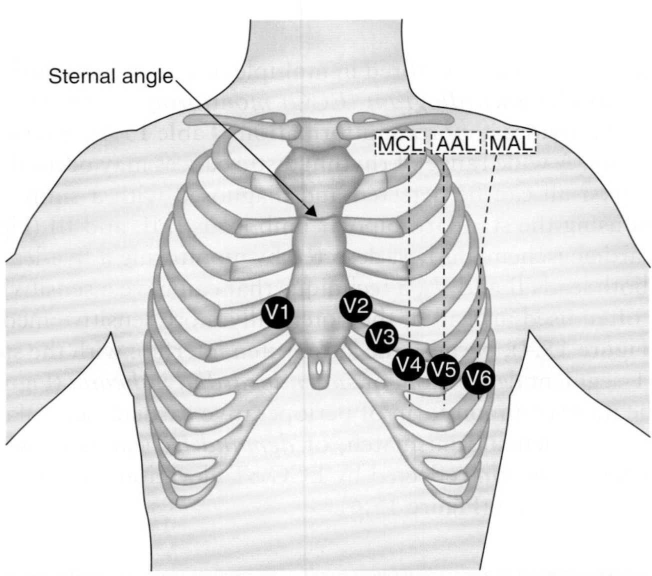

Figure 15.4 Precordial electrocardiogram lead placement. V_3 or V_4 may be more sensitive for detecting cardiac ischemia; however, V_5 is often used, as it is more likely to avoid the surgical field. AAL, anterior axillary line; MAL, mid-axillary line; MCL, mid-clavicular line. (Derived from Mark JB. *Atlas of Cardiovascular Monitoring*. Churchill Livingstone; 1998.)

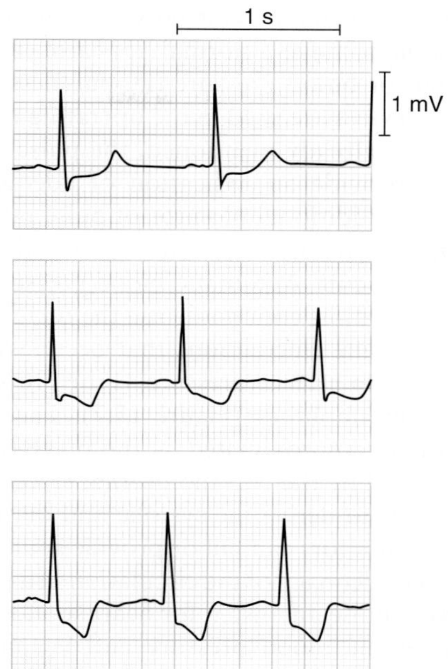

Figure 15.5 Electrocardiogram changes displaying horizontal or downsloping ST-segment depression may indicate "demand ischemia." (Derived from Mark JB. *Atlas of Cardiovascular Monitoring*. Churchill Livingstone; 1998.)

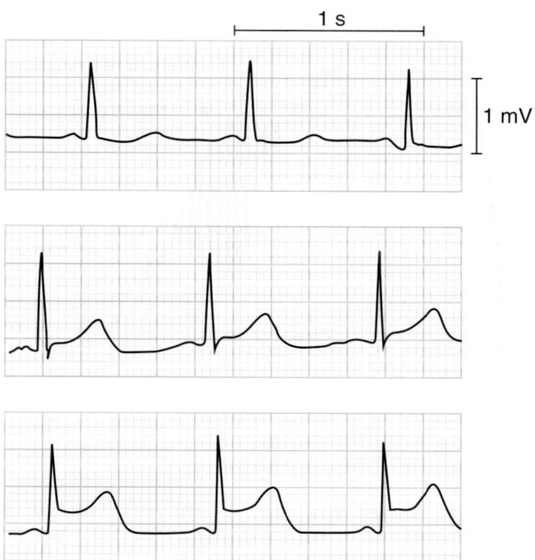

Figure 15.6 Electrocardiogram changes displaying ST-segment elevation, usually the result of coronary artery occlusion. (Derived from Mark JB. *Atlas of Cardiovascular Monitoring*. Churchill Livingstone; 1998.)

It is important to note that the ECG is only a monitor of cardiac electrical activity, and it is possible to have a normal-appearing ECG tracing with little or no cardiac output or blood pressure (ie, pulseless electrical activity or PEA). Therefore, other devices are used in the operating room to further assess a patient's circulation. As already mentioned, the pulse oximeter plethysmographic waveform can provide an indication of adequate perfusion to an extremity and displays an additional monitor of pulse rate.

Blood pressure should, at the very least, be monitored every 5 minutes via a noninvasive blood pressure cuff. Automatic blood pressure cuffs differ slightly between manufacturers but most commonly use the ***oscillometric method***. This method measures the pressure fluctuations that occur with arterial pulsation and usually measures a mean arterial pressure as the pressure at which arterial pulsations are maximal in amplitude (**Figure 15.7**). The systolic and diastolic blood pressures are usually approximated as the pressure at onset and offset of arterial pulsations sensed by the cuff monitoring system, but most monitors use proprietary algorithms to derive the systolic and diastolic pressure values. Given that all electronic monitors can fail or provide spurious values, whenever there is concern about the adequacy of the circulation in a patient, the anesthesia provider should feel for a pulse and listen for heart sounds.

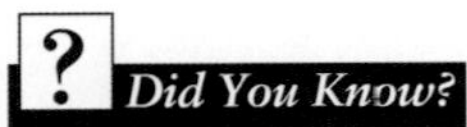

Most noninvasive blood pressure devices use an oscillometric technique, which explains why they are so sensitive to movement artifact.

Appropriate sizing of the blood pressure cuff is important for accurate blood pressure measurement. Inappropriate cuff size is the most common error in blood pressure measurement. A correctly sized blood pressure cuff should have a bladder width at least 40% the circumference of the extremity and bladder length at least 80% the circumference of the extremity (Table 15.5).[4] To aid correct sizing, most cuffs have a line to indicate when the correct size is applied to the patient's arm. Overestimation of blood pressure can

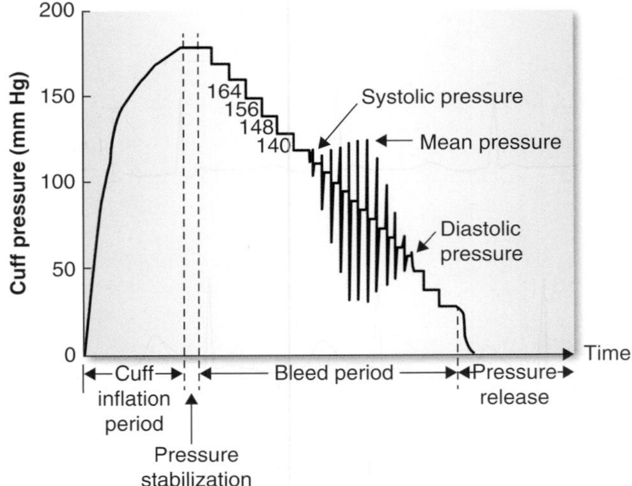

Figure 15.7 Noninvasive blood pressure measurement via the oscillometric method. The cuff is automatically inflated above systolic pressure (no pressure fluctuations present) and then decrementally deflated. Sensors measure the magnitude of the pressure oscillations in the surrounding cuff, which initially increase in magnitude and then decrease. Maximal oscillations occur at the mean arterial blood pressure, and proprietary device algorithms are used to measure the systolic and diastolic pressure values. (Adapted from Dorsch JA, Dorsch SE. *Understanding Anesthesia Equipment.* 4th ed. Williams & Wilkins; 1999 and From Connor CW, Conley CM. Commonly used monitoring techniques. In: Barash PG, Cahalan MK, Cullen BF, et al, eds. *Clinical Anesthesia.* 8th ed. Wolters Kluwer; 2018:706-730, Figure 26.5.)

Table 15.5 Recommended Cuff Sizes for Accurate Measurement of Blood Pressure

Arm Circumference		Recommended Cuff Size (width × length in cm)
cm	in	
22-26	8.7-10.2	12 × 22 (small adult)
27-34	10.6-13.4	16 × 30 (adult)
35-44	13.8-17.3	16 × 36 (large adult)
45-52	17.7-20.5	16 × 42 (extra-large adult)

occur if the cuff is too small, while underestimation may occur with a cuff that is too large. In obese patients, cuff placement may be difficult owing, in part, to the noncylindrical shape of the upper arm, which on occasion might require cuff placement on the forearm or calf.

A second common error in noninvasive blood pressure measurement occurs when the patient is not supine and the cuff is not aligned at the level of the heart.[5] While this is important when the patient is in the lateral position, and the arm is either above or below heart level (leading to blood pressure underestimation or overestimation, respectively), it is extremely important when the patient is in a sitting or "beach chair" position for an operation and the blood pressure cuff is applied to the calf (eg, for shoulder surgery in a patient with a contralateral dialysis shunt, which would preclude using either arm for pressure measurement). In this instance, it should be recognized that the measured lower extremity blood pressure will read *higher* (by as much as 30-40 mm Hg) ***than the central aortic pressure and cerebral perfusion pressure***, which could lead to patient harm if unrecognized.

D. Temperature

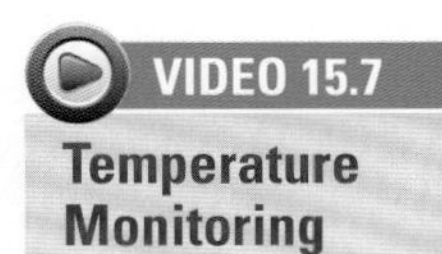

Anesthesia impairs the body's ability to maintain normal body temperature, and *hypothermia* is not only common, but is also associated with adverse outcomes (**Table 15.6**). On the other hand, although very rare, hyperthermia can alert the provider to rare but serious complications of anesthesia, such as malignant hyperthermia, or other metabolic disturbances, such as sepsis, thyroid storm, or neuroleptic malignant syndrome. Therefore, ***temperature should be monitored during anesthesia*** whenever clinically significant changes in body temperature are anticipated or suspected. Several methods, each with their advantages and disadvantages, are available for temperature monitoring (**Table 15.7**).

Table 15.6 Major Consequences of Mild Perioperative Hypothermia

- Increased incidence of surgical wound infection
- Increased number of adverse myocardial outcomes
- Increased incidence of ventricular arrhythmias
- Coagulopathy
- Increased intraoperative blood loss
- Increased requirement for allogeneic transfusion
- Increased duration of action of some muscle relaxants
- Postoperative shivering
- Increased duration of post–anesthetic care unit stay
- Increased duration of hospital stay

Table 15.7 Common Methods for Body Temperature Monitoring during Anesthesia and Potential Advantages and Disadvantages of Each Method

Method	Advantages	Disadvantages	Notes
Skin	Simple, noninvasive	Variable depending on site, and inaccurate; does not correlate well with core temperature	Only use for screening or when other methods are not available or indicated
Esophageal	Accurate in lower third of esophagus	Only used during general anesthesia and tracheal intubation	Most common
Nasopharyngeal	Accurate when resting on posterior nasopharyngeal wall	Only used during general anesthesia and tracheal intubation	Can cause epistaxis
Pulmonary artery catheter	Considered a core temperature	Invasive; any complications associated with a pulmonary artery catheter	Thermistor at the tip of the catheter
Bladder	Reasonable accuracy	Slow response time; influenced by urine flow	Not recommended for routine use
Rectal	Reasonable accuracy	Slow response time; influenced by stool	Not recommended for routine use

In general, monitoring of nasopharyngeal or esophageal temperature is preferred, as this reflects the temperature of the major, highly perfused organs.[6]

II. Common Additional Monitors

In addition to the standard monitoring for anesthesia care previously mentioned, a few other monitors are commonly used during anesthesia.

A. Urine Output

Adequate production of urine is often used as a surrogate marker for adequate perfusion to the rest of the body. Therefore, during major surgery, or even minor surgery of long duration, a urinary (Foley) catheter is often placed to measure urine output. Many anesthesia providers will target 0.5 mL/kg/h of urine production as a sign of adequate overall body perfusion, although the significance of urine output below this threshold has been questioned. Although urine output is not a good monitor of blood volume, intraoperative oliguria or anuria should be taken seriously and investigated in the context of the overall clinical picture.

B. Neuromuscular Blockade

Pharmacologically induced ***muscle paralysis*** during anesthesia and major surgery is common, because muscle paralysis facilitates tracheal intubation and may improve operating conditions. The degree of neuromuscular blockade is usually assessed by stimulation of a peripheral nerve and subsequent measurement of the muscle response. Varying sites for measurement are available (**Table 15.8**) as well as various stimulation patterns.[7,8] Assessment may be visual, tactile, or more accurately measured using a quantitative device such as accelerometry. The most commonly used stimulation pattern is the ***train-of-four (TOF):*** Each train consists of four stimuli (T1, T2, T3, T4) applied at 2 Hz (two twitches per second). With increasing nondepolarizing neuromuscular blockade, the "height" or amplitude of the twitch response decreases, and each twitch in the TOF sequence has a smaller height than the one before it. The TOF ratio, which is the ratio of the amplitude of the fourth and first twitches (T4/T1), should be >0.9 at the end of surgery for neuromuscular blockade to be considered fully reversed (see **Figure 15.8** and Chapter 11). Monitoring the level of neuromuscular blockade during anesthesia is important not only for optimizing operating conditions but also for avoiding postoperative weakness. Residual and often subclinical muscle weakness following reversal of neuromuscular blockade is surprisingly common, and it is a significant contributing factor to postoperative adverse respiratory events.

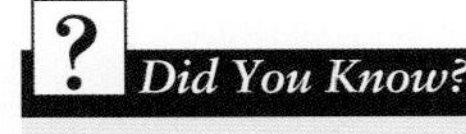

Postoperative residual neuromuscular blockade is quite common and is associated with postoperative respiratory events.

C. Neurologic Monitoring

Monitoring the ***electrical activity of the brain*** via a processed electroencephalogram (ie, BIS monitor, Aspect Medical Systems, Norwood, MA) has become a common way to measure the depth of general anesthesia. The ***bispectral index*** (***BIS***) is a dimensionless number between 0 and 100, with different ranges purported to correlate with different stages of alertness (**Table 15.9**). The main goal of the BIS monitor is to guide titration of anesthetic depth and thereby decrease the risk of intraoperative awareness; however, studies are conflicting as to the ability of the BIS monitor to accomplish this goal.[9]

III. Advanced Hemodynamic Monitors

If patient or surgical factors dictate, more advanced monitoring may be needed to deliver safe and effective anesthesia care. The majority of these advanced monitors focus on hemodynamic measurements, including blood pressure, cardiac output, and blood volume. Many of these monitors are considered "invasive" and employ a catheter to be placed within a blood vessel and connected, via a stiff fluid-filled tubing, to an electromechanical transducer, which will produce a waveform. The data derived from these measurements need to be correctly obtained and interpreted, and both the technical and physiologic aspects of the monitor need to be understood. There are two particularly important technical features that must be addressed for accurate monitoring: (1) establishing the appropriate transducer

VIDEO 15.8
Fallen Transducer

Table 15.8 Potential Sites for Monitoring Neuromuscular Blockade

Nerve	Muscle
Ulnar	Adductor pollicis (preferred)
Posterior tibial	Flexor hallucis brevis
Facial nerve	Orbicularis oculi or corrugator supercilii

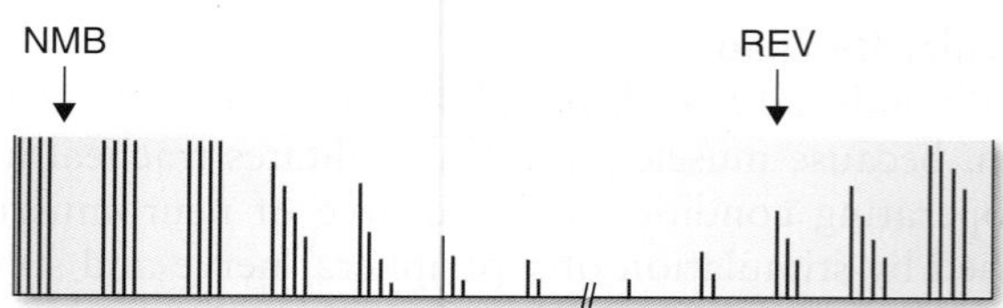

Figure 15.8 Train-of-four monitoring at onset of nondepolarizing neuromuscular blockade (NMB), followed by reversal (REV) with neostigmine.

reference level relative to the patient and (2) "zeroing" or balancing the transducer against atmospheric pressure. In most cases, pressure transducers should be placed at the level of the heart, and in the supine patient, this position is most often the mid-axillary line in the fourth intercostal space.[10] To zero or balance the transducer, it is exposed to atmospheric pressure by opening an adjacent stopcock, exposing the transducer to atmospheric pressure, and then pressing the monitor "zero" control (or its equivalent), which thereby assigns atmospheric pressure a value of zero. All monitored intravascular pressures are subsequently measured in reference to ambient atmospheric pressure.

? Did You Know?

Invasive blood pressure monitoring is subject to artifacts, including under- and overdamping.

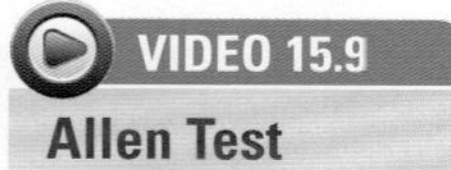

Allen Test

A. Invasive Monitoring of Systemic Blood Pressure

Invasive blood pressure measurement with an ***intra-arterial catheter*** is commonly performed for certain patient, surgical, or anesthetic reasons (**Table 15.10**). The radial artery is the most commonly used site, although ulnar, brachial, axillary, femoral, or dorsalis pedis arteries may also be used. For an individual patient, the anesthesia provider needs to assess whether the benefits of having an arterial line outweigh the risks (**Table 15.11**).

A normal intra-arterial waveform is shown in **Figure 15.9A**. The measurements obtained include the systolic blood pressure at the peak of the upstroke, diastolic blood pressure at the nadir, and mean arterial pressure (MAP), which is average pressure during the cardiac cycle. In addition, the dicrotic notch can often be seen after the systolic peak, during the down stroke, and represents the pressure reflection from closure of the aortic valve (arrow in **Figure 15.9A**). ***Overdamping*** of the waveform (**Figure 15.9B**) attenuates the peaks and troughs and is commonly caused by air bubbles or blood clots in the catheter or tubing. This results in underestimation of the true arterial systolic blood pressure. ***Underdamping*** of the pressure waveform is also possible (**Figure 15.9C**) and is a result of the dynamic response characteristics of the fluid-filled catheter tubing system. An underdamped arterial pressure waveform will cause overestimation of true arterial systolic pressure. Owing to these common artifacts, the MAP pressure is the

Table 15.9 Bispectral Index Monitor Values and Corresponding Levels of Sedation and Anesthesia

BIS Number	Effect
0	EEG silence
1-40	Deep anesthesia
41-60	Desired range for general anesthesia
61-90	Light anesthesia
91-100	Awake

BIS, bispectral index; EEG, electroencephalogram.

Table 15.10 Indications for Intra-arterial Blood Pressure Monitoring

Indication	Examples
Rapid changes or extremes in BP expected	• High-risk patients undergoing vascular, trauma, neurologic, cardiac, thoracic operations • Deliberate hyper- or hypotension
Patient intolerance of hemodynamic instability	• Significant cardiac disease or risk of cardiac ischemia • Cerebrovascular disease • Hemodynamically unstable patients (ie, sepsis)
Patient intolerance of expected respiratory or ventilator changes; impaired oxygenation/ventilation expected	• Pulmonary comorbidities (ie, ARDS), severe COPD, or pulmonary hypertension • One-lung ventilation
Expected metabolic abnormalities	• Anticipated large intravascular volume shifts • Expected acid-base abnormalities (ie, sepsis, hemorrhage)
Miscellaneous	• Failure of or inability to obtain indirect blood pressure measurement • Determination of volume responsiveness from systolic pressure or pulse pressure variation • Need to obtain multiple blood samples

ARDS, acute respiratory distress syndrome; BP, blood pressure; COPD, chronic obstructive pulmonary disease.

most reliable measurement for most monitoring purposes. In clinical practice, it is common to approximate MAP as diastolic blood pressure plus one-third the pulse pressure. This formula is only accurate at low heart rates because the time spent in systole increases at higher heart rates. Note that the MAP derived from direct arterial monitoring is not calculated but directly measured. Before treating abnormal blood pressure, the anesthesia provider should quickly assess whether the tracing appears to be under- or overdamped. In addition, the provider should check that the transducer is at the correct level and confirm the abnormal pressure by comparison with a noninvasive blood pressure measurement.

Table 15.11 Risks of Intra-arterial Catheter Placement

Bleeding Complications • Hemorrhage, hematoma
Vascular Complications • Ischemia, thrombosis, embolism, aneurysm, fistula formation
Other • Nerve damage/injury • Skin necrosis • Infection • Misinterpretation of data

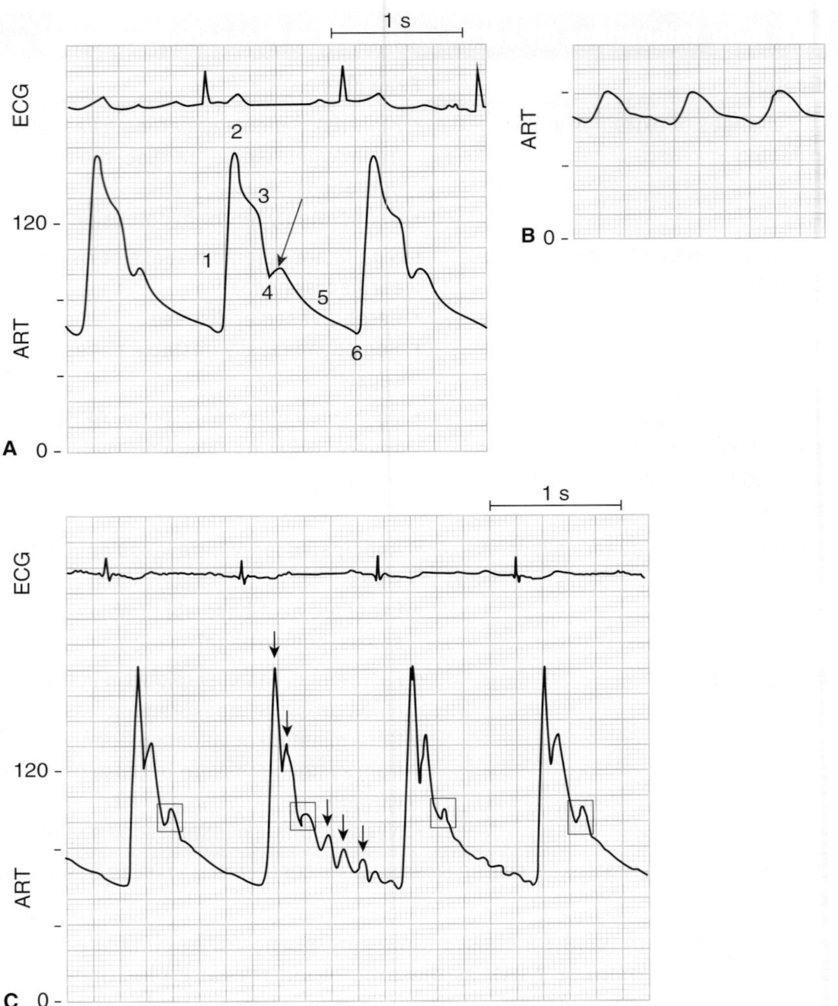

Figure 15.9 Arterial pressure waveforms. A, Normal arterial blood pressure tracing. 1, systolic upstroke; 2, systolic peak; 3, systolic decline; 4, dicrotic notch (*red arrow*) indicating closure of the aortic valve; 5, diastolic run-off; 6, end-diastolic pressure. B, Overdamped waveform, characterized by a prolonged upstroke, loss of the dicrotic notch, and loss of fine detail. C, An underdamped waveform, characterized by systolic pressure overshoot and additional small, nonphysiologic pressure waves (*arrows*) that distort the waveform and make it hard to discern the dicrotic notch (*boxes*). ART, arterial line pressure scale; ECG, electrocardiogram. (Derived from Mark JB. *Atlas of Cardiovascular Monitoring.* Churchill Livingstone; 1998.)

B. Central Venous Pressure Monitoring

Central venous catheterization and monitoring of ***central venous pressure*** (***CVP***) remains a common procedure during anesthesia, especially for patients who undergo high-risk surgical procedures. Indications for central venous catheter placement and well-recognized complications can be found in **Tables 15.12** and **15.13**, respectively. Multiple sites are available for central venous access, but the most common include the internal jugular (usually the right), subclavian, or femoral veins.

Table 15.12 Common Indications for Central Venous Catheterization

• Administration of drugs/solutions
  • Vasopressor/inotropic drugs
  • Parenteral nutrition
  • Long-term infusions

• Patient factors
  • Poor peripheral IV access
  • Pulmonary artery catheter or temporary pacemaker placement

• Surgical factors   • Need for large volume administration, transfusion
• Central venous pressure monitoring

IV, intravenous.

CVP monitoring can occur when a central line is in place. The normal CVP waveform consists of three peaks (a, c, v) and two descents (x, y) (**Figure 15.10; Table 15.14**). For many years, the CVP was thought to reflect the overall "volume status" of a patient. If the CVP was low, the patient was hypovolemic and required fluid administration, and conversely, if the CVP was high, the patient was volume overloaded and required diuresis. However, this physiologic reasoning has proven invalid in clinical practice, owing to the many factors that confound accurate and reproducible measurement and interpretation of CVP, including the complex nonlinear relation between cardiac chamber pressure and volume.[11] For patients with relatively normal heart function undergoing noncardiac surgery, following the ***change*** in CVP resulting from a fluid bolus may be more useful than single pressure measurements. Although CVP has its limitations as an assessment of intravascular volume, the CVP waveform can provide additional information to help diagnose other conditions (**Table 15.15**).

C. Pulmonary Artery Catheter

The ***pulmonary artery catheter (PAC), or Swan-Ganz catheter,*** is a balloon-tipped catheter that is advanced, assisted by the blood flow through the right atrium, across the tricuspid valve, through the right ventricle, across the pulmonic valve, and finally into the pulmonary artery. PAC monitoring has been

Table 15.13 Common Complications of Central Venous Catheterization

• **Bleeding**
  • Adjacent arterial injury
  • Hematoma formation
  • Airway compromise
  • Cardiac tamponade

• **Pneumothorax, hemothorax, or chylothorax**
• **Nerve injury**

• **Infection**
  • Bacteremia, sepsis
  • Endocarditis

• **Venous thromboembolism**
• **Venous (and paradoxical) air embolism**

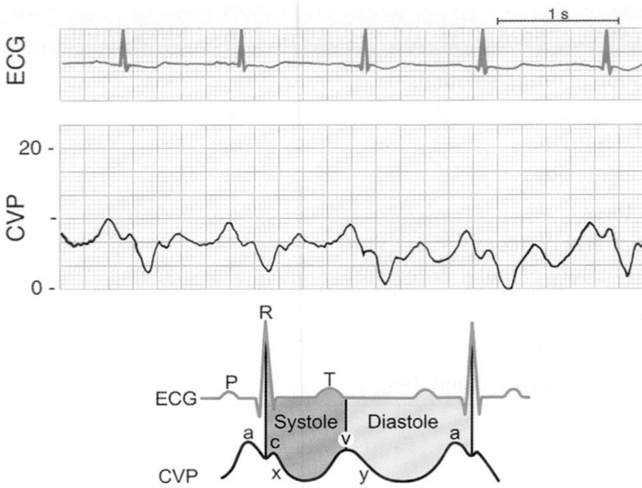

Figure 15.10 Normal central venous pressure (CVP) waveform, showing the timing of waveform components in relation to the electrocardiogram (ECG). See **Table 15.14** for descriptions of the peaks and descents. (Derived from Mark JB. *Atlas of Cardiovascular Monitoring*. Churchill Livingstone; 1998.)

widely used by anesthesia providers and critical care physicians caring for acutely and severely ill patients because of its ability to continually monitor a number of important hemodynamic variables (**Table 15.16**). However, the PAC is not without its risks, which include those for central venous catheterization (**Table 15.13**) as well as additional potential complications specifically related to the PAC (**Table 15.17**). Currently, PAC monitoring is mainly reserved for patients undergoing complicated cardiac operations and critically ill patients requiring advanced cardiopulmonary support therapies.

During flotation of a PAC through the right heart chambers, typical pressure waveforms are recorded as the catheter tip traverses the right side of the heart (**Figure 15.11**). Occasionally, distinguishing right ventricular from

Table 15.14 Physiologic Basis of a Normal Central Venous Pressure Waveform

Waveform Component	Cardiac Cycle Phase	Causative Mechanical Event
a wave	End diastole	Atrial contraction; end-diastolic atrial kick that loads the right ventricle through the open tricuspid valve
c wave	Early systole	Isovolumetric ventricular contraction, closure of tricuspid valve
x descent	Mid-systole	Atrial relaxation and descent of the base of the heart
v wave	Late systole	Venous filling of the right atrium, tricuspid valve closed
y descent	Early diastole	Blood flow from the right atrium to right ventricle after tricuspid valve opens

Table 15.15 Abnormalities of the Central Venous Pressure Waveform

Condition	Change in Central Venous Pressure Waveform	Reason for Change
Atrial fibrillation	• a wave disappears • c wave becomes more prominent	• No atrial contraction • Atrial volume is greater at end diastole and onset of systole
Junctional rhythm	• Tall cannon a wave	• Atrial contraction occurs during ventricular systole, when the tricuspid valve is closed
Tricuspid regurgitation	• Broad, tall systolic c-v wave	• Abnormal systolic filling of the right atrium through the incompetent valve

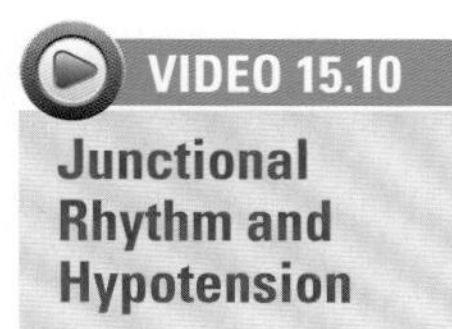

pulmonary artery pressure is difficult, but careful examination of the diastolic portion of these two pressure waveforms clarifies the different locations of the catheter tip. During diastole, filling of the right ventricle results in a pressure increase in that chamber, while diastolic flow from the pulmonary artery toward the lung results in a pressure decrease (**Figure 15.11**, red arrows).

Advancing the balloon-tipped PAC further into the pulmonary artery will allow the catheter to "wedge" and record the ***pulmonary artery wedge pressure***, or ***pulmonary artery occlusion pressure***. The pulmonary artery wedge pressure provides an indirect measurement of ***left atrial pressure***, and the wedge waveform is a slightly delayed and damped reflection of left atrial pressure.

D. Noninvasive Cardiac Output and Volume Assessment

Given the complications and complexity associated with the PAC, a number of minimally invasive cardiac output monitors have been developed (**Table 15.18**). These monitors use a range of fundamental technologies (ultrasound, indicator dilution, pulse contour analysis) to provide estimates of cardiac output, stroke volume, and other derived parameters, such as the variation in pulse pressure during the respiratory cycle. Many of these monitors provide "dynamic" indicators of a patient's volume status by measuring changes that occur during the respiratory cycle in a patient who is receiving positive pressure mechanical ventilation. Thus, they are specifically designed to be used

Table 15.16 Standard Variables Measured With a Pulmonary Artery Catheter

- **Intracardiac pressures**
  - Central venous pressure/right atrial pressure
  - Right ventricular pressure
  - Pulmonary artery pressure
  - Pulmonary artery wedge pressure/left atrial pressure
- **Cardiac output**
- **Mixed venous oxygen saturation**
- **Core body temperature**

Table 15.17 Complications of Pulmonary Artery Catheterization

- Atrial and ventricular dysrhythmias, including ventricular fibrillation
- Right bundle-branch block
- Pulmonary infarction
- Pulmonary artery rupture
- Damage to tricuspid or pulmonic valve(s)
- Misinterpretation of derived data

intraoperatively for patients under general anesthesia. These dynamic variables have been shown to be superior to static indices such as CVP in predicting volume responsiveness, thereby providing a clinically useful guide to perioperative fluid administration.[12]

E. Transesophageal Echocardiography

Transesophageal echocardiography (*TEE*) has been used for many years in cardiac surgery, but its use has expanded to include other major operations (ie, abdominal transplant, major vascular surgery). TEE is really a diagnostic tool as well as a monitoring modality, and it can provide accurate information about volume status, ventricular and valvular function, and a wide range of other cardiac conditions. In current anesthesiology practice, diagnostic TEE is generally used by physicians specifically trained and credentialed in its use. There are simpler disposable TEE monitors available for limited monitoring, and in the future their perioperative use may increase.

Basic anesthesia monitoring is required to safely administer anesthetic care. More advanced monitoring may be required, depending on the clinical situation, including patient and surgical factors. There are a wide array of monitors

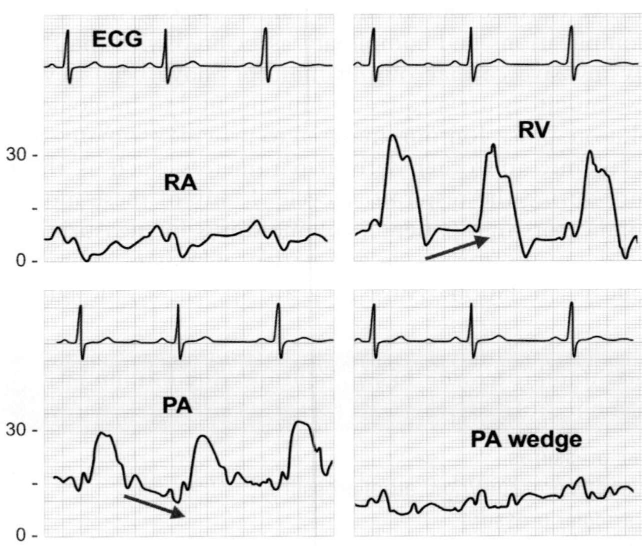

Figure 15.11 Pulmonary artery catheter waveforms as the tip of the catheter advances through the cardiac chambers. The *red arrows* highlight the different pattern of diastolic pressure in the right ventricle (RV) and pulmonary artery (PA). ECG, electrocardiogram; PA wedge, pulmonary artery wedge pressure; RA, right atrium. (Courtesy of Jonathan B. Marks and redrawn from Mark JB. *Atlas of Cardiovascular Monitoring*. New York: Churchill Livingstone; 1998.)

Table 15.18 Noninvasive Cardiac Output Monitors
• Esophageal Doppler
• Carbon dioxide rebreathing systems
• Indicator dilution methods
• Thoracic bioimpedance
• Pulse contour analysis • Invasive (ie, arterial line required) • Noninvasive (ie, finger cuff)

available for use, and over time, the specialty of anesthesiology has seen a trend toward use of less-invasive monitors that often rely on complex algorithms. Despite these sophisticated monitors, a competent and vigilant anesthesia provider is absolutely essential to choose and use these monitors correctly.

Acknowledgment

The authors would like to acknowledge with thanks the contributions of Ryan J. Fink, MD, to the first edition of this chapter.

For further review and interactivities, please see the associated Interactive Video Lectures and "A Closer Look" infographic accessible in the complimentary eBook bundled with this text. Access instructions are located in the inside front cover.

References

1. American Society of Anesthesiologists. Standards for Basic Anesthetic Monitoring. Accessed June 1, 2020. https://www.asahq.org/standards-and-guidelines/standards-for-basic-anesthetic-monitoring
2. Tusman G, Bohm SH, Suarez-Sipmann F. Advanced uses of pulse oximetry for monitoring mechanically ventilated patients. *Anesth Analg*. 2017;124(1):62-71. PMID: 27183375.
3. Ortega R, Mazzini M, Xue K, et al. Electrocardiographic monitoring in adults. *N Engl J Med*. 2015;372:e11.
4. Pickering TG, Hall JE, Appel LJ, et al. Recommendations for blood pressure measurement in humans and experimental animals. Part 1: blood pressure measurement in humans – a statement for professionals from the Subcommittee of Professional and Public Education of the American Heart Association Council on High Blood Pressure Research. *Circulation*. 2005;111(5):697-716. PMID: 15699287.
5. Kuck K, Baker PD. Perioperative noninvasive blood pressure monitoring. *Anesth Analg*. 2018;127:408-11. PMID: 29189276.
6. Sessler DI. Perioperative thermoregulation and heat balance. *Lancet*. 2016;387(10038): 2655-2664. PMID: 26775126.
7. Naguib M, Brull SJ, Kopman AF, et al. Consensus statement on perioperative use of neuromuscular monitoring. *Anesth Analg*. 2018;127(1):71. PMID: 29200077.
8. Ortega R, Brull SJ, Prielipp R, et al. Monitoring neuromuscular function. *N Engl J Med*. 2018;378(4):e6. PMID: 29365307.
9. Lewis SR, Pritchard MW, Fawcett LJ, et al. Bispectral index for improving intraoperative awareness and early postoperative recovery in adults. *Cochrane Database Syst Rev*. 2019;9:CD003843. PMID: 31557307.
10. Ortega R, Connor C, Kotova F, Deng W, Lacerra C. Use of pressure transducers. *N Engl J Med*. 2017;376(14):e26. PMID: 28379806.
11. Magder S. Central venous pressure: a useful but not so simple measurement. *Crit Care Med*. 2006;34(8):2224-2227. PMID: 16763509.
12. Pinsky MR. Cardiopulmonary Interactions: physiologic basis and clinical applications. *Ann Am Thorac Soc*. 2018;15(suppl 1):S45-S48. PMID: 28820609.

BLOOD PRESSURE MONITORING

A CLOSER LOOK

Illustrated below is the distinction between noninvasive blood pressure (NIBP) and arterial line monitors and the influence of arterial hydrostatic pressure.

NIBP—ARM SUPINE

The arm is in the same plane as the central circulation; it is neither elevated nor below the heart, so there is *no change in hydrostatic pressure* within the brachial artery. If the heart produces a blood pressure of 120/80 mm Hg, the brachial artery will also have a blood pressure of 120/80 mm Hg.

Arterial Line—ARM SUPINE

The arm is in the same plane as the central circulation; it is neither elevated nor below the heart, so there is *no change in hydrostatic pressure within the radial artery.* If the heart produces a blood pressure of 120/80 mm Hg, the radial artery will also have a blood pressure of 120/80 mm Hg.

Neither NIBP nor arterial lines are more accurate than the other. They are both prone to error or misinterpretation.

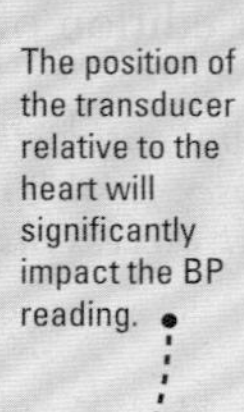

The position of the transducer relative to the heart will significantly impact the BP reading.

NIBP—ARM ELEVATED

The arm is NOT in the same plane as the central circulation; it is elevated relative to the heart, so there is *a decrease in hydrostatic pressure* within the brachial artery. If the heart produces a blood pressure of 120/80 mm Hg, *the brachial artery will have a blood pressure LESS than 120/80 mm Hg.*

Arterial Line—ARM ELEVATED

Think of the radial arterial line tubing as an "extension" of the radial artery. Therefore, *even though there is a dramatic loss of hydrostatic pressure in the radial artery,* this is offset by an equivalent *increase in hydrostatic pressure in the tubing,* which terminates at the monitoring transducer. This transducer is located in the same plane as the central circulation. It is neither elevated nor below the heart, so if the heart produces a blood pressure of 120/80 mm Hg, *the radial artery monitor will show a blood pressure of 120/80 mm Hg, provided that the transducer is correctly leveled.*

Infographic by: Naveen Nathan MD

Questions

1. **Which two wavelengths are employed by the pulse oximeter?**

   A. Red and near-infrared
   B. Red and infrared
   C. Infrared and blue
   D. Near-infrared and blue
   E. None of the above

2. **A sudden large decrease in the end-tidal carbon dioxide concentration most likely indicates:**

   A. Hypovolemia
   B. Hypothermia
   C. Sepsis
   D. Pulmonary embolism
   E. None of the above

3. **Which two leads of the electrocardiogram provide a sensitivity of 80% for the detection of myocardial ischemia?**

   A. Leads I and II
   B. Leads I and V_5
   C. Leads II and V_5
   D. Leads II and V_3
   E. None of the above

4. **When an electromechanical transducer is zeroed, the actual pressure it is measuring is:**

   A. Zero pressure
   B. Ambient atmospheric pressure
   C. The pressure of the fluid in the attached monitoring catheter
   D. The pressure of the fluid in the transducer flush system
   E. None of the above

5. **The x descent of the central venous pressure trace is caused by:**

   A. The opening of the tricuspid valve
   B. Isovolumetric ventricular contraction
   C. The descent of the base of the heart
   D. Atrial diastasis
   E. None of the above

Answers

1. A

These two wavelengths are absorbed differently by oxygenated and deoxygenated blood.

2. D

All of the above can increase alveolar dead space and thus decrease end-tidal carbon dioxide concentration, but a pulmonary embolism would be the most likely to produce a sudden large decrease.

3. C

Cardiac ischemia is best detected by monitoring a five-lead ECG and displaying both leads II and V_5, a technique that can have a sensitivity of up to 80%. V_3 and V_4 may provide sensitivity as good or better than V_5, but their placement may interfere with the surgical field.

4. B

The transducer is zeroed by opening it to atmospheric pressure. Thus, the pressures it measures subsequently are relative to ambient atmospheric pressure.

5. C

The x descent occurs during mid-ventricular systole as the base of the heart descends, pulling the tricuspid and mitral valves with it and thereby expanding the potential volume of the atria and lowering their pressure.

III Clinical Practice of Anesthesia

16 Preoperative Evaluation and Management

Thomas R. Hickey and Natalie F. Holt

Preoperative evaluation of the patient by an anesthesiologist is a cornerstone of perioperative patient care. The main purpose is to obtain information about a patient's medical, surgical, and anesthetic history and to perform a focused physical examination that will help determine whether the patient is in optimum medical condition to proceed with the planned procedure. Increased efficiency can be achieved when need-based preoperative laboratory and other tests are ordered by an anesthesia provider in a dedicated preoperative evaluation clinic, rather than by surgeons or primary care doctors. Anesthesia preoperative clinics also enhance operating room efficiency by reducing day-of-surgery cancellations or delays due to incomplete workups.[1,2] Anesthesia preoperative clinics can alleviate patient anxiety by providing education and counseling, as well as reduce the risk of perioperative morbidity and mortality.[3]

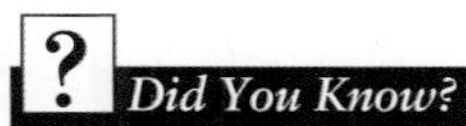

The letter "E" after the American Society of Anesthesiologists (ASA) physical status classification is used to indicate an emergency surgery. Emergency surgeries generally need to be performed within 6 hours in order to save life, limb, or vital organ. Emergency surgery is a risk factor for increased morbidity and mortality.

I. Approach to the Patient

Key elements of the preanesthetic evaluation include a review of (1) the planned surgical procedure and its indication; (2) the patient's present and past medical history; (3) current medications and drug allergies; (4) social history, including use of alcohol, tobacco, or illicit drugs; (5) complications related to previous anesthetics; and (6) performance of a focused physical examination (**Table 16.1**). By convention, anesthesiologists use the ASA's physical status classification system to summarize the health status of the patient and communicate a risk assessment (**Table 16.2**).[4] Information obtained during the preoperative evaluation guides the development of anesthetic and postoperative pain management plans. Most preanesthetic clinics use standardized evaluation templates to guide patient evaluations; use of these forms also increases reporting consistency and limits the risk of missing information. Electronic health records also facilitate consistency in preanesthetic evaluation.

A. Planned Surgery and Its Indication

The planned surgical procedure is an important determinant of the type of anesthesia that will be required for the procedure and the expected level of postoperative pain. The planned procedure also dictates the anticipated patient positioning, duration, blood loss, and intraoperative and postoperative monitoring requirements. Procedures performed for urgent conditions (eg, small bowel obstruction, limb ischemia) are associated with an increased risk of perioperative morbidity and mortality.

Table 16.1 Components of the Preanesthetic Evaluation

I. Review of planned surgical procedure and its indication

II. Review of systems
   a. Head, ears, eyes, throat (glaucoma, dental care, implanted jewelry)
   b. Cardiovascular (exercise tolerance, angina, dyspnea on exertion, hypertension)
   c. Vascular (peripheral vascular, aneurysm)
   d. Pulmonary (smoking, COPD, asthma)
   e. Gastrointestinal (reflux, obstruction)
   f. Hepatic (liver disease, alcohol abuse)
   g. Endocrine (diabetes, thyroid disease)
   h. Renal (chronic kidney disease, dialysis)
   i. Genitourinary (benign prostatic hypertrophy, hematuria)
   j. Musculoskeletal (rheumatoid arthritis)
   k. Neurologic (neuropathy, stroke, seizure)
   l. Psychiatric (bipolar disorder, substance abuse)
   m. Other (dermatologic diseases, chronic pain, etc.)

III. Medication history

IV. Drug/latex allergies (including reactions, if known)

V. Social history
   a. Tobacco use—past and present
   b. Alcohol use
   c. Illicit substance use

VI. Past surgeries and anesthetics (including complications, personal and familial)

VII. Physical examination
   a. Vital signs: blood pressure, heart rate, temperature, height, weight
   b. Heart
   c. Lungs
   d. Neurologic examination: peripheral neuropathies, asymmetries
   e. Airway: oral aperture, Mallampati score, dentition, thyromental distance, neck range of motion

VIII. Laboratory tests (blood, ECG, chest x-ray) as needed based on history and physical examination and planned surgical procedure

COPD, chronic obstructive pulmonary disease; ECG, electrocardiogram.

Table 16.2 American Society of Anesthesiologists' (ASA) Physical Status Classification System

ASA Physical Status Classification	
1	Normal healthy person
2	Mild systemic disease that results in no functional limitation
3	Severe systemic disease that results in functional limitation
4	Severe systemic disease that causes a constant threat to life
5	Moribund patient not expected to live without the planned surgery
6	Brain-dead person whose organs are being removed for donation
E	Qualifier used for emergency procedures

Modified from American Society of Anesthesiologists: new classification of physical status. *Anesthesiology*. 1963;24:111.

B. Present and Past Medical History

Medical history is best addressed using a systems-based approach. A useful way to screen for occult cardiovascular disease is to estimate the patient's functional capacity. Functional capacity is described in terms of metabolic equivalents (METs), where 1 MET is the resting oxygen consumption of a 40-year-old, 70 kg man. A functional capacity less than 4 METs predicts increased perioperative cardiac and long-term risks. An example of an activity that uses about 4 METs is climbing one to two flights of stairs (**Table 16.3**). Instruments such as the Duke Activity Status Index (DASI) can also be used to assess functional status.

Pulmonary evaluation should take into account a history of asthma or recent upper respiratory infection (URI) and signs and symptoms suggestive of obstructive sleep apnea (OSA). Asthma or recent URI may predispose the patient to bronchospasm with airway instrumentation. OSA may signal difficulty with ventilation and suggest the need to use sedative drugs cautiously, as well as consider postoperative noninvasive positive pressure ventilation and a higher level of respiratory monitoring.

When an undiagnosed or uncontrolled medical condition is identified, the patient should be referred to a primary care practitioner for evaluation and management. Whether this workup needs to be completed prior to surgery is at the discretion of the anesthesiologist and surgeon and is often dependent on the urgency and invasiveness of the planned surgical procedure.

C. Current Medications and Drug Allergies

Review of current medications, including over-the-counter and herbal or complementary drugs, is an essential component of the preanesthetic assessment, as many drugs used in the perioperative period have important interactions with commonly prescribed pharmaceuticals. For example, patients who take monoamine oxidase inhibitors (MAOIs) are at increased risk for serotonin syndrome if exposed to meperidine. Those who take gabapentin are especially sensitive to the sedative effects of opioids.

Table 16.3 Metabolic Equivalents for Common Physical Activities

Metabolic Equivalents	Examples
1	Watching television
|	Eating, dressing
|	Walking on level ground at 2-3 mph
∨	Doing light housework (eg, dusting)
4	Climbing a flight of stairs
|	Walking on level ground at 4 mph
∨	Doing heavy chores (eg, scrubbing floors)
>10	Playing strenuous sports (eg, tennis)

Adapted from Fleisher LA, Beckman JA, Brown KA, et al. American College of Cardiology American Heart Association Task Force on practice guidelines; American Society of Echocardiography. ACC/AHA 2007 guidelines on perioperative cardiovascular evaluation and care for noncardiac surgery. *J Am Coll Cardiol.* 2007;50(17):e170.

Cardiovascular Medications

Patients on chronic β-blocker therapy should continue their medications perioperatively, as abrupt withdrawal may precipitate angina, ischemia, or dysrhythmias. Several randomized trials including the POISE-1 (Perioperative Ischemic Evaluation) and DECREASE (Dutch Echocardiographic Cardiac Risk Evaluation Applying Stress Echocardiography) trials have attempted to address the effect of initiation of β-blocker therapy prior to noncardiac surgery in patients with risk factors for cardiovascular complications.[5-7] A review of randomized trials on this subject found that while β-blockade was associated with a reduced risk of nonfatal myocardial infarction (MI), this came at the price of an increased risk of nonfatal stroke, hypotension, and bradycardia.[8]

Patients who take centrally acting sympatholytics, such as clonidine, may experience rebound hypertension with abrupt discontinuation. Therefore, it is recommended that these drugs be continued in patients who take them chronically.

In various studies, calcium channel–blocking drugs have been purported to reduce perioperative ischemia; conversely, they have been associated with an increased risk of surgical bleeding. However, none of these results have been substantiated in large randomized trials, and it is generally agreed that calcium channel blockers should be continued perioperatively. Angiotensin-converting enzyme (ACE) inhibitors and angiotensin II receptor–blocking drugs (ARBs) have been associated with refractory intraoperative hypotension. For this reason, they are generally discontinued the night prior to major surgery except for procedures with a very low risk of hemodynamic instability. There is some evidence to suggest that delay in reinstituting ACE inhibitor or ARB therapy postoperatively is associated with increased mortality. Therefore, preoperative medications should be resumed as soon as possible. Loop diuretics are also generally held on the day of major surgery to avoid intraoperative hypotension. Continuation of diuretics may be appropriate for patients with severe heart failure with frequent exacerbations.

Perioperative use of 3-hydroxy-3-methyl-glutaryl-coenzyme A reductase inhibitors (known as statins) has been shown to reduce cardiovascular morbidity and mortality, especially for patients undergoing vascular surgery.[9] Therefore, it is recommended that statins be continued perioperatively. Furthermore, consideration should be given to initiating statin therapy in patients with cardiac risk factors who will be undergoing vascular surgery.

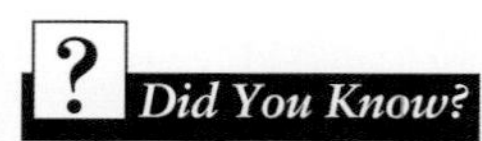

The use of etomidate should be avoided in patients at risk for adrenal suppression, as it interferes with steroid synthesis and may precipitate an adrenal crisis.

Endocrine Medications

Patients who take glucocorticoids should continue these medications perioperatively. The risk of clinically significant adrenal suppression in these patients is estimated based on steroid duration and dose. Patients who have been on a chronic dose equivalent to prednisone ≤5 mg/d for ≤3 weeks are at low risk of adrenal suppression; patients on ≥20 mg/d for ≥3 weeks are at high risk; and patients on intermediate doses are at unknown or intermediate risk. These patients can be evaluated with cosyntropin stimulation testing if time permits. Supplemental "stress dose" glucocorticoids are typically administered based on risk and the anticipated degree of surgical stress. **Table 16.4** summarizes an approach to glucocorticoid supplementation in patients on chronic steroids.

The management of patients with diabetes should be individualized. However, in general, oral hypoglycemic drugs and short-acting insulin preparations should be withheld on the morning of surgery. Metformin is associated

Table 16.4 An Approach to Perioperative Corticosteroid Coverage

For minor surgeries, take usual morning steroid dose. No supplementation is needed.
For moderate surgeries, take usual morning steroid dose. Administer 50 mg hydrocortisone IV prior to induction and 25 mg IV every 8 h for 24 h.
For major surgeries, take usual morning steroid dose. Administer 100 mg IV hydrocortisone IV prior to induction and 50 mg IV every 8 h for 24 h.

IV, intravenous.

with an increased risk of renal hypoperfusion and lactic acidosis in the context of severe dehydration; therefore, most clinicians discontinue its use a full 24 hours prior to major surgery and do not resume it until the patient is well hydrated.

For patients on once-daily dosing of a long-acting insulin, 50% to 75% of the usual dose is usually advised on the night before and/or morning of surgery, depending on the patient's usual dosing regimen. For those who take intermediate-acting insulin, a 25% to 50% dose reduction the night prior and day of surgery is usually sufficient.

It is important to note that type 1 diabetics are dependent on insulin. For patients with insulin pumps, the basal infusion rate is typically continued. For those without insulin pumps, a low-dose insulin infusion along with glucose-containing intravenous fluids and routine capillary "fingerstick" glucose monitoring is appropriate. **Table 16.5** presents general guidelines for the perioperative management of oral hypoglycemic drugs and insulin in diabetic patients.

Women who take oral contraceptives, hormone replacement therapy, and selective estrogen receptor modulators (ie, tamoxifen) are at increased risk for venous thrombosis. Therefore, consideration should be given to discontinuing these medications 4 weeks preoperatively for surgeries associated with a high risk of venous thromboembolism.

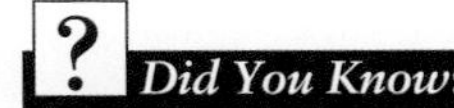

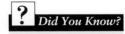

The manifestations of severe hypoglycemia can be masked during general anesthesia. While it is desirable to keep blood glucose at near-normal levels during anesthesia, the consequences of overtreatment with insulin are significant. Frequent perioperative measurement of blood glucose is essential. A target glucose between 140 and 180 mg/dL is recommended.

Psychotropic Medications

Although many psychotropic medications have interactions with anesthetic and analgesic agents, most are continued in the perioperative period, owing to the potential consequences of withdrawing these agents in patients with serious mood disorders. Tricyclic antidepressants may cause QTc prolongation and are associated with anticholinergic effects that may be exacerbated by drugs used during anesthesia. Nonselective MAOIs, such as phenelzine and tranylcypromine, though rarely used today, pose a special concern in the context of anesthesia. They inhibit the breakdown of monoamine neurotransmitters including dopamine, serotonin, epinephrine, and norepinephrine. In patients taking MAOIs, coadministration of indirect-acting sympathomimetic agents such as ephedrine may cause a hypertensive crisis. In addition, concomitant administration of drugs with anticholinergic properties, such as meperidine and dextromethorphan, may cause ***serotonin syndrome,*** a condition marked by agitation, hyperthermia, and muscular rigidity and caused by an excess of serotonergic activity in the central nervous system. For these reasons, many providers will taper and discontinue MAOIs in the weeks prior to surgery, in conjunction with the patient's medication provider.

Mood-stabilizing agents, antipsychotics, antianxiety medications, and antiseizure drugs may be continued perioperatively. However, if patients are taking

Table 16.5 Guidelines for the Perioperative Management of Patients With Diabetes

Schedule as the first case of the day to avoid prolonged fasting, if possible.
Hold oral hypoglycemic drugs and short-acting insulin on the day of surgery; hold metformin for 24 h prior to surgery.
Continue usual insulin regimen through the evening prior to surgery; if there is a history of hypoglycemia, consider reducing the nightly basal insulin dose.
For patients with type 1 diabetes, administer half the usual morning dose of intermediate- or long-acting insulin on the day of surgery; for patients with an insulin pump, continue infusion at a basal rate. For long surgeries, pumps should be stopped and replaced with dextrose and insulin infusions.
For patients with type 2 diabetes, administer 1/3-2/3 the usual morning dose of intermediate- or long-acting insulin on the day of surgery, depending on the patient's usual morning fasting blood glucose measurement. Hold short-acting insulin preparations.
Measure blood glucose level every 1-2 h during surgery.

medications with a narrow therapeutic window, such as lithium and valproate, perioperative monitoring of drug blood levels may be appropriate, as drug absorption may be affected by surgery. Patients on lithium should have electrolyte and drug levels monitored, given the increased risk of nephrogenic diabetes insipidus.

Drugs Affecting Platelet Function

Aspirin irreversibly inhibits the platelet cyclooxygenase (COX) enzyme, which is responsible for prostaglandin and thromboxane production. Among its many effects, aspirin inhibits platelet aggregation. For this reason, aspirin is widely used for prevention of clotting in patients at risk for cardiovascular disease, as well as those with a history of angina, myocardial infarction, stroke, and peripheral vascular disease. Daily aspirin therapy is also necessary for patients with coronary artery stents to prevent in-stent thrombosis. In the context of surgery, however, decreased platelet aggregation predisposes patients on aspirin to increased surgical bleeding. Therefore, decisions about perioperative aspirin use must weigh the risk of perioperative hemorrhage against that of cardiovascular complications. POISE-2 was a large randomized trial that found no difference in cardiovascular or mortality outcomes and an increased bleeding risk in patients who continued perioperative aspirin use.[10] It is generally agreed that aspirin should be withheld for 7 to 10 days prior to surgeries where bleeding would have catastrophic consequences (eg, intracranial, intraocular, middle ear, prostate, and intramedullary spine surgeries) or where the likelihood of major blood loss is high.

Platelet P2Y12 receptor blockers (eg, clopidogrel, prasugrel, ticagrelor, cangrelor) are another class of antiplatelet agents commonly used in patients following an ischemic cerebrovascular event (eg, acute myocardial infarction) or in patients who have undergone placement of coronary artery stents. Combined use of aspirin and a platelet P2Y12 receptor blocker (dual antiplatelet therapy, or DAPT) markedly reduces the risk of in-stent thrombosis in patients with vascular stents. The optimal duration of DAPT in these patients is unknown. The

2016 ACC/AHA Guideline Focused Update on Duration of Dual Antiplatelet Therapy in Patients with Coronary Artery Disease recommends that elective noncardiac surgery should be delayed for 30 days after bare-metal stent (BMS) and at least 3 but preferably 6 months after drug-eluting stent (DES) placement.[11] Clopidogrel, ticagrelor, and prasugrel should be stopped about 7 days before surgery. Cangrelor is a reversible P2Y12 receptor blocker available by infusion that is unique because of its rapid metabolism by plasma enzymes. Discontinuation of cangrelor for as little as 1 hour prior to surgery provides return to near-normal platelet function. Perioperative medical management in this population should be interdisciplinary, allowing both the cardiology and surgery teams to weigh in on the risks and benefits.

It is generally recommended that nonsteroidal anti-inflammatory drugs (NSAIDs) be discontinued for 3 to 5 days preoperatively, owing to their effects on platelet aggregation. Patients are advised to use acetaminophen as the pain reliever of choice preoperatively, as it has no effect on platelet function.

Oral Anticoagulants

Oral anticoagulants include warfarin, which blocks the production of vitamin K–dependent clotting factors, direct thrombin inhibitors, such as dabigatran, and direct Xa inhibitors, such as rivaroxaban and apixaban. Indications for anticoagulant therapy include prevention of clots in patients with atrial fibrillation, prosthetic heart valves, or a history of arterial or venous thromboembolism. Perioperative interruption of anticoagulant therapy involves weighing the risk of thrombosis against the risk of bleeding. Interactive algorithms such as Thrombosis Canada[a] are useful in developing a perioperative anticoagulation management plan. The CHA2DS2-VASc risk stratification score is a way to estimate stroke risk in patients with atrial fibrillation.[12] It is also helpful in identifying high-risk patients in whom interruption of anticoagulant therapy would be most detrimental (**Table 16.6**).

Because its half-life is long, it is recommended that warfarin be stopped 5 days prior to elective surgery. Low-dose oral vitamin K may be used to accelerate normalization of international normalized ratio (INR) in patients on warfarin. When there is a desire to minimize the duration that the patient is without anticoagulation, bridging therapy may be used. This generally involves the subcutaneous administration of low-molecular-weight heparin beginning 3 days prior to surgery, with the last dose administered 24 hours before the start of the procedure. Bridging therapy is typically reserved for patients at high-risk for thrombosis, including those with a (1) history of stroke, thromboembolism, or coronary artery stent placement within 3 months; (2) presence of a mechanical aortic or mitral valve; and (3) atrial fibrillation with a CHA2DS2-VASc > 5.

Dabigatran is used primarily to prevent stroke in patients with atrial fibrillation. Dabigatran is notable in that its half-life is about 12 hours in patients with normal renal function but more than 24 hours in patients with significant kidney disease. In patients with normal renal function, dabigatran should be stopped 2 to 4 days prior to surgery; in patients with a creatinine clearance of <50 mL/min, it should be stopped 3 to 5 days prior to surgery. Rivaroxaban and apixaban are less dependent on renal function for clearance and may be stopped 2 to 3 days

[a]https://thrombosiscanada.ca/tools/?calc=perioperativeAnticoagulantAlgorithm.

Table 16.6 CHA2DS2-VASc Score for Estimating Stroke, Transient Ischemic Attack, and Systemic Embolism Risk

CHA2DS2-VASc Risk Factor	Points
Congestive heart failure	+1
Hypertension	+1
Age 75 y or older	+2
Diabetes mellitus	+1
Previous stroke, transient ischemic attack, or thromboembolism	+2
Vascular disease	+1
Age 65-74 y	+1
Female sex	+1
CHA2DS2-VASc Score	**Stroke/Thromboembolism Event Rate at 1 y (%)**
0	0.78
1	2.01
2	3.71
3	5.92
4	9.27
5	15.26
6	19.74
7	21.50
8	22.38
9	23.64

Adapted from Kirchhof P, Benussi S, Kotecha D, et al. 2016 ESC guidelines for the management of atrial fibrillation developed in collaboration with EACTS. *Europace*. 2016;18(11):1609-1678.

prior to surgery. Because of their relatively short half-life, bridging therapy is not usually required for the direct thrombin and factor Xa inhibitors.

In the past 10 years, there have been significant advances in the development of reversal agents directed at the novel oral anticoagulants (NOACs). Idarucizumab was the first U.S. Food and Drug Administration (FDA)–approved reversal agent of its kind. Idarucizumab is a specific reversal agent for the direct thrombin inhibitor dabigatran. It binds to dabigatran with 350 times the affinity of thrombin and then creates an irreversible complex with dabigatran that is eventually excreted by the kidneys. Andexanet alfa is the second NOAC reversal agent to be approved by the FDA. This drug has the ability to reverse the effects of all of factor Xa inhibitors as well as heparin. However, its official approved use is only for the reversal of rivaroxaban and apixaban. Ciraparantag is the latest drug in this category, being touted as a universal antidote to most of the oral anticoagulants and heparin. However, its use remains investigational. Although there is concern that these agents may increase the risk of thrombotic complications, so far this appears not to be the case.

Antiplatelet and Anticoagulation Agents and Neuraxial Anesthesia

Both the American Society of Regional Anesthesia and Pain Therapy (ASRA) and the European Society of Anesthesiology (ESA) have developed guidelines for the management of antiplatelet and anticoagulant drugs in the context of neuraxial anesthesia.[13] It is important to note that not only the times of insertion but also manipulation and removal of a catheter from the epidural space constitute increased bleeding risks. Therefore, the timing of each should be carefully considered in the context of time since administration of the last dose of an anticoagulant or antiplatelet drug.

Neither NSAIDs nor aspirin therapy alone is believed to pose an increased risk of bleeding in patients undergoing neuraxial anesthesia. **Table 16.7** summarizes the recommendations of the ESA regarding the timing of neuraxial puncture or catheter manipulation/removal in patients on anticoagulant or antiplatelet medications.

Table 16.7 Recommended Time Interval Between Neuraxial Puncture or Epidural Catheter Removal[a]

Drug	Time Before Puncture/ Catheter Manipulation or Removal	Time After Puncture/ Catheter Manipulation or Removal
Unfractionated heparin (for prophylaxis, <15,000 IU/d)	4-6 h PTT<40 s	1 h
Unfractionated heparin (for treatment)	4-6 h (IV) 8-12 h (SC)	1 h
Low-molecular-weight heparin (for prophylaxis)	12 h	4 h
Low-molecular-weight heparin (for treatment)	24 h	4 h
Rivaroxaban (for prophylaxis, 10 mg/d)	22-26 h	4-6 h
Apixaban (for prophylaxis, 2.5 mg BID)	26-30 h	4-6 h
Dabigatran (150-220 mg/d)	72 h	6 h
Warfarin	INR <1.5	After catheter removal
Clopidogrel	7 d	After catheter removal
Prasugrel	7-10 d	6 h after catheter removal
Ticagrelor	5 d	6 h after catheter removal
Ticlopidine	10 d	After catheter removal
Aspirin	None	None
Nonsteroidal anti-inflammatory drugs	None	None

BID, two times a day; INR, international normalized ratio; IU, international units; IV, intravenous; PTT, prothrombin time; SC, subcutaneous.

[a]All time intervals refer to patients with normal renal function.

Note: No delay required in patients receiving only subcutaneous heparin for DVT prophylaxis.

Adapted from Gogarten W, Vandermeulen E, Van Aken H. Regional anaesthesia and antithrombotic agents: recommendations of the European Society of Anaesthesiology. *Eur J Anaesthesiol.* 2010;27(12):1002.

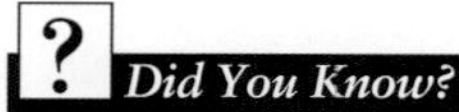

Multimodal anesthesia is the cornerstone of minimizing postoperative reliance on opioids. This strategy involves the use of regional and neuraxial anesthetics, as well as nonopioid medications, including NSAIDs, ketamine, and gabapentin.

Opioids and Medications Used to Treat Addiction

Patients who take opioids for chronic pain should continue these medications perioperatively and often benefit from a pain management plan that includes multimodal treatments such as intraoperative ketamine infusions, NSAIDs, acetaminophen, and regional anesthetic techniques. Patients recovering from opioid or alcohol addiction are sometimes prescribed partial opioid agonists, such as buprenorphine, or opioid antagonists such as naltrexone. These drugs are helpful in addiction recovery because they block the euphoric effects associated with opioid use; however, in the context of surgery, high doses limit the effectiveness of full opioid agonists. In the recent past, conventional wisdom supported the discontinuation of partial opioid agonists preoperatively for patients whose postoperative course was likely to require opioid therapy. However, more recent studies have demonstrated no adverse consequences from the continuation of these medications and a possible reduction in the risk of perioperative relapse and opioid withdrawal. A typical approach is to reduce the daily buprenorphine dose to 16 mg or less in the 48 to 72 hours prior to surgery.[14,15] Decisions regarding perioperative buprenorphine management should be made collaboratively with the prescribing provider.

Herbal or Complementary Supplements

Owing to concerns about their purity and the potential for adverse effects, it is safest to advise that all herbal or complementary drugs be discontinued 1 week prior to surgery. Specific supplements have been associated with particular complications. For example, garlic, ginger, and ginseng may increase bleeding risk. **Table 16.8** summarizes the potential side effects of common herbal supplements.

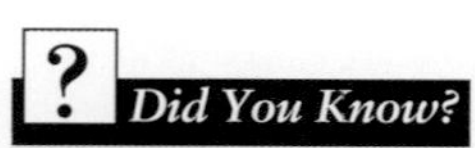

Risk factors for latex allergy include neural tube defects, occupational exposure, as well as a history of atopy and allergies to foods, such as bananas, known to have allergens that cross-react with latex.

Drug Allergies

Information about drug allergies should be elicited during the preanesthetic interview. It has been reported that 10% of the population reports a penicillin allergy; however, based on prior studies, up to 98% of these patients do not have a true penicillin allergy. Signs and symptoms suggestive of true type 1 immunoglobulin-E–mediated allergy include urticaria, angioedema, and wheezing. Although the potential for cross-reactivity exists between allergy to penicillin and the cephalosporins because of the common β-lactam ring, only about 2% of patients with a documented penicillin allergy will have an allergic reaction to a cephalosporin.[16,17]

Patients should also be asked about a history of allergy to latex, as this allergy requires advance preparation of the operating suite with latex-free equipment.

D. Social History

It is useful to inquire about tobacco, alcohol, and illicit drug habits, as patients who abuse these substances may be at risk of specific postoperative complications, including withdrawal. The CAGE questionnaire is a common method used to evaluate for potential alcohol problems (**Table 16.9**). A "yes" response to any of the CAGE questions is a marker of potentially problematic drinking. Abrupt alcohol cessation in patients who screen positive by the CAGE questionnaire may trigger alcohol withdrawal syndrome, which is manifested by agitation, hypertension, and tachycardia, and if untreated, carries a mortality of up to 15%.

Smoking is associated with an increased risk of perioperative respiratory complications, including airway hyperreactivity, and impaired wound healing.

Table 16.8 Perioperative Effects of Common Herbal Supplements

Name	Perioperative Effects
Echinacea	Hepatotoxicity; allergic reactions
Ephedra	Enhanced sympathomimetic effects with other sympathomimetic agents, dysrhythmias
Feverfew	Inhibits platelet activity
Garlic	Inhibits platelet aggregation
Ginkgo	Inhibits platelet-activating factor
Ginseng	Hypoglycemia; inhibits platelet aggregation and coagulation cascade
Goldenseal	Inhibits cytochrome P450 enzymes, which may cause changes in blood concentration of other prescribed drugs; may increase bleeding risk
Kava	Hepatotoxicity, decreased MAC
Licorice	Increased blood pressure, hypokalemia
St. John's wort	Inhibits serotonin, norepinephrine, and dopamine reuptake; induction of cytochrome P450 enzyme, leading to increased drug metabolism
Vitamin E	Increased bleeding when taken with other anticoagulant or antithrombotic medications

MAC, minimum alveolar concentration.

Derived from ASA Physician Brochure. *What You Should Know About Your Patients' Use of Herbal Medicines and Other Dietary Supplements*. 2003. www.asahq.org. https://ecommerce.asahq.org/p-147-what-you-should-know-about-herbal-and-dietary-supplement-use-and-anesthesia.aspx

While greater than 8 weeks of abstinence is ideal, all smokers should be encouraged to quit smoking. It has been shown that patients who quit smoking in the context of an acute medical event (eg, acute myocardial infarction) have high 1-year abstinence rates compared to those who quit without such a context. As a result, it is widely considered that the preoperative period should serve as a "teachable moment," and anesthesiologists should encourage patients to quit smoking as part of a program of preanesthetic optimization.

If substance abuse is known or strongly suspected, associated diseases and end-organ damage may be further investigated. However, a positive urine drug screen only confirms the presence of recent not active substance abuse, and the significance of this information for determining whether anesthesia can be administered safely remains controversial.

Table 16.9 CAGE Questionnaire for the Evaluation of Problem Alcohol Use

Have you ever felt you needed to **C**ut down on your drinking?
Have people **A**nnoyed you by criticizing your drinking?
Have you ever felt **G**uilty about drinking?
Have you ever felt you needed a drink first thing in the morning (**E**ye-opener) to steady your nerves or to get rid of a hangover?

Adapted from Ewing JA. Detecting alcoholism: the CAGE questionnaire. *J Am Med Assoc.* 1984;252:1905-1907.

E. Response to Prior Anesthetics

The preanesthetic interview should include a discussion of any personal or familial history of complications related to anesthesia. Patients should be queried about a history of difficult tracheal intubation, prolonged postoperative nausea or vomiting, difficulty associated with the administration of neuraxial anesthesia, and so forth. ***Malignant hyperthermia*** is a rare but potentially life-threatening anesthetic-triggered disorder of skeletal muscle metabolism that is often inherited in an autosomal dominant fashion. Patients may relate a personal or family history of high fever after surgery requiring hospitalization. Patients heterozygous or homozygous for the atypical plasma cholinesterase gene may describe prolonged hospital stays or ventilator dependence after brief surgical procedures. Advanced planning for these patients is a must; and suspicion or confirmation of these conditions should be flagged in the patient's medical record.

F. Focused Physical Examination

Components of the physical examination of main interest to the anesthesiologist involve the neurologic system, heart, lungs, and airway. Notation of blood pressure and heart rate is useful in screening for undiagnosed or poorly treated hypertension. Auscultation of the heart may reveal murmurs suggestive of cardiac valve abnormalities that may require further workup prior to surgery. Wheezing, rhonchi, or other abnormal lung sounds may require additional workup or indicate patients who may benefit from pretreatment with bronchodilators or steroids. In patients with a history of congestive heart failure, wheezing may also be indicative of decompensation. It is also important to note preexisting neuropathies, central nervous system deficits, and skeletal muscle weakness, as these affect the ability to position patients intraoperatively and may affect the decision to perform neuraxial or regional blockades. Examination of peripheral veins and pulses informs the plan for obtaining vascular access.

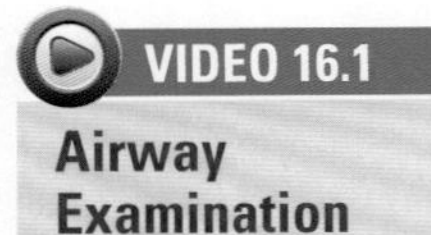

Evaluation of the neck and oral airway helps to determine the potential for difficult ventilation or tracheal intubation and, therefore, the preferred method of and desired equipment for perioperative airway management. Basic components of the airway examination include measurement of the oral aperture, Mallampati score, thyromental distance, range of neck motion, as well as examination of dentition and neck circumference. The ***Mallampati score*** evaluates the size of the tongue in relation to the oral cavity, and the test is performed by having the patient protrude the tongue while keeping his or her head in a neutral position.[18] The anesthesiologist then grades the view on a 4-point scale based on visualization of the uvula and the soft and hard palate (**Table 16.10**). Thyromental distance is measured from the tip of the chin (mentum) to the thyroid cartilage, while the patient's head is maximally extended. A thyromental distance less than 6 cm is suggestive of possible difficult intubation. The patient should also be asked to extend the neck as far as possible (normal is 35°). Significant limitation of neck extension is also a risk factor for difficult intubation. Inability of the lower incisors to extend to reach the upper lip (upper lip bite test) is also a predictor of difficult airway. Preoperative evaluation of dentition is important to determine the presence of prosthetics that should be removed prior to anesthesia and to identify preexisting loose, chipped, or fractured teeth that might later be erroneously attributed to airway manipulation.

Table 16.10 Modified Mallampati Airway Classification

Class	Direct Visualization
I	Soft palate, uvula, tonsillar pillars
II	Soft palate, upper portion of the uvula
III	Soft palate
IV	Only hard palate

Adapted from Mallampati RS, Gatt SP, Gugino LD, et al. A clinical sign to predict difficult tracheal intubation. A prospective study. *Can Anaesth Soc J.* 1985;32:429.

II. Evaluation of the Patient With Known Systemic Disease

A. Cardiovascular Disease

Cardiac Risk Assessment

Cardiovascular complications are a significant source of perioperative morbidity and mortality. Therefore, identifying patients at risk for these complications and finding ways to mitigate these risks preoperatively is a major objective of the preanesthetic workup. The risk of a perioperative major adverse cardiac event (MACE) or death is related to patient factors and the planned surgery. Several validated risk prediction tools have been developed to estimate risk. The Revised Cardiac Risk Index (RCRI) is among the most popular. Based on a retrospective review of over 4000 patients presenting for noncardiac surgery, this index identified six independent predictors of cardiac complications: history of ischemic heart disease; history of congestive heart failure; history of stroke of transient ischemic attack (TIA); preoperative insulin-requiring diabetes; creatinine >2.0 mg/dL; and those presenting for high-risk surgery (intraperitoneal, intrathoracic, or suprainguinal vascular surgery). Two or greater of these factors predict elevated risk. Two newer risk tools have been created by the American College of Surgeon's National Surgical Quality Improvement Program (NSQIP). These incorporate additional factors such as age and functional status. NSQIP has used the information from these tools to create calculators that estimate the risk of MACE and death based on the value of the input variables[b].

Regarding preoperative testing, baseline electrocardiogram (ECG) is reasonable in patients with known ischemic vascular disease (ie, coronary artery, cerebrovascular or peripheral artery disease, significant arrhythmias, or major structural heart disease). Age triggers for ECG vary from institution to institution, as do acceptable time intervals from the last ECG in an otherwise stable patient. In general, preoperative noninvasive cardiac stress testing should be reserved for patients with elevated cardiac risk who demonstrate poor (<4 METs) or unknown functional capacity and are undergoing anything other than low-risk surgery (MACE risk ≥1%).

Regarding the decision to undertake coronary revascularization before surgery, the Coronary Artery Revascularization Prophylaxis (CARP) trial was the first large, randomized study designed to evaluate whether prophylactic coronary revascularization prior to major vascular surgery reduced perioperative cardiac events relative to optimal pharmacologic management. The main finding was no difference in all-cause mortality at a median follow-up of

[b]www.riskcalculator.facs.org and http://www.surgicalriskcalculator.com/microcardiacarrest.

2.7 years. A secondary finding was no difference in the incidence of postoperative myocardial infarction. A criticism that has been rendered against the CARP trial was that selection criteria resulted in the exclusion of too many high-risk patients. However, for the majority of patients, current evidence supports pharmacologic optimization as the best cardiac risk reduction strategy prior to surgery. The 2014 American College of Cardiology/American Heart Association "Perioperative Cardiovascular Evaluation and Management of Patients Undergoing Noncardiac Surgery" guideline presents an algorithmic approach to perioperative cardiac assessment aimed at helping clinicians in the evaluation of these patients (**Figure 16.1**).[19,20]

Perioperative Coronary Stents

Patients with indwelling coronary stents, especially those that have been inserted recently, present a treatment dilemma, as these patients are frequently on lifelong antiplatelet therapy to prevent in-stent thrombosis. Information that should be obtained during the preanesthetic interview includes the type of stent, time since placement, and input from the consulting cardiologist as to whether antiplatelet therapy can be discontinued in the perioperative period. Current recommendations from the American Heart Association/American College of Cardiology call for postponing elective surgery for a minimum of 4 weeks after placement of a BMS and 6 months after placement of a DES (**Figure 16.2**). Time-sensitive surgeries can be considered only after at least 3 months of DAPT after DES placement, with the risks and benefits considered by both the cardiology and surgery teams. If possible, DAPT, or at least aspirin, should be continued throughout the perioperative period.

Figure 16.1 Stepwise approach to perioperative cardiac assessment for coronary artery disease. The American College of Cardiology/American Heart Association (ACC/AHA) guideline calls for stepwise cardiac risk assessment involving consideration of the patient's cardiac risk factors, functional capacity, and the planned surgical procedure. If emergent, surgery should proceed and cardiac risk be mitigated with appropriate intraoperative monitoring and pharmacologic techniques. If surgery is nonemergent and an acute coronary syndrome (eg, unstable angina) is identified, surgery should be delayed and the patient should receive appropriate medical treatment. In general, during preanesthetic evaluation, all patients should receive a cardiac risk assessment using a validated risk tool (RCRI or NSQIP risk calculator). If the risk of MACE is ≥1% and the patient's functional capacity is ≥4 METs, no further testing is indicated. If, however, the risk of MACE is ≥1% and the patient's functional capacity is <4 METs or unknown, pharmacological stress testing should be considered. If the result is abnormal, consideration may be given to PCI or CABG. Pharmacological stress testing is not advised for patients undergoing low-risk surgery (MACE <1%). In addition, pharmacological stress testing should only be undertaken if it is expected to change management. An alternative to stress testing is guideline-directed medical therapy, for example, β-blockers and statins. Colors correspond to class of recommendation based on level of evidence, with green indicating the greatest strength of evidence supporting benefits >>> risks; yellow indicating benefits >> risks but based on weaker evidence; and red indicating no benefit or risks > benefits based on the best available evidence. ACS, acute coronary syndrome; CABG, coronary artery bypass graft; CAD, coronary artery disease; CPG, clinical practice guideline; GDMT, guideline-directed medical therapy; MACE, major adverse cardiac event; MET, metabolic equivalent; NSQIP, National Surgical Quality Improvement Program; PCI, percutaneous coronary intervention; RCRI, Revised Cardiac Risk Index. (From Fleisher LA, Fleischmann KE, Auerbach AD, et al. 2014 ACC/AHA guideline on perioperative cardiovascular evaluation and management of patients undergoing noncardiac surgery: a report of the American College of Cardiology/American Heart Association Task Force on practice guidelines. *J Am Coll Cardiol.* 2014;64(22):e77-e137.)

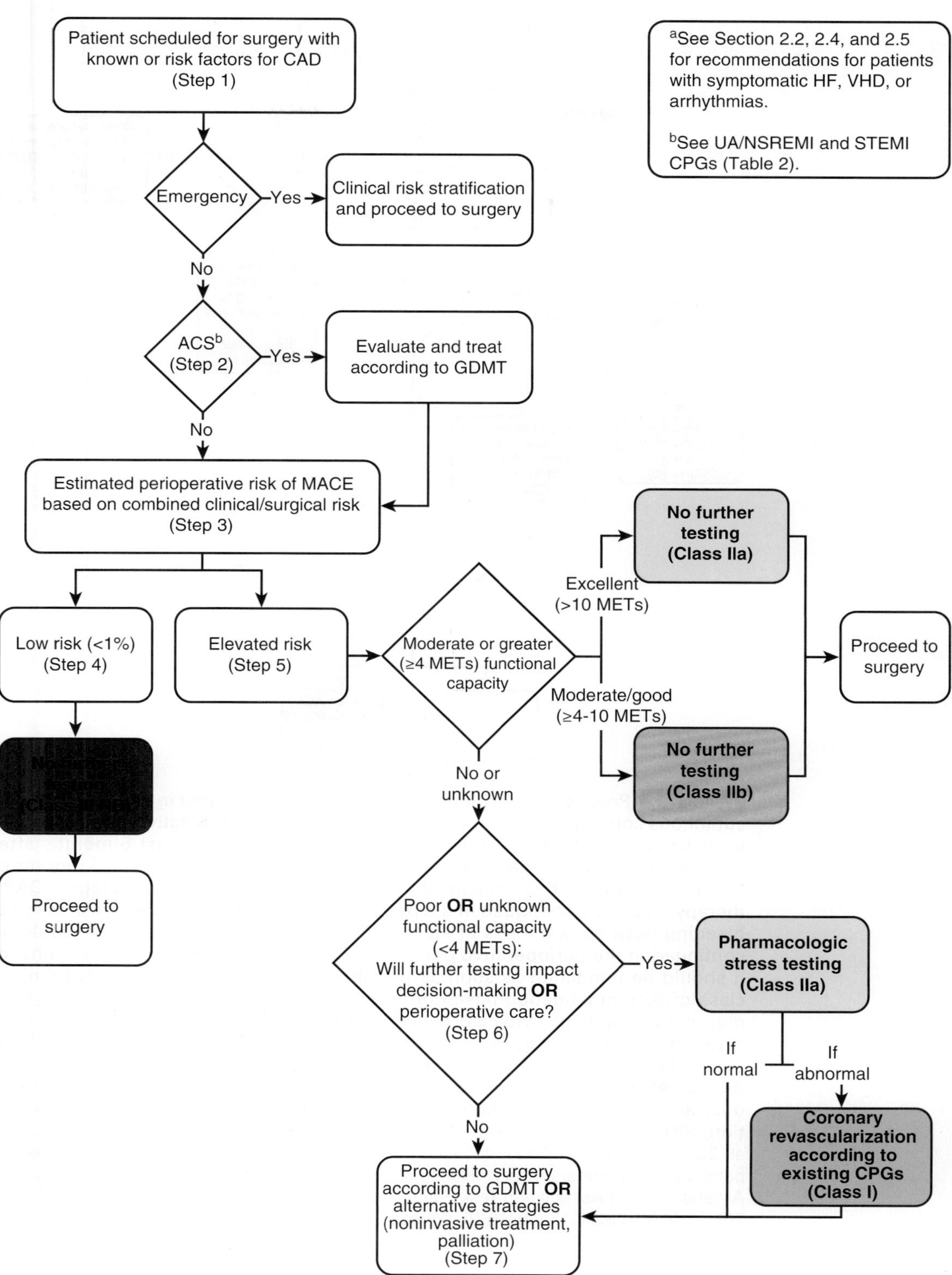

Patient scheduled for surgery with known or risk factors for CAD (Step 1)
Emergency
Yes
Clinical risk stratification and proceed to surgery
No
ACS[b] (Step 2)
Yes
Evaluate and treat according to GDMT
No
Estimated perioperative risk of MACE based on combined clinical/surgical risk (Step 3)
Low risk (<1%) (Step 4)
Elevated risk (Step 5)
Proceed to surgery
Moderate or greater (≥4 METs) functional capacity
Excellent (>10 METs)
No further testing (Class IIa)
Moderate/good (≥4-10 METs)
No further testing (Class IIb)
Proceed to surgery
No or unknown
Poor OR unknown functional capacity (<4 METs): Will further testing impact decision-making OR perioperative care? (Step 6)
Yes
Pharmacologic stress testing (Class IIa)
If normal
If abnormal
Coronary revascularization according to existing CPGs (Class I)
No
Proceed to surgery according to GDMT OR alternative strategies (noninvasive treatment, palliation) (Step 7)
[a]See Section 2.2, 2.4, and 2.5 for recommendations for patients with symptomatic HF, VHD, or arrhythmias.
[b]See UA/NSREMI and STEMI CPGs (Table 2).

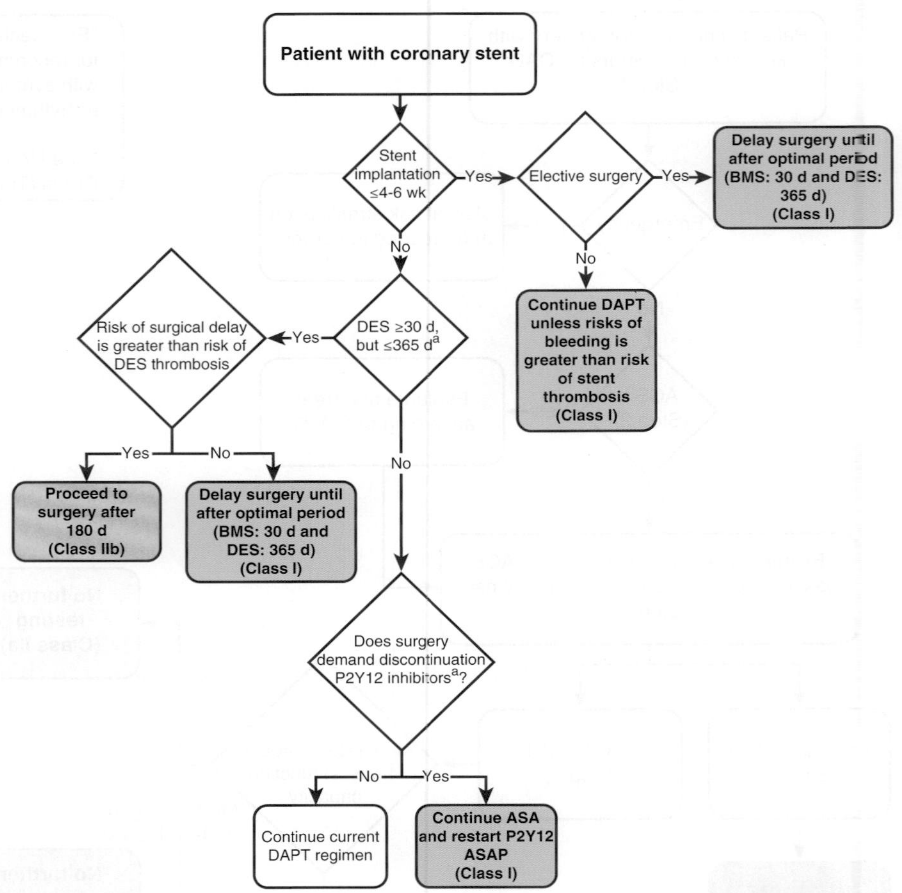

Figure 16.2 Proposed algorithm for antiplatelet management in patients with percutaneous coronary intervention and noncardiac surgery. Elective surgery should be delayed until 30 days after placement of a BMS and at least 6 months after placement of a DES. Time-sensitive surgeries can be considered after 3 months of DAPT therapy after DES, in consultation with the prescribing cardiologist. DAPT therapy should be continued in the perioperative period unless the risk of surgical bleeding outweighs the risk of stent thrombosis; at minimum, aspirin should be continued in the perioperative period. If P2Y12-inhibitor therapy is discontinued, it should be reinitiated as soon as possible after surgery. Colors correspond to class of recommendation based on level of evidence, with green indicating the greatest strength of evidence supporting benefits >>> risks; yellow indicating benefits >> risks but based on weaker evidence; and red indicating no benefit or risks > benefits based on the best available evidence. ACS, acute coronary syndrome; ASA, aspirin; ASAP, as soon as possible; BMS, bare-metal stent; DAPT, dual antiplatelet therapy; DES, drug-eluting stent; PCI, percutaneous intervention; SIHD, stable ischemic heart disease. (From Levine GN, Bates ER, Bittl JA, et al. 2016 ACC/AHA Guideline focused update on duration of dual antiplatelet therapy in patients with coronary artery disease. A report of the American College of Cardiology/American Heart Association Task Force on clinical practice guidelines. *J Am Coll Cardiol.* 2016;68(10):1082-1115. doi:10.1016/j.jacc.2016.03.513)

Patients With CIEDs

Patients with CIEDs are presenting for surgery with increasing frequency, as the indications for these devices increase and the population ages. Traditionally, implantable cardioverter-defibrillator (ICD) therapy has been delivered via transvenous systems which deliver shock therapy via intracardiac leads. More recently, subcutaneous ICD systems have been developed. These systems consist of a pulse generator and a single subcutaneous lead which senses, detects, and delivers treatment when a life-threatening dysrhythmia is detected. Unlike the transvenous systems, subcutaneous ICD systems must be placed in the right chest.

EMI from devices in the operating suite—most commonly monopolar electrocautery—can cause malfunction of these devices. Subcutaneous systems may be even more susceptible to this interference. Specifically, EMI may be interpreted as intrinsic cardiac activity and thereby lead to inappropriate antitachycardia therapy (defibrillation or pacing). In 2011, the Heart Rhythm Society and the ASA published a consensus statement in collaboration with the American Heart Association, American College of Cardiology, and Society of Thoracic Surgeons to provide guidance on the perioperative management of these devices.[21] In 2020, the ASA published similar guidelines.[22] Essential information that should be obtained about the CIED during the anesthesia evaluation includes the reason for device implantation, device type and manufacturer, date of last interrogation and report, current programming, whether the patient is pacemaker dependent, and the device's response to application of a magnet (**Table 16.11**). For most ICDs, external application of a magnet will disable tachycardic therapy but will have no effect on pacemaker settings. This is also true of the subcutaneous systems. Magnet application to a pacemaker will initiate asynchronous pacing.

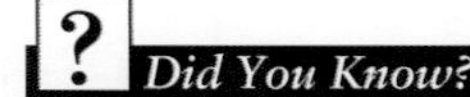

The risk of electromagnetic interference (EMI) affecting the function of a cardiovascular implantable electronic device (CIED) decreases as the distance of the procedure from the CIED increases. For patients having surgery below the umbilicus, surgery may safely proceed without alteration of the CIED or the application of a magnet.

Surgical aspects should also be considered, including accessibility of the pulse generator for magnet application and removal and the risk of EMI. A separation of the monopolar cautery current path and device pulse generator and leads of at least 6 in (15 cm) has traditionally been thought to be the distance at which EMI is unlikely. Practically, surgery below the umbilicus is very unlikely to cause EMI for devices implanted in the upper chest. If monopolar cautery is required, the dispersion pad should be placed to direct current as far from the generator and leads as possible. If EMI is deemed likely, permanent pacemaker function should be altered to an asynchronous mode, particularly in the pacemaker-dependent patient. The antitachycardia function of a defibrillator should be suspended. This can be accomplished by application of a magnet or device reprogramming. Note that in some devices, the magnet response asynchronous ventricular rate for some devices is as high as 100 bpm, which may not be desirable for some patients. In any case, there should be a very low threshold to seek advice on perioperative CIED management from the managing cardiology team. Pacemakers should have been interrogated within 12 months and defibrillators within 6 months of contemplated surgery. **Table 16.11** presents an approach to the perioperative management of the patient with a CIED.

Hypertension

Hypertension is highly prevalent, with over 40% of adults in the United States carrying the diagnosis. From a perioperative perspective, the main concerns in the hypertensive patient are the presence of hypertensive end-organ damage

Table 16.11 Important Information to be Determined About Cardiovascular Implantable Electronic Devices During the Preanesthetic Evaluation
Reason for placement
Device type, manufacturer, model
Date of last interrogation and results (6 mo for defibrillator, 12 mo for pacemaker)
Is the patient pacemaker dependent?
Device programming and response to magnet

and overall cardiovascular risk. Induction of anesthesia results in sympathetic stimulation that manifests as a rise in blood pressure of about 20 to 30 mm Hg and heart rate of about 15 to 20 bpm. This response is exaggerated in patients with preexisting hypertension, especially those who are untreated or poorly controlled. Patients with undiagnosed hypertension are also more likely to exhibit intraoperative blood pressure lability.

Whether to postpone elective surgery in patients with poorly controlled hypertension is controversial. Some anesthesiologists postpone elective surgery in patients who exhibit a sustained systolic blood pressure of >180 mm Hg or diastolic blood pressure of >110 mm Hg or who have signs or symptoms of unrecognized or untreated end-organ damage. The concern in these cases would be an increased risk of perioperative complications including dysrhythmias, myocardial ischemia, neurologic complications, and kidney injury.[23]

B. Pulmonary Disease

Postoperative pulmonary complications occur in an estimated 5% to 10% of surgeries and may account for as many as one in four deaths that occur within 1 week of surgery.[24] The risk of their occurrence is related to both patient and surgical factors (**Table 16.12**). What constitutes a pulmonary complication is not well defined, but it is generally taken to mean any clinically significant pulmonary dysfunction that adversely affects a patient's clinical course. Examples include pneumonia, pneumonitis, hypoventilation, hypoxemia, prolonged mechanical ventilation, reintubation, exacerbation of underlying lung disease, and bronchospasm.

If pulmonary function testing exists, it is useful to consider the risk stratification often employed prior to thoracic surgery. This includes an assessment of (1) respiratory mechanics (ie, forced expiratory volume in 1 second [FEV1]); (2) cardiopulmonary reserve (ie, maximum oxygen consumption [VO_{2max}], as approximated by METs); and (3) gas exchange (ie, diffusing capacity, DLCO).

Table 16.12 Potential Risk Factors for Perioperative Pulmonary Complications

Patient Factors	Surgical Factors
Older age Smoking Chronic obstructive pulmonary disease Obesity Obstructive sleep apnea	Incisions close to the diaphragm (eg, thoracic, upper abdominal procedures, abdominal aortic aneurysm repair) Longer duration procedures General (vs neuraxial, regional) anesthesia

An FEV1 < 40%, DLCO < 40%, and VO_{2max} < 4 METs all predict an increased risk of pulmonary complications.

Patient Factors

As expected, patients with preexisting lung disease, including obstructive diseases, such as asthma or chronic obstructive pulmonary disease, and restrictive diseases such as pulmonary fibrosis, have an increased risk of pulmonary complications compared with healthy adults. Various risk indices have been created to predict postoperative pulmonary complications. One such index is the ARISCAT (Assess Respiratory Risk in Surgical Patients in Catalonia), which includes the following factors: advanced age; low preoperative oxygen saturation; recent (<1 month) respiratory infection, preoperative anemia, or upper abdominal or thoracic surgery; surgery duration > 2 hours; and emergency surgery.

Smoking

Tobacco and nicotine increase sputum production, reduce ciliary function, stimulate the cardiovascular system, and increase carboxyhemoglobin levels. Although smoking cessation for as little as 2 days decreases carboxyhemoglobin levels and improves mucociliary clearance, most studies suggest it takes at least 8 weeks of smoking cessation to reduce the rate of postoperative pulmonary complications. Nevertheless, it is still reasonable to encourage smoking cessation preoperatively owing to its positive implications on a patient's overall health.

Obstructive Sleep Apnea

OSA is a syndrome marked by periodic upper airway obstruction during sleep, which leads to oxygen desaturation and carbon dioxide retention, sleep deprivation, and daytime somnolence. The prevalence of OSA is estimated to be 10% to 15% in women and 10% to 30% in men. Patients with OSA are particularly susceptible to the respiratory depressant effects of inhaled anesthetics and opioids and, therefore, are more likely to suffer critical respiratory events. Patients with OSA have an approximately threefold risk of perioperative complications including difficult mask ventilation and airway management; systemic and pulmonary hypertension; cardiac dysrhythmias; coronary artery disease; delirium; and postoperative respiratory failure and reintubation.[25] For these reasons, screening for OSA is an important part of the preanesthetic examination. There are a number of screening tools used to evaluate for the presence of OSA, including the STOP-Bang questionnaire and one published by the ASA (**Table 16.13**).[26] Symptoms suggestive of OSA include a history of snoring, daytime sleepiness, and headaches. Physical signs include body mass index >35 kg/m^2, neck circumference >17 in in men or >16 in in women, and tonsillar hyperplasia.

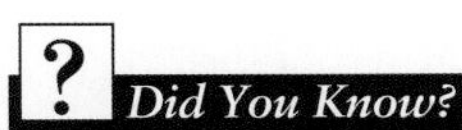

The majority of people with OSA are undiagnosed.

Preoperative and postoperative use of continuous positive airway pressure or noninvasive positive pressure ventilation have been shown to reduce serious perioperative complications. These patients should receive postoperative respiratory monitoring in a setting with continuous pulse oximetry. When contemplating outpatient surgery, the perioperative team should consider the sleep apnea severity, relevant comorbidities, nature of surgery, expectations of postoperative opioid requirements, patient age, and patient support structure at home. If outpatient surgery is planned, discharge should be delayed until postoperative respiratory function has returned to baseline. Opioid use should be minimized in favor of nonnarcotic analgesics and regional anesthetic techniques.

Table 16.13 STOP-Bang Questionnaire

Yes	No	**Snoring?** Do you Snore loudly (loud enough to be heard through closed doors or your bed-partner elbows you for snoring at night)?
Yes	No	**Tired?** Do you often feel Tired, Fatigued, or Sleepy during the daytime (such as falling asleep during driving or talking to someone)?
Yes	No	**Observed?** Has anyone Observed you Stop Breathing or Choking/Gasping during your sleep?
Yes	No	**Pressure?** Do you have or are being treated for High Blood Pressure?
Yes	No	**B**ody Mass Index more than 35 kg/m^2?
Yes	No	**A**ge older than 50 y?
Yes	No	**N**eck size large? (Measured around Adam's apple) For male, is your shirt collar 17 in/43 cm or larger? For female, is your shirt collar 16 in/41 cm or larger?
Yes	No	**G**ender = Male?

For general population
OSA—Low risk: Yes to 0-2 questions
OSA—Intermediate risk: Yes to 3-4 questions
OSA—High risk: Yes to 5-8 questions or Yes to 2 or more of 4 STOP questions + male gender or Yes to 2 or more of 4 STOP questions + BMI > 35 kg/m^2 or Yes to 2 or more of 4 STOP questions + neck circumference 17 in/43 cm in male or 16 in/41 cm in female

Derived from Chung F, Yegneswaran B, Liao P, Chung SA, Vairavanathan S, Islam S, Khajehdehi A, Shapiro CM. STOP questionnaire: a tool to screen patients for obstructive sleep apnea. *Anesthesiology*. 2008 May;108(5):812-21; Chung F, Subramanyam R, Liao P, Sasaki E, Shapiro C, Sun Y. High STOP-Bang score indicates a high probability of obstructive sleep apnoea. *Br J Anaesth*. 2012 May;108(5):768-75; Chung F, Yang Y, Brown R, Liao P. Alternative scoring models of STOP-bang questionnaire improve specificity to detect undiagnosed obstructive sleep apnea. *J Clin Sleep Med*. 2014 Sep 15;10(9):951-8; and The Official STOP-Bang Questionnaire. Available at: http://www.stopbang.ca/osa/screening.php. Accessed June 21, 2021.

Surgical Factors

The site of surgery is the most important factor related to the risk of developing pulmonary complications postoperatively. Patients having thoracic and upper abdominal surgeries are far more likely to suffer pulmonary complications relative to those having lower abdominal or extremity procedures. Abdominal aortic aneurysm repair, head and neck surgery, and neurosurgical procedures are also associated with a higher risk of pulmonary complications relative to other surgeries. This is related mostly to effects on the muscles of the upper airway, accessory respiratory muscles, and diaphragmatic function. Duration of surgery is also important, with longer procedures leading to a higher risk of complications. General anesthesia is associated with a higher rate of clinically significant pulmonary complications relative to neuraxial or regional anesthesia.

C. Endocrine Disease

Diabetes Mellitus

Diabetes is the most common endocrinopathy, affecting nearly 10% of the population. Patients with diabetes have an accelerated rate of atherosclerosis and are susceptible to microvascular complications that manifest as retinopathy, neuropathy, cerebrovascular, peripheral vascular, and kidney diseases. Autonomic neuropathy may predispose those with diabetes to intraoperative hemodynamic instability. Gastroparesis increases the risk of pulmonary aspiration. Poorly controlled diabetic patients are also at greater risk of developing postoperative infections.

Factors including preoperative fasting and the surgical stress response result in large swings in blood glucose levels perioperatively, which make tight glucose control extremely challenging. Overly aggressive glycemic control introduces the risk of life-threatening hypoglycemia, which can go unrecognized under anesthesia. Therefore, in general, guidelines recommend a perioperative glycemic target between 140 and 180 mg/dL.[27-29] Recommendations for preoperative management of oral hypoglycemics and insulin regimens vary by institution. **Table 16.5** presents a suggested approach.

Thyroid and Parathyroid Disorders

Hypothyroidism is more common in women; signs and symptoms include bradycardia, cold intolerance, hypoventilation, and hyponatremia. Hyperthyroidism is marked by tachycardia, tremor, weight loss, and heat intolerance. Patients may also exhibit dysrhythmias such as atrial fibrillation. In symptomatic patients, it may be prudent to delay elective surgery. In addition, thyroid masses may cause distortion of upper airway anatomy. A computed tomography scan of the neck is often useful to evaluate the upper airway and identify tracheal deviation or compression.

The overall prevalence of hyperparathyroidism is about 1%, but the prevalence increases with advancing age. Symptoms include weight loss, polydipsia, hypertension, heart block, lethargy, bone pain, kidney stones, and constipation. In patients with suspected hyperparathyroidism, preoperative determination of serum calcium concentration is prudent.

Adrenal Disorders

Pheochromocytoma, though rare, should be considered in any patient who relates a history of paroxysmal hypertension, headache, and tachycardia. The preoperative evaluation should assess for end-organ damage. Preoperative pharmacologic preparation prior to surgery varies but typically includes combined alpha-blockade followed by β-blockade, intended to reduce intra- and postoperative hemodynamic instability and arrhythmias. Invasive cardiovascular monitoring and central venous access may be indicated.

Adrenal suppression should be considered in any patient who has taken steroids chronically in a dose equivalent to prednisone ≥5 mg/d for at least 3 weeks within 6 to 12 months of surgery. Patients taking a daily prednisone dose ≥20 mg for at least 3 weeks are considered to be suppressed. Patients taking intermediate doses are at intermediate risk of adrenal suppression. Regimens for steroid supplementation perioperatively vary by institution. For minor surgeries, supplementation is rarely needed. For major procedures, one option is to administer 100 mg of hydrocortisone intravenously prior to induction of anesthesia and then 50 mg intravenously every 8 hours for 24 hours (**Table 16.4**).

Other Organ Systems and Conditions

Patients with ***rheumatoid arthritis*** (***RA***) have a higher risk of cardiovascular disease compared with the general population. In addition, they are prone to cervical joint instability, which must be taken into consideration during intubation. Patients are often maintained on long-term glucocorticoid therapy and may require supplementation perioperatively. Biologic agents used to treat RA may adversely affect the immune response and may predispose patients to perioperative infectious complications and poor wound healing. Surgery is ideally planned to occur just before the patient is due for the next dose to minimize wound complications. Patients with significant osteoarthritis or osteoporosis should be positioned with care, as should patients with indwelling artificial joints.

Various neurologic conditions have implications for anesthesia and surgery. For patients with a history of seizures, antiepileptic medications should be continued in the perioperative period and drug levels should be carefully monitored, as surgery and no food by mouth status may affect drug absorption and metabolism. Patients with Parkinson disease have an increased risk of orthostatic hypotension, aspiration, and postoperative pulmonary complications. Drugs used to treat Parkinson disease should be continued perioperatively in an attempt to reduce symptom exacerbation. Patients with a history of stroke are at increased risk of perioperative stroke. Patients with spinal injury and denervation, such as quadriplegia or a history of significant burn injuries, are at risk for hyperkalemia and cardiac arrest if given succinylcholine.

Risk factors suggestive of liver disease include a history of heavy alcohol use, hepatitis, illicit drug use, or sexual promiscuity. Signs on examination include increased abdominal girth, spider telangiectasias, jaundice, gynecomastia, and splenomegaly. Signs of renal disease may be difficult to identify on examination but include hypertension, edema, and lethargy. Of note, patients who are dialysis dependent should ideally be dialyzed within 24 hours of surgery to optimize volume and metabolic status.

Obesity is increasingly common, affecting approximately 40% of the US population. Obesity creates challenges for the perioperative care team in nearly every respect; notably, it increases the risk of cardiovascular disease, restrictive lung disease, atelectasis, sleep apnea, challenging IV access, difficult mask ventilation and intubation, reactive airway disease, pulmonary hypertension, diabetes, liver disease, gastroesophageal reflux disease (GERD), venous thrombosis, and nerve injury.

III. Perioperative Laboratory Testing

There is no benefit to "routine" preanesthetic laboratory testing in patients presenting for elective surgery. Furthermore, this approach is extremely inefficient. Routine preoperative testing has been estimated to cost $3 billion per year.[30,31] Owing to the intrinsic characteristic of screening tests, especially when a panel of tests is ordered, there is a high likelihood that one result will return as abnormal. However, in a person with no risk factors, this result is more likely to be a false positive than a true positive. The ASA's "Practice Advisory for Preanesthetic Evaluation" (2012) and the American Board of Internal Medicine's "Choosing Wisely Campaign" support this view.[32,33] Nevertheless, selective preanesthetic laboratory testing is appropriate for some patients, based on their medical conditions, symptomatology elicited on interview, and the nature of the planned surgery.[34,35] **Table 16.14** summarizes the general principles of preoperative laboratory testing in patients undergoing elective noncardiac surgery.

Table 16.14 General Principles on Preoperative Testing in Adults Undergoing Elective Noncardiac Surgery

Factor	Comment
ASA physical status	ASA PS 1 or 2 patients generally do not require preoperative testing before low-risk surgeries.
Very-low-risk procedures (eg, colonoscopy, cataract surgery) in patients with ≥METs	No testing is generally needed except point-of-care urine pregnancy and blood glucose if the patient is diabetic.
Pregnancy testing	Should be conducted on females of reproductive age unless the patient has had hysterectomy or is confirmed to be postmenopausal.
Point-of-care blood glucose	In diabetic patients.
Cardiac workup	According to ACC/AHA guidelines.
Pulmonary function testing	It is performed for risk stratification prior to lung resection and some cardiac surgeries. Consider in patients with unexplained dyspnea.
Chest x-ray	Consider in patients with significant cardiopulmonary disease, new-onset symptoms plausibly referable to cardiopulmonary disease, or as a baseline in patients undergoing major upper abdominal or thoracic surgery. No need to repeat if one has been completed within 12 mo, results were within normal limits, and there has been no change in clinical status.
Polysomnography	Consider in patients at very high risk of sleep apnea being considered for high-risk procedures.
Intermediate- to high-risk procedures	Serum chemistries, complete blood count, and coagulation profile should be obtained based on the patient's comorbidities. No need to repeat within 6 mo if results were within normal limits, there has been no change in clinical status, and the patient is not on medication likely to significantly change laboratory tests (eg, anticoagulant, diuretic).

ACC/AHA, American College of Cardiology/American Heart Association; ASA, American Society of Anesthesiologists; ECG, electrocardiogram; METs, metabolic equivalents; PS, physical status.

IV. Preparation for Anesthesia

A. Fasting Guidelines

Preoperative fasting is the mainstay of preparation for anesthesia and is designed mainly for minimizing the risk of pulmonary aspiration of gastric contents. Pulmonary aspiration is estimated to occur in 1 in 3000 to 1 in 6000 elective anesthetics but up to 1 in 600 emergency anesthetics. Risk factors for aspiration include emergency surgery, obesity, difficult airway, reflux, hiatal hernia, and inadequate anesthesia. The ASA has developed the "Practice Guidelines for Preoperative Fasting and Pharmacologic Intervention for Prevention of Perioperative Aspiration: Application to Healthy Patients Undergoing Elective Procedures" (**Table 16.15**).[36] These guidelines advise that clear liquids should be stopped at least 2 hours prior to surgery, breast milk at least 4 hours, and nonhuman milk and solids at least 6 hours before surgery. Examples of clear liquids include water, tea, black coffee, and fruit juices without pulp. Fried or fatty foods should be stopped at least 8 hours prior to surgery, as these require longer gastric emptying times. Note that these guidelines may need modification in patients with comorbidities affecting gastric emptying or gastric volume.

B. Pharmacologic Agents to Reduce the Risk of Pulmonary Aspiration

Routine use of drugs to prevent pulmonary aspiration is not advised, but they are effective when used in patients with risk factors for pulmonary aspiration. Several agents with varying mechanisms of action are available (**Table 16.16**).

V. Preoperative Medication

Several medications may be used prior to anesthetic induction to help reduce the patient's anxiety about anesthesia, improve conditions for intubation, reduce complications such as nausea and vomiting, and improve postoperative pain control.

A. Benzodiazepines

In many cases, patient education and informed consent conducted during the preanesthetic interview replace the need for pharmacologic anxiolysis prior to anesthetic induction. However, benzodiazepines are useful for producing moderate sedation and reducing anxiety, as well as providing some degree of anterograde amnesia and postoperative nausea and vomiting (PONV) prophylaxis. Midazolam is commonly used, owing to its rapid onset of action (1-2 minutes) and relatively short half-life (1-4 hours). It can be administered orally as a fluid or in a "lollipop" sponge as well as intravenously.

B. Antihistamines

Diphenhydramine is a histamine-1 antagonist that has sedative, antiemetic, and anticholinergic properties. Although still used in some conscious sedation protocols, it is rarely used as premedication, owing to its long half-life (3-6 hours), which tends to prolong recovery times. Diphenhydramine, along with

Table 16.15 Summary of Fasting Guidelines as Prophylaxis for Pulmonary Aspiration

Ingested Substance	Minimum Fasting Period (h)
Clear liquids	2
Breast milk	4
Infant formula	6
Nonhuman milk	6
Light meal (toast, clear liquids)	6
Heavy meal (fatty foods)	8

From ASA practice guidelines for preoperative fasting and the use of pharmacologic agents to reduce the risk of pulmonary aspiration: application to healthy ptients undergoing elective procedures. *Anesthesiology*. 2017;126(3):376-393.

Table 16.16 Drugs Used to Reduce the Risk of Pulmonary Aspiration

Drug	Onset	Effect	Comment
Antacids (eg, sodium citrate, aluminum or magnesium hydroxide, calcium carbonate)	15-30 min	Raise gastric pH	Nonparticulate antacids (sodium citrate) do not cause pulmonary damage if aspirated, in contrast to particulate antacids (calcium carbonate, aluminum hydroxide)
Histamine-2 receptor antagonists (eg, ranitidine, famotidine)	60 min	Reduce gastric volume Increase gastric pH	
Proton-pump inhibitors (eg, omeprazole, pantoprazole)	30 min	Reduce gastric acid secretion Reduce gastric volume	Block proton pump on gastric parietal cells
Prokinetic agents (eg, metoclopramide)	15-30 min	Increase gastric motility Increase gastroesophageal sphincter tone	Useful for patients with known or suspected large gastric volume or delayed gastric emptying, such as obese patients, parturients, and diabetics Contraindicated in patients with a known bowel obstruction and should be used with caution in the elderly because they are more likely to experience side effects such as confusion and drowsiness

a histamine-2 antagonist and steroids, may be given to patients with a history of latex allergy or chronic atopy or patients undergoing procedures requiring administration of radiocontrast dye as prophylaxis against allergic reactions.

C. Antisialagogues

It is often helpful to administer an anticholinergic agent to reduce upper airway secretions when a fiberoptic-assisted tracheal intubation is expected. Glycopyrrolate is a potent antisialagogue and produces less tachycardia compared to scopolamine or atropine. In addition, glycopyrrolate does not cross the blood-brain barrier; therefore, it does not have central nervous system side effects.

D. Antiemetics

The prophylactic administration of antiemetic agents is not a cost-effective strategy. However, selective premedication of patients with a history of PONV and those with risk factors for PONV (females, history of motion sickness, those likely to receive opioids, and those undergoing gynecologic, ophthalmologic, or cosmetic procedures) may be of benefit. Agents used for this purpose include serotonin antagonists such as ondansetron, phenothiazines such as perphenazine, butyrophenones such as droperidol, and antihistamines such as dimenhydrinate. Most of these drugs are best administered just prior to the end of surgery for optimal onset of action. However, the glucocorticoid dexamethasone is best given at the time of induction, and scopolamine, an anticholinergic drug, is routinely applied as a transdermal patch in the preoperative area. Scopolamine is especially useful in patients with a history of motion sickness. The neurokinin 1 receptor antagonist aprepitant is a representative from the newest class of antiemetics; like scopolamine, it is best given orally in the preoperative area.

E. Preemptive Analgesia

Preemptive analgesia involves the administration of analgesics prior to an expected noxious stimulus. This strategy may not only help improve acute postoperative pain control but also prevent central sensitization that contributes to the development of chronic postoperative pain. Examples of preemptive analgesia include the use of oral acetaminophen; NSAIDs; gabapentinoids; neuraxial techniques (with or without concomitant use of general anesthesia); infiltration with local anesthetics; and the administration of intravenous agents such as ketamine, local anesthetic, or opioids.

IV. Antibiotic Prophylaxis

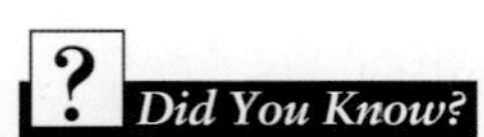

Skin flora such as *Staphylococcus aureus* and *Staphylococcus epidermidis* are the most common causes of SSI.

Antibiotics are administered prior to surgical procedures in order to prevent surgical site infections (SSIs), which occur in 2% to 5% of surgical patients. Documentation of the administration of antibiotic prophylaxis is a commonly used process measure by which anesthesia departments and hospitals are evaluated (eg, Surgical Care Improvement Program, Joint Commission). Surgical wounds are classified into four categories based on the degree of expected microbial contamination: clean, clean-contaminated, contaminated, and dirty. Although there is a moderate correlation between wound classification and SSI risk, other factors are also important. These include length of surgery, health status of the patient, and operative technique.

The microbial flora associated with SSIs vary based on surgical procedure and have also changed over time. For clean wounds, SSIs are usually caused by gram-positive skin flora such as *Staphylococcus aureus, Staphylococcus epidermidis,* and streptococcal species. For clean-contaminated wounds, gram-negative organisms are more commonly involved. In recent years, the proportion of SSIs caused by gram-negative bacteria has decreased. *S. aureus* is currently the most common cause of SSIs, accounting for about 30% of SSIs. Methicillin-resistant *S. aureus* (MRSA) species are isolated from about half of these cases. In addition, fungi such as *Candida albicans* have been isolated from SSIs with growing frequency.

Cefazolin, a first-generation cephalosporin, is the most commonly used antibiotic for prophylaxis against SSIs. It has coverage against gram-positive cocci (except *Enterococcus*) as well as many gram-negative organisms such as *Escherichia coli, Proteus,* and *Klebsiella.* For most adults, an initial dose of 2 g is advised; 3 g is recommended for patients weighing ≥120 kg, and weight-based dosing is used for pediatric patients. Clindamycin or vancomycin is recommended in patients with a true immunoglobulin-E–mediated β-lactam antibiotic allergy. For patients known to be colonized with MRSA, a single dose of vancomycin may also be added preoperatively, as cefazolin does not cover MRSA. Antibiotic infusions should be administered within 1 hour of incision, with the exception of vancomycin and fluoroquinolones, which may be administered within 2 hours of incision. Infusions should be completed prior to incision and prior to the inflation of surgical tourniquets. Intraoperative redosing of antibiotics is recommended at intervals of approximately 2 drug half-lives. Redosing is also recommended in surgeries where blood loss is excessive (>1500 mL) and when duration of drug half-life is shortened, such as through drug-drug interaction or in the setting of extensive burns. In general, antibiotics initiated solely for the purpose of prophylaxis against SSI need only be given intraoperatively; they should certainly be discontinued within 24 hours of surgery. There is no need to continue antibiotic prophylaxis based on the presence of indwelling catheters or surgical drains.

Colonization with *S. aureus,* which usually occurs in the nose, occurs in about 25% of the population and is a risk factor for SSI.[37] For this reason, preoperative screening and eradication of *S. aureus* has been recommended to reduce the rate of SSI, especially in high-risk groups such as cardiac and orthopedic surgery patients. Mupirocin is an intranasal ointment used to treat MRSA colonization.[38] When used preoperatively, it is generally administered 5 days prior to surgery.

A. Surgical Prehabilitation

A relatively new concept in perioperative medicine is that of surgical prehabilitation.[39] With the recognition that complications after surgery often lead to a significant decline in quality of life and the aging of the population, meaning that surgical patients are presenting at older ages than ever before, increasing attention is being given to the prevention of complications through preoperative optimization. Improved nutrition and physical fitness are the cornerstones of care. An exercise program that aims to improve both cardiovascular fitness and muscle mass and strength is ideal.

Malnutrition affects up to 40% of elderly patients and is especially common in patients with cancer. Preoperative nutritional assessments are useful in identifying high-risk patients. Albumin measurement can be useful in determining the severity of malnutrition. The goals of nutritional prehabilitation are not only to optimize weight but also to prevent stress-induced catabolism and maximize immune system function.

For further review and interactivities, please see the associated Interactive Video Lectures and "A Closer Look" infographic accessible in the complimentary eBook bundled with this text. Access instructions are located in the inside front cover.

References

1. Correll DJ, Bader AM, Hull MW, Hsu C, Tsen LC, Hepner DL. Value of preoperative clinic visits in identifying issues with potential impact on operating room efficiency. *Anesthesiology*. 2006;105(6):1254-1259.
2. Ferschl MB, Tung A, Sweitzer B, et al. Preoperative clinic visits reduce operating room cancellations and delays. *Anesthesiology*. 2005;103(4):855-859.
3. Blitz JD, Kendale SM, Jain SK, et al. Preoperative evaluation clinic visit is associated with decreased risk of in-hospital postoperative mortality. *Anesthesiology*. 2016;125(2):280-294.
4. ASA Physical Status Classification System. Accessed March 4, 2020. https://www.asahq.org/standards-and-guidelines/asa-physical-status-classification-system
5. Devereaux PJ, Yang H, Yusuf S, et al. Effects of extended-release metoprolol succinate in patients undergoing non-cardiac surgery (POISE trial): a randomized controlled trial. *Lancet*. 2008;371:1839-1847.
6. Poldermans D, Boersma E, Bax JJ, et al. The effect of bisoprolol on perioperative mortality and myocardial infarction in high-risk patients undergoing vascular surgery. Dutch Echocardiographic Cardiac Risk Evaluation Applying Stress Echocardiography Study Group. *N Engl J Med*. 1999;341:1789-1794.
7. Dunkelgrun M, Boersma E, Schouten O, et al. Bisoprolol and fluvastatin for the reduction of perioperative cardiac mortality and myocardial infarction in intermediate-risk patients undergoing noncardiovascular surgery: a randomized controlled trial (DECREASE-IV). *Ann Surg*. 2009;249:921-926.

8. Wijeysundera DN, Duncan D, Nkonde-Price C, et al. Perioperative beta blockade in noncardiac surgery: a systematic review for the 2014 ACC/AHA guideline on perioperative cardiovascular evaluation and management of patients undergoing noncardiac surgery. a report of the American College of Cardiology/American Heart Association Task Force on practice guidelines. *Circulation*. 2014;130:2246-2264.
9. London MJ, Schwartz GG, Hur K, Henderson WG. Association of perioperative statin use with mortality and morbidity after major noncardiac surgery. *JAMA Intern Med*. 2017;177:231-242.
10. Devereaux PJ, Mrkobrada M, Sessler DI, et al. Aspirin in patients undergoing noncardiac surgery. *N Engl J Med*. 2014;370(16):1494-1503.
11. Levine GN, Bates ER, Bittl JA, et al. 2016 ACC/AHA guideline focused update on duration of dual antiplatelet therapy in patients with coronary artery disease: a report of the American College of Cardiology/American Heart Association Task Force on clinical practice guidelines. *J Am Coll Cardiol*. 2016;68(10):1082-1115.
12. Kirchhof P, Benussi S, Kotecha D, et al. 2016 ESC guidelines for the management of atrial fibrillation developed in collaboration with EACTS. *Europace*. 2016;18(11):1609-1678.
13. Horlocker TT, Vandermeulen E, Kopp SL, et al. Regional anesthesia in the patient receiving antithrombotic or thrombolytic therapy: American Society of Regional Anesthesia and Pain Medicine evidence-based guidelines (fourth edition). *Reg Anesth Pain Med*. 2018;43(3):263-309.
14. Acampora GA, Nisavic M, Zhang Y. Perioperative buprenorphine continuous maintenance and administration simultaneous with full opioid agonist: patient priority at the interface between medical disciplines. *J Clin Psychiatry*. 2020;7(1):81.
15. Quaye AN, Zhang Y. Perioperative management of buprenorphine: solving the conundrum. *Pain Med*. 2019;20(7):1395-1408.
16. Savic LC, Khan DA, Kopac P. Management of a surgical patient with a label of penicillin allergy: narrative review and consensus recommendations. *Br J Anaesth*. 2019;123(1):e82-e94.
17. Shenoy ES, Macy E, Rowe T, et al. Evaluation and management of penicillin allergy: a review. *J Am Med Assoc*. 2019;321(2):188-199.
18. Mallampati RS, Gatt SP, Gugino LD, et al. A clinical sign to predict difficult tracheal intubation. A prospective study. *Can Anaesth Soc J*. 1985;32:429.
19. Fleisher LA, Fleischmann KE, Auerbach AD, et al. 2014 ACC/AHA guideline on perioperative cardiovascular evaluation and management of patients undergoing noncardiac surgery: executive summary. A report of the American College of Cardiology/American Heart Association Task Force on practice guidelines. *Circulation*. 2014;130:e278-e333.
20. Longrois D, Hoeft A, De Hert S. 2014 European Society of Cardiology/European Society of Anaesthesiology guidelines on non-cardiac surgery: cardiovascular assessment and management. A short explanatory statement from the European Society of Anaesthesiology members who participated in the European Task Force. *Eur J Anaesthesiol*. 2014;31(10):513-516.
21. Crossley GH, Poole JE, Rozner MA, et al. The Heart Rhythm Society (HRS)/American Society of Anesthesiologists (ASA) Expert Consensus Statement on the perioperative management of patients with implantable defibrillators, pacemakers and arrhythmia monitors: facilities and patient management this document was developed as a joint project with the American Society of Anesthesiologists (ASA), and in collaboration with the American Heart Association (AHA), and the Society of Thoracic Surgeons (STS). *Heart Rhythm*. 2011;8:1114-1154.
22. Practice advisory for the perioperative management of patients with cardiac implantable electronic devices: pacemakers and implantable cardioverter–defibrillators 2020. An updated report by the American Society of Anesthesiologists Task Force on Perioperative Management of Patients with Cardiac Implantable Electronic Devices. *Anesthesiology*. 2020;132:225-252.
23. Lapage KG, Wouters PF. The patient with hypertension undergoing surgery. *Curr Opin Anaesthesiol*. 2016;29(3):397-402.
24. Yang CK, Teng A, Lee DY, et al. Pulmonary complications after major abdominal surgery: National Surgical Quality Improvement Program analysis. *J Surg Res*. 2015;198:441-449.
25. Chan MTV, Wang CY, Seet E, et al. Association of unrecognized obstructive sleep apnea with postoperative cardiovascular events in patients undergoing major noncardiac surgery. *J Am Med Assoc*. 2019;321(18):1788-1798.

26. American Society of Anesthesiologists. Practice guidelines for the perioperative management of patients with obstructive sleep apnea. *Anesthesiology*. 2014;120:268-286.
27. Joshi GP, Chung F, Vann MA, et al. Society for Ambulatory Anesthesia consensus statement on perioperative blood glucose management in diabetic patients undergoing ambulatory surgery. *Anesth Analg*. 2010;111:1378-1387.
28. Moghissi ES, Korytkowski MT, DiNardo M, et al. American Association of Clinical Endocrinologists and American Diabetes Association consensus statement on inpatient glycemic control. *Endocr Pract*. 2009;15:353-369.
29. Sebranek JJ, Kopp Lugli A, Coursin DB. Glycaemic control in the perioperative period. *Br J Anaesth*. 2013;111:18.
30. Benarroch-Gampel J, Sheffield KM, Duncan CB, et al. Preoperative laboratory testing in patients undergoing elective, low-risk ambulatory surgery. *Ann Surg*. 2012;256:518.
31. Finegan BA, Rashiq S, McAlister FA, O'Connor P. Selective ordering of preoperative investigations by anesthesiologists reduces the number and cost of tests. *Can J Anaesth*. 2005;52(6):575-580.
32. Committee on Standards and Practice Parameters; Apfelbaum JL, Connis RT, Nickinovich DG, et al. Practice advisory for preanesthesia evaluation: an updated report by the American Society of Anesthesiologists Task Force on preanesthesia evaluation. *Anesthesiology*. 2012;116(3):522-538.
33. Colla CH, Mainor AJ. Choosing Wisely Campaign: valuable for providers who knew about it, but awareness remained constant, 2014-17. *Health Aff (Millwood)*. 2017;36(11):2005-2011.
34. Martin SK, Cifu AS. Routine preoperative laboratory tests for elective surgery. *J Am Med Assoc*. 2017;318:567-568.
35. Edwards AF, Forest DJ. Preoperative laboratory testing. *Anesthesiol Clin*. 2018;36(4):493-507.
36. Saraswat MK, Magruder JT, Crawford TC, et al. Preoperative *Staphylococcus aureus* screening and targeted decolonization in cardiac surgery. *Ann Thorac Surg*. 2017;104(4):1349-1356.
37. American Society of Anesthesiologists. Practice guidelines for preoperative fasting and the use of pharmacologic agents to reduce the risk of pulmonary aspiration: application to healthy patients undergoing elective procedures. An updated report by the American Society of Anesthesiologists Task Force on preoperative fasting and the use of pharmacologic agents to reduce the risk of pulmonary aspiration. *Anesthesiology*. 2017;126(3):376-393.
38. Jernigan JA, Pullen AL, Partin C, Jarvis WR. Prevalence of and risk factors for colonization with methicillin-resistant *Staphylococcus aureus* in an outpatient clinic population. *Infect Control Hosp Epidemiol*. 2003;24(6):445-450.
39. Whittle J, Wischmeyer PE, Grocott MPW, Miller TE. Surgical prehabilitation: nutrition and exercise. *Anesthesiol Clin*. 2018;36(4):567-580.

PREOPERATIVE CARDIAC ULTRASOUND

A CLOSER LOOK

Patients with undiagnosed cardiovascular disease, or those with an established diagnosis with a change in symptoms can be assessed quickly with bedside ultrasound. The illustration below shows the basic views obtained with focused cardiac ultrasound (PoCUS).

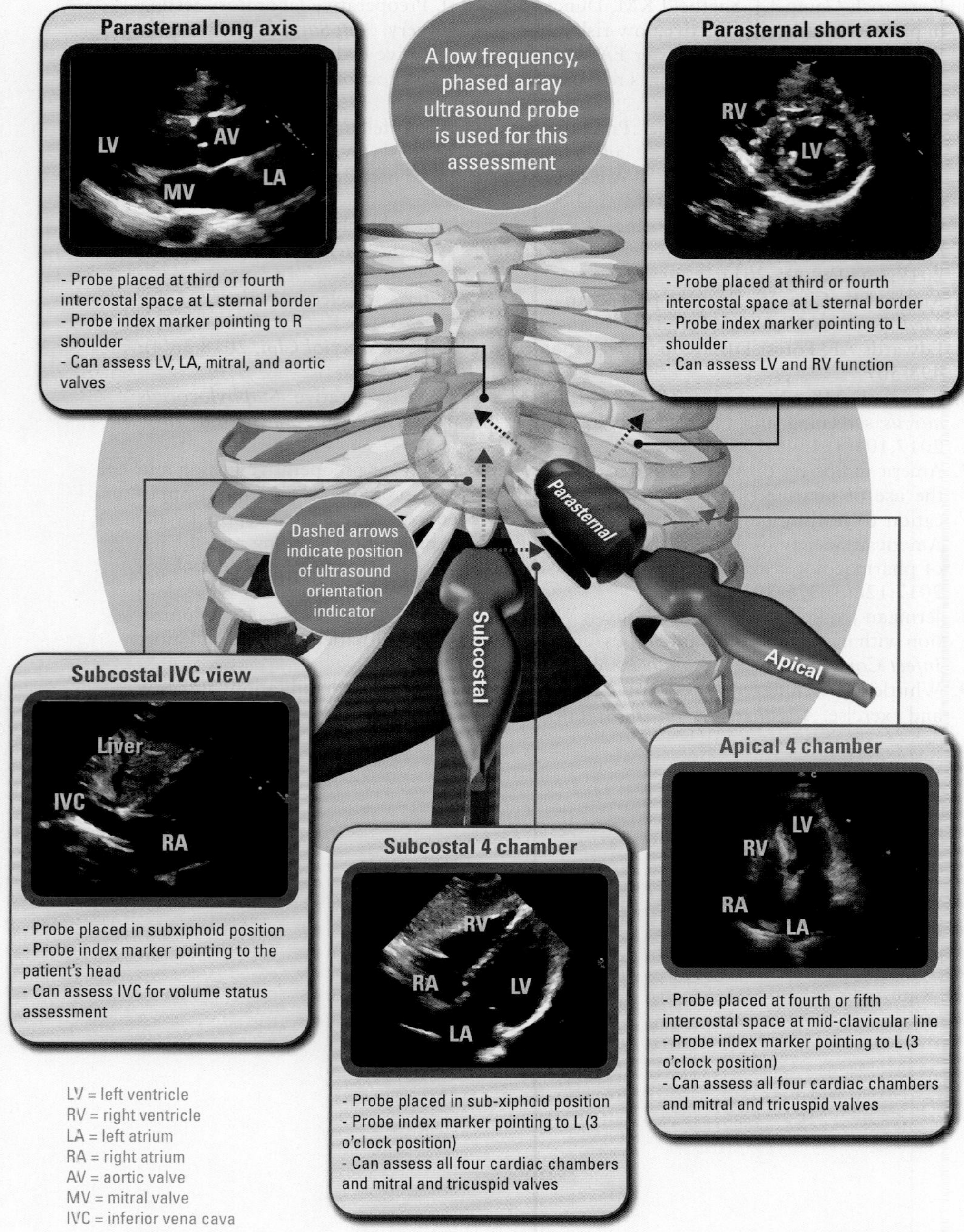

Parasternal long axis
LV
AV
MV
LA
- Probe placed at third or fourth intercostal space at L sternal border
- Probe index marker pointing to R shoulder
- Can assess LV, LA, mitral, and aortic valves
A low frequency, phased array ultrasound probe is used for this assessment
Parasternal short axis
RV
LV
- Probe placed at third or fourth intercostal space at L sternal border
- Probe index marker pointing to L shoulder
- Can assess LV and RV function
Parasternal
Dashed arrows indicate position of ultrasound orientation indicator
Subcostal
Apical
Subcostal IVC view
Liver
IVC
RA
- Probe placed in subxiphoid position
- Probe index marker pointing to the patient's head
- Can assess IVC for volume status assessment
Subcostal 4 chamber
RV
RA
LV
LA
- Probe placed in sub-xiphoid position
- Probe index marker pointing to L (3 o'clock position)
- Can assess all four cardiac chambers and mitral and tricuspid valves
Apical 4 chamber
LV
RV
RA
LA
- Probe placed at fourth or fifth intercostal space at mid-clavicular line
- Probe index marker pointing to L (3 o'clock position)
- Can assess all four cardiac chambers and mitral and tricuspid valves
LV = left ventricle
RV = right ventricle
LA = left atrium
RA = right atrium
AV = aortic valve
MV = mitral valve
IVC = inferior vena cava
Infographic by: Naveen Nathan MD

Questions

1. **A 69-year-old man is scheduled for left knee arthroscopy. His only limitation for moderate exercise is mild arthritis. Past medical history includes glaucoma and hypertension. Medications include aspirin 80 mg/d, timolol eye drops every day, and lisinopril 10 mg every day. An ECG 8 months ago showed sinus bradycardia. Heart rate 60 bpm, blood pressure 150/90 mm Hg, weight 200 lb, and hemoglobin 14 g/dL. Based on this information, what is his ASA physical status?**

   A. I
   B. II
   C. III
   D. IV

2. **Which of the following is a risk factor for PONV?**

   A. Age > 60 years
   B. Smoking
   C. Female sex
   D. Morbid obesity

3. **Discontinuation of daily low-dose aspirin therapy is most appropriate prior to which of the following surgical procedures?**

   A. Coronary artery bypass graft surgery
   B. Tympanoplasty
   C. Cystoscopy with bladder tumor resection
   D. Vaginal hysterectomy

4. **Which of the following dietary supplements has been associated with an increased risk of perioperative bleeding?**

   A. Echinacea
   B. Ephedra
   C. Kava
   D. Garlic

5. **On mouth opening, the soft palate is visible but not the uvula or tonsillar pillars. What is the Mallampati score?**

   A. I
   B. II
   C. III
   D. IV

6. **According to the RCRI, which of the following is NOT a risk factor for cardiac complications after noncardiac surgery?**

   A. High-risk surgery (intrathoracic, intraperitoneal, or suprainguinal vascular)
   B. Uncontrolled hypertension
   C. Diabetes mellitus requiring insulin
   D. History of cerebrovascular disease

7. **Application of a magnet on a pacemaker is MOST likely to do which of the following?**

   A. Initiate asynchronous pacing
   B. Initiate arrhythmia detection
   C. Initiate synchronous pacing
   D. Suspend pacing function

8. **A 26-month-old boy is having myringotomy tube placement. Breastfeeding should be discontinued how many hours prior to surgery?**

   A. 2
   B. 4
   C. 6
   D. 8

9. **Sugammadex administration is NOT recommended for which of the following patients?**

   A. A 20-year-old man with myotonic dystrophy and a history of malignant hyperthermia
   B. A 30-year-old woman of child-bearing age
   C. A 70-year-old man with chronic liver insufficiency
   D. A 50-year-old woman with end-stage kidney disease just about to start dialysis

10. **A 58-year-old man is undergoing debridement of a wound colonized with methicillin-resistant *Staphylococcus aureus*. Administration of which of the following preincision antibiotics is MOST appropriate?**

    A. Cefazolin
    B. Ceftriaxone
    C. Clindamycin
    D. Vancomycin

Answers

1. B

ASA describes ASA Physical Status Classification II as "a patient with mild systemic disease." This includes patients with well-controlled conditions such as hypertension or diabetes mellitus that cause no substantial limitations. To be considered ASA III, a patient should have "severe systemic disease." Examples include patients with poorly controlled diabetes, hypertension, or COPD; BMI >40 kg/m^2; or moderately reduced ejection fraction.

2. C

Known patient risk factors for postoperative nausea and vomiting (PONV) include preprocedural nausea and vomiting, female gender, age <50 years, history of PONV or motion sickness, nonsmoking status, and administration of opioid analgesics.

3. B

Perioperative management of aspirin must weigh the risk of surgical bleeding against that of cardiovascular complications. It is generally agreed that aspirin should be withheld for 7 to 10 days prior to surgeries where bleeding would have catastrophic consequences (e.g., intracranial, intraocular, middle ear, prostate, and intramedullary spine surgeries) or where the likelihood of major blood loss is high.

4. D

Remember that the "three Gs," garlic, ginkgo, and ginseng may increase bleeding risk. Many preoperative clinics advise patients to stop herbal or complementary drugs one week prior to surgery, in part due the possible increased risk of bleeding.

5. C

The Mallampati Airway classification is one of the best known physical exam indications of airway difficulty. It essentially evaluates the size of the tongue in relation to the oral cavity. A Mallampati III airway is one where the soft palate but not the tonsillar pillars or uvula are present on mouth opening.

6. B

The Revised Cardiac Risk Index (RCRI) is a validated tool to estimate the risk of perioperative major adverse cardiac events. Such tools are a key component of employing a stepwise approach to preoperative risk assessments in noncardiac elective surgeries. Elements of the RCRI include surgery-specific risk, history of ischemic heart disease, history of heart failure, history of stroke or transient ischemic attack (TIA), insulin-dependent diabetes mellitus, and preoperative serum creatinine ≥2.0 mg/dL.

7. A

Cardiovascular implantable electronic devices (CIEDs) are increasingly encountered in patients presenting for surgery. Thorough evaluation of these patients and their devices is critical to developing a perioperative plan that will minimize risk of device malfunction, including as a result of electromagnetic interference (EMI) from equipment in the operating suite. Essential information that should be obtained about the CIED during the anesthesia evaluation includes the reason for device implantation, device type and manufacturer, date of last interrogation and report, current programming, whether the patient is pacemaker dependent, and the device's response to application of a magnet. For most CIEDs, external application of a magnet will disable tachycardic therapy but will have no effect on pacemaker settings. Magnet application to a pacemaker will initiate asynchronous pacing.

8. B

American Society of Anesthesiologists' guidelines on fasting prior to elective procedures suggests 2 hours for clear fluids, 4 hours for breast milk, 6 hours for infant formula and nonhuman milk, 6 hours for a light meal, and at least 8 hours for a heavy meal.

9. D

Sugammadex is a modified gamma cyclodextrin that complexes with rocuronium or vecuronium, resulting in a dose-dependent reversal of neuromuscular blockade. It is not metabolized and undergoes renal elimination. Its use is not recommended for patients with a creatinine clearance <30 mL/min.

10. D

Antibiotics are administered prior to surgical procedures in order to prevent surgical site infections (SSIs). SSIs are typically caused by gram-positive skin flora, notably *Staphylococcus aureus*, *Staphylococcus epidermidis*, and streptococcal species. First-generation cephalosporins such as cefazolin remain the mainstay of SSI prophylaxis, given their coverage against most gram-positive cocci and many gram-negative organisms. Patients known to be colonized with methicillin-resistant *Staphylococcus aureus* (MRSA) require alternative antibiotic coverage, for example vancomycin, as cefazolin does not cover MRSA.

17 Coexisting Diseases Impacting Anesthetic Management

Gerardo Rodriguez

Many conditions impact anesthetic management. Some are rare and are unlikely to be encountered during an anesthesiologist's career. It is essential to always investigate thoroughly how to properly manage a rare disorder. When encountering a patient with an uncommon condition, it is advisable to review sources detailing each topic.

I. Duchenne Muscular Dystrophy

Duchenne muscular dystrophy is an X-linked disorder leading to a loss of functional dystrophin, a protein integral to muscle membrane cytoskeleton stability. It presents in childhood and is characterized by proximal muscle weakness and painless muscle atrophy in boys. Serum creatine kinase levels are used for screening in newborns and assessment of muscle degeneration. Patients succumb to cardiopulmonary complications by middle age.

Cardiomyopathy and rhythm disorders are common. Surveillance with electrocardiography and echocardiography and treatment with angiotensin-converting enzyme inhibitors and beta-blockers are routine. Dysrhythmias should be periodically assessed with Holter monitoring.

Recurrent pneumonia occurs due to poor cough effort and inadequate secretion clearance. Derangements in gastric motility result in delayed gastric emptying.

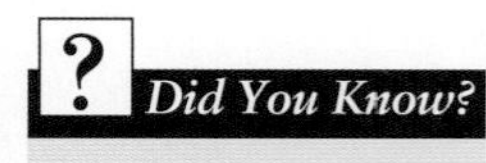

In Duchenne muscular dystrophy, succinylcholine is contraindicated due to risk of hyperkalemia and rhabdomyolysis.

A. Management of Anesthesia

Gastric dysmotility increases the risk of aspiration. Succinylcholine is contraindicated due to risk of hyperkalemia and rhabdomyolysis. Prolonged muscle relaxation may occur with nondepolarizing agents. Potent volatile anesthetics should be used with caution, since exposure may trigger rhabdomyolysis and cardiac complications. Postoperative ventilatory support may be needed especially if there is poor preoperative pulmonary function.[1]

II. The Myotonias

Myotonic dystrophy is an autosomal dominant disorder caused by gene mutations that lead to RNA toxicity, ion channel dysfunction, and myotonias or impaired skeletal muscle relaxation. Progressive muscle wasting with weakness combined with multisystem involvement characterizes this disorder. Myotonic dystrophy is divided into two chief genetic entities. Myotonic dystrophy type 1 (DM1), the predominant major type, is subdivided into congenital, child, and adult onset. Myotonic dystrophy type 2 is rare, with a highly variable, late adult-onset presentation.

Adult-onset DM1, the most common subtype, is characterized by muscle weakness, myotonias, and cataracts. Facial, neck, and distal limb weakness progress to muscle wasting, immobility, and bulbar palsies. Respiratory dysfunction is compounded by aspiration and respiratory muscle weakness.

Functional and anatomical brain dysfunction is manifested by cognitive dysfunction and diffuse white matter atrophy. Systolic and diastolic cardiac failure are complicated by conduction defects, such as atrioventricular conduction blocks and tachyarrhythmias. ***Sudden cardiac death*** due to dysrhythmias is common. Gastrointestinal signs include constipation and diarrhea. Impaired endocrine function results in hypothyroidism and insulin resistance. Treatment is primarily supportive.

A. Management of Anesthesia

Cardiopulmonary abnormalities, muscle weakness, and clinical myotonia are the primary causes of perioperative risk in adult-onset DM1, regardless of anesthetic technique. Sedatives should be used with caution due to potential exaggerated response to their respiratory depression side effects. Succinylcholine should be avoided due to its potential to trigger a severe myotonic muscle contraction. Both nondepolarizing and reversal agents may exacerbate muscle weakness and should be avoided. Respiratory insufficiency can occur. Transcutaneous pacing pads should be considered.

There is potential for prolonged labor, postpartum hemorrhage, and congenital myotonic dystrophy of the neonate.

III. Familial Periodic Paralysis

Channelopathies are a heterogenous group of defects in ion channel function that result in a spectrum of anomalies. Familial periodic paralysis is a subgroup of inherited defects comprising hyperkalemic and hypokalemic periodic paralysis.

A. Hyperkalemic Periodic Paralysis

Hyperkalemic periodic paralysis is an autosomal-dominant inherited disease characterized by episodes of hyperkalemia-related muscle weakness and myotonia. The episodes are triggered by transient hyperkalemia from exercise, fasting, or consumption of potassium-rich foods.

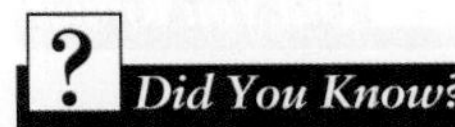

Hypokalemic periodic paralysis is the most common periodic paralysis disease, characterized by recurrent episodes of hypokalemia-related flaccid paralysis, which can last hours to days.

B. Hypokalemic Periodic Paralysis

Hypokalemic periodic paralysis, the most common periodic paralysis disease, is an autosomal dominant disease characterized by recurrent episodes of hypokalemia-related flaccid paralysis, lasting hours to days. Respiratory insufficiency and cardiac arrhythmias can occur during acute attacks. Chronic proximal myopathy is a common outcome in many cases.

C. Management of Anesthesia

Potassium homeostasis is the goal of perioperative management. Electrolyte levels should be monitored and corrected with an emphasis on avoiding metabolic states or medications that may alter serum potassium levels, either directly or indirectly. Nondepolarizing muscle relaxants are best avoided due to unpredictable patient sensitivities. Succinylcholine should be avoided, because it may cause transient hyperkalemia.[2]

? Did You Know?

Myasthenia gravis is caused by a decrease in the number of functional postsynaptic, acetylcholine receptors in the neuromuscular junction available for acetylcholine binding.

? Did You Know?

The newborn of a mother with myasthenia gravis can suffer from a condition known as transient neonatal myasthenia, which may present with feeding problems and respiratory distress at birth.

? Did You Know?

The Lambert-Eaton myasthenic syndrome is associated with small cell lung cancer, and in contrast to myasthenia gravis, exercise might improve the muscle weakness-related symptoms.

IV. Myasthenia Gravis

Myasthenia gravis (MG) is a neuromuscular autoimmune disease characterized by skeletal muscle weakness worsened by exertion and improved with rest. Extraocular muscles are affected primarily, with less frequent impact on limb and respiratory muscles strength.

The etiology is a decrease in the number of functional postsynaptic, acetylcholine receptors (AChRs) in the neuromuscular junction available for acetylcholine binding. Direct antibody receptor blockade, increased antibody-mediated receptor turnover, and postsynaptic membrane complement–mediated injury can contribute to AChR decline. Abnormal thymus tissue is frequently involved.

Signs include ptosis, blurred vision, diplopia, dysphagia, dysarthria, and generalized limb weakness. ***Myasthenic crisis*** is a progression to severe muscle weakness and respiratory failure, usually requiring ventilatory support. Cardiac abnormalities include bundle branch blocks, atrial fibrillation, and focal myocarditis.

Transient neonatal myasthenia is known to occur in newborns of women with active MG, with feeding problems and respiratory distress immediately postpartum. Edrophonium testing is used to diagnosis MG with high sensitivity. Serologic testing, tomographic imaging, and electrophysiological testing comprise a comprehensive MG workup. Treatment is aimed at both symptom management and immunomodulation.

Acetylcholinesterase inhibitors, such as pyridostigmine, minimize MG symptoms by increasing the acetylcholine available at neuromuscular junction sites. Excessive drug administration can result in severe cholinergic side effects, or ***cholinergic crisis***, characterized by hypersalivation, abdominal cramping, bradycardia, and weakness. Plasmapheresis and intravenous immunoglobulin can provide short-term relief. Chronic therapy includes steroids and nonsteroidal immunosuppressants. ***Thymectomy*** is recommended for MG patients with thymomas.[3]

A. Myasthenic Syndrome (Lambert-Eaton Syndrome)

Lambert-Eaton myasthenic syndrome (LEMS) is an autoimmune, neuromuscular disorder of transmission mediated by antibodies to voltage-gated calcium channels at the presynaptic, motor nerve terminal, resulting in acetylcholine release reduction. It is characterized by proximal limb weakness, autonomic dysfunction such as dry mouth, and diminished deep tendon reflexes. In contrast to MG, exercise in LEMS might suddenly improve symptoms. LEMS is a paraneoplastic condition, often associated with small cell lung cancer. Increasing presynaptic, neurotransmitter release with 3,4-diaminopyridine is considered the mainstay of treatment.

V. Guillain-Barre Syndrome (Polyradiculoneuritis)

Guillain-Barre syndrome (GBS) is an autoimmune disorder characterized by the acute or subacute onset of ascending skeletal muscle weakness or paralysis of the legs occurring in the context of a viral or bacterial infection. This inflammatory, multifocal demyelinating disease usually produces varying degrees of autonomic dysfunction. Respiratory muscle weakness is common during severe cases of GBS. Treatment is primarily supportive.[4]

A. Management of Anesthesia

Multifocal demyelination and muscle disuse atrophy in GBS prohibit the use of succinylcholine due to the risk of life-threatening hyperkalemia. Expected muscle relaxation from nondepolarizing agents may be highly variable and unpredictable and should be avoided. Autonomic nervous system lability is common, which can result in hyperdynamic and hypodynamic responses to stimuli or transient preload changes, respectively; therefore, hemodynamic support should be judicious.

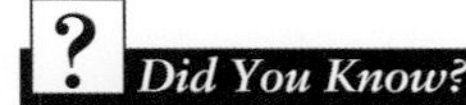

Did You Know?

In addition to respiratory muscle weakness, GBS is accompanied by autonomic nervous system lability, which can result in hyperdynamic and hypodynamic responses.

VI. Central Nervous System Diseases

A. Multiple Sclerosis

Multiple sclerosis (MS) is an inflammatory multifocal demyelinating disorder caused by autoimmune neurodegenerative changes leading to progressively irreversible neurologic deficits. The clinical course is characterized by subacute, relapsing-remitting changes that correlate to activated T-cell blood-brain barrier penetration with subsequent multifocal gray and white matter demyelination and edema (**Figure 17.1**).

MS has a peak incidence at the age 20 to 40 years. Signs and symptoms can be vague or specific, usually determined by the neurologic site focally affected. Symptoms include headache, fatigue, and depression. Sensory symptoms such

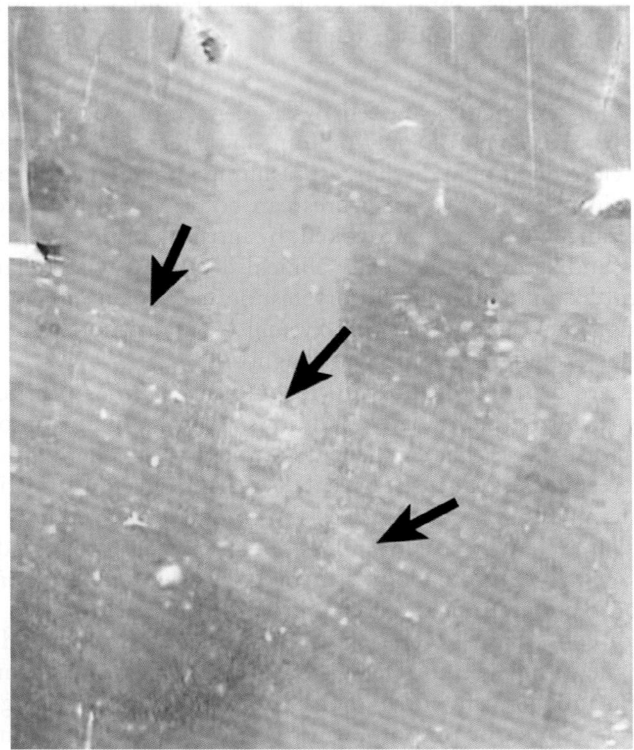

Figure 17.1 The subcortical white matter of a patient with multiple sclerosis showing multiple, small, irregular, partially confluent areas of demyelination (*arrows*). Normal intact myelin stains blue in this Luxol fast blue–stained section. (From Strayer DS, Saffitz JE, Rubin E. *Rubin's Pathology.* 8th ed. Philadelphia, PA: Wolters Kluwer; 2020. Figure 32.74.)

as numbness and paresthesias are common. Partial paralysis of the lower limbs is a common motor symptom that usually correlates to anterior column spinal cord lesions. Visual loss, diplopia, nystagmus, and papillary abnormalities reflect cranial nerve involvement. Diagnosis is based on history and clinical examination with reliance on magnetic resonance imaging to characterize demyelinating, often clinically silent, focal lesions. Cerebral spinal fluid may demonstrate intrathecal immunoglobulin production.

Management strategies are evolving to target acute relapse and symptomatic control. Corticosteroids can hasten acute clinical recovery. Plasma exchange removes harmful antibodies to treat relapses. Interferon-beta and glatiramer acetate block antigen presentation to minimize relapsing-remitting events. Mitoxantrone, an antineoplastic agent, reduces lymphocyte counts to delay progression to secondary degenerative phase. Symptomatic management is usually determined by the diffuse nature of MS. Severe fatigue is common and should be treated promptly with central nervous system stimulants, such as amantadine. Routine depression screening and early treatment are important given the propensity to affect quality of life in this disease. Spasticity treatment requires both physical therapy and antispasticity medications. Intrathecal baclofen pump implantation is reserved for severe cases. Pain is usually due to varied factors, such as neuropathic pain, indirect pain from MS, and treatment-related pain. As a result, pain management is multimodal, potentially involving antiepileptics, tricyclic antidepressants, nonsteroidal anti-inflammatory drugs (NSAIDs), and antispastic agents.

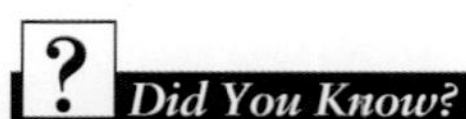

In multiple sclerosis, pain is caused by a variety of mechanisms; therefore, the best treatment is using multimodal analgesia.

B. Epilepsy

Epilepsy is a disorder characterized by sudden, unprovoked, and recurrent seizures. A seizure is a neurologic symptom characterized by a transient attack of rhythmic electroneuronal discharges, resulting in altered consciousness and disturbances in brain function. Seizures can be provoked by factors such as metabolic derangements, or unprovoked, by intrinsic brain disease.

Epilepsies and seizures are mostly clinical diagnoses with reliance on history, physical examination, laboratory testing, electroencephalography, and neuroimaging. Investigating the paroxysmal event, triggers, and recurrence potential helps exclude or confirm the diagnosis.

Epilepsies are broadly divided into ***focal*** and ***generalized.*** In focal epilepsies, usually localized pathologic conditions, such as brain tumors, lead to focal cortical discharges that can generalize and recruit other cortical regions. In generalized epilepsies, diffuse cortical discharges develop, affecting the cortex and bilaterally. ***Grand mal seizure*** is the most recognized type of generalized epilepsy. It is characterized by a loss of consciousness followed by several minutes of a ***tonic phase*** of body stiffening, followed by a ***clonic phase*** of repetitive contractions, and ending in a prolonged ***postictal phase*** of lethargy and return of consciousness. During the tonic phase, breath-holding, incontinence, tongue biting, tremors, and sinus tachycardia may occur. Trauma, aspiration pneumonia, and arrhythmias may also occur during these seizures. Benzodiazepines or propofol can be used to terminate seizure activity. Ventilatory support may be needed. ***Status epilepticus*** is a potentially fatal convulsive disorder marked by serial tonic-clonic phases occurring without return of consciousness. Untreated, hyperpyrexia, hypoxia, and shock can develop acutely. Multiple precipitating risk factors exist, including brain tumor and drug intoxication. Treatment goals should be supportive care, seizure termination, and prevention. Endotracheal intubation should be performed for airway protection. Intravenous phenytoin can be used for seizure recurrence prophylaxis. Refractory seizures may require benzodiazepine or propofol infusion; general anesthesia may even be necessary.[5]

C. Alzheimer Disease

Dementia is an irreversible, chronic, neurodegenerative disease marked by a constant decline in cognitive function, affecting memory, behavior, and executive function that, over time, degrades daily activities and social interaction. ***Alzheimer disease (AD)*** is the most common cause of dementia. Senile plaques and neurofibrillary tangles are the hallmarks of AD. Acetylcholinesterase inhibitors (AChEIs) are considered the first line of pharmacotherapy to treat the central cholinergic deficiency–related cognitive decline in AD. Side effects from cholinergic stimulation during AChEI therapy include hypotension, bradycardia, and bronchoconstriction. Drug interactions with AChEI and muscle relaxants may result in prolonged paralysis with succinylcholine and resistance to muscle relaxation with *N*-methyl-D-aspartates.[6]

D. Parkinson Disease

VIDEO 17.1
Parkinson Disease

Parkinson disease (PD) is a neurodegenerative movement disorder marked by an acetylcholine-dopamine imbalance caused by loss of dopamine-producing cells within the substantia nigra. It is a clinical diagnosis confirmed by motor and nonmotor features in the absence of a pertinent drug history. Common motor features of PD are "pill-rolling" tremors at rest, rigidity, bradykinesia, postural instability, flexed posture, or incapacity to move. Nonmotor features include cognitive impairment, neuropsychiatric disorders, sensory disturbances, sleep disorders, and autonomic dysfunction.

Medical management is determined by factors such as age of onset, symptom fluctuations, dopamine responsiveness, and end-stage disease. ***Levodopa*** remains the most effective form of oral therapy for motor symptoms. It is highly metabolized and can cause nausea and hypotension. Long-term levodopa use can result in confusion, dyskinesia, and poor symptom relief. Hepatic metabolism and peripheral side effects are commonly reduced by combining levodopa with carbidopa, a ***decarboxylase inhibitor***. Pramipexole, ropinirole, and bromocriptine are ***dopamine agonists*** used when levodopa response decreases. Side effects include hallucinations and confusion. Selegiline and rasagiline are ***monoamine oxidase-B inhibitors*** used to augment dopamine concentrations. ***Deep brain stimulation*** via implanted generator electrodes is a surgical treatment option.

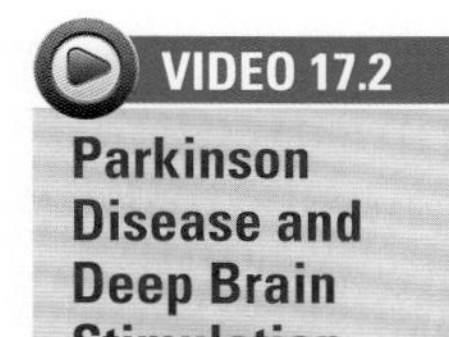

VII. Inherited Disorders

A. Malignant Hyperthermia

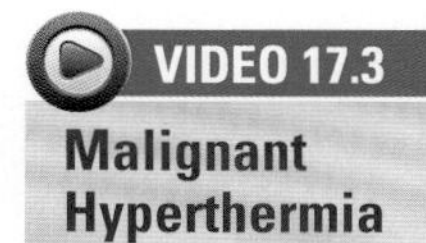

Malignant hyperthermia (MH) is an autosomal dominant, hypermetabolic disorder triggered by halogenated volatile anesthetics and succinylcholine. The principal diagnostic features of MH are unexplained hypercapnia, tachycardia, muscle rigidity, acidosis, hyperthermia, and hyperkalemia. The disorder is variable in its presentation. A ryanodine receptor (RYR) gene mutation is the etiology in the majority of cases. Precipitation of MH in genetically susceptible patients occurs when the RYR, a type of calcium channel located in the sarcoplasmic reticulum membrane, is activated during an exposure to a triggering agent, resulting in a tremendous release of intracellular calcium within skeletal muscle.

Detection and treatment are critical for survival. If MH is suspected, triggering agents should be discontinued immediately. Dantrolene should be administered intravenously, with an initial dose of 2.5 mg/kg, with repeat dosing as needed. MH can be lethal if untreated. Rhabdomyolysis and hyperkalemia should be managed with volume resuscitation and diuresis. Cooling should be instituted immediately with monitoring for coagulopathy. Ventilatory support should be maintained until the patient is stabilized. Once stabilized, the Malignant Hyperthermia Association of the United States hotline should be contacted. Recurrence of MH is possible, and patients should be monitored for up to 72 hours.

The in vitro contracture test is used to analyze the presence of muscle fiber contraction during halothane and caffeine exposure. It is the standard for diagnosis of MH susceptibility. Genetic testing may be pursued with appropriate counseling for patients about the implications of testing results. MH-susceptible patients planning to undergo surgery should have a thoroughly purged anesthesia machine available for use, whether or not the patient is to receive a general anesthetic. Triggering agents should be avoided. Total intravenous general anesthesia should be considered if regional anesthesia is not possible.[7]

B. Porphyria

Porphyrias are a group of enzyme deficiencies that result in heme and P450 cytochrome biosynthesis impairment and a concomitant accumulation of harmful metabolites. ***Acute intermittent porphyria (AIP)*** is among the most severe of the porphyrias. It is a deficiency in porphobilinogen deaminase that leads to nonspecific neuropsychiatric and abdominal complaints. Symptoms include severe abdominal pain, vomiting, seizures, tachycardia, and generalized weakness. Triggers include infection, fasting, ethanol, and medications, including barbiturates, etomidate, and phenytoin. Treatment of symptoms entails the discontinuation of triggers and infusion of hemin. Liver transplantation is reserved for AIP patients with severe, recurrent attacks (**Figure 17.2**).

C. Cholinesterase Disorders

Pseudocholinesterase (PChE) deficiency is an inherited or acquired disorder that results in an inability to efficiently metabolize specific ester substrates.

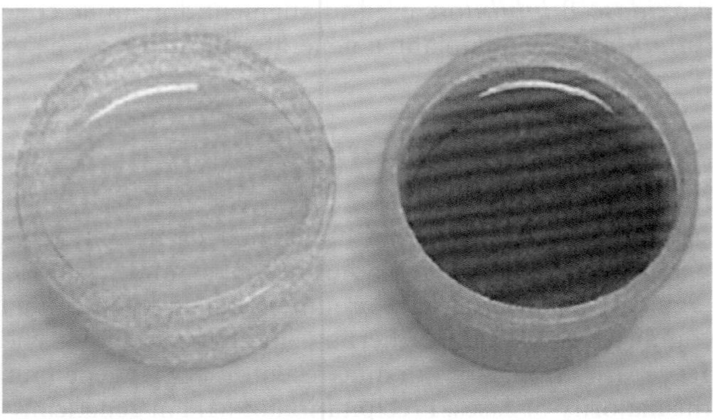

Figure 17.2 Urine from a patient with porphyria cutanea tarda (*right*) and from a patient with normal porphyrin excretion (*left*). (From Rich MW. *Porphyria cutanea tarda*. Postgrad Med. 1999;105:208–214.)

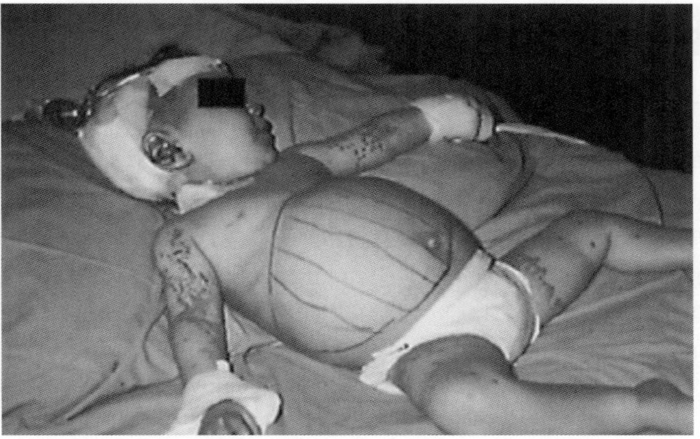

Figure 17.3 A 25-month-old child with von Gierke disease. Note the hepatomegaly and eruptive xanthomas on the arms and legs. The child is in the third percentile for height and weight, indicating a failure to thrive. (From Lieberman MA, Ricer R. *Lippincott's Illustrated Q&A Review of Biochemistry.* Wolters Kluwer Health/Lippincott Williams & Wilkins; 2010, with permission.)

Prolonged paralysis after an anesthetic procedure using succinylcholine usually reveals this deficiency. Delayed metabolism is also seen with use of mivacurium, cocaine, chloroprocaine, procaine, and tetracaine. Deficiency of this hepatic esterase can be due to PChE gene mutations or systemic disease, such as severe liver disease, renal failure, carcinomas, and severe malnutrition. PChE activity and dibucaine inhibition testing can be used to identify individuals at high risk for prolonged paralysis following succinylcholine administration.

D. Glycogen Storage Diseases

Glycogen storage diseases (GSDs) are a rare group of inherited disorders of glycogen production and metabolism that result in excess glycogen storage. Hypoglycemia, metabolic ketoacidosis, and infiltrative organ dysfunction are common among most types of GSD. There are numerous types of GSD, each with a unique set of characteristics based on factors such as enzyme mutation and clinical features (**Figure 17.3**, **Table 17.1**).

E. Osteogenesis Imperfecta

Osteogenesis imperfecta (OI) is an inherited connective tissue disorder that produces a defect in type I collagen synthesis, which is critical to bone and tissue strength. Pediatric bone fractures from minimal trauma, blue sclera, and a family history of OI are usually adequate for diagnosis. Cardiovascular manifestations of OI include arterial dissections and aortic and mitral valve regurgitation. Several types of OI exist, classified by type, inheritance pattern, and clinical features.

VIII. Anemias

A. Nutritional Deficiency Anemias

Nutritional deficiency anemias are due to an insufficiency of any food component necessary for growth and development, with complex vitamin B and iron deficiencies being the most common. Megaloblastic anemia is a characteristic of folate and vitamin B12 (cobalamin) deficiencies. ***Folate deficiency*** is associated with malnutrition, chronic alcohol abuse, and medications that interfere

Table 17.1 Types of Glycogen Storage Diseases

Type	Enzyme Mutation	Clinical Features
Type I (von Gierke disease)	Glucose-6-phosphatase deficiency	Hypoglycemia, acidosis, and seizures
Type II (Pompe disease)	Lysosomal acid glucosidase deficiency	Infantile; cardiac infiltrative cardiomyopathy
Type III (Forbes or Cori disease)	Glycogen debranching enzyme deficiency	Hepatomegaly, muscle weakness, and cardiomyopathy
Type IV (Andersen disease)	Branching enzyme deficiency	Hepatosplenomegaly, cirrhosis, cardiomyopathy, hypotonia, and failure to thrive
Type V (McArdle disease)	Muscle glycogen phosphorylase deficiency	Rhabdomyolysis and myoglobinuria after exercise or succinylcholine
Type VI (Hers disease)	Hepatic phosphorylase deficiency	Benign; mild hypoglycemia, hepatomegaly
Type VII (Tarui disease)	Muscle phosphofructokinase deficiency	Muscle cramps, exercise intolerance, and episodic myoglobinuria
Type IX	Hepatic glycogen phosphorylase kinase deficiency	Hypotonia, short stature, and exertional myoglobinuria
Type XI (Fanconi-Bickel syndrome)	Glucose transporter enzyme deficiency	Hepatomegaly, fasting hypoglycemia, short stature, and proximal renal tubular acidosis
Type 0	Hepatic glycogen synthase deficiency	Severe fasting ketotic hypoglycemia, short stature, seizures, and severe developmental delay

with folate metabolism. Clinically evident ***cobalamin deficiency*** presents with signs of demyelinating disease. Features include peripheral neuropathy with lower extremity loss of proprioception and vibratory sensation. Clinically evident cobalamin deficiency is most often due to ***pernicious anemia***, an autoimmune loss of intrinsic factor from gastric parietal cells needed for cobalamin binding. Nitrous oxide exposure can interfere with cobalamin metabolism in susceptible patients. ***Iron deficiency*** leads to a microcytic, hypochromic anemia, associated with poor iron intake, impaired iron absorption, chronic blood loss, or systemic inflammation. Treatment for all three nutritional deficiency anemias entails supplementation and reversal of contributing causes.

B. Hemolytic Anemias

Hemolytic anemias are any inherited or acquired anemias caused by hemolysis of red blood cells (RBCs). The common presenting features of all hemolytic anemias are jaundice, splenomegaly, increased reticulocyte count, and hyperbilirubinemia. ***Hereditary spherocytosis*** is an inherited disorder characterized by fragile, spherical RBCs that are prone to rupture during transit and spleen sequestration. Another manifestation is cholelithiasis. Treatment recommendations include splenectomy, antipneumococcal vaccination presplenectomy, and prophylactic cholecystectomy.

Immune hemolytic anemias can be caused by autoimmunity, alloimmunity, and drug reactions. ***Autoimmune hemolytic anemias (AIHAs)*** can be caused primarily, usually idiopathic, or secondarily, which is divided into warm and cold agglutinin diseases. Warm AIHA can be caused by leukemias, lymphomas, scleroderma, and rheumatoid arthritis. Cold AIHA can be triggered by infections and cold temperature exposure. ***Drug-induced immune hemolysis anemias*** can be subdivided into type II and type III hypersensitivity reactions. Penicillin and α-methyldopa can result in a type II reaction, where the drug binds to RBCs, triggering antibody-mediated destruction. Drugs known to potentially trigger a type III immune complex reaction include cephalosporins, hydrochlorothiazides, isoniazid, and tetracycline. Hemolytic disease of the newborn, or Rh incompatibility, is the most recognized example of an ***alloimmunity hemolytic disease.***

C. Glucose-6-Phosphate Dehydrogenase Deficiency

Glucose-6-phosphate dehydrogenase (G6PD) is an ubiquitous, X-linked maintenance enzyme present in RBCs and other cell types, which is essential to the pentose phosphate pathway that generates nicotinamide adenine dinucleotide phosphate for oxidative stress resistance. An acute, nonimmune hemolytic anemia reaction to ordinary infections, medications, or fava bean ingestion may be the presenting sign of G6PD deficiency. Aminoester local anesthetics and nitroprusside may trigger ***methemoglobinemia*** in patients with G6PD deficiency.

D. Hemoglobinopathies

Hemoglobinopathies are a group of predominantly genetic RBC diseases caused by aberrant hemoglobin production. Sickle cell disease and thalassemia are the most clinically relevant hemoglobinopathies. ***Sickle cell disease (SCD)*** is caused by an autosomal recessive β-globin gene defect that leads to structurally abnormal hemoglobin, called hemoglobin-S (HbS). RBCs affected with HbS have a propensity for "sickling" and for premature destruction. SCD produces acute and chronic multisystem complications. Acute, painful, and life-threatening attacks of SCD, called ***sickle cell crisis***, can occur spontaneously or be triggered by systemic stressors, such as dehydration, hypoxia, and infections.

Manifestations of sickle cell crisis include vaso-occlusive crisis, acute chest syndrome, splenic sequestration crisis, and aplastic crisis. Sickled RBCs clump together to obstruct capillaries and cause painful tissue ischemia and infarction, called a ***vaso-occlusive crisis***. This is the most common complication of SCD. Treatment consists of intravenous opioids, fluid replacement, and blood transfusion. Acute chest syndrome is a life-threatening manifestation of SCD, where pulmonary inflammation or infection triggers localized pulmonary infarctions that progress to death without appropriate supportive therapy. Clinical signs include acute dyspnea, chest pain, cough, and hypoxia. Aggressive fluid therapy, intravenous opioids, and exchange transfusion should be instituted promptly. Severe hypoxia may require ventilatory support. ***Splenic sequestration crisis*** is an acute splenic enlargement from sequestered abnormal RBCs, resulting in severe abdominal pain, anemia, and hypotension. Treatment is mainly supportive with fluid therapy and blood transfusion. Parvovirus B19 infection, a predominantly pediatric disease, can trigger an ***aplastic crisis*** in adults with SCD, characterized by profound depression of erythropoiesis resulting in life-threatening anemia.

Prophylactic treatment in SCD with oral penicillin, pneumococcal vaccination, and hydroxyurea is intended to reduce infections and recurrence of sickle cell crises.

Thalassemia is a diverse group of autosomal recessive disorders caused by insufficient α- or β-globin synthesis. The β-thalassemias in order of clinical severity include thalassemia major, thalassemia intermedia, and thalassemia minor. ***Thalassemia major*** usually presents by early childhood with anemia and failure to thrive. In time, young adult survivors go on to develop severe anemia, hypertrophic facial and long bone deformities, and secondary multi-organ dysfunction from severe transfusion-related hemochromatosis. Cardiac siderosis can lead to congestive heart failure and arrhythmias. Extensive endocrine dysfunction can present as hypopituitarism, hypothyroidism, hypoparathyroidism, diabetes, and adrenal insufficiency. Infections are common due to secondary immunodeficiency of hemochromatosis, blood-borne infections, and splenomegaly. Primary treatment includes periodic blood transfusions and iron chelating therapy.

IX. Collagen Vascular Diseases

A. Rheumatoid Arthritis

Rheumatoid arthritis (RA) is a chronic, autoimmune disease marked by systemic inflammation that primarily affects peripheral synovial joints, leading to symmetric painful arthritis. Eventual joint deformity, cartilage erosion, and ankylosing, or joint stiffening, develop in patients. ***Atlantoaxial subluxation*** is a common occult radiographic finding. Clinical signs of prolonged joint involvement, synovial fluid analysis, imaging, the presence of RA serology markers, such as rheumatoid factor, and nonspecific inflammatory markers, such as erythrocyte sedimentation rate and C-reactive protein, support the diagnosis. Extra-articular involvement is common and unpredictable. Chronic inflammation likely contributes to accelerated atherosclerotic disease, myocarditis, pericarditis, and valvulopathies. Ischemic heart disease is the most common cause of death. Rheumatoid lung disease can manifest as pleurisy, pulmonary nodules, interstitial lung disease, and pulmonary hypertension. Rheumatoid vasculitis can cause widespread organ injury, specifically renal failure and ischemic stroke.

Therapeutics for RA are broadly divided into NSAIDs, corticosteroids, disease-modifying antirheumatic drugs (DMARDs), and biologic DMARDs. ***Prednisone*** is used during flare-ups or until DMARD therapy is optimized. Despite the risks of long-term corticosteroid use, many RA patients remain on chronic prednisone therapy. ***Methotrexate*** is the mainstay drug of DMARD therapy. Drug-induced interstitial lung disease is a known risk of methotrexate in RA therapy. Other DMARDs include leflunomide, hydroxychloroquine, and sulfasalazine. Biologic DMARDs are intended to target cell surface molecules and cytokines to block the inflammation cascade. Infection and hypersensitivity reactions are the most serious complications associated with DMARD therapy.[8]

B. Systemic Lupus Erythematosus

Systemic lupus erythematosus (SLE) is an autoimmune disorder in which immune complexes formed by autoantibodies and soluble antigens, also known as ***type III hypersensitivity***, deposit in various organs, producing inflammation and tissue injury. Clinical features of SLE and detection of antinuclear antibody most often confirm diagnosis.

The presenting time course and symptoms are variable. Myalgias and fatigue are common symptoms. A photosensitive "butterfly rash" over the malar eminence is characteristic of SLE. Most patients experience mild to severely debilitating polyarthritis. Lupus glomerulonephritis, if untreated, can lead to end-stage renal disease and death. Pericarditis and pleuritis are common manifestations of SLE. Vascular occlusive disease may present with Raynaud phenomenon, acute ischemic stroke, or myocardial infarction.

Current treatment options have reduced morbidity and mortality. Corticosteroids and hydroxychloroquine are first-line therapies for acute flare-ups. Inflammation, chronic pain, and arthralgias are usually controlled with NSAIDs. Potent immunosuppressive agents, such as cyclophosphamide or mycophenolate, are used to treat severe glomerulonephritis.

C. Systemic Sclerosis

Systemic sclerosis (SSc), or scleroderma, is a rare autoimmune disorder marked by destructive, multisystem microvasculopathy, and organ fibrosis. Skin thickening is the most obvious physical sign, whereas Raynaud phenomenon is usually the presenting sign associated with scleroderma. Traditionally, the presence of CREST syndrome (*C*alcinosis, *R*aynaud phenomenon, *E*sophageal dysmotility, *S*clerodactyly, *T*elangiectasia) has been used for diagnosis. Quality-of-life optimization, organ injury prevention, and delay of disease progression are the focuses of treatment. Painful ischemic digits are treated with calcium channel blockers, stress management, and cold temperature avoidance. Active skin disease can be treated with immunosuppressants, such as mycophenolate or cyclophosphamide. Corticosteroids for skin disease should be avoided, because they can lead to a scleroderma renal crisis, manifested by acute hypertension and oliguric renal failure. The most common problem in scleroderma is gastrointestinal dysfunction. Dysphagia, esophageal dysmotility, esophageal strictures, gastroesophageal reflux, and delayed gastric emptying are treated with proton-pump inhibitors and prokinetics. Myocarditis and conduction abnormalities are usually silent. Calcium channel blockers and other vasodilators may be used to preserve cardiac function. Lung disease is the primary cause of death in scleroderma.

D. Inflammatory Myopathies

Inflammatory myopathies are a rare group of muscle disorders typified by muscle inflammation and weakness. ***Dermatomyositis (DM)*** and ***polymyositis (PM)*** are the predominant subtypes of inflammatory myopathies. Both conditions are considered autoimmune disorders, with an acute to subacute presentation usually after a systemic infection. Presenting features of PM include muscle pain and weakness that typically affects muscles of the proximal limbs, posterior neck, pharynx, and larynx. Ocular muscles are spared. DM has a similar presentation, except that onset can be more severe with additional dermal features: heliotropic eyelid discoloration, periorbital edema, and erythematous scaly rash involving the face and the extensor surface of limbs. Muscle necrosis and inflammatory cells on muscle tissue biopsy confirms diagnosis. Complications of both PM and DM include cardiomyopathy, respiratory insufficiency, dysphagia, and aspiration pneumonia.

X. Skin Disorders

A. Epidermolysis Bullosa

Epidermolysis bullosa (EB) is a group of rare, acquired, and inherited skin disorders that result in epidermal fragility due to abnormalities in basement membrane integrity within skin and mucosa. Shear stress across skin can result in epidermal layer detachment and painful bullae formation. Multiorgan dysfunction, such as cardiomyopathy, may develop depending on EB subtype. Esophageal strictures can be disabling, leading to malnutrition and dysphagia. Patients with EB are at risk for secondary bacterial infection and squamous cell carcinoma.[9]

B. Pemphigus Vulgaris

Pemphigus vulgaris (PV) is an autoimmune skin disorder that results in keratinocytes adhesion loss due to antibodies directed at desmoglein-1 and -3. The disorder is characterized by painful, epidermal blistering that develops immediately after minimal skin rubbing. This hypersensitivity reaction can be triggered by many medications, such as angiotensin-converting enzyme inhibitors, nifedipine, and penicillin. Painful, oral lesions are common. Corticosteroids are effective therapy for PV.

For further review and interactivities, please see the associated Interactive Video Lectures and "A Closer Look" infographic accessible in the complimentary eBook bundled with this text. Access instructions are located in the inside front cover.

References

1. Segura LG, Lorenz JD, Weingarten TN, et al. Anesthesia and Duchenne or Becker muscular dystrophy: review of 117 anesthetic exposures. *Paediatr Anaesth*. 2013;23(9):855-864.
2. Bandschapp O, Iaizzo PA. Pathophysiologic and anesthetic considerations for patients with myotonia congenita or periodic paralyses. *Paediatr Anaesth*. 2013;23(9):824-833.
3. Blichfeldt-Lauridsen L, Hansen BD. Anesthesia and myasthenia gravis. *Acta Anaesthesiol Scand*. 2012;56(1):17-22.
4. Turakhia P, Barrick B, Berman J. Pre-operative management of the patient with chronic disease: patients with neuromuscular disorder. *Med Clin North Am*. 2013;97(6):1015-1032.
5. Shorvon S. The historical evolution of, and the paradigms shifts in, the therapy of convulsive status epilepticus over the past 150 years. *Epilepsia*. 2013;54(6):64-67.
6. Seitz DP, Shah PS, Herrmann N, Beyene J, Siddiqui N. Exposure to general anesthesia and risk of Alzheimer's disease: a systematic review and meta-analysis. *BMC Geriatr*. 2011;11:83.
7. Stowell KM. DNA testing for malignant hyperthermia: the reality and the dream. *Anesth Analg*. 2014;118(2):397-406.
8. Samanta R, Shoukrey K, Griffiths R. Rheumatoid arthritis and anaesthesia. *Anaesthesia*. 2011;66(12):1146-1159.
9. Nandi R, Howard R. Anesthesia and epidermolysis bullosa. *Dermatol Clin*. 2010;28(2):319-324.

MALIGNANT HYPERTHERMIA

A CLOSER LOOK

Malignant hyperthermia (MH) is a genetic disorder in which the patient will develop a lethal hypermetabolic state when exposed to either volatile anesthetics or succinylcholine.

Signs and symptoms of MH

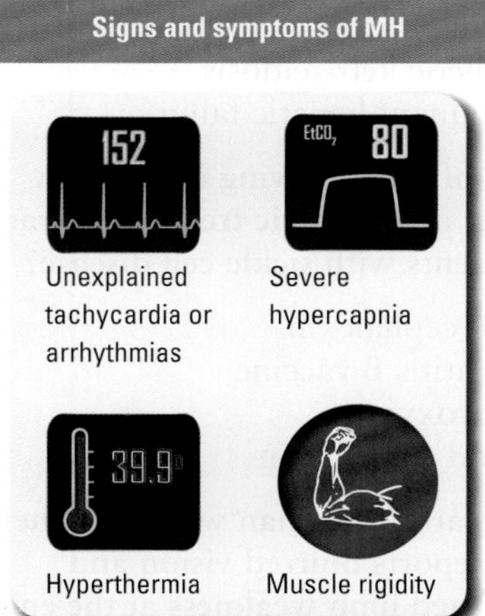

Unexplained tachycardia or arrhythmias
Severe hypercapnia

This syndrome is caused by an abnormal ryanodine receptor in skeletal muscle which, when activated by a triggering agent, results in massive intracellular Ca^{2+} release. This manifests as muscle rigidity and eventually muscle breakdown causing rhabdomyolysis.

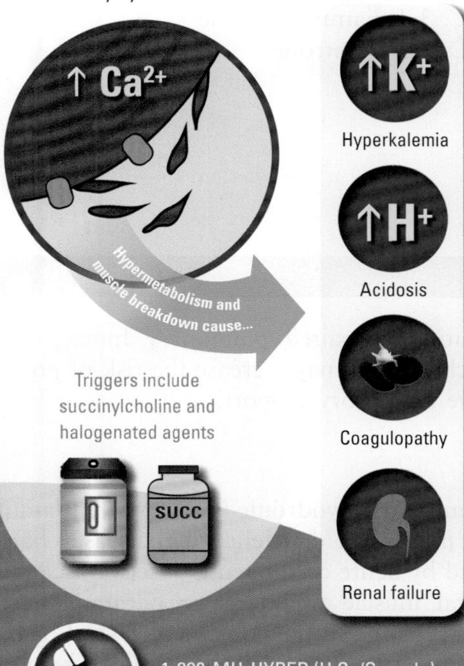

Triggers include succinylcholine and halogenated agents

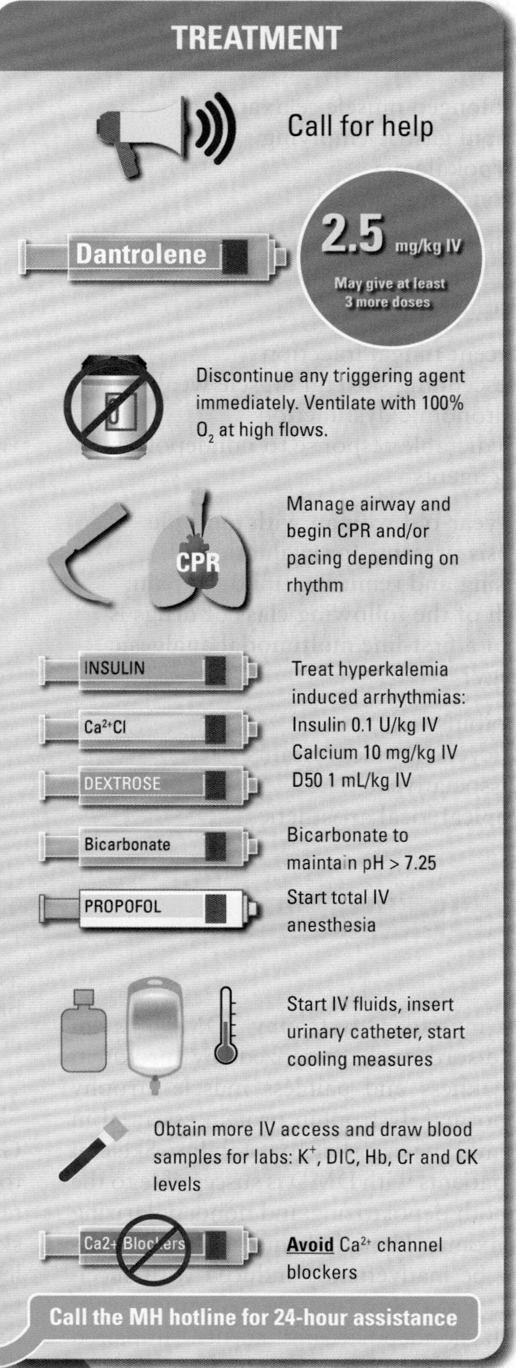

TREATMENT
Call for help
Dantrolene
2.5 mg/kg IV
May give at least 3 more doses
Discontinue any triggering agent immediately. Ventilate with 100% O2 at high flows.
CPR
Manage airway and begin CPR and/or pacing depending on rhythm
INSULIN
Ca2+Cl
DEXTROSE
Treat hyperkalemia induced arrhythmias:
Insulin 0.1 U/kg IV
Calcium 10 mg/kg IV
D50 1 mL/kg IV
Bicarbonate
Bicarbonate to maintain pH > 7.25
PROPOFOL
Start total IV anesthesia
Start IV fluids, insert urinary catheter, start cooling measures
Obtain more IV access and draw blood samples for labs: K+, DIC, Hb, Cr and CK levels
Ca2+ Blockers
Avoid Ca2+ channel blockers
Call the MH hotline for 24-hour assistance

1-800-MH-HYPER (U.S. /Canada)
001-209-417-3722 (worldwide)

Infographic by: Naveen Nathan MD

Questions

1. **A 9-year-old boy with Duchenne muscular dystrophy is undergoing appendectomy. The patient receives vecuronium during general anesthesia. Which of the following conditions may occur in the immediate postoperative period?**

   A. Prolonged muscle relaxation
   B. Rapid gastric emptying
   C. Hypokalemia
   D. Bronchospasm

2. **Which of the following is a common finding in patients with Guillain-Barre syndrome?**

   A. Recent fungal infection
   B. Descending skeletal muscle weakness
   C. Autonomic dysfunction
   D. Predictable response to nondepolarizing agents

3. **A 33-year-old woman with multiple sclerosis presents for evaluation of relapsing and remitting, mild leg pain. Which of the following class of drugs is part of a first-line multimodal analgesic strategy?**

   A. Opioids
   B. Tricyclic antidepressants
   C. Dissociatives
   D. Topical local anesthetic

4. **Which of the following systemic diseases can induce an acquired pseudocholinesterase deficiency?**

   A. Community-acquired pneumonia
   B. Seizure
   C. Diabetic ketoacidosis
   D. Fulminant hepatic failure

5. **Which of the following is part of a routine, prophylactic treatment strategy for patients with sickle cell disease?**

   A. Oral cephalexin
   B. Hepatitis B vaccine
   C. Hydroxyurea
   D. Blood transfusion

6. **A 32-year-old woman with myasthenia gravis reports blurred vision and generalized limb weakness at the end of the day. Administration of which of the following medications is most appropriate?**

   A. Caffeine
   B. Pyridostigmine
   C. 3,4-diaminopyridine
   D. Mitoxantrone

Answers

1. A

Duchenne muscular dystrophy (DMD) is an X-linked disorder characterized by proximal muscle weakness and painless muscle atrophy due to abnormal dystrophin protein essential in muscle membrane cytoskeleton stability. Skeletal muscle in patients with DMD is susceptible to the effects of both depolarizing and nondepolarizing muscle relaxants. Hyperkalemia and rhabdomyolysis may be inadvertently induced with succinylcholine. Prolonged muscle relaxation may occur with nondepolarizing agents. Impaired gastrointestinal function is common, leading to delayed gastric emptying and increased risk of aspiration. Impaired pulmonary function, not bronchospasm, may increase the risk of postoperative ventilatory support.

2. C

Guillain-Barre syndrome (GBS) is an inflammatory, multifocal demyelinating disease characterized by acute or subacute onset of ascending skeletal muscle weakness or paralysis of the legs, occurring in the context of a viral or bacterial infection. In severe cases of GBS, hemodynamic instability may occur due to autonomic dysfunction. Response to nondepolarizing muscle relaxants may be unpredictable.

3. B

A multimodal analgesic strategy using medications with varying mechanisms of action is integral to pain management in multiple sclerosis (MS). Tricyclic antidepressants, antiepileptics, NSAIDs, and antispastic agents are the common class of drugs used in this analgesic strategy. Opioids are generally not recommended as first-line therapy for neuropathic pain syndromes, such as MS. Depression is common in patients with MS. Dissociatives, such as ketamine, have been used as alternative therapy for treatment resistant depression. Topical local anesthetics have a limited role in neuropathic syndromes.

4. D

Acquired pseudocholinesterase deficiency impairs ester substrates metabolism via a reduction in pseudocholinesterase activity. The liver is an important source of this hepatic esterase. Fulminant hepatic failure leads to significant reduction in hepatic function and, therefore, prolonged metabolism of administered esters. Neither pneumonia, seizure, nor diabetic ketoacidosis result in hepatic esterase reduction.

5. C

Sickle cell disease (SCD) is an inherited hemoglobinopathy that results in acute and chronic multisystem complications due to a structurally abnormal hemoglobin called hemoglobin-S or sickle-hemoglobin. Oral penicillin, pneumococcal vaccination, and hydroxyurea are preventative treatments in SCD to reduce infections and sickle crises recurrence. Blood transfusion is the mainstay of treatment for acute complications of SCD. Hepatitis B vaccine, though recommended for high-risk patients such as those with chronic liver disease, is not considered prophylactic therapy for SCD patients. Oral cephalexin is a cephalosporin used for active infection.

6. B

Myasthenia gravis (MG) is an autoimmune disease characterized by skeletal muscle weakness due to a reduction in functional postsynaptic, acetylcholine receptors in the neuromuscular junction. Pyridostigmine is an acetylcholinesterase inhibitor that reduces symptoms by increasing the concentration of acetylcholine available at neuromuscular junction sites. 3,4-diaminopyridine is used as a first-line treatment for patients with LEMS. Mitoxantrone is an antineoplastic agent used to delay progression to secondary degenerative phase of multiple sclerosis. Caffeine is a commonly consumed central nervous system stimulant that is not considered to be treatment for autoimmune diseases.

18 Endocrine Function

Shamsuddin Akhtar

I. Integrated Physiology

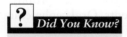

Thyroid hormone is a nonsteroid hormone, but behaves more like a steroid hormone.

Hormones play an essential role in maintaining homeostasis.[1-3] Hormones are divided chemically into either steroids or nonsteroids. Steroid hormones are lipophilic and able to cross the cell membrane to act directly on cytoplasmic pathways (**Figure 18.1**). They are transported in the plasma bound to specific globulins, albumin, and other plasma proteins and have longer half-lives (hours to even days) compared to nonsteroid hormones.

Nonsteroid hormones include catecholamines, peptides, proteins, or glycoproteins. They are hydrophilic and thus unable to cross the cell membrane and require specific cell membrane receptors to exert their effect. These hormones are typically not bound to plasma proteins, have rapid onsets of action (minutes), shorter half-lives (minutes), and faster metabolism. Some hormones are secreted continuously, whereas others are secreted in a pulsatile manner (cortisol).

II. Hypothalamus-Pituitary Complex

? *Did You Know?*

Excessive secretion of growth hormone (GH), usually from a pituitary adenoma, results in acromegaly or gigantism. Acromegaly occurs if excess GH is produced ***after*** epiphyseal closure. Gigantism occurs if excess GH is produced ***before*** epiphyseal closure (**Table 18.1**).

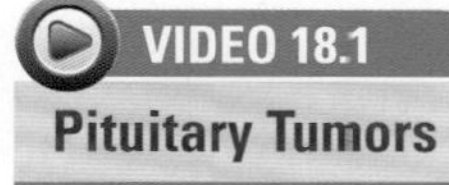

Pituitary Tumors

In conjunction with the hypothalamus, the ***pituitary gland*** is considered a master endocrine gland. Input from various regions of the brain is relayed to specific nuclei in the hypothalamus, which secrete specific releasing factors or hormones that regulate pituitary function[5]. The pituitary gland is composed of two parts: the anterior and posterior pituitary.

A. Anterior Pituitary

The anterior pituitary secretes thyroid stimulating hormone, adrenocorticotrophic hormone, gonadotropins (luteinizing hormone and follicle-stimulating hormone), growth hormone, and prolactin. These hormones in turn affect the thyroid gland, adrenal cortex, gonads, bones, and mammary glands, respectively. The production and release of anterior pituitary hormones are controlled by ***releasing hormones*** (eg, thyroid-stimulating releasing hormone), which are produced by the hypothalamus. The anterior pituitary hormones are released into the systemic circulation and exert their effects on their target organs (**Figure 18.2**).

B. Posterior Pituitary

The posterior pituitary gland is an extension of the hypothalamus. It produces two hormones: ***oxytocin*** and ***vasopressin*** (***antidiuretic hormone*** [ADH]) (**Figure 18.2**).[1]

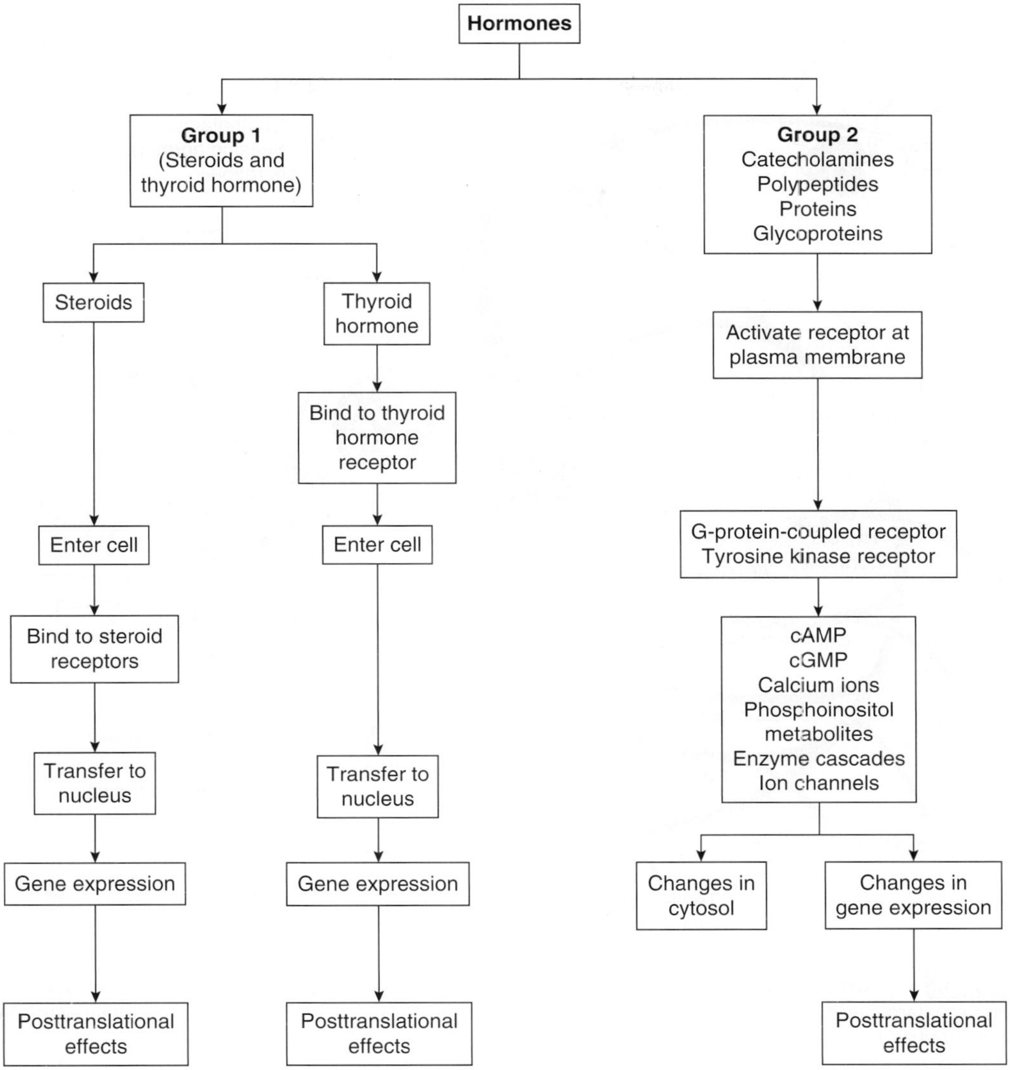

Hormones

Group 1 (Steroids and thyroid hormone)

Steroids → Enter cell → Bind to steroid receptors → Transfer to nucleus → Gene expression → Posttranslational effects

Thyroid hormone → Bind to thyroid hormone receptor → Enter cell → Transfer to nucleus → Gene expression → Posttranslational effects

Group 2 Catecholamines Polypeptides Proteins Glycoproteins

Activate receptor at plasma membrane → G-protein-coupled receptor Tyrosine kinase receptor → cAMP cGMP Calcium ions Phosphoinositol metabolites Enzyme cascades Ion channels → Changes in cytosol; Changes in gene expression → Posttranslational effects

Figure 18.1 Integrated physiology of steroid and nonsteroid hormones.

1. Diabetes Insipidus

Deficiency of vasopressin (***central diabetes insipidus [DI]***) or resistance to its effects on renal tubules (nephrogenic diabetes insipidus) causes an inability to absorb water in the renal tubules and collecting ducts.[2,3] The patient produces liters of dilute urine per day. Central DI can develop acutely after intracranial surgery, head trauma, intracranial tumors, and infections. If the water loss is not supplemented, either by increased water intake or by exogenous supplementation, severe dehydration, hyperosmolality, hypernatremia, cardiovascular collapse, stupor, and coma can result. In central DI, administration of desmopressin, a vasopressin analog, leads to water absorption in the renal tubules and collecting ducts and concentration of urine. This is not seen in nephrogenic DI as kidneys are resistant to the effect of desmopressin. Central DI can be managed by administration of the desmopressin. Perioperative considerations are detailed in **Table 18.2**.

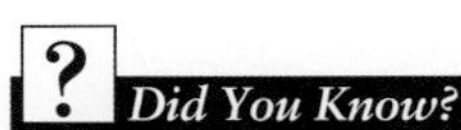

Drugs such as lithium and the antiviral medication foscarnet can cause nephrogenic diabetes insipidus.

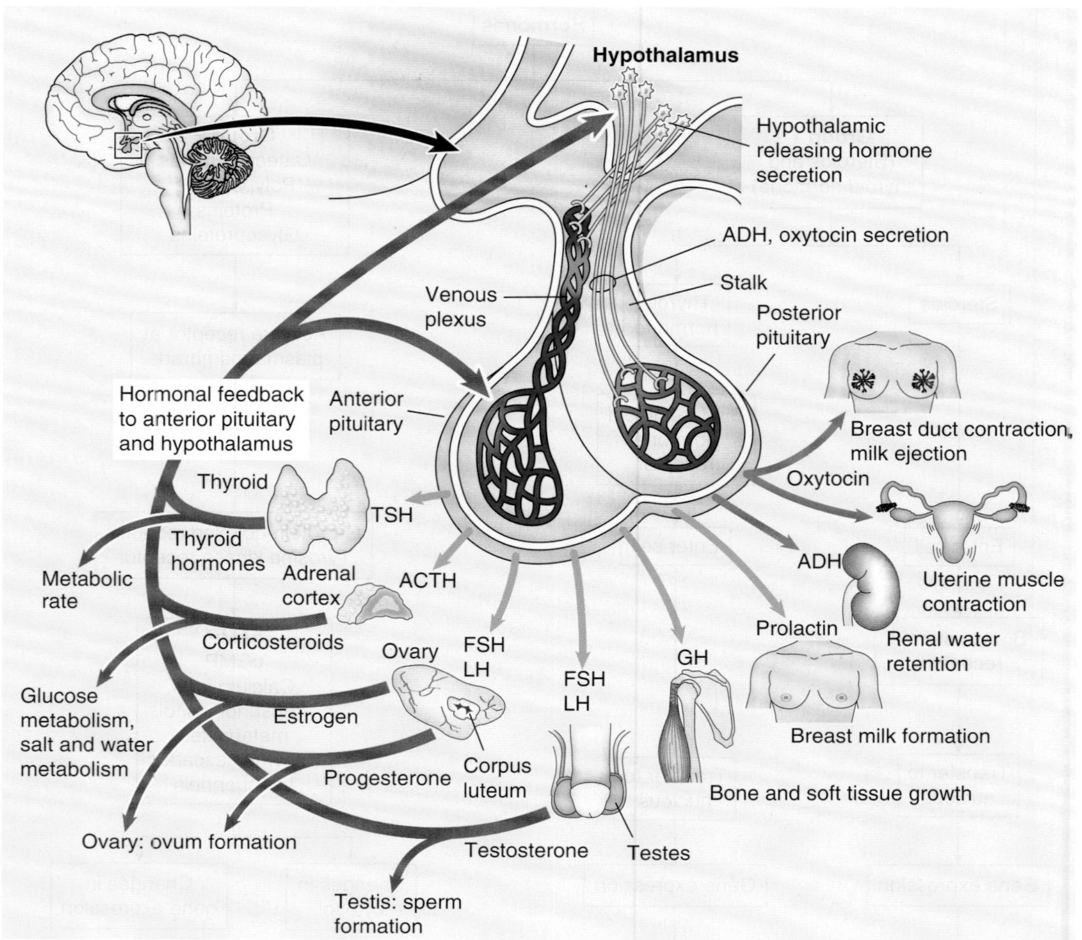

Figure 18.2 **Hypothalamus, pituitary gland, and endocrine target organs.** (From Turbow SD, Patterson BC. Hypothalamic and pituitary disorders. In: Felner EI, Umpierrez GF, eds. *Endocrine Pathophysiology*. Wolters Kluwer; 2014:17.)

Table 18.1 Anesthetic Problems Associated With Acromegaly
Hypertrophy of skeletal, connective, and soft tissues
Enlarged tongue and epiglottis (upper airway obstruction)
Increased incidence of difficult intubation
Thickening of the vocal cords (hoarseness; consider awake tracheal intubation)
Paralysis of the recurrent laryngeal nerve (stretching)
Dyspnea or stridor (subglottic narrowing)
Peripheral nerve or artery entrapment
Hypertension
Diabetes mellitus

Derived from Endocrine function. In: Barash PG, Cullen BF, Stoelting RK, et al, eds. *Handbook of Clinical Anesthesia*. 7th ed. Wolters Kluwer/Lippincott Williams & Wilkins; 2013.

Table 18.2 Diabetes Insipidus: Anesthesia Implications

Clinical picture: Hypovolemia, hyperosmolality, electrolyte disturbances, hypotension, and cardiac dysrhythmias
Treatment: Fluids (hypotonic saline), electrolyte replacement as indicated
Pharmacologic: vasopressin 0.1-0.2 U/h IV, desmopressin 2-4 µg/d: 10 µg intranasally in 1 nostril daily, up to 40 µg/d or 40 µg divided into 2 or 3 daily doses IV

IV, intravenous.

2. Syndrome of Inappropriate Antidiuretic Hormone Secretion

Excess (or inappropriate) vasopressin secretion is a ubiquitous response after trauma and surgery and leads to excess absorption of water by the kidneys. Water absorption in excess of sodium causes dilution of serum sodium (hyponatremia), decreased serum osmolality, and concentrated urine. In certain pathologic states (ie, congestive heart failure or cirrhosis), activation of the renin-angiotensin system can lead to the ***syndrome of inappropriate antidiuretic hormone secretion (SIADH)***. Hyponatremia in the setting of concentrated urine strongly suggests SIADH. Typical management is free water restriction, diuretics, and control of any precipitating conditions. Severe hyponatremia (levels < 120 mEq/L) is a medical emergency. It causes mental status changes (confusion, drowsiness, seizures). Patients with acute severe hyponatremia are usually treated with small boluses of hypertonic (3%) saline. Arginine vasopressin antagonists (tolvaptan, conivaptan) are available but have a limited role in the treatment of SIADH. Perioperative considerations are detailed in **Table 18.3**.

III. Thyroid Gland

The thyroid gland is one of the largest endocrine glands. It secretes three hormones: thyroxine (T_4), triiodothyronine (T_3), and calcitonin (involved in calcium homeostasis). ***Thyroxine*** (***T_4***) and ***triiodothyronine*** (***T_3***) are under tight control of thyroid-stimulating hormone (TSH) from the pituitary gland (**Figure 18.3**).[3]

A. Thyroid Hormone Metabolism

Tyrosine and iodine are needed to form T_4 and T_3 (**Figure 18.3**). Iodine absorbed from the gastrointestinal tract is converted to iodide and transported and concentrated in the thyroid gland. Tyrosine, which is attached to thyroglobulin, is then iodinated by a complex process to yield T_4 and, to a less extent, T_3 (**Figure 18.3**). The majority of T_3 is produced outside the thyroid gland by the conversion of T_4. T_4 feeds back to the pituitary and hypothalamus and decreases the secretion of TSH, which then leads in thyroid hormones. T_4 and T_3 are lipophilic

Table 18.3 Syndrome of Inappropriate Antidiuretic Hormone Secretion: Anesthesia Implications

Clinical picture: Hyponatremia, increased urinary sodium, and osmolarity. Serum sodium <115 mEq/L leads to seizures.
Treatment: Restrict IV fluids, diuretics, use normal or hypertonic saline, and correct serum Na^+ concentration slowly (<12 mEq/24 h).

IV, intravenous.

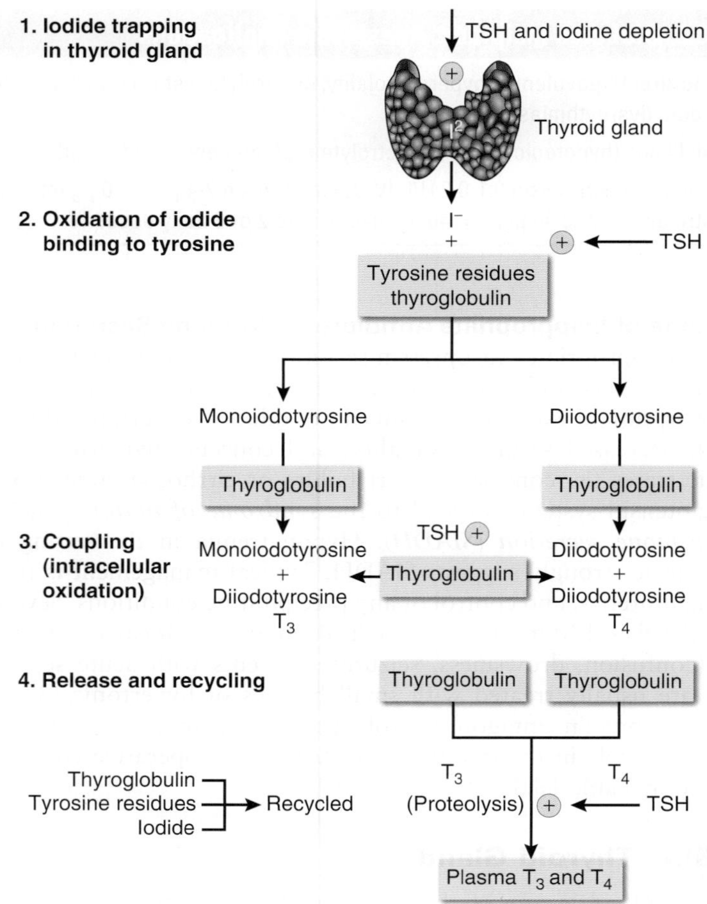

Figure 18.3 **Thyroid hormone biosynthesis consists of four stages: (1) organification, (2) binding, (3) coupling, and (4) release. T_3, triiodothyronine; T_4, thyroxine; TSH, thyroid-stimulating hormone.** (From Schwartz JJ, Akhtar S, Rosenbaum SH. Endocrine function. In: Barash PG, Cahalan MK, Cullen BF, et al, eds. *Clinical Anesthesia*. 8th ed. Wolters Kluwer; 2018:1327-1356, Figure 47.1.)

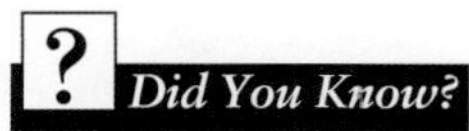

Twenty times more T_4 is produced by the thyroid gland than T_3. However, T_3 is the more potent and less protein-bound form that produces the preponderance of clinical effects.

and are 99.8% bound to albumin, thyroxine-binding globulin, and prealbumin. It is only the small free fraction of hormone that exerts a biologic effect. T_4 and T_3 are metabolized in the liver, kidney, and many other tissues. Glucocorticoids, dopamine, somatostatin, and stress decrease TSH secretion.

B. Physiologic Effects of Thyroid Hormone

T_3 and T_4 increase oxygen consumption of target organs. Thyroid hormones increase carbohydrate, fat, and protein metabolism and are essential for normal growth. They increase cardiac output by increasing heart rate and myocardial contraction and enhance the effect of circulatory catecholamines. β-Adrenergic receptors are increased, and cardiac α-adrenergic receptors are decreased.

C. Tests of Thyroid Function

Abnormalities in thyroid function are seen in both thyroid and nonthyroid diseases (**Table 18.4**). The initial step in evaluating thyroid function is

Table 18.4 Tests of Thyroid Function

	Free Thyroxine	Free Triiodothyronine	Thyroid Stimulating Hormone
Hyperthyroidism	Elevated	Elevated	Normal to low
Primary hypothyroidism	Low	Normal to low	Elevated
Secondary hypothyroidism	Low	Low	Low
Sick euthyroidism	Normal	Low	Normal
Pregnancy	Elevated	Normal	Normal

Derived from Endocrine function. In: Barash PG, Cullen BF, Stoelting RK, et al, eds. *Handbook of Clinical Anesthesia*. 7th ed. Wolters Kluwer/Lippincott Williams & Wilkins; 2013.

to measure TSH and free T_4 (fT_4).[3] Extremely low TSH in the setting of high fT_4 suggests hyperthyroidism, while high TSH and low fT_4 suggest hypothyroidism.

D. Hyperthyroidism

Hyperthyroidism is characterized by nervousness, weight loss, diarrhea, heat intolerance, sweating, tachycardia, and an increase in pulse pressure (because of vasodilation). Patients who present with uncontrolled hyperthyroid symptoms should be managed medically before elective surgery. Medical management consists of decreasing thyroid hormone production and blunting the hyperadrenergic symptoms. Beta-blockers decrease adrenergic symptoms (tachycardia, increased cardiac output), while propylthiouracil and methimazole compete with tyrosine for iodide and thus block T_3 and T_4 production. In acute situations, exogenous iodine can be administered, which depresses thyroid hormone production. Acute thyroid storm is a medical emergency. Patients can present with or develop it intraoperatively. Management of thyrotoxicosis is detailed in **Table 18.5**.

After adequate control of hyperthyroid symptoms, surgical excision of the thyroid gland can be performed. Radioactive iodine ablates the thyroid gland and leads to a progressive loss of function. Loss of thyroid function must be treated with exogenous levothyroxine.

E. Hypothyroidism

Patients with ***hypothyroidism*** present with peripheral vasoconstriction, poor mentation, cold intolerance, and weight gain. Hypothyroidism is treated with exogenous levothyroxine. Patients with severe symptoms should be treated prior to elective procedures. In this situation, T_3 can be used, which has a faster onset of action. These patients are exquisitely sensitive to sedative medications and can quickly develop cardiorespiratory collapse. Management of myxedema coma requires inotropic agents, administration of intravenous T_4 or T_3, fluids, hydrocortisone, and respiratory support (**Table 18.5**).

F. Anesthetic Priorities in Thyroid Surgery

General anesthesia with an endotracheal tube is used for thyroid surgery.[2,3] Anesthesiologists may encounter unexpected difficult airway in 5% to 8% of cases. During thyroid gland resection, ***recurrent laryngeal nerve injury*** is a risk. Unilateral nerve injury usually manifests as hoarseness and can be treated conservatively. Bilateral recurrent laryngeal nerve injury may cause aphonia and

Table 18.5 Perioperative Thyroid Emergencies (Thyrotoxicosis and Myxedema Coma)

Management of Thyroid Storm
IV fluids
Sodium iodide: 250 mg orally or IV every 6 h
Propylthiouracil: 500-1000 mg loading dose orally or via nasogastric tube, then 250 mg every 4 h orally or via nasogastric tube
Hydrocortisone: 300 mg IV bolus, then 100 mg IV every 8 h
Propranolol: 60-80 mg every 4 h orally or esmolol infusion titrated to effect
Cooling blankets and acetaminophen: 25 mg IV of meperidine every 4-6 h may be used to treat or prevent shivering
Diltiazem: Congestive heart failure with atrial fibrillation and rapid ventricular response
Management of Myxedema Coma
Tracheal intubation and controlled ventilation of the lungs as needed
Levothyroxine: 200-300 µg IV over 5-10 min, then 100 µg IV q 24 h
Hydrocortisone: 100 mg IV, then 25 mg IV every 6 h
Fluid and electrolyte therapy as guided by serum electrolyte measurements
Warm environment to conserve body heat

IV, intravenous.

Derived from Endocrine function. In: Barash PG, Cullen BF, Stoelting RK, et al, eds. *Handbook of Clinical Anesthesia*. 7th ed. Wolters Kluwer/Lippincott Williams & Wilkins; 2013.

respiratory distress (**Table 18.6**). Tracheal compression due to hematoma or tracheomalacia (after excision of a large thyroid) is an emergency that may require reintubation (see Chapter 20). If the parathyroid glands have been inadvertently resected or injured, hypocalcemia may develop within 24 to 96 hours after surgery. Signs and symptoms of hypocalcemia include skeletal muscle spasms or seizures.

? *Did You Know?*

A Chvostek sign is contracture of the facial muscle produced by tapping the facial nerve as it crosses the parotid gland. A Trousseau sign is a contraction of the fingers and wrist after application of a blood pressure cuff inflated above systolic blood pressure. Both are signs of hypocalcemia.

IV. Adrenal Gland

A. Adrenal Cortex

The adrenal gland is composed of two parts: the outer cortex and the inner medulla. The cortex is divided into three zones—the ***zona glomerulosa***, ***zona fasciculata***, and ***zona reticularis***—which produce ***mineralocorticoids***,

Table 18.6 Complications of Thyroid Surgery

Thyroid storm: Should be distinguished from malignant hyperthermia, pheochromocytoma, and inadequate anesthesia; it most often develops in undiagnosed or untreated hyperthyroid patients because of the stress of surgery.
Airway obstruction: Hematoma in the neck or tracheomalacia causing airway obstruction.
Recurrent laryngeal nerve damage: Hoarseness may be present if the damage is unilateral, and aphonia may be present if the damage is bilateral.
Hypoparathyroidism: Symptoms of hypocalcemia develop within 24-48 h and include laryngospasm.

Derived from Endocrine function. In: Barash PG, Cullen BF, Stoelting RK, et al, eds. *Handbook of Clinical Anesthesia*. 7th ed. Wolters Kluwer/Lippincott Williams & Wilkins; 2013.

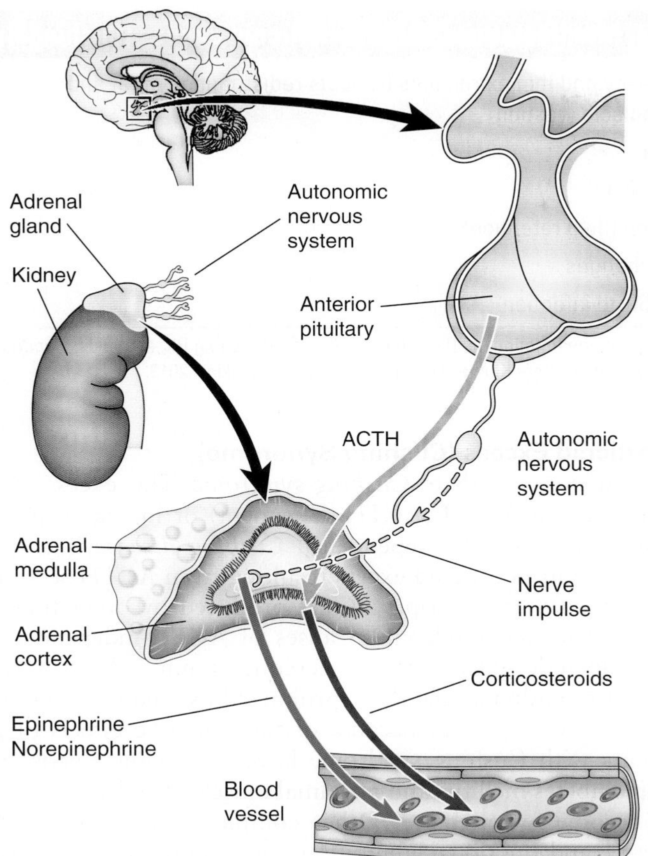

Figure 18.4 The hypothalamic-pituitary axis controls many of the functions of the normal adrenal gland. The cortex is responsive to corticotropin, while the medulla is under control of the autonomic nervous system. (From Hammel JA, Umpierrez GE. Adrenal gland disorders. In: Felner EI, Umpierrez GF, eds. *Endocrine Pathophysiology.* Wolters Kluwer; 2014:480.)

glucocorticoids, and ***androgens***, respectively (**Figure 18.4**).[4-6] The precursor of all steroid hormones is cholesterol, which is converted to pregnenolone in the mitochondria. Pregnenolone is transported to the cytoplasm and then converted by various enzymes into specific steroid hormones. The signs and symptoms of abnormal adrenal cortical function are typically the result of cortisol or aldosterone excess or deficiency.

1. Physiologic Effects of Glucocorticoids

Glucocorticoid production and secretion is controlled by ***corticotropin*** (adrenocorticotropic hormone, ACTH) from the pituitary gland. Glucocorticoids increase protein catabolism, glycogenolysis, and gluconeogenesis and have anti-inflammatory and anti-insulin effects. They are required for glucagon and catecholamines to have their metabolic effects, as well as for normal vascular reactivity, neurologic function, and water excretion.[7]

Table 18.7 Manifestations of Glucocorticoid Excess (Cushing Syndrome)

Truncal obesity and thin extremities (reflects redistribution of fat and skeletal muscle wasting)
Osteopenia
Hyperglycemia
Hypertension (fluid retention)
Emotional changes
Susceptibility to infection

Derived from Endocrine function. In: Barash PG, Cullen BF, Stoelting RK, et al, eds. *Handbook of Clinical Anesthesia*. 7th ed. Wolters Kluwer/Lippincott Williams & Wilkins; 2013.

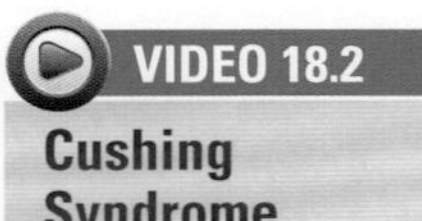

2. Glucocorticoid Excess (Cushing Syndrome)

Glucocorticoid excess leads to ***Cushing syndrome***. This excess can be due to either an increase in ACTH (ACTH-dependent) or increased production by the adrenal gland (ACTH-independent). ***Cushing disease*** is a specific term used to describe glucocorticoid excess resulting from ACTH-secreting tumors in the anterior pituitary. Ectopic ACTH produced by other tumors (eg, the lung) leads to Cushing syndrome. Causes of ACTH-independent glucocorticoid excess include glucocorticoid-secreting tumors of the adrenal gland, hyperplasia of the adrenal gland, or prolonged exogenous administration of glucocorticoids. As expected, because of the catabolic effects of glucocorticoids, patients with Cushing syndrome have significant glucose intolerance and develop diabetes mellitus and proximal muscle atrophy. They retain water and often become hypertensive. Other complications include osteoporosis, truncal obesity, and emotional lability. Anesthetic implications for patients with Cushing syndrome undergoing an adrenalectomy are detailed in **Table 18.7.**

3. Adrenal Insufficiency (Addison Disease)

Adrenal deficiency can occur because of primary adrenal failure or lack of sufficient corticotropin from the pituitary gland (secondary). Patients may present with nonspecific symptoms (chronic fatigue, muscle weakness, anorexia, weight loss, nausea, vomiting, diarrhea). ***Chronic adrenal insufficiency*** is diagnosed by determining the plasma cortisol response to a corticotropin stimulation test. ***Addison disease*** is treated with daily exogenous glucocorticoids and mineralocorticoids. ***Acute adrenal insufficiency (Addisonian crisis)*** frequently presents with hypotension, decreased consciousness, and shock and requires intravenous hydrocortisone. Perioperative implications for patients with Addisonian crisis are detailed in **Table 18.8.**

Table 18.8 Adrenal Insufficiency (Addisonian Crisis): Anesthesia Implications

Clinical picture: In Addisonian crisis, recurrent hypotension requiring multiple doses of vasopressors, hypovolemia, hypokalemia, and hyponatremia. In chronic Addison disease due to primary adrenal insufficiency, hyperpigmentation is seen.
Treatment: Hydrocortisone 100 mg IV, then 100 mg every 8 h or by continuous infusion.

IV, intravenous.

Table 18.9 Comparative Pharmacology of Corticosteroids

	Anti-Inflammatory[a]	Mineralocorticoid[a]	Approximate Equivalent Dose (mg)	Plasma Half-Life (min)	Duration of Action (h)
Short Acting					
Hydrocortisone (cortisol)	1.0	1.0	20	90	8-12
Prednisone	4.0	0.25	5.0	60	12-36
Methylprednisolone	5.0	+/–	4.0	180	12-36
Long Acting					
Dexamethasone	30	+/–	0.75	200	36-54

[a]Relative milligram comparison with hydrocortisone. The glucocorticoid and mineralocorticoid properties are set to 1.0.
Derived from Endocrine function. In: Barash PG, Cullen BF, Stoelting RK, et al, eds. *Handbook of Clinical Anesthesia.* 7th ed. Wolters Kluwer/Lippincott Williams & Wilkins; 2013 and Felner EI, Umpierrez GE. *Endocrine Pathophysiology.* Lippincott Williams & Wilkins; 2014:480.

4. Exogenous Glucocorticoid Therapy

Anesthesiologists should be familiar with the different preparations of synthetic steroids that are used therapeutically (**Table 18.9**). Dexamethasone, betamethasone, and triamcinolone have no mineralocorticoid activity and are typically used for their anti-inflammatory properties. Fludrocortisone has 12 times more mineralocorticoid activity than anti-inflammatory activity and is used to supplement mineralocorticoid activity in adrenal deficiency. Cortisol (hydrocortisone) and cortisone have equal mineralocorticoid and glucocorticoid activity. Prednisone and methylprednisone are typically used for immunologic and inflammatory diseases.

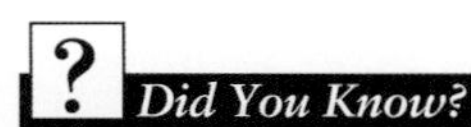

The normal daily production of cortisol is 10 to 20 mg/d but can reach 200 to 500 mg/d under periods of extreme stress (trauma).

5. Steroid Replacement During the Perioperative Period

One of the major consequences of administering exogenous steroids is suppression of the ***hypothalamic-pituitary axis (HPA)***.[2,4,8] Suppression of the HPA is unlikely to develop in a patient who has received <1 week of lower-dose exogenous steroid therapy. Patients who receive >3 weeks of steroid therapy can be considered to have a suppressed HPA, especially if they are consuming more than 20 mg/d of prednisone (or equivalent doses of other steroids). It can take up to 6 to 9 months for the HPA to normalize. If patients do not receive steroid supplementation in the perioperative period, they can present in Addisonian crisis. Patients who receive ≤5 mg/d of prednisolone usually do not require additional supplementation if they have taken their usual morning dose prior to surgery. Perioperative supplementation of steroids is based on expected physiologic stress induced by surgery.[8,9] For high-risk surgeries, usual daily dose plus hydrocortisone 100 mg IV before incision followed by continuous IV infusion of 200 mg of hydrocortisone in 24 hours, is recommended, while for moderate to low-risk surgeries, 50 mg at induction, followed by 25 mg every 8 hours in the next 24 hours, may be sufficient (**Table 18.10**).

6. Physiological Effects of Mineralocorticoids

Aldosterone is the predominant and most potent mineralocorticoid produced by the adrenal gland. Its release is controlled by ***angiotensin II***, ACTH, and serum potassium (**Figure 18.5**). Aldosterone is responsible for sodium and water absorption from the kidney to maintain adequate intravascular volume. Decreased intravascular volume leads to a decrease in afferent arteriolar

Table 18.10 Supplemental Steroid Coverage

For Minor to Moderate Risk Surgery: Hydrocortisone 50 mg IV before induction of anesthesia followed by 25 mg every 8 h for 24 h
For High Risk Surgery: Usual daily dose plus Hydrocortisone 100 mg IV before incision followed by continuous IV infusion of 200 mg of hydrocortisone in 24 h

IV, intravenous.
Derived from Endocrine function. In: Barash PG, Cullen BF, Stoelting RK, et al, eds. *Handbook of Clinical Anesthesia.* 7th ed. Wolters Kluwer/Lippincott Williams & Wilkins; 2013.

pressure in the nephron. This is sensed by the juxtaglomerular apparatus, which secretes renin. ***Renin*** converts circulating angiotensinogen to angiotensin I, which is further converted to angiotensin II by angiotensin-converting enzyme in the lungs. Angiotensin II is a potent stimulus for aldosterone secretion. Aldosterone acts on the distal renal tubules and promotes sodium and water absorption, which leads to restitution of intravascular volume. Sodium is exchanged for potassium or hydrogen ions in the distal tubules.

7. Mineralocorticoid Excess

Mineralocorticoid (aldosterone) excess leads to sodium absorption and potassium or hydrogen ion excretion in the renal tubules. This causes hypertension, muscle weakness (due to contractile dysfunction of skeletal muscle), polyuria, tetany, hypokalemia, and metabolic alkalosis. Aldosterone excess can be broadly classified as primary or secondary hyperaldosteronism. In primary hyperaldosteronism, high levels of aldosterone are caused by increased production by the adrenal cortex. Aldosterone excess can be a result of primary adrenal disease (***Conn syndrome***), adrenal hyperplasia, adrenal adenoma or carcinoma, or a genetic disorder involving corticotropin. In primary hyperaldosteronism, renin activity is depressed and patients rarely exhibit edema. In secondary hyperaldosteronism, which is commonly seen in heart failure, cirrhosis, and nephrosis, aldosterone excess is caused by increased renin levels. In these conditions, the kidneys sense a low intravascular volume, which triggers

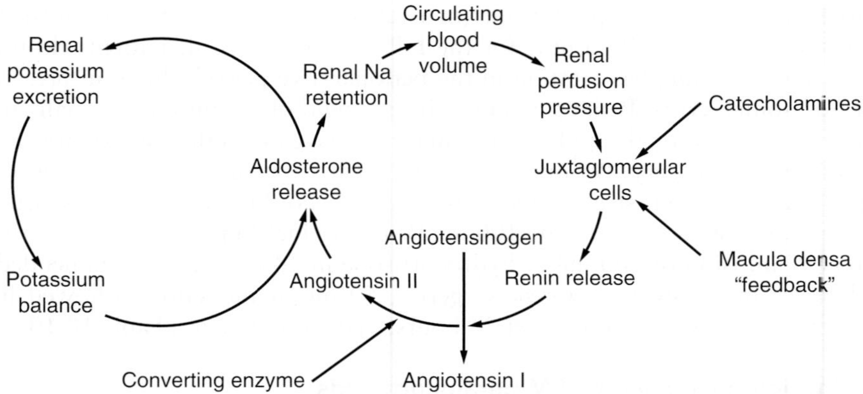

Figure 18.5 **Interrelationship of the volume and potassium feedback loops on aldosterone secretion.** (From Schwartz JJ, Akhtar S, Rosenbaum SH. Endocrine function. In: Barash PG, Cahalan MK, Cullen BF, et al, eds. *Clinical Anesthesia.* 8th ed. Wolters Kluwer; 2018:1327-1356, Figure 47.3 and adapted from Petersdorf RG, ed. *Harrison's Principles of Internal Medicine.* 10th ed. McGraw-Hill; 1983.)

Table 18.11 Hyperaldostonerism (Conn Syndrome): Anesthesia Implications

Clinical picture: Hypertension, hypokalemia, hypernatremia, hypomagnesaemia, hypervolemia, and suppression of renin excretion. Hypokalemia potentiate the effects of nondepolarizing neuromuscular blockers.
Treatment: Potassium-sparing diuretics

renin release and ultimately leads to increased angiotensin II production and aldosterone secretion. Patients retain sodium and water to compensate for low intravascular volume and develop significant edema (**Table 18.11**).

? *Did You Know?*

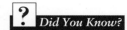

Only the brain and adrenal gland have the specific enzyme phenylethanolamine *N*-methyltransferase, which can convert norepinephrine to epinephrine.

B. Adrenal Medulla

The adrenal medulla predominantly produces ***epinephrine*** and small amounts of ***norepinephrine and dopamine.*** All three catecholamines are derived from the amino acid tyrosine. Adrenal phenylethanolamine *N*-methyltransferase is the enzyme responsible for conversion of norepinephrine to epinephrine. This enzyme is induced by glucocorticoids; thus, glucocorticoids are intricately involved in catecholamine production and function. Epinephrine and norepinephrine levels are significantly increased during and after surgery (**Figure 18.6**).[10] Catecholamines have a very short half-life (2 minutes) and are metabolized to ***vanillylmandelic acid***, metanephrines, or normetanephrine and excreted in the urine (**Figure 18.7**).

1. Pheochromocytoma

Pheochromocytoma is a rare tumor of the adrenal gland that produces catecholamines—mainly norepinephrine. Patients present with sustained or

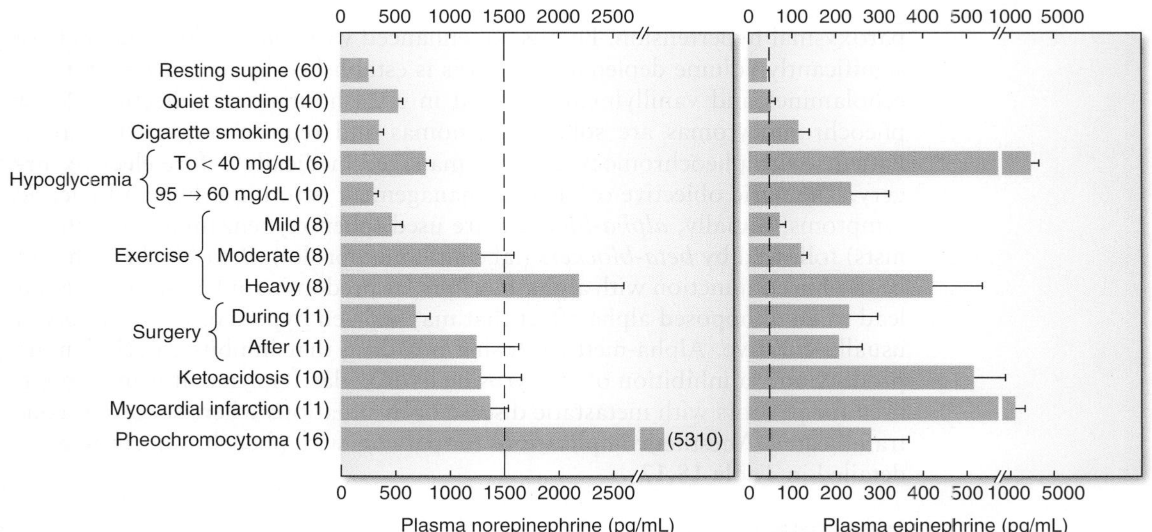

Figure 18.6 Norepinephrine and epinephrine levels in human venous blood in various physiologic and pathologic states. Note that the horizontal scales are different. The numbers to the left in parentheses are the numbers of subjects tested. In each case, the vertical dashed line identifies the threshold plasma concentration at which detectable physiologic changes are observed. (From Barrett KE, Barman SM, Boitano S, Brooks H. *Ganong's Review of Medical Physiology.* 24th ed. McGraw Hill Professional; 2012.)

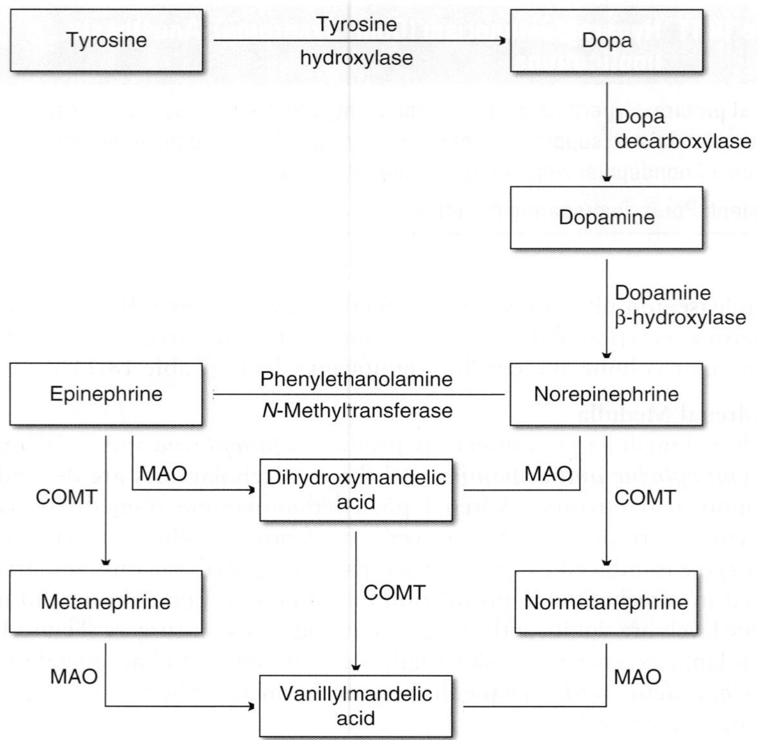

Figure 18.7 Synthesis and metabolism of endogenous catecholamines. COMT, catechol-O-methyltransferase; MAO, monoamine oxidase. (From Schwartz JJ, Akhtar S, Rosenbaum SH. Endocrine function. In: Barash PG, Cahalan MK, Cullen BF, et al, eds. *Clinical Anesthesia*. 8th ed. Wolters Kluwer; 2018:1327-1356, Figure 47.5.)

paroxysmal hypertension. Because of enhanced vasoconstriction, patients are significantly volume depleted. Diagnosis is established by measuring free catecholamines and vanillylmandelic acid in a 24-hour urine collection. Most pheochromocytomas are solitary adenomas and require surgical resection. Patients with pheochromocytoma are managed medically before elective surgery. The basic objective of medical management is to blunt hyperadrenergic symptoms. Initially, ***alpha-blockers*** are used (phenoxybenzamine, α_1 antagonists) followed by ***beta-blockers*** (labetalol, metoprolol). Beta-blockers should be used in conjunction with alpha-blockers, as predominant beta-blockade can lead to an unopposed alpha effect that may worsen hypertension.[11] Surgery is usually curative. Alpha-methyltyrosine is a drug that inhibits catecholamine production via inhibition of the tyrosine hydroxylase enzyme. It is most often used for patients with metastatic disease or in situations where surgery is contraindicated. Anesthetic implications for patients with pheochromocytoma are detailed in **Table 18.12**.

V. Calcium Homeostasis

Calcium is found in plasma in three states: bound to albumin (50%); bound to phosphate, bicarbonate, or citrate (5%-10%); and free ionized calcium (40%-45%) (**Figure 18.8**).[4] It is the ***ionized calcium*** that plays a critical role in regulating muscle contraction, coagulation, neurotransmitter release, and

Table 18.12 Pheochromocytoma

Manifestations
Sustained (occasionally paroxysmal) hypertension (headaches)
Cardiac dysrhythmias
Orthostatic hypotension (decreased blood volume)
Congestive heart failure
Cardiomyopathy
Anesthetic Management of Patients
Continue preoperative medical therapy
Invasive monitoring (arterial central venous catheter, TEE)
Ensure an adequate depth of anesthesia before initiating direct laryngoscopy for tracheal intubation
Maintain anesthesia with opioids and a volatile anesthetic
Control systemic blood pressure with nitroprusside or phentolamine (magnesium, nitroglycerin, and calcium channel blockers may be alternative vasodilator drugs)
Control tachydysrhythmias with propranolol, esmolol, or labetalol
Anticipate hypotension with ligation of the tumor's venous blood supply (initially treat with IV fluids and vasopressors; continuous infusion of norepinephrine is an option if necessary)

IV, intravenous; TEE, transesophageal echocardiography.

Derived from Endocrine function. In: Barash PG, Cullen BF, Stoelting RK, et al, eds. *Handbook of Clinical Anesthesia.* 7th ed. Wolters Kluwer/Lippincott Williams & Wilkins; 2013.

second messenger intracellular functions. Ionized calcium concentration is affected by blood pH and temperature, both of which alter Ca^{2+} binding to albumin. Alkalosis causes a decrease in ionized calcium, while acidosis causes an increase in ionized calcium.

Parathyroid hormone (PTH) is secreted by the parathyroid glands and is intricately involved in the regulation of plasma calcium (**Figure 18.9**). PTH maintains extracellular Ca^{2+} concentration through direct effects on the bone and kidneys. PTH triggers osteoclastic activity in bones, leading to Ca^{2+} and phosphate release. In the kidneys, PTH promotes Ca^{2+} resorption and phosphate excretion in the distal tubule. It also promotes the synthesis of

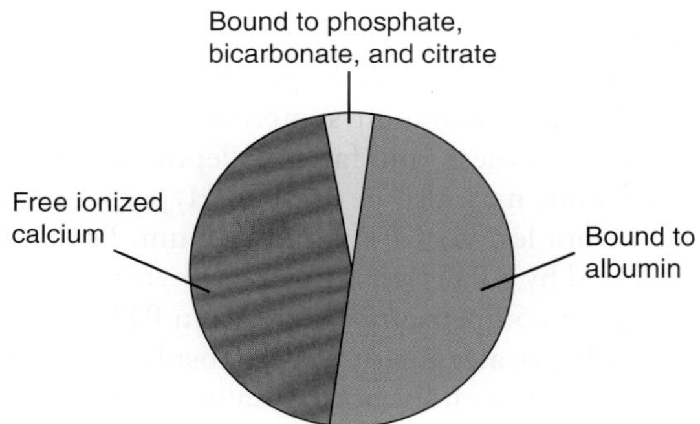

Figure 18.8 Calcium is found in plasma in three states: bound to both albumin and phosphate, as well as ionized calcium.

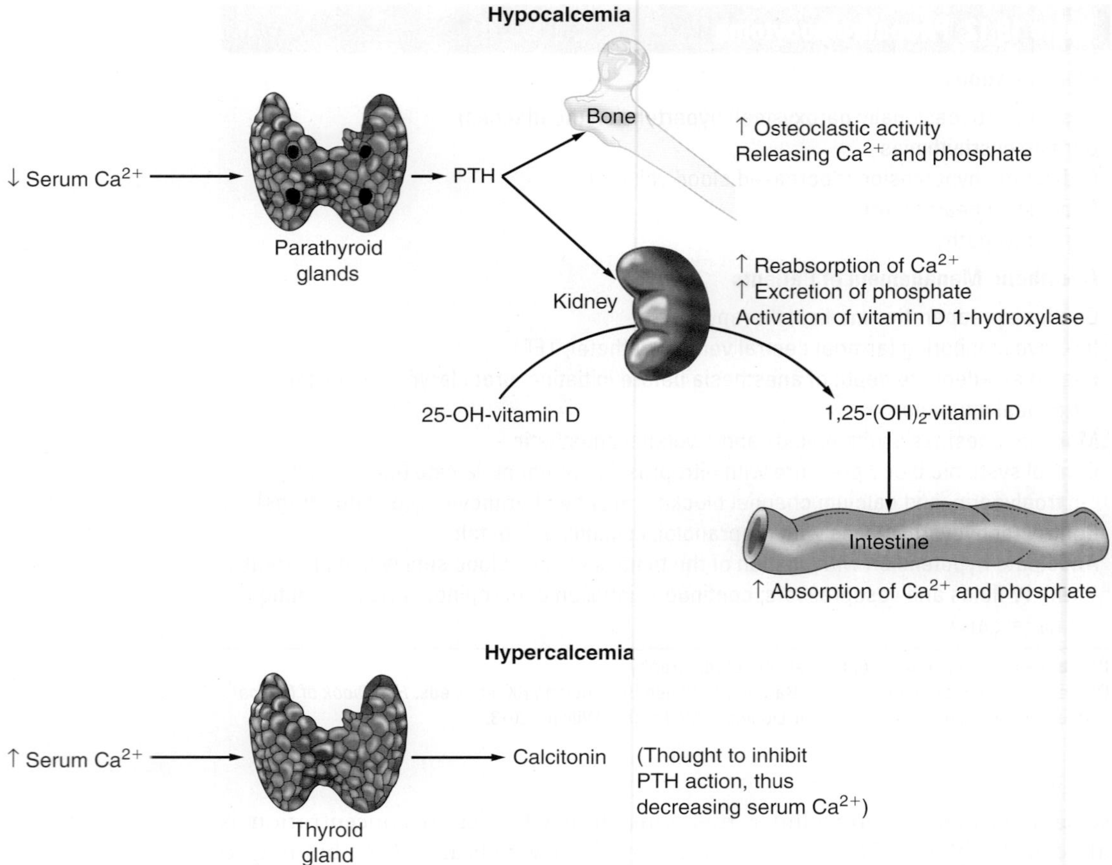

Figure 18.9 **Parathyroid hormone (PTH) and vitamin D metabolism and action. 25-OH, 25-hydroxycholecalciferol; 1,25-$(OH)_2$, 1,25-dihydroxycholecalciferol.** (From Schwartz JJ, Akhtar S, Rosenbaum SH. Endocrine function. In: Barash PG, Cahalan MK, Cullen BF, et al, eds. *Clinical Anesthesia*. 8th ed. Wolters Kluwer; 2018:1327-1356, Figure 47.2.)

1,25-dihydroxyvitamin D, which increases intestinal absorption of calcium and phosphate. PTH secretion is primarily regulated by the serum ionized Ca^{2+} concentration.

A. Hyperparathyroidism

Excess PTH leads to ***hypercalcemia***. Nephrolithiasis is the most common presenting complaint. Other common symptoms include polyuria, polydipsia, generalized muscle weakness, and fatigue. Peptic ulceration, constipation, and psychiatric complaints may also be present. Hyperparathyroidism is diagnosed by increased serum levels of PTH and calcium. Primary hyperparathyroidism is usually caused by a PTH-secreting parathyroid adenoma. Secondary hyperparathyroidism is a compensatory increase in PTH and is seen in conditions that cause either hypocalcemia or hyperphosphatemia (eg, chronic renal failure). Hydration with intravenous normal saline is the first step in the treatment of hypercalcemia. Loop diuretics can be used to enhance renal calcium excretion; however, this intervention rarely is used in contemporary practice. Calcitonin inhibits PTH secretion and osteoclastic bone resorption and is

Table 18.13 Hyperparathyroidism: Anesthesia Implications
Clinical picture: Hypercalcemia, hypophosphatemia, hypovolemia, cardiac dysrhythmias, and pathologic fractures.
Treatment: Correct hypercalcemia (preop Ca^{2+} >14 mEq/L) may require fluids, diuretics, dialysis, and medications (calcitonin, bisphosphonates, or glucocorticoids). Follow electrocardiogram for signs of Ca^{2+} levels.

effective for 24 to 48 hours, after which resistance develops. Bisphosphonates, which decrease osteoclastic activity, may also be used. Glucocorticoids are effective in reducing serum calcium concentration in some conditions (sarcoidosis, malignancy), but have little role in the treatment of primary hypercalcemia. Severe hypercalcemia should be treated prior to elective surgery. In cases of benign adenoma, surgical excision is curative. Anesthetic implications of hypercalcemia are detailed in **Table 18.13**.

B. Hypoparathyroidism

Hypoparathyroidism is a relatively uncommon condition. In infants and children, it is usually the result of a genetic condition. In adults, hypoparathyroidism is most often acquired from iatrogenic or autoimmune damage to the parathyroid gland. Patients with ***hypoparathyroidism*** may present with numbness, paresthesias, muscle spasms, altered mental status, or behavioral disturbances. Rarely, seizures may occur. Cardiovascular manifestations reflect the effects of hypocalcemia and include congestive heart failure, hypotension, and prolonged QT interval. Hypocalcemia in the setting of a low PTH confirms the diagnosis. Treatment involves replacement of electrolytes with oral or intravenous calcium and vitamin D analogues. Clinical manifestations of hypocalcemia are detailed in **Table 18.14**.

> **? Did You Know?**
>
> Propofol can interfere with rapid PTH assay and should not be used for at least 15 minutes prior to measurement of a serum PTH level.

C. Anesthetic Implications of Parathyroid Surgery

General anesthesia with endotracheal tube or a laryngeal mask airway is most often used for parathyroid surgery. Regional anesthesia can be used for minimally invasive parathyroidectomies. In some cases, a rapid PTH assay is used intraoperatively to allow confirmation that the hyperfunctioning gland has been removed successfully. As during thyroid surgery, ***recurrent laryngeal nerve injury*** is a concern and may cause postoperative hoarseness or airway compromise. ***Hypocalcemia*** due to ***hypoparathyroidism*** can develop after parathyroid surgery and may require intravenous calcium supplementation.

Table 18.14 Hypoparathyroidism: Clinical Manifestations
Neuronal irritability
Skeletal muscle spasms
Congestive heart failure
Prolonged QT interval on the electrocardiogram

Derived from Endocrine function. In: Barash PG, Cullen BF, Stoelting RK, et al, eds. *Handbook of Clinical Anesthesia*. 7th ed. Wolters Kluwer/Lippincott Williams & Wilkins; 2013.

VI. Diabetes Mellitus

A. Physiology

Diabetes mellitus is a disease caused by dysfunction of glucose metabolism as a result of either an absolute or a relative (lack of effect) insulin deficiency.[4,12,13] Insulin is produced in the pancreas by β ***cells in the islets of Langerhans.*** Factors that increase insulin secretion include increased levels of plasma glucose, gastrointestinal hormones (incretin hormones), autonomic stimulation (vagal and β adrenergic), α blockade, and nitric oxide. Hypoglycemia and hypokalemia decrease insulin secretion. Insulin is metabolized in the liver and kidneys.

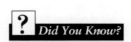

> **? Did You Know?**
>
> Only skeletal and adipose tissue require insulin for glucose entry into cells. Other organs, such as the liver and brain, do not rely on insulin for glucose transport.

The principal effect of insulin is to increase glucose uptake in insulin-sensitive cells (skeletal and adipose tissue). In the absence of effective insulin, lipids and proteins are metabolized to produce glucose, and ketones (ketoacids) are generated as a byproduct.

Insulin secretion or action is opposed by counterregulatory hormones (glucagon, glucocorticoids, catecholamines, growth hormone) and cytokines, which are typically released under stress (trauma, surgery, sepsis) and lead to stress-induced hyperglycemia. Hyperglycemia (defined as >180 mg/dL) leads to osmotic diuresis and fluid and electrolyte disturbances. Diabetes is associated with micro- and macrovascular diseases, neuropathy, nephropathy, retinopathy, impaired wound healing, and deficient immunocompetence.

B. Classification

Diabetes is classified into four broad categories: type 1, type 2, gestational diabetes, and diabetes due to other causes (**Table 18.15**).[4,13] ***Type 1 diabetes*** results from an absolute lack of insulin, typically due to autoimmune destruction of the islets of Langerhans. It presents early in life and requires treatment with exogenous insulin. Patients with type 1 diabetes are also prone to diabetic ketoacidosis.

Type 2 diabetes accounts for 90% of all patients with diabetes. They are typically older and overweight and have developed a resistance to the effects of insulin. Initially, hyperglycemia causes a compensatory increase in insulin production. As the disease progresses, many patients require exogenous insulin to control hyperglycemia.

> **? Did You Know?**
>
> An oral glucose tolerance test involves the administration of 75 g anhydrous glucose dissolved in water. A 2-hour plasma glucose ≥200 mg/dL is diagnostic of diabetes.

C. Diagnosis

A fasting blood glucose of <100 mg/dL is considered normal, while a fasting glucose of ≥126 mg/dL on two occasions confirms the diagnosis of diabetes (**Table 18.15**).[12,13] Patients with fasting glucose levels between 101 and 125 mg/dL are considered ***prediabetic***. An abnormal glucose tolerance test or severe hyperglycemia (>200 mg/dL) in the presence of symptoms of hyperglycemia also fulfills the criteria for diabetes, as does a hemoglobin A1c level of ≥6.5%.[4,12]

D. Treatment

Type 1 diabetics require ***insulin*** treatment. This typically involves a regimen of intermediate- or long-acting insulin plus short-acting insulin with meals titrated to blood glucose level. Alternatively, patients may be managed with an indwelling insulin pump. Insulin pumps are programmed to release a basal amount of insulin continuously and boluses with meals.

Type 2 diabetics are typically started on a regimen that involves diet management, weight control, exercise, and metformin. Metformin is a biguanide

Table 18.15 Diabetes Mellitus Classification and Diagnosis

Classification
Type 1 (Insulin Dependent)
Childhood onset
Thin
Prone to ketoacidosis
Always requires exogenous insulin
Type 2 (Noninsulin Dependent)
Maturity onset
Obese
Not prone to ketoacidosis
May be controlled by diet or oral hypoglycemic drugs
Gestational Diabetes
May presage future type 2 diabetes mellitus
Diabetes From Other Causes
Pancreatic surgery
Chronic pancreatitis
Endocrine diseases (pheochromocytoma, acromegaly, Cushing disease, exogenous steroids)
Treatment of HIV/AIDS
Diagnosis
Hemoglobin A1c ≥6.5%
Fasting plasma glucose ≥126 mg/dL (7.0 mmol/L)
2-Hour plasma glucose ≥200 mg/dL (11.1 mmol/L) during a 75 g OGTT
Random plasma glucose ≥200 mg/dL (11.1 mmol/L) in a patient with symptoms of hyperglycemia

OGTT, oral glucose tolerance test.

Derived from Endocrine function. In: Barash PG, Cullen BF, Stoelting RK, et al, eds. *Handbook of Clinical Anesthesia*. 7th ed. Wolters Kluwer/Lippincott Williams & Wilkins; 2013.

that decreases hepatic glucose production and increases the sensitivity of hepatic and peripheral tissues to insulin. Biguanides are just one class of ***oral hypoglycemics*** used in the treatment of type 2 diabetes. There are several other classes of oral hypoglycemics that increase insulin secretion (sulfonylureas); increase peripheral insulin sensitivity (glitazones); enhance or mimic the action of gastrointestinal hormones that increase insulin secretion (gliptins); decrease carbohydrate absorption from the gastrointestinal tract (alpha-glucosidase inhibitors); or enhance renal excretion of glucose (sodium-glucose transport-2 inhibitors). These may be used in combination or with exogenous insulin. The goal is a HbA1c <7%.[14] Bariatric surgery is a consideration for type 2 diabetics with a body mass index >35 kg/m^2.

E. Anesthetic Management

Diabetes is associated with micro- and macrovascular disease, neuropathy, nephropathy, retinopathy, and impaired wound healing.[2,4] Patients are particularly prone to coronary artery disease, cerebrovascular disease, and peripheral vascular disease. They have a higher incidence of perioperative major adverse cardiovascular events. Management of an oral hypoglycemic

Table 18.16 Diabetes Mellitus Preoperative Evaluation

History and physical examination (detect symptoms of cerebrovascular disease, coronary artery disease, peripheral neuropathy)
Laboratory tests (electrocardiography; blood glucose, creatinine, and potassium levels; urinalysis [glucose, ketones, albumin])
Evidence of stiff joint syndrome (may signal difficult intubation)
Evidence of cardiac autonomic nervous system neuropathy (resting tachycardia, orthostatic hypotension)
Evidence of vagal autonomic nervous system neuropathy (gastroparesis slows emptying of solids but probably not clear fluids)
Autonomic neuropathy predisposes the patient to intraoperative hypothermia

Derived from Endocrine function. In: Barash PG, Cullen BF, Stoelting RK, et al, eds. *Handbook of Clinical Anesthesia.* 7th ed. Wolters Kluwer/Lippincott Williams & Wilkins; 2013.

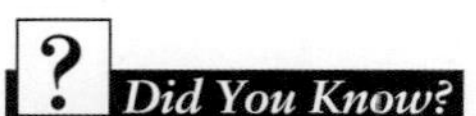

Type 1 diabetics require exogenous insulin during surgery to prevent ketoacidosis. A basal insulin infusion (0.5-2 units/h) in combination with a slow glucose infusion (5% dextrose in water at 75-125 mL/h) is commonly employed.

and insulin regimen is of particular concern in the perioperative period, as nil per os status significantly impacts exogenous glucose consumption (**Table 18.16**). Oral hypoglycemics are typically not administered on the day of surgery and withheld until the patient resumes eating. The insulin regimen has to be modified in the perioperative period. Patients who take both morning and evening doses of insulin should take their usual evening dose of short-acting insulin, but reduce their intermediate- or long acting insulin dose by 20%, the night before surgery. On the morning of surgery, they should omit their morning dose of short-acting insulin and reduce intermediate- or long acting insulin dose by 50% (as long as glucose is greater than 120 mg/dL).

Initially, tight intraoperative glucose control was advocated by some experts. However, subsequent studies demonstrated no significant benefit of tight glucose control (80-110 mg/dL) when compared with modest control (140-180 mg/dL). Owing to an increased risk of hypoglycemia obscured by the effects of anesthesia, tight glucose control is no longer advocated. Frequent glucose monitoring is recommended to prevent inadvertent hypoglycemia (**Table 18.17**).

F. Diabetic Emergencies

Severe hypoglycemia (blood glucose <60 mg/dL) requires a rapid response.[4,12] Anesthetic drugs and adjuvants (eg, beta-blockers) can obscure the signs of a hypoglycemic reaction (**Table 18.17**).

Two other life-threatening emergencies are encountered in diabetic patients. Lack of insulin leads to poor utilization of glucose by insulin-dependent tissues, and the body responds by generating alternative sources of energy. Breakdown of lipids leads to the formation and accumulation of ketoacids, which causes severe metabolic acidosis in the setting of hyperglycemia. This condition is called ***diabetic ketoacidosis (DKA)*** and it is a metabolic emergency. It carries a significant mortality if not recognized and treated promptly. Management consists of brisk fluid administration and exogenous insulin therapy.

Severe hyperglycemia (>600 mg/dL) ***without*** ketoacidosis can also occur (***hyperglycemic hyperosmolar state*** or ***hyperglycemic nonketotic coma***). This condition typically presents in older type 2 diabetics who produce enough

Table 18.17 Treatment of Diabetic Emergencies

Hypoglycemia
Treatment: Moderate to severe hypoglycemia: Dextrose 25 g IV (1 amp $D_{50}W$) followed by D_5W or $D_{10}W$. Continue to monitor and treat blood glucose until >100 mg/dL. If no IV, glucagon 1 mg intramuscular.
Nonketotic Hyperosmolar Coma
Treatment: Significant fluid and electrolyte replacement, insulin therapy after 1-2 L of fluid replacement. Monitor for hemodynamic instability. Mental status improves slowly. (regular insulin).
Diabetic Ketoacidosis
Treatment: 10 U IV of regular insulin followed by a continuous IV infusion (insulin in U/h = blood glucose/150) IV fluids (isotonic) as guided by vital signs and urine output (anticipate a 4- to 10-L deficit) 10-40 mEq/h IV of potassium chloride when urine output exceeds 0.5 mL/kg/h Glucose 5% 100 mL/h when serum glucose concentration decreases to <250 mg/dL Consider IV sodium bicarbonate to correct pH below 6.9

IV, intravenous.

Derived from Endocrine function. In: Barash PG, Cullen BF, Stoelting RK, et al, eds. *Handbook of Clinical Anesthesia*. 7th ed. Wolters Kluwer/Lippincott Williams & Wilkins; 2013.

insulin to blunt fat breakdown and the formation of ketones. The body requires only one-tenth the amount of insulin to prevent lipolysis and ketone production as it does to stimulate glucose utilization. Although metabolic acidosis due to ketoacids does not occur, osmotic diuresis, fluid and electrolyte disturbances, and severe hyperosmolarity lead to altered mental status leading to coma. Treatment involves hydration followed by insulin therapy.

Diabetic ketoacidosis and hyperosmotic hyperglycemic state should be treated prior to elective surgery. Anesthetic implications of diabetic emergencies are detailed in **Table 18.17.**

VII. Endocrine Response to Surgery

Trauma, surgery, and psychological stress elicit a generalized activation of the neuroendocrine system.[4,13] Plasma levels of catecholamines, vasopressin, cortisol, and glucagon increase significantly. This leads to hypertension, tachycardia, fluid retention, and stress-induced hyperglycemia. Protein breakdown is significant after surgery and trauma. Concurrently, endogenous endorphins are released to counteract the stress response. Endorphins act at opioid receptors in the brain and spinal cord and modulate the body's response to pain. General anesthesia and regional anesthesia can blunt this stress response to a variable extent. Insulin resistance is seen for up 14 days following major surgery; therefore, diabetic patients may temporarily require higher doses of insulin compared to their preoperative regimens. Excellent pain control can also assist in blunting some aspects of the stress response.

For further review, please see the associated Interactive Video Lectures accessible in complimentary eBook bundled with this text. Access instructions are located on the inside front cover.

References

1. Barret KE, Boitano S, Barman SM, et al. *Basic concepts of endocrine regulation*. In: *Ganong's Review of Medical Physiology*. 24th ed. McGraw-Hill; 2012:299-306.
2. Russell TW. Endocrine disease. In: Hines RL, Marschall KE, eds. *Stoelting's Anesthesia and Co-existing Disease*. 6th ed. Elsevier; 2012:376-406.
3. Robertson GL. Disorders of neurohypophysis. In: Jameson JL, Fauci AS, Kasper DL, et al, eds. *Harrison's Principles of Internal Medicine*. 20th ed. McGraw-Hill; 2018:2684-2692.
4. Schwartz JJ, Akhtar S, Rosenbaum SH. Endocrine function. In: Barash PG, Cahalan MK, Cullen BF, et al, eds. *Clinical Anesthesia*. 8th ed. Wolters Kluwer; 2018:1327-1356.
5. Felner EI, Umpierrez GE. *Endocrine Pathophysiology*. Wolters Kluwer Health/ Lippincott Williams & Wilkins; 2014:480.
6. Molina PE. *Adrenal gland*. In: *Endocrine Physiology*. 4th ed. McGraw-Hill; 2013:49-72.
7. White BA, Portfield SP. *The adrenal gland*. In: *Endocrine and Reproductive Physiology*. 4th ed. Elsevier; 2013:147-176.
8. Coursin DE, Wood KE. Corticosteroid supplementation for adrenal insufficiency. *J Am Med Assoc*. 2002;287:236-240. PMID: 11779267.
9. Liu MM, Reidy AB, Saatee S, Collard CD. Perioperative steroid management: approaches based on current evidence. *Anesthesiology*. 2017;127:166-172. doi:10.1097/ ALN.0000000000001659
10. Deegnan RJ, Furman WR. Cardiovascular manifestations of endocrine dysfunction. *J Cardiothorac Vasc Anesth*. 2011;25:705-720. PMID: 21330154.
11. Akhtar S. Anesthesia for the adult with pheochromocytoma. *UpToDate, Inc*. Updated May 07, 2020.
12. Umpierrez G, Korytkowski M. Diabetic emergencies—ketoacidosis, hyperglycaemic hyperosmolar state and hypoglycaemia. *Nat Rev Endocrinol*. 2016;12:222-232.
13. Akhtar S, Barash PG, Inzucchi SE. Perioperative hyperglycemia: scientific principles, clinical applications. *Anes Analg*. 2010;110:478-497. PMID: 28121636.
14. Powers AC, D'Alessio D. Endocrine pancreas and pharmacotherapy of diabetes mellitus and hypoglycemia. In: Brunton LL, Hilal-Dandan R, Knollmann BC, eds. *Goodman and Gilman's the Pharmacological Basis of Therapeutics*. 13th ed. McGraw-Hill; 2018:863-886.

Questions

1. **A side effect of lithium therapy is the development of:**

   A. Central diabetes insipidus.
   B. Nephrogenic diabetes insipidus.
   C. Type 1 diabetes mellitus.
   D. Type 2 diabetes mellitus.

2. **Which of the following correctly summaries the action of aldosterone in the kidney?**

   A. Promotes sodium absorption and potassium excretion
   B. Promotes sodium excretion and potassium absorption
   C. Promotes sodium and potassium excretion
   D. Promotes sodium and potassium absorption

3. **An inability to abduct the vocal cord is most often associated with injury to what nerve?**

   A. Vagus nerve
   B. Hypoglossal nerve
   C. Recurrent laryngeal nerve
   D. Phrenic nerve

4. **Most pheochromocytomas predominantly secrete:**

   A. Dopamine.
   B. Epinephrine.
   C. Norepinephrine.
   D. Normetanephrine.

5. **Manifestations of an Addisonian crisis include all of the following EXCEPT:**

   A. Hypertension.
   B. Hypotension.
   C. Hypokalemia.
   D. Hyponatremia.

Answers

1. B

Chronic lithium use can lead to the kidneys becoming resistant to ADH, producing nephrogenic diabetes insipidus. Central diabetes mellitus results from a deficiency of ADH, usually caused by central tumors or head injury. Type 1 diabetes mellitus results from absence of insulin, which is usually inherited. Type 2 diabetes mellitus usually occurs in adulthood and is associated with obesity.

2. A

Aldosterone acts in the distal renal tubule, promoting the absorption of sodium in exchange for the excretion of potassium and hydrogen.

3. C

The recurrent laryngeal nerve is responsible for abduction of the vocal cord. Unilateral injury may produce vocal hoarseness, while bilateral injury can cause aphonia and difficulty breathing. The vagus nerve has sensory and motor functions in the pharynx and larynx. It also stimulates parasympathetic activity in the heart, leading to bradycardia. The hypoglossal nerve innervates muscles of the tongue. The phrenic nerve innervates the diaphragm.

4. C

Pheochromocytomas predominantly release norepinephrine; dopamine and epinephrine may be secreted in lesser quantities. Normetaphrine is a catecholamine metabolite. Elevated levels of normetanephrine, as well as other metabolites such as vanillylmandelic acid, are diagnostic of a pheochromocytoma.

5. A

An Addisonian crisis is the result of corticosteroid and mineralocorticoid deficiency. Signs include hypokalemia, hyponatremia, and severe hypotension, which may lead to circulatory collapse. Hypertension is associated with states of mineralocorticoid excess such as pheochromocytoma.

19 General Anesthesia

Mark C. Norris and Nicholas Flores-Conner

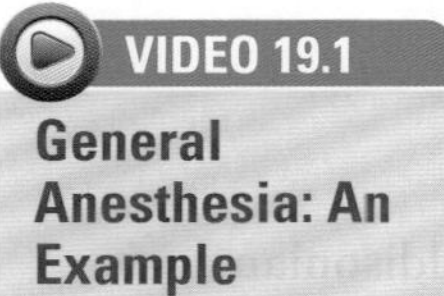

The operating room is a complex environment full of bright lights, sharp instruments, and elaborate equipment, with people speaking a strange language (**Table 19.1**). Modern surgery can remove, repair, or even replace almost every body part. Anesthesia makes these interventions possible, but anesthesia itself can be complicated and overwhelming. This chapter follows a "typical" patient through the planning and conducting of a general anesthetic, highlighting many of the decisions involved. This chapter's purpose is to demystify anesthetic care and provide a basic understanding of the steps involved in planning and conducting a safe procedure.

I. Purpose/Goals of an Anesthetic

A. What Is Anesthesia?

General anesthesia is a process whereby the patient is rendered unconscious and immobile in a reversible, controlled manner. Anesthetics induce unconsciousness by binding to specific receptors throughout the brain, brainstem, and spinal cord. Emerging evidence suggests that anesthetics interrupt the neural networks that underlie consciousness. General anesthetics also produce ***immobility***. Although anesthetics most likely make patients unconscious by acting on the brain, immobility appears to result from effects on the brainstem.

> **? Did You Know?**
>
> Anesthetics most likely produce unconsciousness by acting on the brain. However, immobility appears to result from their effects on the brainstem.

Some operations require skeletal muscle relaxation. Complete muscle paralysis can produce immobility in response to surgical stimulation, although paralysis without unconsciousness can lead to awareness with recall, an uncommon but potentially horrifying complication. In addition, muscle relaxation provides optimal conditions for endotracheal intubation and improves surgical exposure during intra-abdominal and intrathoracic procedures. Although a patient may not move, the body can mount a robust ***sympathetic response*** to surgical stimulation with hypertension, tachycardia, and tachypnea. The last element of general anesthesia aims at controlling these changes. Some drugs provide all of the elements of anesthesia, while others have more specific roles. **Table 19.2** shows the actions of some commonly used anesthetic drugs.

B. Who Gives Anesthesia?

There are a variety of medical professionals who will be encountered on an anesthesia rotation (**Table 19.3**). These people are known as ***qualified anesthesia care providers***. They have different backgrounds and training and may work alone or as part of an anesthesia care team.

C. What Are the Risks of Anesthesia?

Most anesthesia consent forms include a list of possible complications. Some of these, such as sore throat and postoperative nausea or vomiting, are common but transient. Others, such as dental damage or corneal abrasion, are

Table 19.1 Common Anesthesia-Related Terms and Acronyms

Term/Acronym	Definition
MAC	Minimum alveolar concentration: The concentration of inhaled anesthetic that will keep half the patients immobile in response to surgical stimulation. Ninety-five percent of patients will be immobilized at 1.3 MAC.
MAC	Monitored anesthesia care: Monitoring plus varying amounts of sedation
TIVA	Total intravenous anesthesia
GA	General anesthesia
Reversal	A combination of anticholinesterase and anticholinergic drugs used to terminate the effect of certain paralytic drugs
LMA	Laryngeal mask airway
ET tube	Endotracheal tube
TOF	Train-of-four: a measurement of the degree of neuromuscular blockade
PACU	Postanesthesia care unit (or recovery room)

less common but self-limited or repairable. A few, including awareness, brain damage, or death, are rare but catastrophic. About 1 in 10,000 patients will have awareness during anesthesia. Patients with a previous episode of ***awareness*** with recall are at increased risk of this complication after a subsequent anesthetic.[1] Death solely due to anesthesia is very rare, occurring in approximately 1 in 250,000 healthy patients but rising to 1 in 10,000 to 15,000 in patients with comorbidities.[2]

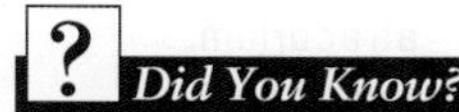
Did You Know?

Awareness during anesthesia is rare, occurring in about 1 in 10,000 cases.

II. Preoperative Evaluation

A. Patient Assessment

Surgery stresses the body, and anesthetics have significant physiologic effects. Therefore, before giving any anesthetic, the anesthesiologist evaluates the patient, looking for problems that might increase risk. This assessment requires knowledge of the patient's past and current medical and surgical conditions. The preoperative evaluation may be completed in person by the anesthesiologist, by a nurse in a preoperative clinic or via a phone interview, or by the patient via a web-based questionnaire. In many centers, healthy patients presenting for outpatient surgery and any patient needing emergency surgery may be evaluated on the day of the operation.

The preanesthetic evaluation begins with the chief complaint: In this case, what surgery is needed and why. Although this information should be available in the medical record, confirming the site and side of surgery directly with the patient is an important safeguard against wrong-site, wrong-side surgery. Next the patient's age, height, and weight are reviewed. Extremes in any of these values can present unique concerns (see Chapters 28 and 33). Reviewing the patient's surgical history can alert the anesthesiologist to significant medical problems. Questions about previous anesthetics can help prepare for a

Table 19.2 Actions of Commonly Used Anesthetic Drugs

Drug	Amnesia/ Unconsciousness	Immobility	Muscle Relaxation	Suppression of Sympathetic Reflexes
Potent inhaled agents (isoflurane, sevoflurane, desflurane)	+++	+++	+ (Dose-dependent muscle relaxation. Unacceptably low blood pressure can accompany profound relaxation.)	+ (Dose-dependent. Isoflurane and desflurane can initially produce tachycardia.)
Nitrous oxide	± (Not potent enough to produce anesthesia but can supplement the potent agents.)	±	–	+
Intravenous anesthetics (propofol, barbiturates, benzodiazepines, ketamine)	+++	+++	–	± (Some efficacy at higher doses.)
Paralytics (succinylcholine, atracurium, rocuronium, vecuronium)	–	–	+++	–
Opioids (fentanyl, remifentanil, hydromorphone, etc)	– (Do not produce unconsciousness or immobility but potentiate the effects of inhaled and intravenous anesthetics.)	–	– (Fentanyl and remifentanil can cause chest wall rigidity.)	++ (Longer acting opioids can also provide postoperative analgesia.)
Sympatholytic drugs (labetalol, esmolol, metoprolol)	–	–	–	++ (No analgesic effects, but can blunt the hemodynamic response to surgical stimulation.)

+, weak effect; ++, moderate effect; +++, strong effect; –, no effect.

difficult airway, postoperative nausea and vomiting, and other possible complications. Even if a patient has never had anesthesia, the family history might reveal malignant hyperthermia, pseudo-cholinesterase deficiency, or other heritable problems. The anesthesiologist also checks the patient's medications and allergies and asks targeted questions about the patient's medical problems and systems review.

On the day of surgery, the anesthesiologist reviews the patient's history and conducts a focused physical examination with emphasis on the heart, lungs,

Table 19.3 Who's Who in the Operating Room

Qualified Anesthesia Providers	Training	Role	Professional Organization
Anesthesiologist (MD/DO)	Bachelor's degree + medical school + 1-y internship + 3-y residency ± 1- or 2-y fellowship	Can personally provide anesthesia care or "medically direct" up to four qualified anesthesia providers or two trainees	American Society of Anesthesiologists (www.asahq.org)
Nurse anesthetist (CRNA)	Bachelor's degree in nursing (BSN), at least 1-y critical care nursing experience + 2- or 3-y nurse anesthesia program	Depending on the state, may personally provide anesthesia care, may be supervised by a physician (ie, a surgeon), or may be medically directed by an anesthesiologist as a member of the anesthesia care team	American Association of Nurse Anesthetists (www.aana.com)
Anesthesiologist assistant (AA)	Bachelor's degree + 2- or 3-y master's of medical science program	AAs only work under the medical direction of an anesthesiologist as a member of the anesthesia care team	American Academy of Anesthesiologist Assistants (www.anesthetist.org)

airway and, if regional anesthesia is planned, the site of the regional anesthetic. Most patients need only this focused history and physical examination before undergoing anesthesia. Some, because of coexisting diseases, and others, because of the proposed surgery, will need additional evaluation.

B. Anesthetic Plan

Anesthesia is often viewed as "putting the patients to sleep." However, there are multiple ways to provide an anesthetic. Choosing the best approach requires an understanding of each patient, his or her medical history, and the proposed procedure. Ideally, an anesthetic should produce the minimum physiologic trespass, optimal surgical conditions, and a comfortable and expeditious recovery.

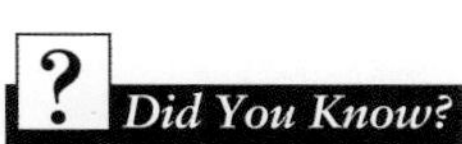

The duration of required fasting (NPO) before an anesthetic depends on the type of food or liquid ingested. For clear liquids, it is as short as 2 hours, but for fatty foods, it is at least 8 hours.

C. Nil Per Os Status

General anesthesia and sedation place patients at risk for regurgitation and aspiration of gastric contents. This complication can produce problems ranging from mild *chemical pneumonitis* and pneumonia to death (see Chapter 40). To minimize this risk, a patient should fast before an elective anesthetic.

Table 19.4 Duration of Preoperative Fasting

Duration of Fasting	Type of Food or Fluid
≥2 h	Clear liquids
≥4 h	Breast milk
≥6 h	Infant formula Light meal Nonhuman milk
≥8 h	Fried or fatty food

From Practice guidelines for preoperative fasting and the use of pharmacologic agents to reduce the risk of pulmonary aspiration: Application to healthy patients undergoing elective procedures. An updated report by the American Society of Anesthesiologists Committee on Standards and Practice Parameters. *Anesthesiology.* 2011;114:495-511, with permission.

The duration of fasting (nil per os [NPO]) depends on the type of food or liquid ingested (**Table 19.4**). Despite these NPO guidelines, patients may take oral medications with a sip of water on the day of surgery (see Chapter 16).

There are exceptions to these rules. Emergency surgeries must begin regardless of the duration of fasting. Trauma patients, those in severe pain, and those with nausea and vomiting or intestinal obstruction may have full stomachs regardless of how long they have been NPO. For these patients, the anesthesiologist may choose a ***rapid sequence*** induction to quickly secure the airway and minimize the risk of aspiration. Also, due to the physiologic changes of pregnancy, parturients are treated as having a full stomach regardless of their last food or liquid intake (see Chapter 31).

D. Informed Consent

The last step in the preoperative evaluation is obtaining informed consent, which should be targeted to the patient's specific risks and concerns. Disclose pertinent risks and allow the patient to ask questions. In some cases (ie, minors), a legal guardian or medical proxy will give consent. Regardless, it is important for the patient to understand and agree with the anesthetic plan. Rarely, in a life-threatening emergency, anesthesia and surgery may proceed without informed consent.

E. Premedication

Many patients are anxious when they are getting ready to have surgery. A thorough preoperative consultation with an anesthesiologist is the best way to relieve a patient's anxiety.[3] In addition, patients sometimes receive a small dose of intravenous benzodiazepine (ie, midazolam) for additional anxiolysis before entering the operating room. Midazolam should be used carefully. Oversedated patients may not cooperate with moving and positioning in the operating room. In outpatient settings, even small doses of midazolam can delay discharge. The elderly are especially sensitive to its sedating effects.

III. Intraoperative Management

Although complications can occur at any time during an anesthetic, ***induction*** and ***emergence*** are especially fraught. During induction, the anesthesiologist administers drugs that render the patient unconscious and have significant cardiac and respiratory effects. Anesthetics can lower the patient's blood pressure by dilating arteries and (mostly) veins, depressing cardiac function, or both. Unconscious patients have diminished upper airway muscle tone, which can obstruct breathing. Many anesthetics act at the brainstem to decrease respiratory drive. Paralytic agents directly affect respiratory muscles. The anesthesiologist gauges and mitigates these effects with careful monitoring and appropriate interventions.

A. Monitoring

Because most anesthetics depress cardiorespiratory function and surgery can increase heart rate and blood pressure, anesthesiologists use both noninvasive and invasive methods to monitor the patient. The most important of these monitors are looking at the patient to help assess oxygenation and perfusion; listening to breath sounds to detect airway problems, bronchospasm, and pulmonary edema; and touching the patient's skin for clues about perfusion and body temperature.

Routine noninvasive monitors include electrocardiogram, blood pressure, pulse oximetry, capnography, and temperature. The electrocardiogram provides information about cardiac rate and rhythm and may detect myocardial ischemia. Blood pressure can vary depending on the depth of anesthesia, the degree of surgical stimulation, and the patient's volume status. Pulse oximetry provides critical information about the adequacy of oxygenation and detects the presence of pulsatile blood flow. Capnometry and capnography detect the presence and adequacy of ventilation. Lastly, changes in body temperature occur routinely during anesthesia, and hypo- and hyperthermia are possible (**Figure 19.1**).

When paralytic agents are used during an anesthetic, neuromuscular function should be evaluated with a ***twitch monitor***. This device consists of a pair of electrodes placed over a motor nerve (usually the ulnar or facial nerve). The electrodes are connected to a device that delivers a reproducible electrical stimulus. The most commonly used stimulus pattern is called a train-of-four (TOF), consisting of four equal pulses delivered at half-second intervals. In patients with normal neuromuscular function, these four pulses will elicit four equal muscular twitches. Stimulating the ulnar nerve will trigger finger flexion and thumb adduction. If the electrodes are on the facial nerve, the orbicularis oculi muscle causes the patient to wink. During onset of muscle paralysis, all four twitches will decrease at the same time and may completely disappear. As the effects of the nondepolarizing muscle relaxant begin to wane, the twitches reappear in a different pattern. Initially, only the first twitch appears. As neuromuscular function recovers further, the other twitches reappear. However, the first twitch (T1) is stronger than the subsequent twitches. The ratio of the fourth twitch (T4) to T1 is a measure of neuromuscular function. When T4:T1 is ≥0.9, the patient should be able to breathe normally and have intact upper airway reflexes (see Chapter 11). Incomplete recovery of neuromuscular function happens in approximately 30% of young and 60% of elderly individuals and is associated with hypoxemia, airway obstruction, and an increased risk of postoperative pulmonary complications.[4,5]

Some operations risk major blood loss. Hemodynamically unstable patients can be sensitive to the effects of anesthetic drugs. In these situations, the anesthesiologist may choose invasive methods such as intra-arterial catheters for blood pressure monitoring, central venous or pulmonary artery catheters to follow changes in blood volume and cardiac output, and transesophageal echocardiography to evaluate cardiac filling and function.

? *Did You Know?*

Using a train-of-four stimulus pattern during the onset of muscle paralysis with a nondepolarizing agent, all four twitches decrease or disappear at the same time. However, as the muscle relaxant effects wear off, the twitches reappear gradually beginning with only one twitch.

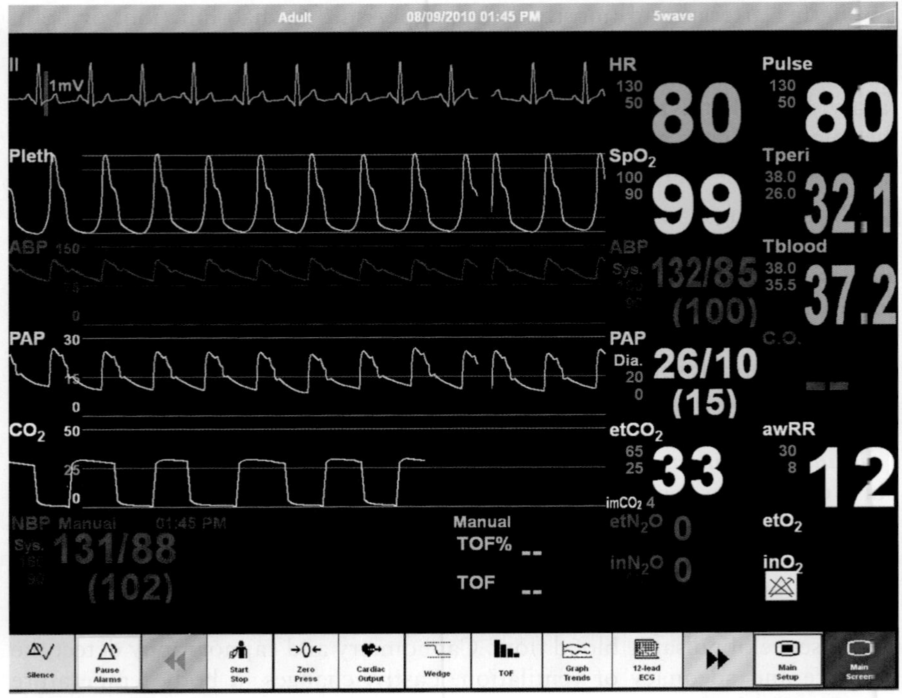

Figure 19.1 Image of an operating room monitor. From top to bottom: ECG with lead II and heart rate, pulse oximeter with plethysmograph (SpO_2), invasive blood pressure monitoring with arterial line tracing (ABP), pulmonary artery pressure with its respective tracing (PAP), end tidal CO_2 with capnograph, noninvasive blood pressure (NBP). On the far right side of the image, from top to bottom are the heart rate (Pulse) determined by the pulse oximetry, temperature (in the periphery [Tperi] and in the blood [Tblood] as determined by the pulmonary artery catheter), and respiratory rate (awRR). Other parameters can be seen in the monitor including inspired and end tidal oxygen and nitrous oxide (N_2O).

B. Time Out

Wrong-site, wrong-side, and wrong-patient surgeries still occur. A universal protocol has been developed by the Joint Commission on Accreditation of Healthcare Organizations and numerous professional organizations to help prevent these errors. Although each institution will have its own version of the ***universal protocol***, three elements remain standard. First, a preprocedure verification confirms the patient's identity, the type of surgery, and the site or side of the procedure. Second, the physician performing the surgery or procedure places a clearly visible, distinctive marking on the site of incision. Lastly, a "time out" occurs immediately before beginning the procedure to confirm that steps one and two have been performed correctly and the incision is about to occur at the correct site and side.

The World Health Organization (WHO) has developed a checklist, "the WHO Surgical Safety Checklist" (**Figure 19.2**), for use in operating rooms worldwide to increase safety and reliability. Implementation of this checklist may decrease surgical complications and deaths. Poor implementation and incomplete compliance with a surgical safety checklist may limit its benefits.[6-8] Many hospitals have expanded their universal protocol to include some iteration of this surgical safety checklist. There are two key elements that help

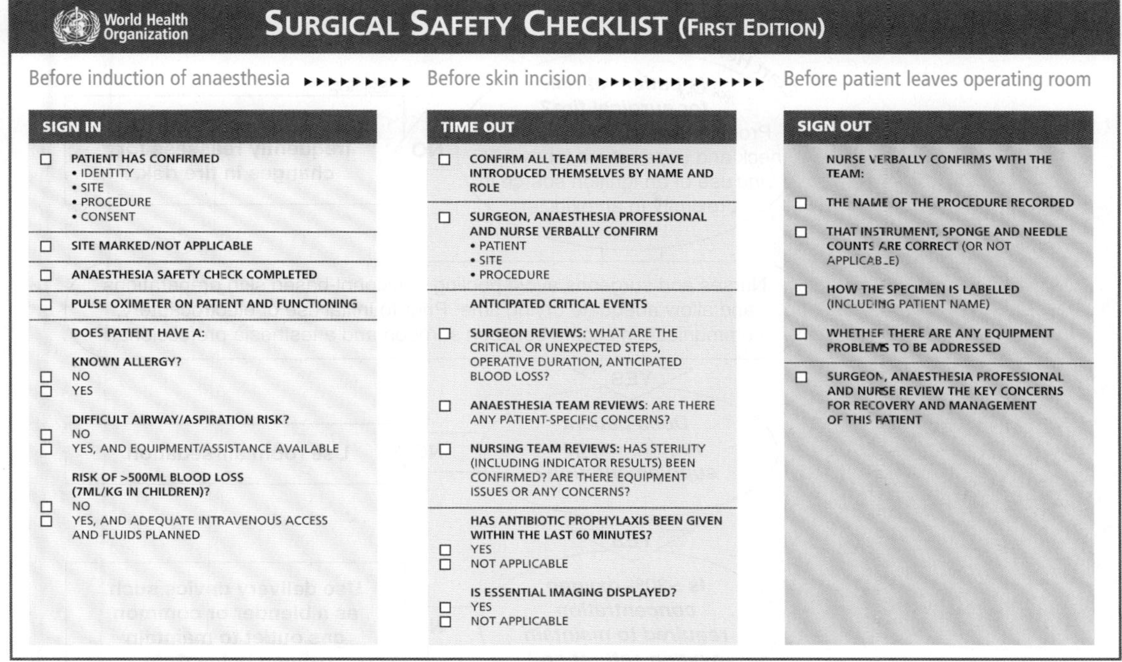

World Health Organization

SURGICAL SAFETY CHECKLIST (FIRST EDITION)

Before induction of anaesthesia ▸▸▸▸▸▸▸▸▸ Before skin incision ▸▸▸▸▸▸▸▸▸▸▸▸▸▸ Before patient leaves operating room

SIGN IN

- ☐ PATIENT HAS CONFIRMED
  - IDENTITY
  - SITE
  - PROCEDURE
  - CONSENT
- ☐ SITE MARKED/NOT APPLICABLE
- ☐ ANAESTHESIA SAFETY CHECK COMPLETED
- ☐ PULSE OXIMETER ON PATIENT AND FUNCTIONING

DOES PATIENT HAVE A:

KNOWN ALLERGY?
- ☐ NO
- ☐ YES

DIFFICULT AIRWAY/ASPIRATION RISK?
- ☐ NO
- ☐ YES, AND EQUIPMENT/ASSISTANCE AVAILABLE

RISK OF >500ML BLOOD LOSS (7ML/KG IN CHILDREN)?
- ☐ NO
- ☐ YES, AND ADEQUATE INTRAVENOUS ACCESS AND FLUIDS PLANNED

TIME OUT

- ☐ CONFIRM ALL TEAM MEMBERS HAVE INTRODUCED THEMSELVES BY NAME AND ROLE
- ☐ SURGEON, ANAESTHESIA PROFESSIONAL AND NURSE VERBALLY CONFIRM
  - PATIENT
  - SITE
  - PROCEDURE

ANTICIPATED CRITICAL EVENTS
- ☐ SURGEON REVIEWS: WHAT ARE THE CRITICAL OR UNEXPECTED STEPS, OPERATIVE DURATION, ANTICIPATED BLOOD LOSS?
- ☐ ANAESTHESIA TEAM REVIEWS: ARE THERE ANY PATIENT-SPECIFIC CONCERNS?
- ☐ NURSING TEAM REVIEWS: HAS STERILITY (INCLUDING INDICATOR RESULTS) BEEN CONFIRMED? ARE THERE EQUIPMENT ISSUES OR ANY CONCERNS?

HAS ANTIBIOTIC PROPHYLAXIS BEEN GIVEN WITHIN THE LAST 60 MINUTES?
- ☐ YES
- ☐ NOT APPLICABLE

IS ESSENTIAL IMAGING DISPLAYED?
- ☐ YES
- ☐ NOT APPLICABLE

SIGN OUT

NURSE VERBALLY CONFIRMS WITH THE TEAM:
- ☐ THE NAME OF THE PROCEDURE RECORDED
- ☐ THAT INSTRUMENT, SPONGE AND NEEDLE COUNTS ARE CORRECT (OR NOT APPLICABLE)
- ☐ HOW THE SPECIMEN IS LABELLED (INCLUDING PATIENT NAME)
- ☐ WHETHER THERE ARE ANY EQUIPMENT PROBLEMS TO BE ADDRESSED
- ☐ SURGEON, ANAESTHESIA PROFESSIONAL AND NURSE REVIEW THE KEY CONCERNS FOR RECOVERY AND MANAGEMENT OF THIS PATIENT

THIS CHECKLIST IS NOT INTENDED TO BE COMPREHENSIVE. ADDITIONS AND MODIFICATIONS TO FIT LOCAL PRACTICE ARE ENCOURAGED.

Figure 19.2 World Health Organization surgical safety checklist. (From http://www.who.int/patientsafety/safesurgery/tools_resources/SSSL_Checklist_finalJun08.pdf?ua=1. Accessed March 17, 2014.)

ensure successful use of the universal protocol and the surgical safety checklist. First, everyone in the operating room stops whatever they are doing and actively participates. Second, ***anyone*** in the room can stop the process and voice questions or concerns.

Several organizations, including the United States Food and Drug Administration, the Joint Commission and the Association of Perioperative Registered Nurses (AORN), have recently emphasized the dangers of surgical fires. A surgical fire can occur when three specific elements are present: an oxidizer (oxygen or nitrous oxide), an ignition source (electrocautery devices, lasers, and fiber-optic illumination systems), and a fuel source (surgical drapes, alcohol-based skin preparations, or the patient's tissue, hair, or skin). Including a Fire Risk Assessment (**Figure 19.3**) in the time out/universal protocol can alert the surgical team to the degree of fire risk and allow advanced preparations to prevent and treat surgical fires.

C. Induction

General anesthesia begins with induction. Babies and small children commonly undergo an inhalation induction (see Chapter 33). Here, the patient breathes increasing amounts of anesthetic through a facemask until he or she becomes unconscious. This approach avoids the need for intravenous access while the child is awake. Inhalation induction can also be used in adults. It may be chosen for patients who are needle phobic or those with poor peripheral venous access.

Because intravenous induction is rapid and reliable, it is the more common choice for older children and adults. The anesthetist usually injects a

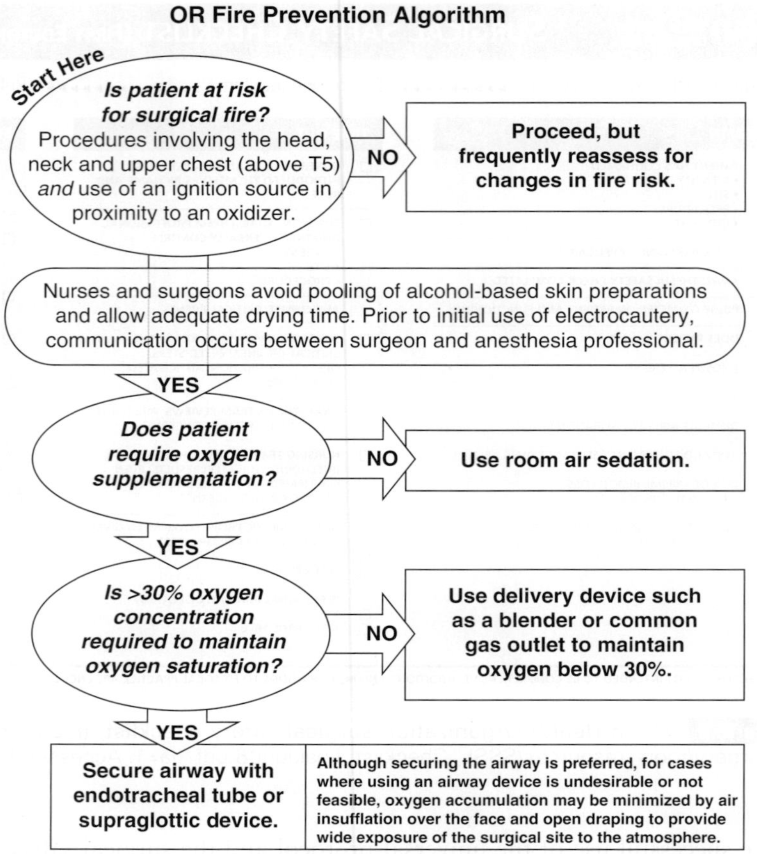

OR Fire Prevention Algorithm
Start Here
Is patient at risk for surgical fire?
Procedures involving the head, neck and upper chest (above T5) and use of an ignition source in proximity to an oxidizer.
NO
Proceed, but frequently reassess for changes in fire risk.
Nurses and surgeons avoid pooling of alcohol-based skin preparations and allow adequate drying time. Prior to initial use of electrocautery, communication occurs between surgeon and anesthesia professional.
YES
Does patient require oxygen supplementation?
NO
Use room air sedation.
YES
Is >30% oxygen concentration required to maintain oxygen saturation?
NO
Use delivery device such as a blender or common gas outlet to maintain oxygen below 30%.
YES
Secure airway with endotracheal tube or supraglottic device.
Although securing the airway is preferred, for cases where using an airway device is undesirable or not feasible, oxygen accumulation may be minimized by air insufflation over the face and open draping to provide wide exposure of the surgical site to the atmosphere.

Figure 19.3 **OR fire prevention algorithm.** (Reproduced from the Anesthesia Patient Safety Foundation Clinical Safety Tools. Copyright © 2014 Anesthesia Patient Safety Foundation.)

VIDEO 19.2
Drawing Medication From a Vial

combination of drugs chosen to quickly anesthetize the patient and provide optimal conditions for airway management and surgery. Today, propofol is the most commonly used intravenous induction agent. This drug has a rapid onset (<60 seconds). Small doses provide sedation and anxiolysis. Larger doses cause loss of consciousness. The patient will remain unconscious for 3 to 5 minutes after an induction dose of propofol. Other induction agents include methohexital, etomidate, and ketamine (**Table 19.5**).

Propofol often burns when injected and does a poor job of blunting the hemodynamic responses to painful stimuli like endotracheal intubation. Intravenous lidocaine can dull the burning and limit the blood pressure and heart rate response to laryngoscopy and intubation. Fast-acting opioids like fentanyl, sufentanil, or remifentanil also are effective at blocking the cardiovascular responses to laryngoscopy and surgery. Less commonly, ***β-adrenergic blocking drugs*** also can be used for this purpose.

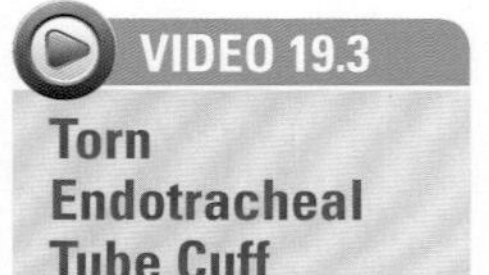

Some operations require endotracheal intubation and skeletal muscle relaxation. In commonly used doses, propofol does not induce skeletal muscle relaxation. So, after the patient loses consciousness, the anesthetist will often inject a paralytic agent (**Table 19.6**). These drugs act at the neuromuscular junction to produce muscle weakness or total paralysis.

Table 19.5 Induction Agents

Agent	Advantages	Disadvantages	Comments
Propofol	• Rapid onset • Short duration • Rapid recovery • No residual effects	• Burns on injection • Hypotension • Can cause respiratory depression, especially when given with opioids • Not an analgesic	Most commonly used induction agent
Methohexital	• Rapid onset • Short duration	• Postoperative nausea and vomiting more likely vs propofol • Contraindicated in patients with acute intermittent porphyria	Often used to induce anesthesia for electroconvulsive shock treatment
Etomidate	• Minimal hemodynamic effects	• Adrenal suppression • May increase mortality	
Ketamine	• Minimal hemodynamic depression (releases catecholamines) • Maintains respiration and airway reflexes • Has analgesic effects	• Dysphoria and hallucinations • Hypertension and tachycardia	

Table 19.6 Inhaled Anesthetics

Agent	Comment
Desflurane	Most insoluble of the potent agents. Most rapid wake up. Pungent aroma can irritate airway. Causes sympathetic stimulation during induction.
Isoflurane	Most potent and most soluble of the currently used agents. Slowest emergence, especially after longer cases. Pungent aroma. Can cause tachycardia during induction.
Nitrous oxide	Not potent enough to produce anesthesia on its own. Often used in combination with other potent agents.
Sevoflurane	Pleasant aroma. Good choice for inhalation induction. No sympathetic stimulation.

D. Airway

Anesthetics impair respiration in many ways. Sedatives like midazolam and propofol relax oropharyngeal muscles and can produce airway obstruction, especially in patients with obstructive sleep apnea. Opioids, like fentanyl, and potent inhaled agents, like sevoflurane, depress the ventilatory response to carbon dioxide. Patients who receive propofol and fentanyl often stop breathing altogether. Potent inhaled agents may also obliterate the respiratory response to hypoxemia. ***Paralytic drugs***, such as succinylcholine and rocuronium, relax oropharyngeal muscles, impair airway protective reflexes, and can paralyze respiratory muscles. For these reasons, the anesthetist must be ready to assist or control the patient's breathing.

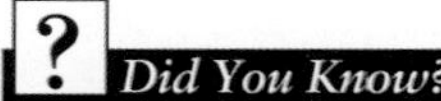

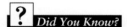

VIDEO 19.4

Nitrogen Expansion During Cryoablation

? *Did You Know?*

Preoxygenation is also referred to as denitrogenation because the administration of 100% oxygen causes the nitrogen in the lungs to be completely replaced by oxygen.

Because of these effects on the airway and respiration, patients usually breathe 100% oxygen for a few minutes before induction of anesthesia. This step, used to replace the nitrogen in a patient's lungs with oxygen, is called ***preoxygenation*** or ***denitrogenation***. This extra oxygen in the patient's lungs helps maintain oxygenation of the blood during the periods of apnea and airway obstruction that can occur during induction of anesthesia. In normal circumstances, the anesthetist will allow 3 minutes for complete denitrogenation. However, in emergencies, four tidal breaths of 100% oxygen will suffice.

If induction of anesthesia merely causes airway obstruction, chin lift and jaw thrust maneuvers may open the airway and allow spontaneous ventilation to resume. If respiration is significantly depressed or the patient is apneic, the anesthetist must begin providing artificial respirations. Initially, the facemask and breathing bag attached to the anesthesia machine are used. An oral or nasal airway may be inserted to help relieve upper airway obstruction and improve ventilation. A ***supraglottic airway*** or an endotracheal tube provides a hands-free airway and allows assisted or controlled ventilation. The most commonly used supraglottic airway is the laryngeal mask airway (LMA) (**Figure 19.4**). This device sits in the posterior pharynx and separates the larynx from the rest of the upper airway. It can be used in spontaneously breathing patients, and, in certain circumstances, to provide controlled ventilation.

? *Did You Know?*

The laryngeal mask airway was invented in 1982 by a British anesthetist named Archie Brain. The original prototype was modeled after plaster casts of the glottic area of cadavers.

Endotracheal (ET) tubes are inserted through the larynx and into the trachea (**Figure 19.5**). Most ET tubes used in adults have a cuff at their tracheal end to separate the lungs from the pharynx. This cuff allows positive pressure ventilation and can protect the lungs against aspiration of gastric contents.

? *Did You Know?*

Advantages of the LMA are that it can be inserted without using paralytic agents and that it is less stimulating than an ET tube, requiring less anesthesia before insertion.

For many surgeries, either the LMA or the ET tube can be safely used. Advantages of the LMA include the following:

- It can be inserted without using paralytic agents.
- It can be inserted blindly.
- It is unlikely to damage teeth, gums, or vocal cords.
- It is less likely than an ET tube to cause hoarseness, coughing, sore throat, or laryngospasm.
- It is less stimulating than an ET tube, so less anesthesia is required to put it in or keep it in.

The main advantage of the ET tube is that it allows higher inflation pressures during controlled ventilation.

E. The Anesthesia Record

Medical students and others with no formal training often performed early anesthetics. Complications were routine and mortality was all too common. In 1895, one such medical student was Harvey Cushing (later a well-known

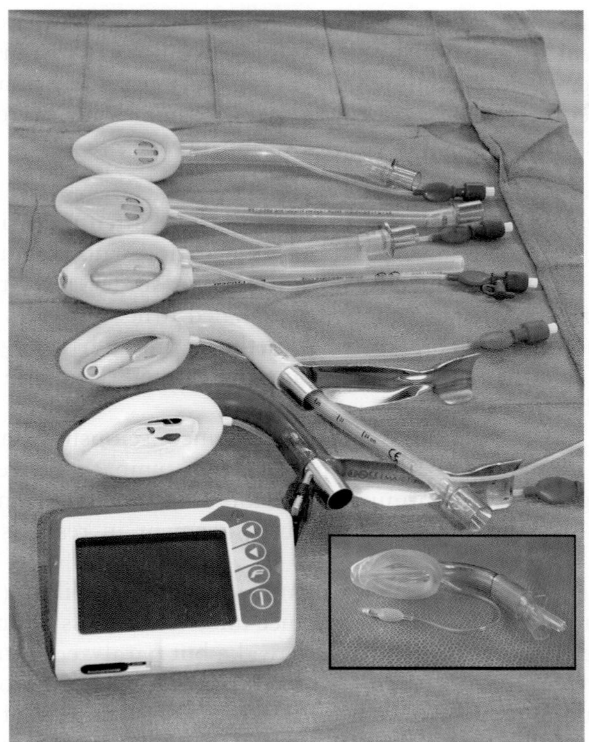

Figure 19.4 The family of laryngeal mask airways (from top): Classic, Flexible, ProSeal, Fastrach, CTrach with CTrach monitor, and Supreme (inset). (From Rosenblatt WH, Sukhupragarn W. Airway management. In: Barash PG, Cullen BF, Stoelting RK, Cahalan M, Stock MC, eds. *Clinical Anesthesia*. 6th ed. Wolters Kluwer; 2010: 751-792, Figure 29.3.)

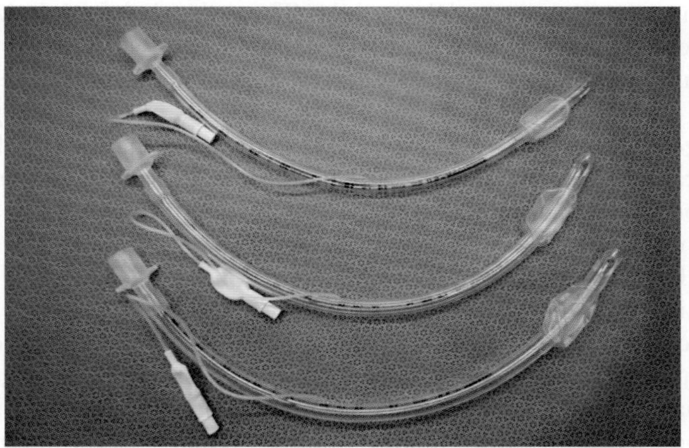

Figure 19.5 Single-lumen cuffed endotracheal tubes of different sizes. (From Torres NE, Stoltenberg A, Woodworth G. Airway equipment setup, operation, and maintenance. In: Woodworth G, Kirsch JR, Sayers-Rana S, eds. *The Anesthesia Technician and Technologist's Manual*. Wolters Kluwer; 2012:330-355, Figure 35.22.)

neurosurgeon). Cushing hoped that by keeping a record of the drugs he used and the patient's pulse and respirations, he would learn from his mistakes and administer anesthetics more safely. From Cushing's idea came the modern anesthesia record. Today's anesthesia record contains far more information but still serves much the same purpose as in Cushing's time.

F. Maintenance

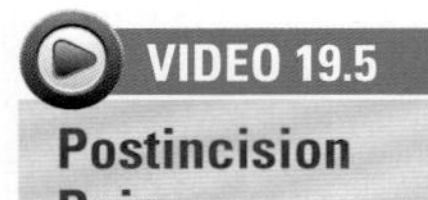

The *maintenance* phase of the anesthetic begins after induction when the airway is secured. The anesthetist may use various intravenous or inhaled agents to keep a patient unconscious throughout surgery. Most often, a balanced combination of intravenous and inhaled drugs provides the elements of general anesthesia (**Table 19.2**).[9] Sometimes, only inhaled agents are used (**Table 19.6**). In other situations, the anesthetist might only use a total intravenous anesthetic.

The goal of anesthesia is to ensure unconsciousness and amnesia, immobility, muscle relaxation, and blunted sympathetic reflexes. Both propofol, if given as a continuous infusion, and the potent inhaled agents provide amnesia and block purposeful movement in response to surgical stimulation.

Paralytic agents (muscle relaxants) produce immobility (**Table 19.7**). However, paralytic agents do not produce unconsciousness or amnesia and, if used improperly, can leave the patient awake but paralyzed. Intra-abdominal and intrathoracic surgeries often require skeletal muscle relaxation for optimal operating conditions. Muscle relaxants are useful in this situation but must be titrated carefully. If they are not enough, the surgeon may have difficulty exposing the operative site or the patient may cough or move during a delicate part of the procedure. If they are given too much, the patient may still be paralyzed at the end of the surgery. The anesthesiologist decides how much muscle relaxant to give by following the TOF. A patient with two or three of the four twitches should be adequately relaxed for most operations but not so paralyzed that the neuromuscular blocking drug cannot be reversed at the end of the surgery.

Opioids are commonly given during general anesthesia (**Table 19.8**). They decrease the dose of potent inhaled agent (or propofol) needed to keep the patient unconscious and immobile. They also help minimize the cardiac depression associated with these drugs. During induction, isoflurane and desflurane often produce tachycardia. Small intravenous doses of opioid can block this effect. Lastly, intraoperative opioids may provide ***postoperative analgesia*** but may cause respiratory depression, nausea, and vomiting. Paradoxically, intraoperative opioids can produce hyperalgesia and actually increase postoperative pain, leading to higher requirements for postoperative pain medications.[10,11]

Surgical stimulation can produce hypertension and tachycardia, even when a patient is adequately anesthetized. Because some patients may not tolerate this increased cardiac workload, the anesthetist will often try to minimize these sympathetic responses by deepening the anesthetic. Either giving more potent inhaled agent or injecting intravenous opioids should blunt the sympathetic response to surgical stimulation. In some situations, the anesthesiologist may numb the affected area with a peripheral nerve block or the surgeon may inject local anesthetic directly into the operative site. Lastly, sympathetic

Table 19.7 Muscle Relaxants

Agent	Mechanism of Action	Onset	Duration	Side Effects	Comments
Succinyl-choline	Depolarizing[a]	Rapid: 30-60 s	Short: 10-15 min Can cause prolonged blockade if given as an infusion, in repeat doses, or to patients with atypical or absent pseudocholinesterase	• Tachycardia • Bradycardia • Myalgia • Hyperkalemia • Rhabdomyolysis • Malignant hyperthermia • Increased intraocular pressure	Almost never used in children
Pancuronium	Nondepolarizing[b]	4-5 min	75-90 min	• Hypertension • Tachycardia	
Vecuronium	Nondepolarizing[b]	3 min	30-45 min		Duration may increase with repeat doses in patients with renal failure
Rocuronium	Nondepolarizing[b]	1-2 min	30-45 min		
Cisatracurium	Nondepolarizing[b]	2-3 min	45 min		Self-destructs in plasma (Hoffman elimination)

[a] Depolarizing muscle relaxants produce noncompetitive neuromuscular blockade. Their actions cannot be reversed by anticholinesterases.

[b] Nondepolarizing muscle relaxants produce competitive neuromuscular blockade. Their residual actions can be reversed by an anticholinesterase.

blocking drugs such as labetalol, esmolol, or metoprolol can blunt these hemodynamic responses and may decrease postoperative pain compared with the more commonly used opioids.[12]

G. Fluid Management

Almost all patients receiving general anesthesia will have at least one intravenous catheter inserted. This catheter is used both to give medications and to infuse fluids (see Chapter 23). Most patients need only enough fluids to keep their intravenous catheters patent. However, many surgeries cause significant bleeding. Trauma victims also may suffer considerable blood loss even before arriving in the operating room. These patients need additional intravenous fluid.

The most commonly used intravenous fluids are called ***crystalloids.*** These fluids are isotonic solutions formulated to mimic the body's electrolyte

Table 19.8 Opioids

Opioid	Onset	Duration	Comment
Remifentanil	Rapid	Brief	Rapidly hydrolyzed by nonspecific esterases. Does not accumulate even with prolonged administration.
Fentanyl	1-2 min (maximum effect within 30 min)	15-20 min	Small doses have a short duration because they are rapidly redistributed from central to peripheral tissues. Larger doses or repeat injection causes accumulation of drug in the peripheral tissues producing longer duration of analgesia.
Hydromorphone	15-30 min (maximum effect may not occur for up to 150 min)	Duration 3-5 h	

composition. Crystalloids are inexpensive and do not require special storage. Although crystalloids can be life-saving when given to a patient suffering significant bleeding, they are inefficient volume expanders. Crystalloids are isotonic, but they are hypo-osmolar. Only about one-third of infused crystalloid stays within the vascular system. The remainder leaks out of the vasculature and causes interstitial edema throughout the body.

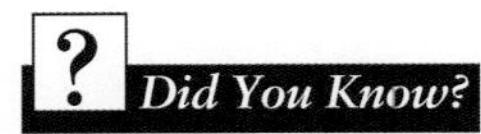

Crystalloids are isotonic, but they are also hypo-osmolar. Only about one-third of infused crystalloid stays within the vascular system with the remainder leaking into the tissues.

An alternate class of fluids, ***colloids*** contain protein (albumin) or starch to maintain osmotic pressure within the blood vessels. Colloids are better volume expanders than crystalloids, but they are expensive and have undesirable side effects (eg, platelet inhibition and possible renal toxicity). Despite years of study, colloids have never been shown to improve outcome compared with the less-expensive but less-efficient crystalloids.[13] As long as volume status is maintained, most patients can tolerate a remarkable degree of anemia. However, some will require blood and blood products (see Chapter 24).

H. Temperature

Anesthesia impairs the body's ability to maintain temperature. After induction, core temperature drops as widespread vasodilation causes core body heat to transfer to peripheral tissues. Furthering this heat transfer, anesthetics lower the temperature at which peripheral blood vessels constrict in response to cold. In addition, the operating room environment offers several avenues for heat loss: ***radiation, conduction, convection, and evaporation.*** Patients lose most heat through radiation from their exposed skin to the surrounding cold environment. Conductive heat loss occurs through contact between the patient and the cold operating room table, other equipment, and the air layer surrounding the skin. The body loses heat through convection when this warmed air circulates away from the patient and more heat transfers to the new layer of colder air. Evaporation from skin and respiratory mucosa also drains heat from the body. Together, these events cause core body temperature to decrease about 1° shortly after induction of anesthesia. Body temperature will continue to fall for the next 3 to 5 hours until a new equilibrium is established.

There are many ways to help maintain the patient's temperature. Prewarming can help prevent the initial redistribution of heat from core to periphery. Warming the operating room is another option. This step is often taken for especially vulnerable patients like small children and trauma victims. However, an operating room that is warm enough for patient comfort is often too warm for the surgical team. One of the most effective ways to maintain a patient's body temperature is with a forced-air warming blanket. These devices blow warmed air across the patient's skin, helping to prevent conductive and convective heat loss. These devices do not prevent the initial redistribution of body heat and can burn the patient's skin if misused. Radiant heat lamps can be helpful, especially when caring for infants and small children.

I. Emergence

As surgery winds down, anesthesiologists prepare the patient for emergence. They review the patient's hemodynamics and temperature, evaluate the degree of residual neuromuscular blockade, and ensure adequate analgesia for the transition to recovery. At the end of the anesthetic, the patient must be hemodynamically stable and normothermic. Hypothermia can increase oxygen consumption, impair hemostasis, and delay emergence. The unstable patient is better left intubated, ventilated, and sedated until his or her vital signs are normal.

If the patient has received a nondepolarizing muscle relaxant (**Table 19.6**), the anesthetist will use an anticholinesterase or sugammadex to reverse residual neuromuscular blockade (see Chapter 11). TOF monitoring can help determine the amount of reversal agent needed.

In addition to assessing the patient's readiness for emergence, the anesthetist begins to decrease or discontinue any intravenous or inhaled anesthetics. The timing of these changes depends on the type of drugs given and the duration of their administration. For example, remifentanil is rapidly broken down by plasma esterases. Its action terminates promptly and predictably no matter how long the anesthetic. On the other hand, isoflurane and sevoflurane are fat soluble and accumulate in the patient's adipose tissues (isoflurane more so than sevoflurane). With these drugs, the longer the anesthetic, the longer the emergence. The anesthetist uses his or her knowledge of the drug kinetics to time the end of the anesthetic.

Removing the endotracheal tube (extubation) is the trickiest part of the emergence process. Before the patient can be extubated, he or she must have reestablished adequate ventilation and respiration. In addition, the patient must have appropriate protective airway reflexes. Some patients can be extubated "deep" before protective airway reflexes have fully recovered, as long as they are ventilating adequately and the anesthetist is prepared to help maintain an open airway. Others should remain intubated until they are awake and can follow commands. Risks of extubating too soon include airway obstruction, aspiration, and ***laryngospasm***. Delaying extubation too long can cause hypertension and tachycardia, increased intracranial pressure, and bleeding, especially in patients who have undergone surgery about the head and neck. Vigorous coughing with an endotracheal tube in place can disrupt abdominal surgical sutures. Once the patient is extubated and ventilating adequately, it is time to go to the recovery room or postanesthesia care unit (PACU).

IV. Postoperative Care

Once the patient arrives in the PACU, the anesthetist must safely transfer care to the recovery room nurse. This transfer of care, or handoff, requires clear and effective communication between health care providers. Lapses in communication during patient care handoffs can lead to errors and harm. Mnemonics have been developed to try to standardize handoff communication. Two such mnemonics are I-PASS (**Table 19.9**) and ISBAR (***I***ntroduction, ***S***ituation, ***B***ackground, ***A***ssessment, and ***R***esponse). A key part of these structured communication tools is the response. The person assuming care for the patient (ie, the PACU nurse) responds to the person transferring care (ie, the anesthetist) to confirm that he or she heard and understands the relayed information. As with the "WHO Safe Surgery Checklist," using a structured handoff tool can improve patient safety.[14,15]

Table 19.9 The I-PASS Mnemonic

I	Illness severity	• Stable, "watcher," unstable
P	Patient summary	• Summary statement • Events leading to admission • Hospital course • Assessment • Plan
A	Action list	• To do list • Timeline and ownership
S	Situation awareness and contingency planning	• Know what is going on • Plan for what might happen
S	Synthesis by receiver	• Receiver summarizes what was heard • Asks questions • Restates key action items

Modified from Starmer AJ, Spector ND, Srivastava R, et al. I-PASS, a mnemonic to standardize verbal handoffs. *Pediatrics.* 2012;129:201-205.

V. Summary

Although the drugs and techniques may differ from anesthetist to anesthetist, some things remain constant with all anesthetics. The anesthesiologist and anesthetist strive to guide the patient's safe passage through the surgical experience by understanding the patient's medical and surgical history. They use their knowledge of physiology and pharmacology to plan and conduct a safe and effective anesthetic. Throughout the perioperative period, they maintain constant vigilance to ensure the patient's well-being.

For further review, please see the associated Interactive Video Lectures accessible in complimentary eBook bundled with this text. Access instructions are located on the inside front cover.

References

1. Aranake A, Gradwohl S, Ben-Abdallah A, et al. Increased risk of intraoperative awareness in patients with a history of awareness. *Anesthesiology*. 2013;119:1275-1283.
2. Botney R. Improving patient safety in anesthesia: a success story? *Int J Radiat Oncol Biol Phys*. 2008;71(1 suppl):S182-S186. doi:10.1016/j.ijrobp.2007.05.095. PMID: 18406924.
3. Egbert LD, Jackson SH. Therapeutic benefit of the anesthesiologist–patient relationship. *Anesthesiology*. 2013;119:1465-1468.
4. Murphy GS, Brull SJ. Residual neuromuscular block: lessons unlearned. Part I. Definitions, incidence, and adverse physiologic effects of residual neuromuscular block. *Anesth Analg*. 2010;111:120-128.
5. Murphy GS, Szokol JW, Avram MJ, et al. Residual neuromuscular Block in the elderly: incidence and clinical implications. *Anesthesiology*. 2015;123(6):1322-1336. doi:10.1097/ALN.0000000000000865. PMID: 26448469.
6. de Vries EN, Prins HA, Crolla RM, et al. Effect of a comprehensive surgical safety system on patient outcomes. *N Engl J Med*. 2010;363:1928-1937.
7. Haynes AB, Edmondson L, Lipsitz SR, et al. Mortality trends after a voluntary checklist-based surgical safety collaborative. *Ann Surg*. 2017;266(6):923-929. doi:10.1097/SLA.0000000000002249. PMID: 29140848.
8. Igaga EN, Sendagire C, Kizito S, et al. World health organization surgical safety checklist, compliance and associated surgical outcomes in Uganda's referral hospitals. *Anesth Analg*. 2018;127(6):1427-1433 doi:10.1213/ANE.0000000000003672. PMID: 30059396.
9. Brown EN, Pavone KJ, Naranjo M. Multimodal general anesthesia theory and practice. *Anesth Analg*. 2018;127(5):1246-1258. doi:10.1213/ANE.0000000000003668. PMID: 30252709.
10. Guignard B, Bossard AE, Coste C, et al. Acute opioid tolerance: intraoperative remifentanil increases postoperative pain and morphine requirement. *Anesthesiology*. 2000;93:409-417.
11. Fletcher D, Martinez V. Opioid-induced hyperalgesia in patients after surgery: a systematic review and a meta-analysis. *Br J Anaesth*. 2014;112(6):991-1004. PMID: 24829420.
12. Bahr MP, Williams BA. Esmolol, antinociception, and its potential opioid-sparing role in routine anesthesia care. *Reg Anesth Pain Med*. 2018;43:815-818. PMID: 30216240.
13. Hemming N, Lamothe L, Jaber S, et al. Morbidity and mortality of crystalloids compared to colloids in critically ill surgical patients: a subgroup analysis of a randomized trial. *Anesthesiology*. 2018;129:1149-1158. doi:10.1097/ALN0000000000002413. PMID: 30212412.
14. Starmer AJ, Sectish TC, Simon DW, et al. Rates of medical errors and preventable adverse events among hospitalized children following implementation of a resident handoff bundle. *J Am Med Assoc*. 2013;310:2262-2270.
15. Sheth S, McCarthy E, Kipps AK, et al. Changes in efficiency and safety culture after integration of an I-PASS–Supported handoff process. *Pediatrics*. 2016;137(2):e20150166. doi:10.1542/peds.2015-0166. PMID: 26743818.

Questions

1. **An otherwise healthy 50-year-old patient presents for elective surgery. Upon your evaluation you determine the patient had a cup of coffee with no milk or sugar approximately 3 hours ago. Considering the above information, determine the appropriateness to pursue surgery in this patient.**

   A. Postpone surgery until a later date given that the patient has not followed the NPO instructions and it presents a risk to his health.
   B. Proceed with surgery in 3 hours because the patient only had coffee, which is considered a light meal, and can safely undergo anesthesia.
   C. Postpone surgery as the patient must have 8 hours of NPO time regardless of the type of food ingested.
   D. Proceed with surgery as coffee with no milk or sugar is considered a clear liquid and should be stopped 2 hours prior to surgery.

2. **You induced your 20-year-old patient using rocuronium prior to intubation. The procedure is finished significantly faster than you anticipated and your patient has no twitches when using your twitch monitor on the ulnar nerve. After confirming appropriate placement of the electrodes and that the monitor is functioning appropriately, you proceed in the following way:**

   A. You give maximum dose of neostigmine and glycopyrrolate and remove the tube as soon as the patient has clinical signs of recovered strength.
   B. You wait until the patient has sufficient twitches before you administer neostigmine and glycopyrrolate for reversal.
   C. You transfer the patient to the postanesthesia care unit and await for the patient to regain clinical strength before you remove the tube.
   D. You call the intensive care unit and have the patient transferred there to be extubated the morning after.

3. **The patient arrives at the operating room for a right total knee arthroplasty and the anesthesiology team start their anesthetic. The patient is unconscious, immobile, and intubated. The surgeon walks into the room, cleans the skin in the left knee, and proceeds with surgery. When the patient regains consciousness in the PACU, they alert the team that the surgery was performed in the wrong side. Which of the following would have decreased the risk of this event?**

   A. Preprocedure verification of the patient's identity, type, site, and side of the procedure.
   B. Surgeon marking of the surgical site.
   C. Surgical timeout prior to the beginning of the procedure to verify that the team is in agreement for the type, site, and side of the procedure as well as the identity of the patient and the surgical marking.
   D. A, B, and C are correct.
   E. There is nothing the team or the institution could have done to prevent this event.

4. **After denitrogenation was performed, the anesthesiologist administers medications and the patient loses consciousness, becomes immobile and apneic. The anesthesiology resident proceeds with intubation, and once the endotracheal tube is inserted in the trachea, the patient's blood pressure and heart rate increase significantly. Of the medications listed below, which one has no role in blunting the sympathetic response to intubation?**

   A. Fentanyl
   B. Lidocaine
   C. Propofol
   D. Esmolol

5. **A patient presents to the operating room for an open abdominal procedure that is expected to last 8 hours. The anesthesiology team does not provide active rewarming and by the end of the surgery the patient's temperature has dropped to 35 °C. What method would have been the most appropriate to prevent heat loss in this patient?**

A. Forced-air warming blanket
B. Warmed fluid administration
C. Rewarming by going on cardiopulmonary bypass
D. Warmed saline bags applied to the patient's skin

Answers

1. D

Intake of coffee with no milk or sugar constitutes a clear liquid. The ASA recommendations noted on **Table 19.4** point to appropriate NPO time for clear liquids to be 2 hours, which allows this patient to undergo surgery safely. Answer A is incorrect given that this approach is not following the ASA recommendations and is unnecessarily postponing a procedure that could be safely performed. Answer B is incorrect as it assumes that coffee with no sugar or milk constitutes a light meal. This answer would be correct if the patient had taken milk with their coffee. Answer C is incorrect because, as we mentioned before, the time for NPO is dependent on the type of food that was ingested, and in this particular case the patient may proceed with surgery safely.

2. B

This is a common situation that occurs with overdosing of nondepolarizing neuromuscular blockers. With the advent of sugammadex, this situation can be rapidly solved by the administration of this medication. Nonetheless, some surgical centers or hospitals with limited resources will not have access to this medication, which reinforces the need to understand the appropriate use of neostigmine and glycopyrrolate as reversal agents. Answer A is incorrect because if these medications are administered prior to the patient having sufficient twitches, the patient may be able to regain clinical signs of strength but lose that strength in the PACU, where they will be less monitored and prone to have complications undiagnosed. Answer C is incorrect because it does not state that the patient would receive reversal agents. The incidence of residual neuromuscular blockade is high even in young patients and it could lead to respiratory complications. Answer D is incorrect because there are other options that are quicker, less expensive, and likely to result in the same outcome without need of incurring on additional expenses. To summarize, reversal agents should be given once the patient has sufficient twitches and full reversal confirmed after the administration of the medications.

3. D

The World Health Organization Surgical Safety Checklist is applied by the characteristics mentioned in answers A, B, and C. None of those options would have been sufficient on their own. The surgical safety checklist should be applied as an institutional policy for the best results to be achieved. Applying it in a case-by-case basis will not have the same effect and errors may continue to be made. Answer E is incorrect because the stem does not show the surgical or anesthesia team performing the appropriate surgical checklist steps and this could have led to the mistake being prevented.

4. C

Propofol has no effect in blunting the sympathetic response but can cause a patient to be sedated with lower doses and lose consciousness with higher doses. Answers A, B, and D are incorrect because all of the medications listed can blunt the sympathetic response to intubation (**Table 19.2**). Fentanyl is routinely used prior to surgical stimulation with the intention of decreasing said response. Lidocaine has the same use when given at higher doses than normally used for prevention of pain on injection from propofol. Esmolol is a selective beta-1-blocker that can be used instead of narcotics or lidocaine and can be given in a bolus or through an infusion resulting in the decrease of narcotic requirements.

5. A

The most effective method to prevent heat-loss for patients undergoing surgery is through forced air warming. This method creates a bubble of warm air around the patient and prevents this air from moving away and loosing heat to the much cooler operating room environment. Although other methods exist, this is the least invasive and safer method of doing it. Answer B is incorrect because administering warmed fluids is not proven to be sufficient or necessary. This is not the case with blood products that should be warmed up prior to administration as they are kept refrigerated prior to use and would cause a decrease in the temperature if administered without warming. Answer C is incorrect because it is unnecessarily invasive when other methods like using a forced-air warming blanket would be sufficient. Answer D is incorrect because placing warmed bags of saline in contact with the patient may warm up the patient, but it will also place the patient at risk of possible burns as the patient is unable to react to the noxious temperature stimulus while they remain under anesthesia.

20 Airway Management

Ron O. Abrons and William H. Rosenblatt

I. Airway Anatomy

? Did You Know?

The glottic opening is the narrowest portion of the airway in infants, children, and adults.

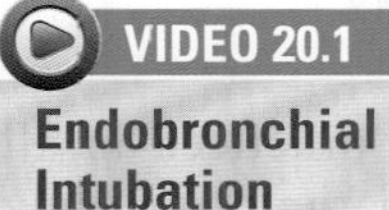

VIDEO 20.1

Endobronchial Intubation

The term ***airway*** refers to the upper airway—consisting of the nasal and oral cavities, pharynx, larynx, trachea, and principal bronchi. The laryngeal skeleton houses and protects the vocal folds, which extend in an anterior-posterior plane from the thyroid cartilage to the arytenoid cartilages. The cricothyroid membrane is an important, externally identifiable structure. In an adult, it typically is identified 1 to 1.5 fingerbreadths below the laryngeal prominence (thyroid notch) (**Figure 20.1**).

The signet ring–shaped cricoid cartilage is located at the base of the larynx, suspended by the underside of the cricothyroid ligament. Inferiorly, the trachea measures approximately 15 cm and ends at the carina where it bifurcates into the principal bronchi. Aspirated materials, as well as a deeply inserted ***endotracheal tube*** (*ETT*), tend to gain entry into the right principal bronchus due to it's less acute angle of divergence from the midline.

There are three clinically important neural innervations of the upper airway. The glossopharyngeal nerve (cranial nerve IX) supplies sensory innervation to the base of the tongue, rostral surface of the epiglottis, and pharynx. The superior laryngeal nerve (a branch of cranial nerve X, the vagus nerve) supplies sensation from the underside of the epiglottis to the surface of the vocal cords and motor innervation to the cricothyroid muscle. The recurrent laryngeal nerve, also a branch of the vagus nerve, supplies motor innervation to the remaining muscles of the larynx and sensation to the mucosal surface of the larynx and trachea (**Table 20.1**; **Figure 20.2**).

II. Patient History and Physical Examination

Airway management always begins with a thorough airway-relevant history, including a search for documentation of airway-related events during previous anesthetics. Signs and symptoms related to potentially difficult airway management, including aspiration risk, should be sought (**Table 20.2**) as many congenital and acquired syndromes are associated with difficult airway management (**Table 20.3**).

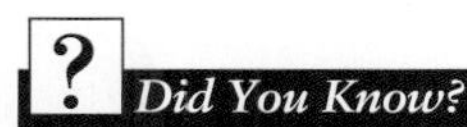

? Did You Know?

The positive predictive value of the Mallampati score in predicting a difficult laryngoscopy is only 40%.

Table 20.4 lists the commonly documented airway examination features. Historically, airway assessment (eg, Mallampati score) has been synonymous with evaluation for the ease of ***direct laryngoscopy*** (*DL*), with the endpoint being the anticipated degree of laryngeal visualization (**Figure 20.3**). Unfortunately, efforts to identify attributes that place patients at high risk for difficult laryngoscopy have been only modestly successful (**Table 20.5**).[1]

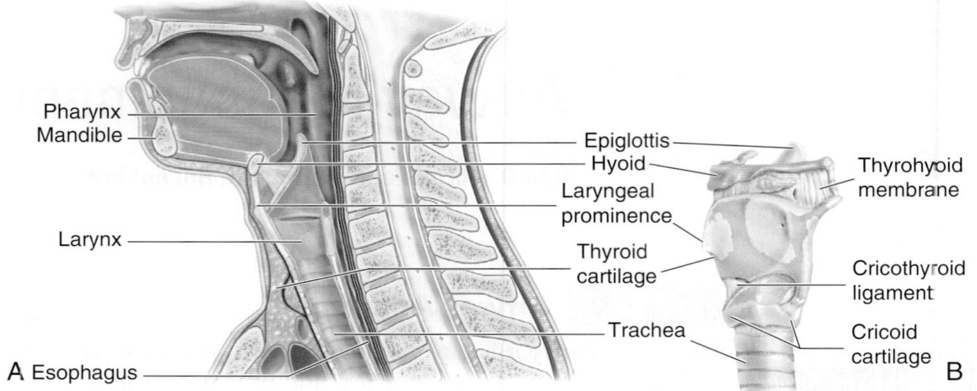

Figure 20.1 Sagittal view of upper airway anatomy (A) and lateral view of laryngeal skeleton (B). (Redrawn from Moore KL, Agur AMR, Dalley AF. *Clinically Oriented Anatomy.* 8th ed. Philadelphia, PA: Wolters Kluwer; 2018. Figure 8.83.)

III. Clinical Management of the Airway

A. Preoxygenation

Preoxygenation (also termed ***denitrogenation***) should be practiced in all cases when time allows. Under ideal conditions, a healthy patient breathing room air (fraction of inspired oxygen [FIO_2] = 0.21) will experience oxyhemoglobin desaturation to a level of <90% after approximately 1 to 2 minutes of apnea. In the same patient, several minutes of preoxygenation with 100% oxygen (O_2) via a tight-fitting facemask may support ≥8 minutes of apnea before desaturation occurs. Patients with pulmonary disease, obesity, or conditions affecting metabolism frequently evidence desaturation

Table 20.1 Innervation of the Laryngotracheal Airway

Nerve	Motor[a]	Sensory[a]
Glossopharyngeal nerve (cranial nerve IX)	None	Posterior 1/3 of tongue Epiglottis (rostral) Pharynx
Vagus nerve—recurrent laryngeal nerve (cranial nerve X)	Larynx (except cricothyroid)	Larynx: mucosal surface Trachea: mucosal surface
Vagus nerve—internal branch of the superior laryngeal nerve (cranial nerve X)	None	Epiglottis (dorsal) Vocal cords
Vagus nerve—external branch of the superior laryngeal nerve (cranial nerve X)	Cricothyroid	None

[a]Predominant action.

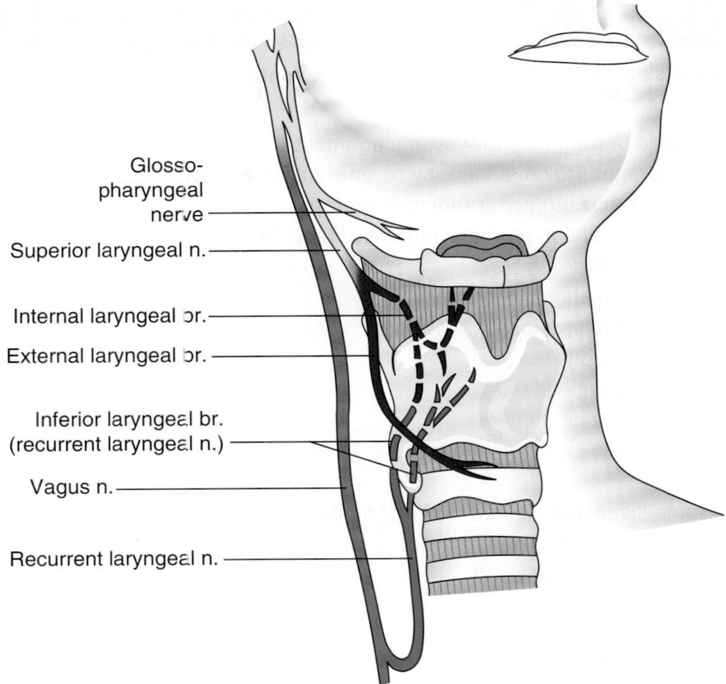

Figure 20.2 **Laryngeal innervation. The dashed lines are nerve branches within the laryngeal-tracheal tree from the branches of the glossopharyngeal and vagus cranial nerves.** (From Rosenblatt WH, Sukhupragarn W. Airway management. In: Barash PG, Cullen BF, Stoelting RK, et al, eds. *Clinical Anesthesia*. 7th ed. Lippincott Williams & Wilkins; 2013:790, Figure 27.22.)

sooner, owing to increased O_2 extraction, decreased functional residual capacity, or right-to-left transpulmonary shunting. The most common reason for suboptimal preoxygenation is a loose-fitting mask, which allows entrainment of room air.

B. Facemask Ventilation

The anesthesia facemask is gently held on the patient's face with the thumb and first finger of the left hand, leaving the right hand free for other tasks. Air leak around the edges of the mask can be prevented by gentle downward pressure. A two-handed grip or an elastic "mask strap" may be used to complement the left-hand grip.

C. Patient Positioning

Appropriate positioning of the patient is paramount for delivering ***positive pressure ventilation*** via facemask. With the patient supine, "ramped," or in reverse Trendelenburg position, the neck is flexed by 35° and the head extended by 15°. This ***sniffing position*** improves mask ventilation by anteriorizing the base of the tongue and the epiglottis.

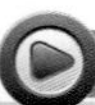
VIDEO 20.2
Vocal Cord Polyp Ball-Valve Effect

VIDEO 20.3
Temporomandibular Joint Assessment

Table 20.2 Conditions With Airway Management Implications

Increased Risk of Difficult Laryngoscopy, Mask Ventilation, or Supraglottic Airway Ventilation
History of failed or traumatic airway management
Dental damage or prolonged airway soreness after a previous anesthetic
History of head/neck surgery or radiation therapy
Various congenital and acquired syndromes (**Table 20.3**)
Supraglottic pathology
Obstructive sleep apnea
Lingual tonsillar hyperplasia
Acute airway pathology
Tongue edema (angioedema)
Airway cyst or tumor
Airway bleeding
Stridor
Cervical spine disease or limited range of motion
Temporomandibular joint disease
Increased Aspiration Risk
Recent meal
Acute trauma
Acute gastrointestinal pathology
Acute narcotic therapy
Significant gastroesophageal reflux
Current intensive care unit admission
Pregnancy (gestational age ≥12 wk)
Immediate postpartum (before second postpartum day)
Systemic disease–associated gastroparesis: diabetes mellitus, collagen vascular disease, advanced Parkinson disease

Dentures left in place may improve the mask seal for an edentulous patient. The advantage of this must be weighed against the risk of denture displacement or damage. Dentures should be removed after the airway is secured.

D. Difficult Mask Ventilation

Table 20.6 describes six independent clinical predictors for difficult mask ventilation.[2,3] Under normal conditions, no more than 20 to 25 cm water (H_2O) pressure in the anesthesia circuit (created by squeezing the reservoir bag) is needed to inflate the lungs. If more pressure is required to produce adequate lung inflation, the anesthesiologist should reevaluate the situation. This evaluation includes adjusting the mask fit, seeking aid with the mask hold, or considering adjuncts such as oral and nasal airways. Oral and nasal airways can bypass obstruction by creating an artificial passage through the pharynx and hypopharynx. Nasal airways are less likely to stimulate cough, gag, or vomiting in the lightly anesthetized patient but more likely to cause epistaxis, thus typically avoided in patients at high risk for nasal bleeding.

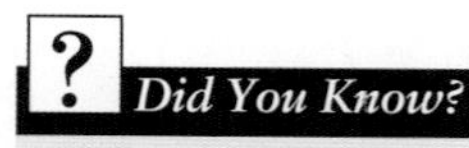
Did You Know?

The leading cause of airway obstruction during induction of anesthesia is the tongue.

Obstruction to mask ventilation may be caused by ***laryngospasm***, a local reflex closure of the vocal folds. Laryngospasm may be triggered by a foreign

Table 20.3 Syndromes Associated With Difficult Airway Management

Pathologic Condition	Features Affecting Airway Management
Congenital	
Pierre Robin sequence	Micrognathia, macroglossia, glossoptosis, cleft soft palate
Treacher Collins syndrome	Malar and mandibular hypoplasia, microstomia, choanal atresia
Down syndrome	Macroglossia, microcephaly, cervical spine abnormalities
Klippel-Feil syndrome	Congenital fusion of cervical vertebrae, decreased cervical range of motion
Cretinism	Macroglossia, compression or deviation of larynx/trachea by goiter
Cri du chat syndrome	Micrognathia, laryngomalacia, stridor
Acquired Infections	
Epiglottitis	Epiglottal edema
Croup	Laryngeal edema
Papillomatosis	Obstructive papillomas
Intraoral/retropharyngeal abscess	Airway distortion/stenosis, trismus
Ludwig angina	Airway distortion/stenosis, trismus
Arthritis	
Rheumatoid arthritis	Restricted cervical spine mobility, atlantoaxial instability
Ankylosing spondylitis	Ankylosis/immobility of cervical spine and temporomandibular joints
Tumors	
Cystic hygroma, lipoma, adenoma, goiter	Airway distortion or stenosis
Carcinoma of tongue/larynx/thyroid	Airway distortion or stenosis, fixation of larynx or adjacent tissues
Trauma	
Head/facial/cervical spine	Airway edema or hemorrhage, unstable facial or mandibular fractures, intralaryngeal damage
Miscellaneous Conditions	
Morbid obesity	Short, thick neck, large tongue, and obstructive sleep apnea are likely
Acromegaly	Macroglossia, prognathism
Acute burns	Airway edema, bronchospasm, decreased apnea tolerance

VIDEO 20.4
Bronchospasm Under Anesthesia

body (eg, oral or nasal airway), saliva, blood, or vomitus touching the glottis. It may also result from pain or visceral stimulation. Management of laryngospasm consists of removing the offending stimulus (if identified), administering oxygen with continuous positive airway pressure, deepening the plane of the anesthesia and, if other maneuvers are unsuccessful, using a rapid-acting muscle relaxant.[4]

E. Supraglottic Airways

Airway devices that isolate the airway above the vocal cords are referred to as ***supraglottic airways*** (SGAs). These devices may be advantageous in patients with reactive airway disease as they lead to reversible bronchospasm than ETTs. A wide variety of SGA devices are currently available. The original SGA, the laryngeal mask airway (LMA), is composed of a perilaryngeal mask and an airway barrel. The mask has an inflatable cuff, which fills the hypopharyngeal space, creating a seal that allows positive pressure ventilation with up to 20 cmH_2O pressure. The following description of the LMA can be applied to all commercially available SGAs, although it should be noted that the iGel does not have an inflatable cuff.

Table 20.4 Physical Examination Features With Airway Management Implications

Physical Examination Feature	Significance
Mouth opening	Difficult blade insertion/tongue displacement if limited
Jaw protrusion	Difficult tongue displacement if limited
Dentition	Obstructed view (if large central incisors), increased risk of dental trauma (if poor or restored dentition), difficult mask ventilation (if edentulous)
Retrognathia	Difficult tongue displacement
Thyromental distance	Reflects neck mobility and degree of retrognathia
Mallampati grade	Describes the relationship between mouth opening, tongue size, and pharyngeal space
Presence of beard	Difficult mask seal
Airway pathology	Potential for difficult mask ventilation (obstructive masses/tissue, atypical facial contours) and laryngoscopy (friable tissue, atypical or absent landmarks, and limited mouth opening, jaw protrusion, tongue displacement, and neck mobility)

VIDEO 20.5

Torus Mandibularis

The manufacturer recommends that the clinician choose the largest size LMA that fits comfortably within the oral cavity. For use, the LMA mask is completely deflated. The patient's neck is extended and the superior surface of the mask is placed against the hard palate. Force is applied by the index finger in an upward direction toward the top of the patient's head, and the mask is allowed to follow the palate into the pharynx and hypopharynx. Next, the LMA is inflated to the minimum pressure that allows ventilation to 20 cmH_2O without an air leak. The intracuff pressure should remain below 44 mm Hg (60 cmH_2O) and should be periodically monitored, especially if nitrous oxide is used.[5] When an adequate seal cannot be obtained with 60 cmH_2O cuff pressure, the LMA's positioning or sizing should be reevaluated. Light anesthesia and laryngospasm also may contribute to poor seal.

Positive pressure ventilation can be used safely with the LMA.[6] There is no difference in gastric inflation with positive pressure ventilation (<17 cmH_2O) when comparing the LMA and ETT.[7] With the classic LMA, tidal volumes should be limited to 8 mL/kg and airway pressure to 20 cmH_2O.

If at any time gastric contents are noted in the LMA barrel, the LMA should be left in place. The patient is placed in a Trendelenburg position, 100% oxygen is administered, and the LMA barrel is suctioned.

SGA Removal

SGAs should be removed either when the patient is deeply anesthetized or after protective reflexes have returned and the patient is able to open his or her mouth on command. Many clinicians remove the LMA fully inflated so that it acts as a "scoop" for secretions above the mask, bringing them out of the airway.

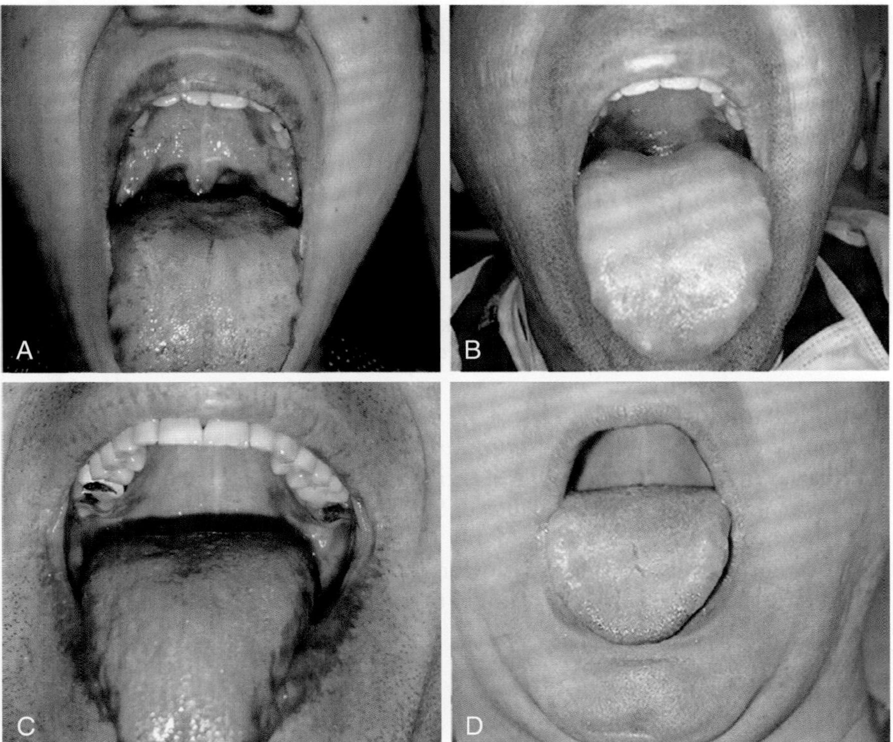

Figure 20.3 Mallampati/Samsoon-Young classification of the oropharyngeal view. A, Class I: Uvula, faucial pillars, soft palate visible. B, Class II: Faucial pillars, soft palate visible. C, Class III: Soft and hard palate visible. D, Class IV: Hard palate visible only (added by Samsoon and Young). (From Rosenblatt WH, Abrons RO, Sukhupragarn W. Airway management. In: Barash PG, Cahalan M, Cullen BF, et al, eds. *Clinical Anesthesia*. 8th ed. Wolters Kluwer; 2018:767-808, Figure 28.8.)

Table 20.5 Summary of Pooled Sensitivity and Specificity of Commonly Used Methods of Airway Evaluation

Examination	Sensitivity (%)	Specificity (%)
Mouth opening	46	89
Thyromental distance	20	94
Mallampati classification	49	86

From Shiga T, Wajima Z, Inoue T, et al. Predicting difficult intubation in apparently normal patients: a meta-analysis of bedside screening test performance. *Anesthesiology*. 2005;103:429.

Contraindications to SGA Use

The primary contraindication to elective use of an SGA is the clinical scenario where there is an increased risk of aspiration of gastric contents (**Table 20.2**). Other contraindications include airway resistance greater than the seal pressure of the device, glottic or subglottic airway obstruction, and limited mouth opening (<1.5 cm).[8]

Table 20.6 Independent Risk Factors for Difficult Mask Ventilation

Older age
Higher BMI
Full beard
Head/neck irradiation
Sleep apnea
Male gender

Data from Lundstrom LH, Rosenstock CV, Wetterslev J, Norskov AK. The DIFFMASK score for predicting difficult facemask ventilation: a cohort study of 46,804 patients. *Anaesthesia.* 2019;74:1267-1276. and Kheterpal S, Martin L, Shanks AM, Tremper KK. Prediction and outcomes of impossible mask ventilation: a review of 50,000 anesthetics. *Anesthesiology.* 2009;110(4):891-897.

Complications of SGA Use

Apart from gastroesophageal reflux and aspiration, reported complications include laryngospasm, coughing, gagging, and other events characteristic of airway manipulation. The incidence of SGA-induced postoperative sore throat varies from 4% to 50% and is highly dependent on the study methods. No single device shows a consistently lower rate of dysphagia, although all appear to be better than tracheal intubation in this regard.[9] Rare reports exist of nerve injury associated with SGA use.

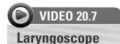

VIDEO 20.6
Cough Reflex

Second-Generation SGAs

Many modern SGAs now incorporate a second lumen which, when properly placed, sits within the upper esophageal opening. Second-generation SGAs tend to allow higher airway positive pressure than first-generation SGAs ($\geq$40 cmH_2O), as well as passive (regurgitation) and active (gastric tube insertion) emptying of the stomach.

F. Tracheal Intubation

Direct Laryngoscopy

The ultimate goal of DL is to produce a direct line of sight from the operator's eye to the glottic opening. This view of the larynx is generally described in terms of the Cormack-Lehane grade (grades 1-4), which correlate with increasingly difficult intubation (**Figure 20.4**). No single preoperative measure is adequate to predict difficulty of DL. Unanticipated failure of DL is primarily a problem of tongue displacement, and lingual tonsil hyperplasia is the most common cause of unanticipated difficult DL (**Figure 20.5**).

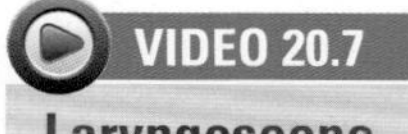
Laryngoscope

Direct Laryngoscope Blades

Two blades, each with a unique manner of application, are in common use. The ***Macintosh*** (curved) ***blade*** is used to displace the epiglottis out of the line of sight by placement in the vallecula and tensing of the glossoepiglottic ligament. The ***Miller*** (straight) ***blade*** reveals the glottis by compressing the epiglottis against the base of the tongue (**Figure 20.6**). Both blades include a flange along the left side of their length, which is used to sweep the tongue to the left. As a generalization, the Macintosh blade is considered advantageous when there is little room to pass an ETT (eg, small mouth). The Miller blade is considered superior in the patient who has a small mandibular space, large incisors, or a large epiglottis.

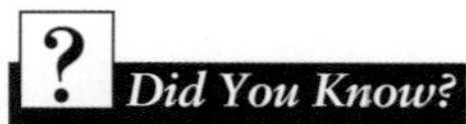
Did You Know?

Application of the Miller blade stimulates the vagus cranial nerve (X), while the Macintosh blade stimulates the glossopharyngeal cranial nerve (IX). Thus, there is a greater risk of bradycardia with the Miller blade.

With either blade, the laryngoscopist must strive to avoid rotating the laryngoscope handle in a cephalad direction, bringing the blade against the upper

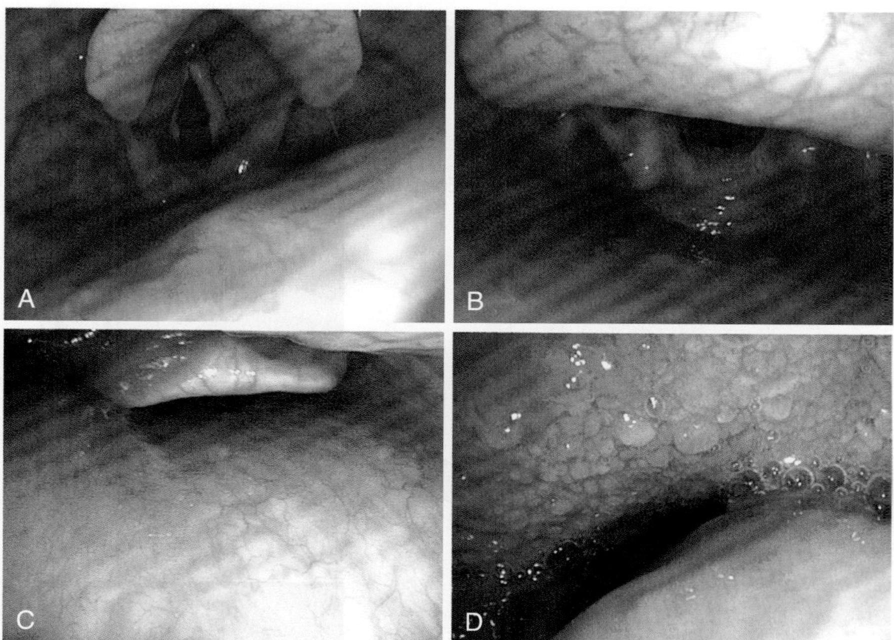

Figure 20.4 The Cormack-Lehane laryngeal view scoring system: grade 1 (A), grade 2 (B), grade 3 (C), and grade 4 (D). (From Rosenblatt WH, Abrons RO, Sukhupragarn W. Airway management. In: Barash PG, Cahalan M, Cullen BF, et al, eds. *Clinical Anesthesia*. 8th ed. Wolters Kluwer; 2018:767-808, Figure 28.11.)

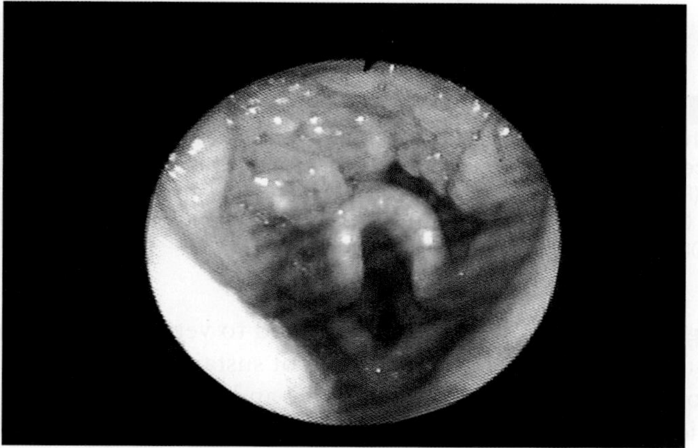

Figure 20.5 **Lingual tonsil hyperplasia: The vallecula is filled with hyperplastic lymphoid tissue in a patient who had an unanticipated difficult direct laryngoscopy.** (From Rosenblatt WH, Abrons RO, Sukhupragarn W. Airway management. In: Barash PG, Cahalan M, Cullen BF, et al, eds. *Clinical Anesthesia*. 8th ed. Wolters Kluwer; 2018:767-808, Figure 28.9.)

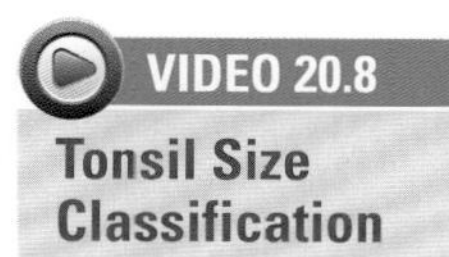

incisors. Extending either blade style too deeply can bring the tip of the blade to rest under the larynx itself, so that forward pressure lifts the airway from view. If a satisfactory laryngeal view is not achieved, the BURP maneuver may be applied. In this maneuver, the larynx is displaced (B) backward, (U) upward, and (R) to the right, using pressure (P) over the cricoid cartilage.[10]

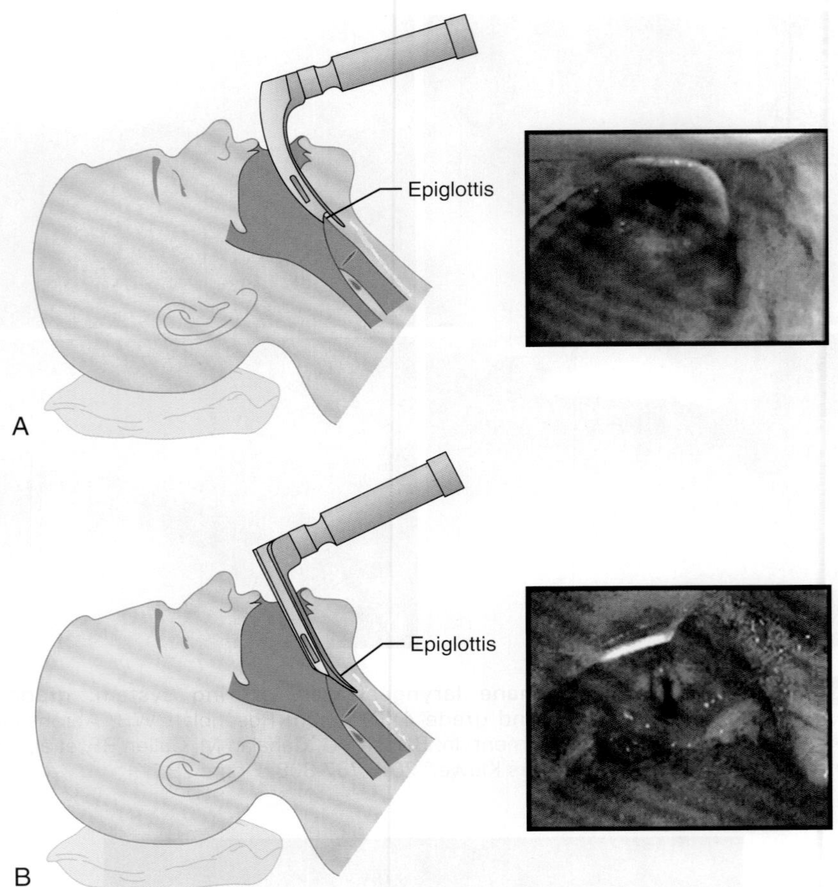

Figure 20.6 A, When a curved laryngoscope blade is used, the tip of the blade is placed in the vallecula, the space between the base of the tongue and the pharyngeal surface of the epiglottis. B, The tip of a straight blade is advanced beneath the epiglottis. (From Rosenblatt WH, Abrons RO, Sukhupragarn W. Airway management. In: Barash PG, Cahalan M, Cullen BF, et al, eds. *Clinical Anesthesia*. 8th ed. Wolters Kluwer; 2018:767-808, Figure 28.10.)

Although a variety of methods can be used to verify that the tracheal tube has been successfully placed, the detection of sustained end-tidal carbon dioxide is the only method considered definitive and should be sought in all cases. Other indicators of endotracheal placement include humidity in the tracheal tube, chest rise and fall, full return of the tidal volume during expiration, and auscultation of breath sounds over the lungs but not the stomach.

Airway Bougies

Airway bougies (or introducers) are low-cost adjuncts that can aid with intubation when a poor laryngeal view (Cormack-Lehane grade 3 or 4) is obtained. These semiflexible stylets can be blindly manipulated under the epiglottis and into the trachea. The operator often feels “clicks” as the bougies’ tip passes over the tracheal rings. An ETT is then “threaded” over the bougie and into the trachea.

Optical Stylets

Optical stylets incorporate both optical and light source elements into a single styletlike stainless steel shaft.

Videolaryngoscopy

Videolaryngoscopy (*VL*) mimics the actions of a traditional laryngoscope but, by placing an imaging device toward the distal end of a laryngoscope blade, removes the need for a direct line of sight to the glottis. The first widely available videolaryngoscope was the Glidescope, which has a 60-degree angulated blade. The "channel configuration" VLs incorporate a semicircular channel alongside the optical elements. These scopes have an anatomic shape with a near right angle between the handle-oral segment and the pharyngeal-hypopharyngeal segment. The channels are aligned with the laryngoscopic view so that, once the glottis is visualized, a preloaded, lubricated tube is advanced through the channel.

The American Society of Anesthesiologists (ASA) Difficult Airway Taskforce recommends that a videolaryngoscope be available as a first attempt or rescue device for all patients being intubated.[11] VL improves the ability to visualize the larynx, and intubation success approaches 97% to 98%. An added benefit is decreased cervical motion when compared with DL, which appears to be more pronounced with the channeled devices.

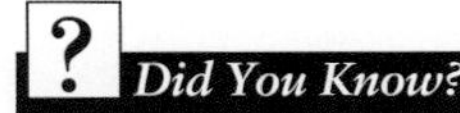

As many as 96% of failed attempts at intubation with direct laryngoscopy can be rescued with a videolaryngoscope.

G. Control of Gastric Contents

Risk of Aspiration

Preventing pulmonary ***aspiration*** of gastric contents is a primary concern during airway management. Altered physiologic states (eg, pregnancy and diabetes mellitus) and gastrointestinal pathology (eg, bowel obstruction and peritonitis) adversely affect the rate of gastric emptying, thereby increasing aspiration risk. The ASA recommends a fasting period of 4 hours for breast milk and 6 hours for nonhuman milk, infant formula, and a light solid meal. Clear liquids can be administered up to 2 hours prior to anesthesia without increased risk for regurgitation and aspiration.[12]

Reduction of gastric acidity can be achieved with the aid of H_2 receptor antagonists and proton pump inhibitors, which also reduce gastric volume.[12] Sodium citrate oral solution increases gastric pH (more alkaline) and is best administered within 1 hour preoperatively.[13] A nasogastric tube can be used to reduce gastric volume prior to anesthesia in patients at high risk of regurgitation.

Rapid-Sequence Induction

Rapid-sequence induction (***RSI***) is indicated when aspiration of gastric contents poses a significant risk. The goal of RSI is to gain control of the airway in the shortest amount of time after the ablation of protective airway reflexes with the induction of anesthesia. In the RSI technique, an intravenous anesthetic induction agent is administered and immediately followed by a rapidly acting neuromuscular blocking drug. Laryngoscopy and intubation are performed as soon as muscle relaxation is confirmed. ***Cricoid pressure may be*** employed (Sellick maneuver), which entails the downward displacement of the cricoid cartilage against the vertebral bodies in an attempt to ablate the

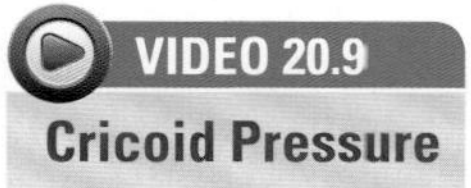

esophageal lumen. The effectiveness of cricoid pressure is in question and it may make laryngoscopy more difficult. Historically, face mask ventilation is not undertaken prior to intubation, but little evidence supports this. Many practicing clinicians have abandoned these latter two practices for lack of evidence-based support.

H. Intubating SGAs

A variety of SGAs specifically designed to facilitate intubation are available. These SGAs are inserted using a similar technique to the classic LMA. Once seated, the mask is inflated and ventilation is attempted. After adequate ventilation is achieved, an ETT is advanced through the barrel of the SGA. Although the Fastrach LMA excels at blind intubation, a fiberscope should be used with the other varieties. Once successful intubation is confirmed, an intubating SGA may be removed, leaving the ETT in place. When rescuing the airway after failed laryngoscopy, intubating SGAs are preferred as they can facilitate a later exchange for an ETT. Nonintubating SGAs, such as the second-generation, single-use, LMA-supreme, will not accept an adult ETT and an exchange procedure, with removal of the SGA prior to endotracheal intubation, may be necessary.

I. Extubation of the Trachea

Criteria for routine postsurgical extubation are outlined in **Table 20.7**. After the patient is asked to open their mouth, a suction catheter is used to remove supraglottic secretions or blood. Some clinicians prefer to allow the airway pressure to rise to 5 to 15 cm of H_2O to facilitate a "passive cough," and the ETT is removed after the cuff (if present) is deflated. If coughing or straining is contraindicated or hazardous (eg, in the presence of an increased intracranial pressure), extubation may be performed with the patient in a surgical plane of anesthesia and breathing spontaneously ("deep" extubation). There are three requirements for deep extubation: (1) excellent mask fit and ventilation during induction, (2) no surgical manipulation of the

Table 20.7 Criteria for Routine "Awake" Postsurgical Extubation

Subjective Clinical Criteria:
Breathing spontaneously
Following commands
Five-second sustained head lift
Intact gag reflex
Airway clear of debris
Adequate pain control
Minimal end expiratory concentration of inhaled anesthetics
Objective Criteria:
Vital capacity: ≥10 mL/kg
Peak voluntary negative inspiratory pressure: –20 cmH_2O or more negative
Tidal volume >6 mL/kg
Sustained tetanic contraction (5 s)
T4/T1 ratio >0.9

Table 20.8 Complications of Tracheal Extubation

Respiratory drive failure (eg, residual anesthetic)
Hypoxia (eg, atelectasis)
Upper airway obstruction (eg, edema, residual anesthetic/reduced upper airway tone)
Vocal fold–related obstruction (eg, laryngospasm, vocal cord paralysis)
Tracheal obstruction (eg, subglottic edema)
Bronchospasm (airway irritation from endotracheal tube)
Aspiration (from decreased gag and swallow reflexes)
Hypertension
Increased intracranial pressure
Increased ocular pressure
Increased abdominal wall pressure (risk of wound dehiscence)

airway, and (3) absence of a full stomach. Extubation of the trachea has its own set of potential complications and may prove more perilous than the act of intubation[13] (**Table 20.8**).

Difficult Extubation

Airway obstruction is a common cause of extubation failure. Incomplete recovery from neuromuscular relaxation, aspirated blood, and edema of the uvula, soft palate, tongue, and glottic structures all may contribute to the obstruction.[13] Laryngospasm upon ETT removal may also cause extubation failure and accounts for 23% of all critical postoperative respiratory events in adults.[4] Unilateral vocal cord paralysis may result from trauma to the recurrent laryngeal nerve during surgery in the neck. Airway obstruction can occur if the contralateral nerve has been damaged previously. Transient vocal cord and swallowing dysfunction has been demonstrated in the absence of injury, placing even healthy patients at risk of aspiration after general anesthesia.

Pharmacologic agents used during the maintenance and emergence phases of the anesthetic also may affect the success of extubation. Although low concentrations of inhalation anesthetics (eg, 0.2 minimal alveolar concentration) do not alter the respiratory response to carbon dioxide, they may blunt hypoxic drive. Opiates, and to a lesser extent benzodiazepines, affect both hypercarbic and hypoxic respiratory drives. Some nondepolarizing muscle relaxants may also reduce the hypoxic ventilatory drive.

Identification of Patients at Risk for Complications at Time of Extubation

All patients should be evaluated for the potential of difficult extubation just as they are evaluated for potential difficult intubation. A number of well-known clinical situations may place patients at increased risk for difficulty with oxygenation or ventilation at the time of extubation (**Table 20.9**). Management strategies range from continued ventilation to the preparation of standby reintubation equipment to the active establishment of a bridge or guide for reintubation or oxygenation. A number of obturators, which

Table 20.9 Clinical Situations Presenting Increased Risk for Complications at Time of Extubation

Edema (local, generalized, or angioneurotic)	Airway narrowing
Thyroid surgery	Risk of recurrent laryngeal nerve injury
Laryngoscopy (diagnostic)	Edema, laryngospasm (especially after biopsy)
Uvulopalatoplasty	Palatal and oropharyngeal edema
Obstructive sleep apnea	Upper airway obstruction
Carotid endarterectomy	Wound hematoma, glottic edema, nerve palsies
Maxillofacial trauma	Laryngeal fracture, mandibular/maxillary wires
Cervical vertebrae decompression/fixation	Supraglottic and hypopharyngeal edema
Anaphylaxis	Laryngotracheal narrowing
Hypopharyngeal infections	Laryngotracheal narrowing
Hypoventilation syndromes	Residual anesthetic, central sleep apnea, myasthenia gravis, morbid obesity, severe chronic obstructive pulmonary disease
Hypoxemic syndromes	Ventilation-perfusion mismatch, increased oxygen consumption, impaired alveolar oxygen diffusion, severe anemia
Inadequate airway-protective reflexes	Increased aspiration risk

VIDEO 20.10
Anaphylaxis

may be left in the airway for extended periods, are available for use in trial extubation. These devices are generally referred to as airway exchange catheters (AECs). The success of first-pass reintubation is significantly higher, and the incidence of hypoxia is lower, in patients with a retained exchange catheter.[14] AECs have been associated with significant morbidity, though, including loss of airway control, mucosal trauma, pneumothorax, esophageal intubation, and death.

J. The Difficult Airway Algorithm

The ASA Difficult Airway Algorithm

Difficult and failed airway management accounts for 2.3% of anesthetic deaths in the United States. The ASA defines the difficult airway as the situation in which the "conventionally trained anesthesiologist experiences difficulty with intubation, mask ventilation, or both" and has designed the ***difficult airway algorithm*** (ASA-DAA, **Figure 20.7**) to address such a scenario.[11]

Entry into the algorithm begins with the evaluation of the airway, which should direct the clinician to enter the ASA-DAA at one of its two root points: awake intubation (**Figure 20.7**, Box A) or intubation attempts after the induction of general anesthesia (**Figure 20.7**, Box B). Awake intubation is chosen when difficulty is anticipated that will place the patient's life in jeopardy, while the airway management after induction is chosen when an uncorrectable situation is not expected.

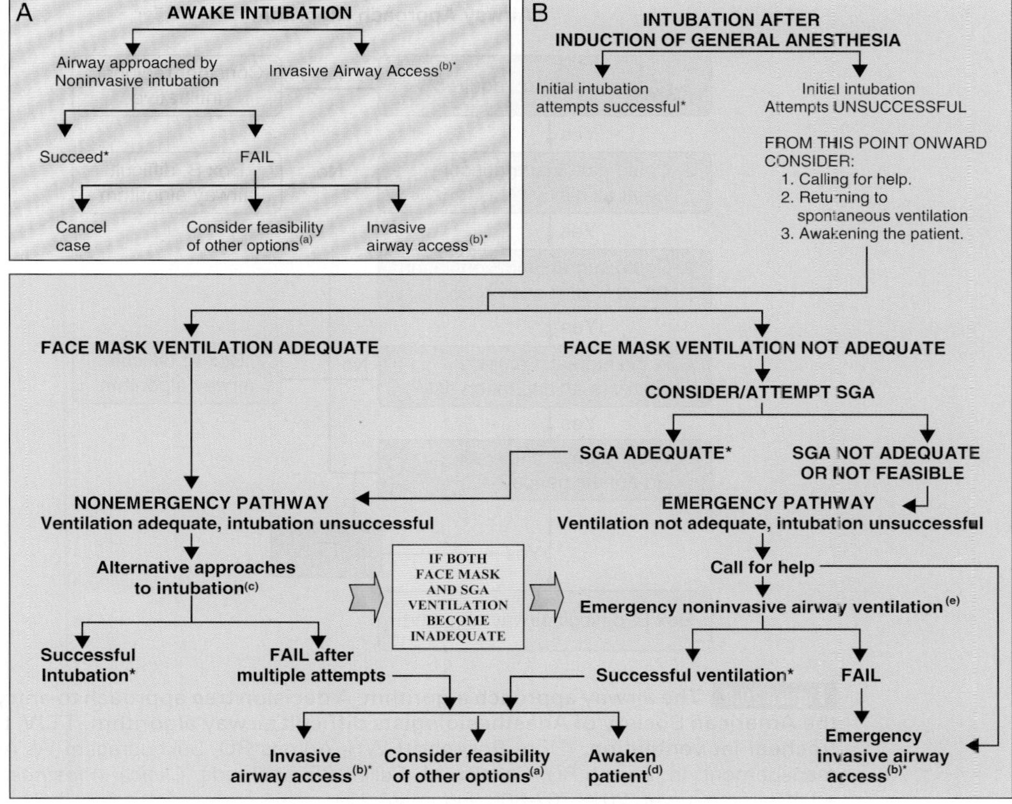

Figure 20.7 **The American Society of Anesthesiologists difficult airway algorithm. A, Awake intubation. B, Intubation after induction of general anesthesia.** (From Apfelbaum JL, Hagberg CA, Caplan RA, et al; American Society of Anesthesiologists Task Force on Management of the Difficult Airway. Practice guidelines for management of the difficult airway: an updated report by the American Society of Anesthesiologists Task Force on Management of the Difficult Airway. *Anesthesiology.* 2013;118(2):251-270, with permission.)

The Airway Approach Algorithm

This has been further delineated in a preoperative decision tree by Rosenblatt[15] known as the ***airway approach algorithm*** (***AAA***). **Figure 20.8** outlines the AAA, a simple one-pathway algorithm for entering the ASA-DAA, which follows five steps:

1. ***Is airway control necessary?*** Can regional or infiltrative anesthesia be applied?
2. ***Could tracheal intubation be (at all) difficult?*** Based on the airway evaluation.
3. ***Can supraglottic ventilation be used if needed?*** If both intubation and ventilation may be difficult, an awake intubation is chosen (**Figure 20.7A**).

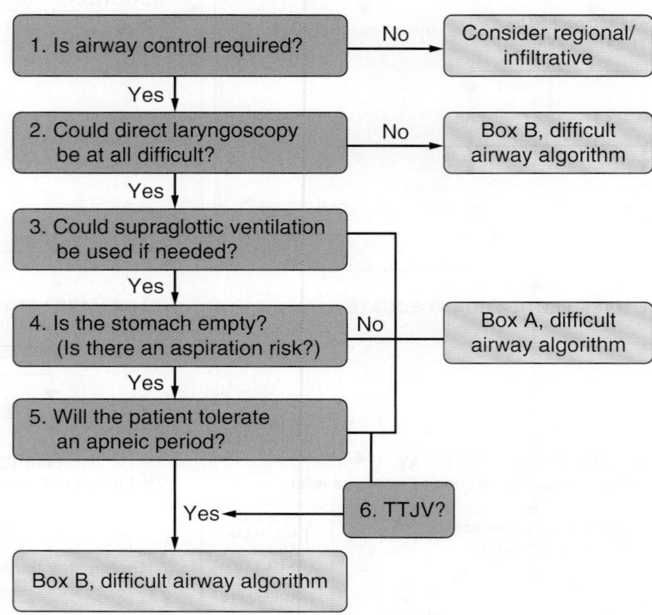

Figure 20.8 The airway approach algorithm: A decision tree approach to entry into the American Society of Anesthesiologists difficult airway algorithm. TTJV, transtracheal jet ventilation. (From Rosenblatt WH, Abrons RO, Sukhupragarn W. Airway management. In: Barash PG, Cahalan M, Cullen BF, et al, eds. *Clinical Anesthesia*. 8th ed. Wolters Kluwer; 2018:767-808, Figure 28.21.)

4. ***Is there an aspiration risk?*** The patient at risk for aspiration is not a candidate for elective SGA use. If intubation is also evaluated to be difficult, **Figure 20.7A** is chosen.
5. ***Will the patient tolerate an apneic period?*** Should intubation fail and SGA ventilation is inadequate, will the patient rapidly desaturate? If so, awake intubation is the better choice (**Figure 20.7A**).

The ASA-DAA becomes truly useful with the unanticipated difficult airway. When initial attempts fail, the airway is supported via mask ventilation. Then, if needed, the clinician may turn to the most convenient or appropriate technique for establishing tracheal intubation. The number of laryngoscopy attempts should be limited as serial attempts increase the incidence of complications.[16] This is because laryngoscopy can result in soft-tissue trauma, which may diminish the efficacy of a rescue facemask or supraglottic ventilation. When mask ventilation fails, the algorithm suggests supraglottic ventilation via an SGA. Should SGA ventilation fail to sustain the patient adequately, the emergency pathway is entered and the ASA-DAA suggests the use of transtracheal oxygenation or a surgical airway. Although several commercial kits are available for such situations, data suggest that a scalpel-based technique, with or without a bougie, may be optimal.[13]

K. Awake Airway Management

Awake airway management provides maintenance of spontaneous ventilation and airway protection in the event that the airway cannot be secured rapidly. A sedative agent can be used during awake intubation, but the clinician must remember that producing obstruction or apnea in the patient with a difficult airway can be devastating. Administration of an antisialagogue, commonly atropine or

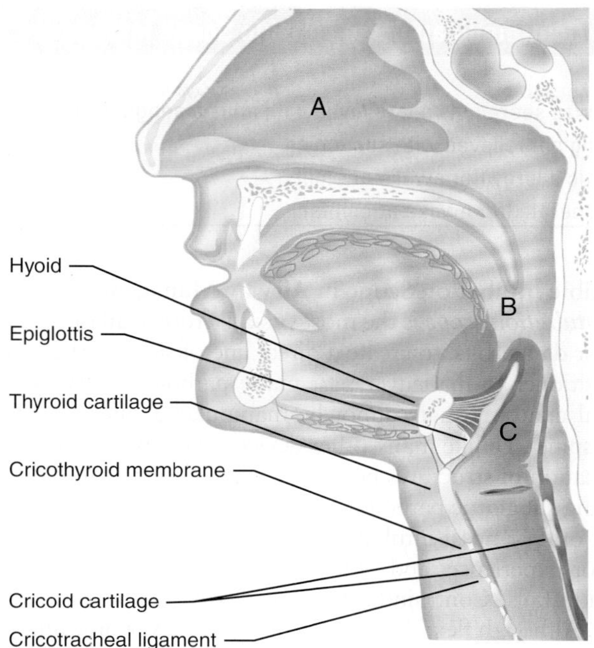

Figure 20.9 Areas of local anesthetic delivery for awake airway management: The nasal cavity/nasopharynx (A), pharynx/base of tongue (B), hypopharynx, and (C) larynx/trachea.

glycopyrrolate, is important to the success of awake intubation techniques as even small amounts of liquid can obscure the objective lens of indirect optical instruments (eg, flexible or rigid intubating scope, videolaryngoscope). Vasoconstriction of the nasal passages is also required for instrumentation of this part of the airway.

Local anesthetics are a cornerstone of awake airway control techniques (see Chapter 12). Both topical anesthesia and injected nerve block techniques are commonly used to blunt airway reflexes and provide analgesia. This chapter focuses on the noninvasive options.

The clinician directs local anesthetic therapy to three anatomic areas: the nasal cavity/nasopharynx, the pharynx/base of tongue, and the hypopharynx/larynx/trachea (**Figure 20.9**). To address the nasopharynx, cotton-tipped applicators soaked in local anesthetic are passed along the lower border of the nasal cavity until the posterior wall of the nasopharynx is reached and are left in place for 5 to 10 minutes.

The glossopharyngeal nerve can be blocked as its branches transverse behind the palatoglossal folds. These folds are seen as soft-tissue ridges that extend from the posterior border of the soft palate to the base of the tongue. A noninvasive technique employs anesthetic-soaked cotton-tipped applicators positioned against the inferior-most aspect of the folds and left in place for 3 to 5 minutes. In many instances, topical application of anesthetics in the pharyngeal/hypopharyngeal cavities provides adequate analgesia of the hypopharynx, larynx, and trachea. Additional anesthetic agents can also be injected down the working channel of a flexible intubation scope.

When awake intubation fails, the clinician has a number of options. They include cancellation of a nonemergent surgical case until specialized equipment or personnel can be arranged for, the use of regional anesthetic techniques or, if demanded by the situation, a surgical airway (eg, tracheostomy).

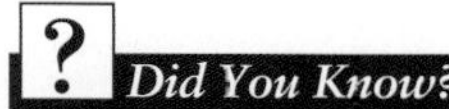

Elective awake intubation is relatively contraindicated by inability to cooperate (eg, child, profound mental retardation, intoxication) and allergy to local anesthetics.

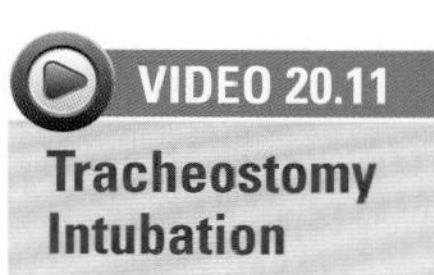

Table 20.10 Contraindications to Flexible Scope Intubation
Hypoxia
Significant airway secretions not relieved with antisialagogues and suction
Airway bleeding not relieved with suctioning
Local anesthetic allergy (for awake attempts)
Inability to cooperate (for awake attempts)

L. The Flexible Intubation Scope in Airway Management

The *flexible intubation scope* is the most versatile tool available in situations when it is difficult, or dangerous, to create a direct line of sight to the glottis. The scope allows a practitioner to maneuver past many pathologic airway obstructions as well as normal anatomy that cannot be manipulated safely (eg, the unstable or fixed cervical spine). Unlike many other devices, the flexible intubation scope also allows visualization of structures below the level of the vocal folds. This is helpful in characterizing subglottic pathology as well as verifying tracheal tube placement. The choice of oral or nasal intubation is based on clinical requirements, surgical needs, operator experience, and other intubation techniques available if flexible scope intubation fails. Contraindications to flexible scope intubation are relative (**Table 20.10**). Although flexible scope intubation is a versatile and vital technique, there are several pitfalls. **Table 20.11** lists the most common reasons for failure.

M. The SGAs in the Failed Airway

Failed intubations and failed mask ventilation can be rescued with SGA insertion. The major disadvantage of the SGAs in resuscitation is the lack of mechanical protection from regurgitation and aspiration, which is a secondary concern in the face of life-threatening hypoxemia.

N. Transtracheal Procedures

When intubation and mask and SGA ventilation fail, airway access via the extrathoracic trachea may be warranted (**Table 20.12**). These techniques range from minimally invasive (eg, retrograde wire–aided intubation and percutaneous translaryngeal jet ventilation) to surgical (eg, cricothyrotomy and open tracheostomy). Although these techniques are beyond the scope of this chapter, it is important to be aware of their presence at the terminal end of the DAA.

Although the ASA's Taskforce on the difficult airway has given the medical community an immensely valuable tool in the approach to the patient with the difficult airway, the ASA's algorithm must be viewed as a starting point only.

Table 20.11 Common Reasons for Failure of Flexible Scope Intubation
Lack of provider experience
Failure to adequately dry the airway: Antisialagogue underdose, rushed technique
Failure to adequately anesthetize the airway (awake patient)
Nasal cavity bleeding: Inadequate vasoconstriction/lubrication, rushed technique
Obstructing base of tongue: Insufficient tongue displacement (may require jaw thrust/tongue extrusion/concurrent laryngoscopy)
Hang-up: Endotracheal tube/scope diameter ratio too large
Flexible scope fogging: Suction or oxygen not attached to working channel, cold bronchoscope

Table 20.12 Criteria for Establishment of an Emergent Invasive Airway

When all five criteria are met, an emergent invasive airway is indicated:
Cannot intubate
Cannot ventilate
Cannot awaken patient
Supraglottic airway has failed
Clinically significant hypoxemia

Did You Know?

The clinician does not need to be expert with all airway equipment and techniques. No one device can be considered superior to another for all tasks. A broad range of approaches should be mastered so that the failure of one does not preclude safe airway management and emergency rescue.

Judgment, experience, the clinical situation, and available resources all affect the appropriateness of the chosen pathway through, or divergence from, the algorithm. When managing the difficult airway, flexibility, not rigidity, prevails.

For further review and interactivities, please see the associated Interactive Video Lectures and "At a Glance" infographic accessible in the complimentary eBook bundled with this text. Access instructions are located in the inside front cover.

References

1. Shiga T, Wajima Z, Inoue T, et al. Predicting difficult intubation in apparently normal patients: a meta-analysis of bedside screening test performance. *Anesthesiology*. 2005;103:429. PMID: 16052126.
2. Lundstrom LH, Rosenstock CV, Wetterslev J, Norskov AK. The DIFFMASK score for predicting difficult facemask ventilation: a cohort study of 46,804 patients. *Anaesthesia*. 2019;74:1267-1276. PMID: 31106851.
3. Kheterpal S, Martin L, Shanks AM, Tremper KK. Prediction and outcomes of impossible mask ventilation: a review of 50,000 anesthetics. *Anesthesiology*. 2009;110(4):891-897.
4. Hagberg CA, ed. *Benumof's Airway Management: Principles and Practice*. Mosby; 2007.
5. Seet E, Yousaf F, Gupta S, et al. Use of manometry for laryngeal mask airway reduces postoperative pharyngolaryngeal adverse events. *Anesthesiology*. 2010;112:652. PMID: 20179502.
6. Idrees A, Khan FA. A comparative study of positive pressure ventilation via laryngeal mask airway and endotracheal tube. *J Pak Med Assoc*. 2000;50:333. PMID: 11109752.
7. Brimacombe JR, Brain AI, Berry AM, et al. Gastric insufflation and the laryngeal mask. *Anesth Analg*. 1998;86:914. PMID: 9539625.
8. Brimacombe JR. Advanced uses: clinical situations. In: Brimacombe JR, Brain AIJ, eds. *The Laryngeal Mask Airway. A Review and Practical Guide*. Saunders; 2004:138.
9. Yu SH, Ross Beirne O. Laryngeal mask airways have a lower risk of airway complications compared with endotracheal intubation: a systematic review. *J Oral Maxillofac Surg*. 2010;68:2359-2376.
10. Ulrich B, Listyo R, Gerig HJ, et al. The difficult intubation: the value of BURP and 3 predictive tests of difficult intubation. *Anaesthesist*. 1998;47:45. PMID: 9530446.
11. Practice guidelines for management of the difficult airway. *Anesthesiology*. 2013;118(2):251-270. PMID: 23364566.
12. Practice guidelines for preoperative fasting and the use of pharmacologic agents to reduce the risk of pulmonary aspiration. Application to healthy patients undergoing elective procedures: an updated report by the American Society of Anesthesiologists Task Force on preoperative fasting and the use of pharmacologic agents to reduce the risk of pulmonary aspiration. *Anesthesiology*. 2017;126:376. PMID: 28045707.
13. Cook TM, Woodall N, Frerk C; Fourth National Audit Project. Major complications of airway management in the UK. Results of the Fourth National Audit Project of the Royal College of Anaesthetists and the Difficult Airway Society. Part 1: anaesthesia. *Br J Anaesth*. 2011;106(5):617-631. PMID: 21447488.
14. Mort TC. Continuous airway access for the difficult extubation: the efficacy of the airway exchange catheter. *Anesth Analg*. 2007;105:1357. PMID: 17959966.
15. Rosenblatt W. The airway approach algorithm. *J Clin Anesth*. 2004;16:312. PMID: 15261328.
16. Mort TC. Emergency tracheal intubation: complications associated with repeated laryngoscopic attempts. *Anesth Analg*. 2004;99:607. PMID: 15271750.

AIRWAY MANAGEMENT

AT A GLANCE

Below is a visual representation of the ASA difficult airway algorithm.

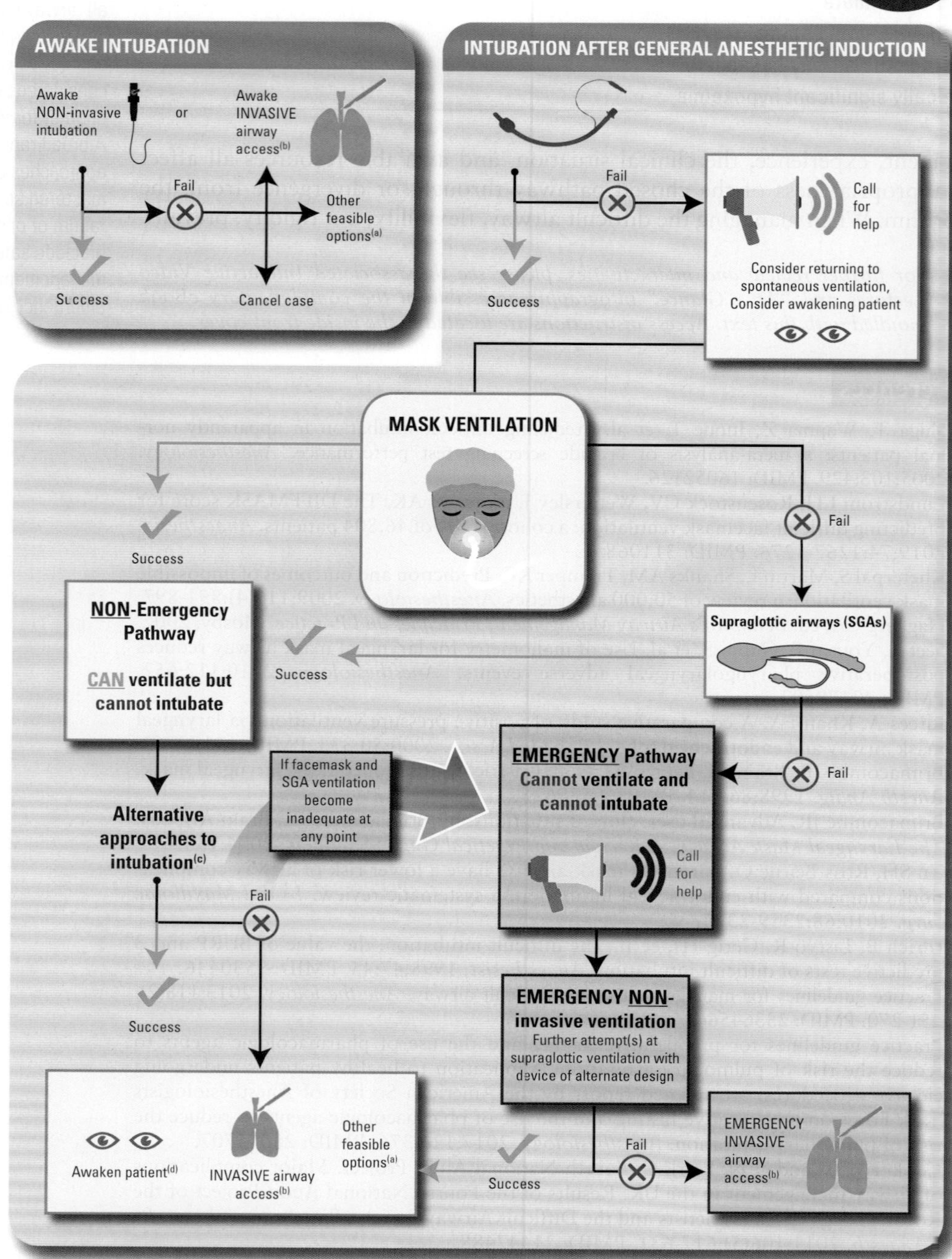

(a) If ventilation can be established and is adequate, one may consider utilizing facemask/SGA, or local or regional techniques for the procedure. These options may not be feasible if reached through the emergency pathway. **(b)** Includes surgical or percutaneous airway (tracheotomy, cricothyrotomy, or retrograde intubation) and bronchoscopy with jet ventilation. **(c)** Includes video laryngoscopy, alternate laryngoscope blades, SGA as an intubating conduit, fiberoptic intubation, intubating stylet, light wand, and blind oral or nasal intubation. **(d)** Consider pursuing awake intubation or cancelling surgery.

Infographic by: Naveen Nathan MD

Questions

1. **Which cranial nerve (CN) must be anesthetized to prevent the gag reflex during awake intubation?**

   A. Facial nerve (CN VII)
   B. Glossopharyngeal nerve (CN IX)
   C. Superior laryngeal nerve (branch of CN X)
   D. Recurrent laryngeal nerve (branch of CN X)

2. **Inflation of an LMA cuff should be limited to what pressure?**

   A. <20 cmH_2O
   B. <40 cmH_2O
   C. <60 cmH_2O
   D. <80 cmH_2O

3. **What is the most reliable verification of successful endotracheal tube placement?**

   A. Humidity ("fogging") in the tube
   B. Chest rise with positive pressure breaths
   C. Continued end-tidal CO_2 over serial breaths
   D. Chest radiograph showing the tube within the outline of the trachea

4. **Which of the following is true about rescue needle cricothyrotomy?**

   A. It should be performed with an angiocatheter.
   B. Kinking of the catheter is unlikely.
   C. A high pressure, though regulated oxygen source, is necessary.
   D. A scalpel is needed.

5. **Which of the following is an absolute indication for use of an awake technique in a patient who requires tracheal intubation?**

   A. Assessment of difficulty with face mask ventilation only
   B. Assessment of difficulty with intubation and ventilation
   C. Assessment of difficulty with surgical airway
   D. Assessment of difficulty with intubation only

Answers

1. B

The glossopharyngeal nerve (CN IX) innervates the base of tongue, pharynx, and rostral surface of the epiglottis. Stimulation of any of these surfaces may elicit a gag reflex.

2. C

Maintaining an LMA intracuff pressure <60 cmH_2O (44 mm Hg) is associated with decreased postoperative pharyngolaryngeal complications.

3. C

The only definitive method of verifying successful endotracheal tube placement is persistent end-tidal CO_2 over serial breaths. Humidity in the tube and small, transient end-tidal CO_2 waveforms can be seen with esophageal intubation, as can an overlying (underlying) outline on chest radiograph.

4. C

Cannula over the needle cricothyrotomy should only be performed with a designated translaryngeal catheter. Kinking of angiocatheters has long been known to be a serious problem when used for this purpose. When using cannula over the needle technique, a high-pressure source of oxygen must be available, but overpressurization can lead to barotrauma.

5. B

Any assessed difficulty with intubation, ventilation, aspiration risk, or surgical airway can justify awake intubation, but there are only three distinct situations of absolute indication: assessed cannot intubate and cannot ventilate, assessed cannot intubate and significant aspiration risk, and assessed cannot intubate and significantly reduced safe apneic period.

21 Regional Anesthesia

Alexander M. DeLeon and Yogen Girish Asher

I. General Principles and Equipment

Utilized alone or in conjunction with general anesthesia, regional anesthesia provides clinicians vital tools to reduce pain after various types of painful surgeries. Not only do these techniques improve patient satisfaction, but they also serve to decrease postoperative complications such as nausea, respiratory depression, and recovery room time. Application of regional anesthesia requires knowledge of indications, contraindications, and local anesthetic pharmacology as well as practiced technical skills before it can be offered. This chapter will briefly review basic concepts of peripheral nerve blockade prior to describing specific block technique for some commonly performed blocks.

A. Setup and Monitoring

Peripheral nerve blocks are often performed outside of the operating room, typically preoperatively so that they may take effect prior to surgical incision. They must be performed with the American Society of Anesthesiologists (ASA) standard monitors including pulse oximetry, continuous electrocardiogram, and blood pressure cuff. If mild sedation is used, oxygen should be applied via nasal cannula. A "block cart" should be in the immediate vicinity and contain airway equipment, emergency supplies, and medications, such as lipid emulsion.

B. Peripheral Nerve Stimulators

A peripheral nerve stimulator can be used to identify nerves and guide placement of local anesthetic, with or without ultrasound. An insulted needle that only allows the tip of the needle to conduct electric current must be used for this purpose. The closer the tip of the needle is to a nerve, the less current is required to stimulate it. Dose ranges are typically 0.1 to 1mA for elicited motor response (EMR). Longer duration impulses (>0.3 ms) are more likely to cause pain by stimulating sensory nerves, while shorter duration impulses (0.1 ms) cause significantly less discomfort because the motor component of the nerve is primarily stimulated.

> **? Did You Know?**
>
> Ultrasound guidance has not definitively been proven to be safer or more effective, yet evidence is emerging showing that ultrasound allows for faster onset, lower doses of local anesthetics, and fewer needle passes.

C. Ultrasound Guidance

The prevalence of ***ultrasound guidance*** has increased the popularity of regional anesthesia. Ultrasound allows for the visualization of nerve structures, vascular structures, and local anesthetic spread. Ultrasound guidance has not definitively been proven to be safer or more effective, yet evidence is emerging showing that ultrasound allows for faster onset, lower doses of local anesthetics, and fewer needle passes.[1] To obtain the optimal view of a target nerve, a basic understanding of ultrasound physics is useful.

Ultrasound beams are sound waves beyond the threshold of hearing (>20,000 MHz). Images are created when these waves are reflected back to the sensor (located within the probe) and then processed by a computer. ***Acoustic impedance*** is the quality of structures allowing for visualization using ultrasound. Differences in acoustic impedance of a structure relative to its surrounding tissue dictate whether the structure will be visible. Certain structures are more likely to attenuate an ultrasound beam. For example, ultrasound waves pass easily through blood vessels (ie, minimal attenuation), compared with bone and air, which cause a high degree of attenuation.

Probes differ in frequency ranges. Higher frequency probes have less penetration but greater resolution and are useful for superficial structures, including most peripheral nerves. Lower frequency probes are useful for deeper structures such as the heart and liver.

Once the appropriate depth is set when viewing an ultrasound image, the *gain* can be adjusted to brighten or darken the image. Color flow Doppler can help to identify blood vessels due to the turbulent nature of blood flow toward and away from the probe.

When orienting the needle to the probe, two different techniques have been defined: in plane versus out of plane (**Figure 21.1**). The benefit of an in-plane approach is that it allows for the entire needle, including the tip, to be visualized at all times.

> **? Did You Know?**
>
> Differences in acoustic impedance of a structure relative to its surrounding tissue dictate whether the structure will be visible during ultrasound examination.

> **? Did You Know?**
>
> Higher frequency ultrasound probes have less penetration but greater resolution and are therefore useful for visualizing superficial structures including most peripheral nerves.

D. Other Related Equipment

Insulated needles must be used when nerve stimulation is desired. Needles designed for peripheral nerve blocks are usually short beveled to decrease the likelihood of injuring nerves and vascular structures, in contrast to long-beveled needles intended for intramuscular injections. Although a standard insulated needle can be seen with ultrasound, specifically produced hyperechoic needles are considerably easier to view.

> **? Did You Know?**
>
> The best needles to use for peripheral nerve blocks are insulated, short beveled, and hyperechoic needles.

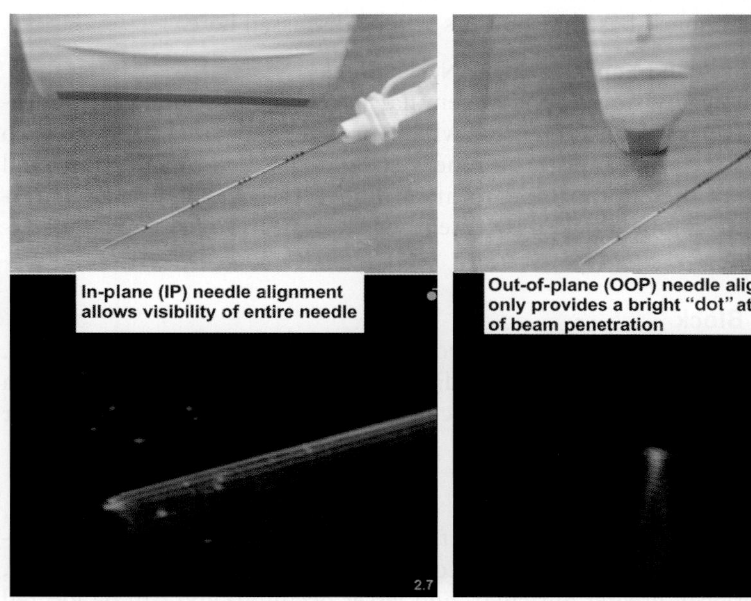
In-plane (IP) needle alignment allows visibility of entire needle
Out-of-plane (OOP) needle alignment only provides a bright "dot" at the point of beam penetration
2.7
2.7

Figure 21.1 **In-plane versus out-of-plane approaches.** (From Tsui BCH, Rosenquist RW. Peripheral nerve blockade. In: Barash PG, Cahalan M, Cullen BF, et al, eds. *Clinical Anesthesia*. 8th ed. Wolters Kluwer; 2018:945-1002, Figure 36.3.)

II. Avoiding Complications

Complications from peripheral nerve blocks include local anesthetic toxicity, nerve injury, bleeding, infection, and damage to adjacent structures. ***Local anesthetic toxicity*** is discussed in Chapter 12. Techniques to reduce the risk of local anesthetic systemic toxicity include reducing the dose to the lowest effective dose, intermittent aspiration during injection, adding an intravascular marker (epinephrine) to the local anesthetic, and maintaining communication with the patient to assess for central nervous system symptoms (eg, perioral numbness, tinnitus).

Avoidance of ***nerve injury*** can theoretically be reduced with ultrasound imaging, yet ultrasound has not been conclusively shown to reduce such complications. Mechanisms include mechanical injury, chemical toxicity, ischemia, or compression. Injuries can range in severity, but most resolve with time.

Adherence to the American Society of Regional Anesthesia's guidelines on peripheral nerve blocks should minimize risk of ***bleeding***, especially for patients on antiplatelet or anticoagulant medications.[2]

Infectious complications are rare but can be minimized with sterile technique, especially during placement of an indwelling catheter. Damage to adjacent structures can be minimized through identification of such structures (eg, pleura, blood vessels).

III. Specific Techniques for the Head, Neck, Upper Extremities, and Trunk

A. Head and Neck

Head and neck blocks can be used for a variety of procedures including carotid endarterectomy, awake craniotomy, and plastic and maxillofacial surgeries. Only a few landmark-based techniques will be discussed here.

B. Supraorbital and Supratrochlear Nerve Blocks

The ophthalmic division of the trigeminal nerve (V1) supplies the supraorbital and supratrochlear nerves, which provide sensory innervation to the anterior scalp. The supraorbital nerve can be blocked by injecting local anesthetic near the supraorbital foramen above the eyebrow. The supratrochlear nerve can be blocked by extending this injection medially approximately 1 cm.

Infraorbital Block

The infraorbital block is useful for providing analgesia after cleft lip repair. This terminal branch of the maxillary division of the trigeminal nerve (V2) can be blocked by injecting local anesthetic near the infraorbital foramen inferior to the eye.

Superficial Cervical Plexus Block

The ventral rami of the C2-C4 form the superficial and deep cervical plexuses. The superficial cervical plexus comprises four nerves (supraclavicular, transverse cervical, greater auricular, and lesser occipital) and can be located posterolateral to the sternocleidomastoid at the level of the cricoid cartilage. The greater auricular and lesser occipital nerves provide sensory innervation to the lateral and posterolateral scalp, respectively.

Figure 21.2 Levels of the brachial plexus. A, Anatomic relationship of brachial plexus to surrounding structures. B, Detailed description of brachial plexus anatomy. C, Relevant scapular anatomy. (From Moore KL, Agur AMR, Dalley AF. *Clinically Oriented Anatomy*. 8th ed. Philadelphia, PA: Wolters Kluwer; 2018. Figure 3.44.)

Greater Occipital Nerve Block

To provide analgesia for the posterior scalp, the greater occipital nerve (dorsal rami C2) can be blocked along the superior nuchal line lateral to the occipital protuberance and adjacent (typically medial) to the occipital artery.

C. Brachial Plexus Blockade

The brachial plexus consists of spinal roots C5-T1 with a variable contribution from C4 and T2. There are four major approaches to blockade of the brachial plexus: interscalene, supraclavicular, infraclavicular, and axillary (**Figure 21.2**).

Interscalene Block

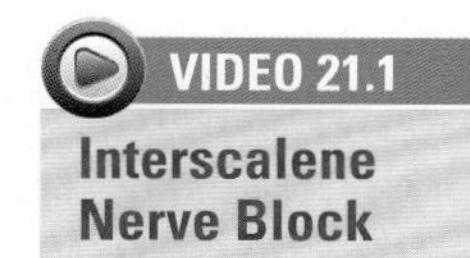

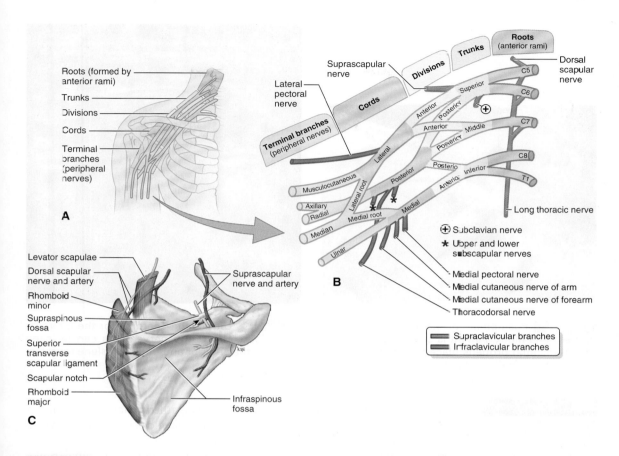

The primary use of the interscalene block is for shoulder surgery (eg, total shoulder arthroplasty, rotator cuff repair, arthroscopic shoulder surgery). The interscalene approach targets the nerves of the upper brachial plexus (C5-C7). Inferior nerve roots of the brachial plexus (C8-T1) are least likely to be blocked (**Figure 21.2**).

Known side effects of the interscalene block include phrenic nerve paralysis, Horner syndrome, and recurrent laryngeal nerve paralysis. Phrenic nerve paralysis has been reported in up to 100% of patients, yet with the introduction of ultrasound, the incidence has been reduced considerably to as low as 13%.[3,4] Horner

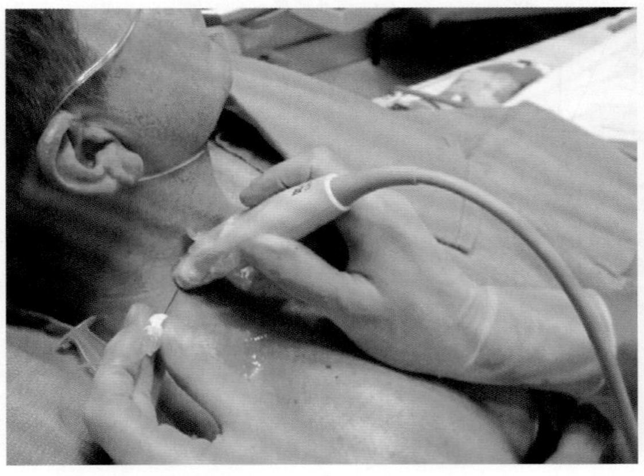

Figure 21.3 Positioning for the ultrasound-guided interscalene block. Patient is seated at 70° to 90°. The ultrasound probe is placed at the level of the cricoid cartilage (C6) in the transverse plane with a slightly downward angle.

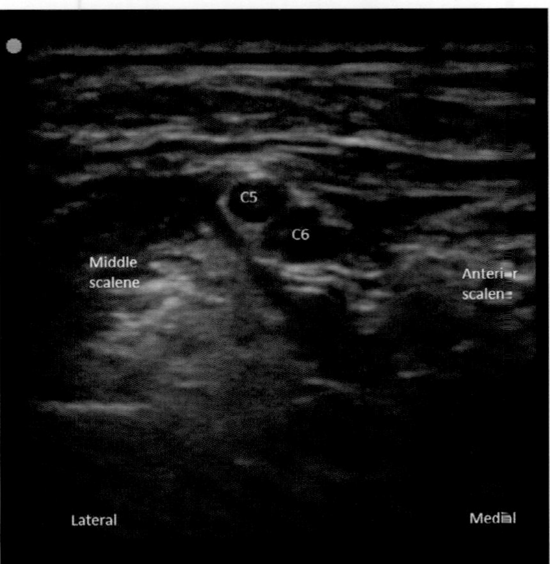

Figure 21.4 Ultrasound anatomy for the interscalene block. The C5-C6 nerve roots can be seen between the anterior and middle scalene muscles.

? Did You Know?

The introduction of ultrasound-guided needle placement has reduced the incidence of phrenic nerve blockade from nearly 100% to as low as 13% during interscalene block.

syndrome results from blockade of the cervical sympathetic chain, as seen in up to half of patients who receive interscalene blocks. The incidence of hoarse voice from recurrent laryngeal nerve block is on the order of 10% to 20%.

The interscalene approach targets the level of the distal roots or proximal trunks of the brachial plexus. Two of the primary nerves of the shoulder derived from the C5-C6 nerve roots, suprascapular nerve and axillary nerve, are blocked by this approach. The supraclavicular nerve (C4), which provides the cutaneous innervation for the top of the shoulder, is often blocked by the interscalene approach.

In order to perform an ultrasound-guided interscalene block, the patient is positioned in a near-seated position of 70° to 90° (**Figure 21.3**). Ultrasound scanning with a high-frequency probe begins above the midpoint of the clavicle where the subclavian artery is located. The nerves of the brachial plexus will be located lateral to the subclavian artery and should be traced to the level of the cricoid cartilage, which corresponds to the level of the C6 vertebrae. The needle is inserted posterior to the ultrasound probe for the in-plane approach (**Figure 21.4**).

When performing a landmark-based interscalene block, the interscalene groove should be palpated lateral to the clavicular head of the sternocleidomastoid at the level of the cricoid cartilage (C6). The needle should be advanced 60° to the sagittal plane until motor response is obtained at the deltoid, biceps, or triceps at <0.5 mA.

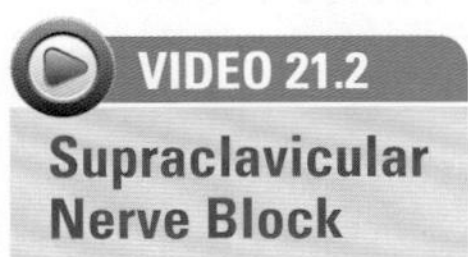

Supraclavicular Block

The supraclavicular block is indicated for elbow, wrist, and hand surgery. The supraclavicular block can also be used for shoulder surgery. But it tends to miss the C4 distribution and may require a superficial cervical plexus block if anesthesia of the top of the shoulder is needed. The supraclavicular block targets the distal trunks and divisions (**Figure 21.2**).

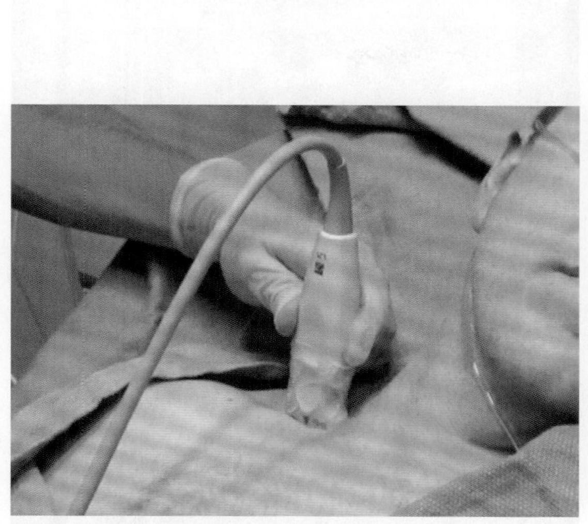

Figure 21.5 Positioning for the ultrasound-guided supraclavicular block.

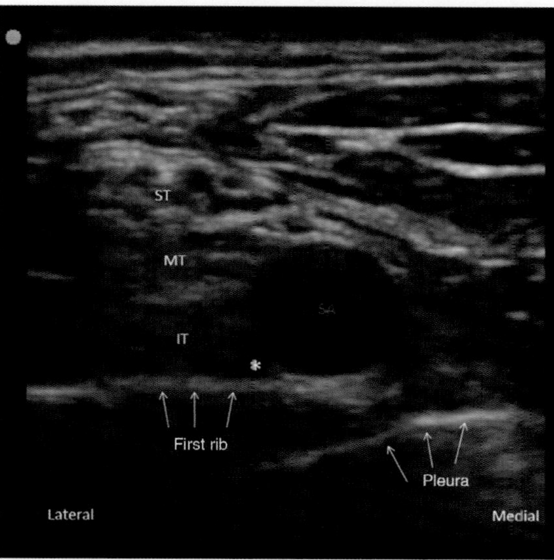

Figure 21.6 Ultrasound anatomy for the supraclavicular block. MT, middle trunk; IT, inferior trunk; SA, subclavian artery; ST, superior trunk. The asterisk (*) signifies the "corner pocket" injection target.

Side effects are similar to the interscalene block. Phrenic nerve paralysis is possible, although it occurs about half as often as with an interscalene block. Pneumothorax is possible, but it is less common when ultrasound is used.

To perform an ultrasound-guided supraclavicular block, ultrasound scanning begins with a high-frequency ultrasound probe at the midpoint of the clavicle with the ultrasound probe angled vertically, similar to the start of the interscalene block (**Figure 21.5**). The brachial plexus appears as a "bundle of grapes" lateral and superficial to the subclavian artery (**Figure 21.6**). The target location for the needle tip is posterior and slightly lateral to the subclavian artery and has been described as the "corner pocket" location.[5]

Due to the risk of pneumothorax being as high as 6% with the landmark technique, other blocks such as the axillary or infraclavicular block can be utilized when ultrasound is not available.[6]

Infraclavicular Block

The infraclavicular block can be used interchangeably with the supraclavicular block for wrist and hand surgery but often spares the suprascapular nerve distribution necessary for shoulder surgery. Compared with the supraclavicular block, the infraclavicular block has virtually no risk of phrenic nerve paralysis and can be used in patients with preexisting lung disease. The infraclavicular block targets the level of the medial, lateral, and posterior cords (**Figure 21.2**).

When performing an ultrasound-guided infraclavicular block, scanning should begin in the parasagittal plane medial to the coracoid process and inferior to the clavicle (**Figure 21.7**). The axillary artery is located deep to the pectoralis major and minor muscles. The target is the posterior cord, which is immediately deep to the subclavian artery (**Figure 21.8**).

A landmark-based technique can be alternatively used. The needle insertion site is immediately inferior to the clavicle, 1 to 2 cm medial to the coracoid process. The needle angle is perpendicular to the skin with a slight (15°-30°)

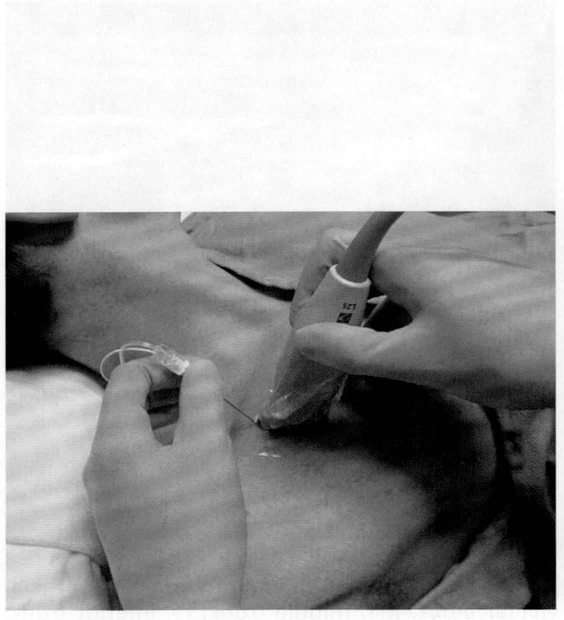

Figure 21.7 Positioning and needle placement for the ultrasound-guided infraclavicular block.

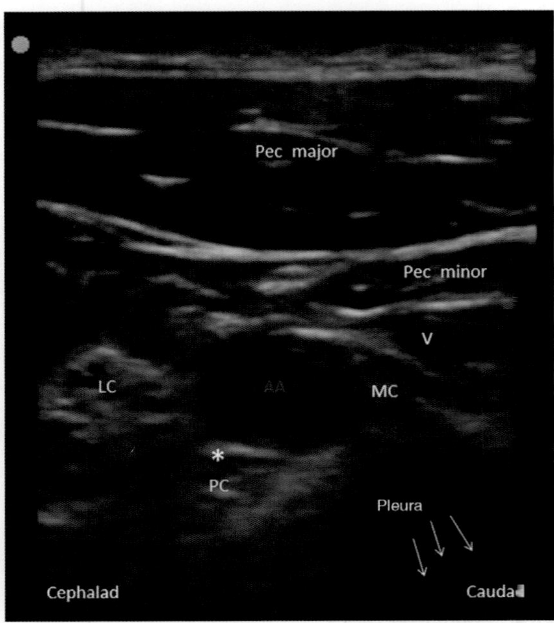

Figure 21.8 Ultrasound anatomy for the infraclavicular block. AA, axillary artery; LC, lateral cord; MC, medial cord; PC, posterior cord; V, subclavian vein. The asterisk (*) signifies the injection target.

caudad angle. The desired end points are either extension of the hand- or elbow-indicated posterior cord stimulation or flexion at the fingers, indicating medial cord stimulation. Biceps flexion indicates lateral cord stimulation and has been associated with a high failure rate of the block.[7]

Axillary Block

The axillary block is a more distal approach to the brachial plexus when compared with the infraclavicular and supraclavicular blocks. The axillary block is performed at the level of the terminal branches of the brachial plexus (**Figure 21.2**). The musculocutaneous, median, ulnar, and radial nerves are blocked, although the musculocutaneous nerve may require a separate injection. Given that the terminal branches are individually visible when using ultrasound, the axillary block can be used as a rescue block when a particular distribution is missed with an infraclavicular or supraclavicular block (**Figures 21.9** and **21.10**). The musculocutaneous nerve terminates as the lateral cutaneous nerve of the forearm and may be missed by the axillary block. For this reason, a separate injection targeting the musculocutaneous nerve may be necessary for surgery involving the lateral wrist.

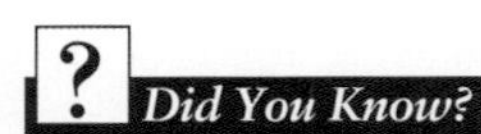

The musculocutaneous nerve terminates as the lateral cutaneous nerve of the forearm and may be missed by the axillary block.

D. Terminal Upper Extremity Nerve Blocks

The terminal branches of the brachial plexus can be blocked individually using more distal approaches. The use of ultrasound to specifically target terminal branches with the axillary approach has made the use of distal rescue blocks less common. Specific circumstances can make these blocks ideal, such as a patient requiring a rescue block from an inadequate supraclavicular block who cannot abduct his or her arm.

Using ultrasound, the median nerve can be blocked at the antecubital fossa. The median nerve appears as a hypoechoic structure medial to the brachial

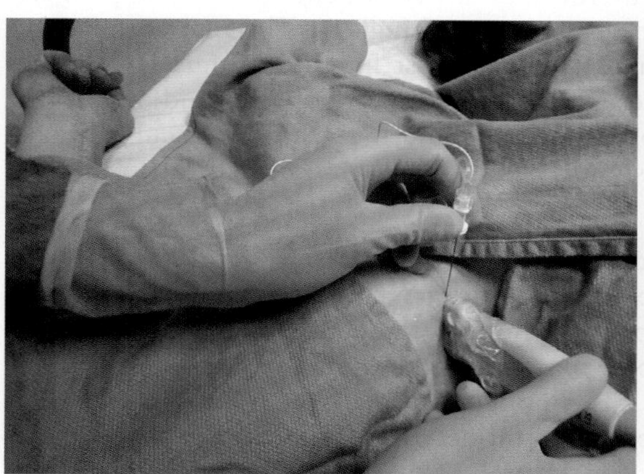

Figure 21.9 Positioning and needle placement for the ultrasound-guided axillary block.

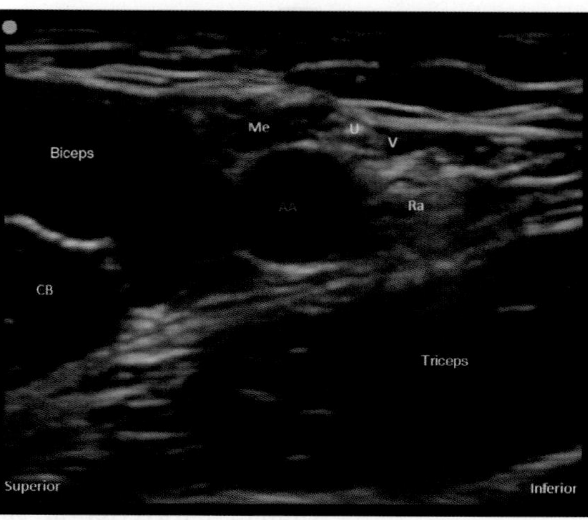

Figure 21.10 Ultrasound anatomy for the axillary block. AA, axillary artery; CB, coracobrachialis; Me, median nerve; Ra, radial nerve; U, ulnar nerve.

artery. The radial nerve can be located on the anterior surface of the elbow, 1 to 2 cm lateral to the biceps tendon, and appears hypoechoic, similar to the median nerve. Nerve stimulation can be used to confirm identification by eliciting a radial nerve response such as wrist or finger extension. The ulnar nerve can be localized at the mid-forearm. The nerve will appear hyperechoic, just medial to the pulsating ulnar artery.

E. Intravenous Regional Anesthesia

Commonly known as a ***Bier block***, the ***intravenous regional anesthesia (IVRA)*** duration of action is mainly limited by a patient's ability to tolerate tourniquet pain. Therefore, IVRA is indicated for surgeries lasting approximately 40 minutes or less that do not require a block for postoperative analgesia. IVRA is commonly used for carpal tunnel releases, trigger finger releases, and wrist arthroscopy.

An intravenous (IV) catheter is placed at a distal location of the operative hand. A double tourniquet is placed on the upper arm with the proximal and distal tourniquets clearly identified. An elastic bandage is then used to exsanguinate the arm, followed by inflation of the distal tourniquet to 250 mm Hg. Next, the proximal tourniquet is inflated, followed by deflation of the distal tourniquet. The elastic bandage is removed, and a dose of 3 mg/kg of lidocaine is then injected. The IV catheter is removed prior to surgery.

The patient will often begin to complain of dull tourniquet pain between 20 and 40 minutes after tourniquet inflation. Treatment of tourniquet pain may require inflation of the distal tourniquet followed by deflation of the proximal tourniquet. If surgery is completed prior to 20 minutes, the tourniquet should remain inflated until at least 20 minutes have passed due to the association with toxic IV concentration of local anesthetic when tourniquets are released after less than 20 minutes. If a patient begins to experience symptoms of local anesthetic systemic neurotoxicity (eg, tinnitus, perioral numbness), the tourniquet should be reinflated and deflated in a cyclic manner until symptoms no longer occur with deflation. After 45 minutes, the tourniquet can be released with minimal risk of systemic neurotoxicity.

F. Intercostal Nerve Blocks

Intercostal nerve blocks are useful in an array of acute or chronic pain settings from rib fractures to herpes zoster "shingles". The intercostal nerve travels in between the internal and innermost intercostal muscles and lies inferior to the intercostal artery and vein, which are inferior and deep to the rib. Due to the proximity to these vessels and high rate of vascular uptake of local anesthetic, patients should be adequately monitored for local anesthetic systemic toxicity.

G. Paravertebral Nerve Blocks

Bounded medially by the intervertebral foramina and lateral spine, anteriorly by the parietal pleura, and posteriorly by the superior costotransverse ligament, the thoracic paravertebral space houses the spinal nerve root as it splits into dorsal and ventral rami. It is contiguous medially with the epidural space via foramina, laterally to the intercostal nerve and vessels, and the cephalocaudad paravertebral spaces (**Figure 21.11**). When unilateral analgesia is desired (eg, for breast or thoracic surgery), local anesthetic can be injected via one large volume injection or multiple smaller volume injections at adjacent levels. When performed under ultrasound guidance, the parietal pleura appears to be "pushed down" by the spread of local anesthetic during injection. Potential complications include pneumothorax, epidural or intrathecal spread of local anesthetic, bleeding, and infection.

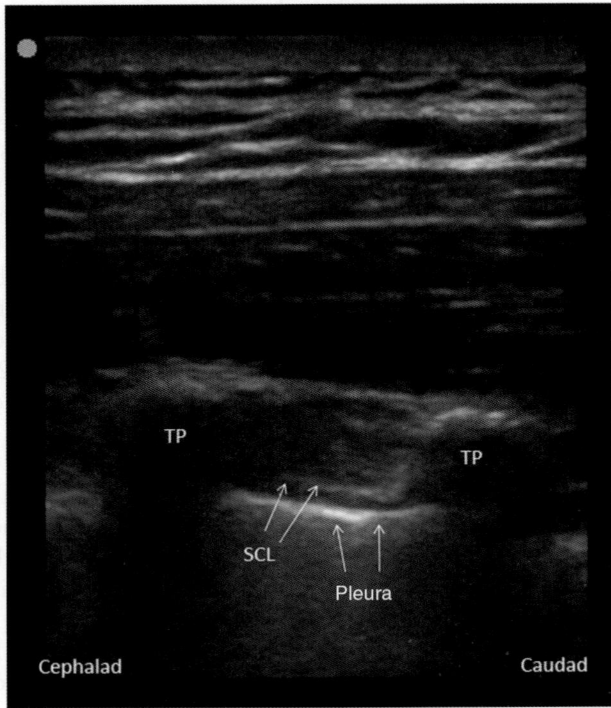

Figure 21.11 Ultrasound anatomy for the paravertebral block. The probe is oriented in the parasagittal plane at the T2-T3 level, 5 cm lateral to the midline. SCL, superior costotransverse ligament; TP, transverse process of thoracic vertebrae.

H. Erector Spinae Plane Block

Similar to the paravertebral block, the erector spinae plane (ESP) block can provide unilateral analgesia for pain located at the cervical, thoracic, or lumbar levels but has been most utilized for thoracic or abdominal surgeries.[8] It is performed by locating the erector spinae muscle lateral to the spine and injecting local anesthetic deep to the muscle, superficial to the transverse process. The local anesthetic will spread to a few craniocaudal dermatomes depending on volume and dose. In contrast with the paravertebral block, the ESP block is technically less challenging but cannot be used for surgical anesthesia.

I. Transversus Abdominis Plane Block

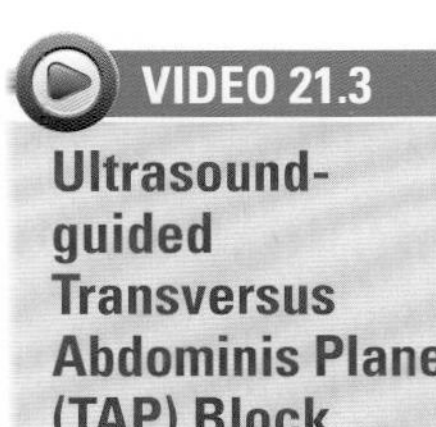

VIDEO 21.3
Ultrasound-guided Transversus Abdominis Plane (TAP) Block

In the anterior abdomen, deep to a fascial plane that lies between the transversus abdominis and internal oblique muscles, there is a network of terminal branches of the ventral rami of the T7-L1 nerve roots and their communicating nerves (**Figure 21.12**). The plane extends medially to the rectus sheath, laterally to the latissimus dorsi, cranially to the rib cage, and caudally to the iliac crest. Injection of local anesthetic at this location provides analgesia to the abdominal wall and skin and can be useful following or preceding laparoscopic or umbilical surgery. This block is most often performed under ultrasound guidance, shown in **Figure 21.13** lateral to the rectus sheath in the T10 dermatome. Care must be taken not to traverse the peritoneum, which lies deep to the transversus muscle.

J. Inguinal Nerve Block

The ilioinguinal and iliohypogastric nerves are also located in the transversus plane in the anterior abdomen, which originate from L1. Injection around

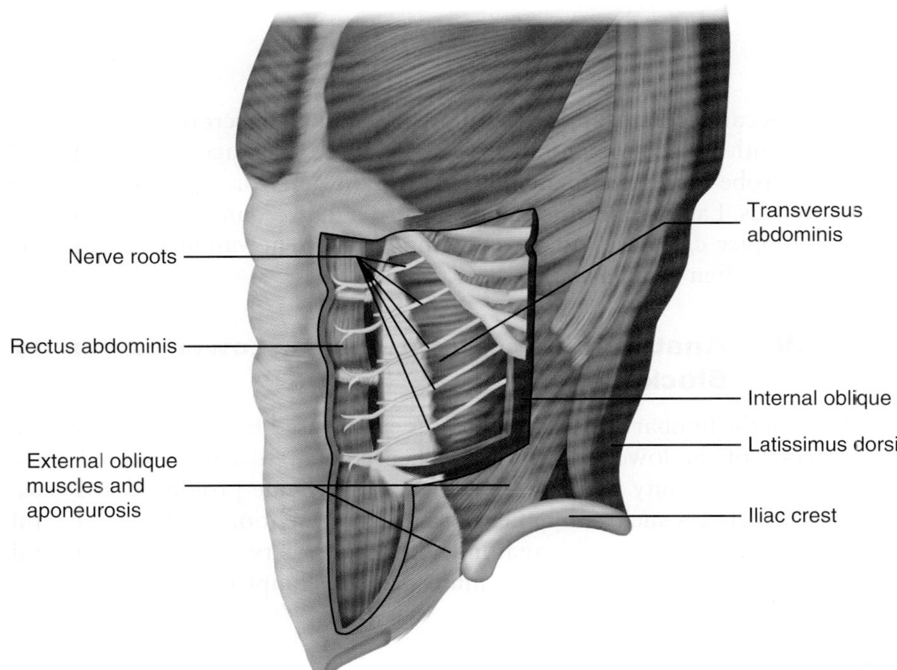

Figure 21.12 Anatomy for the transversus abdominis plane block. The nerves (T7-L1) are located in the fascial layer between the internal oblique and the transversus abdominis muscles.

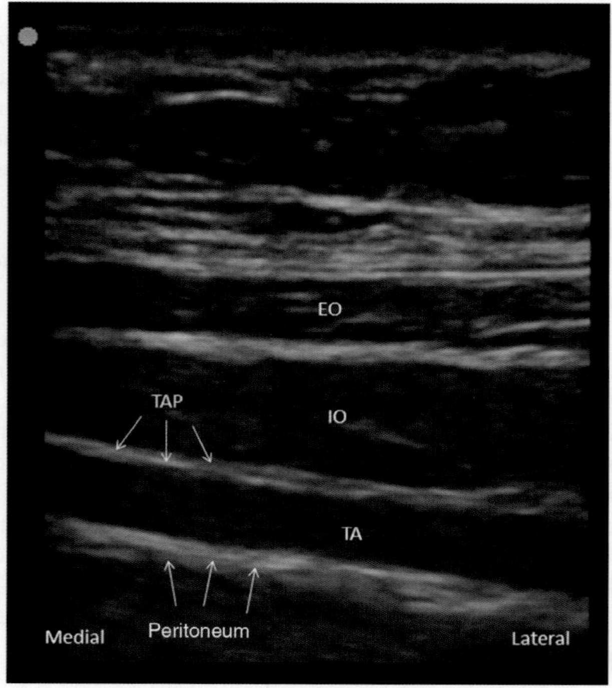

Figure 21.13 Ultrasound anatomy for the transversus abdominis plane block. EO, external oblique; IO, internal oblique; TA, transversus abdominis. The transversus abdominal plane (TAP) label indicates the injection target.

these nerves can facilitate analgesia following inguinal or scrotal surgery when combined with the genitofemoral nerve block. Optimal image view is obtained when the probe is aligned on an axis between the anterior superior iliac spine and umbilicus. Lateral injection can be preferred to avoid incidental peritoneal injury. Doppler can be useful in avoiding inadvertent vascular injection as small vessels often lie adjacent to these nerves.

IV. Anatomic Considerations for Lower Extremity Blockade

Blockade of the lumbar and sacral plexuses can be used for surgical anesthesia or analgesia of the lower extremities. When compared with neuraxial anesthesia, lower extremity peripheral nerve blocks provide prolonged analgesia without side effects such as hypotension, urinary retention, and contralateral muscle weakness. Due to the anatomic separation between the lumbar and sacral plexuses, a single injection cannot provide complete anesthesia of the entire lower extremity.

A. Lumbar Plexus

The lumbar plexus is formed from the ventral rami of nerve roots of T12 and L1-L4 bilaterally and gives rise to six major nerves: the femoral, obturator, lateral cutaneous, ilioinguinal, iliohypogastric, and genitofemoral nerves (**Figure 21.14**).

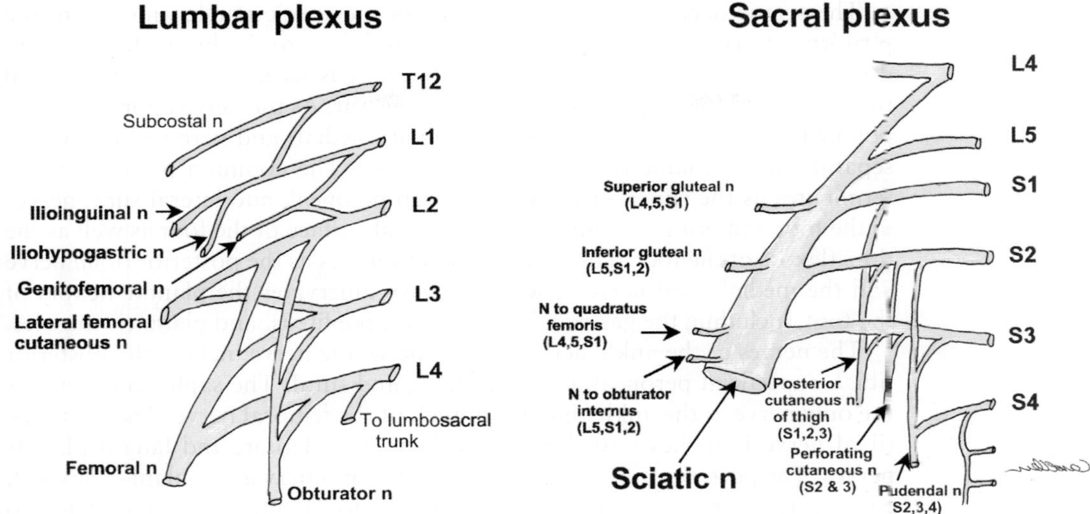

Figure 21.14 Anatomy of the lumbar and sacral plexuses. (From Tsui BCH, Rosenquist RW. Peripheral nerve blockade. In: Barash PG, Cahalan M, Cullen BF, et al, eds. *Clinical Anesthesia*. 8th ed. Wolters Kluwer; 2018:945-1002, Figure 36.13.)

The femoral nerve (L2-L4) is the largest nerve of the lumbar plexus. It provides the primary innervation to the knee and can be used for postoperative analgesia for total knee arthroplasty, anterior cruciate ligament repair, as well as surgery involving the patellar tendon. The femoral nerve sends motor branches to the quadriceps muscles and provides the cutaneous innervation for the anterior thigh and knee. The femoral nerve is located approximately 1 to 2 cm lateral to the femoral artery at the level of the inguinal crease. The terminal branch of the femoral nerve is the saphenous nerve, which innervates the skin of the medial knee, calf, and ankle, and can be blocked in the adductor canal with minimal motor weakness.

The obturator nerve (L2-L4) supplies the cutaneous innervation to the medial thigh and knee. The motor innervation of adductors of the leg (adductor longus, gracilis, adductor brevis, and pectineus) is to a variable extent supplied by the obturator nerve. The medial knee can be supplied by articular branches of the obturator nerve. The obturator nerve courses from the medial border of the psoas major muscle and then courses along the lateral wall of the pelvic cavity toward the obturator canal.

The genitofemoral nerve (L1-L2) supplies the cremaster muscle and skin over the scrotum in men and the anterior part of the labium majorus and mons pubis in women. The lateral cutaneous nerve (L2-L3) supplies the cutaneous innervation to the lateral thigh.

B. Sacral Plexus

The anterior rami of S1-S4 join the lumbosacral trunk after exiting the sacral foramina toward the sacral plexus. Various nerves are derived from the sacral plexus including the pudendal nerve, gluteal nerves, and pelvic splanchnic nerves, yet the nerves most relevant to lower extremity surgery are the sciatic nerve and the posterior cutaneous nerve of the thigh (**Figure 21.14**).

The sciatic nerve (L4-S3) passes through the sciatic notch, anterior to the piriformis muscle, and then travels lateral and deep to the biceps femoris tendon at the gluteal crease. At this level, the nerve is located between the ischial tuberosity and the greater trochanter of the femur. As the nerve approaches the popliteal fossa, the two components—tibial (medial) and peroneal (lateral)—separate at a variable distance from the knee. The common peroneal nerve terminates as the superficial peroneal, deep peroneal, and lateral sural nerves in the foot and primarily innervates the dorsal surface of the foot as well as the dorsiflexors of the foot. The tibial nerve terminates as the posterior tibial nerve and the medial sural nerve. The tibial nerve innervates the plantar flexors of the foot, including the gastrocnemius, soleus, popliteus, and plantaris muscles.

The nerves at the ankle derived from the sciatic nerve include the posterior tibial, superficial peroneal, deep peroneal, and sural. The saphenous nerve is the only nerve at the ankle that is a branch of the femoral nerve. The posterior tibial nerve branches into the calcaneal, medial plantar, and lateral plantar nerves. The posterior tibial nerve provides motor innervation (plantar flexors), cutaneous innervation (plantar surface of the foot), and bony innervation to the foot. The deep peroneal nerve provides cutaneous innervation to the web space between the first and second toe and terminates as the second, third, and fourth dorsal interosseous nerves. The superficial peroneal nerve provides the cutaneous innervation to the dorsum of the foot except for the lateral aspect of the dorsum, which is supplied by the sural nerve. The saphenous nerve supplies the cutaneous innervation to the medial ankle and foot.

V. Specific Techniques for the Lower Extremities

A. Psoas Compartment Block

The ***psoas compartment block*** is useful for unilateral hip or anterior leg surgery in combination with sciatic nerve block and is often performed with guidance of a nerve stimulator to obtain a quadriceps twitch response. This response is often obtained when a 100-mm insulated block needle is inserted 1 to 2 cm deep to the L4 (sometimes L3) transverse process. Due to the concern of hematoma, retroperitoneal bleeding, or epidural spread, careful consideration and monitoring in addition to an experienced practitioner are mandatory for safe and effective completion of this advanced block.

VIDEO 21.4
Ultrasound-guided Femoral Nerve Block

B. Femoral Nerve Block

The femoral nerve can be blocked at the level of the inguinal crease with or without ultrasound guidance. With the patient in the supine position, the femoral artery pulse is palpated. The needle insertion site for the landmark approach is 1 to 1.5 cm lateral to the femoral pulse with a slight cephalad trajectory of about 30°. The goal is to obtain a patellar or quadriceps response at <0.5 mA.

When performing the ***femoral nerve block*** with ultrasound, the femoral artery is visualized at the inguinal crease. The femoral nerve appears as a hyperechoic triangular structure lateral to the artery (**Figure 21.15**). Nerve stimulation can be used in combination with ultrasound to confirm a patellar or quadriceps response.

C. Saphenous Nerve Block

A ***saphenous nerve block*** can be performed for anesthesia of the medial calf and ankle. This block can be performed at the anterior midthigh level using ultrasound guidance by locating a hyperechoic structure adjacent to the superficial femoral artery, deep to the sartorius muscle (**Figure 21.16**).

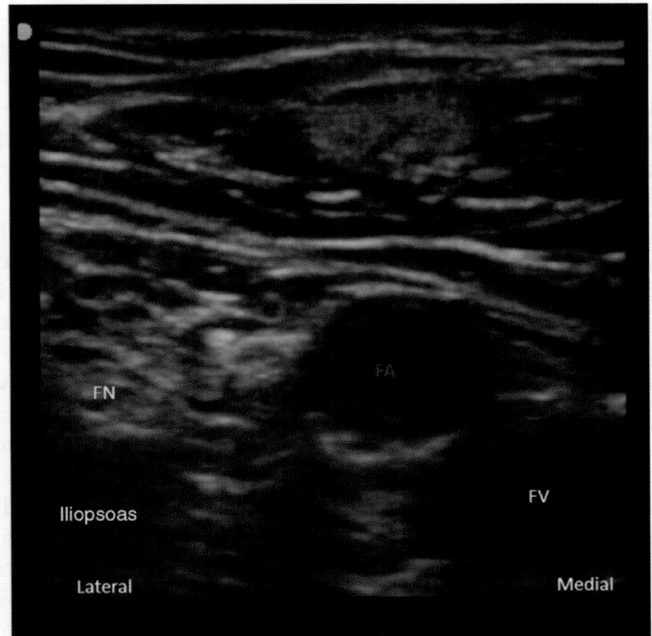

Figure 21.15 Ultrasound anatomy for the femoral nerve block. FA, femoral artery; FN, femoral nerve; FV, femoral vein.

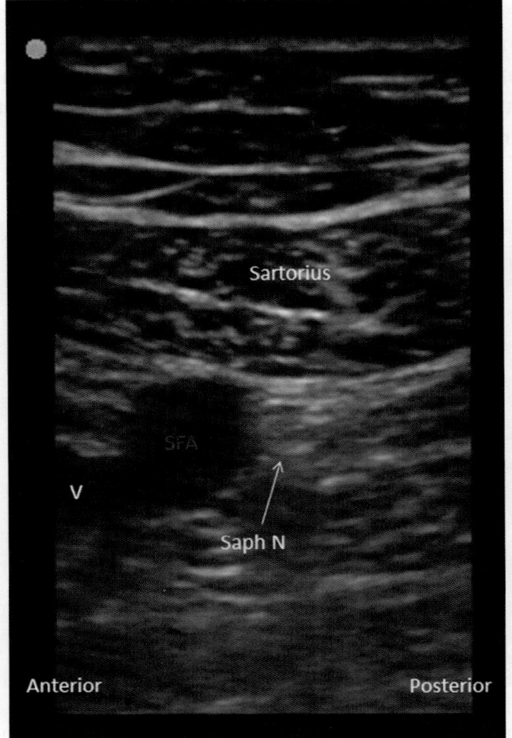

Figure 21.16 Ultrasound anatomy for the midthigh saphenous nerve block. SaphN, saphenous nerve; SFA, superficial femoral artery.

D. Sciatic Nerve Block

The ***sciatic nerve block*** provides complete anesthesia to the ankle and foot when combined with a saphenous nerve block. Surgeries such as mid- and hindfoot fusions, open reductions and internal fixations of ankle fractures, Achilles tendon repairs, and total ankle arthroplasties can all be performed with sciatic-saphenous nerve anesthesia with minimal intraoperative sedation required.

Classically the gluteal approach (Labat) has been used, but with the popularity of ultrasound and the ease of visualization of the sciatic nerve at the level of the gluteal crease, more distal approaches have come into favor. The landmarks for the gluteal approach include an oblique line from the posterior superior iliac spine to the greater trochanter of the femur with the patient in a semiprone position with the hip and knee flexed and the operative side up. A second line from the greater trochanter of the femur to the sacral hiatus is drawn. A third line, perpendicular to the first line, will cross the second line at the approximate needle entry point (**Figure 21.17**).

An ultrasound-guided subgluteal approach can be performed with the patient either lateral or prone. Either a high-frequency probe or a lower frequency probe can be used. Many high-frequency probes penetrate up to 6 cm, and thus, the vast majority of sciatic nerves may be visible with a high-frequency probe, reducing the need to switch probes between various blocks. The nerve is visualized slightly deep and lateral to the biceps femoris muscle (**Figure 21.18**). A nerve stimulator can be used to confirm proper identification of the sciatic nerve. A plantar flexion motor response in the foot indicates that the medial (tibial) component of the nerve is being stimulated. A dorsiflexion (common peroneal) or an eversion (superficial peroneal) response indicates the lateral components of the nerve are being stimulated. An inversion response is considered optimal and signifies that both components (tibial and peroneal) are being stimulated. Regardless of stimulation, local anesthetic spread should be visualized surrounding both components of the sciatic nerve.

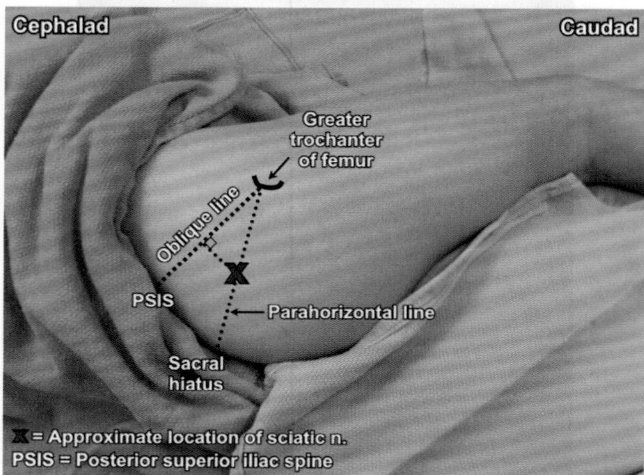

Figure 21.17 Surface anatomy for the gluteal (Labat) approach to the sciatic nerve. (From Tsui BCH, Rosenquist RW. Peripheral nerve blockade. In: Barash PG, Cahalan M, Cullen BF, et al, eds. *Clinical Anesthesia*. 8th ed. Wolters Kluwer; 2018:945-1002, Figure 36.38.)

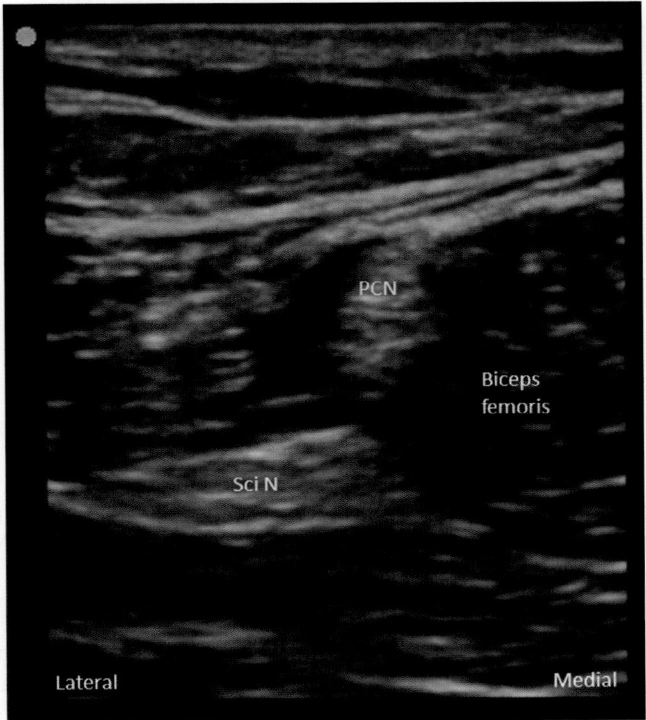

Figure 21.18 Ultrasound anatomy for the infragluteal sciatic nerve block. PCN, posterior cutaneous nerve of the thigh; SciN, sciatic nerve.

The popliteal block is a distal sciatic block performed proximal to the popliteal fossa. The nerve may be more superficial with the distal approaches, yet if the block is attempted distal to the bifurcation of the tibial and peroneal nerves, one of the two components may be missed. Blocking approximately 10 to 15 cm proximal to the popliteal crease usually ensures that the two components have joined. A simple technique to locate the sciatic nerve for a distal (popliteal) approach is to begin by visualizing the popliteal artery at the popliteal fossa. The tibial nerve will be located superficial and slightly lateral to the artery and appears hyperechoic. The tibial nerve can then be traced proximally, and the peroneal nerve can be seen joining the tibial component.

E. Ankle Block

Surgery on the distal foot, including bunion surgeries, can be performed with ***ankle block*** anesthesia. Many clinicians considered the ankle block to be a "field" block in the past, but the use of ultrasound has made ankle block anesthesia more precise.

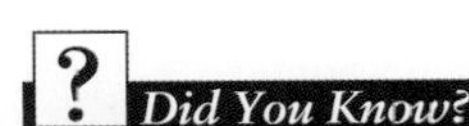

Did You Know?

Many clinicians formerly considered the ankle block to be a "field" block, but the use of ultrasound has made ankle block anesthesia more precise.

The posterior tibial nerve can be blocked using a high-frequency ultrasound probe. Scanning posterior to the medial malleolus, the posterior tibial nerve will be located slightly posterior and deep to the posterior tibial artery (**Figure 21.19**). The needle can be placed out of plane either superior or inferior to the probe. A nerve stimulator can be used to confirm identification of the nerve with toe flexion.

The deep peroneal nerve can be blocked between the upper borders of the medial and lateral malleoli, lateral to the anterior tibial artery (under

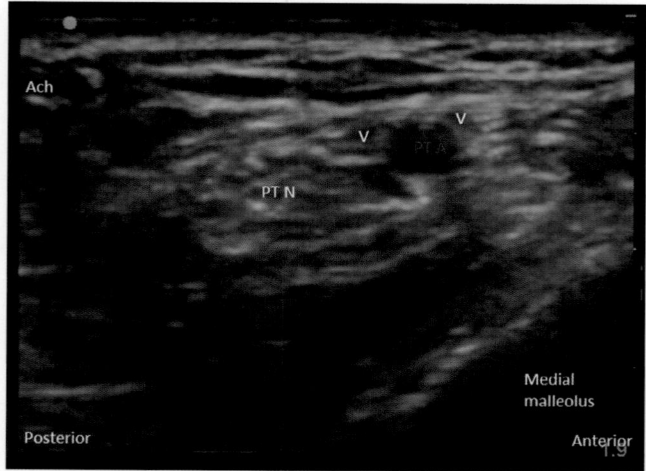

Figure 21.19 Ultrasound anatomy for the posterior tibial nerve at the level of the medial malleolus. Ach, Achilles tendon; PTA, posterior tibial artery; PTN, posterior tibial nerve; V, vein.

ultrasound). The superficial peroneal nerve can be blocked via subcutaneous ring between the medial and lateral malleoli. The saphenous and sural nerves are adjacent to the greater and lesser saphenous veins, respectively, and can be blocked by subcutaneous ring or ultrasound.

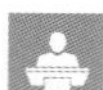

For further review and interactivities, please see the associated Interactive Video Lectures and "A Closer Look" infographic accessible in the complimentary eBook bundled with this text. Access instructions are located in the inside front cover

References

1. Liu SS, Ngeow JE, Yadeau JT. Ultrasound-guided regional anesthesia and analgesia: a qualitative systematic review. *Reg Anesth Pain Med.* 2009;34(1):47-59. PMID: 19258988.
2. Horlocker TT, Vandermeulen E, Kopp SL, Gogarten W, Leffert LR, Benzon HT. Regional anesthesia in the patient receiving antithrombotic or thrombolytic therapy American Society of Regional Anesthesia and Pain Medicine evidence-based guidelines (fourth edition). *Reg Anesth Pain Med.* 2018;43:263-309. PMID: 29561531.
3. Renes SH, Rettig HC, Gielen MJ, et al. Ultrasound-guided low-dose interscalene brachial plexus block reduces the incidence of hemidiaphragmatic paresis. *Reg Anesth Pain Med.* 2009;34(5):498-502. PMID: 19920426.
4. Urmey WF, Talts KH, Sharrock NE. One hundred percent incidence of hemidiaphragmatic paresis associated with interscalene brachial plexus anesthesia as diagnosed by ultrasonography. *Anesth Analg.* 1991;72(4):498-503. PMID: 2006740.
5. Soares LG, Brull R, Lai J, et al. Eight ball, corner pocket: the optimal needle position for ultrasound-guided supraclavicular block. *Reg Anesth Pain Med.* 2007;32(1):94-95. PMID: 17196502.
6. Brown DL, Cahill DR, Bridenbaugh LD. Supraclavicular nerve block: anatomic analysis of a method to prevent pneumothorax. *Anesth Analg.* 1993;76(3):530-534. PMID: 8452261.
7. Rodriguez J, Barcena M, Alvarez J. Restricted infraclavicular distribution of the local anesthetic solution after infraclavicular brachial plexus block. *Reg Anesth Pain Med.* 2003;28(1):33-36. PMID: 12567341.
8. Tsui BCH, Fonseca A, Munshey F, McFadyen G, Caruso TJ. The Erector Spinae Plane (ESP) block: a pooled review of 242 cases. *J Clin Anesth.* 2019;53:29-34. PMID: 30292068.

INTRAVENOUS REGIONAL ANESTHESIA

A CLOSER LOOK

Intravenous regional anesthesia (also referred to as a Bier block) is a simple, effective anesthetic plan for brief hand and forearm procedures limited to soft tissue dissection.

Remember to use only: **0.5% PRESERVATIVE - FREE LIDOCAINE**

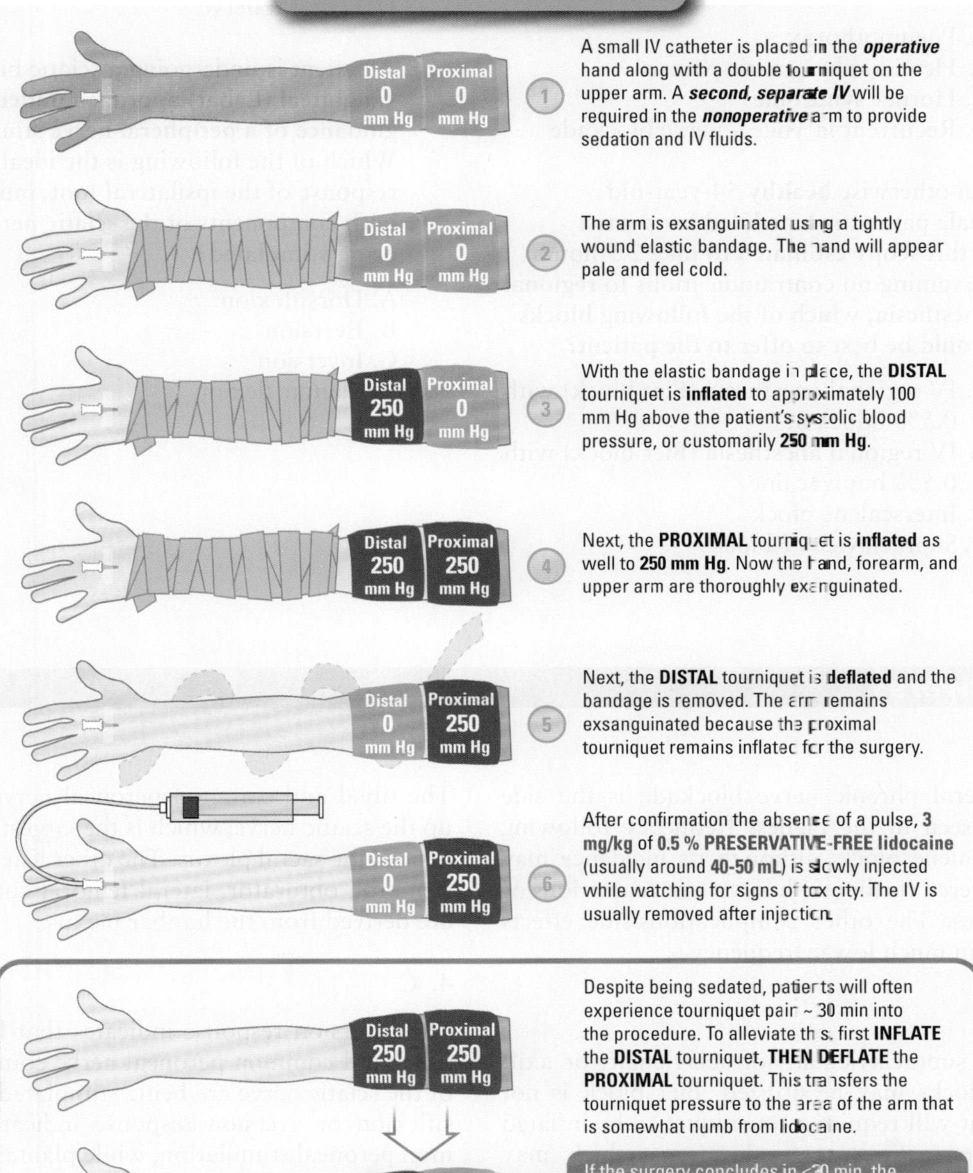

Distal
0
mm Hg
Proximal
0
mm Hg
1
A small IV catheter is placed in the operative hand along with a double tourniquet on the upper arm. A second, separate IV will be required in the nonoperative arm to provide sedation and IV fluids.
Distal
0
mm Hg
Proximal
0
mm Hg
2
The arm is exsanguinated using a tightly wound elastic bandage. The hand will appear pale and feel cold.
Distal
250
mm Hg
Proximal
0
mm Hg
3
With the elastic bandage in place, the DISTAL tourniquet is inflated to approximately 100 mm Hg above the patient's systolic blood pressure, or customarily 250 mm Hg.
Distal
250
mm Hg
Proximal
250
mm Hg
4
Next, the PROXIMAL tourniquet is inflated as well to 250 mm Hg. Now the hand, forearm, and upper arm are thoroughly exsanguinated.
Distal
0
mm Hg
Proximal
250
mm Hg
5
Next, the DISTAL tourniquet is deflated and the bandage is removed. The arm remains exsanguinated because the proximal tourniquet remains inflated for the surgery.
Distal
0
mm Hg
Proximal
250
mm Hg
6
After confirmation the absence of a pulse, 3 mg/kg of 0.5 % PRESERVATIVE-FREE lidocaine (usually around 40-50 mL) is slowly injected while watching for signs of toxicity. The IV is usually removed after injection.
Distal
250
mm Hg
Proximal
250
mm Hg
Distal
250
mm Hg
Proximal
0
mm Hg
Despite being sedated, patients will often experience tourniquet pain ~ 30 min into the procedure. To alleviate this, first INFLATE the DISTAL tourniquet, THEN DEFLATE the PROXIMAL tourniquet. This transfers the tourniquet pressure to the area of the arm that is somewhat numb from lidocaine.
If the surgery concludes in <20 min, the tourniquet should remain inflated for AT LEAST 20 min total. Afterward, repeated deflation/inflation of the tourniquet will slow the release of lidocaine into circulation.

Infographic by: Naveen Nathan MD

Questions

1. **An ultrasound-guided interscalene block is performed using 25 mL of 0.5% bupivacaine with a 22-gauge short-bevel stimulating needle. Which of the following side effects or complications is MOST likely to occur?**

   A. Pneumothorax
   B. Hemidiaphragmatic paresis
   C. Horner syndrome
   D. Recurrent laryngeal nerve blockade

2. **An otherwise healthy 54-year-old male patient is scheduled for a wrist arthroscopy estimated to take 2.5 hours. Assuming no contraindications to regional anesthesia, which of the following blocks would be best to offer to the patient?**

   A. IV regional anesthesia (Bier block) with 0.5% lidocaine
   B. IV regional anesthesia (Bier block) with 0.5% bupivacaine
   C. Interscalene block
   D. Supraclavicular block

3. **Which of the following nerves is originally derived from the sacral plexus?**

   A. Tibial and common peroneal nerves
   B. Obturator nerve
   C. Lateral femoral cutaneous nerve
   D. Femoral nerve

4. **A patient is undergoing a sciatic block via gluteal (Labat) approach under the guidance of a peripheral nerve stimulator. Which of the following is the ideal motor response of the ipsilateral foot, indicating both components of the sciatic nerve are being stimulated?**

   A. Dorsiflexion
   B. Eversion
   C. Inversion
   D. Plantar flexion

Answers

1. B

Unilateral phrenic nerve blockade is the side effect seen in the highest frequency following interscalene block, although its incidence may be lowered further with lower concentrations or volumes. The other complications/side effects occur in much lower frequency.

2. D

Either supraclavicular, infraclavicular, or axillary blocks may be utilized. Bier block is not ideal; it will require a tourniquet to be inflated for the entire surgery duration, which may place the patient at risk for limb ischemia. Bupivacaine should NEVER be injected intravascularly. Interscalene block, typically utilized for upper arm/shoulder surgery, will likely miss the inferior brachial plexus blockade (ulnar sparing) needed for this operation.

3. A

The tibial and common peroneal nerves make up the sciatic nerve, which is the largest component of the sacral plexus. The other listed nerves (femoral, obturator, lateral femoral cutaneous) are derived from the lumbar plexus.

4. C

The inversion response indicates that both the tibial and common peroneal nerve components of the sciatic nerve are being stimulated. A dorsiflexion or eversion response indicates common peroneal stimulation, while plantar flexion indicates tibial stimulation.

22 Patient Positioning and Potential Injuries

Bridget P. Pulos, Rebecca L. Johnson, and Mary E. Warner

The single most important principle of patient positioning is "to do no harm." Anesthesiologists often reduce or eliminate the ability of patients to sense the positions in which they have been placed for procedures by giving amnesic, analgesic, and anesthetic drugs. Thus, it is the responsibility of anesthesiologists, as well as other members of the surgical team, to ensure that patients are not placed into positions that may lead to injury.

I. Anesthesia and Sedation: So Different Than Regular Sleep

Many of us develop mild neuropathy or soft tissue injury when we sleep. We may awaken from sleep with tingling in the arm and hand due to ulnar nerve compression. The buttock soft tissues may be sore after awaking from prolonged sleep in a sitting position after a long air flight. Awakening allows us to reposition, reducing the tissue stretch and compression forces that caused our symptoms. Anesthesia and analgesics blunt the ability of patients to sense these symptoms and react by repositioning. Prolonged immobilization leads to the development of interstitial edema and inflammation in compressed tissue. These two factors exacerbate stretch and compression forces and, over time, may cause ischemia and more significant tissue damage.

Although most common, not all patient positioning problems involve mechanical forces on tissues. Some of the most catastrophic positioning injuries occur during procedures that require positions other than supine. For instance, the head elevated, "beach chair" position required for some shoulder or neurosurgical procedures may cause decreased brain perfusion, leading to stroke. Procedures performed in the prone positioning are associated with an increased risk of postoperative vision loss due to ischemic optic neuropathy, which may be caused by venous congestion in the optic canal. The lithotomy position is associated with the highest incidence of positioning-related lower extremity nerve injuries. Common peroneal injury may be caused by compression where the nerve wraps around the fibula; stretch-related sciatic nerve injury may be caused by excessive hip extension. Less commonly, venous engorgement of the lower extremities may cause hypoxic tissue damage and clinical compartment syndrome.

> **? Did You Know?**
>
> Based on data from the Anesthesia Closed Claims Project, peripheral nerve injury claims represent approximately 12% of claims since 1990.[1]

Perioperative positioning problems have not been well studied, and etiologic factors are not well defined. Although some etiologies are clear (eg, direct compression of a stoma in a prone-positioned patient that causes ischemia to

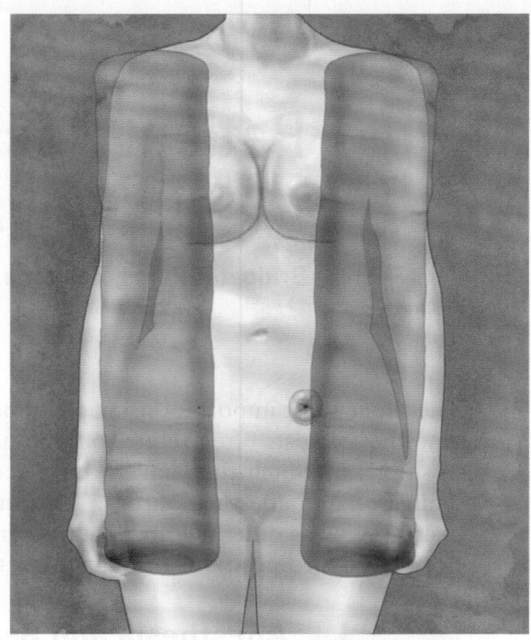

Figure 22.1 Soft tissues can be compressed and even become ischemic if there is too much pressure on them for long periods of time. This figure illustrates how chest rolls may compress the lateral aspects of large breasts or a stoma in prone-positioned patients.

the externalized stomal tissues), others are not as evident (**Figure 22.1**). Most patients who develop perioperative ulnar neuropathy do not become symptomatic until 2 to 5 days after their procedures.[2] However, direct compression to nerves should cause immediate ischemia and symptoms of neuropathy. Thus, it appears that factors beyond intraoperative positioning may be at play. Recent evidence indicates that many patients with new-onset ulnar neuropathy have systemic lymphatic microvasculitis of their peripheral nerves, which is treatable with corticosteroids.[3] These findings suggest that the perioperative inflammatory response associated with most surgical procedures may be a factor in the development of injuries formerly attributed to pressure-related positioning injury. This chapter explains the mechanisms common to perioperative soft tissue injuries.

II. Mechanisms of Soft Tissue Injury

A. Stretch

Peripheral nerves are vascularized by a complex of short nutrient arteries called the vasa nervosum (**Figure 22.2**). These minute arteries profusely anastomose to form an unbroken intraneural net. This net rarely leaves any particular segment of a peripheral nerve dependent on a single vessel for nutrient support. This net is not seen as commonly in central nerve tissue.

Stretch of nerve tissue, especially to more than 5% of resting length, may kink or reduce the lumens of feeding arterioles and draining venules.[4] This phenomenon can lead to direct ischemia from reduced arteriole blood flow, as well as indirect ischemia from venous congestion, increased intraneural pressure, and the need for high driving pressures for arteriolar blood flow. Prolonged periods of ischemia may cause transient or permanent nerve injury. The lack of extensive vascular nets in central nervous tissue suggests that stretch may be less well tolerated.

Soft tissue is usually less susceptible to stretch injury than nervous tissue. Soft tissue is often more compliant and elastic, and many peripheral soft tissues do not need the same level of blood flow as nervous tissue. Nonetheless, prolonged stretch of any soft tissue may result in ischemia and tissue injury. Unique perioperative patient positions may increase the risk of soft tissue stretch (eg, prone positions and their impact on breast tissue) (**Figure 22.1**).

B. Compression

Direct pressure on soft and nerve tissues may reduce local blood flow and disrupt cellular integrity, resulting in tissue edema, ischemia, and, if prolonged, necrosis. The impact is especially damaging to ischemic-susceptible tissue (eg, stomas associated with gastrointestinal diversions into cutaneous stomas) (**Figure 22.1**).

III. Common Perioperative Neuropathies

A. Upper Extremity Neuropathies

1. Ulnar Neuropathy

Ulnar neuropathy is the most common perioperative peripheral neuropathy (**Table 22.1**).[5] There are a number of factors that may be associated with ulnar neuropathy, including direct extrinsic nerve compression (often on the medial aspect of the elbow), intrinsic nerve compression (associated with prolonged elbow flexion), and inflammation. Key points of interest are as follows:

- ***Timing of postoperative symptoms:*** Most patients experience their first symptoms at least 24 hours postoperatively. This suggests that the mechanism of acute injury occurs primarily outside the operating room. Importantly, medical patients also develop ulnar neuropathies during hospitalization.
- ***Impact of elbow flexion:*** The ulnar nerve is the only major peripheral nerve in the body that always passes on the extensor side of a joint, in this case, the elbow. All other major peripheral nerves primarily pass on the flexion side of joints (eg, median and femoral nerves). This anatomic difference may contribute to the relatively higher rate of perioperative injury involving the ulnar nerve. In general, peripheral nerves begin to lose function and develop foci of ischemia when they are stretched >5% of their resting lengths. Elbow flexion, particularly >90°, stretches the ulnar nerve. Prolonged elbow flexion and stretch of the ulnar nerve can result in ischemia sufficient to cause symptoms in awake patients.

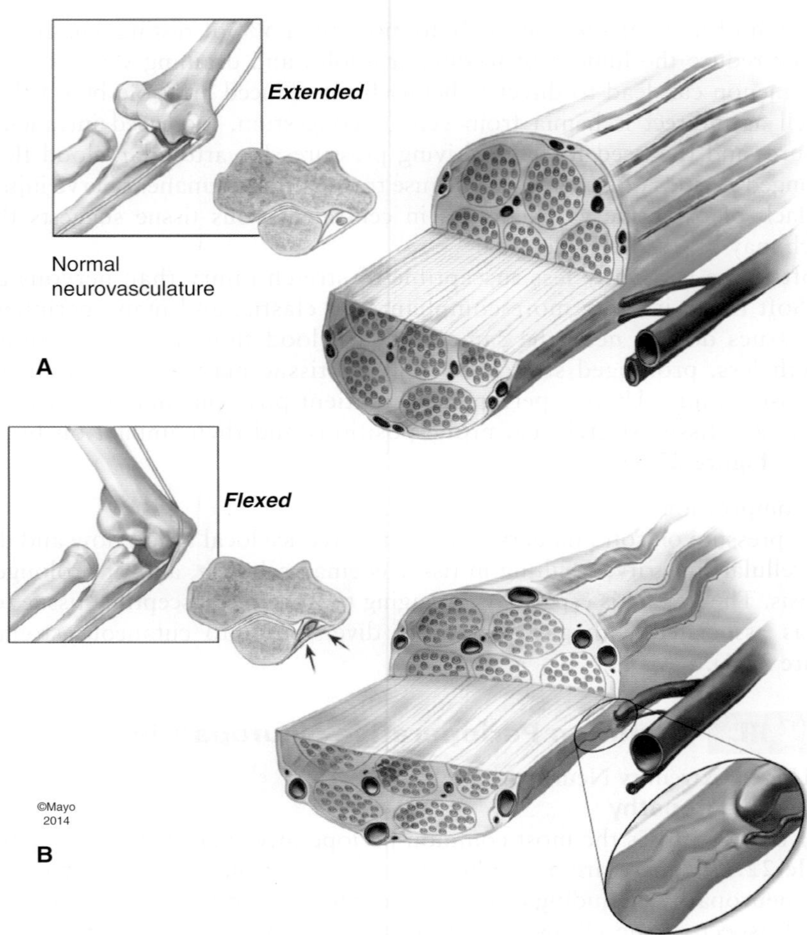

Figure 22.2 Effect of tissue stretch and compression on nerve vasa nervosum. This example shows potential ulnar nerve injury with elbow flexion. A, Extended elbow and relaxed ulnar nerve, noting patent perforating arterioles and venules. B, Flexed elbow, noting that stretch of the penetrating arterioles and venules from elongation of the ulnar nerve or compression by the cubital tunnel retinaculum can lead to vessel kinking and result in reduced arteriole blood flow from outside to inside the nerve (causing direct ischemia) and venous congestion from reduced venule outflow as vessel exits the nerve (leading to indirect ischemia). Prolonged ischemia can lead to nerve injury.

- *Anatomy and intrinsic pressure:* Prolonged elbow flexion of >90° increases intrinsic pressure on the nerve and may be as important an etiologic factor as prolonged extrinsic pressure.[6,7] The ulnar nerve passes behind the medial epicondyle and then runs under the aponeurosis that holds the two muscle bodies of the flexor carpi ulnaris together. The proximal edge of this aponeurosis is sufficiently thick, especially in men, to be separately named the cubital tunnel retinaculum. This retinaculum stretches from the medial epicondyle to the olecranon. Flexion of the elbow stretches the retinaculum and generates high pressures intrinsically on the nerve as it passes underneath (**Figures 22.3** and **22.4**).

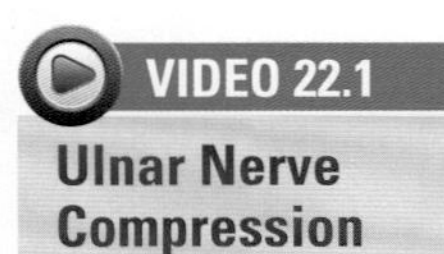

Table 22.1 Common Upper Extremity Neuropathies

Nerve	Presentation	Mechanism of Injury	Comments
Ulnar	• Numbness and tingling in fourth and fifth digits • Overall hand weakness, specifically weak opposition of thumb and fifth digit	• Mechanism often unknown • Potential factors include direct compression (medial aspect of elbow), intrinsic compression (associated with prolonged elbow flexion), or inflammation	• Most common upper extremity neuropathy • Most develop during postoperative rather than intraoperative period • More common in men, due to anatomic differences • Good prognosis for recovery if sensory symptoms only
Radial	• Numbness, tingling, and burning pain in the first through third digits • Weak hand grip and extension of the hand at the wrist and forearm at the elbow	• Most commonly thought to be due to direct compression in mid-humerus region • May also occur in supine position if arm slips off arm board and is unsupported	• Lateral positioning may increase pressure in mid-humerus region from overhead arm board • Relatively good prognosis
Median	• Numbness and tingling in the forearm, thumb, and second through fourth digits • Weak hand grip, flexion of the hand at the wrist, and pronation	• Often due to stretching of nerve with full extension of elbow in patients with shortened median nerve (eg, in body builders)	• More common in men, particularly patients with large biceps/reduced flexibility at the elbow • Providing forearm support for these patients to prevent full extension of elbow is key • Often involves motor symptoms with prolonged recovery
Brachial plexus	• Depending on the neural divisions most impacted, numbness and tingling of shoulder, arm, and/or hand • Weakness of the muscles of the shoulder and arm, along with reduced hand grip strength and weak hand flexion or extension at the wrist	• Susceptible to both stretch and compression • Can be caused by hyperextension of the shoulders • Prone and lateral positions may cause brachial plexus entrapment	• Most common after sternotomy • Often seen in patients with multiple risk factors, difficult to differentiate from surgical factors versus other causes

Data from Chui J, Murkin JM, Posner KL, Domino KB. Perioperative peripheral nerve injury after general anesthesia: a qualitative systematic review. *Anesth Analg*. 2018;127:134-143.

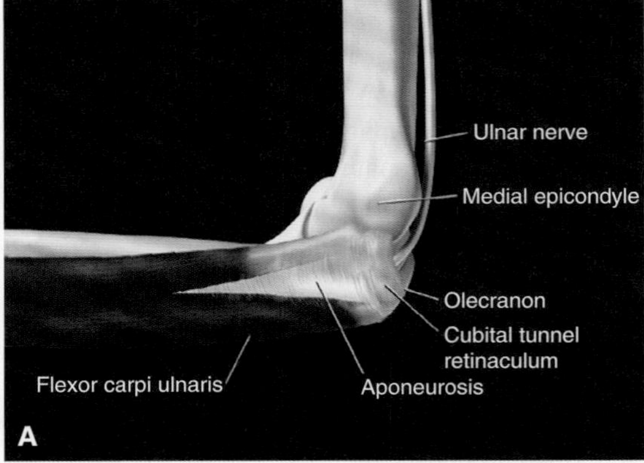

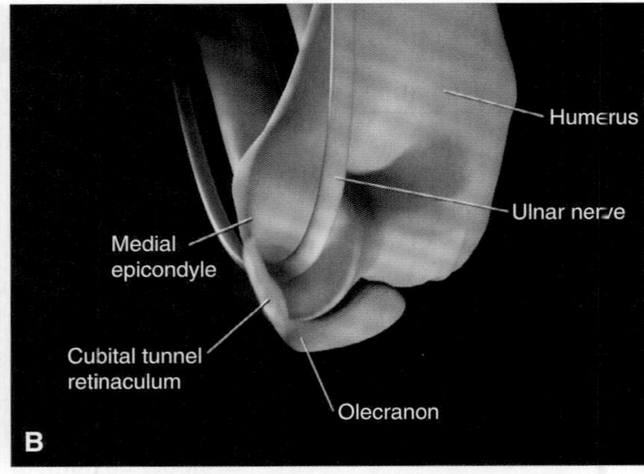

Figure 22.3 A, The ulnar nerve of the right arm passes distally behind the medial epicondyle and underneath the aponeurosis that holds the two heads of the flexor carpi ulnaris together. The proximal edge of the aponeurosis is sufficiently thick in 80% of men and 20% of women to be distinct anatomically from the remainder of the tissue. It is commonly called the cubital tunnel retinaculum. B, Viewed from behind, the cubital tunnel retinaculum intrinsically compresses the ulnar nerve when the elbow is progressively flexed beyond 90° and the distance between the olecranon and the medial epicondyle increases.

- *Forearm supination and ulnar neuropathy:* Supination of the forearm and hand does not, by itself, reduce the risk of ulnar neuropathy. The action of forearm supination occurs distal to the elbow. Supination is typically used when positioning arms on arm boards or at the patient's sides because of the impact it has on humerus rotation. That is, with forearm supination there will be external rotation of the humerus. It is this external rotation of the humerus that lifts the medical aspect of the elbow, including the ulnar nerve, from directly resting on the table or arm board surface. This rotation helps reduce extrinsic pressure on the ulnar nerve.
- *Outcomes of ulnar neuropathy:* Forty percent of sensory-only ulnar neuropathies resolve within 5 days; 80% resolve within 6 months. Few combined sensory and motor ulnar neuropathies resolve within 5 days, only 20% resolve within 6 months, and most result in permanent motor dysfunction and pain. The motor fibers in the ulnar nerve are primarily located in its middle. Injury at this depth of the nerve is likely associated with a more significant ischemic or pressure-related insult.

? *Did You Know?*

Ulnar neuropathy with sensory-only symptoms has a good prognosis. Most cases resolve spontaneously within a few days or months.

2. Median Neuropathies

Median neuropathies primarily occur in men between the ages of 20 and 40 years. These men often have large biceps and reduced flexibility (eg, as in the case of weightlifters) which compromise complete extension at the elbow. This limitation in range of motion results in shortening of the median nerve over time. Median neuropathies typically involve motor dysfunction and do not resolve readily. In fact, up to 80% of median neuropathies with motor dysfunction are sustained 2 years after initial onset. Key points of interest are as follows:

- *Stretch:* As mentioned previously, nerves become ischemic when stretched >5% of their resting length. This amount of stretch tends to kink penetrating arterioles and exiting venules, both of which decrease perfusion pressure.

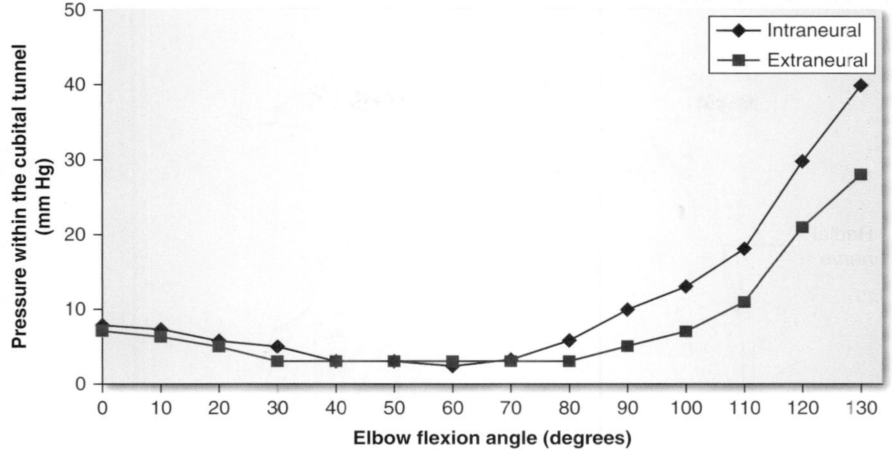

Figure 22.4 Pressure within the cubital reticulum at the elbow escalates once the angle of elbow flexion reaches and exceeds 90°. (From Gelberman RH, Yamaguchi K, Hollstien SB, et al. Changes in interstitial pressure and cross-sectional area of the cubital tunnel and of the ulnar nerve with flexion of the elbow. An experimental study in human cadavera. *J Bone Joint Surg.* 1998;80(4):492-501, with permission.)

- *Arm support:* Full extension at the elbow stretches chronically contracted median nerves and promotes ischemia. Thus, it is important that the forearm and hand be supported to prevent full extension, especially in men who have large, bulky biceps and who cannot fully extend their elbows because of a lack of flexibility.

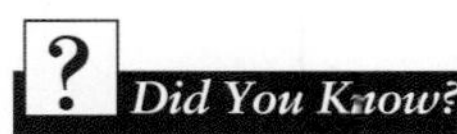

Muscular men with large biceps are susceptible to median nerve injury if the arm is fully extended during surgery.

3. Radial Neuropathies

Radial neuropathies occur more often than median neuropathies. The radial nerve appears to be injured by direct compression. The important factor appears to be compression of the nerve in the mid-humerus region, where it wraps posteriorly around the bone (**Figure 22.5**). Radial neuropathies tend to have a better prognosis than ulnar or median neuropathies. Approximately half get better within 6 months, and 70% appear to resolve completely within 2 years. Key points of interest are as follows:

- *Surgical retractors:* A case series reported several radial neuropathies associated with compression of the radial nerve by the vertical bars of upper abdominal retractor holders. These vertical support bars reportedly impinged the arms (**Figure 22.5A**).
- *Lateral positions:* The radial nerve may be impinged by overhead arm boards when they protrude into the mid-humerus soft tissue (**Figure 22.5D**).
- *An unsupported arm:* Compression of the radial nerve by the weight of the humerus may occur when a previously supported arm (either at the patient's side or on an arm board) slips and loses support particularly where vulnerable in the mid-humeral region. (**Figure 22.5E**).

4. Brachial Plexopathies

Brachial plexopathies occur most often in patients undergoing sternotomy, particularly with internal mammary artery mobilization. This finding is presumed to be associated with excessive concentric retraction on the chest wall and compression or stretch of the plexus between the clavicle and rib cage.

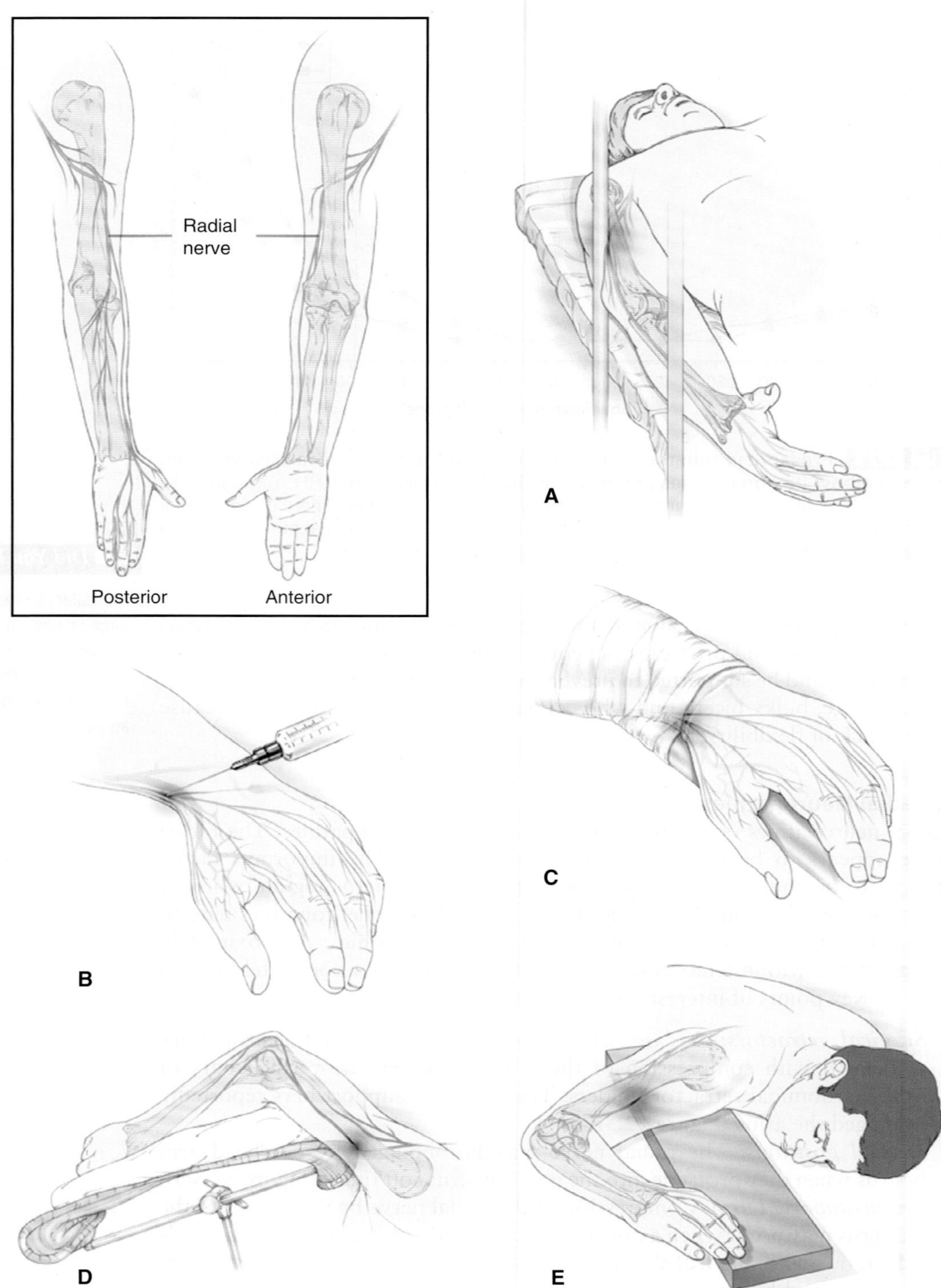

Figure 22.5 The anatomy of the radial nerve is shown in the upper left corner, illustrating how it wraps around the mid-humerus. Reported mechanisms of perioperative injury include (A) compression by surgical retractor support bar; (B) direct needle trauma at the wrist; (C) compressive tourniquet effect by a draw sheet at the wrist; (D) impingement by an overhead arm board; and (E) compression in the mid-humerus level as the arm supports much of the weight of the upper extremity.

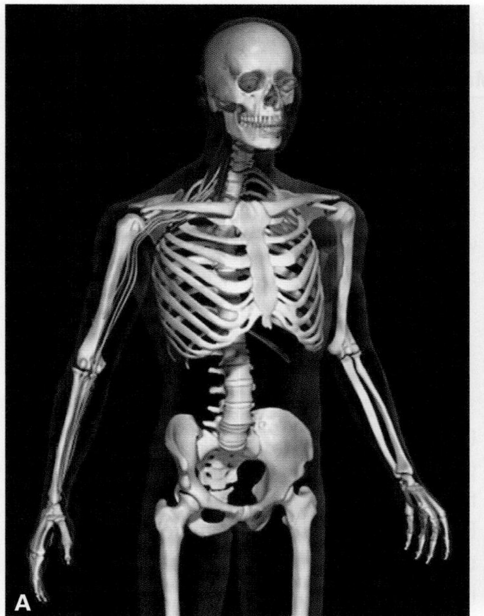

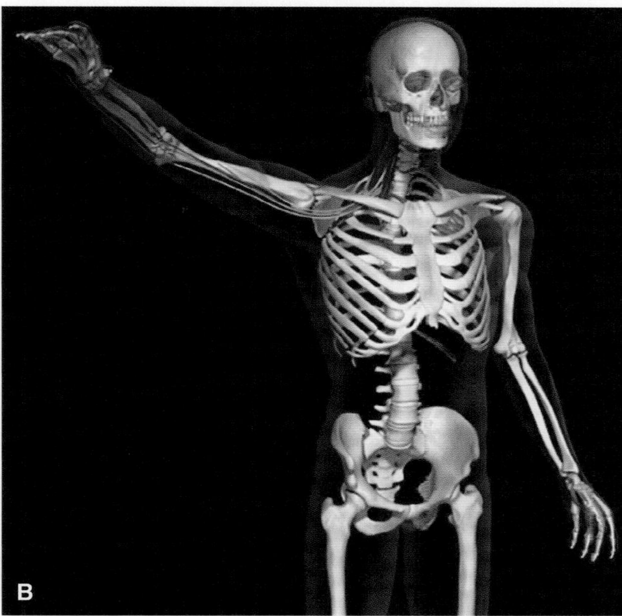

Figure 22.6 A, The neurovascular bundle to the upper extremity passes on the flexion side of the shoulder joint when the arm is at the side or abducted <90°. B, Abduction of the arm beyond 90° transitions the neurovascular bundle to where it now lies on the extension side of the shoulder joint. Progressive abduction >90° increases stretch on the nerves at the shoulder joint.

With the exception of sternotomy surgeries, brachial plexus injury is more common in surgeries performed in the prone or lateral position rather than the supine position. Key points of interest are as follows:

- ***Brachial plexus entrapment:*** The brachial plexus can become entrapped between the clavicle and the rib cage. Special attention should be given to altering positions that might exacerbate this potential problem.
- ***Prone positioning:*** In surgeries requiring the prone position, it is prudent to tuck the arms at the side if possible, as many patients have somatosensory-evoked potential changes when their arms are abducted (eg, a "surrender" position).
- ***Anatomy of shoulder abduction:*** Abduction of the shoulder >90° places the distal plexus on the extensor side of the joint and potentially stretches the plexus (**Figure 22.6**). Therefore, it is best to avoid abduction >90°, especially for extended periods.

B. Lower Extremity Neuropathies

Although common peroneal/fibular, and sciatic neuropathies have the most impact on ambulation, the most common perioperative neuropathies in the lower extremities involve the obturator and lateral femoral cutaneous nerves (**Table 22.2**). Key points of interest are as follows:

- ***Obturator neuropathy:*** Hip abduction >30° results in significant strain on the obturator nerve.[8] The nerve passes through the pelvis and out the obturator foramen. With hip abduction, the superior and lateral rim of the foramen serves as a fulcrum (**Figure 22.7**). The nerve stretches along

Table 22.2 Common Lower Extremity Neuropathies

Nerve	Presentation	Mechanism of Injury	Comments
Obturator	• Numbness, tingling, and pain in the medial thigh and groin, often extending to the medial aspect of the knee • Weak adduction	• Often due to nerve stretch as well as compression via obturator foramen when hip abducted >30°	• Most common lower extremity neuropathy • Most injuries are present immediately after emergence from anesthesia • Motor dysfunction is common and often long-lasting
Lateral femoral cutaneous	• Burning pain, itching, numbness, and tingling on the anterolateral aspect of the thigh	• Often due to prolonged hip flexion >90°, • Excess hip flexion causes stretch of inguinal ligament and compression of penetrating nerve fibers, resulting in nerve ischemia	• Nerve is sensory only, no motor disability • Pain/dysesthesia can be severe
Common peroneal/ fibular	• Pain, numbness, and tingling on the lateral lower limb and dorsal foot • Weak dorsiflexion of the foot and foot drop	• Most commonly associated with direct pressure on lateral leg • Potentially caused by leg holders, ie "candy canes"	• In severe cases, may cause permanent foot drop • Often causes devastating injury due to effects on ambulation

Data from Chui J, Murkin JM, Posner KL, Domino KB. Perioperative peripheral nerve injury after general anesthesia: a qualitative systematic review. *Anesth Analg*. 2018;127:134-143.

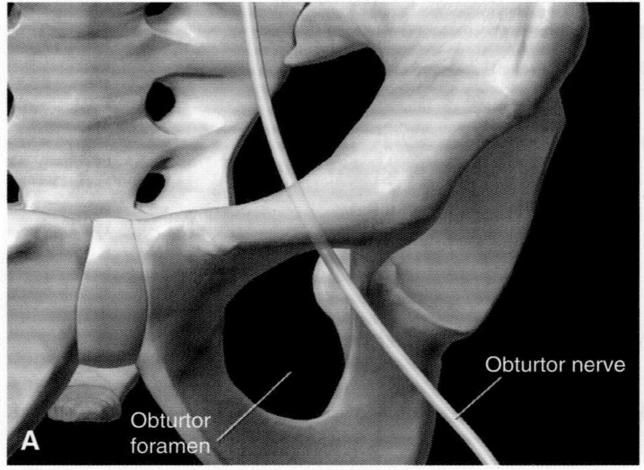

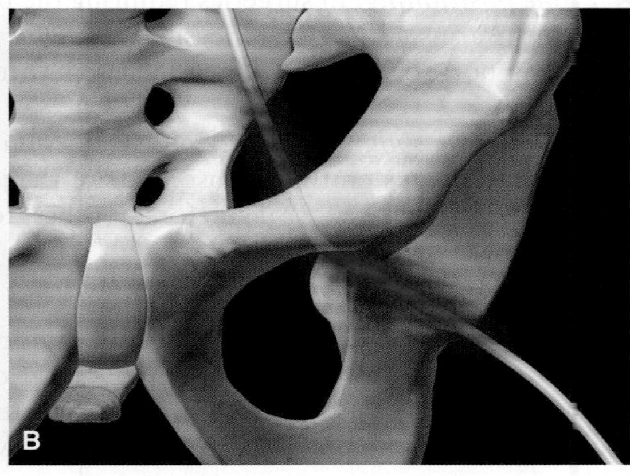

Figure 22.7 A, The obturator nerve passes through the pelvis and exits out the superior and lateral corner of the obturator foramen as it continues distally down the inner thigh. B, Abduction of the hip stretches the obturator nerve and can provoke ischemia, especially at the exit point of the obturator foramen. The point serves as a fulcrum for the nerve during hip abduction.

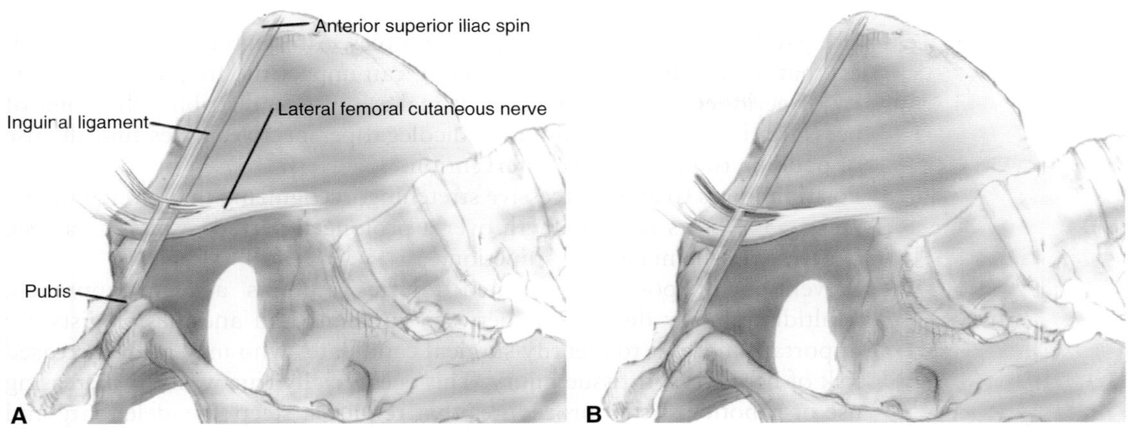

Figure 22.8 A, Approximately one-third of the lateral femoral cutaneous nerve fibers penetrate the inguinal ligament as the nerve passes out of the pelvis and distally into the lateral thigh. B, Hip flexion, especially when >90°, leads to stretch of the inguinal ligament as the ilium is displaced laterally. This stretch causes the intraligament pressure to increase and compresses the nerve fibers as they pass through the ligament.

its full length and is also compressed at this fulcrum point. Thus, excessive hip abduction should be avoided. With obturator neuropathy, motor dysfunction is common. Although it is usually not painful, it can be crippling. Approximately 50% of patients who have motor dysfunction in the perioperative period will continue to have it 2 years later.

- *Lateral femoral cutaneous neuropathy:* Prolonged hip flexion >90° increases ischemia on fibers of the lateral femoral cutaneous nerve. One-third of this nerve's fibers pass through the inguinal ligament as they enter the thigh (**Figure 22.8**). Hip flexion >90° results in lateral displacement of the anterior superior iliac spine and stretch of the inguinal ligament. The penetrating nerve fibers are compressed by this stretch and, with time, become ischemic and dysfunctional. The lateral femoral cutaneous nerve carries only sensory fibers, so there is no motor disability when it is injured. However, patients with this perioperative neuropathy can have disabling pain and dysesthesias of the lateral thigh. Approximately 40% of these patients have dysesthesias that last longer than 1 year.

- *Common peroneal/fibular neuropathy:* Most common peroneal/fibular neuropathies appear to be associated with direct pressure on the lateral leg just below the knee, where the common peroneal nerve wraps around the head of the fibula. Leg positioners, which include a range of styles ("candy cane," "crutch," and "stirrups") can impinge on the nerve as it wraps around the head of the fibula. Common peroneal/fibular neuropathy can have devastating results, including prolonged foot drop and difficulty ambulating.

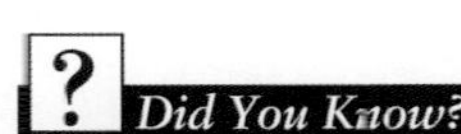

Great care must be exercised when positioning the lower extremities of an anesthetized patient. Excessive flexion or abduction of the hip can injure the lateral femoral cutaneous or obturator nerves, respectively.

IV. Practical Considerations to Prevent Perioperative Peripheral Neuropathies

There are several practical considerations that should be taken to prevent perioperative peripheral neuropathies. These include:

- Use padding to distribute compressive forces. Although there are few studies that demonstrate generous padding can impact the frequency or severity of perioperative neuropathies, it makes sense to distribute the point of pressure. Furthermore, from a medicolegal perspective, juries find the use of padding to be a positive intervention.
- Position joints to avoid excessive stretching, recognizing that stretch of any nerve >5% of its resting length over a prolonged period results in varying degrees of ischemia and dysfunction.
- Prevention of positioning-related injuries requires a team approach. Multidisciplinary discussions between surgeons and anesthesiologists are important in order to identify surgical candidates who may be at increased risk of nerve or soft tissue injury. This is especially true with the increasing use of robotic-assisted procedures that require a steep Trendelenburg and lithotomy positioning. Mills and colleagues have shown injuries to be more likely for case with median durations of ≥5.5 hours.[9] Teams should have heightened consideration for returning patients to the supine position as soon as possible after undocking of robotic arms.

The management of the patient with a new-onset peripheral neuropathy after surgery depends on the nature of the symptoms. If the loss is sensory only, it is reasonable to follow up with the patient daily for up to 5 days. Many sensory deficits in the immediate postoperative period will resolve during this time. If the deficit persists for longer than 5 days, it is likely that the neuropathy will have an extended impact. It is appropriate at that point to get a family physician, internist, or neurologist involved to provide long-term care. If the loss is motor or combined sensory and motor, it is prudent to get a neurologist involved early. These patients likely have a significant neuropathy and will need prolonged rehabilitative care.

V. Unique Positioning Problems With Catastrophic Results

A. Spinal Cord Ischemia With Hyperlordosis

This rare event occurs when patients undergoing pelvic procedures (eg, prostatectomy) are placed in a hyperlordotic position, with >15° of hyperflexion at the L2-3 interspace. This results in spinal cord ischemia, infarction, and devastating neurologic deficit. Magnetic resonance imaging is the most useful at detecting this condition. Operating room tables made in the United States are designed to limit hyperlordosis in supine patients, even when the table is maximally retroflexed with the kidney rest elevated. In almost all reported cases the table has been maximally retroflexed, the kidney rest has been elevated, and towels or blankets have been placed under the lower back to promote further anterior or forward pelvic tilt (to improve vision of deep pelvic structures). In general, anesthesiologists should not allow placement of materials under the lower back for this purpose.

B. Thoracic Outlet Obstruction

Thoracic outlet obstruction is a rare event that occurs when patients with this syndrome are positioned prone or, less commonly, laterally. In almost all reported cases, the shoulder has been abducted >90°. In that position, the vasculature to the upper extremity is either compressed between the clavicle and rib cage or between the anterior and middle scalene muscles. This entrapment of the vasculature leads to upper extremity ischemia. When prolonged, the results range from minor disability to severe tissue loss that requires forequarter amputation. Simple preoperative questions such as "Can you use your arms to work above your head for more than a minute?" can elicit a history of thoracic outlet obstruction and reduce the risk of this potentially devastating complication.

C. Steep Head-Down Positions

As surgeons gain experience with new technologies (eg, robotics for pelvic procedures), they often request steep head-down positions. These positions can be associated with cephalad shifting of the anesthetized patient on an operating room table. Cephalad shifting can lead to cervical plexopathies from stretch and subclavian vessel obstruction from compression. There are reports of patients sliding off operating room tables when they are placed in steep head-down positions and not properly secured. The cervical spine and cerebral injuries have been devastating to both patients and members of the surgical team. Although intracranial pressure also increases, it rarely results in a negative outcome. However, orofacial edema requires careful attention as it may compromise the airway. In addition, permanent vision loss may be caused by venous congestion in the optic canal leading to optic nerve ischemia.

D. Steep Head-Up Positions

The steep head-up position—also called the "beach chair" position—is used to facilitate surgeries involving the posterior cranial fossa and cervical spine as well as many shoulder procedures. In addition to the well-known risk of venous air embolism in the craniotomy patient, this position can have considerable hemodynamic impact, specifically on systemic and cerebral blood pressures.[10] Measuring mean arterial pressure at the level of the circle of Willis has been advised to maintain adequate cerebral perfusion pressure. In addition, a number of severe cases of brachial and cervical plexopathies have been reported. It appears that at least some of these plexopathies have been associated with nerve stretch or compression when patients have their heads fixated laterally during procedures.

E. Soft Tissue Problems

Skin and soft tissues are particularly vulnerable to sustained pressure, resulting in ischemia. Although there are many examples of this, several related to the prone position deserve special mention. Tissues in direct contact with rolls that extend from the shoulder girdle across the chest and to the pelvis may become ischemic with prolonged pressure (**Figure 22.1**). There are multiple cases of women with large breasts who have developed severe ischemia of one or both breasts because they had been pushed in between chest rolls. This pressure was sufficient to cause necrosis and sloughing. In most of these reported cases, the women subsequently underwent mastectomies. Similarly, ostomies have developed ischemia from pressure after they were placed in direct contact with these rolls.

VI. Summary

There are many potential etiologies of positioning injuries during surgery. Peripheral nerve injuries due to compression, stretch, or generalized ischemia are among the most common. Surgeries requiring a position other than supine are associated with an increased risk of nerve injury. Prevention is the most reliable way to reduce the risk of injuries. When possible, patients should position themselves while awake before administering sedatives or anesthesia. Pressure points should be carefully padded. Vigilance of the entire surgical team is required to minimize patient risk.

For further review and interactivities, please see the associated Interactive Video Lectures and "At a Glance" infographic accessible in the complimentary eBook bundled with this text. Access instructions are located in the inside front cover.

References

1. Chui J, Murkin JM, Posner KL, Domino KB. Perioperative peripheral nerve injury after general anesthesia: a qualitative systematic review. *Anesth Analg*. 2018;127:134-143. PMID: 29787414.
2. Warner MA, Warner DO, Matsumoto JY, et al. Ulnar neuropathy in surgical patients. *Anesthesiology*. 1999;90:54-59. PMID: 9915312.
3. Staff NP, Engelstad J, Klein CJ, et al. Post-surgical inflammatory neuropathy. *Brain*. 2010;133:2866-2880. PMID: 20846945.
4. Warner ME, Johnson RL. Patient positioning and related injuries. In: Barash PG, Cullen BF, Stoelting RK, et al, eds. *Clinical Anesthesia*. 8th ed. Wolters Kluwer; 2017:809-825.
5. Practice advisory for the prevention of perioperative peripheral neuropathies 2018. An updated report by the American Society of Anesthesiologists Task Force on prevention of perioperative peripheral neuropathies. *Anesthesiology*. 2018;128:11-26. PMID: 29116945.
6. Contreras MG, Warner MA, Charboneau WJ, et al. Anatomy of the ulnar nerve at the elbow: potential relationship of acute ulnar neuropathy to gender differences. *Clin Anat*. 1998;11:372-378. PMID: 9800916.
7. Gelberman RH, Yamaguchi K, Hollstien SB, et al. Changes in interstitial pressure and cross-sectional area of the cubital tunnel and of the ulnar nerve with flexion of the elbow. An experimental study in human cadavera. *J Bone Joint Surg*. 1998;80(4):492-501. PMID: 9563378.
8. Litwiller JP, Wells RE, Halliwill JR, et al. Effect of lithotomy positions on strain of the obturator and lateral femoral cutaneous nerves. *Clin Anat*. 2004;17:45-49. PMID: 14695587.
9. Mills JT, Burris MB, Warburton DJ, et al. Positioning injuries with robotic assisted urological surgery. *J Urol*. 2013;190:580-584. PMID: 23466240.
10. Lee LA, Caplan RA. APSF workshop: cerebral perfusion experts share views on management of head-up cases. *APSF Newsletter*. 2009-2010;24(4):45-48.

PERIOPERATIVE NERVE INJURIES

AT A GLANCE

Perioperatively, nerves are injured primarily through excessive stretch or compression.

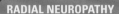

Compression injury

Stretch injury

Nerves become ischemic when stretched greater than **5%** of their resting length.

BRACHIAL PLEXOPATHY

- ↑ risk in prone and lateral positions
- High risk in patients undergoing sternotomy
- Plexus entrapped between clavicle and ribs
- AVOID arm abduction >90 °

RADIAL NEUROPATHY

- Compression in the midhumerus region
- Consider this with overhead arm boards in the lateral position
- Better chance of recovery than ulnar or median injuries

ULNAR NEUROPATHY

The most common neuropathy

- Symptoms typically appear >24 h
- Most likely occurs outside of the OR
- ↑ risk with elbow flexion >90°
- Nerve is stretched and compressed in cubital tunnel
- External rotation of humerus ↓ risk
- 80% of sensory-only neuropathies resolve in 6 m

MEDIAN NEUROPATHY

- Men between ages 20-40 y
- ↑ risk when the patient has large biceps and arm is extended
- Low chance of recovery
- Motor dysfunction common

LATERAL FEMORAL CUTANEOUS NEUROPATHY

- AVOID hip flexion >90°
- No motor dysfunction but quite painful

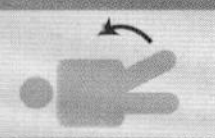

OBTURATOR NEUROPATHY

- AVOID hip abduction >30°
- Motor dysfunction common

PERONEAL NEUROPATHY

- AVOID pressure on head of fibula in leg holders
- Results in foot drop

Infographic by: Naveen Nathan MD

Questions

1. **Which of the following statements about ulnar neuropathies is NOT accurate?**

   A. Most ulnar neuropathies are caused by stretch of the nerve.
   B. More men than women experience postoperative ulnar neuropathies.
   C. A mild paresthesia (sensory-only) injury to the ulnar nerve will most likely resolve within 5 days after the injury.
   D. Many ulnar neuropathies may occur after surgery, rather than intraoperatively.

2. **Performing which action during surgical positioning could have the MOST potential detrimental consequences?**

   A. Removing the standard padding on the arm boards and replacing it with blankets when positioning a patient in the prone "surrender" position
   B. Adding a blanket on top of the kidney rest to further retroflex the patient
   C. Using bed extenders for obese patients
   D. Using gel pads on arm boards

3. **A 59-year-old develops foot drop after a gynecological procedure performed in the lithotomy position with "candy cane" leg holders. What nerve is most likely injured?**

   A. Obturator nerve
   B. Peroneal nerve
   C. Femoral nerve
   D. Lateral femoral cutaneous nerve

4. **A 43-year-old man undergoing nephrectomy for kidney donation awakens from general anesthesia experiencing numbness and tingling in his fourth and fifth fingers, which evolves over several hours to include an inability to oppose his fifth digit to this thumb. What is the most likely prognosis?**

   A. Full recovery within 5 days
   B. Full recovery within 6 months
   C. Recovery of motor but persistent sensory deficit
   D. A combined motor and sensory deficit that may be permanent

5. **A 73-year-old woman undergoing laparoscopic-assisted hysterectomy in lithotomy position complains of numbness (sensory-only) involving the outside of her left thigh. Which of the following nerves is MOST likely to have sustained injury?**

   A. Sciatic nerve
   B. Spinal cord
   C. Lateral femoral cutaneous nerve
   D. Ulnar nerve

6. **The mechanism of action most commonly associated with median nerve injury is:**

   A. Stretch.
   B. Compression.
   C. Ischemia.
   D. Inflammation.

7. **Brachial plexopathies are most commonly associated with what type of surgery?**

   A. Lumbar spine surgery in the prone position
   B. Total hip arthroplasty in the lateral position
   C. Vaginal hysterectomy in the lithotomy position
   D. Median sternotomy in the supine position

Answers

1. A

Ulnar neuropathy is the most common perioperative peripheral neuropathy. Compression rather than stretching appears to be the cause of most cases of perioperative ulnar neuropathy. Ulnar neuropathy is more common in men than women. Most patients experience symptoms within the first 24 hours after surgery, suggesting the mechanism of injury may occur outside the operating room. Patients who experience only mild sensory symptoms have a good prognosis.

2. B

Operating room tables are designed to limit hyperlordosis in supine patients, even when the table is maximally retroflexed with the kidney rest elevated. However, when extra padding is placed on top of the kidney rest, then hyperlordosis may be accentuated enough to cause spinal cord ischemia. All of the other interventions may be used to allow proper padding of pressure points.

3. B

Foot drop is a sign of peroneal neuropathy, which can develop as a complication of surgeries performed with leg holders, due to direct pressure of the lateral leg below the knee, where the peroneal nerve wraps around the head of the fibula. Obturator nerve injury is associated with impaired hip adduction. Femoral nerve damage is rarely associated with positioning but rather direct trauma to the nerve caused by surgical manipulation. Femoral nerve injury can cause numbness in the thighs and weakness of the leg muscles. Lateral femoral cutaneous nerve injury manifests as numbness and dysesthesias in the lateral thigh. This injury is most commonly caused by prolonged hip flexion >90°.

4. D

The patient's presentation is consistent with ulnar neuropathy. Few combined sensory and motor ulnar neuropathies resolve within 5 days, only 20% resolve within 6 months, and most result in permanent motor dysfunction and pain.

5. C

Pain and dysesthesias of the lateral thigh are suggestive of injury to the lateral femoral cutaneous nerve. This is a relatively common lower extremity neuropathy that may develop during procedures that require prolonged hip flexion beyond 90°.

6. A

Median nerve injury is most commonly caused by excessive stretching, which causes ischemia to the nerve.

7. D

Brachial plexopathies are most commonly associated with sternotomy procedures.

23 Fluids and Electrolytes

Trefan Archibald and Aaron M. Joffe

I. Acid-Base Interpretation and Treatment

A. Overview of Acid-Base Equilibrium

Precise regulation of ***blood pH*** is necessary for maintaining physiologic homeostasis. Outside of the normal physiologic range (7.35-7.45), vital functions such as oxygen transport, organ perfusion, and cellular metabolism may become impaired. At extremes of pH (<6.8 or >7.8), basic cellular processes are so impaired as to be incompatible with life.

The body is presented with significant acid and alkali loads daily, largely a consequence of nutrient intake and cellular metabolism. Nonetheless the blood pH remains stable through buffering of ***hydrogen ions (H^+)*** in the blood, their excretion by the kidneys (see Chapter 5), and elimination of ***carbon dioxide (CO_2)*** by the lungs (see Chapter 2). The amount of H^+ in the blood is determined by the ratio of CO_2 and ***bicarbonate*** (hydrogen carbonate, HCO_3^-) as represented by the ***Henderson-Hasselbalch equation*** (**Equation 23.1**):

$$H^+ = (24 \times PCO_2)/HCO_3^- \tag{23.1}$$

> **? Did You Know?**
>
> Acidemia and alkalemia refer to a low or high blood pH irrespective of the cause of the acid-base disturbance. Acidosis or alkalosis refers to the primary processes responsible for the alterations in pH, such as metabolic acidosis or respiratory alkalosis.

Accumulation of H^+ or HCO_3^- due to exhaustion of body buffers or dysregulation by the kidneys results in ***metabolic*** disturbances, whereas high or low arterial CO_2 results from ***respiratory*** disturbances. Note the semantic difference between an "***–emia***" and an "***–osis.***" ***Acidemia*** and ***alkalemia*** refer to a low or high blood pH, respectively. ***Acidosis*** or ***alkalosis*** refers to the primary processes responsible for the alterations in pH (**Figure 23.1**). Only one ***–emia*** can ever be present at one time, while more than one ***–osis*** can coexist.

B. Metabolic Acidosis

Primary ***metabolic acidosis*** is characterized by an arterial pH <7.35 and HCO_3^- <22 mEq/L and occurs as a result of either accumulation of H^+ or a loss of HCO_3^-. The nature of the acidosis can be further characterized by the presence or absence of a greater than expected concentration of unmeasured anions (high gap or normal gap, respectively). Because the plasma normally contains more unmeasured anions than cations, an ***anion gap (AG)*** in the 6 to 11 mEq/L range is normally present. Calculation of the AG is determined with the following equation:

$$AG = Na^+ - \left(Cl^- + HCO_3^-\right) \tag{23.2}$$

where Na^+ is the sodium ion and Cl^- is the chloride ion.

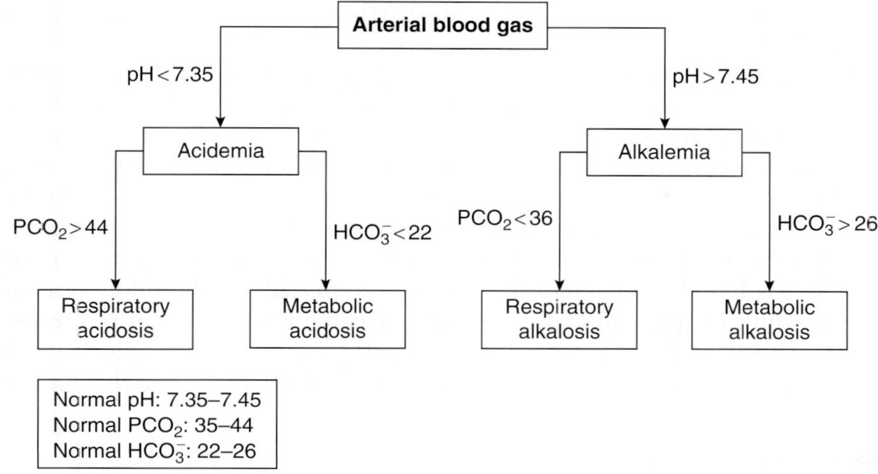

Figure 23.1 Derangements in acid-base status can be derived from arterial blood gas analysis by first determining acidemia or alkalemia from the pH, and then assessing the respiratory and metabolic components of the derangement from the P_{CO_2} and HCO_3^- values (see text and **Table 23.6** for details). HCO_3^-, hydrogen carbonate; P_{CO_2}, partial pressure of carbon dioxide.

An elevated AG develops when an acid accumulates and then dissociates into a proton (H^+) and the unmeasured anion (UA^-). The proton is titrated by HCO_3^-, decreasing its concentration, while the UA^- remains in the plasma. Because neither the Na^+ nor the Cl^- changes, the AG increases (**Equations** 23.2 and 23.3):

$$H^+ + HCO_3^- \rightarrow H_2O + CO_2 \quad (23.3)$$

The most common causes of ***high AG metabolic acidosis (HAGMA)*** include ketoacidosis, uremia, lactic acidosis, and a variety of toxins including methanol, salicylates, paraldehydes, and ethylene glycol (**Table 23.1**). ***Nonanion gap metabolic acidosis (NAGMA)*** results when HCO_3^- is lost from the gastrointestinal tract or kidneys or due to an inability of the kidneys to excrete protons. Because electroneutrality is maintained by Cl^- retention, the AG remains unchanged. The most common causes of NAGMA are excessive

Table 23.1 Causes of Metabolic Acidosis

High Anion Gap
Ketones—diabetes, starvation **U**remia **L**actate—sepsis, hypovolemia, congestive heart failure **T**oxins—methanol, ethylene glycol, paraldehydes, salicylates, isoniazid
Nonanion Gap
Hyperchloremia (excessive saline administration) Renal tubular acidosis Gastrointestinal losses (diarrhea, ileostomy)

administration of 0.9% NaCl solution, diarrhea, and renal tubular acidosis (**Table 23.1**).

Treatment of metabolic acidosis should be directed toward correcting the underlying cause. For example, in the case of a NAGMA due to 0.9% NaCl administration, the Cl^- load can be reduced with balanced lactate solutions for resuscitation or by adding 150 mL of 8.4% $NaHCO_3$ to a 1000-mL bag of 5% dextrose in water. Antidiarrheal medications can be given, and in cases of severe diarrhea where HCO_3^- losses are significant, administration of sodium bicarbonate can be considered. Treatment for HAGMA is based on the underlying cause. ***Ketoacidosis*** should be treated with insulin therapy, and ***lactic acidosis*** is treated with oxygenation, resuscitation, and cardiovascular support. Treatment of lactic acidosis with sodium bicarbonate is not recommended unless pH is <7.15 and the patient is clinically deteriorating.[1,2]

C. Metabolic Alkalosis

Metabolic alkalosis is characterized by an arterial pH >7.45 (alkalemia) and HCO_3^- >26 mEq/L. This disorder results from a net gain of HCO_3^- or loss of H^+ ions. The kidney has a tremendous ability to excrete HCO_3^-, so metabolic alkalosis must not only be generated but also maintained, usually by obligatory $NaHCO_3^-$ reabsorption in the proximal tubule in the setting of hypovolemia. Severe hypokalemia from any cause may also lead to HCO_3^- retention. Loss of H^+ ions usually results from significant vomiting or renal excretion, as suggested by a history of vomiting or diuretic use. Urine electrolytes (notably urine Cl^-) are used to further characterize the metabolic alkalosis. Low urine Cl^- is considered saline responsive, whereas normal or high urine Cl^- is saline unresponsive. The most common causes of metabolic alkalosis are listed in **Table 23.2**.

Treatment of metabolic alkalosis is based on correcting the underlying cause. Saline responsive metabolic alkalosis should receive resuscitation with sodium and potassium chloride to enable to kidneys to resume HCO_3^- excretion.

D. Respiratory Acidosis

Respiratory acidosis is defined as an arterial pH <7.35 and partial pressure of CO_2 (Pco_2) >44 mm Hg. An increase in CO_2 will result in more H^+ ions, decreasing the pH (**Equation 23.3**). Arterial CO_2 levels reflect the balance between CO_2 production via cellular respiration and its excretion through alveolar ventilation. It should be noted that increased production alone would rarely be the cause of respiratory acidosis, as healthy spontaneously breathing individuals have the ability to increase their alveolar ventilation. The most common causes of respiratory acidosis are listed in **Table 23.3**. Respiratory acidosis can be further classified as acute or chronic based on the presence and extent of renal compensation (see the section that follows).

Table 23.2 Causes of Metabolic Alkalosis

Low Urine Cl^- (Saline Responsive)	Normal or High Urine Cl^- (Saline Unresponsive)
Vomiting	Primary aldosteronism
Nasogastric suctioning	Renal failure
Hypokalemia	Cushing syndrome
Diuretic use	Hypomagnesemia

Table 23.3 Causes of Respiratory Acidosis
Decreased CO_2 Elimination
Pulmonary disease (acute respiratory distress syndrome, pneumonia)
Airway obstruction (laryngospasm, asthma, obstructive sleep apnea)
Central nervous system depression (opioids, anesthetics)
Neuromuscular weakness (amyotrophic lateral sclerosis, Guillain-Barre syndrome, residual drug-induced paralysis)
Increased CO_2 Production
Laparoscopy
Exhausted soda lime
Sepsis
Fever
Hyperthyroidism
Overfeeding
Malignant hyperthermia
Neuroleptic malignant syndrome
Increased Inspired CO_2
Exhausted soda lime (circle breathing system)

Treatment of respiratory acidosis relies on identification of the underlying cause. The most common interventions include supporting increased alveolar ventilation by institution of noninvasive or invasive mechanical ventilation or reversal of respiratory depressant medications. Avoiding high carbohydrate foods and providing sedative medications will decrease metabolic CO_2 production. Sodium bicarbonate is not recommended, as it offers no proven benefit and can worsen the hypercapnea by producing more CO_2 (**Equation 23.3**).

E. Respiratory Alkalosis

Respiratory alkalosis is defined as an arterial pH >7.45 and P_{CO_2} <36 mm Hg. Because arterial partial pressure of CO_2 (Pa_{CO_2}) is inversely proportional to alveolar ventilation, respiratory alkalosis results from low Pa_{CO_2} due to inappropriate alveolar hyperventilation. **Equation 23.3** demonstrates that a decrease in CO_2 results in fewer H^+ ions and therefore an increase in pH. The most common causes of respiratory alkalosis are listed in **Table 23.4**. Treatment is to identify the underlying cause and provide appropriate treatment.

Table 23.4 Causes of Respiratory Alkalosis
Pain
Hyperventilation
Pregnancy
Hypoxia
Central nervous system disease
Medications
Liver disease

Table 23.5 Physiologic Compensation for Acid-Base Disturbances

Primary Disorder	Disturbance	Compensation
Metabolic alkalosis	↑ HCO_3	P_{CO_2} ↑ 0.5-0.7 mm Hg per 1 mEq/L ↑ HCO_3^-
Metabolic acidosis	↓ HCO_3	P_{CO_2} ↓ 1.2 mm Hg per 1 mEq/L ↓ HCO_3^-
Respiratory alkalosis		
Acute	↓ P_{CO_2}	HCO_3^- ↓ 2 mEq/L per 10 mm Hg
Chronic	↓ P_{CO_2}	↓ P_{CO_2} HCO_3^- ↓ 5-6 mEq/L per 10 mm Hg ↓ P_{CO_2}
Respiratory acidosis		
Acute	↑ P_{CO_2}	HCO_3^- ↑ 1 mEq/L per 10 mm Hg
Chronic	↑ P_{CO_2}	↑ P_{CO_2} HCO_3^- ↑ 4-5 mEq/L per 10 mm Hg ↑ P_{CO_2}

HCO_3^-, hydrogen carbonate; P_{CO_2}, partial pressure of carbon dioxide.

F. Physiologic Compensation of Acid-Base Disorders

Primary metabolic disorders lead to ***respiratory compensation*** and vice versa. Respiratory compensation is quite swift. Rapid increases in alveolar ventilation can normalize pH in a matter of minutes. Conversely, ***metabolic compensation*** for respiratory disorders takes hours to days, as it requires the kidneys to alter plasma HCO_3^- levels. Most compensatory responses are quite effective, although respiratory compensation for metabolic alkalosis requires alveolar hypoventilation to increase P_{CO_2}, but it is limited to a maximum of 75% due to the resulting hypoxemia that occurs. A list of the normal compensatory responses expected for the acid-base disturbances is provided in **Table 23.5**.

II. Practical Approach to Acid-Base Interpretation

Arterial blood gas (ABG) analysis is primarily used to assess adequacy of gas exchange and oxygen delivery. It is the most frequently ordered test in anesthetized and critically ill patients to guide ventilation and treatment, and it provides data including pH, arterial partial pressure of oxygen (Pa_{O_2}), Pa_{CO_2}, and HCO_3^-. Analysis of these values can be used to determine whether an acid-base disturbance exists, what the disturbance is, and its possible etiologies. Thus, the understanding and ability to quickly analyze ABG data are crucial for every anesthesiologist.

A simple acid-base disorder, typically one of the metabolic or respiratory disturbances occurring in isolation, is the most common clinical presentation. However, critically ill patients can have multiple acid-base disorders. Physiologic compensation is never complete; thus the pH will never be completely normal in a simple acid-base disorder. However, in the presence of multiple acid-base disturbances, the pH can normalize or reach life-threatening extremes.

ABG analysis is best approached systematically to ensure rapid and precise interpretation. One common, stepwise method is based on the Henderson-Hasselbalch equation; it analyzes the pH, Pa_{CO_2}, HCO_3^-, AG, and presence of compensation (**Table 23.6**).

Table 23.6 Stepwise Approach to Arterial Blood Gas Analysis

Step 1: Examine the pH to determine whether academia or alkalemia is present: If the pH is <7.35, a primary acidemia present If the pH is >7.45, a primary alkalemia is present
Step 2: Examine the $Paco_2$ to determine if the primary disturbance is respiratory or metabolic: If acidemia is present: $Paco_2$ >40 mm Hg = respiratory acidosis; $Paco_2$ <40 mm Hg = metabolic acidosis (proceed to Step 3) If alkalemia is present: $Paco_2$ >40 mm Hg = metabolic alkalosis; $Paco_2$ <40 mm Hg = respiratory alkalosis (proceed to Step 4)
Step 3 (acidemia only): Calculate the anion gap (AG): AG = $Na^+ - (Cl^- + HCO_3^-)$; if AG >11, then a "high anion gap metabolic acidosis" is present (see **Table 23.1**)
Step 4: Determine if appropriate compensation is present to assess whether the disturbance is acute or chronic: See **Table 23.5**
Step 5: Determine likely etiologies of the acid-base disturbance: See **Tables 23.1-23.4**

Cl, chlorine; HCO_3^-, hydrogen carbonate; Na, sodium; $Paco_2$, arterial partial pressure of carbon dioxide.

A typical perioperative clinical scenario illustrating the application of this stepwise method is shown in the *Clinical Scenario* that follows.

Clinical Scenario: Arterial Blood Gas Interpretation

A 52-year-old, morbidly obese woman with diabetes presents to the operating room for emergent debridement of a necrotizing soft tissue infection of her left foot, with the following preoperative ABG (room air):

ABG: pH 7.10, $Paco_2$ 28 mm Hg, Pao_2 88 mm Hg, HCO_3^- 11 mEq/L, Na^+ 136 mEq/L, K^+ 5.5 mEq/L, Cl^- 99 mEq/L, lactate 14 mmol/L

Step 1: because the pH is <7.35, acidemia is present.

Step 2: because the $Paco_2$ is <40, a primary metabolic acidosis is present.

Step 3: because the anion gap is [136 − (99 + 11)] 26, a "high anion gap" metabolic acidosis is present.

Step 4: because the $Paco_2$ is appropriately decreased (HCO_3^- is 13 mEq/L below the normal of 24 mEq/L; 13 × 1.2 mm Hg = 15.6 mm Hg; 28 + 15.6 = 43.6 mm Hg), a compensated metabolic acidosis is present.

Step 5: The patient has a severe soft tissue infection and systemic sepsis, with impaired tissue oxygen use resulting in anaerobic metabolism and accumulation of lactic acid, leading to a compensated, high anion gap, metabolic acidosis.

III. Physiology of Fluid Management

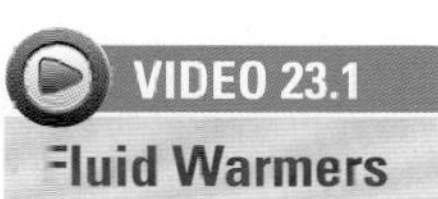

The kidneys play several key roles in maintaining homeostasis in the human body. In addition to maintaining normal acid-base status, the kidneys must regulate total body water and solute because daily intake of each is variable. Improper regulation can result in too little body water (cellular dehydration) or too much body water (tissue edema). Similar regulation occurs when patients have no oral intake and instead are receiving intravenous fluid (ie, water with dissolved solute). A thorough knowledge of how administered fluids are distributed among the various body compartments, as well as their individual components, is essential. Intravenous fluid should be considered like any other pharmaceutics insofar as there are specific indications and clinical contexts that determine proper fluid therapy. For example, patients residing in the intensive care unit or presenting to the operating room may have low extracellular fluid volume, cellular dehydration, or both as a result of major trauma, hemorrhage, prolonged fasting or malnutrition, or protracted vomiting or diarrhea. Both the choice of fluid composition and its infusion rate are dictated accordingly, in this case, most likely high-volume resuscitation with isotonic crystalloid. The anesthesiologist must take into account such clinical contexts and pathophysiologies when tailoring fluid management for a given patient.

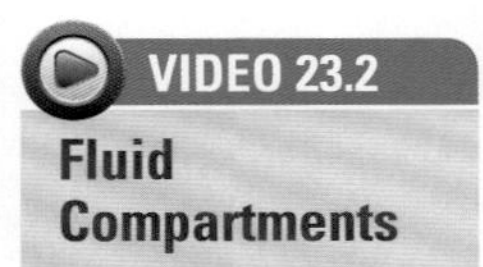

A. Body Fluid Compartments

Total body water (TBW) is estimated to comprise 60% and 50% of the lean body mass of adult males and females, respectively. TBW is distributed throughout various body compartments with roughly 66% making up the ***intracellular fluid (ICF)*** and 33% making up the ***extracellular fluid (ECF)***. ECF is further divided into interstitial fluid and plasma, which account for approximately 24% and 8% of the TBW, respectively (**Figure 23.2**). Thus, for an adult male weighing 70 kg, the TBW is estimated to be 42 L. Of this amount, only 3.5 L is plasma, with the remainder of the circulating blood volume being red blood cells (see also Chapter 3).

B. Regulation of Extracellular Fluid Volume

The control of ECF concentration and volume is important for cellular function, transfer of molecules between ICF and ECF, and maintenance of circulating blood volume. Normal serum osmolarity is 285 to 295 mOsm/L and is calculated from measured concentrations of sodium, glucose, and urea (blood urea nitrogen [BUN]) as follows:

$$\text{Serum osmolarity} = \left(2 \times \text{Na}^{+}\right) + \left(\text{Glucose}/18\right) + \left(\text{BUN}/2.8\right) \quad (23.4)$$

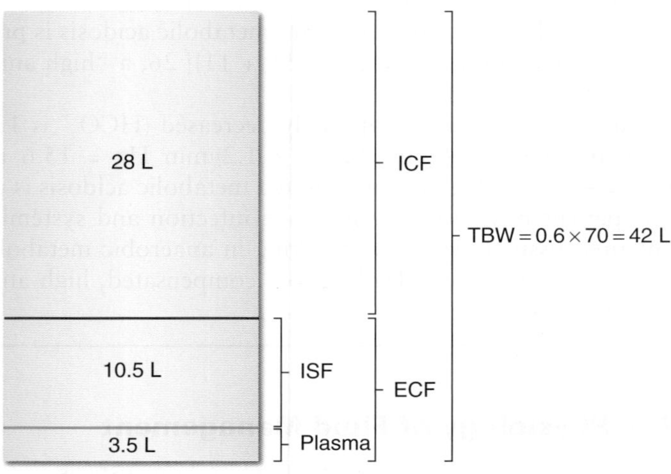

Figure 23.2 The approximate distribution of total body water (TBW) in the various body compartments is shown for a 70-kg adult man. ECF, extracellular fluid; ICF, intracellular fluid; ISF, interstitial fluid.

It should be noted, however, that a difference exists between ***osmolarity*** (the concentration of particles dissolved per unit of serum volume) and ***tonicity*** (the effective osmolarity that can exert an osmotic force across a membrane). Tonic molecules (eg, Na^+) are considered "effective osmoles" because they do not move freely across a membrane. They are able to cause water movement down a concentration gradient. In contrast, because urea freely diffuses across biologic membranes and distributes itself throughout the TBW, it is not ***tonic.*** Thus, under conditions of relative normoglycemia, the major contributor to serum osmolarity and tonicity is the Na^+ concentration.

The concentration and volume of the ECF are maintained by both thirst and the hormonal actions of the ***renin-angiotensin-aldosterone system (RAAS)*** and ***antidiuretic hormone (ADH)*** on the kidneys, which alter the amount of Na^+ and water excreted in urine. ADH is released (ie, nontonic release) from the posterior pituitary in response to small changes (2%-3%) in serum tonicity or >10% decreases in effective circulating volume. The RAAS is activated by hypotension, the sympathetic nervous system, and decreased Na^+ delivery to the kidneys (**Figure 23.3**). The end result is increased thirst (increased water intake), increased renal retention of Na^+

? *Did You Know?*

Osmolarity is the number of solute particles per liter of solution, whereas osmolality is the number of particles per kilogram of solvent. Both terms describe the solute concentration of a solution, and due to the negligible difference in their values, are often used interchangeably.

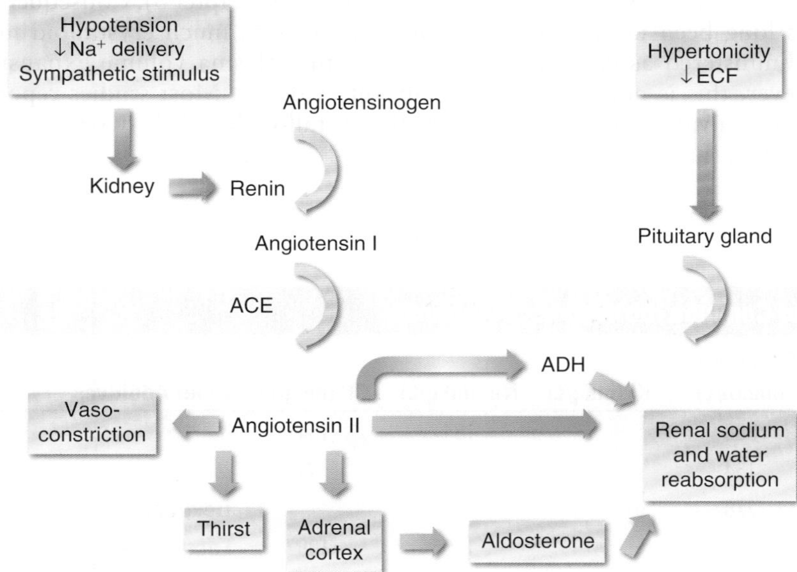

Figure 23.3 Neurohormonal regulation of extracellular volume, arterial blood pressure, and sodium/water balance is modulated by the renin-angiotensin-aldosterone system (RAAS) and the hypothalamic-pituitary-adrenal (HPA) axis. The RAAS is activated by hypotension, decreased sodium intake, or sympathetic nervous system activity, resulting in the release of renin from the kidneys, leading to increased angiotensin II. Angiotensin II promotes vasoconstriction, thirst, aldosterone secretion from the adrenal cortex, and increased renal sodium and water reabsorption. The HPA axis secretes antidiuretic hormone (ADH) in response to increased plasma osmolarity, decreased extracellular fluid (ECF), or decreased plasma angiotensin and leads to increased renal free water absorption in the kidneys and further vasoconstriction. ACE, angiotensin converting enzyme.

and water, and vasoconstriction, all of which act to maintain effective circulating volume and perfusion of vital organs.

C. Distribution of Infused Fluids

There are two types of fluids commonly used for intravenous administration that are categorized by their ability to diffuse through a semipermeable membrane: ***crystalloids*** and ***colloids***. Crystalloids readily diffuse across a semipermeable membrane, whereas colloids do not. Crystalloids are generally a base of sterile water in which various electrolytes are dissolved. They may be further categorized by their tonicity relative to serum: ***hypotonic***, ***isotonic***, and ***hypertonic*** solutions. The composition of several commonly used intravenous solutions is presented in **Table 23.7**.

Renal excretion notwithstanding, the tonicity of a given crystalloid will determine across which body compartments the solution will initially distribute. Hypotonic and isotonic solutions generally equilibrate across TBW and ECF, respectively. An estimation of the initial volume distribution following the rapid infusion of 1000 mL of various crystalloids and colloids is presented in **Table 23.8**.

Traditional teaching is that colloids are unable to move across an intact endothelial barrier and therefore remain entirely within the plasma. Additionally, the maintenance of normal plasma colloid oncotic pressure allows for maximal reabsorption of interstitial fluid back into the vascular tree on the venular side of the microcirculation (see Chapter 3). Consequently, it has long been taught that three or four times as much crystalloid must be administered as colloid to achieve the same plasma volume expansion. However, this is not supported by current evidence. Most studies report a volume equivalence of colloid to isotonic crystalloid less than two to one (see the section that follows).

Table 23.7 Composition of Common Intravenous Solutions

Solution	pH	Osmolarity (mmol/L)	K^+ (mEq/L)	Na^+ (mEq/L)	Cl^- (mEq/L)	Other Additives
0.9% NS	4.5-7	308		154	154	
0.45% NS	4.5-7	154		77	77	
D5W	5.0	278				Dextrose
Ringer's lactate	6-7.5	273	4	130	109	Lactate, calcium
Plasmalyte	6.5-7.6	294	5	140	98	Acetate, gluconate, magnesium
Albumin 5%	6.9	300		145	145	
Albumin 25%	6.9	1500		145	145	
HES 450/0.7 (Hespan)	5.9	309		154	154	
HES 130/0.4 (Voluven)	4-5.5	309		154	154	

Cl^-, chlorine; D5W, 5% dextrose in water; K^+, potassium; Na^+, sodium; NS, normal saline.

Table 23.8 Comparison of Body Compartment Distribution of 1000 mL Intravenous Fluid

Hypotonic	Isotonic	Hypertonic	Colloids
Dextrose 5% water	0.9% normal saline	3% NaCl	Blood
0.45% normal saline	Ringer's lactate		Albumin
	Plasmalyte		
Distribution	**Distribution**	**Distribution**	**Distribution**
ICF—650 mL	ICF—None	ICF—None	ICF—None
ISF—250 mL	ISF—750 mL	ISF—None	ISF—None
IVF—100 mL	IVF—250 mL	IVF—1000 mL	IVF—>1000 mL

ICF, intracellular fluid; ISF, interstitial fluid; IVF, intravascular fluid.

IV. Fluid Replacement Therapy

Maintenance of sufficient intravascular volume to support organ perfusion is the chief goal of perioperative fluid administration. Perioperative intravascular volume depletion (ie, ***hypovolemia***) is common for various reasons, including prolonged preoperative starvation (NPO) status, sepsis, hyperthermia, chronic diuretic use, uncontrolled hyperglycemia, vomiting, and diarrhea. Hypovolemia results in organ hypoperfusion, tissue hypoxia, acidosis, and arterial hypotension. Replacing any existing fluid deficit and administering maintenance intravenous fluids to achieve normovolemia both promote adequate organ perfusion pressure and tissue oxygenation, thereby improving surgical outcomes.[3,4] Although hypovolemia is often the main concern perioperatively, excessive fluid administration leading to volume overload has been shown to increase postoperative complications. ***Hypervolemia*** increases the risk for bowel edema, nausea, vomiting, pulmonary edema, and decompensated heart failure. Thus, obtaining a detailed history and accurate preoperative assessment of volume status (see below) are important factors when managing fluid perioperatively.

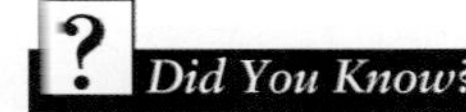

Maintenance of sufficient intravascular volume to support organ perfusion, tissue oxygenation, and aerobic metabolism is the chief goal of perioperative fluid administration.

A. Maintenance Requirements for Water, Sodium, and Potassium

Under normal physiologic conditions, the average adult loses approximately 1500 mL of water daily from perspiration, respiration, feces, and urine. Sodium and potassium losses are minimal and replacement is roughly 1 mmol/kg daily. Generally these daily water and electrolyte requirements are easily achieved with oral intake. However, various disease states alter normal electrolyte balance, resulting in severe abnormalities, and can pose great challenges to perioperative fluid administration.

B. Glucose Requirements and Dextrose

Blood glucose is under tight hormonal control, such that a healthy adult is capable of maintaining normal blood glucose levels for weeks without caloric intake. Thus, blood glucose is not routinely monitored in healthy adults, nor are dextrose-containing fluids routinely administered. However, patients with insulin-dependent diabetes mellitus are susceptible to both *hypoglycemia* and *hyperglycemia*; therefore, blood glucose should be carefully monitored in these patients perioperatively. In addition, infants younger than 6 months have limited glycogen stores, are susceptible to hypoglycemia after short periods of fasting, and typically receive dextrose-containing fluids perioperatively.

C. Surgical Fluid Requirements

Traditional teaching surrounding the estimation of perioperative fluid deficit and the calculation of maintenance intravenous fluid has relied upon a seminal 1957 study by Holliday and Segar that generated the often-quoted "4-2-1 rule" of maintenance fluid management based on body weight (ie, hourly hypotonic fluid requirement is 4 mL/kg for the first 10 kg, 2 mL/kg for the second 10 kg, and 1 mL/kg for all remaining kilograms).[5] However, application of this method fails to account for a number of physiologic factors and can lead to hypervolemia and hyponatremia that are associated with increased postoperative complications, including longer hospital stay, pulmonary edema, pneumonia, and ileus. Thus, current practice is to use isotonic solutions for maintenance fluid, with superior outcomes demonstrated for balanced electrolyte solutions over normal saline.

Despite numerous studies, controversy still exists over optimal perioperative fluid management. However, recent studies have demonstrated improved outcomes when fluid therapy is based on specific clinical criteria. Notably, consensus guidelines from the Enhanced Recovery Partnership recommend the use of ***goal-directed fluid management*** for patients who are acutely ill, undergoing major surgery, or have comorbidities that warrant cardiac output monitoring, but not for patients undergoing low-risk surgery.[6] However, evidence does not support a single, specific hemodynamic goal or method of measurement. The authors advocate for using the related measures of "pulse pressure variation" and "stroke volume variation" (discussed below) when performing goal-directed fluid management as outlined above. This approach treats fluid therapy as a medication that is administered using the "five rights" rule-of-thumb: administer the right drug, at the right dose, to the right patient, via the right route, and at the right time. Furthermore, intraoperative maintenance fluids should be limited to 2 mL/kg/h (including drug infusions). Postoperatively, intravenous fluids should be limited and oral hydration resumed as soon as possible.

V. Colloids, Crystalloid, and Hypertonic Solutions

The ideal resuscitative fluid would have a similar composition to plasma, have predictable and reliable effects on circulating blood volume, be free of undesired side effects, be inexpensive, and lead to improvements in patient-centered outcomes (morbidity, mortality, or length of stay). However, as one might expect, such a fluid does not exist, thus, the ongoing controversy between crystalloid and colloid solutions. The most commonly used resuscitation fluids are isotonic salt solutions and colloids, whose compositions are listed in **Table 23.7**.

A. Physiology and Pharmacology

The efficacy of any intravenous fluid in expanding the plasma volume is dependent on the proportion of administered fluid that remains in the intravascular space. Traditionally, net transcapillary fluid flux within the ECF space—from plasma to interstitial fluid—is described by the ***Starling equation:***

$$F = Kf \times ([Pc - Pt] - \sigma[\pi c - \pi i]), \quad (23.5)$$

where F is the net fluid movement between compartments, Kf is a filtration coefficient, Pc is the capillary hydrostatic pressure, Pt is the tissue hydrostatic pressure, σ is the reflection coefficient (a measure of leakiness to a particular substance), πc is the capillary oncotic pressure, and πi the interstitial oncotic pressure.

Based on the traditional Starling equation (described in detail in Chapter 3), fluid moves from the plasma to the interstitium at the arteriolar level driven by the dominant hydrostatic pressure gradient. On the venular side of the circulation, the colloid oncotic pressure within the vasculature promotes fluid reabsorption back into circulation (see Figure 3.18). In order to exploit these basic physiologic mechanisms, hypertonic salt and colloidal solutions were introduced into clinical practice.

However, in clinical practice, volume expansion as a result of administered intravenous resuscitative fluids cannot be reliably predicted by the traditional Starling equation. This is especially true in states of inflammation, physiologic stress, and shock, in which capillary permeability is altered. In these situations, intravascular fluid loss (including both crystalloid and colloid solutions) to the interstitium is greater than would be expected. This signals the emerging importance of multiple capillary components (eg, endothelial glycocalyx, capillary basement membrane, and extracellular matrix) in driving diffusion physiology, as well as highlights the importance of the lymphatic circulation in returning interstitial fluid to the intravascular compartment. Thus, the actual volume equivalence of colloids to crystalloids observed in clinical practice is actually closer to two to one rather than the predicted three or four to one.[7]

B. Clinical Implications of Choosing Crystalloid or Colloid

The debate over crystalloid and colloid fluid administration is long-standing, and an overwhelming number of studies in the literature have compared their benefits and liabilities. For example, crystalloid resuscitation is generally associated with greater weight gain, which itself is associated with various negative clinical outcomes. However, this association is not causation and the literature still lacks strong evidence supporting one fluid type over the other. Studies suggest, however, that there are subsets of patients in whom the use of albumin and synthetic colloids appears to confer a worse outcome. **Table 23.9** summarizes selected literature comparing clinical outcomes with colloid and crystalloid resuscitation. Additional characteristics should also factor into the decision. Crystalloids are inexpensive, nonallergenic, and do not inhibit coagulation. However, their administration results in tissue edema, leading to gut flora translocation, poor wound healing, impairment of alveolar gas exchange, limited intravascular volume expansion, and metabolic derangements. Conversely, colloids are expensive, allergenic, and linked to renal failure and coagulopathy, and their theoretic benefit of remaining in the intravascular space is not supported by evidence.

C. Implications of Crystalloid and Colloid Solutions on Intracranial Pressure

Based on the discussion above, it could be expected that colloid solutions increase ***intracranial pressure (ICP)*** less than crystalloid, thus improving outcomes in ***traumatic brain injury (TBI)*** patients. This theory, however, assumes ideal physiologic conditions in which the ***blood-brain barrier*** remains intact. Unfortunately, as demonstrated in the SAFE trial (**Table 23.9**), this theory does not hold true clinically, and TBI patients resuscitated with colloids demonstrated increased mortality. A subgroup analysis of the SAFE trial further indicated that albumin resuscitation in TBI patients is associated with

Table 23.9 Summary of Literature Comparing Colloid and Crystalloid as Primary Resuscitative Fluids

Study	Findings
Cochrane Injuries Group Albumin Reviewers. Human albumin administration in critically ill patients: systematic review of randomised controlled trials. *Br Med J.* 1998;317(7153):235-240.	• Albumin increased overall rate of death in patients with hypovolemia, burns, hypoalbuminemia
Finfer S, Bellomo R, Boyce N, et al. A comparison of albumin and saline for fluid resuscitation in the intensive care unit. *N Engl J Med.* 2004;350(22):2247-2256.	• No statistically significant difference in 28-d mortality • Subgroup analysis showed increased rates of death at 2 y with the use of colloid in TBI but decreased risk of death at 28 d in severe sepsis
Myburgh JA, Finfer S, Bellomo R, et al. Hydroxyethyl starch or saline for fluid resuscitation in intensive care. *N Engl J Med.* 2012;367(20):1901-1911.	• Mortality higher in HES group but not statistically significant • AKI higher in Saline group • Need for RRT higher in HES group • HES was associated with significantly more adverse events
Bayer O, Reinhart K, Kohl M, et al. Effects of fluid resuscitation with synthetic colloids or crystalloids alone on shock reversal, fluid balance, and patient outcomes in patients with severe sepsis; a prospective sequential analysis. *Crit Care Med.* 2012;40(9):2543-2551.	• PRAC concluded that the benefits of HES no longer outweighed the risks, and it was withdrawn from the market in Europe • FDA recommends HES not be used in critically ill patients or those with preexisting renal dysfunction
Perel P, Roberts I, Ker K. Colloids versus crystalloids for fluid resuscitation in critically ill patients. *Cochrane Database Syst Rev.* 2013;2:CD000567.	• Time to shock reversal was equal in both groups • Similar in-hospital mortality, total LOS, and ICU LOS • HES and gelatin were independent risk factors for AKI • Crystalloid volume equivalence 1.4:1 with HES; 1.1:1 with gelatin • Fluid balance more negative in crystalloid group by HD 5
Rhodes A, Evans LE, Alhazzani W, et al. Surviving Sepsis Campaign: International Guidelines for Management of Sepsis and Septic Shock: 2016. *Intensive Care Med.* 2017;43(3):304-377.	Authors' conclusion: "The absence of any clear benefit following the administration of colloid compared to crystalloid solutions in the combined subgroups of sepsis, in conjunction with the expense of albumin, supports a strong recommendation for the use of crystalloid solutions in the initial resuscitation of patients with sepsis and septic shock." • Crystalloids supported as primary resuscitative fluid for severe sepsis and septic shock • There are safety concern for HES use in sepsis • Albumin resuscitation for severe sepsis and septic shock supported when patients require substantial amounts of crystalloids

AKI, acute kidney injury; FDA, Food and Drug Administration; HD, hospital day; HES, hydroxyethyl starch; LOS, length of stay; PRAC, Pharmacovigilance Risk Assessment Committee; RRT, renal replacement therapy; TBI, traumatic brain injury.

significantly higher ICPs in the first week postinjury than for those receiving crystalloids. The mechanism is not fully elucidated, but it is thought to involve a disruption in the blood-brain barrier, resulting in colloid leaking into brain parenchyma and rebound intracranial hypertension. Thus, colloid administration should be avoided in patients with suspected or known TBI.

D. Implications of Isotonic Fluid Choice

The choice of isotonic fluid remains somewhat unclear. Normal saline has historically been the default fluid for volume resuscitation, although it is technically slightly hypertonic and hyperchloremic. It has long been observed that administration of 0.9% normal saline has been associated with hyperchloremic metabolic acidosis, the full mechanisms of which are still being elucidated.[8] Given the deleterious effects observed from other types of acidosis, concern for harm from 0.9% normal saline administration has grown.

Other fluid solutions that more closely mimic the soluble component of plasma through the lowering of NaCl content and the addition of other physiologically important solutes, such as potassium, calcium, magnesium, and buffers, were developed. These are referred to as "buffered" or "balanced" solutions (eg, lactated Ringer's, Plasmalyte). Numerous studies have compared normal saline to buffered solutions to identify harm in the form of death, acute kidney injury, renal replacement therapy needs, coagulopathy, damage to other organs, and so on. A 2019 Cochrane Review of this topic in the setting of critically ill adults and children showed that compared to 0.9% saline, buffered isotonic solutions were associated with higher pH, higher bicarb, and lower chloride levels; However, in-hospital mortality and/or renal injury did not differ, with the caveat that evidence certainty was low.[9] This same review also reported insufficient evidence for differences in coagulopathy, transfusion requirements, or damage to other organs. Despite this lack of evidence of harm, it is the opinion of the authors that differing clinical scenarios may dictate that one fluid type is more appropriate. For example, in patients with TBI and elevated ICP, the lower sodium content of buffered solutions may not be desired. In contrast, in patients with hyperchloremia and acidosis a buffered solution may be beneficial. However, for the many patients without specific indication for one fluid type over the other, there is likely to be ongoing debate and controversy until more definitive research is available.

E. Clinical Implications of Hypertonic Fluid Administration

Hypertonic fluids commonly used in clinical practice include hypertonic saline and mannitol. Hypertonic saline is most commonly used to treat symptomatic hyponatremia, whereas hypertonic mannitol is used primarily to reduce increased ICP. Theoretically, administration of a hypertonic fluid creates a large osmotic gradient between ECF and ICF, drawing interstitial fluid into the intravascular space. The rapid increase in intravascular volume is the rationale behind giving hypertonic salt solutions for volume resuscitation. Initial successful studies of low-volume, hypertonic saline resuscitation in hemorrhagic shock were conducted in military environments where medical supply weight is of significant importance. Subsequent trials in civilian settings comparing hypertonic saline to isotonic fluid for resuscitation in trauma patients are sparse in number but have failed to show significant clinical improvement and, in fact, may worsen outcomes.

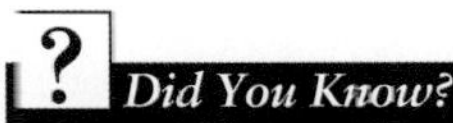

Hypertonic crystalloids can be administered in smaller volumes than isotonic crystalloids to achieve the same effect in intravascular fluid expansion, making hypertonic solutions attractive for use in low-resource settings such as military combat care.

Hypertonic mannitol is used as a temporizing measure to decrease ICP until the primary pathology can be addressed. Mannitol remains intravascular and rapidly decreases ICP by drawing fluid into the intravascular space from brain interstitium and parenchyma. Additionally, mannitol inhibits reabsorption of free water and sodium in the kidneys, resulting in a rapid and large volume diuresis. However, a recent meta-analysis reviewing the studies comparing hypertonic saline and mannitol for treatment of elevated ICP concludes that hypertonic saline may be superior.[10] Unfortunately, only limited trials exist assessing long-term neurologic outcomes and adverse events associated with hypertonic saline administration, warranting further investigation.

VI. Fluid Status: Assessment and Monitoring

A. Conventional Clinical Assessment

Hypovolemia, defined as inadequate circulating blood volume, results from either volume depletion (ECF sodium deficit) or dehydration (ECF water deficit). Prolonged hypovolemia increases patient morbidity and mortality, yet can be rapidly corrected with fluid resuscitation. However, evidence also demonstrates poor patient outcomes with excessive fluid administration. Although the goal of fluid management and resuscitation is to maintain an effective circulating volume, many of the conventional metrics used to assess volume status do not accurately reflect intravascular volume. **Table 23.10** lists the most commonly used noninvasive tools for clinical assessment of volume status.

Physical examination findings and body weight changes are all potentially useful tools in the assessment of volume status. Caution must be used in their application, however, as concomitant pharmacotherapy (eg, beta-blockade, diuretics), comorbid conditions (congestive heart failure, chronic hepatic or renal impairment), and interobserver bias can limit the use of these clinical signs. Similarly, laboratory values, including serum electrolytes, BUN, and creatinine, are important components of volume assessment, but premorbid states can complicate their interpretation. Despite these limitations, tachycardia, oliguria, and eventually hypotension are normal physiologic responses to intravascular volume depletion. Considered together in the appropriate clinical setting, these signs frequently indicate hypovolemia and warrant an isotonic crystalloid fluid bolus challenge for both diagnostic and therapeutic purposes. Initially, a 20 to 30 mL/kg fluid bolus should be administered. Serial reassessment of vital signs and laboratory values is essential to evaluate the progress of resuscitation efforts and determine whether hypovolemia is indeed the underlying problem and if further resuscitation is indicated.

Table 23.10 Conventional Methods of Volume Assessment

Physical Examination
Jugular venous distension
Skin turgor, dry mucous membranes, dry axilla
Inspiratory crackles
Tissue edema
S3 heart sound
Capillary refill
Vital signs (including orthostatic changes)
Body weight changes
Fluid intake/output balance
Laboratory Values
Hematocrit
Serum sodium
Serum blood urea nitrogen (BUN)
Serum creatinine
Urine electrolytes
Acid-base status

B. Intraoperative Clinical Assessment

Although physical examination and laboratory assessment also play a role in the evaluation of volume status in the operating room, the increased acuity and frequent changes in intravascular volume in this setting make invasive measures of volume status of paramount importance. Static measures of volume status that are used intraoperatively include central venous pressure, pulmonary artery occlusion pressure, and inferior vena cava diameter. Once thought to be highly accurate measurements of intravascular volume status, recent evidence has shown these static measurements to be neither accurate measures of intravascular volume nor accurate predictors of fluid responsiveness. Coupled with the fact that these measures are heavily influenced by mechanical ventilation and perturbations in cardiac function, they have fallen out of favor as primary measures of volume status.

Dynamic measures of volume status, however, take into account fluctuations of the cardiopulmonary system across a period of time and have been shown to be more accurate for predicting fluid responsiveness (see Chapter 15). One increasingly popular dynamic measure that has been shown to be useful is ***pulse pressure variation (PPV)***, the variation in pulse pressure with the respiratory cycle. PPV is easily obtained from an arterial blood pressure waveform, provided the patient is mechanically ventilated and in sinus rhythm (**Figure 23.4**). PPV is calculated as a percentage, as shown in **Equation 23.6**, with values >12% over at least three respiratory cycles predictive of both hypovolemia and fluid responsiveness:

$$PPV = \left(PP_{max} - PP_{min}/PP_{mean}\right) \times 100 \tag{23.6}$$

Both PPV and the related measure of stroke volume variation (SVV) have been shown to be highly predictive of responsiveness to fluid resuscitation,[11] an important observation because up to 50% of hypovolemic patients may not respond to fluid resuscitation. That PPV and SVV may accurately identify those patients who will benefit from volume repletion makes them both valuable clinical tools.

? Did You Know?

Static measures of intravascular volume status, such as central venous pressure, do not adequately account for cardiovascular and pulmonary fluctuations over time. In contrast, dynamic measures, such as pulse pressure variation, may more accurately predict patients who will respond to volume resuscitation.

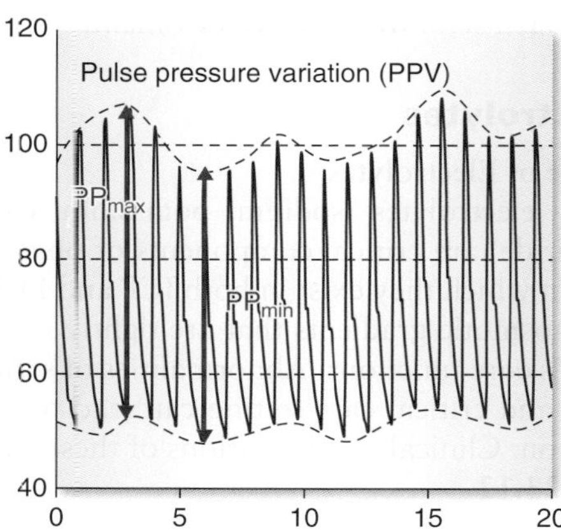

Figure 23.4 Pulse pressure variation (PPV) is identified on the arterial blood pressure waveform by first determining the maximum pulse pressure (PP_{max}) and the minimum pulse pressure (PP_{min}), and then comparing their difference to the mean pulse pressure, as described in **Equation 23.6**.

Table 23.11 Markers of Tissue Perfusion and Organ Dysfunction

Markers of End Organ Dysfunction
Hypoxemia: P_{IO_2}/F_{IO_2} ratio <300
Oliguria: urine output <0.5 kg/h × 2 h despite fluid resuscitation
Serum creatinine increase >0.5 mg/dL
Coagulopathy: INR >1.5 or PTT >60 s
Thrombocytopenia: platelet count <100,000 platelets/µL
Hyperbilirubinemia: total serum bilirubin >4 mg/dL
Ileus
Evidence of Tissue Hypoperfusion
Base deficit >2 mEq/L
Lactate >2.5 mmol/L
Capillary refill >2 s
Cold mottled skin
Mixed venous oxygen saturation <65%
Central venous oxygen saturation <70%

F_{IO_2}, fraction of inspired oxygen; INR, international normalized ratio; O_2, oxygen.; P_{IO_2}, partial pressure of inspired oxygen; PTT, partial thromboplastin time.

C. Oxygen Delivery as a Goal of Management

The primary concern in the setting of depleted intravascular volume is impaired tissue oxygen delivery due to poor end-organ perfusion. If this impairment becomes severe enough, oxidative phosphorylation cannot occur, and tissues must rely on inefficient anaerobic respiration and simple glycolysis for energy production, ultimately resulting in end-organ dysfunction. Furthermore, prolonged impaired oxygen delivery is associated with significant morbidity and mortality. The adequacy of oxygen delivery is determined by measuring markers of end-organ perfusion that act as a surrogate for effective circulating volume. Commonly utilized markers of the adequacy of global tissue perfusion as well as signs of organ dysfunction are listed in **Table 23.11**. Over the past decade, improvements in morbidity and mortality have been attributed to the adoption of early and aggressive therapy directed toward such markers, using an algorithmic approach with frequent reassessment.[12,13]

VII. Electrolytes

A. Physiologic Role of Electrolytes

The body's primary electrolytes (sodium, potassium, calcium, magnesium, phosphate, and chloride) are critical components of physiologic homeostasis. In the ionized form in which they exist in both ICF and ECF, these electrolytes create electrical and osmotic gradients that are tightly regulated and essential to many of the body's core functions. Abnormalities of serum electrolyte levels in the perioperative and critical care setting can lead to severe perturbations in physiologic function. Clinical manifestations of these various abnormalities are shown in **Table 23.12**.

B. Sodium

Sodium is the most prevalent electrolyte in the ECF. Abnormalities of serum sodium are most often due to some form of abnormal renal water regulation. Loss of water by the kidneys or in the gastrointestinal tract, lack of oral intake

Table 23.12 Clinical Manifestations of Electrolyte Abnormalities

Hyponatremia Cerebral edema Impaired thermoregulatory control Lethargy, coma, seizures Nausea Reflex impairments	**Hypernatremia** Weakness Lethargy, seizures, coma Demyelinating lesions Intracerebral or subarachnoid hemorrhage
Hypokalemia Muscle weakness Respiratory failure Rhabdomyolysis Ileus Cardiac arrhythmias ECG changes Nephrogenic diabetes insipidus	**Hyperkalemia** Severe muscle weakness Ascending paralysis Cardiac conduction abnormalities ECG changes Cardiac arrhythmias
Hypomagnesemia Tremors, tetany, convulsions Arrhythmias ECG changes	**Hypermagnesemia** Nausea Flushing Decreased deep tendon reflexes Hypotension Bradycardia Somnolence, coma
Hypocalcemia Tetany Anxiety, depression Papilledema Seizures Hypotension	**Hypercalcemia** Weakness Anxiety, depression Constipation, nausea Dehydration Cardiac conduction abnormalities

ECG, electrocardiogram.

(typically in the setting of an impaired thirst mechanism), or administration of hypertonic salt solutions may all lead to ***hypernatremia***. Clinical manifestations of hypernatremia are varied. Correction of hypernatremia can be achieved with 0.9% saline, 0.45% saline, or 5% dextrose in water, depending on the cause and level of sodium elevation. Great care should be taken to avoid rapid overcorrection of the serum sodium in cases of chronic hypernatremia. Except in emergent circumstances, hypernatremia should not be corrected more quickly than ~0.7 mEq/h, to avoid fluid shifts that can lead to life-threatening cerebral edema.

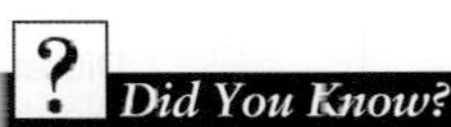

Too rapid correction of both hypernatremia or hyponatremia—particularly when chronic—can result in central nervous system dysfunction, including cerebral edema and central pontine myelinolysis.

The differential diagnosis of ***hyponatremia*** is presented in **Figure 23.5**. Clinical manifestations can be mild to severe, and at its extreme, cerebral edema, coma, or seizures may develop. As a general rule, patients cannot become more hyponatremic than they already are if hypotonic fluid is not administered. Thus, fluid restriction to an amount less than the previous day's urine output is a reasonable initial measure. In cases of symptomatic hyponatremia (severely altered mentation or seizures), correction with hypertonic saline is recommended. Overzealous correction, however, as with the

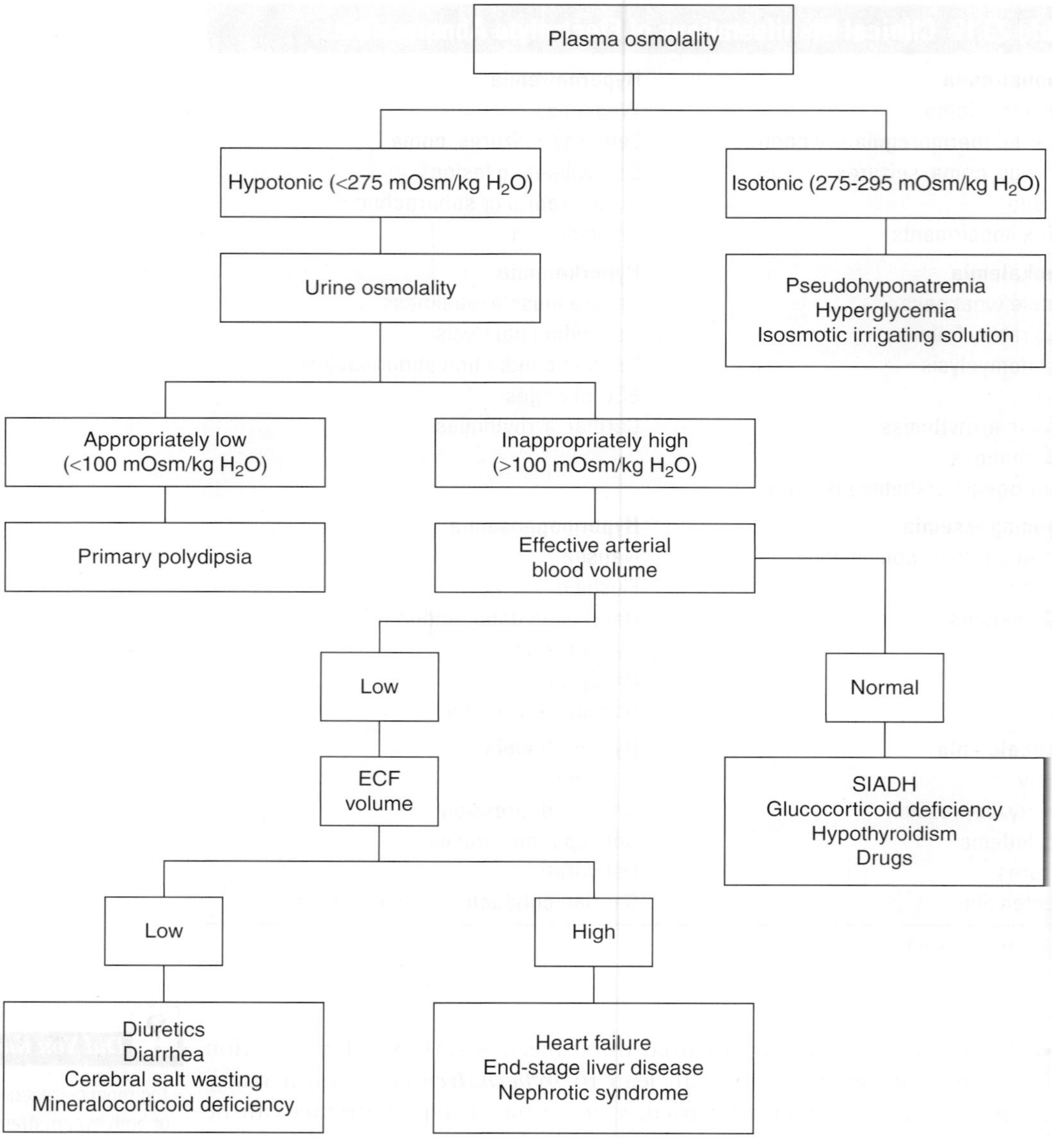

Plasma osmolality

Hypotonic (<275 mOsm/kg H_2O)

Isotonic (275-295 mOsm/kg H_2O)

Urine osmolality

Pseudohyponatremia
Hyperglycemia
Isosmotic irrigating solution

Appropriately low (<100 mOsm/kg H_2O)

Inappropriately high (>100 mOsm/kg H_2O)

Primary polydipsia

Effective arterial blood volume

Low

Normal

ECF volume

SIADH
Glucocorticoid deficiency
Hypothyroidism
Drugs

Low

High

Diuretics
Diarrhea
Cerebral salt wasting
Mineralocorticoid deficiency

Heart failure
End-stage liver disease
Nephrotic syndrome

Figure 23.5 Potential etiologies of hyponatremia can be identified with an algorithm that uses serum osmolarity, urine osmolarity, intravascular fluid volume, and extracellular fluid volume. ECF, extracellular fluid; SIADH, syndrome of inappropriate antidiuretic hormone secretion.

irreversible and devastating neurologic injury of central pontine myelinolysis, can result from too rapid correction of the serum sodium.

C. Potassium

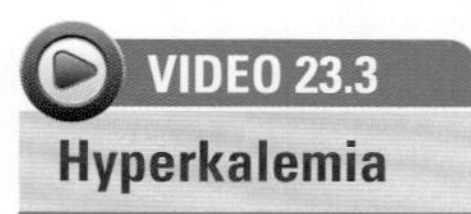

Abnormalities in potassium concentration hold great clinical significance, as *hyperkalemia* may result in severe life-threatening cardiac conduction abnormalities (**Figure 23.6**). Its differential diagnosis includes renal insufficiency or failure, metabolic acidosis, severe tissue injury or rhabdomyolysis, iatrogenic oversupplementation, or drug effect (succinylcholine, nonselective beta-blockers). Symptomatic hyperkalemia is often not present until serum

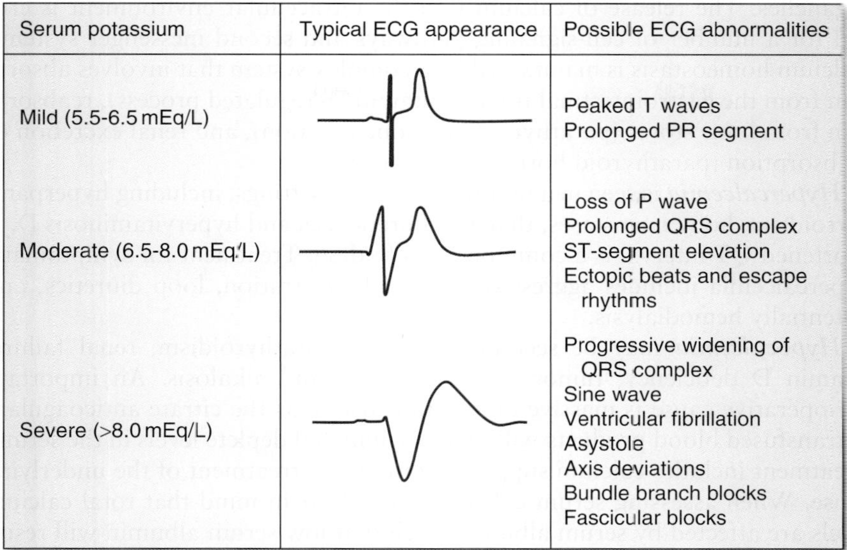

Serum potassium	Typical ECG appearance	Possible ECG abnormalities
Mild (5.5-6.5 mEq/L)		Peaked T waves Prolonged PR segment
Moderate (6.5-8.0 mEq/L)		Loss of P wave Prolonged QRS complex ST-segment elevation Ectopic beats and escape rhythms
Severe (>8.0 mEq/L)		Progressive widening of QRS complex Sine wave Ventricular fibrillation Asystole Axis deviations Bundle branch blocks Fascicular blocks

Figure 23.6 As hyperkalemia progresses from mild to severe, the electrocardiogram tracing evolves in a predictable fashion and may include abnormal T waves, ST segments, QRS duration, and characteristic dysrhythmias.

levels are >6.5 mEq/L, and its treatment should initially include administration of parenteral calcium as a cardiac membrane stabilizer. Reduction in the serum potassium level can be achieved by administration of a combination of dextrose and insulin (the latter forces uptake of potassium into cells), sodium bicarbonate if the patient is acidemic (potassium is forced into cells in exchange for H^+ ion to achieve pH balance), or treatment with furosemide or β-agonists. Ultimately, none of these mechanisms lowers total body potassium definitively, as this requires either potassium-binding resins (eg, Kayexalate) or hemodialysis.

Hypokalemia may be seen in the setting of excessive diuresis or in patients with renal artery stenosis or hyperaldosteronism. Clinically, the condition may also lead to cardiac dysrhythmias, and early electrocardiogram (ECG) findings include blunted T waves and the presence of U waves. Treatment includes potassium supplementation and correction of the underlying condition. Serum potassium does not accurately reflect changes in total body potassium stores, which are equal to ~50 mEq/kg. Depending on the patient's size, it will take 150 to 300 mEq of exogenous potassium to raise the serum potassium 1 mEq/L. However, potassium supplementation is commonly given orally or intravenously in 10, 20, 40, or 80 mEq aliquots. Intravenous potassium is toxic and extremely painful and must be diluted prior to administering. Hypokalemia is rarely life-threatening, and thus standard practice for intravenous potassium replacement is not to exceed 10 mEq/h using a peripheral intravenous line. Using a central venous catheter, however, it may be given at a rate up to 40 mEq/h when necessary.

D. Calcium

Calcium is a divalent cation that exists in both albumin-bound and physiologically active ionized forms in the serum. Within the cells, free calcium ion exists at a very low concentration and is mostly sequestered within specific organelles. The release of calcium into the intracellular environment is critical for a number of cell-signaling pathways and second messenger systems. Calcium homeostasis is maintained by a complex system that involves absorption from the gastrointestinal tract (a vitamin D–regulated process), reabsorption from bone stores (parathyroid hormone function), and renal excretion or reabsorption (parathyroid hormone function).

Hypercalcemia is seen in a number of clinical settings, including hyperparathyroidism, bony metastases, thiazide diuretic use, and hypervitaminosis D. A shortened QT interval is a common ECG finding. Treatment for symptomatic hypercalcemia includes aggressive saline administration, loop diuretics, and potentially hemodialysis.

Hypocalcemia may be secondary to hypoparathyroidism, renal failure, vitamin D deficiency, tumor lysis syndrome, and alkalosis. An important perioperative cause is massive blood transfusion, as the citrate anticoagulant in transfused blood products will bind calcium and deplete levels in the serum. Treatment includes calcium supplementation and treatment of the underlying cause. When assessing serum calcium levels, bear in mind that total calcium levels are affected by serum albumin, such that low serum albumin will result in low total calcium levels. To correct for this, simply measure the ionized calcium levels.

E. Magnesium

Magnesium is the second most important physiologically active divalent cation next to calcium. Magnesium is a critical component of nucleic acid structure and is an important cofactor for numerous enzymatic functions. It also plays a role in the maintenance of normal serum levels of other electrolytes. ***Hypermagnesemia*** may be seen in cases of hemolysis, tumor lysis, renal insufficiency, or in severe burns or trauma. In minor cases, symptoms are similar to those of hypercalcemia. However, if serum levels continue to rise, this may result in progressive atrioventricular block and cardiac arrest. Treatment includes parenteral calcium supplementation as a membrane stabilizer and hemodialysis to definitively decrease serum magnesium levels.

Hypomagnesemia may occur due to renal losses, chronic diarrhea, alcoholism, diuresis, nutritional deficiency, or in cases of refeeding syndrome. Symptoms are similar to those for hypocalcemia. ECG findings may include a wide QRS or long QT segment. Treatment of the underlying condition is key. It is also important to note that repletion of magnesium is essential in order to adequately maintain normal serum potassium and calcium levels.

For further review and interactivities, please see the associated Interactive Video Lectures and "A Closer Look" infographic accessible in the complimentary eBook bundled with this text. Access instructions are located in the inside front cover.

References

1. Boyd JH, Walley KR. Is there a role for sodium bicarbonate in treating lactic acidosis from shock? *Curr Opin Crit Care*. 2008;14(4):379-383. PMID: 18614899.
2. Rhodes A, Evans LE, Alhazzani W, et al. Surviving Sepsis Campaign: International Guidelines for Management of Sepsis and Septic Shock: 2016. *Intensive Care Med*. 2017;43(3):304-377. PMID: 28101605.
3. Joshi GP. Intraoperative fluid restriction improves outcome after major elective gastrointestinal surgery. *Anesth Analg*. 2005;101(2):601. PMID: 16037184.
4. Chappell D, Jacob M, Hofmann-Kiefer K, et al. A rational approach to perioperative fluid management. *Anesthesiology*. 2008;109(4):723. PMID: 18813052.

5. Holiday MA, Segar WE. The maintenance need for water in parenteral fluid therapy. *Pediatrics*. 1957;19(5):823-832. PMID: 13431307.
6. Mythen MG, Swart M, Acheson N, et al. Perioperative fluid management: consensus statement from the enhanced recovery partnership. *Periop Med*. 2012;1:2.PMID: 24764518.
7. Woodcock TE, Woodcock TM. Revised Starling equation and the glycocalyx model of transvascular fluid exchange: an improved paradigm for prescribing intravenous fluid therapy. *Br J Anesth*. 2012;108(3):384-394. PMID: 22290457.
8. Hoorn EJ. Intravenous fluids: balancing solutions. *J Nephrol*. 2016;30(4):485-492. PMID: 27900717.
9. Antequera Martín AM, Barea Mendoza JA, Muriel A, et al. Buffered solutions versus 0.9% saline for resuscitation in critically ill adults and children. *Cochrane Database Syst Rev*. 2019;7(7):CD012247. PMID: 31334842.
10. Kamel H, Navi BB, Nakagawa K, et al. Hypertonic saline versus mannitol for the treatment of elevated intracranial pressure: a meta-analysis of randomized clinical trials. *Crit Care Med*. 2011;39(3):554-559. PMID: 21242790.
11. Marik PE. Techniques for assessment of intravascular volume in critically ill patients. *J Intensive Care Med*. 2009;24:329. PMID: 19648183.
12. Rivers E, Nguyen B, Havstad S, et al. Early goal directed therapy in the treatment of severe sepsis and septic shock. *N Engl J Med*. 2001;345:1368-1377. PMID: 11794169.
13. The ProCESS Investigators; Yealy DM, Kellum JA, Huang DT, et al. A randomized trial of protocol-based care for early septic shock. *N Engl J Med*. 2014;370(18):1683-1693. PMID: 24635773.

METABOLIC ACIDOSIS

A CLOSER LOOK

A metabolic acidosis exists when arterial pH is < 7.35 and HCO_3^- is < 22 mEq/dL. This is further evaluated by calculating the anion gap (AG). The presence or absence of an AG characterizes the type of metabolic acidosis.

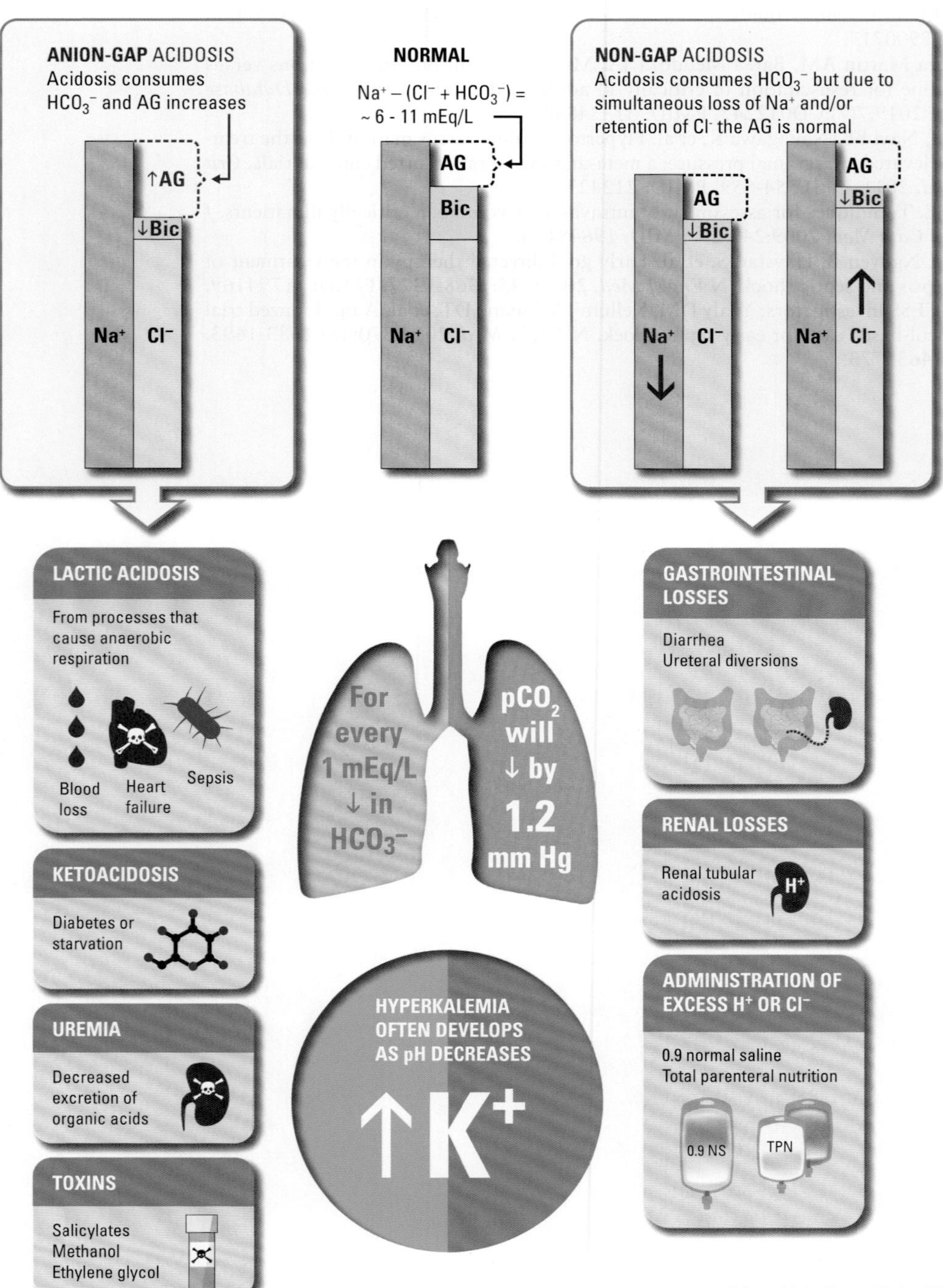

Infographic by: Naveen Nathan MD

Questions

1. An otherwise healthy 18-year-old man breaks his ankle playing football. In the emergency room his work-up is otherwise normal except for a painful and deformed ankle, and the only medication he received was intravenous morphine. On your preoperative evaluation he appears somnolent. His ABG shows $Paco_2$ of 90. Assuming normal baseline values for pH, $Paco_2$, and $[HCO_3^-]$ (7.4, 40 mm Hg, and 24 mEq/L, respectively), what would you estimate his current pH to be?

   A. 6.8
   B. 7.0
   C. 7.2
   D. 7.8

2. A 40-year-old woman with no past medical history suffers a traumatic brain injury in a small, remote, rural location. Due to inclement weather, transport to a tertiary care hospital for definitive treatment was not possible. The outside hospital intubated and hyperventilated the patient to a $Paco_2$ of 25 mm Hg for the past 3 days. Assuming normal baseline $Paco_2$, HCO_3^-, and renal function, what would you estimate her new $[HCO_3^-]$ to be after 3 days?

   A. 16.5 mmol/L
   B. 10 mmol/L
   C. 30.5 mmol/L
   D. 21 mmol/L

3. A 19-year-old man with no past medical history presents with sepsis after bacterial pneumonia. Over the course of his first hospital day, he develops a lactic acidosis and drops his pH from 7.4 to 7.2. He is normotensive and shows no other signs of end organ dysfunction. What is the most likely effect on his serum potassium level due to this decrease in pH?

   A. Decreased 1.2 mEq/L
   B. Increased 1.2 mEq/L
   C. Increased 2.4 mEq/L
   D. Decreased 2.4 mEq/L
   E. Unchanged

4. A 56-year-old man with history of coronary artery disease, diabetes, hypothyroidism, and current tobacco use is admitted after elective total knee arthroplasty. Due to excessive sedation, an arterial blood gas and electrolytes are measured, showing pH 7.32, $Paco_2$ 60 mm Hg, Pao_2 100 mm Hg, $[HCO_3^-]$ 32 mEq/L, Na^+ 140, Cl^- 115, and K^+ 4.2. What is his primary acid-base disturbance, and is it acute or chronic?

   A. Respiratory acidosis; acute
   B. Metabolic alkalosis; acute
   C. Respiratory acidosis; chronic
   D. Metabolic acidosis; acute

5. You are caring for a 50-year-old woman postoperatively after an open cholecystectomy for acute cholecystitis. She is intubated and ventilated, and her noninvasive blood pressure is 85/40. You place an arterial line that confirms this blood pressure. Because you are unsure if she needs fluid resuscitation or inotropic/vasopressor support, you calculate the pulse pressure variation (PPV). Over multiple respiratory cycles, you see her largest pulse pressure was from a blood pressure of 86/40 and her smallest pulse pressure was from a blood pressure of 79/40. What is her PPV and does it predict fluid responsiveness?

   A. 8; No
   B. 10; Yes
   C. 16; Yes
   D. 17; No

Answers

1. B

With acute respiratory acidosis, there will be a decrease in pH of approximately 0.08 pH units for every increase on $Paco_2$ of 10 mm Hg. This patient's $Paco_2$ increased from 40 to 90 mm Hg, or 50 mm Hg total. That increase in $Paco_2$ would decrease his pH 50 mm Hg CO_2 × 0.08 pH units/10 mm Hg CO_2, or 0.4 pH unit. This would give him an estimated pH of 7.0. Answer B is the correct answer. Answers A and C also show acidemia but not the correct magnitude. Answer D shows an alkalemia, which is the opposite of what is expected.

2. A

Respiratory alkalosis is compensated for acutely with buffering by CO_2. This acute compensation will decrease $[HCO_3^-]$ about 2 mmol/L for every 10 mm Hg decrease in CO_2. Chronically, alkalosis causes changes in metabolic and renal physiology that produce more buffer and reabsorb HCO_3^-. This chronic compensation will decrease $[HCO_3^-]$ about 5 mmol/L for every 10 mm Hg decrease in CO_2. Given this patient has been hyperventilated for 3 days, she is likely chronically compensated. Thus, her $Paco_2$ decrease is 40 to 25 mm Hg, or 15 mm Hg. This decrease in 15 mm Hg would decrease her $[HCO_3^-]$ 15 mm Hg CO_2 × 5 mmol/L HCO_3^-/10 mm Hg CO_2, or 7.5 mmol/L HCO_3^-. Her new $[HCO_3^-]$ would then be 24 – 7.5 mmol/L or 16.5 mmol/L. Answer A is the correct answer. Answer D shows the acute compensation. Answer C shows the right magnitude of $[HCO_3^-]$ change but in the wrong direction, that is increased. Answer B is too low and likely represents another process going on.

3. B

Excess hydrogen ions cause a shift of potassium from the intracellular to the extracellular space. As an approximation, for every decrease in pH of 0.1 the plasma potassium increases by 0.6 mEq/L. In the above clinical scenario, the patient's pH decreases 0.2; therefore this plasma potassium would increase 0.2 × 0.6 mEq/L, or 1.2 mEq/L, making B the correct answer. A, D, and E are incorrect as potassium would increase and not decrease or stay unchanged. C is incorrect in the magnitude of potassium increase.

4. C

Using stepwise analysis, the first step in acid-base disturbance evaluation is to assess pH. His pH is below normal which means his primary disturbance is acidosis, making answer B incorrect. Next, assess his $Paco_2$. This patient's $Paco_2$ is elevated, indicating that the main driver for his acidosis is respiratory; this makes answer D incorrect. To determine if his respiratory acidosis is acute or chronic, the magnitude of increase in $[HCO_3^-]$ is evaluated next. Acutely, the body will buffer retained CO_2, which will cause $[HCO_3^-]$ to increase ~1 mEq/L per 10 mm Hg increase in $Paco_2$. Chronically, metabolic and renal physiology change to increase $[HCO_3^-]$ ~4 to 5 mEq/L per 10 mm Hg increase in $Paco_2$. The patient's $Paco_2$ is increased ~20 mm Hg from normal and his $[HCO_3^-]$ is increased ~8 mEq/L from normal. This makes his compensatory increase in $[HCO_3^-]$ 4 mEq/L per 10 mm Hg of $Paco_2$ increase; therefore, he is in the chronic phase of compensation, making C the correct answer.

5. C

$PPV = (PP_{max} - PP_{min})/PP_{mean} \times 100$. This patient's PP_{max} = 86 to 40 = 46, PP_{min} = 79 to 40 = 39, and her PP_{mean} = (46 + 39)/2 = 42.5. Thus her PPV = (46 – 39))/42.5 × 100 = 16.5%. This PPV is above 10% and thus suggestive of fluid responsiveness. Therefore, C is the correct answer.

24 Blood Therapy

Louanne M. Carabini and Glenn Ramsey

Blood component therapy is the mainstay of treatment for hemorrhagic shock, acute or chronic anemia, and acquired or congenital disorders in hemostasis. Anesthesiologists serve a unique role as perioperative physicians frequently charged with the management of patients suffering acute blood loss or coagulopathy. Therefore, it is important to understand the physiologic principles of oxygen delivery and hemostasis, the risks and safety precautions associated with blood-product transfusion, and the pharmacology of anticoagulants, antithrombotics, and procoagulant medications.

I. Blood-Product Transfusion

A. Component Therapy and Indications for Transfusion

> **? Did You Know?**
>
> Transfusion of separated blood components, such as RBCs, plasma, or platelets, allows for targeted treatment and saves a precious resource.

Blood-product transfusion is conventionally performed with individual component therapy targeted to replace the specific deficiencies at hand. Most patients require only a single blood component or a combination of selected components. For example, red blood cells (RBCs) are needed to treat anemia with evidence of tissue hypoxia, whereas plasma is used to treat coagulopathy and factor deficiencies. Separating blood transfusion into component therapies allows for targeted efficient treatment while also minimizing the risks of transfusion reactions and transfusion-transmitted infection. Whole blood transfusion is reserved for initial emergent treatment of trauma or active bleeding.

Packed red blood cells (PRBCs) are the most common blood product transfused worldwide, with over 10.5 million units administered annually in the United States.[1] A unit of PRBCs is obtained from a single donor and consists of about 300 mL, with a hematocrit of approximately 60% to 70% and only about 20 to 30 mL of plasma. One unit of PRBCs generally increases the patient's hemoglobin concentration by 1 g/dL. **Table 24.1** describes blood component storage and preparation.

> **? Did You Know?**
>
> There is no general rule regarding the minimum hemoglobin at which patients should be transfused. The trigger for transfusion should be individualized for each specific patient.

The clearest indication for PRBC transfusion is acute blood loss or anemia with evidence of inadequate oxygen delivery to the tissues. Patients suffering hypovolemic shock secondary to critical bleeding require resuscitation with PRBCs, but they may also require treatment of dilutional coagulopathy and thrombocytopenia. The recommended transfusion threshold during acute hemorrhage in hemodynamically unstable patients is higher to provide oxygen carrying capacity during active bleeding, but still restrictive (hemoglobin goals of >7.0-9.0 g/dL) given the risks associated with allogenic blood-product transfusion.[2] Transfusion for major bleeding should also include replacement

Table 24.1 Blood Component Storage and Preparation

Component	Average Volume per Dose	Comments
PRBCs	300 mL	1-6 °C for 21-35 d or up to 42 d with adenine added to citrate, dextrose, and phosphate preservative
Plasma	250 mL	<–20 °C for up to 1 yr
Platelets, whole blood derived	50 mL/bag pooled to usual dose 4-6 bags	20-24 °C for 5 d
Platelets, apheresis	300 mL	20-24 °C for 5 d
Cryoprecipitate	15 mL/bag pooled to usual dose of 4-6 bags	<–20 °C for up to 1 yr
Whole blood	500 mL	1-6 °C for 14 d

PRBCs, packed red blood cells; plasma may be thawed from fresh frozen plasma (FFP) or plasma frozen within 24 hours (PF24).

of coagulation factors and platelets with consideration given to administration of medications and strategies for blood conservation.

The transfusion threshold for hemodynamically stable patients with anemia has been the topic of many review articles and original studies for over 2 decades. The controversy stems around the balance of the benefits of RBC treatment for anemia and the risks of transfusion. Most international guidelines, including the AABB, formerly the American Association of Blood Banks, the American Society of Anesthesiologists, the British Society for Haematology (BSH), and the Society of Cardiovascular Anesthesiologists, agree that restrictive transfusion practices are indicated for most hemodynamically stable trauma, perioperative, and critically ill patients.[2-6] There are a few circumstances, such as hemorrhagic shock, major orthopedic surgery with a history of cardiovascular disease, and cardiac surgery, where higher transfusion triggers are indicated to maximize oxygen delivery to end organs under stress. Otherwise, hemodynamically stable patients without evidence of tissue hypoxia (elevated lactate levels, low central venous oxygen saturation) generally tolerate hemoglobin levels as low as 7.0 g/dL with compensatory mechanisms to increase cardiac output and oxygen extraction at the tissue level. **Figure 24.1** describes a suggested clinical algorithm based on international guidelines for patient blood managment.[2,5,7]

Plasma contains all the clotting factors, fibrinogen, and plasma proteins from whole blood donation or apheresis. Each unit is collected from a single donor and must be frozen within 6 to 8 hours to be designated fresh frozen plasma (FFP). Most of the plasma currently collected in the United States is frozen within 24 hours (PF24) with minimal detrimental effects on its efficacy. However, it is most appropriate to use the term "plasma" moving forward as opposed to FFP to account for all types of plasma products.[8] The volume of 1 unit of plasma is approximately 250 mL, with physiologic levels of stable clotting factors and approximately 50% to 60% of labile factors VIII and V after 5 days of thawed storage. The most recent report from the National Blood Collection and Utilization Survey (NBCUS) documents significant declines in the transfusion rates of plasma products; however, there are still over 3.2

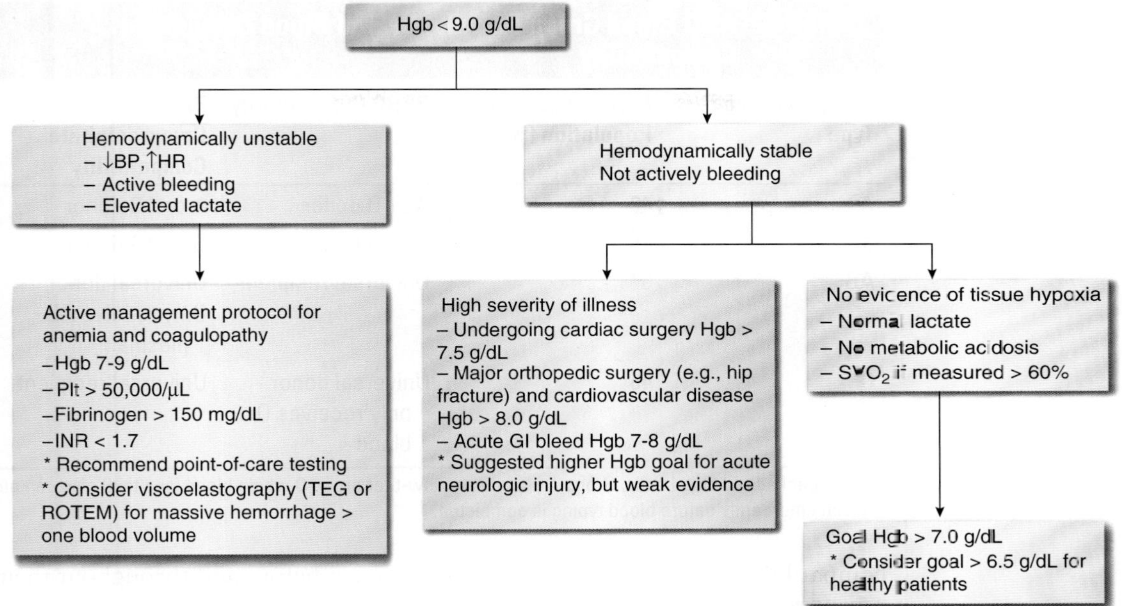

Figure 24.1 Suggested algorithm for red blood cell transfusion in hemodynamically stable and unstable patients with hemorrhagic shock. Stable angina and history of cardiovascular disease do not require transfusion thresholds greater than 7.0 g/dL; although there are recommendations for higher transfusion thresholds for patients with acute severity of illness. BP, blood pressure; GI; gastrointestinal; Hgb, hemoglobin; HR, heart rate; Plt, platelets; ROTEM, rotational thromboelastography; $S\bar{V}O_2$, mixed or central venous oxygen saturation; TEG, thromboelastography.[2,4-7]

million plasma units administered annually in the United States.[1] The most common indications for plasma transfusion are treatment of dilutional coagulopathy and factor deficiency. The current guidelines recommend basing the dose of plasma transfusion therapy on coagulation assay results. However, when testing is not available, the initial recommended dose for factor repletion in a bleeding patient is 10 to 20 mL/kg. Other indications for plasma transfusion include replacement of antithrombin in cases of long-term heparin use or as a second-line agent for warfarin or direct acting oral anticoagulant reversal. There is no indication for the use of plasma as prophylaxis in a patient with abnormal coagulation studies but no bleeding or pending invasive procedure.[8,9]

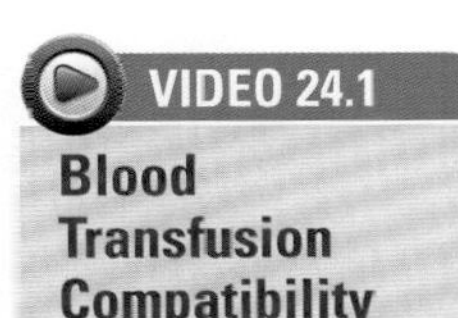

Plasma contains the antibodies to blood type antigens and should therefore be compatible when transfused. **Table 24.2** presents the plasma compatibility profiles as they compare with RBC component compatibility. The ABO blood system is the major carbohydrate-based blood-borne antigen system that induces naturally occurring immunoglobulin-M (IgM) antibodies without the need for RBC exposure. Thus, ABO incompatibility for PRBCs or plasma-containing components carries significant risk of acute hemolytic transfusion reactions (discussed in depth below). Type AB plasma is the universal plasma donor as it does not contain any ABO blood cell antibodies, but limited amounts of group A plasma may be given in emergencies before ABO typing is available. Type O patients are the universal recipient for plasma because there are no A or B antigens in type O blood. The RhD blood group

Table 24.2 ABO Blood Group Prevalence and Blood Component Compatibility

Recipient Blood Type	Prevalence in US Population (%)	PRBC Compatibility	Plasma/ Cryoprecipitate Compatibility
A	40	A or O donor	A or AB donor
B	15	B or O donor	B or AB donor
AB	5	Universal recipient	Universal donor Only receive AB plasma
O	45	Universal donor only receives O blood	Universal recipient

PRBCs, packed red blood cells. Group A plasma and low-titer group O whole blood (see text) also can be given emergently before blood typing is completed.

compatibility is of significant concern in women before and throughout their reproductive age as alloimmunization may result in complications during pregnancy. Alloimmunization is of highest risk in RhD negative patients who receive RhD positive RBCs. Plasma products do not typically contain enough RBCs to cause alloimmunization and may be transfused without concern for RhD compatibility.[9]

Cryoprecipitate (sometimes simply called "cryo") is produced after a controlled thaw and centrifuge of FFP. The yield of cryoproteins that precipitates from 1 unit of FFP is reconstituted in 15 to 20 mL of plasma. It must contain at least 150 mg of fibrinogen and at least 80 international units (IU) of factor VIII. Therefore, a dose of cryoprecipitate is usually pooled from four to six separate donors in approximately 60 to 120 mL and contains a high concentration of fibrinogen relative to plasma, as well as clinically significant amounts of factor VIII, von Willebrand factor, factor XIII, and fibronectin.[8,9] Hypofibrinogenemia and disseminated intravascular coagulopathy (DIC) are the most common indications for cryoprecipitate transfusion. Given the low volume of plasma from each donor in a pooled dose of cryoprecipitate, the overall immune-mediated risks are relatively small.

Platelet transfusions have increased approximately 5% over recent years despite an overall reduction in blood-product administration.[1] This is presumed to be secondary to the aging population and increased incidence of hematopoietic malignancies. Platelets are produced either as a pooled unit from four to six whole blood donors or from a single or double apheresis donation. Unlike other blood components, they have a short shelf life of only 5 to 7 days, and they are stored at room temperature and therefore have carried a higher risk of bacterial contamination. Because of this, pathogen-reduction treatment of platelets, which inactivates bacteria and other pathogens, is being introduced more widely.[8] Typically a single dose of platelets (pool or apheresis) is expected to increase the platelet count initially by 25,000 to 30,000 per microliter. However, the response to platelet transfusion varies greatly depending on the indication, acuity, and systemic syndrome of the patient.

Platelet transfusion may be indicated when platelets are decreased as a result of dilution, bleeding, destruction, or sequestration. Transfusion thresholds for thrombocytopenia depend on whether the patient has clinical signs of bleeding or whether bleeding or the risk of bleeding involves the closed intraorbital, intracranial, or neuraxial spaces. In these high-risk instances, the transfusion threshold is <100,000 per microliter. Otherwise, for surgical patients where bleeding is anticipated and prophylaxis is desired, the threshold is generally <50,000 per microliter. Guideline recommendations for lumbar puncture suggest a threshold of at least 40,000 per microliter prior to performing a lumbar puncture and 80,000 for insertion or removal of an epidural catheter. Patients without clinical signs of bleeding are not at risk of spontaneous hemorrhage until the platelet count drops to <10,000 per microliter.[8,10] Platelet transfusion may also be necessary for patients with qualitative deficiencies that are acquired or congenital. Commonly acquired platelet dysfunction occurs with extracorporeal circulation, such as cardiopulmonary bypass, extracorporeal membrane oxygenation (ECMO), or with medications or systemic illnesses, such as liver disease and uremia. Concerns for platelet dysfunction in a patient with signs of bleeding should prompt a platelet function test or viscoelastography.[5] Cold-stored platelets have very short circulation times but are hemostatically more activated and have been reintroduced by the military because they can be refrigerated for <14 days for remote or prehospital use.[11]

Whole blood, usually given as low-titer group O whole blood (LTOWB), can be used for initial emergency transfusions to rapidly provide RBCs, plasma, and platelets simultaneously.[12] When donors with high anti-A and anti-B ABO antibody titers are avoided, LTOWB can be safely given to non-O patients. Whole blood can be administered as fresh warm units from prescreened walking donors in austere environments or it can be refrigerated for <14 days. Practices vary as to antibody titer cutoffs or limits on numbers of units given.

II. Blood Compatibility

RBC compatibility testing consists of typing for ABO and Rh(D), screening the plasma for non-ABO antibodies, and crossmatching prospective RBC units. Group O, A, and B persons have naturally occurring strong plasma anti-A and/or anti-B to the antigen(s) they lack, and RBC units must be ABO compatible to avoid hemolytic transfusion reactions. D-negative persons can easily make anti-D when exposed to D-positive RBCs and should normally receive D-negative RBCs. This is especially important for girls and women of reproductive age to avoid risk of hemolytic disease of the newborn in future D-positive fetuses. One to 2% of all patients and 5% to 20% of multitransfused patients have non-ABO hemolytic alloantibodies to Rh and other blood group antigens. These antibodies must be identified so that RBC units negative for the target antigens can be given to avoid hemolysis. After these "type and screen" tests, donor RBC units are crossmatched to the patient, either by computer confirmation (electronic crossmatch) or, if significant antibodies are present, by serological crossmatching of plasma versus donor RBCs. Compatibility testing routinely takes 45 to 60 minutes or longer if RBC alloantibodies, warm (IgG), or cold (IgM) autoantibodies are present. If RBCs must be given emergently before testing is completed, uncrossmatched group O RBCs (D-negative for girls and women of reproductive age) are the best choice, after weighing the risk of non-ABO hemolytic RBC antibodies. In an emergency, as a guide to help remember that group O is a "universal donor," think of the "O" in donor.

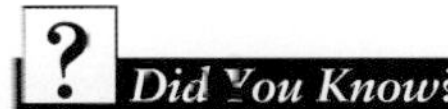

In an emergency, when a bleeding patient's blood type is not known and there is no time to perform a crossmatch, it is best to transfuse RBCs which are type O, and in females <50 years old, RhD-negative.

III. Blood Administration

Before transfusion, it is mandatory that the blood bank's transfusion *tag* on the blood unit be carefully checked against the blood *bag* and the patient's *wristband* identification to avoid a hemolytic reaction from administering the wrong blood or component. All blood components must be administered through a 150- to 260-μm blood filter to prevent clots from entering the patient's bloodstream. Products should be infused within 4 hours of issuance from the blood bank. A blood warmer should be used in rapid large-volume transfusions to avoid hypothermia and may be recommended for transfusing RBCs to patients with cold autoantibodies.[6]

IV. Transfusion Reactions

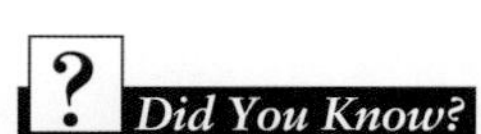

Did You Know?

Acute hemolytic transfusion reactions most often result from errors made by medical personnel. It is critical that blood donors and recipients be properly identified and all labels on blood products be properly matched to those individuals.

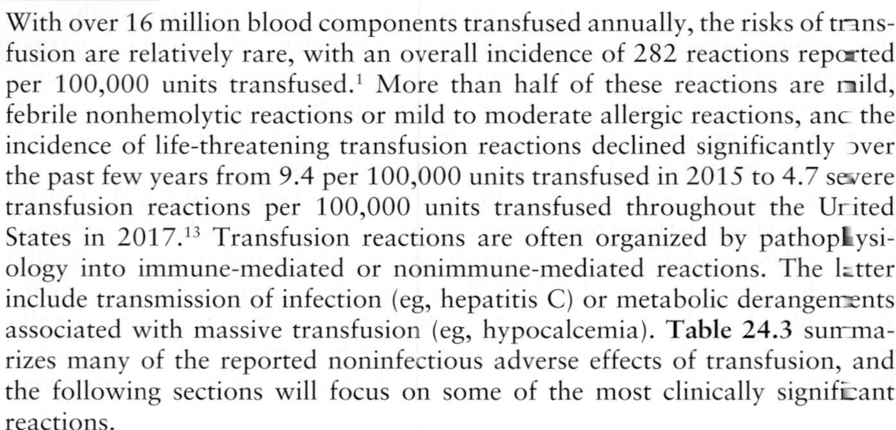

With over 16 million blood components transfused annually, the risks of transfusion are relatively rare, with an overall incidence of 282 reactions reported per 100,000 units transfused.[1] More than half of these reactions are mild, febrile nonhemolytic reactions or mild to moderate allergic reactions, and the incidence of life-threatening transfusion reactions declined significantly over the past few years from 9.4 per 100,000 units transfused in 2015 to 4.7 severe transfusion reactions per 100,000 units transfused throughout the United States in 2017.[13] Transfusion reactions are often organized by pathophysiology into immune-mediated or nonimmune-mediated reactions. The latter include transmission of infection (eg, hepatitis C) or metabolic derangements associated with massive transfusion (eg, hypocalcemia). **Table 24.3** summarizes many of the reported noninfectious adverse effects of transfusion, and the following sections will focus on some of the most clinically significant reactions.

Hemolytic transfusion reactions result from intravascular or extravascular hemolysis of endogenous and transfused RBCs, typically when the recipient expresses antibodies to blood-borne antigens within the donor product. This reaction is acute and severe when transfusion involves the naturally occurring IgM anti-A and anti-B antibodies to the ABO blood cell antigens. Acute hemolytic transfusion reactions (AHTRs) are rare (1:40,000) and almost always result from clerical errors with blood sampling, typing, crossmatch, or erroneous administration of an inappropriate blood product to the wrong patient. Rarely, transfusion of incompatible plasma can also result in acute hemolysis reported less than once every 50,000 transfusions (**Table 24.2**).[8]

Vigilance for the diagnosis of AHTR must remain high because many of the signs and symptoms can be masked during general anesthesia. Responsive patients may complain of chest pain, or abdominal discomfort. Vital signs become unstable, with hemolysis and diffuse bradykinin and histamine release leading to hemoglobinuria, fever, hypotension, tachycardia, and bronchospasm. AHTRs are best treated with supportive care after discontinuing all blood-product transfusions and initiating investigation into the etiology of the incompatibility. The mortality from AHTR remains high with approximately 2% to 7% of mistransfusions being fatal as patients may progress to multiorgan system failure from systemic shock, DIC, acute renal failure, and obstructive hepatic dysfunction.[8]

Delayed hemolytic transfusion reactions (DHTR) often occur days after blood-product administration and are typically less severe, presenting with progressive anemia, jaundice, and hemoglobinuria in the absence of

Table 24.3 Transfusion Reactions

Adverse Reaction	US Reactions per 100,000 Components transfused[a]	Notes
Overall	281.8	No change in overall number, but life-threatening reactions down from 9.4/100,000 in 2015 survey
All life-threatening	4.7	
Immune-Mediated Reactions		
Febrile nonhemolytic reaction	120.5	
Mild-moderate allergic reactions	88.4	
Anaphylaxis, severe allergic reaction	2.5	IgA deficiency increases risk; washing PRBCs may avoid reaction
Delayed hemolytic transfusion reaction	4.8	Alloantibodies to minor RBC antigens
Acute hemolytic transfusion reaction	1.1	ABO incompatibility (0.21/100,000) other antibodies (0.84/100,000)
Posttransfusion purpura	3.7	
Transfusion-related acute lung injury	1.5	Reduced risk with male-predominant donors
Transfusion-associated graft-versus-host	Zero reported in 2017 (0.0058 in 2015)	Avoided with blood irradiation for at-risk patients
Nonimmune Mediated		
Transfusion-associated circulatory overload	11.7	Higher risk in critically ill patients
Metabolic derangements		Hyperkalemia, hypocalcemia, hypothermia, iron overload
Transfusion-Transmitted Infections		
Viral infections	0.039	Estimated: HIV 1:1.5 million units HCV 1:1.2 million units HBV 1:1 million units
Bacterial infections	0.23	Negligible with PRT
Parasitic infections (babesia, Chagas)	0.068	Negligible with PRT

HBV, hepatitis B virus; HCV, hepatitis C virus; HIV, human immunodeficiency virus; IgA, immunoglobulin-A; NBCUS, National Blood Collection and Utilization Survey; PRBCs, packed red blood cells; PRT, pathogen-reduction technology.[8,13]

[a]Numbers reported in the 2017 National Blood Collection and Utilization Survey and from the American Red Cross guidelines.[8,13]

hemodynamic instability. DHTR results from a humoral reaction to antigens in transfused blood products in recipients with a history of alloimmunization to antigens such as Rh, Kell, Kidd, Duffy, among others. ***Alloimmunization*** occurs with pregnancy or exposure to blood-product transfusion as the recipient develops antibodies to blood-borne antigens at a rate of about 1 per 1500 to 3000 RBC transfused. This puts these patients at risk for future hemolytic transfusion reactions and emphasizes the importance of antibody screening and complete crossmatch prior to nonemergency transfusion.[8]

Posttransfusion purpura (PTP) is a rare complication; but PTP carries high risk and mortality as it results in significant thrombocytopenia 7 to 10 days post transfusion. Patients with a history of alloimmunization secondary to pregnancy or previous transfusions are at highest risk of PTP. Treatment includes high-dose intravenous immune globulin (IVIG) and supportive care.[8]

Transfusion-related acute lung injury (TRALI) remains one of the leading causes of transfusion-associated morbidity and mortality. Consensus diagnostic criteria require acute (within 6 hours of transfusion), noncardiogenic pulmonary edema with bilateral infiltrates and a ratio of arterial partial pressure of oxygen to the inspired concentration of oxygen of <300 (eg, 200/0.75). Blood products with high plasma content are generally implicated in the majority of the cases of TRALI, which can be explained by two suggested pathophysiologic mechanisms.

The most likely cause involves antineutrophil (anti-HNA) or anti-HLA antibodies formulated in multiparous female donors during a past pregnancy or as a result of sensitization from previous transfusions or transplantation. In fact, the practice of using male-predominant plasma donors significantly decreases the incidence of TRALI. The second commonly discussed "two hit hypothesis" for TRALI implicates the role of pro-inflammatory biologic response modifiers released in stored blood products that activate primed neutrophils in the recipient. Both pathophysiologic mechanisms result in breakdown of the capillary alveolar membrane, interstitial pulmonary edema, and microscopic alveolar hemorrhage, all of which lead to acute lung injury. The treatment for TRALI focuses on supportive care and lung protective low tidal volume mechanical ventilation as the low-pressure pulmonary edema does not generally respond to diuretic therapy.[8]

Transfusion-associated circulatory overload (TACO) is one of the most frequent serious complications of blood therapy with an incidence of about 1:50 component transfusions. It results from high-pressure cardiogenic pulmonary edema frequently associated with large volume or rapid transfusion. It is not an immune-mediated response and occurs more frequently in critically ill patients or those with a history of cardiopulmonary or renal disease. These patients develop hypoxemia secondary to ventilation perfusion mismatch and intrapulmonary shunt. Furthermore, patients express an elevated level of brain natriuretic peptide in response to ventricular distension. Typically, TACO responds to diuretic treatment and pulmonary alveolar recruitment.[8]

Transfusion-transmitted infections have been a focus of transfusion medicine research for several decades, which has resulted in a significant decrease in the rate of infection for recipients of allogeneic transfusion. The overall rate of transfusion-transmitted infections was significantly lower in the 2017 NBCUS than the number reported in 2015.[13] The greatest fear among blood transfusion recipients usually concerns viral infections such as hepatitis C and human immunodeficiency virus (HIV). However, these are actually a rare result of blood-product transfusion because of the increased sensitivity of donor screening tests now available and a short window of time between donor infection and seroconversion. Transfusion transmission of hepatitis B has also declined because of widespread vaccination. Over the past few years, many blood centers have introduced pathogen-reduction technology to reduce the risk of bacterial contamination especially with apheresis platelet components. Accordingly, the incidence of posttransfusion sepsis, or transfusion-transmitted bacterial infections, is quite rare. **Table 24.3** summarizes the residual risk of transfusion-transmitted infections.

> **? Did You Know?**
>
> Only in unusual circumstances is it appropriate to transfuse an anemic patient prior to elective surgery. The cause for anemia should be found and the patient treated. Alternatives to transfusion, such as perioperative cell salvage, should be considered.

V. Perioperative Alternatives to Transfusion

The risks of transfusion are indisputable. Even 1 unit of PRBCs can significantly increase perioperative morbidity. Fortunately, there are some blood conservation strategies to minimize allogenic RBC transfusion. Experts in transfusion medicine advocate for Patient Blood Management (PBM) programs defined by the AABB as "an evidence-based, multidisciplinary approach to optimizing the care of patients who might need transfusion." PBM uses preventive strategies and active management protocols to optimize patients prior to surgery and mitigate the risks of acute anemia and transfusion during active hemorrhage, while minimizing the incidence of adverse reactions to blood component therapy.[7,8]

Preoperative anemia is an independent risk factor for perioperative blood transfusion, morbidity, and mortality. Thus, strategies to conserve and even increase the patient's hemoglobin concentration prior to surgery should be considered for all elective cases. There should be a thorough preoperative diagnostic workup for the cause of the anemia and, if indicated, aggressive treatment of an iron deficiency or replacement of vitamin deficiencies (eg, vitamin B_{12} or folic acid). With a longer lead time before surgery for diagnosis and treatment of anemia, fewer patients require perioperative transfusion.[7,8]

Iron therapy is an important consideration for patients with preoperative anemia secondary to iron deficiency. Oral formulations for iron replacement are often associated with gastrointestinal upset and therefore poorly tolerated by patients long enough for them to be effective. However, intravenous iron therapy is more readily available as iron sucrose and iron gluconate, which carry far less risk of anaphylaxis than previous formulations.[8]

Erythropoietin is the most common erythropoiesis-stimulating agent (ESA) approved for use in patients with end-stage renal disease, presurgical anemia, and chemotherapy or malignancy-associated anemia. Erythropoietin increases RBC production in the bone marrow and has been shown to reduce allogenic transfusion requirements when used prior to orthopedic and cardiac surgery, especially if administered with iron repletion.[8] However, it carries a significant risk of venous and arterial thromboembolism and therefore should be used conservatively and with close patient monitoring.[7]

Autologous blood donation (collection and saving of the patient's own blood for later use) reduces several of the risks associated with allogenic blood transfusion, including viral infection and immune reactions such as TRALI and alloimmunization. However, preoperative autologous donation has not been shown to reduce perioperative allogenic transfusion due to the resultant lower preoperative hemoglobin concentration. Autologous blood donation still carries the risks associated with clerical error, bacterial contamination, TACO, and storage lesions. Furthermore, there is significant risk of donated blood expiring prior to surgery date if surgery is postponed or delayed for any cause. Certain patients may be candidates for autologous transfusion if they have antibodies to high-prevalence blood antigens, multiple alloantibodies, or they refuse allogenic transfusion and are at risk for significant surgical blood loss; in those cases, ESAs should be used in conjunction with preoperative donation.[8]

Acute normovolemic hemodilution involves the removal of 2 or 3 units of whole blood with volume replacement with intravenous fluids immediately preincision. The blood is typically stored in the operating room but may be preserved for 8 hours prior to reinfusion. This results in the patient losing blood at a lower hematocrit during surgery and for the patient to be resuscitated with autologous whole fresh blood after most of the surgical blood loss has resolved. This method is very efficacious in young healthy patients who can tolerate intraoperative anemia without risk of end-organ hypoxia or for patients who have a higher risk of transfusion reactions from allogenic blood products. It can also be considered for patients who refuse allogenic transfusions including those of the Jehovah's Witness faith as the blood removed can be kept in continuity with the patient at their request.[8]

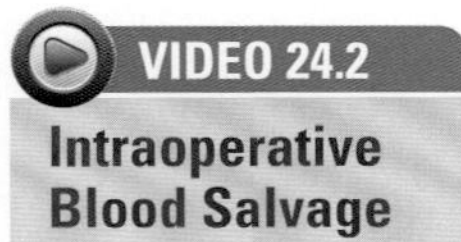

Perioperative blood salvage with intraoperative "cell saver" technology or postoperative intracompartment cell salvage is the most used and efficacious method for perioperative blood conservation. Especially in orthopedic surgery for total knee arthroplasty and hip replacement, perioperative cell salvage has significantly decreased patient risk for blood transfusion. Postoperative cell salvage is generally limited to orthopedic surgery as mediastinal cell salvage after cardiac and thoracic surgery has been associated with worse postoperative bleeding and morbidity.

Intraoperative RBC salvage systems typically involve three phases, all of which must be run by trained operators to optimize RBC return and minimize risks. Shed blood is first anticoagulated and collected with limited variable suctioning to minimize the detrimental effects of sheer forces. Inefficient collection may increase the risk of hemolysis. Suction of wounds contaminated with frank infection, ruptured tumor sections, amniotic fluid, metal, or pharmaceutical compounds may increase the risks associated with cell salvage. Generally, leucodepletion filters limit the white blood cells and contaminants, including tumor cells and amniotic fluid contents, from entering the collection chamber. Thus, intraoperative cell salvage systems remain acceptable in obstetrics, as well as any procedures with anticipated blood loss >1000 mL. Collected blood is centrifuged, washed, filtered, and reconstituted to a resultant hematocrit of 45% to 55%.[8] Meta-analysis of studies using cell salvage in urologic and gynecologic cancer surgery demonstrates that it is safe and is not associated with additional risk of tumor recurrence or metastasis. Risks associated with reinfusion of salvaged RBCs include air embolism and hemolysis. But these risks are minimal when the system is used properly and still negligible when compared with the risk of allogeneic blood transfusion.

Overall, perioperative blood salvage is cost-efficient, low risk, and clinically effective at reducing the need for RBC transfusion. It is particularly important when considering use of perioperative blood conservation strategies for patients requiring rare blood types and those who are Jehovah's Witnesses, who generally refuse any transfusion when RBCs have been removed from the body. Often Jehovah's Witness patients will accept RBC salvage if the salvaged blood remains in continuity with the patient. This is easily established with a primed venous line attached to the reinfusion bag of the cell savage system.

Oxygen carriers as blood substitutes are an attractive alternative to transfusion, eliminating many of the risks associated with RBC administration.

There are no compounds currently approved for human use, although this is an active field of research. Unfortunately, blood substitutes containing recombinant hemoglobin molecules have been associated with hypertension and renal and liver dysfunction, while substitutes containing perfluorocarbon compounds, which increase the fraction of dissolved oxygen, commonly cause thrombocytopenia. Hopefully, further studies will provide an efficient low-risk alternative blood substitute.[8]

VI. Primary Hemostasis

Figure 24.2 shows the three general phases of platelet function: adherence, activation, and stabilization. When the blood vessel is injured, platelets adhere via surface receptors to underlying collagen and to von Willebrand factor (vWF) on endothelium or in a blood clot. These engaged receptors set off signaling pathways mediated via phospholipase C (PLC) to cause platelet activation. In the activation phase, platelets secrete numerous agents to

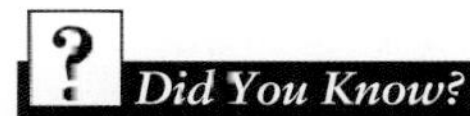

The process of coagulation is complex, involving numerous components and interactive processes. If time permits, the cause for unusual bleeding should be carefully elucidated and therapy precisely targeted. In an emergency, "shotgun" therapy with fresh frozen plasma or platelets may be necessary.

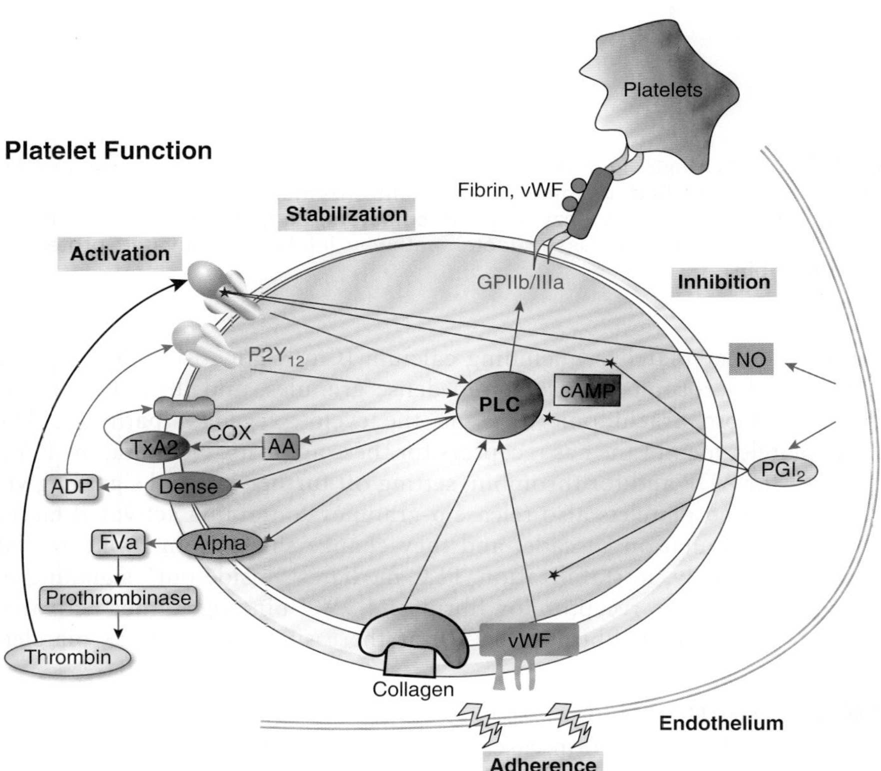

Figure 24.2 Diagram of platelet function. *Blue arrows,* activating signaling pathways. *Red lines,* inhibiting signaling pathways. *Green arrows,* secretion. Adherence: *Yellow lightning bolts,* injury. vWF, von Willebrand factor. Activation: PLC, phospholipase C. Alpha, alpha granules. Dense, dense granules. TxA_2, thromboxane A_2. COX, cyclo-oxygenase. ADP, adenosine diphosphate. FVa, activated factor V. $P2Y_{12}$, ADP receptor. Not all activation elements are shown. Stabilization: GPIIb/IIIa, glycoprotein IIb/IIIa. Inhibition: NO, nitric oxide. PGI_2, prostaglandin I_2 (prostacyclin). cAMP, cyclic adenosine monophosphate. Targets of antiplatelet medications (*blue*): COX, aspirin, and nonsteroidal anti-inflammatory drugs. P_2Y_{12}, clopidogrel class. cAMP, dipyridamole class. GPIIb/IIIa, abciximab class.

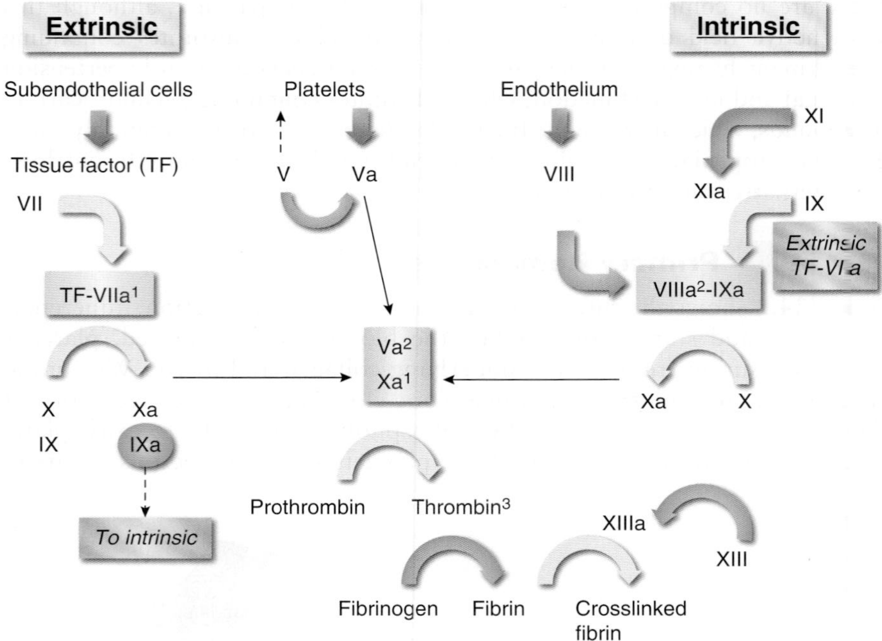

Figure 24.3 Extrinsic and intrinsic pathways for coagulation cascade. *Gray arrows:* secretion. *Red:* vitamin K–dependent enzymes. *Blue arrows:* activation by thrombin. *Solid boxes:* enzymes with cofactors, Ca^{++}, and platelet-membrane phospholipid. Inhibition: [1]tissue factor pathway inhibitor; [2]activated protein C; [3]antithrombin.

stimulate other platelets, including calcium (Ca^{++}), adenosine diphosphate (ADP), and serotonin released from dense granules, and thromboxane A_2 produced from arachidonic acid via the cyclo-oxygenase pathway. The outer platelet membrane has receptors for these agonists, including the P_2Y_{12} receptor for ADP and for thrombin, setting off further internal signaling via PLC. Activated platelets also release α-granules containing activated factor V for the coagulation cascade, and they change shape from round to flat and spiky. Finally, in stabilization, PLC mediates "inside-out" signaling to activate the surface receptor for fibrin and vWF binding. Other activated platelets crosslink to fibrin and vWF at these sites, creating the platelet-fibrin plug.

A. Secondary Hemostasis

Classically, the coagulation cascade is subcategorized into (1) the ***extrinsic pathway***, activated by tissue factor (TF) from cells outside a disrupted blood vessel; (2) the ***intrinsic pathway***, involving only plasma factors; and (3) the ***common pathway***, fed by both the intrinsic and extrinsic to form thrombin, then fibrin (**Figure 24.3**). However, the extrinsic and common pathways also amplify the intrinsic pathway. Each of these three pathways has a central enzyme complex with four parallel elements: a plasma enzyme, a cofactor (mostly cell or platelet derived), the Ca^{++} ion, and a phospholipid (PL) platform provided in vivo by the platelet membrane.

The extrinsic pathway activates factor X to Xa via the extrinsic "ten-ase," comprising enzyme factor VIIa (activated by TF), its cofactor TF, Ca^{++}, and PL. The intrinsic pathway activates Xa with the intrinsic ten-ase, containing enzyme IXa, cofactor VIIIa, Ca^{++}, and PL. In the common pathway, the Xa enzyme formed by these processes combines with cofactor Va, Ca^{++}, and PL to form prothrombinase. Prothrombin is then converted to thrombin, which in turn converts fibrinogen to the end product fibrin.

When thrombin is formed, it also amplifies the intrinsic VIIIa to IXa ten-ase: thrombin activates VIIIa and XIa, which produces IXa. The extrinsic ten-ase also makes some IXa for the intrinsic ten-ase. Thrombin amplifies its own prothrombinase by activating some plasma Va. However, platelets provide most of the Va by taking up plasma factor V, converting it to Va, and then secreting Va during platelet activation. Finally, thrombin also activates factor XIII, which crosslinks and stabilizes the fibrin clot.

B. Fibrinolysis

Fibrin is broken down by plasmin after the need for hemostasis has resolved. Plasmin is activated from plasminogen in several ways: (1) tissue plasminogen activator (tPA) from endothelial cells cleaves plasminogen and is itself activated by plasmin; (2) urokinase from the endothelium and kidney activates plasminogen; (3) factor IXa and the contact factors XIIa and kallikrein, associated with the intrinsic pathway, activate a minor fraction of plasminogen. Contact factors can activate XIa during in vitro testing (partial thromboplastin time) but not in vivo. Fibrinolysis is also regulated. The α_1-antiplasmin and thrombin-activated fibrinolysis inhibitor (TAFI) inhibit plasmin. TAFI and plasminogen activation inhibitor-1 (PAI-1) interfere with tPA function, and PAI-1 promotes clearance of tPA and urokinase.

C. Regulation of Hemostasis

Platelet activation is physiologically inhibited by nitric oxide (NO) and prostaglandin I_2 (PGI_2) secreted by endothelial cells. NO stimulates a pathway leading to inhibition of the thromboxane A_2 receptor. PGI_2 binds to a platelet receptor, which signals for suppression of vWF adherence, PLC function, and thromboxane A_2 activation.

Secondary hemostasis is also regulated at several junctures (**Figure 24.3**). Tissue factor pathway inhibitor, secreted by endothelial cells and facilitated by its cofactor protein S, dampens functions of extrinsic TF-VIIa ten-ase and the common pathway Xa. Antithrombin, particularly when bound to heparin, inhibits thrombin and all the other enzyme factors.

Activated protein C cleaves extrinsic VIIIa and common-pathway Va. Protein C is activated by protein C-ase, comprising the enzyme thrombin, a cofactor thrombomodulin secreted by endothelial cells, Ca^{++}, and PL.

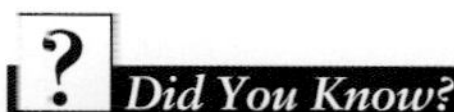

Use of low-dose aspirin is ubiquitous among patients because it is an effective prophylaxis against myocardial infarction. It acts by irreversibly inhibiting cyclo-oxygenase and impairing platelet aggregation. It should be discontinued more than a week before intraocular or intracranial surgery to reduce the risk of devastating hemorrhage.

VII. Pharmacology

Anticoagulant and antiplatelet medications target various points within the hemostatic pathways. Antiplatelet medications prevent platelet activation and aggregation, while anticoagulant medications inhibit coagulation factor activation at various points within secondary hemostasis. **Table 24-4** outlines the specific targets inhibited by each drug along with some details about monitoring their effect and drugs that can be used in the event of bleeding emergencies.

Table 24.4 Anticoagulant and Antiplatelet Medications

Medication	Trade Name	Target/MOA	Monitor Test	Antidote
Anticoagulants				
Heparin		Antithrombin enhanced activity to inhibit Xa and thrombin	aPTT, ACT, or anti-Xa	Protamine
LMWHs				
Enoxaparin	Lovenox	Factor Xa inhibition	Anti-Xa	Protamine has limited effect
Dalteparin	Fragmin	Factor Xa inhibitor	Anti-Xa	Protamine has limited effect
Fondaparinox	Arixtra	Factor Xa inhibition	Anti-Xa	None
Argatroban	Acova	DTI	ACT	None
Bivalirudin	Angiomax	DTI	aPTT or ECT	None but rapid metabolism
Warfarin	Coumadin	Vitamin K antagonist	INR	Vitamin K or 4-factor PCC
DOACs				
Apixaban	Eliquis	Factor Xa inhibition	Calibrated anti-Xa assay	Andexanet alfa
Rivaroxaban	Xarelto	Factor Xa inhibition	Calibrated anti-Xa assay	Andexanet alfa
Edoxaban	Savaysa	Factor Xa inhibition	Calibrated anti-Xa assay	4-Factor PCC
Dabigatran	Pradaxa	DTI	Thrombin time	Idarucizumab
Antiplatelet Drugs				
Aspirin		COX inhibition	Platelet function assay	Platelet transfusion
Clopidogrel	Plavix	P_2Y_{12} antagonist	P_2Y_{12} assay	Platelet transfusion
Abciximab	ReoPro	Monoclonal antibody to GPIIb/IIIa	aPTT or ACT	None

ACT, activated clotting time; aPTT, activated thromboplastin time; COX, cyclo-oxygenase; DTI, direct thrombin inhibitor; ECT, ecarin clotting time; INR, international normalized ratio; LMWHs, low-molecular-weight heparins; MOA, mechanism of action; NOAC, new oral anticoagulants; PCC, prothrombin complex concentrate.

Antiplatelet therapy is the mainstay of treatment for cerebrovascular and cardiovascular disease. Aspirin is an irreversible inhibitor of cyclo-oxygenase, thereby preventing the synthesis of thromboxane, a major stimulant for platelet activation. The second most used class of antiplatelet medications includes clopidogrel and ticlopidine, P_2Y_{12} receptor antagonists, which result in a decreased expression of the glycoprotein IIb/IIIa receptors on the surface of activated platelets, thereby inhibiting platelet adhesion and aggregation. Finally, the direct glycoprotein IIb/IIIa receptor antagonists—abciximab and eptifibatide—prevent platelet aggregation by inhibiting the crosslink of fibrinogen. These agents are only available for intravenous administration and are primarily used in treatment of acute coronary syndrome.

Unfractionated heparin is one of the oldest and most used medications for anticoagulation, especially for emergency treatment of pulmonary embolism, myocardial infarction, vascular thrombosis, or cardiopulmonary bypass. It acts by improving the affinity of antithrombin for thrombin, thereby inhibiting the final step of secondary hemostasis. The therapeutic effects of heparin primarily inhibit the intrinsic and common coagulation pathway and can be monitored with the activated partial thromboplastin time or the activated clotting time. However, it is a large molecule with significant risks of heparin-induced thrombocytopenia (HIT), a disorder characterized by microvascular thrombosis secondary to platelet-activating IgG antibodies to the heparin and platelet factor 4 complexes. Low-molecular-weight heparins such as enoxaparin, fondaparinox, and dalteparin inhibit the activation of factor X as a means of preventing thrombin formation and hemostasis. They are smaller molecules with longer half-lives making them less likely to cause HIT and suitable for intermittent therapeutic dosing that does not require an infusion. Enoxaparin should be used with caution in patients with renal dysfunction and creatinine clearance <30 mL/min. Parenteral direct thrombin inhibitors such as argatroban and bivalirudin bind to free thrombin preventing ongoing hemostatic activity. They are primarily indicated for patients with HIT or those with a heparin allergy and can be monitored with activated clotting times.[14]

Warfarin is a classic oral anticoagulant medication clinically used for treatment and prophylaxis in patients at high risk for stroke or venous thromboembolism such as those with a hypercoagulable disorder (ie, lupus anticoagulant, factor V Leiden, antithrombin deficiency) or a history of deep vein thrombosis, pulmonary embolism, heart valve replacement, or atrial fibrillation. Mechanistically, it is a vitamin K antagonist that prevents the hepatic synthesis of vitamin K–dependent coagulation factors, including factors II, VII, IX, and X. Incidentally, it also prevents the synthesis of protein C, a natural anticoagulant with a short half-life. Therefore, patients initiated on warfarin treatment will be hypercoagulable for the first 1 to 2 days until the available supply of factors is depleted. The effective concentration of warfarin is highly variable between patients and commonly affected by food and drug interactions. Regular monitoring is necessary and facilitated by the international normalized ratio (INR), a hemostatic assay designed to normalize the prothrombin time across different laboratories for patients with a combined deficiency of factors II, VII, IX, and X. For patients on warfarin therapy who experience a bleeding emergency, the warfarin should be reversed with vitamin K supplementation or 4-factor prothrombin complex concentrates (PCCs). Plasma is the second-line therapy indicated for urgent warfarin reversal only if PCCs are not available.[14] The direct oral anticoagulants (DOACs) include dabigatran, a direct thrombin inhibitor, and rivaroxaban, edoxaban, or apixaban, direct factor Xa antagonists. This class of anticoagulants is very popular for patients at risk of venous thromboembolism or stroke related to atrial fibrillation because of their rapid onset, simple dosing, and lack of need for regular laboratory monitoring secondary to a high degree of bioavailability and few significant drug or food interactions.[15]

Table 24.5 Oral Anticoagulant Medications

	Warfarin	Dabigatran	Apixaban	Rivaroxaban	Edoxaban
Target	Vitamin K	Thrombin	Factor Xa	Factor Xa	Factor Xa
Time to peak	72-96 hr	1-2 hr	3 hr	2.5-4 hr	1-2 hr
Half-life	40 hr	9-13 hr	8-15 hr	7-11 hr	10-14 hr
Dose	2-10 mg	150 mg	5 mg	20 mg	30-60 mg
Frequency	Daily or qod	Once or twice daily	Twice daily	Daily	Daily
Metabolism	None	80% renal excretion	Hepatic	Hepatic	Hepatic with 50% renal excretion
Drug interactions	CYP2C9	Few	CYP3A4	CYP3A4	MDR1 P-glycoprotein

qod, every other day.

There is active research around specific antidotes for treatment of critical hemorrhage or bleeding emergencies in patients on DOACs. Dabigatran can be fully reversed with the administration of the monoclonal antibody, idarucizumab.[16] Furthermore, there is widely accepted evidence and FDA approval for the use of andexanet alfa, an inactive recombinant form of coagulation factor Xa, for the blockade of direct acting factor Xa inhibitors including rivaroxaban and apixaban.[17] Andexanet alfa has not been studied for edoxaban, although the mechanism of effect is directed at all factor Xa inhibitors. In the absence of andexanet alfa, current recommendations dictate the use of 4-factor PCCs for treatment of critical bleeding in patients on DOAC therapy.[15] In the stable patient scheduled for surgery, the most recent guidelines suggest waiting four to five half-lives of a DOAC prior to elective procedures, including neuraxial anesthesia, and longer for patients with renal insufficiency. **Table 24.5** outlines the pharmacokinetics and pharmacodynamics of warfarin versus the DOACs.[8,18]

Hemostatic medications serve an integral role in patient blood management and the control of hemorrhage by promoting the formation and stabilization of blood clots. There are several mechanistic targets for procoagulant agents from the initiation of primary hemostasis to the activation of clotting factors. However, it is imperative that these agents target only the site of vascular injury as systemic activation of hemostatic pathways can lead to catastrophic arterial and venous thromboembolism.

Desmopressin (1-deamino-8-D-arginine vasopressin [DDAVP]) is a synthetic analogue of vasopressin with a wide range of hemostatic effects, some of which are still poorly understood. DDAVP is clinically indicated for treatment and prophylaxis of bleeding in patients with platelet dysfunction, often related to uremia, hemophilia, and von Willebrand disease, as it facilitates the cleavage of factor VIII and vWF to increase the activity of both factors, thereby improving platelet function. Additionally, DDAVP provides a modest decrease in bleeding associated with major surgery such as spinal fusion, revision orthopedic procedures, and high-risk cardiac surgery, without a significant increased risk of thromboembolism. Other adverse effects of DDAVP include hyponatremia and resultant cerebral edema, but this is clinically rare in the adult population.[8]

Antifibrinolytics prevent the dissolution of established blood clots, thereby improving vascular integrity at the site of injury and decreasing bleeding. There are two types of antifibrinolytics. Aprotinin is a serine protease inhibitor that directly inhibits plasmin. It is not available in the United States because a large randomized trial demonstrated an association between use of aprotinin and increased morbidity and mortality. However, it has been proven to be effective at decreasing blood loss and transfusion requirements for patients undergoing high-risk surgery and is currently approved for use in Canada and Europe.[8]

The lysine analogue antifibrinolytics, including epsilon-aminocaproic acid (EACA) and tranexamic acid (TXA), inhibit the cleavage of plasminogen to plasmin. They are less potent than aprotinin and in comparative trials less effective, but the incidence of thromboembolism and adverse effects from TXA and EACA are minimal, making them an attractive option for prophylaxis in patients at risk for major bleeding. Large clinical trials in trauma patients, as well as many studies in cardiac and orthopedic surgical patients, have documented the clinical efficacy of these medications especially when used prophylactically.[3,8]

Factor concentrates provide the substrates for the secondary hemostasis phase of the clotting cascade without the transfusion risks associated with plasma administration. Concentrates can be delivered individually when indicated, for example, factor VIII concentrates in classic hemophilia. Recombinant activated factor VII is currently approved for treatment of hemophilia in patients with inhibitors to factors VIII or IX.

PCCs have different compositions, but generally include varied amounts of three to four factor concentrates, including factors II, IX, X, and sometimes VII. For most of the PCCs, these factors are administered inactive and complexed with an anticoagulant such as antithrombin, protein C, or heparin, making the overall therapy less likely to cause unwanted thromboembolism. PCCs are currently indicated for treatment of hemophilia patients with inhibitors to specific factor concentrates. However, they are more frequently used as the first-line reversal agents for warfarin and the DOACs in cases of critical bleeding. It is important to recognize that these medications carry a risk of arterial and venous thromboembolism and should be redosed with extreme caution. They are contraindicated in patients with suspicion of having DIC, a systemic disorder of uncontrolled hemostasis with microvascular clotting, coagulation factor, and platelet consumption that may progress to multiorgan system failure and massive hemorrhage.

For further review and interactivities, please see the associated Interactive Video Lectures and "At a Glance" infographic accessible in the complimentary eBook bundled with this text. Access instructions are located in the inside front cover.

References

1. Jones JM, Sapiano MRP, Savinkina AA, et al. Slowing decline in blood collection and transfusion in the United States - 2017. *Transfusion*. 2020;60(suppl 2):S1-S9. PMID 32086817.
2. Spahn DR, Bouillon B, Cerny V, et al. The European guideline on management of major bleeding and coagulopathy following trauma: fifth edition. *Crit Care*. 2019;23(1):98. PMID 30917843.

3. American Society of Anesthesiologists Task Force on Perioperative Blood Management. Practice guidelines for perioperative blood management: an updated report by the American society of Anesthesiologists task force on perioperative blood management*. *Anesthesiology*. 2015;122(2):241-275. PMID 25545654.
4. Carson JL, Guyatt G, Heddle NM, et al. Clinical practice guidelines from the AABB: red blood cell transfusion thresholds and storage. *J Am Med Assoc*. 2016;316(19):2025-2035. PMID 27732721.
5. Raphael J, Mazer CD, Subramani S, et al. Society of cardiovascular Anesthesiologists clinical practice improvement advisory for management of perioperative bleeding and hemostasis in cardiac surgery patients. *Anesth Analg*. 2019;129(5):1209-1221. PMID 31613811.
6. Robinson S, Harris A, Atkinson S, et al. The administration of blood components: a British Society for Haematology Guideline. *Transfus Med*. 2018;28(1):3-21. PMID 29110357.
7. Mueller MM, Van Remoortel H, Meybohm P, et al. Patient blood management: recommendations from the 2018 frankfurt consensus conference. *J Am Med Assoc*. 2019;321(10):983-997. PMID 30860564.
8. *A Compendium of Transfusion Practice Guidelines*. 3rd ed. American Red Cross; 2017.
9. Green L, Bolton-Maggs P, Beattie C, et al. British Society of Haematology Guidelines on the spectrum of fresh frozen plasma and cryoprecipitate products: their handling and use in various patient groups in the absence of major bleeding. *Br J Haematol*. 2018;181(1):54-67. PMID 29527654.
10. Estcourt LJ, Birchall J, Allard S, et al. Guidelines for the use of platelet transfusions. *Br J Haematol*. 2017;176(3):365-394. PMID 28009056.
11. Cancelas JA. Furture of platelet formulations with improved clotting profile: a short review on human safety and efficicy data. *Transfusion*. 2019;59(suppl 2):1467-1473. PMID 30980736.
12. Yazer MH, Spinella PC. An international survey on the use of low titer group O whole blood for the resuscitation of civilian trauma patients in 2020. *Transfusion*. 2019;60(suppl 3):S176-S179. PMID 32478858.
13. Savinkina AA, Haass KA, Sapiano MRP, et al. Transfusion-associated adverse events and implementation of blood safety measures - findings from the 2017 National Blood Collection and Utilization Survey. *Transfusion*. 2020;60(suppl 2):S10-S16. PMID 32134123.
14. Witt DM, Nieuwlaat R, Clark NP, et al. American Society of Hematology 2018 guidelines for management of venous thromboembolism: optimal management of anticoagulation therapy. *Blood Adv*. 2018;2(22):3257-3291. PMID 30482765.
15. Smith MN, Deloney L, Carter C, Weant KA, Eriksson EA. Safety, efficacy, and cost of four-factor prothrombin complex concentrate (4F-PCC) in patients with factor Xa inhibitor-related bleeding: a retrospective study. *J Thromb Thrombolysis*. 2019;48(2):250-255. PMID 30941571.
16. Pollack Jr CV, Reilly PA, van Ryn J, et al. Idarucizumab for dabigatran reversal—full cohort analysis. *N Engl J Med*. 2017;377(5):431-441. PMID 28693366.
17. Connolly SJ, Crowther M, Eikelboom JW, et al. Full study report of andexanet alfa for bleeding associated with factor Xa inhibitors. *N Engl J Med*. 2019;380(14):1326-1335. PMID 30730782.
18. Shaw JR, Kaplovitch E, Douketis J. Periprocedural management of oral anticoagulation. *Med Clin North Am*. 2020;104(4):709-726. PMID 32505262.

BLOOD THERAPY

AT A GLANCE

Blood product administration is often indicated to manage patients experiencing life-threatening hemorrhage. Important facts about the four most commonly transfused blood products are illustrated below.

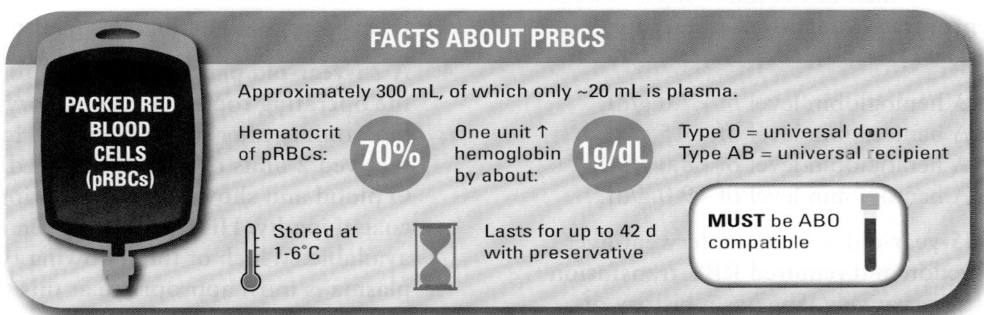

FACTS ABOUT PRBCS
PACKED RED BLOOD CELLS (pRBCs)
Approximately 300 mL, of which only ~20 mL is plasma.
Hematocrit of pRBCs: 70%
One unit ↑ hemoglobin by about: 1g/dL
Type O = universal donor
Type AB = universal recipient
Stored at 1-6°C
Lasts for up to 42 d with preservative
MUST be ABO compatible

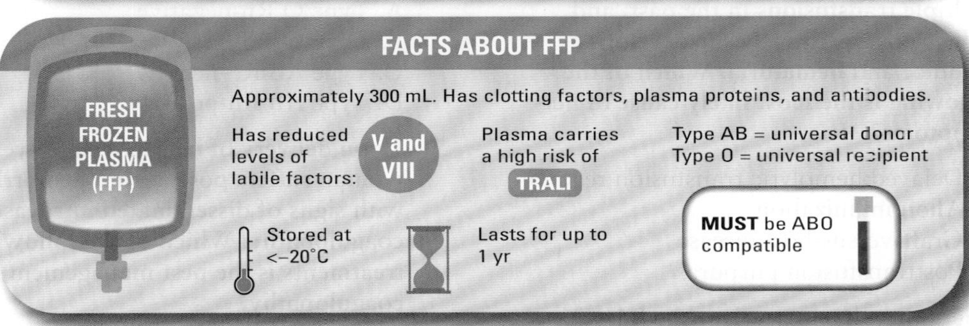

FACTS ABOUT FFP
FRESH FROZEN PLASMA (FFP)
Approximately 300 mL. Has clotting factors, plasma proteins, and antibodies.
Has reduced levels of labile factors: V and VIII
Plasma carries a high risk of TRALI
Type AB = universal donor
Type O = universal recipient
Stored at <–20°C
Lasts for up to 1 yr
MUST be ABO compatible

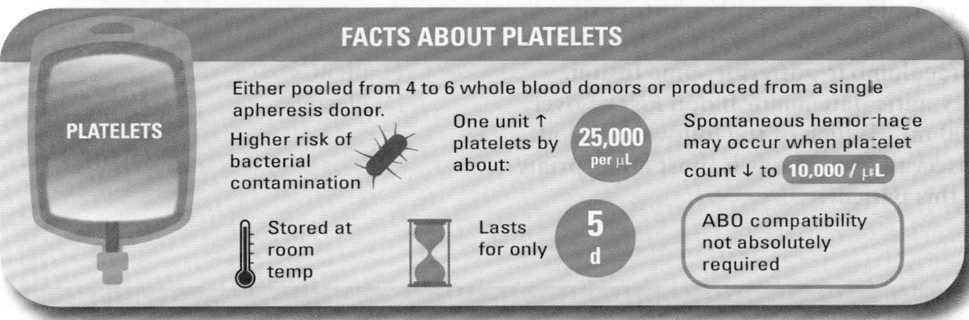

FACTS ABOUT PLATELETS
PLATELETS
Either pooled from 4 to 6 whole blood donors or produced from a single apheresis donor.
Higher risk of bacterial contamination
One unit ↑ platelets by about: 25,000 per μL
Spontaneous hemorrhage may occur when platelet count ↓ to 10,000 / μL
Stored at room temp
Lasts for only 5 d
ABO compatibility not absolutely required

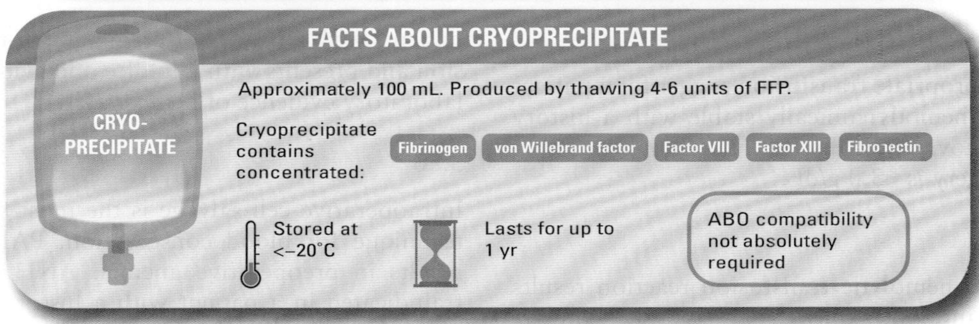

FACTS ABOUT CRYOPRECIPITATE
CRYO-PRECIPITATE
Approximately 100 mL. Produced by thawing 4-6 units of FFP.
Cryoprecipitate contains concentrated:
Fibrinogen
von Willebrand factor
Factor VIII
Factor XIII
Fibronectin
Stored at <–20°C
Lasts for up to 1 yr
ABO compatibility not absolutely required

Infographic by: Naveen Nathan MD

Questions

1. **After a fall from a scaffold, a 50-year-old man is undergoing intramedullary nailing for a femur fracture. He has a history of coronary artery disease and his vitals are stable. Which of the following is the most appropriate transfusion trigger for this patient?**

   A. A hemoglobin level of <7.0 g/dL
   B. A hemoglobin level of <7.5 g/dL
   C. A hemoglobin level of <8.0 g/dL
   D. A hemoglobin level of <9.0 g/dL

2. **A 45-year-old woman underwent liver resection and required RBC transfusion intraoperatively. She has a history of multiple transfusions in the past, and 2 days postoperatively she develops jaundice and hematuria. Which of the following is the most likely cause of her symptoms?**

   A. Delayed hemolytic transfusion reaction
   B. Alloimmunization
   C. Graft-versus-host disease
   D. Posttransfusion purpura

3. **The spine surgery service schedules a 70-year-old woman with a history of coronary artery disease for multilevel thoracolumbar posterior spine fusion. They anticipate major blood loss of over 1500 mL. Which of the following blood conservation methods is most appropriate for this patient?**

   A. Preoperative autologous donation (PAD)
   B. Intraoperative cell salvage
   C. Acute normovolemic hemodilution (ANH)
   D. Erythropoietin-stimulating agent

4. **A 25-year-old patient is brought to the operating room for exploratory laparotomy after major trauma. He received 2 units of uncrossmatched type O blood and shows signs of dilutional coagulopathy. His type and screen is not available. Which of the following types of plasma is most appropriate at this time?**

   A. Type O Rh-negative
   B. Type O Rh-positive
   C. Type AB Rh-negative
   D. Type AB Rh-positive

5. **Upon delivery of her baby, a 33-year-old woman suffers postpartum hemorrhage with signs of disseminated intravascular coagulopathy. Which of the following treatments is the best management of coagulopathy?**

   A. Cryoprecipitate
   B. Platelets
   C. PRBCs
   D. Plasma

Answers

1. C

The appropriate transfusion trigger for a patient who is hemodynamically stable with a history of cardiovascular disease undergoing orthopedic surgery is <8.0 g/dL.

2. A

Delayed hemolytic transfusion reaction results from antibodies in the recipient hemolyzing donor blood cells. It most often occurs in patients with a history of pregnancy or transfusion and presents with jaundice and evidence of laboratory evidence of hemolysis.

3. B

Intraoperative cell salvage is the most efficient technique for blood conservation. PAD often results in preoperative anemia. ANH is contraindicated in a patient with a history of significant cardiovascular disease who will not tolerate acute anemia.

4. D

Type AB Rh-positive plasma does not contain any antibodies to the major ABO and Rh blood antigen groups. It is the universal donor type for plasma similar to the type O Rh-negative, which is the universal donor for PRBCs.

5. A

Cryoprecipitate contains high concentrations of fibrinogen and therefore, it is the blood product most appropriate for a patient with disseminated intravascular coagulopathy.

25 Ambulatory Anesthesia, Monitored Anesthesia Care, and Office-Based Anesthesia

Meghan E. Rodes and Louise Hillen

According to a 2017 National Health Statistics Report from the Centers for Disease Control and Prevention, in 2010, 48.3 million surgical and nonsurgical procedures were performed during 28.6 million ambulatory surgery visits to hospitals and ambulatory surgical centers combined.[1] Self-reports from the American Hospital Association show that roughly 66% of all surgeries performed at community hospitals were performed in the outpatient setting, up from 57% in 1994.[2] According to the Agency for Healthcare Research and Quality, the most common ambulatory procedures were lens and cataract procedures, followed by muscle and tendon repair surgeries, such as rotator cuff repairs.[2] Especially for ambulatory anesthesia, it is important that all anesthesiologists are able to formulate an appropriate anesthetic plan that allows an expeditious return of consciousness and has minimal side effects, thereby permitting timely patient discharge. Many ambulatory procedures are performed under ***monitored anesthesia care (MAC)***. In this chapter, we will discuss techniques and common medications used in ambulatory anesthesia, as well as offer an introduction to the realm of office-based anesthesia.

I. Monitored Anesthesia Care

A. Terminology

According to the American Society of Anesthesiologists (ASA) position statement, MAC is a specific anesthesia service for a diagnostic or therapeutic procedure and may encompass varying levels of sedation.[3] Factors when considering the appropriateness of MAC include the type of procedure, the patient's clinical condition, and the potential need to convert to a general or regional anesthetic.[3] Furthermore, it includes all aspects of anesthetic care, including a preprocedure visit, intraprocedure care, and postprocedure recovery management.[3] The anesthesia provider must be prepared and qualified to convert to general anesthesia when necessary.[4] If the patient is unarousable even with painful stimulus, the anesthesia care is a general anesthetic, irrespective of whether airway instrumentation is required.[3] ASA standard monitoring, which includes electrocardiography (ECG), pulse oximetry, noninvasive blood pressure (NIBP), and end-tidal carbon dioxide ($ETCO_2$) monitoring, must be used for every anesthetic including MAC. MAC should be distinguished from moderate sedation. The term moderate sedation is used to describe a proceduralist-directed service, which does not include a qualified anesthesia provider and is governed by specific institutional policies.

B. Preoperative Assessment

Patients scheduled for MAC should receive a preoperative assessment equivalent to any other preoperative patient. MAC is unique in that it also requires an element of cooperation on the part of the patient. It is important for the patient to accept the possibility of some degree of awareness during the procedure, be able to tolerate the positioning required for surgery, and, in some instances, communicate with the surgeon or proceduralist.

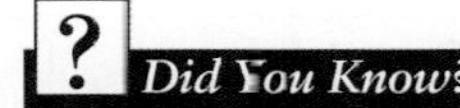

Patients scheduled for MAC should receive preoperative and postoperative assessments equivalent to any other preoperative patient.

C. Techniques of MAC

Successful MAC involves the use of a combination of a sedative-hypnotic and an analgesic agent used in varying doses depending on the goals of the anesthetic and the requirements of the procedure. Regional nerve block performed by an anesthesiologist or local anesthetic administered by the surgeon may improve patient comfort and lower anesthetic requirements. Medications with minimal side effects and short durations of action are preferable in ambulatory anesthesia, where efficiency and rapid recovery are highly desirable.

D. Specific Drugs Used During MAC

This section will provide a brief description of the drugs most commonly utilized during MAC. For a more in-depth discussion of these medications, the reader is referred to Chapters 9 and 10. **Table 25.1** provides a profile of several drugs commonly used in MAC.

Propofol

Propofol is a short-acting, intravenous, sedative-hypnotic agent. It is used for induction and maintenance of general anesthesia, for procedural sedation, and as a sedative for mechanically ventilated patients in the intensive care unit. Propofol has multiple mechanisms of action, including potentiation of γ-aminobutyric acid (GABA) receptor activity and sodium channel blockade. It possesses antiemetic and bronchodilator properties and has a short context-sensitive half-life time that is minimally affected by duration of infusion. Bolus and induction doses of propofol should be based on lean body weight; however, infusion dosing should be based on total body weight. In addition to its desired therapeutic effects, propofol also decreases systemic vascular resistance (SVR), blood pressure (BP), cerebral metabolic rate for oxygen ($CMRO_2$), cerebral blood flow (CBF), and intracranial pressure (ICP). Propofol also produces significant respiratory depression, so it requires that the provider be prepared to support the airway. Propofol may produce a burning sensation on administration, especially when injected into a small vein. The most effective strategy to prevent this symptom is pretreatment with lidocaine (3 mL of 1% lidocaine) while occluding the vein proximal to the intravenous insertion site.[5] Despite the addition of additives, propofol is a lipid emulsion that supports rapid bacterial growth. Strict aseptic technique is critical to minimizing contamination risk. Propofol vials should be discarded within 6 hours of opening. Propofol is metabolized by the liver and excreted by the kidneys.

Fospropofol

Fospropofol is a water-soluble prodrug form of propofol. It is metabolized by alkaline phosphatases to its active metabolite, propofol; therefore, its onset

Table 25.1 Profile of Drugs Frequently Used in Monitored Anesthesia Care

Drug	Route of Administration	Mechanism of Action	Side Effects	Metabolism	Antagonist
Propofol	IV	Potentiation of GABA receptor activity, sodium channel blockade	• Antiemetic • Bronchodilator • Respiratory depression • ↓ SVR, BP, $CMRO_2$, CBF, ICP • Burning sensation on administration	Hepatic	None
Midazolam	IV IM PO	Enhancement of GABA	• ↓ $CMRO_2$, CBF • Anticonvulsant	Hepatic	Flumazenil
Fentanyl	IV Intrathecal Transmucosal	Opioid receptor agonist	• Respiratory depression • ↓ HR, CBF • Delayed gastric emptying • Nausea/vomiting • Urinary retention	Hepatic	Naloxone
Ketamine	IV IM PO	NMDA receptor antagonist	• ↑ $CMRO_2$, CBF, ICP, IOP, HR, BP • Secretions • Hallucinations	Hepatic	None
Dexmedetomidine	IV	$Alpha_2$ receptor agonist	• ↓ $CMRO_2$, CBF, HR, BP	Hepatic	None

BP, blood pressure; CBF, cerebral blood flow; $CMRO_2$, cerebral metabolic rate for oxygen; GABA, γ-aminobutyric acid; HR, heart rate; ICP, intracranial pressure; IM, intramuscular; IOP, intraocular pressure; IV, intravenous; NMDA, *N*-methyl-d-aspartate; PO, by mouth; SVR, systemic vascular resistance.

of action is slower than propofol. Potential advantages over propofol include less chance of bacterial contamination, less pain on injection, and lower risk of hyperlipidemia associated with long-term administration. Although fospropofol has been approved by the Food and Drug Administration for use during MAC, it is not commonly used in clinical practice at this time.

Benzodiazepines

Benzodiazepines, most commonly midazolam, are used to provide anxiolysis and anterograde amnesia. They work by enhancing the effect of GABA at its receptors. Benzodiazepines produce minimal respiratory depression when used alone. They decrease $CMRO_2$ and CBF but have no appreciable impact on ICP. Benzodiazepines are potent anticonvulsants and may be used to treat status epilepticus and seizures related to local anesthetic toxicity or alcohol withdrawal. Midazolam is metabolized by the liver and excreted by the kidneys. In addition to the intravenous route, it can be administered intramuscularly, intranasally, or orally. The oral dose of midazolam is much higher than the intravenous dose due to poor oral bioavailability. Although midazolam has a short elimination half-life, larger doses may be associated with delayed emergence. Benzodiazepines offer a safety advantage compared to propofol in that there is a specific benzodiazepine antagonist, flumazenil. However, the effects of midazolam frequently outlast those of flumazenil. Therefore, resedation is a possibility, and flumazenil redosing may be required.

Opioids

Opioids, most commonly fentanyl, are administered for analgesia. In addition to intravenous administration, opioids may be given by various routes including oral, intramuscular, subcutaneous, transmucosal, and neuraxial. The mechanism of action of opioids is through an agonist action at specific opioid receptors in the central and peripheral nervous systems, which in turn decreases the transmission of pain signals. Side effects of opioids include dose-dependent respiratory depression, decreased CBF, delayed gastric emptying, increased urinary sphincter tone leading to urinary retention, and nausea and vomiting. Opioids may also induce skeletal muscle rigidity when large doses are administered rapidly. Chest wall rigidity can be severe enough to make ventilation difficult, and therefore, large doses should be avoided. It is also important to note that opioids alone do not provide amnesia. Opioids are metabolized by the liver and excreted mainly in the urine. Differences in lipid solubility within this class of drugs account for varying pharmacokinetic profiles. Like benzodiazepines, opioids also have a specific antagonist, naloxone. Naloxone can be given to reverse the respiratory effects of opioids but should be used judiciously due to potential adverse side effects such as tachycardia, hypertension, and pulmonary edema. The half-life of naloxone is shorter than most opioids, so the provider must watch for a recrudescence of overdose symptoms; repeated naloxone doses or an infusion may be necessary.

? *Did You Know?*

Rapid intravenous opioid—especially fentanyl—administration may induce muscle and chest wall rigidity that can be severe enough to make ventilation difficult.

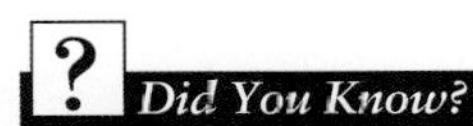

Opioids alone do not provide amnesia.

Ketamine

Ketamine is a phencyclidine derivative that produces intense analgesia and amnesia. While small doses may be used as an adjunct in MAC, larger doses can be used to induce general anesthesia. Its primary mechanism of action is antagonism at the *N*-methyl-D-aspartate (NMDA) receptor. Ketamine can be administered by oral, intramuscular, or intravenous routes. Ketamine has bronchodilator properties, making it beneficial in asthmatic patients. Also, in contrast to other sedatives and opioids, it has minimal effect on respiration. In addition to its therapeutic effects, ketamine has traditionally been associated with increased $CMRO_2$, CBF, ICP, and increased stimulation of the sympathetic nervous system resulting in increased heart rate (HR) and BP. For these reasons, ketamine is best avoided in patients with increased ICP or intraocular pressure (IOP) and those with coronary artery disease. It should be noted that ketamine may have a paradoxical cardiac effect in patients with disease states associated with catecholamine depletion (eg, septic shock), resulting in direct myocardial depression. Ketamine increases secretions; administration of an antisialagogue such as glycopyrrolate is helpful. Ketamine also produces dissociative amnesia, which is a conscious but trance-like state where the patient is disconnected from the sensory, motor, memory, and emotional functions in the brain. This is uncomfortable for patients and may be minimized by prior administration of a benzodiazepine. Ketamine is metabolized in the liver to norketamine, which has approximately one-fifth the potency of ketamine and may contribute to lingering effects.

Dexmedetomidine

Dexmedetomidine is an intravenous centrally active selective alpha$_2$-receptor agonist, which may be used to provide sedation, analgesia, and anxiolysis. Its major benefit is that it has little effect on respiratory drive when used alone. Dexmedetomidine has no intrinsic amnestic properties but can help reduce anesthetic requirements. Side effects of dexmedetomidine include decreased $CMRO_2$ and CBF, as well as a combination of decreased sympathetic outflow and increased vagal activity, which may precipitate hypotension and severe bradycardia. Dexmedetomidine is extensively metabolized in the liver and excreted by the kidneys. The context-sensitive half-time is roughly 4 minutes after a 10-minute infusion but can increase to 250 minutes after an 8-hour infusion. Since dexmedetomidine has no amnestic properties, it must be supplemented with a drug such as propofol or midazolam if amnesia is desired.

> **? Did You Know?**
>
> Ketamine and dexmedetomidine are unique sedative drugs in that they do not suppress ventilatory drive.

E. Patient-Controlled Analgesia and Sedation

Patient-controlled analgesia (PCA) is a familiar technique for the management of postoperative pain. PCA has a favorable safety profile compared with intermittent larger boluses of analgesics. In addition, PCA is associated with increased patient satisfaction compared to provider-driven analgesic administration. Patient-controlled sedation has been shown to be effective for use during procedural sedation; however, it is not widely used owing to the cumbersome nature of the setup and safety concerns.[6]

F. Respiratory Function and Sedative-Hypnotics

Most of the drugs used during MAC are associated with dose-dependent adverse respiratory effects, which include direct respiratory depression, suppression of normal airway reflexes, and an increase in upper airway resistance.

Sedation and the Upper Airway

Successful ventilation requires coordination of all parts of the airway from the oropharynx to the muscles of the thorax. Patients with preexisting sleep-disordered breathing (obstructive sleep apnea, OSA), lung disease, or neuromuscular disorders are particularly susceptible to developing ventilatory problems while receiving sedation.

Sedation and Protective Airway Reflexes

Intact upper airway reflexes are necessary to safeguard against pulmonary aspiration. Many anesthetic drugs have an adverse effect on these protective upper airway reflexes. Patients at risk for aspiration are generally not good candidates for MAC.

Sedation and Respiratory Control

The negative pulmonary effects of anesthetic agents are synergistic when used in combination. Therefore, smaller doses of each must be used. Supplemental oxygen is commonly employed during MAC, as mild hypoventilation and hypoxemia are common.

G. Monitoring During MAC

ASA Standards for Basic Anesthetic Monitoring

The ASA standards for basic monitoring apply to every anesthetic delivered by an anesthesia provider, regardless of anesthetic type, patient condition, and duration or urgency of the procedure.[7] These standards require that qualified anesthesia personnel are present in the room throughout the course of all anesthetics and oxygenation, ventilation, circulation, and temperature are continually evaluated. Oxygenation is most commonly monitored by pulse oximetry. An in-line oxygen analyzer, which monitors inspired oxygen concentration, is required for all general anesthetics with an anesthesia machine. Capnography is used to monitor ventilation when an endotracheal tube or laryngeal mask airway is in place. Although $ETCO_2$ monitoring became an ASA standard monitor in 2011, it has been shown to be a poor indicator of ventilation in the sedated, spontaneously breathing patient, owing to factors such as mouth breathing or dilution from high oxygen flows. Alarms must be in place to detect absence of $ETCO_2$, signifying apnea or a disconnection in components of the breathing system. Circulation is monitored by continuous ECG and pulse oximetry, as well as evaluation of BP and HR at a minimum of 5-minute intervals. Temperature must be monitored when clinically significant changes in body temperature are intended, anticipated, or suspected.

? Did You Know?

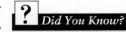

The ASA requires that end-tidal carbon dioxide be measured during all forms of sedation, including MAC.

Communication and Observation

There is no substitute for a meticulous, focused, and attentive anesthesia provider. While basic monitors are applied for all anesthetics, sight and sound are important tools for the assessment of clinical condition, particularly during MAC.

Recognition and Treatment of Local Anesthetic Toxicity

Since MAC is often provided as an adjunct to regional, neuraxial, or local anesthesia, it is important for the anesthesia provider to be aware of toxic dose ranges of local anesthetics, to be able to recognize the signs and symptoms of local anesthetic systemic toxicity (LAST), and to be prepared to treat LAST in an expeditious fashion. Symptoms of LAST often begin with numbness of the tongue or perioral area and a metallic taste in the mouth. As the concentration of local anesthetic in the central nervous system increases, patients may report tinnitus or restlessness, which may progress to slurred speech, muscle twitching, and seizures. Sedation may mask the early signs of LAST. The side effects of sedation such as hypercarbia and acidemia, which result in increased CBF and an increase in the ionized form of local anesthetic crossing into the brain, may aggravate central nervous system and cardiac toxicity. Seizures may be treated with a benzodiazepine or propofol. If arrhythmias are present, amiodarone is the drug of choice. Definitive treatment of LAST is intravenous lipid emulsion (see also Chapter 12).

H. Sedation and Analgesia by Nonanesthesiologists

The spectrum of anesthetic depth is fluid, meaning there are no concrete demarcations between levels of sedation. Furthermore, the level of sedation intended may differ from the level of sedation achieved. **Table 25.2** defines each of the four levels on the continuum of depth of sedation, as developed by the ASA.[8] The table lists observations regarding patient responsiveness, airway, spontaneous ventilation, and cardiovascular function for each of the four levels of sedation. The goal is for the provider to have early recognition of a patient progressing to a deeper level of sedation than intended. The ASA recommends that nonanesthesia providers tasked with the administration of sedation participate in formal training and be able to demonstrate airway rescue skills such as bag-mask ventilation.

Table 25.2 Continuum of Depth of Sedation: Definition of General Anesthesia and Levels of Sedation/Analgesia

	Minimal Sedation, Anxiolysis	Moderate Sedation/ Analgesia "Conscious Sedation"	Deep Sedation/ Analgesia	General Anesthesia
Responsiveness	Normal response to verbal stimulation	Purposeful response to verbal or tactile stimulation	Purposeful response following repeated or painful stimulation	Unarousable even with painful stimulus
Airway	Unaffected	No intervention required	Intervention may be required	Intervention often required
Spontaneous ventilation	Unaffected	Adequate	May be inadequate	Frequently inadequate
Cardiovascular Function	Unaffected	Usually maintained	Usually maintained	May be impaired

Derived from American Society of Anesthesiologists. *Continuum of Depth of Sedation, Definition of General Anesthesia and Levels of Sedation/Analgesia*. 2009. www.asahq.org

II. Ambulatory Anesthesia

A. Patient and Procedure Selection

Ambulatory anesthesia encompasses anesthesia provided in a hospital-based ambulatory surgery unit, freestanding ambulatory surgery center, or physician's office. One advantage of an outpatient site is that costs are generally much lower than in the hospital. Turnaround time is also frequently improved in an ambulatory center, which may be the result of more streamlined processes or financial incentives.

A commonly held misconception is that ambulatory surgery is only appropriate for healthy, ASA physical status (PS) I and II patients. However, ASA PS III and IV patients may be cared for successfully in ambulatory centers provided their comorbidities are stable. Uncomplicated obesity is not necessarily a risk factor for poor outcomes. However, obese patients are more likely to have OSA, which is associated with postoperative respiratory complications. The ASA has published specific guidelines pertaining to the perioperative management of ambulatory surgery patients with OSA. Regardless of age and comorbidities, all patients who undergo ambulatory surgery should have a responsible adult escort them home and assist with postoperative care for the first 24 hours, when needed.

Many institutions and some states have a lower age cutoff for ambulatory surgery. For example, centers may require that infants born at term be at least 1 month of age to be eligible for outpatient surgery. Preterm infants are often required to be older (50-60 weeks postconceptual age) because they have a higher risk of postoperative apnea. Similarly, advanced age is not a contraindication to surgery in an ambulatory center; however, medications are more slowly metabolized in the elderly, and anesthetic plans should be modified accordingly.

Procedure selection is also important. Procedures appropriate for the ambulatory setting should have a low risk of postoperative complications and require minimal postoperative care. Ideally, procedures should be of short duration (<2 hours). It is generally best to perform longer procedures or procedures on higher risk patients early in the day to allow more time for postoperative monitoring.

B. Preoperative Evaluation

Preoperative screening is an important tool to reduce adverse outcomes on the day of surgery. This involves a complete medical history, including surgeries, past anesthetics, medications, and allergies as well as a focused physical examination (at minimum, heart, lungs, and airway). This is also the appropriate occasion to review preoperative fasting and medication instructions, set realistic expectations about the anesthetic and postoperative pain, and confirm postoperative plans for transportation by a responsible adult.

Upper Respiratory Tract Infection

Whether to proceed with anesthesia in a patient with an upper respiratory infection (URI) requires consideration of several factors. If the URI is mild and without constitutional symptoms, surgery may usually proceed, particularly if intubation of the trachea is not expected. If the URI is severe and wheezing or constitutional symptoms are present or if intubation is required, the surgery should probably be postponed for 4 to 6 weeks. The recommendations for children are somewhat different, mainly because children have URIs more frequently than adults and delaying surgery may be infeasible. Most anesthesiologists would proceed with surgery if the child appears well, is afebrile, and is breathing and eating normally.

Restriction of Food and Liquids Prior to Ambulatory Surgery

The ASA has established practice guidelines for preoperative fasting, which are listed in **Table 25.3**.[9] The guidelines are the same regardless of whether the patient is being treated in a hospital or ambulatory setting. These guidelines permit a light meal up to 6 hours prior to elective surgery (8 hours for a fatty meal) and clear liquids such as black coffee or tea without cream or other additives up to 2 hours prior to surgery. In infants, breast milk is permitted up to 4 hours prior to surgery and infant formula up to 6 hours prior to surgery. To the extent possible, fasting duration should be minimized, especially in young children.

Table 25.3 ASA Fasting Guidelines for Elective Surgery

Substance	Fasting Time	Examples
Clear liquids	2 h	Water, transparent juice, coffee/tea without additives
Breast milk	4 h	
Infant formula	6 h	
Light meal	6 h	Dry toast
Fatty meal	8 h	Fried food, butter, cream

ASA, American Society of Anesthesiologists.

From American Society of Anesthesiologists Committee. Practice guidelines for preoperative fasting and the use of pharmacologic agents to reduce the risk of pulmonary aspiration: application to healthy patients undergoing elective procedures. An updated report by the American Society of Anesthesiologists Committee on Standards and Practice Parameters. *Anesthesiology.* 2011;114:495-511.

Anxiety Reduction

Probably the most effective and undervalued way to reduce patient anxiety is through a conversation with an anesthesia provider prior to surgery. For children, parental presence during induction may be of benefit. Involvement of a child life specialist and distraction techniques may also be helpful. Oral and intravenous anxiolytic medications may also be used.

C. Managing the Anesthetic: Premedication

Premedication is not necessarily different in the ambulatory setting, but careful selection of agent and dose is important to facilitate timely discharge.

Benzodiazepines

Midazolam is the most commonly used benzodiazepine for the purpose of anxiolysis. Due to a synergistic effect with other anesthetic agents, it may delay emergence or discharge following very short procedures, and therefore, it is important to assess whether the patient requires or desires preoperative sedation. In addition to its anxiolytic properties, midazolam also has the benefit of inducing amnesia. These effects on memory are independent of the sedative effects, and a patient may appear completely awake yet have no recollection of events afterward.

Opioids and Nonsteroidal Analgesics

In addition to their analgesic effects, opioids are often administered as part of preprocedural sedation or to decrease the hemodynamic response to sympathetic stimulation (eg, laryngoscopy, intubation, or surgical incision). A multimodal approach to pain control is especially important in the ambulatory setting. The addition of nonsteroidal anti-inflammatory drugs (NSAIDs), such as ketorolac and ibuprofen, and acetaminophen help modulate pain through alternative pathways. These drugs effectively decrease narcotic requirements, thereby reducing the adverse side effects related to opioid administration.

D. Intraoperative Management: Choice of Anesthetic Method

Anesthetic Options

The anesthetic choices for ambulatory surgery include general anesthesia, regional or neuraxial anesthesia, MAC, and local anesthesia. Regional and local anesthetic techniques have the potential benefit of requiring minimal sedation. In some situations, the type of surgery dictates the choice of anesthetic; in most situations, a discussion between patient, surgeon, and anesthesiologist is useful to determine the most appropriate choice. Recovery time is an important element in determining the anesthetic technique.

Regional Techniques

The regional anesthetic techniques used in ambulatory surgery include neuraxial anesthesia (spinal or epidural), peripheral nerve blocks (PNBs), intravenous regional anesthesia (such as Bier block), and local anesthetic infiltration, or field and digital blocks performed by the surgeon. The use of local anesthetics with long-acting analgesic effects such as bupivacaine can be especially useful to help with postoperative pain control.

Spinal Anesthesia

Spinal anesthesia is an appropriate choice for surgery on the lower extremities, pelvis, or lower abdomen. The use of a short-acting local anesthetic will result in rapid recovery of motor and sensory function and shortens the time to discharge. Intrathecal opioids are not often administered when spinal anesthesia is performed for ambulatory surgery. Postdural puncture headache is not a common complication when smaller gauge pencil-point noncutting needles are used.

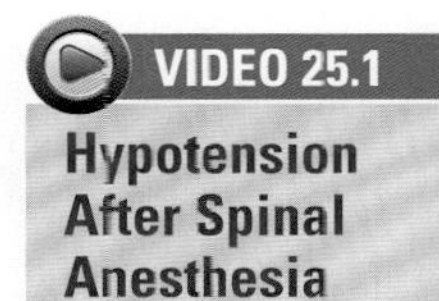

Epidural and Caudal Anesthesia

Epidural anesthesia involves the introduction of a catheter into the epidural space, which may be placed preoperatively and injected with local anesthetic just prior to surgery. Doses of local anesthetic can be repeated intermittently, or the catheter can be connected to an infusion for longer surgeries. Epidural anesthesia is rarely used in adult ambulatory procedures.

Caudal anesthesia is a form of epidural anesthesia often performed in children for urologic surgeries and those in the lower abdomen and involves local anesthetic injection into the caudal canal. It is frequently used in conjunction with general anesthesia since children cannot generally tolerate needle insertion. Caudal anesthesia allows surgery to be performed with minimal perioperative opioids, and postoperative analgesia may last for several hours based on the choice of medication and dose administered. Caudal anesthesia is a great option for pediatric patients who are at high risk for perioperative apnea.

Peripheral Nerve Blocks

The use of peripheral nerve blocks (PNBs) for certain painful procedures such as shoulder surgery has allowed these procedures to be performed in the ambulatory setting. PNBs are associated with reduced pain, nausea, and vomiting and increased patient satisfaction. If postoperative pain is expected to be severe, a peripheral nerve catheter that provides a slow release of local anesthetic can be placed via ultrasound guidance. Patients can go home with the catheters in place and are usually instructed to remove them within 48 to 72 hours. It is important for the patient to receive detailed postoperative instructions. A more in-depth discussion of regional anesthesia can be found in Chapter 21.

Sedation and Analgesia

Intravenous sedation is a common adjunct to local anesthetic techniques. Analgesic agents decrease pain during initial injection of local anesthetic and alleviate discomfort from positioning on an operating table for a prolonged period. Additionally, their amnestic properties ensure that most patients have little recollection of intraoperative events.

General Anesthesia

General anesthesia is commonly performed in the ambulatory setting. Appropriate selection of anesthetic agents is necessary to facilitate rapid awakening and short recovery, while avoiding adverse side effects. The most common agents used for maintenance of general anesthesia are propofol and sevoflurane. Nitrous oxide, while more rapid in recovery than sevoflurane, may be associated with a higher risk of postoperative nausea and vomiting (PONV) when used for long periods of time. It is also contraindicated in patients undergoing middle ear surgery or retinal surgeries involving the creation of an intraocular gas bubble. Nitrous oxide should not be used in pregnant patients due to its effect on vitamin B12 and folate metabolism. Furthermore, while it is not considered flammable, nitrous oxide does support combustion and therefore should not be used in head and neck surgeries in which electrocautery will be used. Although a short-acting neuromuscular blocking agent is often appropriate for intubation, continuous neuromuscular blockade is often not necessary for ambulatory surgeries.

E. Postanesthesia Care

Many potential postoperative adverse events or complications can be anticipated and prevented. Patient selection plays a major role in planning a successful ambulatory surgical experience. The careful selection and titration of anesthetic agents have a significant impact on recovery. Common causes of delayed recovery are pain, nausea, and sedation due to residual anesthetic effects. Early identification and management are paramount. A more thorough discussion of the postoperative recovery can be found in Chapter 40.

Nausea and Vomiting

Postoperative nausea and vomiting (PONV) is a significant cause of delayed discharge and in rare cases may require admission to the hospital. In addition, PONV has a negative impact on patient satisfaction and quality of recovery. Factors predictive of PONV include female gender, history of PONV or motion sickness, nonsmoking, and certain types of surgery such as head and neck, ophthalmic, breast, and laparoscopy. The risk factors have an additive effect; the greater the number of risk factors present, the greater the risk of PONV. Unfortunately, many anesthetic agents contribute to PONV. Volatile anesthetics, nitrous oxide, and opioids all have emetogenic properties. The most commonly used antiemetics are selective serotonin receptor antagonists such as ondansetron. Other classes of drugs used to treat PONV are the dopamine antagonist butyrophenones (droperidol) and phenothiazines (prochlorperazine); antihistamines (dimenhydrinate); and anticholinergics (scopolamine). The glucocorticoid dexamethasone is also commonly used for PONV prevention and treatment and has been shown to improve quality of recovery. It has no appreciable impact on wound healing and little effect on glucose regulation in healthy subjects.[10,11] The most effective method to manage PONV is to identify patients at greatest risk and employ a combination of preventive strategies and avoidance of exposure to agents known to contribute to PONV. Total intravenous anesthesia with propofol is often used in patients with a history of severe PONV, as propofol has intrinsic antiemetic properties.

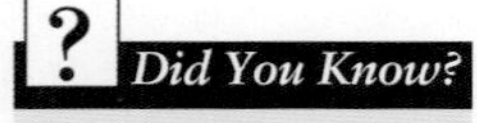

Patient risk factors for PONV include female gender, younger age, and a history of motion sickness or previous PONV.

Pain

A multimodal approach to analgesic management is advised. The multimodal approach involves the concomitant use of analgesic agents with different mechanisms of action and has an opioid-sparing effect. The most commonly used adjuncts include ketorolac, celecoxib, pregabalin, ibuprofen, and acetaminophen.

Reversal of Drug Effect

In the recovery room, it may occasionally become necessary to administer agents such as naloxone or flumazenil to reverse the respiratory depressant effects of opioids or benzodiazepines, respectively. Caution is advised when using these antagonists since they may have serious cardiovascular or central nervous system effects. When reversal agents are administered, discharge should be delayed to allow time to monitor the patient for the development of resedation.

Patient Discharge

Postanesthesia care is typically divided into two phases. In Phase I, the emphasis is on ensuring that the patient has recovered from the effects of anesthesia and vital signs are near baseline. In Phase II, the focus is on preparing the patient for hospital discharge, including education on postoperative care. Most patients who receive MAC are ready for Phase II recovery immediately at the end of surgery. In contrast, most patients who receive general anesthesia require a period of time in Phase I recovery. However, with the use of preemptive analgesia and short-acting anesthetics, some patients who receive general anesthesia may bypass Phase I recovery; this is called "fast-tracking." One recent study demonstrated significantly shortened recovery duration by eliminating Phase I recovery after general anesthesia (based on standardized criteria), without any change in patient outcome.[12]

Several scoring systems have been developed to help determine a patient's readiness for discharge; they have been modified over time to reflect changes in anesthesia techniques and patient management. The original Aldrete score included an evaluation of activity; respiration; circulation; consciousness; and color.[13] The Postanesthetic Discharge Scoring System (PADSS) was initially based on vital signs; ambulation and mental status; pain and nausea/vomiting; surgical bleeding; and fluid input/output. Ability to void and to tolerate oral intake are no longer required for discharge in most institutions. A contemporary version of the PADSS includes these five categories: vital signs; activity; nausea and vomiting; pain; and surgical bleeding. Discharge home typically requires a PADSS score ≥9 (**Table 25.4**).[14] Additional discharge criteria for the patient who receives neuraxial anesthesia should include the return of motor and sensory function and the ability to ambulate independently.

Discharge instructions should be written and explained to the patient and the patient should acknowledge an understanding of these instructions. Patients should be advised not to drive or make any critical decisions for the remainder of the day. The instructions should always include a plan for a contact person or emergency facility should a postoperative issue arise. The patient needs to be discharged home with a responsible adult escort. Most ambulatory facilities conduct a follow-up call the day after surgery to assess the patient's condition.

III. Office-Based Anesthesia

Office-based anesthesia involves anesthesia provided at a location other than a hospital or freestanding surgical facility. It is estimated that 17% to 24% of elective procedures are performed in the office setting.[15] The major incentives for office-based procedures are the financial benefits and convenience to the surgeon and patient. A potential disadvantage of being remote from a hospital is the lack of assistance in the event of an emergency. Current studies and review of closed claims data suggest an increased risk with an office-based anesthetic, with problems ranging from inadequate equipment, monitoring, and evaluation, to poor preparation and response to events. Almost half of the adverse events reported in office settings were classified as preventable.

Table 25.4 Post-Anesthetic Discharge Scoring System (PADSS)

Parameter	Value	Score
Vital signs	BP and pulse within 20% of preoperative level	2
	BP and pulse within 20%-40% of preoperative level	1
	BP and pulse greater than 40% different from preoperative level	0
Activity	Steady gait, no dizziness or meets preoperative level	2
	Requires assistance	1
	Unable to ambulate	0
Nausea and vomiting	Minimal/treated with oral medication	2
	Moderate/treated with parenteral medication	1
	Severe/continues despite treatment	0
Pain	Controlled with oral analgesics and acceptable to patient	2
	Uncontrolled or unacceptable to patient	1
Surgical bleeding	Minimal/no dressing changes	2
	Moderate/up to two dressing changes required	1
	Severe/more than three dressing changes required	0

From Chung F, Chan V, Ong D. A post anesthetic discharge scoring system for home readiness after ambulatory surgery. *J Clin Anesth.* 1995;7:500-506.

Though office-based surgery standards may differ from state to state, it should be clear that the standard of anesthesia care in an office-based setting is no different than anesthesia care completed in a hospital setting. The ASA statement from its Ambulatory Surgical Committee, last updated in October 2019, provides guidelines to assist those intending to perform ambulatory anesthesia in an office-based setting.[16]

A. Patient Selection and Preoperative Management

The anesthesiologist should complete a thorough preoperative evaluation and feel confident that the planned procedure is within the scope of practice for the involved practitioners and the facility. Patients with significant comorbidities who are at risk for anesthetic or surgical complications are not appropriate candidates for office-based procedures and should be referred to an appropriate facility. **Table 25.5** provides suggestions for patients that may not be appropriate for an office-based procedure.[17] Longer surgical procedures have a greater likelihood of postoperative complications and need for hospital admission. Many facilities plan to have procedures completed by early afternoon to provide for complete recovery prior to discharge from the facility.

B. Equipment and Monitoring

Office surgery locations must be equipped appropriately. At a minimum, the facility should have a reliable oxygen source, suction, resuscitation equipment, and emergency drugs. It is mandatory that all machines be current, in functioning order, and serviced as per manufacturer's guidelines. All ASA standard monitors are required, including pulse oximetry, capnography, BP, continuous ECG, and the ability to measure temperature. A selection of suitable

Table 25.5 Patients Not Suitable for Office-Based Anesthesia

Cardiac conditions: • Activity level <4 METs • Unstable angina • MI: 0-3 mo • MI: 3-6 mo, must have evaluation by cardiologist before surgery • Severe cardiomyopathy • Poorly controlled Hypertension • Internal defibrillator or pacemaker • Heart transplant recipient/candidate	Pulmonary conditions: • Obstructive sleep apnea • Severe chronic obstructive pulmonary disease • Airway abnormality • Previous difficult intubation • Asthma: <6 mo since last Emergency department visit/acute exacerbation • Lung transplant recipient/candidate	Central nervous system: • Multiple sclerosis • Stroke <6 mo prior • Para-/quadriplegia • Seizure disorder • Psychological instability • Dementia with disorientation
Renal: • Creatinine > 2 mg/dL • End-stage renal disease on dialysis • On special diet due to renal disease • Kidney transplant candidate	Hepatic: • Elevated bilirubin or transaminases • Liver transplant candidate	Endocrine: • Morbid obesity with BMI >35 mg/kg • Poorly controlled diabetes mellitus • Hemoglobin A1c > 8% • Type I diabetes mellitus
Hematologic: • Sickle cell disease • Anticoagulant therapy • von Willebrand disease • Hemophilia	Musculoskeletal: • History of malignant hyperthermia • Myasthenia gravis • Muscular dystrophy or myopathy	Other: • Alcohol/substance overuse • No adult escort

BMI, body mass index; METs, metabolic equivalents; MI, myocardial infarction.
Adapted from Ahmad S. Office based – is my anesthetic care any different? Assessment and management. *Anesthesiol Clin.* 2010;28:369-384.

airway equipment is needed, including a spectrum of oxygen delivery devices from nasal cannula to intubation equipment, as well as emergency airway supplies such as a self-inflating (Ambu) ventilation bag. Suction must also be available. If pediatrics patients are treated in the facility, appropriately sized equipment and resuscitation devices must be available. Medications for the treatment of malignant hyperthermia must be available when triggering agents (succinylcholine or volatile anesthetics) are used. Emergency medications and a crash cart including a defibrillator are essential. Written protocols need to be in place to ensure the safe and timely transfer of patients who may require extended emergency or in-hospital services.

C. Safety and Organization

Each facility should have a medical director who is in charge of delineating the responsibilities of each staff member. Clear policies and procedures should be available and reviewed annually. All local and federal regulations must be followed, and all practitioners need to hold current and valid licenses appropriate for their assigned duties. It is the responsibility of the anesthesiologist to participate in quality improvement and risk management projects. The building construction should comply with rules pertaining to fire prevention and proper disposal of medical and hazardous waste. At least one member of the staff must be certified in advanced cardiovascular life support (ACLS) and remain present until all patients have been discharged from the facility.

D. Anesthetic Management

Similar to ambulatory anesthesia, the choice of anesthetic in the office setting is based on the need to facilitate rapid discharge and minimize adverse side effects. Cost of anesthetic equipment and medications may also be a factor.

IV. Conclusion

The same standards for preoperative evaluation and preparation, intraoperative monitoring, and postoperative care must be maintained regardless of the patient, setting, or type of anesthetic to be administered. Policies and procedures should be in place to ensure a minimum standard of care across all anesthetizing locations. All persons providing sedation must have knowledge of the pharmacologic properties of sedatives and analgesic drugs, be able to recognize and manage their adverse side effects, and be capable of performing the emergency procedures that may be needed to rescue a patient from a deeper than intended level of sedation. The duration of action of medications used in any individual anesthetic should be based on the patient's condition and the nature of the planned procedure. Follow-up with patients and analysis of outcomes will allow our specialty to continually increase patient safety and satisfaction in all settings where anesthesia is administered.

For further review and interactivities, please see the associated Interactive Video Lectures and "A Closer Look" infographic accessible in the complimentary eBook bundled with this text. Access instructions are located in the inside front cover.

References

1. *Surgeries in Hospital-Based Ambulatory Surgery and Hospital Inpatient Settings* [Internet]. 2014. Accessed October 4, 2020. https://hcup-us.ahrq.gov/reports/statbriefs/sb223-Ambulatory-Inpatient-Surgeries-2014.jsp
2. Hall MJ, Schwartzman A, Zhang J, et al. Ambulatory surgery data from hospitals and ambulatory surgery centers: United States, 2010. *Natl Health Stat Report*. 2017;(102):1-15.
3. American Society of Anesthesiologists. *Position on Monitored Anesthesia Care*. Accessed July 20, 2020. 2008. www.asahq.org
4. American Society of Anesthesiologists. *Distinguishing Monitored Anesthesia Care ("MAC") From Moderate Sedation/analgesia (Conscious Sedation*. 2013. Accessed July 20, 2020. www.asahq.org
5. Jalota L, Kalira V, George E, et al. Prevention of pain on injection of propofol: systematic review and meta-analysis. *Br Med J*. 2011;342:d1110. PMID: 21406529.
6. Mazanikov M, Udd M, Kylänpää L, et al. Patient-controlled sedation for ERCP: a randomized double-blind comparison of alfentanil and remifentanil. *Endoscopy*. 2012;44(5):487-492. PMID: 22450724.
7. American Society of Anesthesiologists. *Standards for Basic Anesthetic Monitoring*. 2011. Accessed July 20, 2020. www.asahq.org
8. American Society of Anesthesiologists. *Continuum of Depth of Sedation, Definition of General Anesthesia and Levels of Sedation/Analgesia*. 2009. Accessed July 20, 2020. www.asahq.org

9. American Society of Anesthesiologists Committee. Practice guidelines for preoperative fasting and the use of pharmacologic agents to reduce the risk of pulmonary aspiration: application to healthy patients undergoing elective procedures. An updated report by the American Society of Anesthesiologists Committee on Standards and Practice Parameters. *Anesthesiology*. 2011;114:495-511.
10. De Oliveira GS, Ahmad S, Fitzgerald PC, et al. Dose ranging study on the effect of preoperative dexamethasone on postoperative quality of recovery and opioid consumption after ambulatory gynaecological surgery. *Br J Anaesth*. 2011;107(3):362-371. PMID: 21669954.
11. Murphy GS, Szokol JW, Avram MJ, et al. The effect of single low-dose dexamethasone on blood glucose concentrations in the perioperative period: a randomized, placebo-controlled investigation in gynecologic surgical patients. *Anesth Analg*. 2014;118(6):1204-1212. PMID: 24299928.
12. Apfelbaum JL, Walawander CA, Grasela TH, et al. Eliminating intensive postoperative care in same-day surgery patients using short-acting anesthetics. *Anesthesiology*. 2002;97(1):66-74. PMID: 12131105.
13. Aldrete JA, Kroulik D. A postanesthetic recovery score. *Anesth Analg*. 1970;49(6): 924-934. PMID: 5534693.
14. Chung F, Chan VW, Ong D. A post-anesthetic discharge scoring system for home readiness after ambulatory surgery. *J Clin Anesth*. 1995;7(6):500-506. PMID: 8534468.
15. Kurrek MM, Twersky RS. Office-based anesthesia: how to start an office-based practice. *Anesthesiol Clin*. 2010;28(2):353-367. PMID: 20488399.
16. *Guidelines for Office-Based Anesthesia* [Internet]. Accessed July 30, 2020. https://www.asahq.org/standards-and-guidelines/guidelines-for-office-based-anesthesia
17. Ahmad S Office based—is my anesthetic care any different? Assessment and management. *Anesthesiol Clin*. 2010;28(2):369-384. PMID: 20488400.

POSTOPERATIVE NAUSEA AND VOMITING

A CLOSER LOOK

Postoperative nausea and vomiting (PONV) is a leading cause of delayed discharge from the postanesthesia care unit and a major source of patient dissatisfaction. Major patient-related risk factors for PONV include:

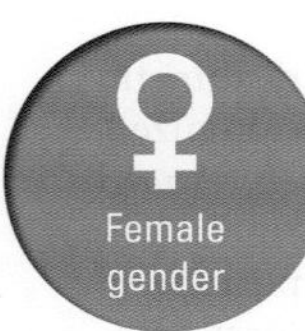

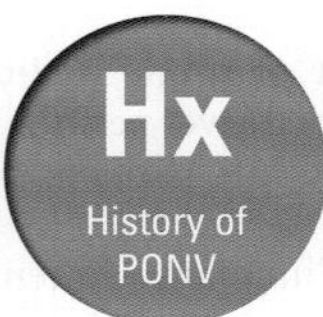

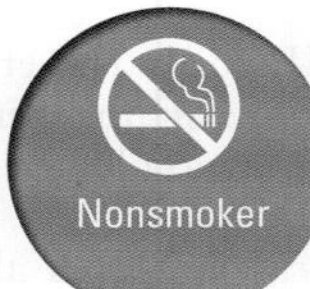

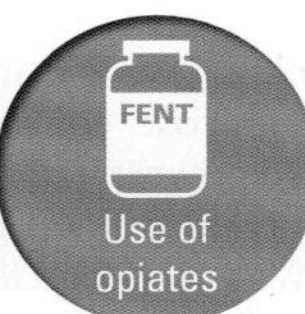

Modify anesthetic technique to reduce risk of PONV

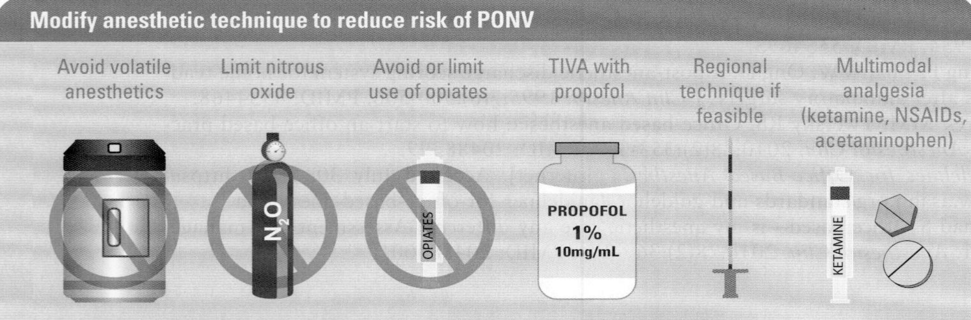

Prophylaxis for patients at higher risk...

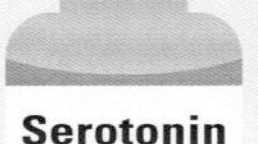

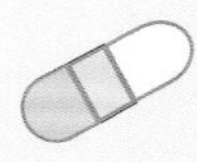

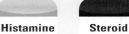

Serotonin antagonist	Dopamine-2 antagonist	Histamine antagonist	Steroid	Neurokinin antagonist	Acetylcholine antagonist
Ondansetron	Haloperidol	Diphenhydramine	Dexamethasone	Aprepitant	Scopolamine
4-8 mg IV	**0.5-1 mg IV**	**12.5-25 mg IV**	**4-10 mg IV**	**40-80 mg PO**	**1 mg transdermal patch**
Administer 30 min prior to emergence Side effects: headache and QT prolongation	Administer 30 min prior to emergence Side effects: sedation, extrapyramidal symptoms and QT prolongation *Avoid in patients with Parkinson disease.*	Administer 30 min prior to emergence Side effects include sedation and dry mucous membranes *Avoid in patients at risk for delirium.*	Administer at any time during anesthetic Avoid rapid IV bolus when patient is awake because this may result in perineal pain May increase blood glucose.	Administer preoperatively May interfere with oral contraceptive medication	Place patch behind the ear preoperatively Side effects: sedation, dry mouth, diplopia, ↑ intraocular pressure and amnesia *Avoid in the elderly and in patients with glaucoma.*

A small 10-20 mg IV dose of propofol can be used to treat resistant PONV

Repeated doses from the same drug class are *ineffective*. Target multiple receptors to treat PONV.

Infographic by: Naveen Nathan MD

Questions

1. **The most common serious side effect of dexmedetomidine is:**

   A. Hypertension.
   B. Respiratory depression.
   C. Increased cerebral blood flow.
   D. Bradycardia.

2. **According to the ASA fasting guidelines for elective surgery, infant formula should be withheld for how many hours before surgery?**

   A. 2
   B. 4
   C. 6
   D. 8

3. **All of the following medications produce amnesia EXCEPT:**

   A. Fentanyl.
   B. Midazolam.
   C. Ketamine.
   D. Propofol.

4. **ASA standards include requirements for monitoring temperature, circulation, oxygenation, and:**

   A. Pain level.
   B. Ventilation.
   C. Consciousness.
   D. Position.

5. **Which of the following patients is the LEAST appropriate candidate for surgery in a freestanding ambulatory surgery center?**

   A. A 95-year-old with well-controlled hypertension undergoing cataract surgery.
   B. A 25-year-old with a BMI of 50 kg/m^2 undergoing tonsillectomy.
   C. A 40-year-old with a history of PONV undergoing carpal tunnel release.
   D. A 2-year-old healthy toddler undergoing tympanoplasty.

Answers

1. D

Dexmedetomidine may cause a decrease in blood pressure and heart rate. Bradycardia is the most serious significant side effect and may be accompanied by profound hypotension. It is fairly unique among sedatives in that it does not cause significant respiratory depression. It decreases cerebral blood flow and cerebral metabolic rate for oxygen.

2. C

Infant formula should be withheld for 6 hours prior to elective surgery in infants. It is only necessary to withhold breast milk for 4 hours prior to elective surgery, because it is digested relatively more quickly than formula. Full, fatty meals require an 8-hour fasting period, while light, low-fat meals require a 6-hour fasting period.

3. A

Opioids have analgesic but not amnestic properties. Midazolam, ketamine, and propofol all have intrinsic amnestic properties.

4. B

Basic anesthesia monitoring should include assessment of temperature, circulation, oxygenation, and ventilation. Ventilation is monitored using capnography.

5. B

Patient selection is an important aspect of ambulatory anesthesia. A morbidly obese patient undergoing upper airway surgery is probably not a good candidate for an ambulatory facility, as respiratory depression is a significant risk that would require prolonged postoperative monitoring. Advanced age is not a contraindication to outpatient surgery, especially in a patient undergoing minor surgery who is otherwise reasonably healthy. A history of PONV increases the risk of PONV during subsequent anesthetics; however, this risk can be mitigated by pretreatment and the use of an anesthetic technique that avoids emetogenic agents. Very young infants may not be suitable for treatment in an ambulatory facility; however, otherwise healthy toddlers can be successfully treated in this environment.

26 Orthopedic Anesthesia

Ian Slade and Arman Dagal

I. Preoperative Assessment

Orthopedic spine and extremity surgeries are generally classified as intermediate risk, although major spine surgery or more limited procedures in patients with preexisting medical conditions (eg, hip arthroplasty in the elderly) can significantly increase perioperative risk. The purpose of the preoperative assessment includes the identification and optimization of modifiable risk factors, explanation of the risks, and formulating the best possible anesthetic plan for the patient. In addition to the standard preoperative assessment (see Chapter 16), focused orthopedic evaluation should include the following:

- Appraisal of the urgency of the planned procedure, to appropriately expedite further testing and optimization (eg, risk of progression of secondary injury, infection risk of open fractures, thromboembolic complications of immobilization while awaiting surgery).
- Airway and cervical spine assessment (eg, rheumatoid arthritis, osteoarthritis, and ankylosing spondylitis could result in limited neck motion, atlantoaxial instability, or limited mouth opening due to the involvement of the temporomandibular joint).
- Assessment of respiratory system (eg, scoliosis-induced restrictive chest defects, impaired diaphragm function due to spinal cord injury).
- Assessment of cardiovascular system. Fitness level is the deciding criterion for the need for further assessment. Spine and orthopedic surgery patients may have limited exercise tolerance due to other reasons (commonly, pain) and therefore complicate this assessment.
- Assessment of neurologic status, including existing neurologic deficiencies and active range of motion of extremities.
- Assessment of pain and psychological burden in order to establish realistic postoperative expectations for pain and function.
- Review of past medical, surgical, and anesthetic history, allergies, and current medications with special attention to chronic opioid use and disease-modifying drugs such as steroids, methotrexate, and nonsteroidal anti-inflammatory drugs.
- Hematologic profile and anticoagulant or antiplatelet drug use. Management of anemia and modification or discontinuation of the drugs affecting coagulation will likely be required.

- Assessment of frailty via standardized frailty instruments, to plan perioperative interventions to mitigate risks of delirium, major deconditioning, and postoperative morbidity (eg, exercise prehabilitation, nutritional optimization, discharge support planning).[1]
- Planning for the postoperative care transition, intensity of care, pain management approaches including multimodal and regional analgesia, and eventual discharge destination.

II. Enhanced Recovery Pathways

Since the late 1990s, a great deal of investigation has been directed to methods of optimizing surgical outcomes and accelerating recovery through enhanced recovery after surgery (ERAS) pathways. ERAS pathways consist of bundles of care elements targeted to specific surgical procedures, combining preoperative optimization, intraoperative measures, and postoperative care goals. ERAS pathways have been described and evaluated for patients undergoing major spine and orthopedic surgery, among many other surgical populations.[2,3] Common aims of such bundles include reducing the risk of major organ dysfunction, improving pain management, improving wound healing, promoting early mobilization to speed surgical recovery, and minimizing risk of venous thromboembolism. All of these objectives support overarching goals of reducing hospital length of stay, morbidity, and mortality.

The anesthesiologist's role in ERAS pathways begins in the preanesthetic assessment phase, helping to clearly identify which patients are candidates for particular pathways and coordinating preoperative medication optimization, correction of anemia, smoking cessation, improving nutritional status, and conducting appropriate testing.

On the day of surgery, preoperative consumption of a clear carbohydrate beverage several hours before surgery is shown to decrease insulin resistance. Multimodal analgesic therapy is frequently initiated shortly before surgery, often combining nonsteroidal anti-inflammatory drugs, acetaminophen, gabapentinoids, and other adjuncts. Regional anesthetic techniques may also be initiated in this phase.

Intraoperative priorities focus on optimizing fluid balance and oxygen delivery by goal-directed fluid management and reducing intraoperative blood loss through use of antifibrinolytics (tranexamic acid [TXA]). Wound healing is promoted by maintaining normothermia and euglycemia perioperatively.

Postoperatively, oral hydration and nutrition are resumed as early as possible while attaining euglycemia. Multimodal analgesics are generally continued in combination with regional blocks, opioids, and nonopioid analgesics. Side effects such as nausea and vomiting are specifically treated, all with the goal of promoting patient comfort to engage in early mobilization, helping to reduce deconditioning and to prepare the patient for discharge.

III. Spine and Spinal Cord Pathology

A. Spinal Cord Injuries

Vehicle crashes are currently the leading cause of traumatic spinal cord injury (TSCI). Injury most commonly affects the cervical column (57.4%), followed by thoracic (21.5%) and lumbosacral (13.8%) levels.[4] The initial trauma can result in irreversible neuronal damage (primary injury) that is "complete" (no spinal cord function distal to the injury) or "incomplete" (partial function

Table 26.1 American Spinal Injury Association (ASIA) Spinal Cord Injury Classification

Grade	Type of Injury	Description
A	Complete	No motor or no sensory function below level of injury, including S4-5
B	Incomplete	Sensory function is preserved below the level of injury, but not motor function, including S4-5
C	Incomplete	Motor and sensory function is preserved below the level of injury (motor strength <3/5 in at least half of the major muscles)
D	Incomplete	Motor and sensory function is preserved below the level of injury (motor strength ≥3/5 in at least half of the major muscles)
E	Normal	Motor and sensory functions are intact

distal to the injury) and is only modifiable by prevention. *Secondary injury* starts within minutes and is exacerbated by inflammation and edema, leading to further ischemia and neurologic deterioration. Focused medical care aims to limit its extent with careful coordinated management strategies.[5] The American Spinal Injury Association score is used to classify the neurologic injury severity (**Table 26.1**). Incomplete neurologic injuries are eight times more common than complete injuries and may have a variety of presentations (**Table 26.2**).

Table 26.2 Incomplete Spinal Cord Injury Syndromes

Type	Description
Central cord syndrome	Common in elderly with hyperextension injury Motor dysfunction in upper extremities greater than lower extremities Sensory dysfunction below the injury Bladder dysfunction
Anterior cord syndrome	Anterior spinal artery or anterior cord injury Impaired motor function, pain and temperature sensation Two-point discrimination and proprioception remains intact
Brown-Sequard syndrome	Typically due to penetrating trauma Section of lateral half of the spinal cord Ipsilateral loss of motor and proprioception Contralateral loss of pain and temperature
Posterior cord syndrome	Loss of touch, proprioception, and vibration with intact motor function
Cauda equina syndrome	Injury below the conus medullaris—below L2 Perineal numbness, urinary retention, fecal incontinence Lower extremity weakness

Hemodynamic Management

Hypotension is common after TSCI and may be associated with intravascular volume depletion, tension pneumothorax, pericardial tamponade, and neurogenic shock. ***Neurogenic shock*** is characterized by hypotension with or without bradycardia due to loss of sympathetic tone when the injury occurs at the level of T6 and above. Chronotropic agents or cardiac pacing may be required for the treatment of associated bradycardia. Optimizing spinal cord perfusion aims to reduce the risk of secondary injury to vulnerable cord tissue in the setting of adjacent injury and edema. This goal is frequently addressed by augmentation of mean arterial blood pressure (MAP) above 85 mm Hg, which may be achieved with a combination of intravenous volume expansion, vasopressors, and inotropes. However, high-quality evidence is lacking to support an ideal management strategy, such as a target MAP or the duration after injury for which a higher cord perfusion pressure might alter neurologic outcome.[6,7]

Decompressive Surgery

Decompression of the injured spinal cord and stabilization of the spinal column is generally required after TSCI. It follows the initial resuscitation and surgical management of other immediate life-threatening conditions such as traumatic brain injury or intra-abdominal hemorrhage. When decompression is performed within 24 hours of injury, evidence suggests neurologic outcome may be better.[8]

B. Scoliosis

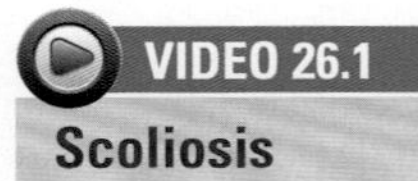

Scoliosis is defined as an abnormal lateral curvature of the spinal column in the coronal plane. It is frequently accompanied by a rotation deformity (**Table 26.3**). Its severity is assessed by the measurement of Cobb angle (**Figure 26.1**). Despite the application of a brace, progression of the curve to a Cobb angle >45° generally requires surgery to stop further deterioration. When untreated, progressive scoliosis may lead to severe back pain, restrictive ventilatory impairment, hypoxia, hypercarbia, and pulmonary hypertension.

Table 26.3 Etiology of Scoliosis

Idiopathic (80%)	Infantile: 0-3 y old Juvenile: 4-10 y old Adolescent: 11-18 y old
Congenital	VATER syndrome
Neuromuscular	Muscular dystrophies Poliomyelitis Cerebral palsy Spina bifida Friedreich ataxia Neurofibromatosis
Neural	Syringomyelia Chiari malformation
Syndromic	Marfan syndrome Neurofibromatosis

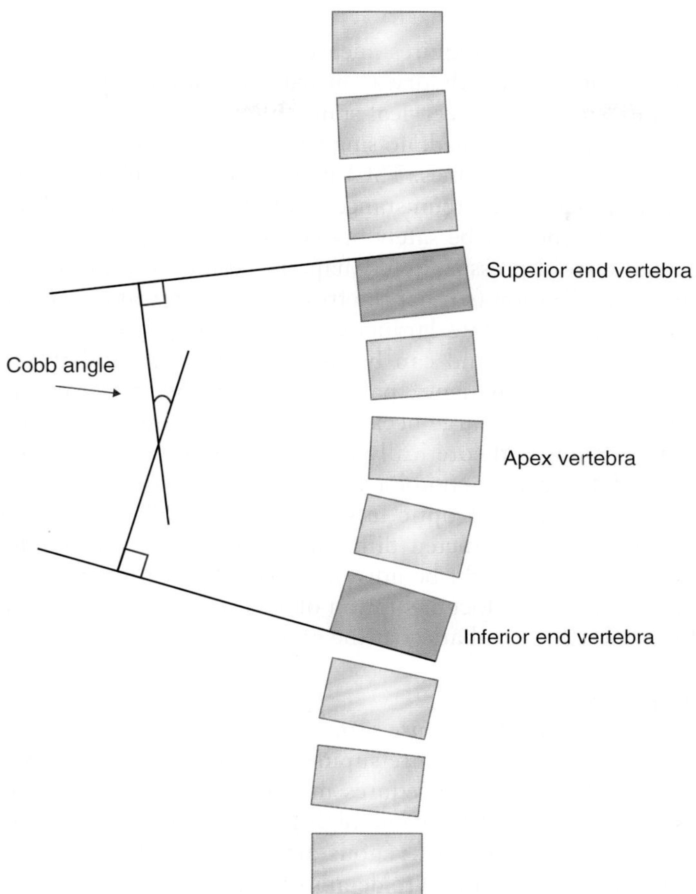

Figure 26.1 Cobb angle is the angle between the two lines drawn (**1**) parallel to the superior border of the superior end vertebra and the (**2**) inferior border of the inferior end vertebra.

C. Degenerative Vertebral Column Disease

Adult degenerative spine disease is a leading cause of chronic pain and disability worldwide. ***Spondylosis*** is a term used to refer to a spectrum of degenerative conditions, including spinal stenosis, osteophyte formation, and intervertebral disc disease, any of which may be asymptomatic or accompanied by radiculopathy or myelopathy. Its etiology is uncertain (>50% due to repetitive spine trauma), and it is generally managed nonoperatively. ***Spondylolisthesis*** refers to a loss of vertebral alignment as a result of forward displacement of one vertebra over another and most commonly affects the lumbosacral region. Management is generally conservative (physical therapy, multimodal analgesia, and epidural steroid injections), although progressive myelopathy, neuropathy, or loss of bowel or bladder control are all indications for surgical decompression with or without fusion.

D. Anesthesia for Spine Surgery

Spine surgery is indicated for the correction of vertebral column deformities and for decompression of nerves and spinal cord due to impingement from diseases of the disc, bone, tumors, and trauma.

Airway

Cervical spine instability requires measures to minimize neck movement during tracheal intubation. All airway instruments and techniques can potentially cause movement in the cervical spine, but these are typically negligible. Thus, when carefully performed, no single technique has been shown superior in terms of neurologic outcomes. TSCI patients who require tracheal intubation in urgent or emergent circumstances and in the absence of other difficult airway issues can generally be safely managed with rapid sequence induction with bimanual cricoid pressure (see Chapters 20 and 32) and manual inline cervical spine stabilization (so that the front of the cervical collar can be temporarily removed to facilitate laryngoscopy). Video laryngoscopy may provide less neck movement and can be used for tracheal intubations in both awake and unconscious patients, particularly those with features predicting difficult laryngoscopy (eg, large neck circumference, limited mouth opening). Fiberoptic intubation is theoretically associated with minimal cervical spine movement, and frequently combined with video laryngoscopy for optimal management. "Awake" fiberoptic intubation is typically reserved for cooperative patients with a predicted difficult intubation where maintenance of spontaneous breathing would be advantageous. After intubation before cuff inflation, assessment and documentation of air leak enables more robust evaluation of readiness for extubation at the end of the surgery.

> **? Did You Know?**
>
> In patients with cervical spine instability, no single airway management technique has been shown superior in preventing rare, tracheal intubation-related spinal cord injury.

Positioning

Most spine surgery patients require prone positioning, although certain cervical and lumbar approaches require supine positioning, and some thoracic or minimally invasive lumbar procedures may require lateral positioning. The sitting position is preferred for some high posterior cervical surgeries, which may slightly increase the risk of venous air embolism (VAE). All such positioning requires careful attention to details of patient anatomy, vascular access lines, and monitoring equipment. This is facilitated by adequate numbers of personnel and proper equipment training for safety (**Figures 26.2** and **26.3**).

The endotracheal tube and all vascular access lines must be secured adequately before turning from the supine to another position. A soft bite block will prevent tongue or endotracheal tube biting. Special spine tables allow the prone abdomen to hang free and reduce intraoperative bleeding by minimizing

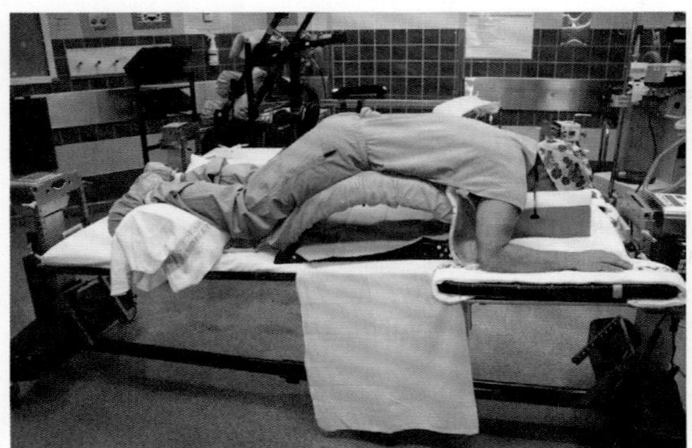

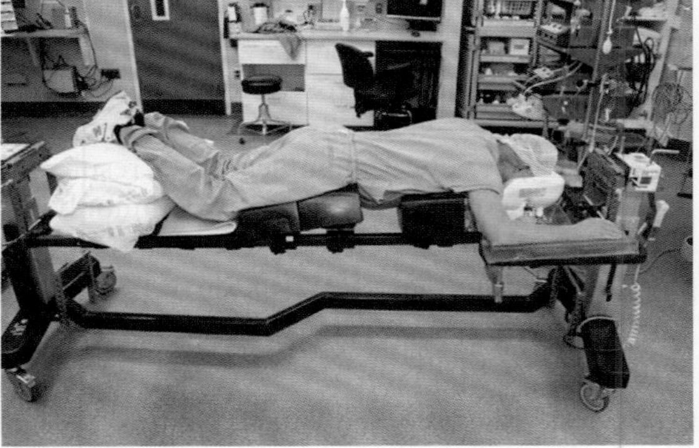

Figure 26.2 Prone positioning on Wilson frame (**left**) and Jackson table (**right**) with foam pillow and prone view headrest, respectively.

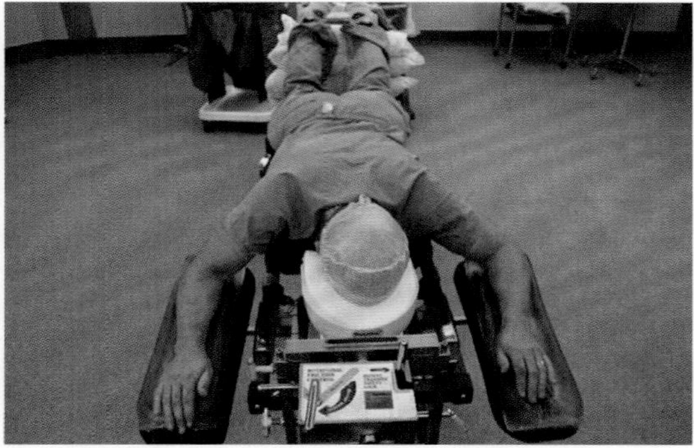
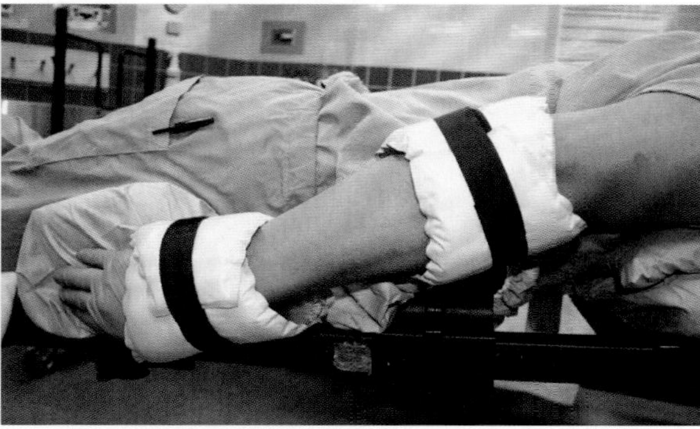

Figure 26.3 Correct placement of the arms in prone position. Arms can be positioned either in swimmer position (**left**) or tucked at the sides (**right**), with the axillae and ulnar grooves free from direct pressure and the wrists and elbows padded.

compression of abdominal contents (and attendant increases in vena cava and epidural venous pressure) as well as facilitating positive pressure ventilation. Slight reverse Trendelenburg tilt also limits the venous back pressure and bleeding. Foam- or gel-based face pillows or Mayfield pins are used to provide pressure-free positioning of the face, with the neck in a neutral position to prevent neurologic injury.

Monitoring and Access

In addition to standard American Society of Anesthesiologists monitors, an arterial catheter provides continuous blood pressure monitoring and facilitates blood sampling in selected cases of anticipated hemodynamic instability or large blood loss. At least two peripheral intravenous lines are ideal due to the restricted intraoperative extremity access that occurs with cervical spine procedures with arms tucked at the sides. Additional robust vascular access must be considered for procedures with higher risks of bleeding, such as scoliosis corrections, anterior lumbar approaches (risk of major vascular injury during exposure), and for resection of hypervascular lesions (such as tumors or infected bone). Central venous catheterization may be helpful for resuscitation and aspiration of intracardiac air if an air embolism occurs.

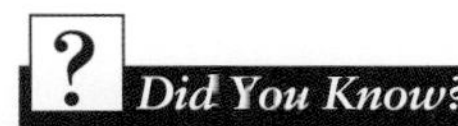

Prior to the advent of modern neurophysiologic monitoring of spinal cord function with motor- or sensory-evoked potentials, intraoperative assessment of spinal cord function was performed by the "wake-up test," transiently reducing anesthetic depth during the surgical procedure to observe patient extremity movement in response to verbal commands.

Anesthetic Technique

General anesthesia is required for most spine procedures. Because volatile anesthetics have variable effects on evoked potential monitoring of spinal cord function, total intravenous anesthesia is usually preferred in such cases, either alone or in combination with a low-dose (<1 minimum alveolar concentration [MAC]) volatile agent (**Table 26.4**).

E. Spinal Cord Monitoring

Intraoperative neurophysiologic monitoring of motor or sensory-evoked potentials in the central nervous system is used during spinal surgery to detect unintended spinal cord injury. It is also used to guide surgical and medical interventions to avoid permanent neurologic injury. Multimodal neurophysiologic monitoring (**Table 26.5**) is sensitive and specific to detect intraoperative neurologic injury, but evidence that it reduces the incidence of new or worsening neurologic deficits is weak.[9]

Table 26.4 Commonly Used Anesthetic Agents in Spine Surgery

		Primary Anesthetic Dosing	Adjunct Dosing
Inhalational Agents	Desflurane	4.5%-6% expired concentration	2%-3% expired concentration
	Sevoflurane	1.5%-2% expired concentration	0.5%-1% expired concentration
Intravenous Agents	Propofol	100-150 μg/kg/min	50-75 μg/kg/min
	Ketamine	2-3 mg/kg/h (may be higher in children)	0.25-2 mg/kg/h Reduce to 8 mg/h for postoperative analgesia; start 45 min before the end of surgery
	Dexmedetomidine	NA	0.2-0.4 μg/kg/h (low dose)
	Remifentanil	NA	0.1-0.4 μg/kg/min

NA, not applicable.

Management of Acute Evoked Potential Signal Changes

If an acute change in neurophysiologic monitoring is detected, the following steps should be taken to identify its cause and reverse the abnormality:

- Rule out surgical- and equipment-related factors; communicate with the surgeon and neuromonitoring team.
- Reposition the patient (maintain natural alignment of spinal column).
- Correct hypotension, metabolic abnormalities, severe anemia, and hypo- or hyperthermia.
- Raise MAP >85 mm Hg to increase spinal cord perfusion.
- Turn off inhalation agent and switch to total intravenous anesthesia.

F. Blood Transfusion Strategies

Blood loss can be significant during spine surgery, with up to 80% of patients requiring an intraoperative transfusion. Perioperative blood loss and blood transfusion have potential negative consequences. Thus, various techniques

Table 26.5 Intraoperative Neurophysiologic Monitoring Modalities

Monitoring Modality	Monitored Region of the Cord	Significance
SSEP	Only measures dorsal ascending column	Amplitude reduction >50% or increased latency >10%
tcMEP	Motor descending tracts	Amplitude reduction >50%
EMG	Nerve roots and peripheral nerves	Impingement on a nerve root by an instrument will cause immediate motor activity

EMG, electromyography; SSEP, somatosensory evoked potentials; tcMEP, transcranial motor evoked potentials.

have been proposed to minimize blood loss and blood product transfusion in this setting.[10] Along with meticulous surgical technique, maintenance of normothermia and avoiding acidosis will reduce bleeding. Goal-directed transfusion strategies by either rapid emergency hemorrhage panel (EHP) including hemoglobin, hematocrit, platelets, prothrombin time, and fibrinogen or point of care testing using viscoelastic hemostatic assays are increasingly used to guide blood product transfusion.

Preoperative Hemoglobin Optimization

Preoperative hemoglobin levels of 12 g/dL for females and 13 g/dL for males serve as thresholds for anemia that generally require further attention in the preoperative period. Laboratory evaluation, diagnosis, and treatment of existing anemia should occur before elective orthopedic procedures through correction of nutritional deficiencies, use of recombinant human erythropoietin, and oral or intravenous iron supplementation. Preoperative autologous blood donation and acute normovolemic hemodilution have been investigated for spine surgery but are not components of routine practice.

Antifibrinolytics

TXA is the most common lysine analogue used as an antifibrinolytic to decrease perioperative blood loss and transfusion requirements through the inhibition of clot degradation. Its use is contraindicated in cases of known allergy, history of thromboembolic disease, and preexisting seizure disorders. Potential adverse effects include thromboembolic events, seizures, and vision changes. The recommended dosing regimen is a 1 g bolus over 10 minutes following by an infusion of 1 g over 8 hours. In acute major trauma, initiation of TXA more than 3 hours after time of injury is associated with increased mortality.

Cell Saver

Evidence supports the use of intraoperative washed erythrocyte salvage in spine surgery, as autologous transfusion significantly lowers donor blood transfusion rates. Its use is controversial, however, during cancer surgery, bacterial infections, wound irrigation with antibiotics, and concurrent use of topical hemostatic agents.

G. Visual Loss After Spine Surgery

Perioperative visual loss (POVL) is a potentially devastating complication that can occur following spine surgery. Its incidence ranges from 0.03% to 0.2%, and it has several different types, presentations, and etiologies (**Table 26.6**).

The following management strategies have been suggested for prevention of POVL in spine surgery patients with the risk factors noted in **Table 26.6**[11]:

- POVL should be discussed as part of the preoperative informed consent.
- Assess patient's baseline blood pressure.
- Continually monitor blood pressure in high-risk patients.
- Avoid deliberate hypotension in high-risk patients.
- The neck should be placed in a neutral position, and the head should be level with or higher than the heart to minimize venous congestion.
- Maintain adequate intravascular volume with balanced combinations of crystalloids, colloids, and blood products.
- For prolonged operations, consideration should be given for staging the surgery.

Table 26.6 Perioperative Visual Loss

	CRAO	AION	PION	CB
Onset	Immediate	First 48 h	Immediate	Immediate
Site	Unilateral	Frequently bilateral	Mostly bilateral	Bilateral
Potential causes/risk factors	Direct pressure Emboli Hypotension	History of vascular diseases (coronary, cerebral, peripheral) Diabetic retinopathy Preoperative anemia Males more often than females Hypotension Long surgery Massive blood loss and large volume shifts Large volume crystalloid use	Venous congestion Anemia	Emboli Hypotension Anemia

AION, anterior ischemic optic neuropathy; CB, cortical blindness; CRAO, central retinal artery occlusion; PION, posterior ischemic optic neuropathy.

H. Venous Air Embolism

Venous air embolism (VAE) results from entrainment of ambient air into the venous circulation through intraosseous vessels or open epidural veins at the surgical site. Procedures above the level of the right atrium that involve opening of large venous structures, including removal of large areas of cortical bone or procedures in sitting position, may carry higher VAE risk. When air accumulation in the right heart reaches a critical level to impact right ventricular output, cardiovascular collapse may occur. The risk of VAE is increased with hypovolemia, hypotension, and spontaneous ventilation and is decreased with positioning to allow epidural veins to remain below the heart level. VAE may be detected by echocardiography, precordial Doppler, or strongly suspected based on clinical presentation. The presentation and management of VAE are summarized in **Table 26.7**.

I. Postoperative Care

One in five spine surgery patients will develop immediate postoperative complications. Independent risk factors include male sex, advanced age, surgical approach (combined anterior and posterior approach being associated with the highest complication rates), and preexisting comorbidities. Hospital mortality rates are 0.2% to 0.5% and are associated most often with concomitant congestive heart failure, liver disease, coagulopathy, neurologic disorders, renal disease, electrolyte imbalances, and pulmonary circulatory diseases.

Decision to Extubate

Anterior cervical fusion surgeries carry the particular risk of hematoma and edema formation up to 36 hours after surgery and tracheal extubation. This may lead to postoperative airway compromise and the need for emergent reintubation. Operative injury to the recurrent laryngeal nerve may also cause vocal cord dysfunction and respiratory difficulty. There are no uniformly accepted criteria to guide extubation decisions. Potential risk factors for postoperative reintubation include advanced age, higher American Society of

Table 26.7 Intraoperative Venous Air Embolus Presentation and Management

Presentation	Sudden reduction in $ETCO_2$ Hypercarbia (increased $Paco_2$) Hypoxemia Hypotension Tachyarrhythmias Elevated CVP or distended neck veins Cardiac murmur, respiratory wheeze Cardiac arrest (>5 mL/kg air accumulation)
Management	Stop operating Stop inhalational anesthetics including N_2O FiO_2 100% Prevent further emboli Flood the field with fluid Advance the central line intracardiac and attempt to aspirate if in situ Level the table Turn the patient to left lateral decubitus position CPR—fluid boluses, hemodynamic agents
Monitoring	Along with standard ASA monitoring requirements, consider precordial or transesophageal Doppler

ASA, American Society of Anesthesiologists; CPR, cardiopulmonary resuscitation; CVP, central venous pressure; $ETCO_2$, end-tidal carbon dioxide; FiO_2, fraction of inspired oxygen; N_2O, nitrous oxide; $PaCO_2$, arterial carbon dioxide partial pressure.

Anesthesiologists' class, extent of the procedure and its duration, administered fluid volume, blood loss >300 mL, combined anterior and posterior cervical approach, and previous spine surgery.

Pain Management

Postoperative pain is a major concern following spine surgery and is frequently complicated by preoperative chronic pain, long-term opioid use, and related psychosocial issues. ***Multimodal analgesic management*** is recommended in such patients. Combining analgesics with different mechanisms of action such as acetaminophen, nonsteroidal anti-inflammatory drugs, gabapentin, dexamethasone, ketamine, and lidocaine facilitates early mobilization, reduces opioid consumption, and improves patient satisfaction. There is no single optimal multimodal analgesic regimen, so individual patient factors must be considered to maximize likely benefits and reduce the risk of serious side effects. For example, while helpful for some patients, gabapentinoids potentiate the respiratory depressant effects of opioids and should be used with caution in vulnerable patients, such as those with obstructive sleep apnea.[12]

J. Neuraxial and Regional Anesthesia for Spine Surgery

Neuraxial (spinal subarachnoid or epidural) anesthesia may be used for lumbar or lower thoracic microdiscectomy or laminectomy surgery that is limited to one or two levels. It has the potential to reduce intraoperative blood loss through the combined effects of sympathetic blockade (leading to vasodilation and relative hypotension) and maintenance of spontaneous ventilation (which lowers intrathoracic ventilation pressures and reduces congestion of the epidural veins). Neuraxial anesthesia also provides postoperative analgesia and can reduce opioid requirements, nausea and vomiting, and urinary retention. Bilateral erector spinae plane blocks or retrolaminar blocks are showing promise as alternative strategies.

IV. Anesthesia for Extremity Surgery

Orthopedic extremity surgery is extremely common. It is performed for both elective and emergent indications and takes place in both inpatient and ambulatory outpatient settings. Furthermore, such surgery spans the age range from newborn (eg, congenital hip dysplasia) to the elderly (eg, traumatic hip fracture), as well as the spectrum of concurrent medical morbidities from the healthy professional athlete to a debilitated nursing facility resident. In addition, the following statements generally apply to anesthesia for extremity orthopedic surgery:

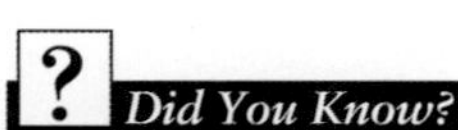

Regional anesthesia, using both single-shot and indwelling catheter techniques, is increasingly common for both inpatient and outpatient orthopedic extremity surgery. It is used not only for intraoperative anesthesia but also for the many benefits of prolonged postoperative analgesia.

- Many orthopedic procedures can potentially use regional anesthesia techniques for intraoperative anesthesia, postoperative pain control, and joint rehabilitation.
- Prevention of positioning-related complications, such as nerve and soft-tissue injuries, requires procedural knowledge and vigilance.
- Significant blood loss can occur and requires familiarity with blood loss–reducing techniques, such as tourniquet use, cell savers, and antifibrinolytics, transfusion triggers, and transfusion-related complications.
- Prolonged immobilization following surgery, particularly involving the knee, hip, or pelvis, is associated with increased risk of deep venous thrombosis and thromboembolism. Conversely, thromboembolism prophylaxis may interfere with regional anesthesia techniques.

A. Choice of Anesthetic Technique

Many orthopedic surgical procedures are well suited for regional anesthesia, the general details of which are described in Chapter 21. Potential clinical benefits of regional anesthesia particular to orthopedic surgery include prolonged analgesia that reduces surgical stress, facilitates joint rehabilitation, and increases patient satisfaction. It can also decrease opioid analgesic use, postoperative nausea and vomiting, cognitive impairment, immunosuppression, and duration of recovery room stay. Thromboembolism reduction may occur with regional anesthesia and result from diminished sympathetic tone that enhances blood flow and prevents venous stasis. Risks of regional anesthesia include local anesthetic toxicity, hematoma formation, bleeding, nerve damage, and infection. With the introduction of ultrasound-guided techniques, both single-shot and indwelling catheter techniques (that enable prolonged analgesia and facilitate functional therapy) have become safe, efficient, and desirable anesthetic choices. Some patients may benefit from continued use of peripheral nerve catheters for 2 to 4 days after discharge, via single-use disposable local anesthetic infusion pumps that are lightweight, portable, and can be taken home.

Alternatively, general anesthesia can be used for virtually any orthopedic extremity procedure and may be required for prolonged procedures, those involving unique positioning, and those performed on the torso. In some cases, combined general and regional anesthesia may be indicated to achieve both

Table 26.8 General Considerations for Specific Surgical Procedures

Type of Surgery	Positioning	Anesthetic	Tourniquet	Blood Loss
Total shoulder arthroplasty	Lateral decubitus or beach chair	GA/interscalene block	–	Moderate
Arthroscopic shoulder surgery	Beach chair	GA/interscalene block	–	Minimal
Total elbow arthroplasty	Supine or lateral	GA/supraclavicular, infraclavicular, or axillary block	+	Limited
Elbow arthroscopy	Prone with sandbags under antecubital fossa	GA/supraclavicular, infraclavicular, or axillary block	±	Minimal
Forearm/wrist/hand	Supine	GA/supraclavicular, infraclavicular, axillary, or selective peripheral nerve block	±	Minimal
Total hip arthroplasty, open	Fracture table, lateral	GA/neuraxial/psoas block	–	Moderate
Nondisplaced hip fractures	Fracture table, supine	GA/neuraxial	–	Limited
Total knee arthroplasty	Supine, possible hip bump	GA/neuraxial/sciatic and femoral (or adductor canal) nerve blocks	+	Moderate
Knee arthroscopy	Supine with operative thigh placed against an arthroscopy post	GA/neuraxial/sciatic and femoral nerve blocks	±	Minimal
Ankle/foot		See **Table 26.10**.		

GA, general anesthesia.

ideal operative conditions and postoperative analgesia. The final choice of anesthetic technique should be tailored to the individual patient's needs based on specific medical conditions, comorbidities, age, type of surgery, and both the surgeon's and patient's preferences (**Table 26.8**).

V. Surgery to the Upper Extremities

Regional anesthesia is an excellent choice for anesthesia and postoperative analgesia for upper extremity surgery from the shoulder to the fingers. Ultrasound guidance may be particularly advantageous for peripheral upper extremity blocks targeting nerves in close proximity to large vascular structures and the lung (eg, supraclavicular, infraclavicular, and interscalene blocks). However, some surgical factors (bilateral procedures or prolonged surgery) and patient factors (severe obstructive sleep apnea, severe pulmonary disease, preexisting neurologic deficits, impaired cognition, or failed regional block) may require general anesthesia. Patients who are considered candidates for regional block may find themselves surprised with the potentially long duration of sensory and motor block following a surgical-density brachial plexus block, and some may find this experience to be unwelcome, despite the excellent analgesia that usually accompanies the block. Therefore, in addition to discussing block risks, the anesthesiologist should try to offer realistic expectations of the post-surgical course when seeking informed consent.[13]

A. Surgery to the Shoulder and Upper Arm

Common shoulder and upper arm procedures include arthroplasty, arthroscopy, subacromial decompression, rotator cuff repair, repair of fracture, and frozen shoulder manipulation. Lateral decubitus and beach chair positions are commonly used with either pharmacologic neuromuscular paralysis or a motor block that facilitates arm traction. Significant blood loss may occur because tourniquet use is not feasible, so careful hemodynamic monitoring is required and serial hemoglobin measurement may be necessary (**Table 26.9; Figures 26.4** and **26.5**). If the patient is in the beach chair position, then blood pressure targets must be chosen to account for the hydrostatic pressure difference between the arm and the brain. The effective mean arterial pressure decreases by 1 mm Hg for every 1.35 cm of elevation of the blood column from the heart to the brain. Severe cerebral hypotension can occur, leading to watershed ischemia and intraoperative stroke.

B. Surgery to the Elbow

Surgeries involving the elbow can be done with either open (eg, total elbow replacement, fracture repair) or endoscopic (elbow arthroscopy) techniques. Minimally invasive surgery and advances in sedation practices have resulted in an increased ability to perform most elbow surgeries on an ambulatory basis

Table 26.9 Comparison of Different Specialized Surgical Positioning

Surgical Positioning	Body Position	Operative Extremity Position	Positioning-Specific Pressure Points	Advantages and Risks
Lateral decubitus (UE, LE)	Lateral, torso stabilized with bean bag or braces	Vertical or on an arm support	Axillary roll under upper chest wall (not in the axilla) to prevent axillary neurovascular compression	Good surgical view Risk of traction arm injury and challenging in obese patients Difficult to access face and nonoperative arm
Beach chair (UE)	Sitting with hips flexed to 45°-90°, knees flexed to 30°	On a Mayo stand or mounted arm positioner	Head holder may cause lesser occipital and greater auricular nerve injuries	Easy surgical access but pressure gradient between surgical site and heart increases risk of VAE. Risk of hypotension/bradycardia with possible cerebral ischemia
Fracture table (LE)	Supine or lateral	In a traction device	Perineal post may compress perineal anatomy	Easy C-arm access; risk of traction and pressure-related nerve injuries

LE, lower extremity surgery; UE, upper extremity surgery; VAE, venous air embolism.

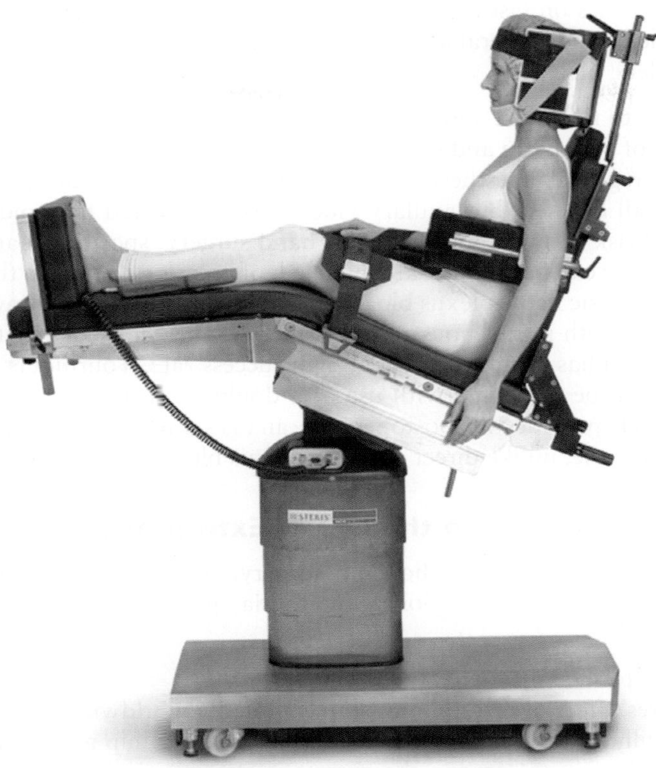

Figure 26.4 Beach chair surgical positioning. (Courtesy of STERIS®.)

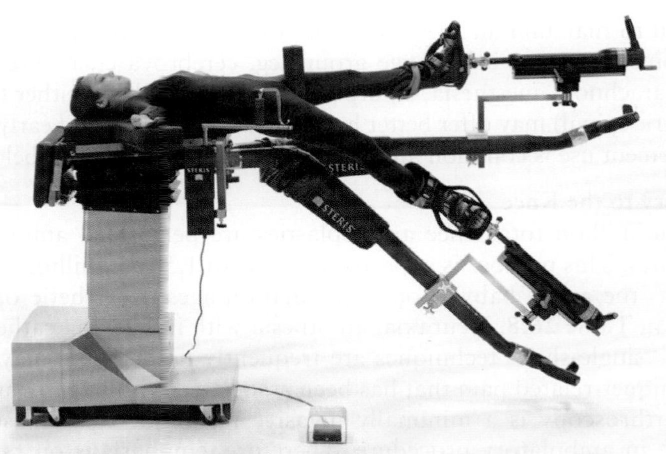

Figure 26.5 Positioning on a fracture table. (Courtesy of STERIS®.)

with an emphasis on fast recovery and excellent analgesia. Such surgeries can be performed under general anesthesia or regional anesthesia (supraclavicular or interscalene block).

C. Surgery to the Wrist and Hand

A majority of distal arm and hand procedures are performed on an outpatient basis with regional anesthesia. Supraclavicular, infraclavicular, or axillary blocks can all be used, but axillary block is often favored to avoid potential (albeit low) risk of pneumothorax. For hand surgery, specific ulnar, median, or radial nerves can be targeted and blocked, often more distally in the extremity than the classic nerve plexus blocks. Brief surgery below the elbow can also be performed with intravenous regional anesthesia (Bier block) that is simple to perform and has rapid onset and a high success rate. Tourniquet pain with Bier block can be alleviated with use of a double-cuff tourniquet. However, the Bier block provides no postoperative analgesia at the surgical site upon tourniquet release, unlike direct nerve or plexus blocks.

VI. Surgery to the Lower Extremities

As with upper extremity orthopedic surgery, lower extremity procedures can be performed under regional anesthesia, general anesthesia, or their combination.[14]

A. Surgery to the Hip

Hip fractures affect over 4 million people annually worldwide and are associated with billions of dollars in health care costs. Total hip arthroplasties and hemiarthroplasties are among the most common surgical procedures in the United States. Three main types of hip fractures based on anatomical location are ***intracapsular, intertrochanteric, and subtrochanteric.***[15]

Intracapsular fracture may cause femoral head ischemia if displaced and often requires hemiarthroplasty. Other types of fractures could be treated with closed or open reduction with percutaneous screw placement or intramedullary nail.

Reduction in bleeding during hip arthroplasty significantly shortens the operating time and decreases thromboembolism risk. Therefore, a controlled hypotensive epidural anesthesia technique may be an option with a hemodynamic goal to maintain an MAP of 60 mm Hg, in the absence of contraindications sometimes seen in this age group (eg, cerebrovascular disease). With spinal subarachnoid anesthesia, a purposeful unilateral block (either hyperbaric or hypobaric spinal) may offer better hemodynamic stability and early recovery. Surgical cement use is common and its implications are described below.

B. Surgery to the Knee

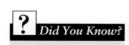

As the active baby boomer generation ages, it is anticipated that 1.5 to 3 million total knee replacements will be performed annually by 2030.

Nearly one million total knee arthroplasties are performed annually in the United States. This number is expected to grow to 1.5 to 3 million procedures by 2030 as the active baby boomer population ages. Anesthetic options are presented in **Table 26.8**. Neuraxial anesthesia with indwelling catheter placement and "single-shot" techniques are frequently used. These may also prevent tourniquet-related pain that has been associated with hypercoagulability.

Knee arthroscopy is a minimally invasive technique that is usually performed as an ambulatory procedure. Therefore, emphasis is on rapid emergence and early ambulation. Reconstruction of anterior cruciate ligament and repair of a torn meniscus are also common procedures of the knee.

Table 26.10 Anesthetic Management of Common Foot and Ankle Procedures

Procedure	Tourniquet Placement	Sciatic (Popliteal) + Saphenous Block + Sedation	Sciatic (Popliteal) Block + GA	NA	Ankle Block	Sciatic + Femoral Blocks
Forefoot: Hallux valgus, hammer toes	Ankle	+	±	±	+	–
Midfoot: Lisfranc fracture transmetatarsal amputations	Ankle/calf	+	+	+	±	+
Hindfoot	Thigh	±	+	+	–	+[a]
Ankle	Thigh	–	+	+	–	+[a]

GA, general anesthesia; NA, neuroaxial anesthesia.
[a]Femoral + high sciatic nerve blocks are generally needed for thigh tourniquet pain relief.

C. Surgery to the Ankle and Foot

With the current advances in surgical techniques and sedation, regional anesthesia is emerging as the anesthetic of choice for foot and ankle surgeries. General anesthesia is administered when regional techniques are contraindicated or for lengthy procedures. The anesthetic management options for the most common foot and ankle surgeries are presented in **Table 26.10**.

VII. Postoperative Regional and Multimodal Analgesia

With regional anesthesia, the pain pathways are blocked at the level of spinal cord and nerve roots, nerve plexus, or peripheral nerve, providing excellent analgesia and facilitating both rapid recovery and functional physical therapy. Multimodal analgesic agents similar to those described previously for spine surgery should also be included in the postoperative care plan to provide comprehensive postoperative analgesia care, particularly for those patients with chronic pain or substance use disorders. Accelerated availability of high-fidelity ultrasound and the relative speed of learning ultrasound-guided approaches to basic peripheral nerve blocks have led to increased popularity of these techniques in the last 10 to 15 years. Coupled with the rapid escalation in opioid use leading to associated public health dangers, the safety of regional analgesic methods offers great promise as a component of care pathways for a variety of surgical procedures, particularly joint replacement. Many acute trauma patients, such as those with extremity fractures, can also benefit from selective early application of regional blocks, achieving superior pain relief with reduced need for opioids and sedatives.

VIII. Pediatric Orthopedic Surgery

Anesthetic management of pediatric orthopedic patients encompasses general pediatric anesthesia considerations (see Chapter 33) but in the specific orthopedic context of traumatic injury, cancer, and unique disease states such as congenital disorders. Fractures, scoliosis, joint abnormalities, clubfoot, and syndactyly can require surgical repair in childhood and demand special anesthetic considerations. Positioning can be challenging due to muscle contractures (cerebral palsy) and bone abnormalities (osteogenesis imperfecta). This is also true in other conditions associated with cervical spine instability (Down syndrome), limited neck range of motion (achondroplasia), and cardiac defects (Marfan syndrome). Children with Charcot-Marie-Tooth disease, Duchenne muscular dystrophy, and myotonic dystrophy are prone to succinylcholine-induced hyperkalemia, rhabdomyolysis, and malignant hyperthermia. In addition, pediatric patients present unique challenges to using regional anesthesia, particularly that the accepted standard of care is to perform blocks under general anesthesia or deep sedation.[16] The same peripheral nerve blocks used in adults with ultrasound guidance can generally be used in children, with appropriate weight-based local anesthetic dose adjustments.[17]

IX. Other Considerations and Complications

A. Tourniquet Management

The use of a pneumatic tourniquet placed proximal to the surgical site and inflated to suprasystemic pressure minimizes blood loss and facilitates surgery by creating a bloodless field. Potential complications can be local, related to tissue pressure and ischemia, or systemic (**Table 26.11**). Extremity exsanguination prior to tourniquet inflation is performed by elevation of the limb or by compression with an elastic bandage to create a bloodless surgical field. Appropriate cuff sizing (cuff width 20% greater than limb diameter) and thorough padding help to reduce local tissue injury. Maximal duration of tourniquet time is not well defined, although 2 hours is generally considered safe to avoid distal tissue ischemia. If surgery duration requires extended tourniquet time, the tourniquet can be briefly deflated for 5 to 10 minutes before reinflation. The inflation pressure should not exceed 100 mm Hg above the systolic pressure for the upper extremity or above 150 mm Hg for the lower extremity. However, higher pressure may be needed in morbidly obese patients to prevent arterial inflow.

B. Fat Embolus Syndrome

Subclinical fat embolism is common with long bone fractures or major joint prostheses. When clinically significant, it manifests as ***fat embolism syndrome*** (FES), which is a potentially lethal condition. The prevailing pathogenesis theory of FES involves the increase in intramedullary pressure as a result of

Table 26.11 Systemic Manifestations With Pneumatic Tourniquet Use

Tourniquet	Hemodynamic Changes	Hematologic Changes	Temperature Changes	Respiratory Changes
Inflation	Increase in core blood volume, CVP, PVR, BP, HR	Systemic hypercoagulation	Increase of core temperature	Increase in RR due to tourniquet pain
Deflation	Temporary decrease of CVP, HR, BP, possible arrhythmias	Temporary increase in thrombolytic activity	Decrease of core temperature	Increase in end-tidal CO_2 due to reperfusion of ischemic tissue

BP, blood pressure; CO_2, carbon dioxide; CVP, central venous pressure; HR, heart rate; RR, respiratory rate; PVR, peripheral vascular resistance.

traumatic swelling, hematoma formation, or expansion with bone cement. When intramedullary pressure exceeds venous pressure, fat globules are forced into the venous circulation. Another theory suggests that fat globules are formed in the blood as a response to acute changes in fatty acid metabolism. Fat macroemboli can cause mechanical obstruction to pulmonary (and occasionally systemic) blood flow and damage capillary endothelium in the lungs and central nervous system. Major criteria for FES diagnosis include pulmonary manifestations (hypoxia, pulmonary edema, and adult respiratory distress syndrome), neurologic impairment ranging from confusion or lethargy to seizures and coma, and petechia on the conjunctiva and upper trunk. Minor diagnostic criteria include fever, tachycardia, fat globules in sputum and urine, and decreased platelets and hematocrit. Early recognition is essential for therapeutic success. Treatment options include early fracture stabilization and aggressive cardiovascular and pulmonary supportive therapy.

C. Methyl Methacrylate

Polymethyl methacrylate is an acrylic bone cement used for securely binding prosthetic devices to bone during joint arthroplasties. Cement expansion during the hardening process may cause an increase in intramedullary pressure followed by systemic embolization of polymer, bone marrow, or air. Although volatile ***methylmethacrylate monomer*** can cause direct systemic toxic effects, the deleterious hemodynamic changes most likely result from embolism. Prevention includes surgical precautions such as creating vent holes or avoiding cement over pressurization as well as maintaining normovolemia.

D. Venous Thromboembolism and Antithrombotic Prophylaxis

The incidence of ***deep venous thrombosis*** can be as high as 60% after major orthopedic procedures if thromboprophylaxis is not used. Although often asymptomatic, it can lead to venous thromboembolism and pulmonary embolism. The incidence of venous thromboembolism is especially high after lower extremity fractures and joint replacements. Mechanical (sequential compression devices), pharmacologic, and ancillary (early mobilization) options can be employed for thromboprophylaxis. Pharmacologic methods include low-molecular-weight heparin, unfractionated heparin, or other anticoagulants such as fondaparinux or vitamin K inhibitors. Various evidence-based guidelines for ***thromboprophylaxis*** have been introduced by the American Association of Orthopedic Surgeons, the American College of Chest Physicians, and the National Institute of Clinical Excellence, most of which recommend a combination of pharmacologic and mechanical prophylaxis measures.[18]

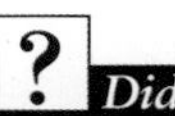

Did You Know?

The incidence of deep venous thrombosis after major orthopedic procedures can be as high as 60%, highlighting the importance of perioperative antithrombotic prophylaxis with mechanical, pharmacologic, or other techniques.

Prophylactic anticoagulation (eg, warfarin for atrial fibrillation) can interfere with regional anesthesia use for orthopedic surgery due to the potential risk of hematoma formation and permanent neurologic damage. Although the actual incidence of neurologic impairment as a result of this complication is unknown and likely low, the American Society of Regional Anesthesia and Pain Medicine has published evidence-based guidelines for regional anesthesia in patients receiving antithrombotic therapy.[19]

For further review and interactivities, please see the associated Interactive Video Lectures and "A Closer Look" infographic accessible in the complimentary eBook bundled with this text. Access instructions are located in the inside front cover.

References

1. McIsaac DI, MacDonald DB, Aucoin SD. Frailty for perioperative clinicians: a narrative review. *Anesth Analg*. 2020;130(6):1450-1460. PMID: 32384334.
2. Dagal A, Bellabarba C, Bransford R, et al. Enhanced perioperative care for major spine surgery. *Spine (Phila Pa 1976)*. 2019;44(13):959-966. PMID: 31205177.
3. Kaye AD, Urman RD, Cornett EM, et al. Enhanced recovery pathways in orthopedic surgery. *J Anaesthesiol Clin Pharmacol*. 2019;35(suppl 1):S35-S39. PMID: 31142957.
4. Selvarajah S, Hammond ER, Haider AH, et al. The burden of acute traumatic spinal cord injury among adults in the United States: an update. *J Neurotrauma*. 2014;31(3):228-238. PMID: 24138672.
5. Walters BC, Hadley MN, Hurlbert RJ, et al. Guidelines for the management of acute cervical spine and spinal cord injuries: 2013 update. *Neurosurgery*. 2013;60(CN_suppl_1):82-91. PMID: 23839357.
6. Evaniew N, Mazlouman SJ, Belley-Cote EP, Jacobs WB, Kwon BK. Interventions to optimize spinal cord perfusion in patients with acute traumatic spinal cord injuries: a systematic review. *J Neurotrauma*. 2020;37(9):1127-1139. PMID: 32024432.
7. Squair JW, Belanger LM, Tsang A, et al. Empirical targets for acute hemodynamic management of individuals with spinal cord injury. *Neurology*. 2019;93(12):e1205-e1211. PMID: 31409736.
8. Wilson JR, Witiw CD, Badhiwala J, Kwon BK, Fehlings MG, Harrop JS. Early surgery for traumatic spinal cord injury: where are we now? *Global Spine J*. 2020;10(1 suppl):84S-91S. PMID: 31934526.
9. Malhotra NR, Shaffrey CI. Intraoperative electrophysiological monitoring in spine surgery. *Spine (Phila Pa 1976)*. 2010;35(25):2167-2179. PMID: 21102290.
10. Bible JE, Mirza M, Knaub MA. Blood-loss management in spine surgery. *J Am Acad Orthop Surg*. 2018;26(2):35-44. PMID: 29303921.
11. Practice advisory for perioperative visual loss associated with spine surgery 2019: an updated report by the American Society of Anesthesiologists Task Force on Perioperative Visual Loss, the North American Neuro-Ophthalmology Society, and the Society for Neuroscience in Anesthesiology and Critical Care. *Anesthesiology*. 2019;130(1):12-30. PMID: 30531555.
12. Cozowicz C, Bekeris J, Poeran J, et al. Multimodal pain management and postoperative outcomes in lumbar spine fusion surgery: a population-based cohort study. *Spine (Phila Pa 1976)*. 2020;45(9):580-589. PMID: 31770340.
13. Droog W, Hoeks SE, van Aggelen GP, et al. Regional anaesthesia is associated with less patient satisfaction compared to general anaesthesia following distal upper extremity surgery: a prospective double centred observational study. *BMC Anesthesiol*. 2019;19(1):115. PMID: 31266454.
14. Memtsoudis SG, Sun X, Chiu YL, et al. Perioperative comparative effectiveness of anesthetic technique in orthopedic patients. *Anesthesiology*. 2013;118(5):1046-1058. PMID: 23612126.
15. Bhandari M, Swiontkowski M. Management of acute hip fracture. *N Engl J Med*. 2017;377(21):2053-2062. PMID: 29166235.
16. Taenzer AH, Walker BJ, Bosenberg AT, et al. Asleep versus awake: does it matter? Pediatric regional block complications by patient state. A report from the Pediatric Regional Anesthesia Network. *Reg Anesth Pain Med*. 2014;39(4):279-283. PMID: 24918334.
17. Suresh S, Ecoffey C, Bosenberg A, et al. The European Society of Regional Anaesthesia and Pain Therapy/American Society of Regional Anesthesia and Pain Medicine recommendations on local anesthetics and adjuvants dosage in pediatric regional anesthesia. *Reg Anesth Pain Med*. 2018;43(2):211-216. PMID: 29319604.
18. Falck-Ytter Y, Francis CW, Johanson NA, et al. Prevention of VTE in orthopedic surgery patients – antithrombotic therapy and prevention of thrombosis, 9th ed: American College of Chest Physicians Evidence-Based Clinical Practice Guidelines. *Chest*. 2012;141(2 suppl):e278S-e325S. PMID: 22315265.
19. Horlocker TT, Vandermeulen E, Kopp SL, Gogarten W, Leffert LR, Benzon HT. Regional anesthesia in the patient receiving antithrombotic or thrombolytic therapy: American Society of Regional Anesthesia and Pain Medicine Evidence-Based Guidelines (fourth edition). *Reg Anesth Pain Med*. 2018;43(3):263-309. PMID: 29561531.

REGIONAL ANESTHESIA & ANTICOAGULATION

A CLOSER LOOK

Neuraxial anesthesia is contraindicated in anticoagulated patients. Guidelines for managing neuraxial anesthesia in heparinized patients is presented below and is based on the 2018 American Society of Regional Anesthesia recommendations.

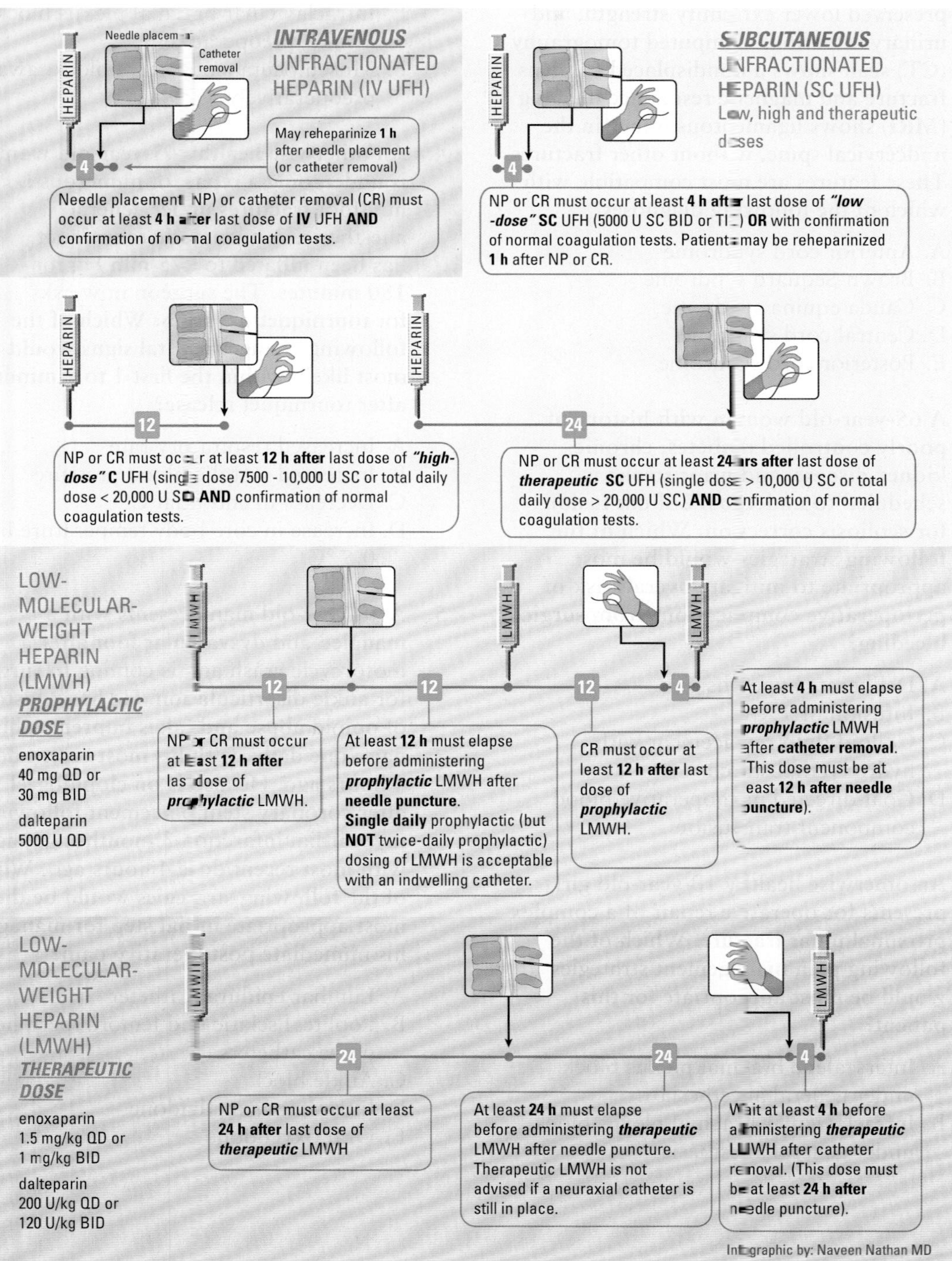

INTRAVENOUS UNFRACTIONATED HEPARIN (IV UFH)
HEPARIN
Needle placement
Catheter removal
May reheparinize 1 h after needle placement (or catheter removal)
4
Needle placement (NP) or catheter removal (CR) must occur at least 4 h after last dose of IV UFH AND confirmation of normal coagulation tests.
SUBCUTANEOUS UNFRACTIONATED HEPARIN (SC UFH)
Low, high and therapeutic doses
NP or CR must occur at least 4 h after last dose of "low-dose" SC UFH (5000 U SC BID or TID) OR with confirmation of normal coagulation tests. Patients may be reheparinized 1 h after NP or CR.
12
NP or CR must occur at least 12 h after last dose of "high-dose" SC UFH (single dose 7500 - 10,000 U SC or total daily dose < 20,000 U SC) AND confirmation of normal coagulation tests.
24
NP or CR must occur at least 24 hrs after last dose of therapeutic SC UFH (single dose > 10,000 U SC or total daily dose > 20,000 U SC) AND confirmation of normal coagulation tests.
LOW-MOLECULAR-WEIGHT HEPARIN (LMWH)
PROPHYLACTIC DOSE
enoxaparin
40 mg QD or
30 mg BID
dalteparin
5000 U QD
LMWH
NP or CR must occur at least 12 h after last dose of prophylactic LMWH.
At least 12 h must elapse before administering prophylactic LMWH after needle puncture. Single daily prophylactic (but NOT twice-daily prophylactic) dosing of LMWH is acceptable with an indwelling catheter.
CR must occur at least 12 h after last dose of prophylactic LMWH.
At least 4 h must elapse before administering prophylactic LMWH after catheter removal. (This dose must be at least 12 h after needle puncture).
LOW-MOLECULAR-WEIGHT HEPARIN (LMWH)
THERAPEUTIC DOSE
enoxaparin
1.5 mg/kg QD or
1 mg/kg BID
dalteparin
200 U/kg QD or
120 U/kg BID
NP or CR must occur at least 24 h after last dose of therapeutic LMWH
At least 24 h must elapse before administering therapeutic LMWH after needle puncture. Therapeutic LMWH is not advised if a neuraxial catheter is still in place.
Wait at least 4 h before administering therapeutic LMWH after catheter removal. (This dose must be at least 24 h after needle puncture).
Infographic by: Naveen Nathan MD

Questions

1. **A 79-year-old man presents after tripping on a rug and falling forward, striking his head on the ground. Examination findings include new upper extremity weakness, preserved lower extremity strength, and urinary retention. Computed tomography (CT) scan shows a nondisplaced C2 dens fracture and magnetic resonance imaging (MRI) shows ligamentous injury in the midcervical spine, without other fractures. These features are most compatible with which of the following diagnoses?**

   A. Anterior cord syndrome
   B. Brown-Sequard syndrome
   C. Cauda equina syndrome
   D. Central cord syndrome
   E. Posterior cord syndrome

2. **A 65-year-old woman with history of poorly controlled diabetes, chronic kidney disease, and prior stroke is scheduled to undergo T2-ilium fusion for scoliosis correction. Which of the following strategies would be most appropriate to mitigate overall risk of perioperative complications from surgical bleeding?**

   A. Deliberate hypotension
   B. Infusion of TXA
   C. Colloid fluid replacement with hydroxyethyl starch
   D. Goal-directed intraoperative blood component transfusion

3. **An otherwise healthy 10-year-old girl presents for operative repair of a complex proximal ulnar fracture. Which of the following pain management strategies would be most appropriate for this patient?**

   A. Interscalene brachial plexus block under general anesthesia
   B. Infraclavicular brachial plexus block under general anesthesia
   C. Musculocutaneous nerve block under general anesthesia
   D. Interscalene brachial plexus block, awake, preoperatively
   E. Infraclavicular brachial plexus block, awake, preoperatively
   F. Musculocutaneous nerve block, awake, preoperatively

4. **An otherwise healthy 45-year-old woman is undergoing a repair of numerous hindfoot fractures under general anesthesia. A pneumatic tourniquet has been inflated to 275 mm Hg for 180 minutes. The surgeon now asks for tourniquet deflation. Which of the following changes in vital signs would be most likely within the first 1 to 2 minutes after tourniquet release?**

   A. Increased respiratory rate
   B. Increased systolic blood pressure
   C. Decrease in end-tidal CO_2
   D. Increase in core body temperature by 0.5 °C

5. **A 48-year-old man presents with a mangled and dysvascular foot after a motorcycle crash and is coming to surgery for ankle disarticulation. He has a history of opioid abuse and takes buprenorphine/naloxone daily, with his most recent dose 4 hours ago. He also is on clopidogrel after coronary stent placement following a myocardial infarction 3 months ago, again with most recent dose 4 hours ago. Which of the following strategies would be the most appropriate initial step for managing his immediate postoperative pain?**

   A. Lumbar epidural catheter
   B. Popliteal sciatic and femoral peripheral nerve catheters
   C. Ankle block
   D. Intravenous methadone
   E. Oral oxycodone

Answers

1. D

The patient's injury mechanism involves likely hyperextension of the cervical spine, and the combination of upper extremity weakness with preserved lower extremity strength is most consistent with central cord syndrome. Anterior cord syndrome would be expected to cause impaired motor function and impaired pain and temperature sensation everywhere below the level of injury. Brown-Sequard syndrome usually results from penetrating trauma injuring just one-half of the spinal cord, with ipsilateral loss of motor function and contralateral loss of pain and temperature sensation. Cauda equina syndrome results from injury to the lower lumbar spine, often accompanied by bowel and bladder dysfunction. Although this patient has urinary retention, cauda equina syndrome would be expected to also have some lower extremity weakness and have a mechanism of injury different than this patient's history, which is more consistent with cervical spinal cord injury. Finally, posterior cord syndrome is associated with isolated loss of touch, proprioception, and vibration, with preservation of motor function; this patient's presentation of new arm weakness is not consistent with posterior cord syndrome.

2. D

A strategy for close hemodynamic monitoring, tracking surgical bleeding, and periodic laboratory assessments of coagulation status is most likely to reduce this patient's risk for postoperative major organ dysfunction, stroke, or vision loss. Deliberate hypotension would be inappropriate with history of prior stroke. TXA is contraindicated for history of cerebrovascular disease due to increased risk of thrombosis, as well as for increased risk of renal injury. Colloid replacement has previously been among the fluid management approaches for spine surgery, but hydroxyethyl starch is associated with greater risk of needing postoperative renal replacement therapy and would be inappropriate for this patient.

3. B

Of the options listed, only the infraclavicular brachial plexus block would provide appropriate coverage of the proximal ulna (other appropriate blocks include supraclavicular or axillary approaches to the brachial plexus). A pediatric patient of this age is unlikely to willingly tolerate a block procedure awake, and the standard of care in pediatric patients is to perform regional blocks under deep sedation or general anesthesia. Of the other block options listed, the interscalene brachial plexus approach would cover the shoulder and proximal humerus but not the ulna, while the musculocutaneous nerve supplies the muscles in the anterior compartment of the upper arm and cutaneous sensation on the lateral aspect of the forearm, not the appropriate regions for the planned procedure.

4. A

Tourniquet release after 3 hours would be expected to result in the systemic circulation of lactic acid and other compounds from reperfusion of the ischemic operative limb. The increased lactic acid will manifest as an increase in arterial and end-tidal CO_2, for which the spontaneously breathing patient will compensate by increasing minute ventilation by both increasing respiratory rate and tidal volume. Even in the presence of neuromuscular blockade, this increase in CO_2 may cause patients to overbreathe the ventilator after tourniquet release. Systolic blood pressure generally falls in the first minutes after tourniquet release due to the resolution of sympathetically driven ischemic pain and circulation of vasodilatory compounds. Core body temperature falls resulting from reperfusion of a cold extremity.

5. B

This patient has a history of opioid tolerance and is taking a mixed opioid agonist/antagonist that will make postoperative pain management challenging if it relies solely on opioids. His use of clopidogrel contraindicates epidural placement. Peripheral nerve blocks, although carrying some risk of bleeding, are likely the most effective option and can be placed safely while being vigilant for potential bleeding complications. Ankle block requires block of multiple nerves at the level of the ankle, which will not be feasible with the level of his amputation. IV methadone, although potentially helpful with NMDA receptor antagonism, is unlikely to be effective as the primary mode of analgesia. Oral oxycodone will not be as effective in his early postoperative course due to his recent dose of buprenorphine/naloxone, though may begin to have efficacy after the first 24 to 48 hours from the last dose of buprenorphine/naloxone.

27 Anesthesia for Laparoscopic and Robotic Surgeries

Lalitha Vani Sundararaman

Laparoscopic surgical techniques have significant benefits over the traditional open approach, including smaller incisions, decreased postoperative pain, faster recovery time, and reduced chance of blood transfusion and wound infection. Potential disadvantages include higher risk of inadvertent vascular and major organ puncture during placement of the access ports as compared with the traditional open approach. Recently, robot-assisted laparoscopy has been introduced to address some of the disadvantages of laparoscopy, including surgeon fatigue, hand tremor, poor ergonomics, and difficult visualization and manipulation of instruments while retaining all the advantages of laparoscopic techniques.[1] Specific disadvantages pertain to the quality and consistency of data connection between the surgeon and the robot and to the high cost of robot-assisted procedures. This chapter reviews laparoscopic and robot-assisted laparoscopic techniques, their physiologic impact on the patient, and the essential perioperative management strategies for patients undergoing these procedures.

I. Surgical Techniques

Laparoscopic surgery has four basic steps: gaining access to the peritoneal cavity, establishing the pneumoperitoneum, the surgical procedure, and the closure. Prior to peritoneal access, the stomach and bladder are decompressed in order to minimize the likelihood of bowel or bladder injury. Then, access can be established using two accepted techniques: an open approach (***Hasson***) or a closed approach (***Veress*** needle). The Hasson technique uses a small incision performed anywhere on the abdomen but is most commonly done periumbilically, followed by placement of the trocar through that incision and insufflation of the abdomen. The Veress needle technique uses blind passage of the needle through the skin into the peritoneal cavity, followed by insufflation. The Veress needle technique is preferred in patients without intra-abdominal adhesions or umbilical hernias and has a higher risk of organ puncture compared with the Hasson approach.

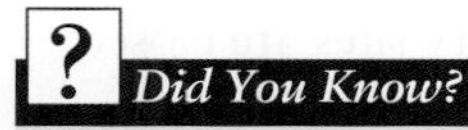

The Hasson technique is preferred to the Veress needle technique in patients with abdominal adhesions.

After accessing the peritoneal cavity, it is slowly insufflated with ***carbon dioxide*** (CO_2) until the intra-abdominal pressure reaches 10 to 15 mm Hg and the abdominal wall is sufficiently distended to allow the surgical procedure. The laparoscopic camera is introduced into the abdomen, and under the visual guidance it provides, additional ports are placed with trocars as needed for the other instruments required for surgery. For robot-assisted procedures, access to the peritoneal cavity is obtained with either technique, followed by laparoscopic exploration of the cavity, placement of the robotic instruments in the

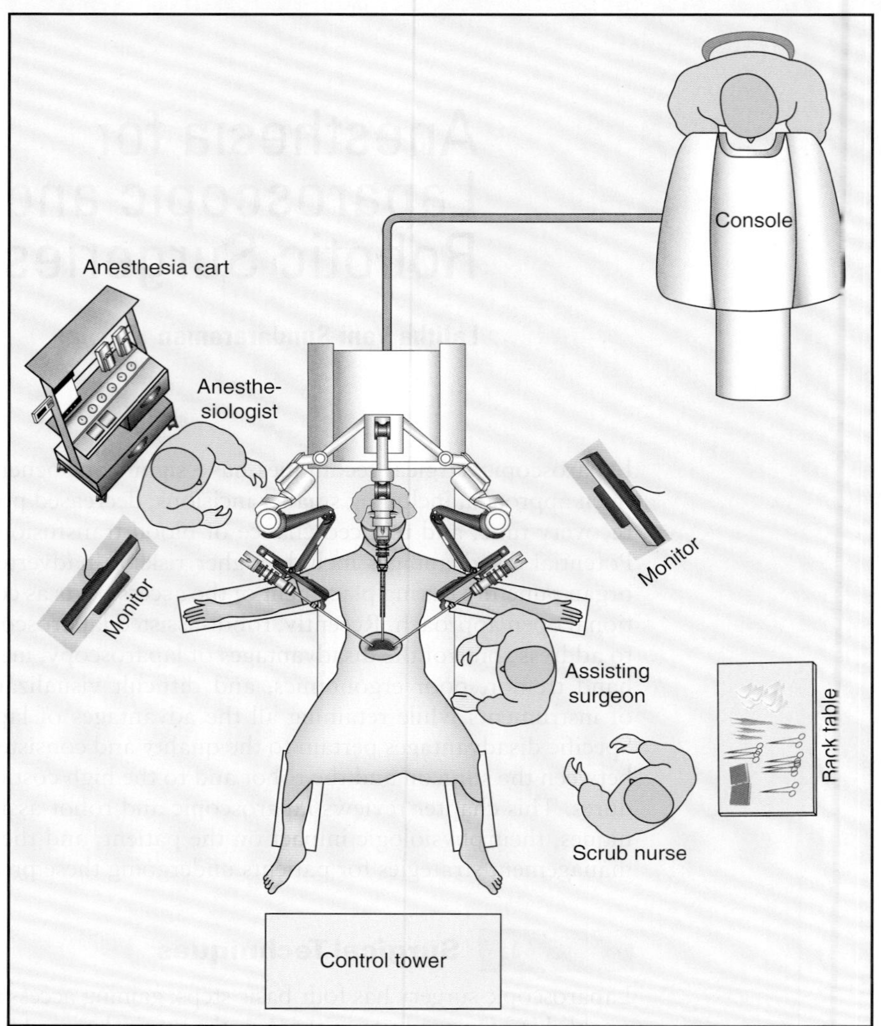

Figure 27.1 **Layout of the operating room during robotic surgery.** (From Horgan S, Sedrak MF. *Robotic surgery.* In: Fischer JE, Jones DB, Pomposelli FB, et al. *Fischer's Mastery of Surgery.* 6th ed. Wolters Kluwer Health/Lippincott Williams & Wilkins; 2012:257, Figure 17.1.)

peritoneum, positioning of the robot, and then attachment of the robotic arms to the instruments (**Figure 27.1**). The surgeon and his first assistant are seated at consoles separate from the operating table, and their hand movements are computer translated into the movement of the robotic arms and instruments (**Figure 27.2**). Following the surgical procedure, the abdominal entry sites are closed.

II. Physiologic Effects

A. Systemic Cardiovascular Effects

Cardiovascular changes during laparoscopy become apparent when the ***intra-abdominal pressure*** exceeds 10 mm Hg, resulting from the combination of increased intra-abdominal pressure, CO_2 absorption, general anesthesia, and patient positioning. ***Cardiac output decreases*** due to decreased venous return,

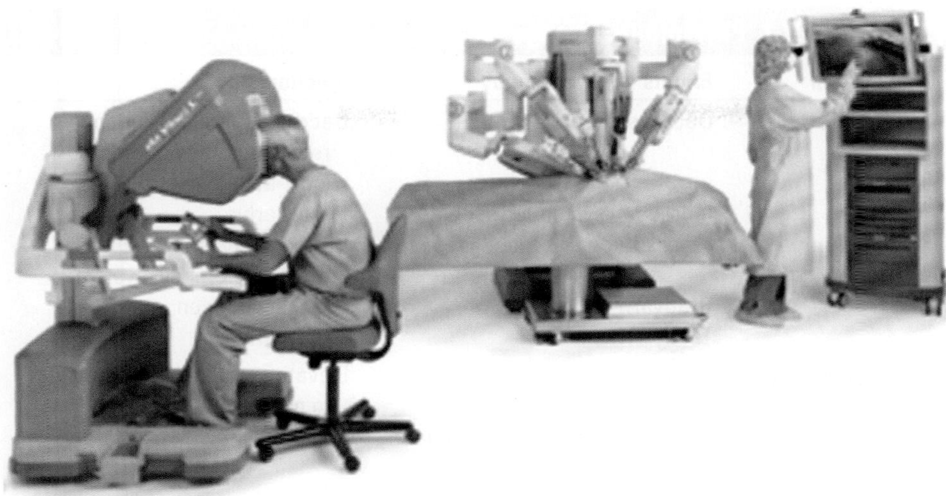

Figure 27.2 A control console where the surgeon is stationed and operates the robotic arms and camera. (© 2012 Intuitive Surgical, Inc, with permission.)

which is secondary to the increased intra-abdominal pressure, causing inferior vena caval compression and pooling of blood in the lower extremities. Systemic vascular resistance increases secondary to the catecholamine release stimulated by the absorbed CO_2 and to the release of vasopressin and activation of the renin-angiotensin system, in part due to the decreased renal blood flow sensed by the juxtaglomerular apparatus and caused by the pneumoperitoneum. Lestar et al reported that a 45° Trendelenburg position with a 12 mm Hg intraperitoneal pressure caused a two- to threefold increase in filling pressures and up to a 35% increase in mean arterial pressure (MAP).[2] In addition, during the insufflation phase of laparoscopy, stretching of the peritoneum stimulates a ***vagal reflex*** and may cause bradycardia or even asystole. These changes occur in the first minutes after establishing the pneumoperitoneum. Subsequently, on desufflation and return to the horizontal position, both cardiac output and systemic vascular resistance normalize within 10 to 15 minutes. When steep Trendelenburg positioning is required, as it is for robot-assisted radical prostatectomies, it increases venous return and cardiac output, thereby opposing the changes due to pneumoperitoneum. In contrast, reverse Trendelenburg and lithotomy positioning further decrease cardiac output by further impairing venous return. These changes can cause significant hemodynamic disturbances in patients with compromised cardiac status.

B. Regional Perfusion

Pneumoperitoneum induces a modest ***splanchnic hyperemia*** due to the vasodilating effects of the absorbed CO_2. CO_2 absorption rapidly increases with insufflation and usually plateaus at 30 minutes of insufflation. Many studies have shown that there is no difference in rise of CO_2 levels between the retroperitoneal and transperitoneal approaches.[3,4] In contrast to the splanchnic hyperemia, pneumoperitoneum ***decreases renal blood flow***, glomerular filtration rate, and urine output by up to 50%. Cerebral blood flow increases during pneumoperitoneum due to an increase in arterial carbon dioxide partial pressure ($Paco_2$). This may be a transient effect if normocarbia is reestablished by increasing minute ventilation

Table 27.1 Physiologic Changes During Laparoscopy

System	Effects of Laparoscopy	Mechanism
Cardiac	Decreased cardiac output	Decreased preload (venous return) due to increased intra-abdominal pressure
	Increased systemic vascular resistance and blood pressure	Hypercarbia Hormones (vasopressin, renin-angiotensin system)
	Bradyarrhythmias	Vagal stimulation
	Tachyarrhythmias	Hypercarbia
Respiratory	Decreased thoracic and respiratory compliance Decreased functional residual capacity Atelectasis Increased peak airway pressures	Elevation of the diaphragm due to pneumoperitoneum
	Hypercarbia	Absorption of carbon dioxide Ventilation/perfusion mismatch
Renal	Decreased renal perfusion, urine output, and glomerular filtration rate	Increased intra-abdominal pressure
Regional circulation	Increased intracerebral and intraocular pressure Modest splanchnic hyperemia	Hypercarbia

appropriately. However, if steep Trendelenburg is employed, it increases intraocular pressure and could further increase intracranial pressure.[5] Patients at risk for ***cerebral hypertension*** and those with poorly controlled ***glaucoma*** may not be appropriate candidates for this positioning (**Table 27.1**).

? Did You Know?

The pneumoperitoneum induced for laparoscopy decreases respiratory compliance and functional residual capacity and worsens pulmonary perfusion and ventilation matching.

C. Respiratory Effects

Intra-abdominal insufflation elevates the diaphragm, causing a ***decrease*** in ***thoracic*** and ***respiratory compliance*** and in functional residual capacity. These changes lead to atelectasis unless countered by positive end-expiratory pressure and periodic recruitment maneuvers. General anesthesia and the combined respiratory effects of pneumoperitoneum increase mismatching of ventilation and perfusion and through that mechanism decrease Pao_2.[6] Postoperative pulmonary function tests demonstrate a reduction in one-second forced expiratory volume (FEV1) and forced vital capacity (FVC) (**Table 27.1**).

III. Anesthetic Management

A. Patient Selection

Patients with cardiac disease, especially severe valvular heart, may not tolerate the cardiovascular effects of pneumoperitoneum. Similarly, morbidly obese patients, patients with severe chronic obstructive pulmonary disease, and those with severe cardiac disease may not be able to compensate for the *steep*

Trendelenburg position often required for some laparoscopic or robotic-assisted surgery. Hence, careful cardiac assessment prior to surgery is required prior to surgery.

For routine laparoscopic cholecystectomy, obesity and even morbid obesity do not seem to increase the rate of significant complications.[7] There are many studies comparing single-site Robotic cholecystectomy (SSRC) and laparoscopic cholecystectomy. While there is no difference in operating time, bleeding, and incidence of complications, the risk of incisional hernia is higher with SSRC. Hence, case selection must be judicious for robotic procedures.[8]

B. Induction of Anesthesia and Airway Management

General endotracheal anesthesia is most often required for laparoscopic procedures because of the discomfort from the pneumoperitoneum and the required ventilatory support. Virtually any well-managed anesthetic induction technique is acceptable, but propofol may be the preferred agent for its antiemetic properties.[9] Use of a laryngeal mask airway instead of endotracheal intubation is reserved for patients undergoing short procedures requiring low insufflation pressures and minimal Trendelenburg.

C. Maintenance of Anesthesia

During positioning after intubation, the anesthesia team should be protective of the chest and face as they may come in contact with the longer than usual robotic instruments. However, they should also avoid cramming the surgical team in a small space. For example, no IV poles should be used that stand caudal to the patient's head, and preferably, the upper drape should fall over the patient's head or be lax enough to accommodate the long robotic instruments and leverage needed in the case. During positioning, the anesthesia provider should also be able to ascertain if there is any subcutaneous emphysema or abnormal sliding of the body on the table in the Trendelenburg position and notify the surgeon immediately if any of these complications occur.

Aggressive use of paralytic agents is essential in robotic surgery: emergency undocking may be needed when patients buck or move under the robot, as this may cause major vessel injury or even death. Intravenous or inhalational anesthetic may be used as per anesthesia provider preference and other patient concerns. However, ***nitrous oxide*** is usually avoided given the risk of worsening postoperative nausea and vomiting (PONV) and its potential for diffusing into and expanding the bowel, worsening surgical conditions. Total intravenous anesthesia can be used if the risk of PONV is significant. Controlled ***normocapnic ventilation*** with positive end-expiratory pressure is required for most laparoscopic and robot-assisted procedures to counter the respiratory impact of the pneumoperitoneum and positioning.

Monitoring other than the American Society of Anesthesiologists standards for general anesthesia should be dictated by each patient's comorbidities. Most cases, however, do not require an arterial or central line.

Hypertension is often seen during laparoscopic surgery due to hypercarbia-induced sympathetic stimulation and activation of the renin-angiotensin axis due to decreased renal blood flow. As this is reversible at the end of the procedure, agents employed to decrease blood pressure should ideally be short-acting and titrated slowly. Often an agent is chosen with the dual purposes of hemodynamic control and analgesic adjuvant potency in mind.[10,11]

Due to the extremes of positioning and case duration sometimes required, adequate padding of the ulnar and common peroneal nerves, appropriate positioning of the arms and padding of the shoulders to avoid ***brachial plexus injury***, and ***safety belt*** securing of the patient to the operating room table must be confirmed prior to incision. If the Trendelenburg or reverse Trendelenburg position is required, it should be achieved slowly to allow for management of hemodynamic changes or migration of the endotracheal tube. Prior to emergence, antiemetic medications should be administered because the incidence of PONV after laparoscopic procedures is high.

IV. Pain Prevention

Pain after laparoscopic procedures is ***far less*** than after comparable procedures performed through open laparotomy. However, the insertion sites of the instruments are painful, and CO_2 insufflation and residual pneumoperitoneum often cause diaphragmatic irritation, leading to referred pain to the shoulder.[12] Local anesthetic infiltration is beneficial at the insertion sites and has very few potential complications. Narcotic doses can be limited if they are combined with other analgesics including nonsteroidal anti-inflammatory drugs (NSAIDs). Prior to administering an NSAID, the surgical team should be consulted to confirm there is no unreasonable risk of bleeding from the NSAID's antiplatelet effect. Rarely would more invasive pain therapy such as regional block be required for adequate pain relief except in patients with chronic pain problems or chronic narcotic use.

V. Intraoperative Complications

A. Cardiopulmonary Complications

Hypotension is quite common during the initial insufflation of the peritoneum due to reduced cardiac output secondary to decreased venous return. Less commonly, a vagal response to stretching of the peritoneum causes significant bradycardia and very ***rarely asystole***. Hypertension or tachycardia can result from hypercarbia-induced catecholamine release or, more commonly, inadequate anesthesia. All of these changes in hemodynamics are readily managed with routine measures and should be quite transient. However, profound, persistent hypotension or cardiovascular collapse can occur very rarely. This should warrant an urgent search and treatment of possible etiologies, including but not limited to excessive intra-abdominal pressure, ***CO_2 embolism***, and ***pneumothorax*** (**Table 27.2**). Although pneumoperitoneum and Trendelenburg positioning increase ventilation and perfusion mismatching, significant hypoxia is uncommon during controlled ventilation with supplemental oxygen unless the patient has preexisting pulmonary disease. Should hypoxia persist despite administration of 100% oxygen, positive end-expiratory pressure, and alveolar recruitment maneuvers; the intra-abdominal pressure should be lowered and other potential etiologies investigated, including endobronchial intubation, pulmonary aspiration, and pneumothorax.

> **? *Did You Know?***
>
> Subcutaneous emphysema with CO_2 is common after laparoscopy and can extend all the way to the neck with potential post-extubation airway compromise.

B. Surgical Complications

1. Carbon Dioxide Extravasation

Subcutaneous emphysema is one of the most common complications of extraperitoneal insufflation of CO_2. This complication is more likely to occur when five or more ports are used for the laparoscopic procedure, during procedures longer than 3.5 hours with intra-abdominal pressures >15 mm Hg, and with improper position of the cannulas. It should be suspected by a rise in end-tidal CO_2 of more than 25% or to more than 50 mm Hg occurring after end-tidal CO_2 has already plateaued. It is confirmed by the presence of crepitus (**Table 27.3**).

Table 27.2 Cardiovascular Complications During Laparoscopy

Complication	Mechanism
Hypotension	Decreased venous return
Hypertension	Hypercarbia Neurohumoral factors
Bradyarrhythmias	Vagal reaction to peritoneal stretching
Tachyarrhythmias	Hypercarbia
Cardiovascular collapse	Arrhythmias (tachy/bradyarrhythmias) Blood loss Gas embolism Capno-/pneumothorax Capnopericardium Cardiac ischemia Excessive intra-abdominal pressure Hypercapnia Deep anesthesia

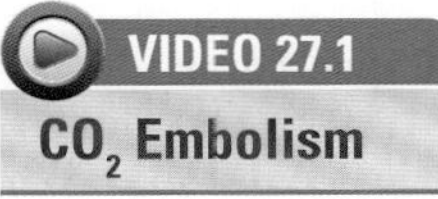

CO_2 **Embolism**

Subcutaneous emphysema can extend into the thorax or mediastinum, as ***capnothorax*** and ***capnomediastinum***, and into the upper torso or neck as well as toward the groin.

Treatment should include deflation of the abdomen and reinflation at lower pressures with confirmation of correct cannula positioning. The presence of subcutaneous emphysema in the neck should raise the question of a possible capnothorax, especially if airway pressures are increased or arterial saturation decreased. Unlike an intraoperative pneumothorax, which presents with increased $PaCO_2$ and decreased end-tidal CO_2, a capnothorax presents with both increased (**Table 27.3**). If blood pressure is well maintained, capnothorax can be treated conservatively by deflation of the abdomen. In the event of a tension capnothorax, as evidenced by tracheal deviation and hypotension, the tension should be vented by a needle thoracostomy and continued mechanical ventilation with positive end-expiratory pressure. Capnopericardium and capnomediastinum are rare complications of laparoscopy; they are diagnosed by chest x ray and treated by deflation of the abdomen and supportive care during spontaneous resolution.

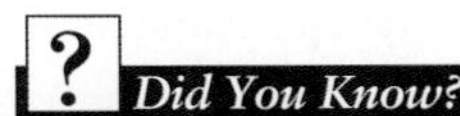

Capnopericardium and capnomediastinum are rare complications of laparoscopy, diagnosed by chest X-ray, and treated by deflation of the abdomen and supportive care during spontaneous resolution.

2. Carbon Dioxide Embolization

CO_2 intravascular embolization is a serious but ***rare complication*** of laparoscopy, usually the consequence of direct insufflation of CO_2 into a vessel or, alternatively, into a solid organ with subsequent intravascular migration. Due to the high blood solubility of CO_2, relatively large amounts of it can be absorbed by the blood and eliminated by the lungs. Thus, a small volume of embolized CO_2 may have no apparent impact except an increase in the end-tidal CO_2. However, a large bolus can impede venous return to the heart, distend the right atrium and ventricle, and produce ***cardiovascular collapse***. The acute increase in the right atrial pressure can lead to paradoxical embolism through a foramen ovale and the potential for neurologic injury. A large intravascular CO_2 embolism should be suspected when sudden, severe hypotension is accompanied by a marked decrease in end-tidal CO_2 occurring during insufflation (**Table 27.3**). Treatment should include immediate cessation of insufflation and deflation of the abdomen, placement of the patient in

Table 27.3 Complications of Pneumoperitoneum

Complication	Mechanism	Diagnosis	Management
CO_2 subcutaneous emphysema	Extraperitoneal insufflation in subcutaneous, preperitoneal, or retroperitoneal tissue Extension of extraperitoneal insufflation	Sudden rise in $ETCO_2$ Crepitus If postoperatively, signs of hypercarbia (increased heart rate, blood pressure), somnolence	Deflation of the abdomen
Capnothorax	Tracking of insufflated CO_2 around the aortic, caval, and esophageal hiatuses of the diaphragm into the mediastinum with subsequent rupture into the pleural space Tracking of CO_2 through diaphragmatic defects Diaphragmatic injury when inserting the laparoscopic needle	High index of suspicion (subcutaneous emphysema of the neck), site of surgical procedure Increased airway pressure Decreased SaO_2 Increased $ETCO_2$ Bulging hemidiaphragm If tension capnothorax, hypotension, decreased $ETCO_2$, and cardiovascular collapse Confirmation by chest x-ray	Discontinuation of N_2O Hyperventilation Apply PEEP
Capnomediastinum **Capnopericardium**	Same as for capnothorax	Hemodynamic changes Confirmation by chest x-ray	Deflation of the abdomen Supportive care Hyperventilation
Endobronchial intubation	Cephalad migration of the carina	Steep increase in peak airway pressure Decrease in SaO_2	Reposition the endotracheal tube
Gas embolism	Placement of the Veress needle into a blood vessel Passage of CO_2 into the abdominal wall and peritoneal vessels	Hypoxemia Hypotension Decreased $ETCO_2$ Arrhythmias or right heart strain on ECG	Deflation of the abdomen Supportive treatment/ cardiovascular resuscitation Hyperventilation

CO_2, carbon dioxide; N_2O, nitrous oxide; PEEP, positive end-expiratory pressure; SaO_2, oxygen saturation; $ETCO_2$, end-tidal carbon dioxide; ECG, electrocardiogram.

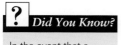

In the event that a trocar punctures a major vessel, it should be left in place to help tamponade the bleeding while the abdomen is open and the vessel repaired.

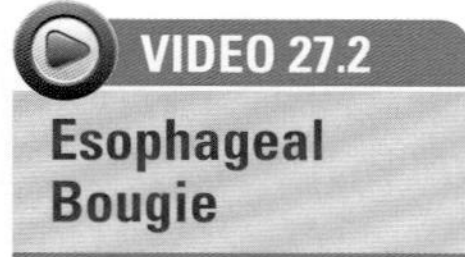

a head-down, left ***lateral decubitus position***, which limits migration of the embolus into the pulmonary artery, hyperventilation in order to speed the elimination of CO_2, and hemodynamic support including cardiac massage if indicated.

3. Other Surgical Complications

Direct injury to vascular structures or the bowel or bladder may occur during trocar or Veress needle placement. Major ***vascular injuries*** have a low incidence (0.02% to 0.03%) but can be catastrophic when a trocar is placed into the aorta, vena cava, or iliac vessels causing ***massive bleeding***. When a major vessel injury occurs, the trocar should be left in place to tamponade bleeding while the surgical team opens the abdomen to control the damage. Bowel and major organ injuries occur in up to 0.4% of laparoscopy cases and are the result of trocar misplacement. Most of the injuries involve the stomach, duodenum, and small and large bowel. Prior abdominal surgery leading to adhesions is a definite risk factor, and most of the bowel injuries go unrecognized until the postoperative period when the patient develops peritonitis.

C. Hypothermia

Severe hypothermia is a significant risk during laparoscopy because, in addition to the usual mechanisms of heat loss during anesthesia (convection, conduction, radiation, and evaporation), insufflation of cold CO_2 (at 23 °C) causes additional heat loss. This loss can be limited by restricting CO_2 flow and leakage and by forced air warming of the patient's upper and lower body.

D. Complications Related to Positioning

Nerve and tissue injuries are serious and preventable complications of positioning, especially in patients undergoing robotic-assisted laparoscopy in the steep Trendelenburg position. Cephalad slippage of the patient can injure nerves and soft tissues by causing pressure points or tissue stretch. If shoulder restraints are used to stabilize the patient, they can apply stretch to the ***brachial plexus***. In addition, over the course of hours, steep Trendelenburg can lead to severe head, neck, and facial swelling, resulting in postextubation airway compromise or, in very rare cases, blindness due to optic nerve ischemia. Chapter 22 provides a detailed discussion of these risks and preventive measures.

? *Did You Know?*

Cephalad slippage of the patient and the cephalad movement of the diaphragm during steep Trendelenburg can result in movement of the endotracheal tube into the right main stem bronchus.

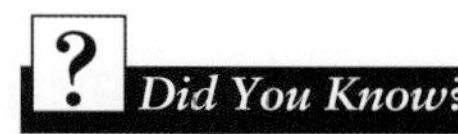

Steep Trendelenburg positioning has been associated with blindness due to optic nerve ischemia.

VI. Postoperative Considerations

Complete clearance of intra-abdominal CO_2 may require longer than 1 hour, and during that time, patients may experience severe shoulder pain referred from diaphragmatic irritation. However, most patients tolerate laparoscopy quite well except those with limited pulmonary reserve or patients with prior diaphragmatic paralysis. These patients may require postoperative respiratory support until the intra-abdominal CO_2 is resorbed fully and pain control is optimized. Postoperative hemorrhage is rare but should be suspected when there is hemodynamic instability, a distended abdomen, or an unexpectedly low hematocrit.

VII. Ambulatory Laparoscopic Procedures

Due to the low complication rate and potential for early ambulation, most uncomplicated laparoscopic procedures (cholecystectomy, gynecologic procedures) in patients with no or very well-controlled comorbidities can be performed on an ***outpatient basis***.[13] Postoperative hospital admission in these patients is rarely needed unless the procedure is complicated by persistent postoperative nausea and vomiting or inadequate pain control. Safety of outpatient laparoscopic bariatric surgery is controversial because of the high incidence of sleep apnea and postoperative surgical complications. Robot-assisted procedures for radical cancer surgery require postoperative hospital admission or admission to the hospital because of their duration and extensive fluid shifts.

VIII. Summary

Laparoscopic and robot-assisted procedures have several advantages over the traditional, open approach, including early mobilization, shorter length of hospital stay, and quicker recovery. The hemodynamic and respiratory consequences of the pneumoperitoneum required for these procedures are generally well tolerated except in patients with severe cardiac or pulmonary disease. General anesthesia is required for the majority of these procedures to ensure adequate ventilation and prevent the pain from peritoneal distension. The majority of complications due to laparoscopy result from insufflation pressures higher than 15 mm Hg or improper placement of trocars. The former complications can be managed most often by decreasing the intra-abdominal pressure, while the latter may require open laparotomy if the trocar has injured a vital organ or major vessel. However, on the whole, laparoscopic techniques have been proven safe and highly effective in reducing surgical morbidity and speeding recovery.

Acknowledgment

The authors gratefully acknowledge the First Edition contributions of Dr Adriana Dana Oprea as portions of the chapter were retained in this update.

For further review and interactivities, please see the associated Interactive Video Lectures and "At a Glance" infographic accessible in the complimentary eBook bundled with this text. Access instructions are located in the inside front cover.

References

1. Liu JJ, Maxwell BG, Panousis P, et al. Perioperative outcomes for laparoscopic and robotic compared with open prostatectomy using the National Surgical Quality Improvement Program (NSQIP) database. *Urology*. 2013;82(3):579-583.
2. Lestar M, Gunnarsson L, Lagerstrand L, Wiklund P, Odeberg-Wernerman S. Hemodynamic perturbations during robot-assisted laparoscopic radical prostatectomy in 45° Trendelenburg position. *Anesth Analg*. 2011;113(5):1069-1075.
3. Kadam P, Marda M, Shah VR. Carbon dioxide absorption during laparoscopic donor nephrectomy: a comparison between retroperitoneal and transperitoneal approaches. *Transplant Proc*. 2008;40(4):1119-1121. doi:10.1016/j.transproceed.2008.03.024
4. Ng CS, Gill IS, Sung GT, Whalley DG, Graham R, Schweizer D. Retroperitoneoscopic surgery is not associated with increased carbon dioxide absorption. *J Urol*. 1999;162(4):1268-1272.
5. Hsu RL, Kaye AD, Urman RD. Anesthetic challenges in robotic-assisted urologic surgery. *Rev Urol*. 2013;15(4):178-184.
6. Grabowski JE, Talamini MA. Physiological effects of pneumoperitoneum. *J Gastrointest Surg*. 2009;13(5):1009-1016.
7. Afaneh C, Abelson J, Rich BS, et al. Obesity does not increase morbidity of laparoscopic cholecystectomy. *J Surg Res*. 2014;19(2):491-497.
8. Sun N, Zhang J, Zhang C, Shi Y. Single-site robotic cholecystectomy versus multiport laparoscopic cholecystectomy: a systematic review and meta-analysis. *Am J Surg*. 2018;216(6):1205-1211. doi:10.1016/j.amjsurg.2018.04.018
9. Vaughan J, Nagendran M, Cooper J, et al. Anaesthetic regimens for day-procedure laparoscopic cholecystectomy. *Cochrane Database Syst Rev*. 2014;1:CD009784.
10. Kamali A, Ashrafi TH, et al. A comparative study on the prophylactic effects of paracetamol and dexmedetomidine for controlling hemodynamics during surgery and postoperative pain in patients with laparoscopic cholecystectomy. *Medicine (Baltimore)*. 2018;97(51):e13330. doi:10.1097/MD.0000000000013330
11. Collard V, Mistraletti G, Taqi A, et al. Intraoperative esmolol infusion in the absence of opioids spares postoperative fentanyl in patients undergoing ambulatory laparoscopic cholecystectomy. *Anesth Analg*. 2007;105(5):1255-1262.
12. Donatsky AM, Bjerrum F, Gogenur I. Surgical techniques to minimize shoulder pain after laparoscopic cholecystectomy. A systematic review. *Surg Endosc*. 2013;27(7):2275-2282.
13. Vaughan J, Gurusamy KS, Davidson BR. Day-surgery versus overnight stay surgery for laparoscopic cholecystectomy. *Cochrane Database Syst Rev*. 2013;7:CD006798.

COMPLICATIONS OF LAPAROSCOPY

AT A GLANCE

Laparoscopic procedures insufflate carbon dioxide into the abdomen. This has profound impact on the patient's physiology.

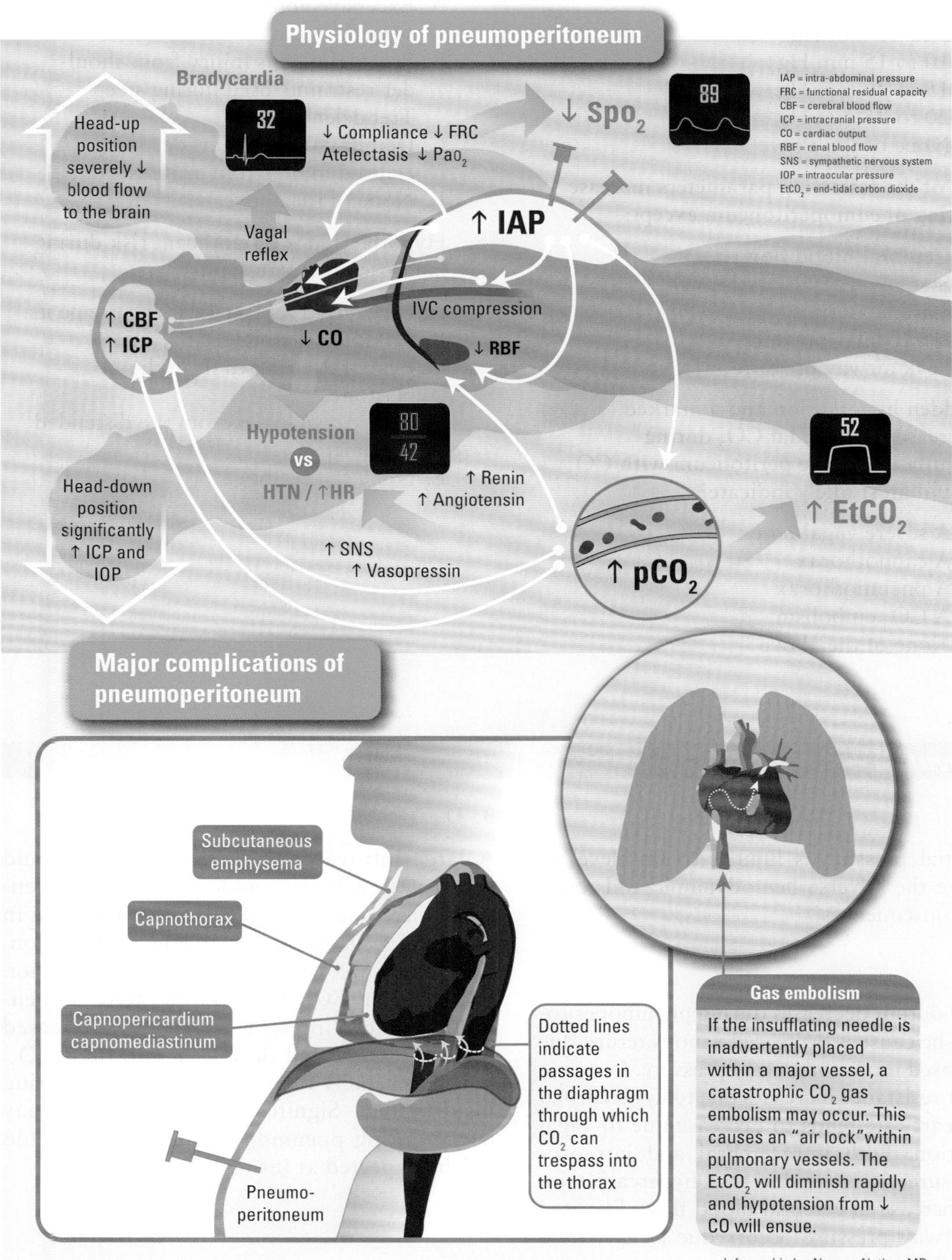

Infographic by: Naveen Nathan MD

Questions

1. **What is the recommended initial intra-abdominal insufflation pressure for laparoscopy?**

   A. 5 to 10 mm Hg
   B. 10 to 15 mm Hg
   C. 15 to 20 mm Hg
   D. 20 to 25 mm Hg
   E. None of the above

2. **All of the following parameters increase during pneumoperitoneum except:**

   A. Cerebral blood flow
   B. Systemic vascular resistance
   C. Cardiac output
   D. Intraocular pressure
   E. Peak airway pressure

3. **Sudden hypotension and a marked decrease in end-tidal CO_2 during insufflation of the peritoneum with CO_2 would most likely indicate?**

   A. A severe vagal reflex
   B. A capnothorax
   C. A pneumothorax
   D. A CO_2 embolism
   E. None of the above

4. **Shoulder pain after laparoscopy is likely the result of:**

   A. Excessive abduction of the arm during surgery.
   B. Brachial plexus injury from shoulder restraints used during steep Trendelenburg.
   C. Diaphragmatic irritation.
   D. Deltoid injury from arm restraints.
   E. None of the above.

5. **Hypothermia is a significant risk during laparoscopy because of:**

   A. Large fluid replacement requirements.
   B. Cold insufflating gas.
   C. Evaporative losses from the peritoneum.
   D. Convective losses from the distended abdomen.
   E. None of the above.

Answers

1. B

The initial pressure is limited to this level to minimize the adverse hemodynamic and respiratory consequences.

2. C

Cardiac output decreases during pneumoperitoneum. The cause is decreased venous return due to increased intra-abdominal pressure. Systemic vascular resistance increases due to hypercarbia, while heart rate tends to decrease due to vagal stimulation. Both intracerebral and intraocular pressures increase due to a hypercarbia-induced increase in cerebral blood flow. Elevated peak airway pressure occurs due to increased intra-abdominal pressure.

3. D

A large intravascular CO_2 embolism should be suspected when sudden, severe hypotension is accompanied by a marked decrease in end-tidal CO_2 occurring during insufflation. A capnothorax can present with hypotension but end-tidal CO_2 should be elevated. A pneumothorax can present with both decreased blood pressure and decreased end-tidal CO_2, but is less likely than a CO_2 embolism during insufflation. Significant bradycardia may occur during pneumoperitoneum, but would not be expected at insufflation.

4. C

Shoulder pain referred from the diaphragm is common after laparoscopy. Complete clearance of intra-abdominal CO_2 may require over 1 hour, and during that time, patients may experience severe shoulder pain referred from diaphragmatic irritation. The other answers are plausible but much less likely.

5. B

Severe hypothermia is a significant risk during laparoscopy because in addition to the usual mechanisms of heat loss during anesthesia (convection, conduction, radiation and evaporation), insufflation of cold CO_2 (at 23 °C) causes additional heat loss.

28 Anesthetic Considerations for Patients With Obesity, Hepatic Disease, and Other Gastrointestinal Issues

Sundar Krishnan, Lovkesh Arora, and Archit Sharma

I. Obesity

Obesity is commonly defined by the patient's body mass index (BMI). The number of obese (BMI >30 kg/m^2) and severe obese (BMI >40 kg/m^2) patients undergoing surgical procedures is steadily increasing. Since obese patients have an increased risk of perioperative morbidity and mortality, several aspects of care need to be tailored to mitigate these risks.[1]

A. Pathophysiology

Respiratory System

Patients with truncal obesity have reduced ventilatory compliance, tidal volume, functional residual capacity (FRC), and vital capacity.[2] As a result, they often become hypoxic much more rapidly than nonobese patients. Additionally, the impact of positioning and surgery on lung function is exaggerated because of the effects of a large abdomen on diaphragmatic position and movement, causing FRC to fall below closing capacity. Resultant small airway closure leads to atelectasis and further hypoxemia.

> **? Did You Know?**
>
> Obese patients become hypoxic rapidly and can tolerate only brief periods of apnea due to reduced functional residual capacity.

The metabolic activity of fat and supportive tissue increases oxygen consumption and carbon dioxide (CO_2) production in obese patients. This is compensated for with increased minute ventilation and cardiac output. Due to the aforementioned mechanical limitations, obese patients are often unable to increase tidal volume at times of increased oxygen need and must rely on tachypnea to improve minute ventilation.[3]

Sleep disordered breathing describes the spectrum of conditions ranging from ***obstructive sleep apnea (OSA)*** through ***obesity hypoventilation syndrome (OHS)***.[4] Airway obstruction occurs in obese patients due to growth of adipose tissue in oral and pharyngeal structures. OSA is characterized by recurrent episodes of upper airway obstruction during sleep, causing hypoxia and hypercarbia. OSA occurs in up to 70% of severely obese patients undergoing bariatric surgery and is a risk factor for adverse perioperative outcomes. OHS—also called Pickwickian syndrome—is seen in 5% to 10% of patients with OSA. It is characterized by daytime hypercapnia, hypoventilation, and sleep disordered breathing. Patients with sleep disordered breathing are at increased risk for sedative- and opioid-related ventilatory impairment because of upper airway obstruction, depressed central respiratory drive, and impaired

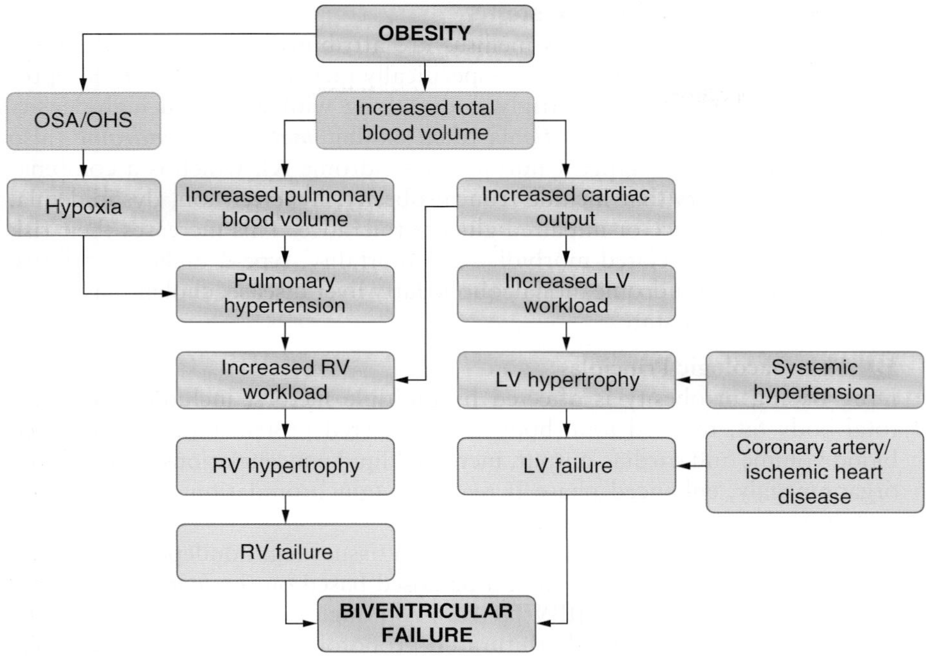

Figure 28.1 Interrelationship of cardiovascular and pulmonary sequelae of obesity. LV, left ventricular; OHS, obesity hypoventilation syndrome; OSA, obstructive sleep apnea; RV, right ventricular. (From Fernandez-Bustamante A, Bucklin BA. Anesthesia and obesity. In: Barash PG, Cahalan MK, Cullen BF, et al, eds. *Clinical Anesthesia*. 8th ed. Wolters Kluwer; 2018:1277-1297, Figure 45.2.)

lung mechanics. Over the long term, OSA and OHS lead to polycythemia, systemic and pulmonary hypertension, left ventricular hypertrophy, cardiac dysrhythmias, right heart strain, and cor pulmonale (**Figure 28.1**).

VIDEO 28.1
Sequelae of Obesity

Cardiovascular System

Obesity is associated with an increase in blood volume, although the weight-based blood volume is reduced (from 70 mL/kg in lean individuals to 50 mL/kg in obese patients). Obese patients are at higher risk for hypertension, left ventricular hypertrophy, diastolic dysfunction, and heart failure. The combination of dyslipidemia, diabetes, and hypertension predisposes obese patients to atherosclerosis and hence coronary and cerebrovascular disease. Obesity also predisposes to a hypercoagulable state because of increased levels of procoagulant factors and decreased fibrinolysis. Obesity has been associated with an increased risk of both deep venous and thrombosis, pulmonary embolism, and stroke.

Gastrointestinal System

Mechanical and hormonal changes increase the risk of gastroesophageal reflux disease (GERD) in obese patients. Obesity-associated liver disease includes fatty infiltration (nonalcoholic fatty liver disease), inflammation (nonalcoholic steatohepatitis), focal necrosis, and cirrhosis. Obese patients are also at risk for cholelithiasis, particularly after intestinal bypass surgery.

Endocrine and Metabolic Systems

Most cases of type 2 diabetes mellitus are attributed to obesity. Obesity is also associated with dyslipidemia—specifically increased low-density lipoprotein (LDL), cholesterol, and triglycerides along with decreased high-density lipoprotein (HDL). Obese patients often exhibit ***metabolic syndrome*** (also known as insulin resistance syndrome or syndrome X), which is a combination of risk factors that include truncal obesity, hypertension, dyslipidemia, and insulin resistance or impaired glucose tolerance. This increases their risk for cardiovascular-related morbidity and mortality, type 2 diabetes mellitus, polycystic ovary syndrome, nonalcoholic fatty liver disease, cholelithiasis, and a proinflammatory state.

B. Pharmacologic Principles

Drug dosing in obesity is affected by multiple factors, including increased total body fat, reduced total body water, altered protein binding, increased blood volume and cardiac output, increased lipid concentrations in the blood, organomegaly, enhanced phase II reactions (glucuronidation and sulfation), and drug absorption in fat stores.[5]

Drugs that are mainly distributed to lean tissues (eg, nondepolarizing neuromuscular blocking agents) should be dosed based on the ***lean body weight*** (LBW ≈ ideal body weight [IBW] × 1.2). Although initial doses for lipophilic drugs (eg, benzodiazepines, barbiturates, propofol) should be based on LBW as well, maintenance doses should be based on ***total body weight (TBW)*** because of the significantly increased volume of distribution. Multiple doses of lipophilic drugs lead to accumulation in fat stores, causing a prolonged response as the drug is released back into circulation.

For inhaled anesthetics, the longer time constants for equilibrium with fat along with poor perfusion of fat tissue counteract the effect of increased fat mass on uptake. As a result, obesity does not influence induction times and only modestly affects the wake-up time with the inhaled anesthetics in routine clinical practice; this is especially for surgeries lasting <4 hours. The principles for administration of commonly used perioperative drugs in obese patients are listed in **Table 28.1**. It must be noted that the dose-response relationships for most drugs in obese patients have not been completely elucidated.

C. Preoperative Evaluation

Preoperative evaluation of the obese patient should include assessment of the risk of airway management difficulties, vascular access options, identification of comorbidities, and education of the patient regarding the perioperative anesthetic plan. Preoperative medical management of the comorbidities, when possible, may help reduce the perioperative risk.

There is a high prevalence of difficult airways in obese patients due to a large tongue, perimandibular and nuchal fat tissue, and redundant pharyngeal soft tissue. OSA independently correlates with difficult mask ventilation. Difficult intubation rates in obese patients range from 5% to 15% and up to 21% in patients with OSA. Male sex, neck circumference, and Mallampati score have been shown to predict difficult intubation in obese patients, although these results are inconsistent across multiple studies and the positive predictive value for each factor is low. Laryngoscopic view is improved in morbidly obese patients with the use of a video laryngoscope. The ramped position, as described later, also improves laryngoscopic view.

Table 28.1 Principles for Administration of Common Perioperative Drugs in Obese Patients

Drug	Initial Dosing Based on	Remarks
Thiopental	LBW	Increased cardiac output in obese patients results in lower peak arterial concentration and more rapid awakening.
Propofol	LBW	TBW-based dosing should be used for continuous infusions and maintenance dosing.
Etomidate	LBW	May have prolonged half-life.
Benzodiazepines	TBW	Longer duration of action due to increased volume of distribution. Higher initial doses may be necessary to achieve adequate sedation, resulting in prolonged sedation.
Dexmedetomidine	TBW	Short-acting sedative infusion that does not cause respiratory depression. Useful for awake fiberoptic intubation and as an anesthetic adjunct. However, bradycardia and hypotension can be significant.
Fentanyl	LBW	Clearance increases with LBW. Dosing based on TBW overestimates dose requirements in obese patients. Titrate doses to clinical response.
Hydromorphone	LBW	
Sufentanil	LBW	Increased volume of distribution and elimination half-life because of high lipophilicity.
Remifentanil	LBW	Rapid hydrolysis in plasma and tissues. Dosing by TBW will result in increased risk of side effects.
Succinylcholine	TBW	Lower doses will result in poor intubating conditions due to increased extracellular volume and increased activity of pseudocholinesterase activity in obese patients. Low incidence of myalgias in obese patients.
Vecuronium	LBW	Dosing by TBW results in prolonged duration of action. Repeat doses should be based on neuromuscular monitoring.
Rocuronium	LBW	Faster onset and prolonged duration of action when dosed by TBW. Repeat doses should be based on neuromuscular monitoring.
Atracurium	LBW	
Cisatracurium	LBW	Dosing by TBW results in prolonged duration of action, while dosing by IBW may result in decreased duration of action.
Pancuronium	BSA	Airway and respiratory derangements in obese patients make this long-acting neuromuscular blocker undesirable.
Sugammadex	IBW + 40%	
Neostigmine	TBW, not exceeding 5 mg	Prolonged time to adequate reversal (TOF ratio 0.9), up to four times slower than that for nonobese patients (26 min vs 7 min).
Heparin	LBW	Dose response in obese patients is not established. Obese patients have a higher risk of deep venous thrombosis and pulmonary embolism perioperatively than nonobese patients.

IBW, ideal body weight; LBW, lean body weight; TBW, total body weight; TOF, train of four.

Preoperative evaluation for OSA and initiation of at-home continuous positive airway pressure (CPAP) for patients with OSA is recommended. In the absence of a formal preoperative sleep study, tools like the ***STOP-BANG*** questionnaire can help identify patients with OSA. The questionnaire consists of questions on *S*noring, *T*iredness, *O*bserved apnea, high blood *P*ressure, *B*MI >35 kg/m^2, *A*ge >50 years, *N*eck circumference >40 cm, and male *G*ender, with positive answers to three or more questions suggesting a higher risk for OSA. Elective surgeries on patients with well-controlled OSA, who are compliant with positive airway pressure (PAP) devices can proceed without further evaluation. For patients with proven OSA not treated with PAP therapy, preoperative cardiopulmonary optimization should be considered. However, urgent and emergency surgery should not be postponed for a formal diagnosis of OSA or to institute treatment. Patients who are on PAP therapy for OSA should continue treatment up to the day of surgery and should bring their PAP device with them on the day of surgery for postoperative use.

The American Heart Association (AHA) Scientific Advisory on Cardiovascular Evaluation and Management of Severely Obese Patients Undergoing Surgery recommends that severely obese patients with at least one risk factor for coronary artery disease (diabetes, smoking, hypertension, or hyperlipidemia) or poor exercise tolerance should have a 12-lead electrocardiogram (ECG) and chest radiograph prior to surgery, since their cardiac symptoms can easily be masked by obesity-related issues. Preoperative cardiac evaluation and management, otherwise, is similar to patients with a normal BMI.

D. Preoperative Planning and Type of Anesthetic

Availability of appropriate weighing scale, gowns, chairs, transport beds, and monitors should be checked prior to arrival. Patients should be asked to trim their beard preoperatively. Operating rooms should be equipped with suitable sized operating tables and gel pads for positioning. Extra personnel should be available to help with patient positioning. An experienced surgeon and anesthesiologist are ideal for severely obese patients.

Monitored Anesthesia Care and Sedation

The risks associated with procedural sedation in the obese patient should not be underestimated. There should be close monitoring of respiratory function because of preexisting respiratory compromise, increased risk of respiratory depression with sedation, and the potential for difficult mask ventilation and intubation. The presence of OSA increases the risk of perioperative hypoxemia and the requirement of airway interventions during sedation. Dexmedetomidine is a selective α_2-adrenergic agonist that provides sedation without respiratory depression. However, its clinical use can be limited because of hemodynamic instability.

Regional Anesthesia

The 2014 American Society of Anesthesiologists' (ASA) practice guidelines for management of patients with OSA recommend that regional analgesic techniques be considered to reduce or eliminate the requirement for systemic opioids.[6] However, excessive sedation used to perform or manage the regional anesthetic may negate the advantages. In addition, obesity may make both neuraxial and peripheral nerve blocks more difficult to perform and may be associated with higher block failure rates. Ultrasound guidance can reduce procedure time and improve procedural success; however, imaging may be suboptimal due to increased depth of target structures. Retraction and taping of excessive soft tissue away from the procedural site allow for sterile preparation and easier access to insertion sites. Local anesthetic dosing for peripheral nerve blocks in obese patients should be based on IBW rather than TBW to avoid systemic toxicity.

Neuraxial Techniques

Spinal or epidural placement in the sitting position allows for easier identification of the vertebral midline. Ultrasound can be used to identify the spinous processes and to reduce the number of needle passes. When longer needles are used, a careful assessment of the midline will avoid injury. Obese patients have decreased cerebrospinal fluid volume due to fatty tissue spread into intervertebral foramina and engorged epidural veins resulting from elevated venous pressure. Additionally, large buttocks can cause a head-down tilt of the vertebral column. Hence during spinal anesthesia, local anesthetics and opioids can have an exaggerated cephalad spread. A ramp under the chest elevates the cervical and thoracic spine, limiting cephalad spread of hyperbaric local anesthetic.

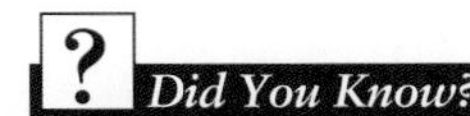

Obese patients require less epidural local anesthetic than normal weight patients to achieve a comparable level of anesthetic block.

Epidural placement can be challenging because needle transit through fat planes can produce a false sense of loss of resistance and difficulty in predicting the depth of the epidural space. There is a higher initial failure rate for epidural catheters in obese laboring patients than in lean patients.

General Anesthesia

Obese patients undergoing sedation should be consented for general anesthesia because of the risk of airway obstruction and respiratory depression and the chances for a failed regional anesthetic nerve block. Deeper levels of sedation should be avoided, and an early plan for general anesthesia should be considered. General anesthesia offers the ability to control ventilation and protect the airway. However, the airway and cardiopulmonary side effects of general anesthesia in obese patients require proper planning and close monitoring.

Ambulatory Versus Inpatient Surgery

Severely obese (BMI >40 kg/m^2) patients undergoing procedures that require general anesthesia and postoperative opioid administration often require overnight admission and observation in an inpatient unit because of an increased risk of perioperative complications.[7] As such, in general, their procedures should not be performed in isolated ambulatory surgery centers but rather in a hospital site that can handle their potentially complicated postoperative course.

E. Intraoperative Considerations

Premedication

Although obesity is a risk factor for GERD, gastric emptying is not delayed by obesity alone. However, comorbid conditions such as diabetes mellitus may cause gastroparesis. In general, standard nil per os (NPO) guidelines should be followed. Antacids, prokinetics, H_2 receptor antagonists, and/or proton-pump inhibitors should be administered prior to induction in patients with an identifiable risk of aspiration but not routinely. Preprocedural sedation should only be given in conjunction with continuous monitoring of respiration and oxygenation.

Positioning

Whenever possible, patients should position themselves on the operating table. In extreme cases, a mechanical lifting device may be required to move the patient. Specially designed tables are required for surgery in the extremely obese. Well-padded sleds or arm boards are often required to position the arms. For surgeries that require tilting or turning of the table, strapping or taping the patient to the table along with stiffened "bean bags" can prevent accidental falls. Gel and foam pads should be used to support pressure points and prevent peripheral neuropathy and skin breakdown. The supine position is associated with reduction in lung volumes and hypoxemia, and venous return may be impeded through caval compression. In the prone position, emphasis should be placed on ensuring free abdominal wall movement, with support for the chest wall and the pelvis. The Trendelenburg position causes the highest degree of respiratory compromise, with a decrease in FRC and lung compliance. Shoulder bars may cause injury to the brachial plexus if incorrectly placed. Lateral positioning and the sitting position allow the weight of the abdominal fat to fall away from the chest and diaphragm (**Figure 28.2**).

Monitoring and Vascular Access

Noninvasive monitoring of blood pressure overestimates the blood pressure in a large proportion of obese patients because of inappropriate cuff size and the conical shape of the obese arm. Also, recording times may be prolonged, leading to delayed recognition of changes in blood pressure. The forearm offers an

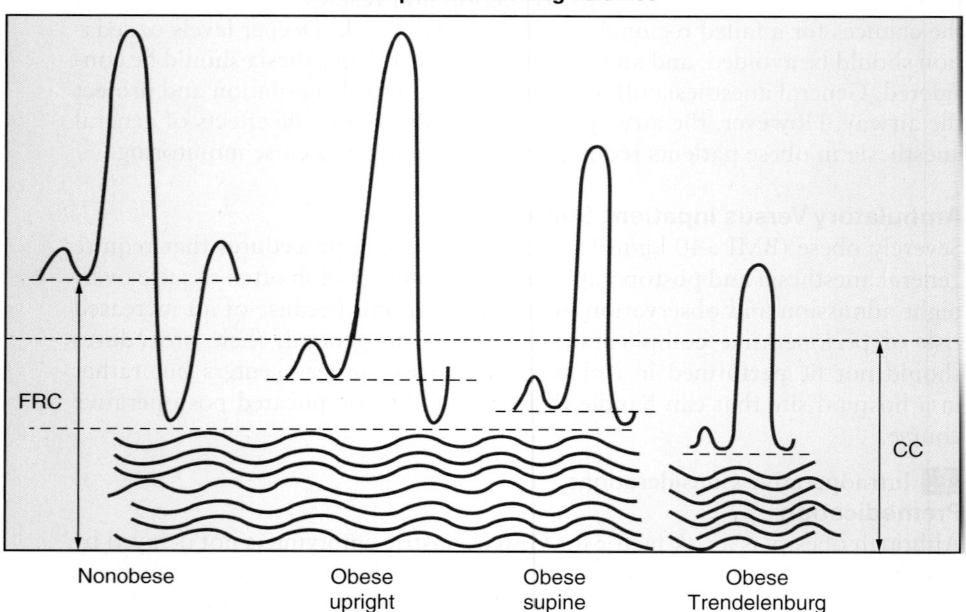

Figure 28.2 Effects of obesity, positioning, and anesthesia on lung volumes. CC, closing capacity; CV, closing volume; FRC, functional residual capacity; RV, residual volume. (From Fernandez-Bustamante A, Bucklin BA. Anesthesia and obesity. In: Barash PG, Cahalan MK, Cullen BF, et al, eds. *Clinical Anesthesia*. 8th ed. Wolters Kluwer; 2018:1277-1297, Figure 45.1.)

alternative site for blood pressure measurement and appears to provide reasonably accurate results. The use of invasive monitoring should be considered, especially in the presence of comorbid conditions. Peripheral venous access can also be challenging and may require ultrasound guidance.

Airway Management

With induction of anesthesia in the supine position, obese patients experience a further reduction of FRC, and oxygen saturation may fall rapidly. Maneuvers that prolong safe apnea times during induction include preoxygenation with 100% oxygen at a high flow rate (approximately twice the minute ventilation), application of 10 cm H_2O CPAP during preoxygenation, positive end-expiratory pressure (PEEP) during mask ventilation, and the use of a 25- to 30-degree reverse Trendelenburg or semisitting beach-chair position. The head-up position also minimizes the risk of passive gastric regurgitation.

Mask ventilation is usually difficult in obese patients. Use of an oral or nasopharyngeal airway, or a two-handed approach is often helpful. Appropriate planning based on the ASA difficult airway algorithm is necessary, particularly before muscle relaxants are administered.

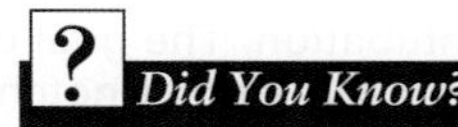

The best position for inducing anesthesia in obese patients is a semisitting position using a ramp to place the patient's ears at the level of the anterior chest wall.

In severely obese patients, supraglottic airways (SGAs) are generally not preferred because of the risk of hypoventilation during spontaneous ventilation. During positive pressure ventilation, an SGA may not maintain a seal at the higher airway pressures needed in obese patients. Decisions about airway choice should be made for individual patients, taking into consideration the grade and distribution of obesity, the type and length of surgery, and the intraoperative patient position. When SGAs are used, second-generation devices, which allow for higher seal pressures and provide a port for gastric decompression, are frequently employed.

Intubation may be more challenging in obese patients. Placing the patient in a ramped position can facilitate laryngoscopic visualization of the vocal cords. Positioning can be achieved with towels or folded blankets under the patient's shoulders and head or with a commercially available device. The head, shoulders, and upper body are elevated above the chest, with the goal of positioning the external auditory meatus at the level of the anterior chest wall (**Figure 28.3**).

Mechanical Ventilation

There is no clear evidence of a benefit to volume-controlled versus pressure-controlled ventilation in obese patients. Tidal volumes of 6 to 8 mL/kg IBW with PEEP are recommended for intraoperative ventilation. Alveolar recruitment maneuvers and subsequent application of moderate PEEP (10 cm H_2O) helps prevent atelectasis, particularly in patients undergoing laparoscopic surgery. Reduced ventilatory compliance can cause high airway pressures, making it difficult to maintain plateau pressures <30 cm H_2O, especially with pneumoperitoneum during laparoscopic surgeries. High airway pressures can cause barotrauma and hypotension. Hypercapnia may have to be tolerated. However, hypercapnia can result in a further increase of pulmonary vascular resistance in patients with preexisting pulmonary hypertension.

Fluid Management

Obese patients may suffer increased perioperative blood loss because of technical difficulties with surgical exposure. It may also be more difficult to

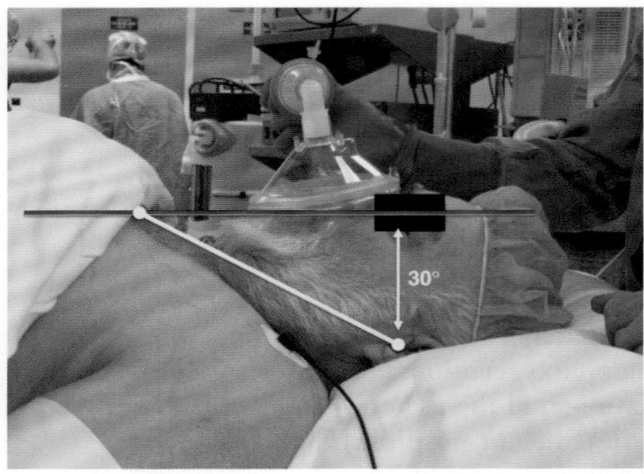

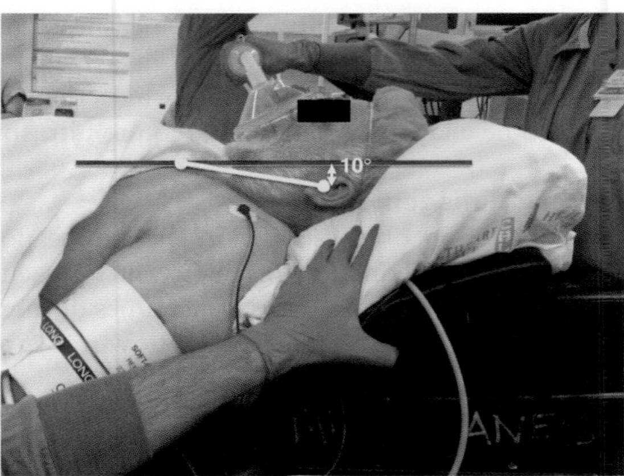

Figure 28.3 Positioning of an obese patient supine on the operating table with use of an upper body (shoulder/head) "ramp" will likely enhance laryngoscopic view of the vocal cords and facilitate tracheal intubation. The goal of such positioning is to bring a line drawn between the external auditory meatus and the sternal notch (*yellow line*) into a position parallel to the horizontal plane (*red line*). Standard supine positioning (*left*) demonstrates a 30° difference between these two lines, whereas proper ramp positioning (*right*) has reduced this angle to only 10°.

estimate fluid balance, adequacy of peripheral perfusion, and blood loss in obese patients. Measurement of urine output, venous pressures, pulse pressure variation, and acid-base status may be helpful.

Analgesia

A multimodal, opioid-sparing approach to analgesia should be used for all obese patients. This includes use of nonsteroidal anti-inflammatory drugs (NSAIDs) such as ketorolac and acetaminophen; local anesthetic wound infiltration; adjuncts like ketamine; alpha-2 agonists (eg, clonidine and dexmedetomidine); magnesium; systemic lidocaine; and gabapentin.

Emergence

Precautions similar to induction should be observed. Patients should be extubated when neuromuscular blockade has been completely reversed (ideally assessed quantitatively) and the patient is awake. Use of a semisitting or reverse Trendelenburg position is helpful. Postoperative lung function is improved with application of some form of noninvasive positive-pressure ventilation (NIPPV) immediately after extubation.

F. Anesthesia for Bariatric Surgery

Surgical treatment of obesity is generally considered if BMI is >40 kg/m^2 (or BMI >35 kg/m^2 with obesity-related comorbidities) and the patient is unable to maintain weight loss with medical management. All of the intraoperative recommendations noted previously should be considered (eg, positioning, padding, extubation, etc.). Continuation of home CPAP therapy in the immediate postoperative period, along with a semiupright position, aids in maintaining oxygenation after surgery. Postoperative nausea and vomiting can cause disruption of gastric repair. In addition to antiemetics, adequate fluid replacement reduces postoperative nausea and vomiting in bariatric surgery patients. An opioid-sparing postoperative analgesia strategy includes local anesthetic wound infiltration, intravenous acetaminophen, NSAIDs, and thoracic epidural infusion of local anesthetics. Implementation of bariatric clinical care pathways improves patient care and reduces cost.

G. Postoperative Management, Critical Care, and Resuscitation

Postoperatively, severely obese patients are at increased risk for prolonged mechanical ventilation and intensive care unit (ICU) stay. Mobilization, incentive spirometry, and judicious handling of analgesia and sedation are required to prevent reintubation in the postanesthesia care unit. NIPPV provides ventilatory support through an external interface such as a nasal or oronasal mask. The provision of positive pressure into the nasopharynx or oropharynx helps keep open the airway, reduce alveolar decruitment, and increase lung volumes. Patients should have continuous pulse oximetry monitoring until they have demonstrated that they can maintain adequate oxygenation when left unstimulated. Patients who cannot maintain adequate oxygenation when left undisturbed should not be discharged from the hospital.

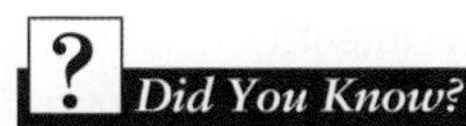

First-line management of postoperative hypoxemia in the obese patient should be some form of noninvasive positive pressure ventilation. Tracheal intubation should be used as a method of last resort.

Postoperative anticoagulation for a prolonged period (eg, heparin 5000-7500 U three times daily for 10 days) is helpful to prevent deep vein thrombosis and pulmonary embolism in obese patients. Early, high-protein, hypocaloric enteral feeding provides an anabolic advantage, reduces infectious complications, and reduces ICU stays. Frequent repositioning of the patient, use of pressure-relief mattresses, and early mobilization will prevent decubitus ulcers. Appropriate antibiotic dosing and redosing, prevention of hyperglycemia, and maintenance of arterial and tissue oxygenation are required to prevent surgical site infections.

Should cardiopulmonary resuscitation be required, it may be difficult to provide effective chest compressions. Repeat defibrillation shocks may be necessary because of the higher transthoracic impedance. Although airway management by conventional means can be challenging, surgical access through a thick neck can also be extremely difficult.

II. Hepatic Disease

Patients with hepatic disease present for hepatic and nonhepatic surgery and are at increased risk of postoperative morbidity and mortality.

A. Assessment of Hepatic Function

Hepatic functions include bile production, protein synthesis, regulation of glucose metabolism, lipid and protein metabolism, hematopoiesis, and drug and metabolite clearance. Clinical evidence of liver disease can be subtle. Risk factors (alcoholism, illicit drug use, sexual promiscuity, blood transfusions) provide clues to possible hepatic disease. Signs and symptoms often include loss of appetite, malaise, pruritus, abdominal pain, indigestion, jaundice, and changes in urine or stool color. Patients with advanced disease may have ascites, palmer erythema, gynecomastia, spider angiomas, or encephalopathy.

Standard liver function tests provide information about hepatocyte integrity, cholestasis, and hepatic synthetic function, while other tests evaluate the extent and nature of hepatic injury. **Table 28.2** lists the various tests commonly used to evaluate the liver.

B. Hepatic and Hepatobiliary Diseases

Drug toxicity and infection are the most common causes of acute liver disease, which may progress to acute liver failure, resolve spontaneously, or develop

Table 28.2 Liver Function Tests

Function	Test	Remarks
Hepatocyte integrity	AST	Formerly, SGOT. Produced in the liver, heart, skeletal muscle, kidney, brain, and red blood cells.
	ALT	Formerly, SGPT. Produced in the liver.
	LDH	Nonspecific, also increased with hemolysis, rhabdomyolysis, tumor necrosis, myocardial infarction.
	GST	Released from cells in the centrilobular region (zone 3). Sensitive marker of centrilobular necrosis in the early stages. Short plasma half-life (30 min).
Synthetic function	Albumin	Protein loss through the gastrointestinal tract and kidneys and increased catabolism can also cause hypoalbuminemia. Long half-life (2–3 wk).
	PT/INR	Both bile salt-mediated vitamin K absorption and hepatic synthesis of coagulation factors are necessary to maintain normal PT/INR. Short half-life of factor VII (4–6 hr) makes PT/INR a sensitive indicator of acute liver disease.
	Ammonia	Markedly elevated in patients with hepatic encephalopathy, when hepatic urea synthesis is disrupted.
Excretory function	Alkaline phosphatase	Present in biliary canaliculi, bone, intestine, liver, and placenta. Lacks specificity for hepatobiliary disease.
	GGT	Elevated in hepatobiliary disease, closely tracks alkaline phosphatase in timeline. Most sensitive laboratory marker of biliary tract disease, but not specific.
	5′ NT	Elevations are specific to hepatobiliary obstruction.
	Bilirubin	Product of heme catabolism. Indirect (unconjugated) hyperbilirubinemia happens in prehepatic disease, while direct (conjugated) hyperbilirubinemia is present in intra- or extrahepatic bile duct obstruction. Hepatic disease causes elevation of both kinds of bilirubin.

5′ NT, 5′-nucleotidase; ALT, alanine aminotransferase; AST, aspartate aminotransferase; GGT, γ-glutamyl transferase; GST, glutathione S-transferase; LDH, lactate dehydrogenase; PT/INR, prothrombin time/international normalized ratio; SGOT, serum glutamic-oxaloacetic transaminase; SGPT, serum glutamic-pyruvic transaminase.

into chronic liver failure. Other causes include alcoholic hepatitis, nonacetaminophen drug toxicity, and pregnancy-related hepatic disease. Chronic liver disease is usually a consequence of viral hepatitis, alcoholic liver disease, or nonalcoholic fatty liver disease. Chronic liver disease can lead to portal hypertension, cirrhosis, and malignancy.

C. Cirrhosis and Portal Hypertension

Cirrhosis describes the pathological transformation of liver tissue into nodules surrounded by fibrous bands. Recurrent episodes of inflammation cause hepatic parenchymal necrosis and fibrosis. These changes also cause an increase in resistance to blood flow through the hepatic capillary bed, causing portal hypertension. The most common cause of cirrhosis in the United States is alcohol. Other causes include viral hepatitis, nonalcoholic steatohepatitis, primary biliary cirrhosis, chronic right heart failure, autoimmune disease, and alpha-1 antitrypsin deficiency. Systemic manifestations of cirrhosis and portal hypertension are listed in **Table 28.3**.

Table 28.3 Clinical Manifestations of Cirrhosis and Portal Hypertension

Cardiovascular	Hyperdynamic circulation Low systemic vascular resistance Low systemic systolic blood pressure Systolic and diastolic dysfunction Reduced effective circulating volume Increased cardiac output
Pulmonary	Decreased functional residual capacity Restrictive ventilation due to ascites and pleural effusion Hepatopulmonary syndrome Portopulmonary hypertension
Gastrointestinal	Ascites Esophageal varices Hemorrhoids Gastrointestinal bleeding
Renal	Salt and water retention due to activation of renin-angiotensin pathway Decreased renal function Hepatorenal syndrome
Hematologic	Anemia Coagulopathy Thrombocytopenia Spontaneous bacterial peritonitis
Metabolic	Sodium, potassium, calcium, and magnesium abnormalities Hypoalbuminemia Hypoglycemia
Neurologic	Hepatic encephalopathy

Hemostasis

Laboratory tests in cirrhotic patients often show alterations in the procoagulant system. However, the anticoagulant system is also altered. Hence, tests of coagulation should be interpreted carefully. Hepatic disease can lead to anemia of chronic disease due to red blood cell destruction and bone marrow suppression. Patients may also have dysfibrinogenemia. Thrombocytopenia develops as a result of decreased production and increased splenic sequestration. Fibrinolysis may occur in cirrhotic patients because of decreased clearance of tissue plasminogen activator.

Cardiac

Cirrhosis and portal hypertension cause an increase in the production of vasodilators, which results in a so-called hyperdynamic circulation with high cardiac output and low systemic vascular resistance. Systolic blood pressure is often <100 mm Hg. A large amount of blood is sequestered in the splanchnic bed, causing a decreased effective circulating volume. Arteriovenous shunts develop, both in systemic and pulmonary circulation, leading to increased cardiac output.

Renal

As cirrhosis progresses, there is an increase in cardiac output and decrease in systemic vascular resistance. There is also activation of the sympathetic, renin-angiotensin-aldosterone, and vasopressin systems. This leads to ascites, peripheral edema, and electrolyte disturbances, including dilutional hyponatremia and hypokalemia (from secondary hypoaldosteronism). Patients are at risk of renal hypoperfusion due to decreased effective circulating volume, systemic hypotension, diuresis, gastrointestinal bleeding, and diarrhea as well as other renal insults, including drug-related nephrotoxicity, sepsis, and immune complex–related nephropathies. Hepatorenal syndrome is an extreme manifestation of the systemic circulatory derangement in cirrhosis and refers to the symptom complex characterized with azotemia, ascites, and oliguria. There is also intense constriction of the renal afferent arteriole, which causes a decrease in renal blood flow and glomerular filtration rate (GFR).

Pulmonary

Ascites and pleural effusion can cause ventilation-perfusion mismatch in cirrhotic patients due to restriction of lung expansion, creation of intrapulmonary arteriovenous channels, and atelectasis. Portal hypertension also causes hepatopulmonary syndrome (liver dysfunction, unexplained hypoxemia, and intrapulmonary vascular dilatation causing right-to-left shunting) and portopulmonary hypertension (pulmonary hypertension with no other known cause in patients with portal hypertension).

Encephalopathy

Hepatic encephalopathy is related to the amount of hepatic parenchymal damage and shunting of portal venous blood into the systemic circulation. Gastrointestinal bleeding, increased oral protein intake, dehydration, infections, and worsening liver function can precipitate this condition. Hyperammonemia caused by cirrhosis can lead to increased intracranial pressure. Neurologic signs include altered mental status with fluctuating asterixis and hyperreflexia, along with characteristic high-voltage, slow-wave activity on electroencephalography. Treatment includes supportive care, amelioration of the precipitating cause, and oral lactulose or neomycin to decrease intestinal ammonia absorption.

Ascites

Portal hypertension, hypoalbuminemia, lymphatic fluid seepage from the diseased liver, and renal fluid retention are all implicated in the development of cirrhotic ascites. Treatment includes salt restriction, diuretics, paracentesis, and, occasionally, a transjugular intrahepatic portosystemic shunting (TIPS) procedure. It is recommended that large-volume (>5 L) ascitic fluid drainage be accompanied with albumin replacement (6-8 g/L). Rapid drainage of a large volume of ascites causes paracentesis-induced circulatory dysfunction (PICD) in up to 80% of patients, when no fluid replacement is used. The incidence is reduced to 15% to 30% when volume expanders are used. Patients with ascites are at increased risk for the development of spontaneous bacterial peritonitis due to bacterial translocation from the bowel flora. Therefore, it is imperative to maintain strict aseptic technique during any procedural interventions.

Varices

Esophageal varices develop as portosystemic shunts because of portal hypertension. They can cause massive bleeding, leading to hypovolemia from blood loss. Treatment includes supportive care, endoscopic sclerotherapy, electrocoagulation or banding, medical therapy (vasopressin, somatostatin, or propranolol), and balloon tamponade (with a Sengstaken-Blakemore tube). Anesthetic challenges include the full stomach, fragile physiology, acute hypovolemia, and encephalopathy. Bleeding from varices into the gastrointestinal track can serve as a nitrogen load and worsen the encephalopathy.

D. Preoperative Evaluation

Preoperatively, the severity of liver disease and the risk of surgery can be estimated using the modified Child-Turcotte Pugh score (commonly known as the Child-Pugh Score) and MELD (model for end-stage liver disease) scoring systems. The Child-Pugh score is described in **Table 28.4**. The MELD score ranks patients according to their risk of death from liver disease, based on a logarithmic calculation of creatinine, bilirubin, and the international normalized ratio of the prothrombin time. The MELD score is typically used to prioritize patients on the liver transplant list. In 2016, serum sodium was also added to the MELD score calculation in recognition of hyponatremia as an additional risk factor. Adding age and ASA classification to MELD score also increases its predictive value for estimating survival after nontransplant surgery in cirrhotic patients.

On preoperative evaluation, minor elevations of liver function tests in asymptomatic patients are most likely irrelevant.[8] More significant elevations and the presence of risk factors or evidence of liver disease should prompt further investigation. Contraindications to elective surgery include fulminant hepatic failure, acute hepatitis, Child-Pugh class C cirrhosis, heart failure, acute kidney injury, and severe coagulopathy (platelet count <50,000/μL).

E. Intraoperative Management

Hemodynamic monitoring for patients with end-stage liver disease should include an arterial catheter and other invasive monitoring, depending on the extent of the surgery and the patient's comorbidities. Neuromuscular blockade monitoring is also recommended since the metabolism and duration of action of many neuromuscular blocking agents is altered by liver failure and associated renal insufficiency. Transesophageal echocardiography should be performed with caution because of the risk of bleeding from esophageal varices, although the data from published case series suggest the risk is low.

Ascites and variceal bleeding can increase the risk of aspiration during anesthetic induction. Induction doses of intravenous induction agents are short acting despite liver disease, because the action is terminated by redistribution. However, with repeat doses or infusions, a prolonged duration of action can be expected. For procedures requiring sedation, propofol is preferable to benzodiazepines, since it has a quicker onset and rapid redistribution. Inhaled anesthetic agents may cause a significant reduction in hepatic blood flow; however, isoflurane, sevoflurane, and desflurane are all considered safe for use. The action of opioid agents is often prolonged due to a higher free fraction in the blood because of reduced circulating albumin levels. In addition, patients with liver disease often have an exaggerated response to sedatives. Cisatracurium is the neuromuscular blocker of choice, owing to its organ-independent metabolism.

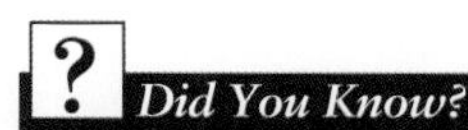

Although many drugs are metabolized in the liver, the duration of action following a single dose may be shorter than expected. This is because cardiac output is high in advanced liver disease and drug action is terminated primarily by redistribution.

Table 28.4 Modified Child-Pugh Score

	Points[a]		
Presentation–	**1**	**2**	**3**
Albumin (g/dL)	>3.5	2.8–3.5	<2.8
Prothrombin time			
Seconds prolonged	<4	4–6	>6
International normalized ratio	<1.7	1.7–2.3	>2.3
Bilirubin (mg/dL)[b]	<2	2–3	>3
Ascites	Absent	Slight to moderate	Tense
Encephalopathy	None	Grades I–II	Grades III–IV

[a] Class A = 5 to 6 points; B = 7 to 9 points; C = 10 to 15 points. Perioperative mortality—Class A: 10%; B: 30%; C: >80%.

[b] For cholestatic diseases, assign 1, 2, and 3 points for bilirubin <4, 4 to 10, and >10 mg/dL, respectively.

From Kamath PS. Clinical approach to the patient with abnormal liver test results. *Mayo Clin Proc.* 1996;71:1089, with permission.

Maintenance of circulating volume as well as hepatic and renal perfusion is important. However, in patients undergoing abdominal surgery, a restrictive fluid strategy helps decrease bleeding by minimizing portal venous pressure. Cirrhotic patients often exhibit a diminished response to endogenous and exogenous vasoconstrictors, necessitating higher doses. Hypotension, high mean airway pressures during mechanical ventilation, and sympathetic stimulation should be avoided.

During major surgery, the utility of standard testing of the coagulation system (eg, prothrombin time, platelet count) is limited. Viscoelastic tests like thromboelastography (TEG) and rotational thromboelastometry (ROTEM) are preferred for the management of bleeding in high-risk patients.

F. Specific Procedures

Transjugular Intrahepatic Portosystemic Shunt Procedure

Transjugular intrahepatic portosystemic shunt (TIPS) is indicated for decompression of portal hypertension in the setting of esophageal varices or intractable ascites. A shunt is placed transvenously, connecting the portal circulation to a hepatic vein (**Figure 28.4**). Monitored anesthesia care or general anesthesia may be used. Acute volume overload due to influx of portal blood into the systemic circulation is a frequent complication, and this may unmask previously undiagnosed heart failure or pulmonary hypertension. Since the shunted blood bypasses the liver, new or worsening hepatic encephalopathy is seen in up to 30% to 35% patients after the procedure, occurring soon after TIPS insertion.

Since TIPS is usually performed for end-stage liver disease, these patients usually have massive ascites and atelectasis, both of which make lying flat difficult. If a general anesthetic is planned, rapid sequence intubation is recommended. In addition to encephalopathy, postprocedural complications include bleeding, pneumothorax, vascular injury, and dysrhythmia.

Hepatic Resection

Hepatic resections are most commonly performed for malignancy (primary hepatobiliary or metastatic) and carry a high perioperative mortality risk.

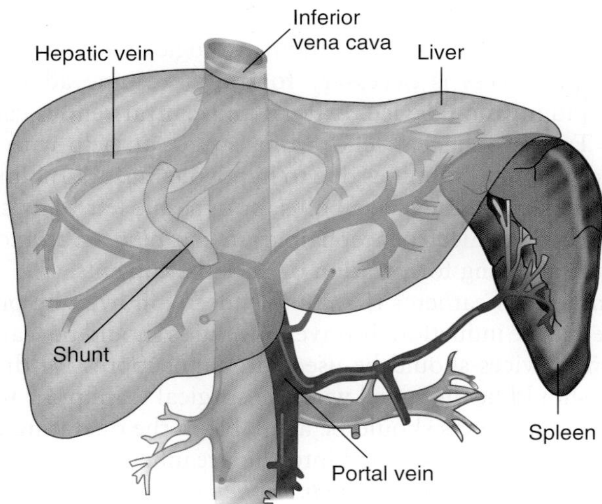

Figure 28.4 Transjugular intrahepatic portosystemic shunt (TIPS) procedure. A stent (or stents) is passed through the internal jugular vein over a wire into the hepatic vein. The wire and stent or stents are then advanced into the portal vein, after which blood can pass through the portal vein into the hepatic vein and bypass and decompress dilated esophageal veins. (From Steadman RH, Braunfeld MY. The liver: surgery and anesthesia. In: Barash PG, Cahalan MK, Cullen BF, et al, eds. *Clinical Anesthesia*. 8th ed. Wolters Kluwer; 2018:1298-1326, Figure 46.2.)

Adequate vascular access and cross-matched blood should be available to combat massive hemorrhage. Prevention of hypothermia is essential to allow normal hemostasis. Blood loss also depends on site of surgery; the right lobe of the liver represents about two-thirds of its total mass and hence is associated with a higher bleeding risk. In the initial stages of the surgery, drainage of ascites can lead to significant fluid shifts, and placement of retractors for exposure can cause respiratory and hemodynamic compromise. Compression of the inferior vena cava (IVC) during exposure and control of vascular supply leads to diminished preload. Liver blood flow can be manipulated with vascular clamping below and above the liver, but this can also cause significant hemodynamic fluctuations. Maintaining a low central venous pressure (CVP) (<5 cm H_2O) with a fluid restrictive strategy and with vasodilators like nitroglycerin helps decrease blood loss and transfusion requirements. The head-up position should not be used to decrease CVP, since it can increase the risk of venous air embolism. An abrupt drop in end-tidal CO_2, with rising pulmonary artery pressures, should raise suspicion of a significant air embolism. Laboratory testing–guided administration of procoagulants is necessary to improve clotting without unwanted thrombotic complications.

G. Hepatic Transplantation

Alcohol- or hepatitis-induced chronic, severe hepatocellular disease is the most common indication for liver transplantation. The MELD scoring system allows for prioritization of organ allocation, with score adjustments for patients with hepatocellular carcinoma and hepatopulmonary syndrome. Fulminant hepatic failure puts patients on the top of the waiting list.

Patients presenting for liver transplantation usually have had an extensive diagnostic workup. Immediate preoperative assessment should include evaluation for a change in functional status since the last assessment, recent oral intake, options for vascular access, and neurologic and renal function.

Large-bore venous access is necessary for rapid volume administration, often through a rapid infusion device. Arterial and central venous catheterization is necessary. Transesophageal echocardiography can help with the management of hemodynamic instabilities due to hypovolemia, IVC manipulation, right ventricular failure, pulmonary embolus, or dynamic left ventricular (LV) outflow tract obstruction. Electroencephalogram can be used to monitor the depth of anesthesia, allowing for titration of anesthetic agents.

A preinduction arterial catheter is recommended, followed by preoxygenation and rapid-sequence induction. Intravenous fluids should be warmed, and forced-air warming devices should be used. Immunosuppressive drugs, their doses, and timing should be discussed with the surgical team prior to surgery. Cross-matched blood products should be available in the operating room.

The intraoperative course is divided into the preanhepatic, anhepatic, and the neohepatic or reperfusion phase. The ***preanhepatic*** phase has similar anesthetic implications as encountered during hepatic resection. Preoperative coagulopathy is managed by administering blood products. Venovenous bypass may be necessary if IVC clamping is performed. The ***anhepatic*** phase begins with clamping of the vascular supply to the liver, usually starting with the hepatic artery. After a period of relative stability, graft reperfusion starts with flushing of the preservative fluid by perfusion through the portal vein to the hepatic vein and the surgical field. Maintenance of euvolemia is important during this phase of controlled bleeding. With reanastomosis of the hepatic vein, acidemia and embolism can cause pulmonary hypertension with severe cardiopulmonary instability. Vasopressors, inotropes, and pulmonary vasodilators are often necessary to support blood pressure. The anesthesiologist also needs to monitor the serum electrolyte, glucose, and acid-base status. Patients are at particular risk of hypocalcemia, due to high volume infusion of citrated blood products, and hyperkalemia, because of underlying renal function, potassium-sparing diuretic use, blood transfusion, splanchnic ischemia, and acidosis.

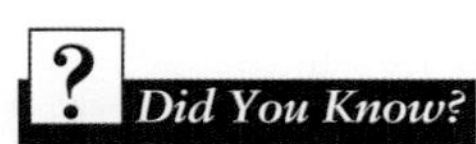

Massive transfusion is associated with hypocalcemia (due to citrate in banked blood) and hyperkalemia (due to K+ leaking out of stored red blood cells).

Early in the ***neohepatic*** phase, patients develop a hypocoagulable, fibrinolytic state. Maintenance of hemostasis is accomplished with guidance from conventional coagulation tests as well as viscoelastic tests (TEG and ROTEM). Postoperatively, patients can develop fluid overload, transfusion-related acute lung injury, and intra-abdominal hypertension related to massive transfusion. Anastomotic leaks or stenosis or thrombosis of a vascular anastomosis may require urgent surgical reexploration.

III. Anesthetic Management for Gastrointestinal Surgery

The care of patients undergoing gastrointestinal surgery forms a significant part of anesthesia practice in most hospitals. Many facilities have developed evidence-based protocols as part of an enhanced recovery after surgery (ERAS) pathway to reduce complications and length of hospital stay in patients undergoing major gastrointestinal procedures.

A. Pharmacology

Opioids decrease lower esophageal sphincter (LES) tone and reduce gastric and bowel motility, often causing ileus and constipation in intensive care patients sedated with opioids. Relaxation of the LES can allow reflux of gastric contents and increase the risk for aspiration. Opioids—particularly morphine—cause contraction of the common bile duct sphincter, which can be problematic if intraoperative cholangiograms are taken. Cholinesterase inhibitors and high neuraxial blockade can cause hyperperistaltic activity because of parasympathetic activation and inhibition of the sympathetic system, respectively. This may be detrimental in patients with bowel obstruction.

Nitrous oxide (N_2O) will diffuse into bowel, particularly if it is already distended with bowel gas. This can result in bowel distension and increased intraluminal pressure, which can impair abdominal closure and, in extreme situations, cause bowel ischemia. Consequently, N_2O should be used rarely, if at all, during surgeries involving ischemic bowel.

B. Pulmonary Function

Patients undergoing upper abdominal surgery are at increased risk for postoperative pulmonary complications, likely related to atelectasis, reduced cough (pain, edema, ileus), and the risk of perioperative aspiration. Intraoperatively, supine or head-down positioning and abdominal retractors can impair diaphragmatic movement and induce atelectasis and hypoxia. Strategies to prevent pulmonary complications include preoperative cessation of smoking and optimization of preexisting pulmonary disease, intraoperative avoidance of long-acting neuromuscular blockers, good postoperative pain control, and nasogastric drainage in selected patients. The evidence in favor of spinal and epidural techniques to reduce postoperative pulmonary complications is suggestive but not conclusive. The impact of laparoscopic surgery on the respiratory system is discussed elsewhere in this book.

C. Mechanical Obstruction and Paralytic Ileus

Mechanical obstruction of the bowel usually requires surgical management. Patients present with pain, distension, vomiting, and obstipation. Up to 7 to 9 L of fluid may be secreted daily into the gut in an adult (approximately 1 L of saliva, 2 L of gastric juice, 1 L of bile, 2 L of pancreatic juice, and 1 L of succus entericus), and patients can present with severe dehydration and electrolyte abnormalities. An abdominal radiograph may show multiple air-fluid levels in small bowel obstruction. Perioperative considerations for the anesthesiologist include the management of aspiration risk, fluid resuscitation, and postoperative analgesia. Gastric decompression via nasogastric tube insertion prior to intubation is often advised. Nitrous oxide should be avoided due to its propensity to diffuse into airspaces and worsen bowel distension.

Following major gastrointestinal surgery, postoperative ileus is common, related to physical manipulation of the abdominal viscera. Small bowel motility recovers within a few hours after surgery, gastric peristalsis returns after 24 to 48 hours, and colonic activity returns after 48 hours. Passage of flatus, cramping, and return of appetite signify the return of peristaltic activity. Conventional surgical wisdom was to withhold enteral feeding until the return of these physical signs of peristalsis. However, more recently, studies suggest that early (within 24 hours) enteral feeding is not associated with increased postoperative nausea, vomiting, or other complications and may reduce hospital length of stay. Paralytic ileus can also develop after blunt abdominal trauma, bowel perforation, bilious peritonitis, intra-abdominal sepsis, or in the context of extra-abdominal pathologies like severe pneumonia, trauma, sepsis and myocardial infarction, and electrolyte abnormalities.

D. Bowel Perforation and Peritonitis

Perforation of the gastrointestinal tract into the peritoneal cavity leads to peritonitis and sepsis. Potential sources for a perforated viscus include peptic ulcer, appendicular lesion, diverticulitis, and small bowel disease. Treatment usually involves surgical repair. Advanced age, delayed presentation (>24 hours), organ failure on presentation, diffuse generalized peritonitis, and fecal contamination of the peritoneum are associated with increased hospital stay and mortality.

Patients with severe peritonitis are often severely hypovolemic and present with metabolic acidosis and reduced perfusion of tissues. Preoperative and intraoperative restoration of hemodynamics with adequate fluid resuscitation and early institution of appropriate antibiotic therapy are essential. Postoperatively, these patients require admission to an ICU.

For further review and interactivities, please see the associated Interactive Video Lectures and "A Closer Look" infographic accessible in the complimentary eBook bundled with this text. Access instructions are located in the inside front cover.

References

1. Sharma S, Arora L. Anesthesia for the morbidly obese patient. *Anesthesiol Clin.* 2020;38(1):197-212. PMID: 32008653.
2. Hodgson LE, Murphy PB, Hart N. Respiratory management of the obese patient undergoing surgery. *J Thorac Dis.* 2015;7(5):943-952. PMID: 26101653.
3. Ortiz VE, Kwo J. Obesity: physiologic changes and implications for preoperative management. *BMC Anesthesiol.* 2015;15:97. PMID: 26141622.
4. Chau EHL, Lam D, Wong J, et al. Obesity hypoventilation syndrome. A review of epidemiology, pathophysiology, and perioperative considerations. *Anesthesiology.* 2012;117:188-205. PMID: 22614131.
5. Willis S, Bordelon GJ, Rana MV. Perioperative pharmacologic considerations in obesity. *Anesthesiol Clin.* 2017;35(2):247-257. PMID: 28526146.
6. Practice guidelines for the perioperative management of patients with obstructive sleep apnea: an updated report by the American Society of Anesthesiologists Task Force on Perioperative Management of patients with obstructive sleep apnea. *Anesthesiology.* 2014;120(2):268-286. PMID: 24346178.
7. Skues MA. Perioperative management of the obese ambulatory patient. *Curr Opin Anaesthesiol.* 2018;31(6):693-699. PMID: 30379735.
8. Giannini EG, Testa R, Savarino V. Liver enzyme alteration: a guide for clinicians. *CMAJ (Can Med Assoc J).* 2005;172:367-379. PMID: 15684121.

LIVER DISEASE AND HEMOSTASIS

A CLOSER LOOK

The liver is the production center for a large array of plasma proteins including not only coagulation factors, but a number of other pro-thrombotic and anti-thrombotic substances. Normal liver function is essential for achieving the complex balance required for hemostasis.

The healthy liver produces factors and proteins that promote ***both*** clot *formation* and clot *breakdown*.

Factors that promote clotting

Factors II, V, VII, VIII, IX, X, XI, XII, XIII and Fibrinogen

Protein C, Protein S, Antithrombin, Plasminogen

Factors promoting clot dissolution

End stage liver disease is characterized by a multitude of complex changes in hemostasis.

CIRRHOSIS

↑ Factor VIII
↓ Protein C
↑ vWF levels
↓ Plasminogen
↑ PAI (plasminogen activator inhibitor)

↓ Platelet count
↓ Platelet function
↓ Factor production

In patients with cirrhosis, ***both*** **abnormal bleeding and clotting can occur**. Careful monitoring of intraoperative blood loss and hemostasis lab tests can guide management.

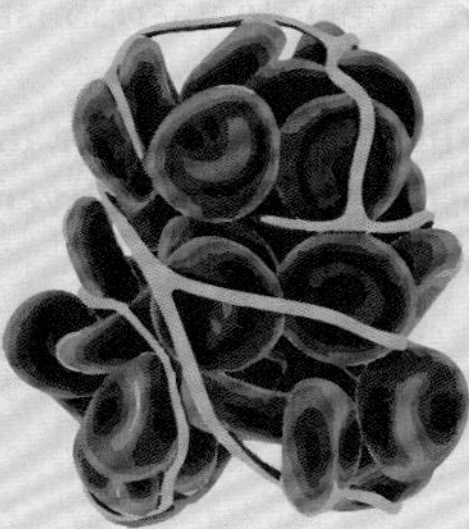

Thrombotic tendency

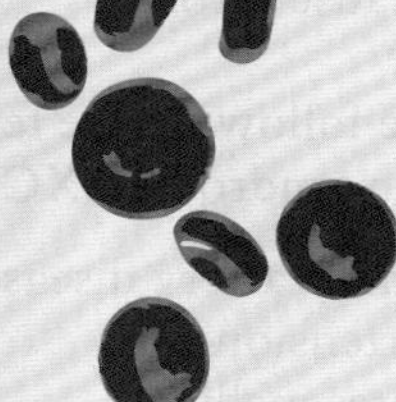

Bleeding tendency

Infographic by: Naveen Nathan MD

Questions

1. **Severe obesity is defined as a BMI greater than:**

   A. 25 kg/m^2
   B. 30 kg/m^2
   C. 40 kg/m^2
   D. 50 kg/m^2

2. **In an obese patient, lean body weight should be used when calculating the initial dose for which of the following drugs?**

   A. Succinylcholine
   B. Midazolam
   C. Dexmedetomidine
   D. Rocuronium

3. **In the obese patient, which of the following positions is associated with the greatest negative impact on ventilation and oxygenation?**

   A. Supine
   B. Lateral
   C. Sitting
   D. Trendelenburg

4. **In the obese patient, all of the following statements regarding blood pressure measurement with a standard automated cuff are true EXCEPT:**

   A. The time required to make blood pressure measurement can be prolonged.
   B. The blood pressure cuff should be longer and narrower.
   C. The forearm is an appropriate site for cuff placement.
   D. The conical shape of the upper arm may cause errors.

5. **All of the following are features of the metabolic syndrome EXCEPT:**

   A. Coronary artery disease
   B. Hypertension
   C. Diabetes mellitus
   D. Dyslipidemia

6. **Which of the following is the most significant early contributor to right ventricular heart failure in obese patients with sleep-disordered breathing?**

   A. Systemic hypertension
   B. Increased cardiac output
   C. Pulmonary hypertension
   D. Left ventricular hypertrophy

7. **Regarding the use of propofol in a patient with advanced hepatic cirrhosis, which of the following is TRUE?**

   A. The duration of action of a single induction dose will be shorter than normal.
   B. The duration of action of a second dose given 5 minutes after induction will be prolonged.
   C. The duration of action of a continuous infusion will be shorter than normal.
   D. None of the above.

8. **A patient is to undergo laparotomy for a bowel obstruction with associated significant bowel distension. Which of the following agents is relatively contraindicated?**

   A. Nitrous oxide
   B. Sevoflurane
   C. Isoflurane
   D. Fentanyl

9. **Which of the following is a feature of the hepatorenal syndrome?**

   A. Increased renal blood flow
   B. Increased glomerular filtration rate
   C. Afferent arteriole vasodilation
   D. Afferent arteriole vasoconstriction

10. **Which of the following liver function tests is most diagnostic of liver excretory dysfunction?**

    A. AST
    B. ALT
    C. GGT
    D. Albumin

Answers

1. C

Severe obesity is defined as a BMI >40 kg/m^2.

2. D

Lean body weight should be used to calculate the initial dose of nondepolarizing muscle relaxants such as vecuronium. For all of the other drugs listed, initial dose should be calculated based on total body water.

3. D

Trendelenburg positioning causes the highest degree of respiratory compromise, with a decrease in functional residual capacity and lung compliance, due in large part to the weight of the abdominal contents and elevation of the diaphragm.

4. B

Whereas a longer cuff may be necessary to encircle a large arm, in an obese patient, the cuff should be wider, not more narrow, than normal in order to produce an accurate result.

5. A

The metabolic syndrome is characterized by obesity (especially in the truncal region), hypertension, diabetes mellitus or insulin resistance, and dyslipidemia.

6. C

Pulmonary hypertension is the most significant early contributor to right ventricular heart failure in obese patients. Pulmonary hypertension is the result of chronic hypoxia and increased pulmonary blood volume.

7. A

Single induction doses of intravenous induction agents are short acting despite liver disease because cardiac output is elevated and drug effect is terminated primarily by redistribution. The duration of action of continuous infusions may be prolonged due to deposition of drug in fat and delayed metabolism.

8. A

Nitrous oxide will diffuse into distended bowel, which can result in increased intraluminal pressure and difficulty with abdominal closure or, in extreme situations, bowel ischemia.

9. D

Cirrhosis causes activation of the sympathetic, renin-angiotensin-aldosterone, and vasopressin systems, causing salt and water retention and intense afferent arteriole vasoconstriction. This causes a decrease in renal blood flow and glomerular filtration rate, which contributes to the development of the hepatorenal syndrome.

10. C

GGT, along with alkaline phosphatase, 5′NT, and bilirubin, are the liver function tests most helpful in diagnosing impaired liver excretory function.

29 Anesthesia for Otolaryngologic and Ophthalmic Surgery

R. Mauricio Gonzalez, Joseph Louca, and Alexander Dekel

ANESTHESIA FOR OTOLARYNGOLOGIC SURGERY

I. General Considerations

The anesthetic management of otolaryngologic (ORL) surgery is complex. Many variables must be considered, including understanding the surgical indications and procedure(s). Depending on the operation, the anesthesiologist may jointly manage the airway with the surgeon. Additionally, airway anatomy may be distorted by tumor, infection, trauma, congenital abnormalities, radiation exposure, or prior surgery. Age-specific differences in anatomy and physiology, along with existing comorbidities, must also be considered.

Assessing the airway extends beyond the physical examination. Familiarity with airway imaging, particularly computed tomography (CT) and magnetic resonance imaging (MRI), is critical. A review of digital videos of airway fiberoptic examinations should be performed if they are available. If not, the anesthesiologist may consider performing fiberoptic examination of the airway under topical anesthesia prior to induction.

The selection and dosage of anesthetics and adjuvant medications should be tailored to the procedure being performed. Patients undergoing ORL procedures must also be carefully monitored for blood loss, which can be underestimated due to spillage onto the surgical field, swallowing, and distance of the surgical field from the anesthesiologist. Ingestion of blood can contribute to postoperative nausea and vomiting (PONV) and should be aspirated via orogastric tube prior to emergence and extubation.

Topical alpha agonists for vasoconstriction (eg, phenylephrine) can cause hypertension and increased blood flow to the pulmonary circulation. This can be associated with pulmonary edema and death, especially if the alpha agonistic effect is combined with pharmacologic beta blockade. Given the short duration of action of topical vasoconstrictors, one can allow moderate hypertension to self-resolve or it can be treated by increasing the dose of vasodilatory anesthetics. Direct vasodilators are the proper treatment for a severe hypertensive response to topical vasoconstrictors.[1] Closed-loop communication with the ORL team is critical in anticipating and responding to the side effects of mucosal vasoconstrictors.

II. Anesthetic Considerations in the Pediatric Population

A. Anatomy and Physiology

Diseases of the ear in children can be best understood by reviewing the anatomy and physiology of the middle ear and adjacent structures. The eardrum is a thin, well-innervated membrane sitting at the deepest part of the external auditory canal. It borders the middle ear laterally. The middle ear drains into the nasopharynx via the Eustachian tube. During infancy, it drains poorly due to its small cross-sectional area, floppy cartilaginous walls, and the low angle it travels toward the nasopharynx. Additionally, its short length increases the proximity of the middle ear to the mucous and bacteria of the nasopharynx. These factors increase the risk of otitis media, with incidence peaking at 1 year of age. Normal growth of these structures reduces the risk of otitis media up through the age of 7 years, where the incidence plateaus at the same level as that of adults.[2]

? Did You Know?

During infancy, the Eustachian tube drains poorly due to its small cross-sectional area, floppy cartilaginous walls, and the low angle it travels toward the nasopharynx. This explains why otitis media has a peak incidence in 1-year-old children.

B. Myringotomy and Tube Insertion

Myringotomy with ear tube placement requires general anesthesia (GA) to provide the surgeon with the immobility suitable for work under an operating microscope. The short length and relatively mild stimulation of the procedure permit the use of inhaled anesthetics alone, and so these procedures are often performed without securing either intravenous (IV) access or the airway. Induction using a face mask with a mixture of oxygen, nitrous oxide, and sevoflurane can be followed by maintenance with sevoflurane. Positioning the head with 30° to 45° of axial rotation provides favorable surgical access. Due to a highly innervated tympanic membrane, an adequate depth of anesthesia must be ensured prior to blade insertion to prevent patient movement and laryngospasm. Rectal acetaminophen (~10 mg/kg) or fentanyl per nostril (1 µg/kg) may be given to reduce postoperative pain and/or emergence agitation.

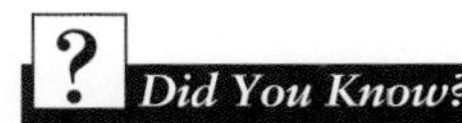

? Did You Know?

Myringotomy and ear tube placement, a short-duration procedure, is frequently performed under general anesthesia using a facemask and without intravenous access.

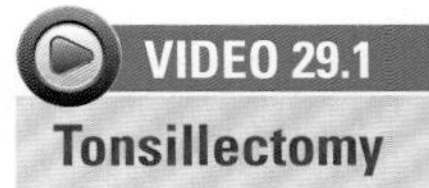

C. Tonsillectomy and Adenoidectomy

Tonsillar hypertrophy may be asymptomatic or lead to obstructive sleep apnea (OSA) and recurrent tonsillitis, which are frequent indications for removal of tonsils and/or adenoids. The tonsils grow rapidly between the ages of 1 through 3 years and are often largest between the ages of 3 to 7 years. Thus, this is the most common age range for this procedure.

The assessment of a child having tonsillectomy should include evaluating the overall respiratory function. If the patient's apnea-hypopnea index, assessed during a sleep study is severe, strong consideration should be given to a postoperative overnight stay in the intensive care unit. The worst cases of OSA may also be complicated by pulmonary hypertension with cor pulmonale and may require pharmacologic cardiovascular support during induction.

In the setting of an upper respiratory tract infection (URI), proceeding with the operation may increase the risk of respiratory complications. However, delaying a procedure for a patient with mild or improving symptoms often results in the patient returning on their next visit with similar or worse symptomology. Therefore, it may be sensible to proceed in the presence of a mild URI because complete optimization is rarely possible.[3]

A variety of regimens exist for improving postoperative analgesia and decreasing the incidence of postoperative delirium and PONV:

- Acetaminophen 10 to 40 mg/kg per rectum can be given prior to incision for analgesia.
- Dexamethasone 0.5 mg/kg is useful in the management of postoperative pain, edema, and PONV.
- If opioids are required, IV fentanyl (0.25-1.0 µg/kg) can provide effective relief while reducing the incidence and/or severity of emergence delirium (ED).
- Dexmedetomidine 0.5 µg/kg can also be bolused as prophylaxis for ED.[4] Ibuprofen PO, given either pre- or postoperatively, is a safe and effective analgesic, though some surgeons are concerned with its impact on postoperative bleeding.[5]

D. Posttonsillectomy Hemorrhage

While rare (<1%-2% of patients), posttonsillectomy hemorrhage can be life-threatening. Risk factors include chronic tonsillitis, older age (>11 years), intraoperative blood loss greater than 50 mL, and hypertension. Primary hemorrhage occurs within 24 hours of the surgery; secondary hemorrhage typically occurs within 5 to 10 days of the surgery, corresponding to the time period when a fibrin clot sloughs off.

The management of posttonsillectomy hemorrhage starts with basic life support: airway, circulation, and breathing. Assess cardiovascular stability and obtain or increase IV access. Examine the airway, look for active bleeding or a clot, and obtain the history of any bleeding expeditiously. Keep the patient leaning forward and face down to drain blood away from the laryngopharynx. When minor or recurrent bleeding is present, there is a significant risk (perhaps > 40%) for severe hemorrhage to ensue, due to relaxation of vasospasm or the displacement/lysis of a clot. One must notify the blood bank and prepare for surgery.

In the operating room (OR), a gauze soaked in 1:10,000 epinephrine should be available. Direct pressure can be applied to tonsillar fossae using a Magill forceps wrapped with gauze. Suction and airway equipment should also be available before the patient is placed supine. Children may not tolerate efforts at hemostasis while awake and may need sedation or GA before attempts are made. Ketamine may be an excellent choice as an induction agent; it is less likely to cause respiratory compromise or to exacerbate hypotension in hypovolemic patients.[6-8]

E. Emergencies/Stridor

Stridor, high-pitched or musical breathing caused by obstruction of the larynx, is a medical emergency that must be considered life-threatening. Common causes include foreign body aspiration (FBA), epiglottitis, and croup (**Table 29.1**).

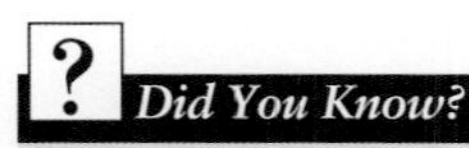

Stridor, a high-pitched or musical breathing caused by obstruction of the larynx, is a medical emergency and must be considered life-threatening.

FBA is a common problem in children, particularly of age 1 to 5 years, which can be difficult to diagnose unless the event was witnessed. FBA may present with wheezing and coughing, decreased breath sounds, and stridor. Also, it may mimic allergic reactions, asthma, OSA, gastroesophageal reflux disease (GERD), bronchiolitis, or airway obstruction due to abscess or congenital anomaly. Radiography of a patient with FBA may detect atelectasis and hyperinflation without detecting the foreign body itself, which is often

Table 29.1 Causes of Stridor

Supraglottic Airway	Larynx	Subglottic Airway
Congenital malformations	Laryngomalacia	Subglottic stenosis
Infection and abscesses	Vocal cord paralysis	Infection
Tumors and cysts	Laryngeal webs, cysts, and clefts	Tracheomalacia
Foreign body		Foreign body
Anaphylaxis and angioedema	Anaphylaxis and angioedema	

radiolucent. If there is a high index of suspicion for FBA, rigid bronchoscopy may be the necessary next step. (See **Figure 29.1**.)

Epiglottitis, a life-threatening condition typically caused by bacterial infection, often affects the epiglottis, aryepiglottic folds, arytenoids, and uvula. Its incidence has declined in the pediatric population due to widespread vaccination against *Haemophilus influenzae B* (Hib). Other bacteria, however, including *Streptococcus pneumoniae*, may also cause epiglottitis.

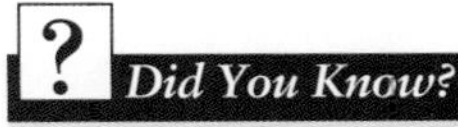

A chest x-ray may detect atelectasis and hyperinflation, but it cannot rule out FBA if the aspirated body is radiolucent. When there is a high index of suspicion for FBA, rigid bronchoscopy may be necessary to establish a diagnosis.

Epiglottitis presents with stridor, drooling, odynophagia, outright avoidance of food and drink, dysphagia, and/or high fever. Other signs include malaise and agitation or a history of rapid symptom onset (within hours); absence of Hib vaccination is of obvious concern. A child growing tired or lethargic suggests impending respiratory failure necessitating that the airway be secured expeditiously. Hypotension, hypoxemia, and bradycardia are also indications for rapid intervention.

It is essential to triage and initiate treatment patients with suspected epiglottitis swiftly. Continuously monitor with pulse oximetry and administer supplemental oxygen. Do not agitate the patient as it may lead to laryngospasm. It is often necessary to forgo radiological imaging and transport to the OR. However, if stable enough for imaging, an x-ray may show the "thumb sign" seen on a lateral film, representing the swollen epiglottis, or the "steeple sign" seen on an AP film representing subglottic tracheal narrowing seen in croup.

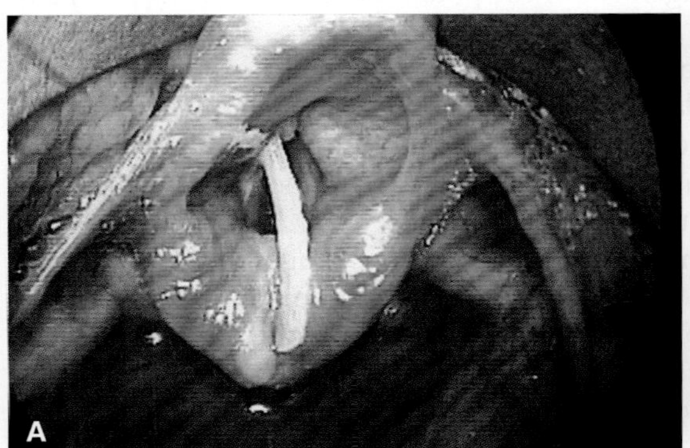

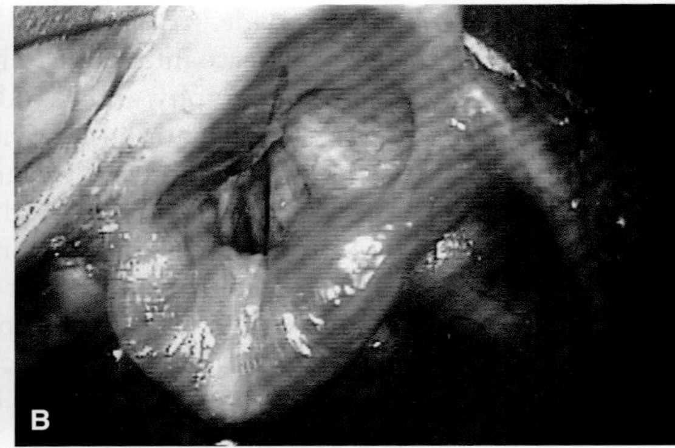

Figure 29.1 A radiolucent plastic strip is visible in the glottic inlet (just above the vocal cords) in a child who presented with inspiratory and expiratory stridor (A). Following foreign body removal, a small endothelial laceration is visible on the posterior surface of the epiglottis (B).

Keep the child upright during transport and proceed directly to the OR for an inhaled anesthetic induction with continuous positive airway pressure ventilation. After induction and IV placement, weigh the benefit of preventing laryngospasm with a neuromuscular blocking agent against the risk of abolishing spontaneous respiration should tracheal intubation fail. For direct laryngoscopy, a curved Macintosh blade placed gently into the vallecula is likely the best approach. Prevent contact with the epiglottis as this may induce bleeding or swelling. An endotracheal tube 0.5 to 1 mm smaller in diameter than would normally be age-appropriate should be placed due to the likelihood that edema has reduced the caliber of the airway. Smaller endotracheal tubes should also be readily available.

Have atropine and succinylcholine ready for IM administration to treat cardiac depression and/or laryngospasm, respectively. Alternative airway management plans are essential, and they include immediate access to rigid bronchoscopy, emergency tracheostomy, or cricothyroidotomy. Thus, concern for epiglottis warrants an ORL consult and early intubation to avoid further airway swelling and loss.

Postoperative sedation and mechanical ventilation allow time for airway inflammation to subside. The infection must also be cultured and treated. Extubation should only occur after visual inspection reveals that the swelling and friability of airway tissues has decreased; a leak test may be helpful in determining readiness.[9]

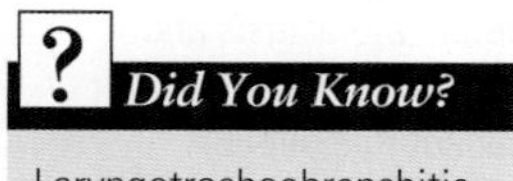

Laryngotracheobronchitis, also known as croup, may cause stridor; however, it tends to have a milder course than epiglottitis.

Laryngotracheobronchitis, or croup, is another cause of stridor, though it tends to have a milder course than epiglottitis. Croup presents with a barking high-pitched cough and less severe systemic involvement. Consider croup in a vigorously coughing, alert toddler with a hoarse voice. For croup in an otherwise healthy child, it is unlikely that tracheal intubation and mechanical ventilation will be necessary.[9]

III. Anesthesia for Adult Otolaryngologic Surgery

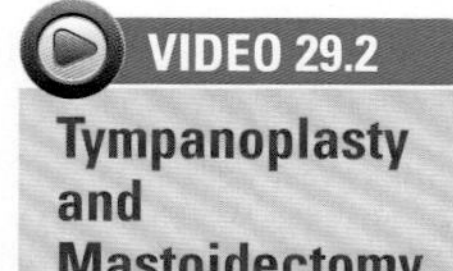

A. Middle Ear and Mastoid

Common procedures include stapedectomy, tympanoplasty, mastoidectomy, and myringotomy. Intraoperative considerations for middle ear and mastoid surgery include preservation of the facial nerve, prevention of brachial plexus or cervical injuries, and management of the potential adverse effects related to nitrous oxide.

Facial nerve integrity can be monitored and maintained with intraoperative electromyography and avoidance of neuromuscular blocking agents. A preoperative evaluation of cervical spine range of motion is essential to prevent injuries to the brachial plexus and cervical spine. Extreme neck extension or rotation should be avoided during surgery.

Nitrous oxide can result in pathological pressure changes in the middle ear if the Eustachian tube is not patent. In particular, sudden discontinuation of nitrous oxide, leading to rapid absorption of nitrous oxide, creates negative pressure and may result in changes to middle ear anatomy, rupture of tympanic membrane, disruption of grafts, and PONV.

B. Nasal and Sinus Surgery

Nasal and sinus surgeries can be performed under local anesthesia with sedation or under GA when there is concern regarding arterial damage or advancing into the intracranial space, the latter being a concern during endoscopic sinus surgery.

Intraoperative bleeding is minimized with intranasal vasoconstriction, elevation of the head to facilitate venous drainage, and induced mild hypotension.[10]

C. Maxillofacial Trauma and Orthognathic Surgery

High-speed impact trauma, with or without external evidence of injury, is frequently associated with life-threatening injuries. The anesthetic plan must consider the possibility of cervical spine injuries and skull fractures. Cervical spine stabilization prior to tracheal intubation and oral versus nasal intubation (contraindicated in LeFort III fracture) are also important considerations. Orthognathic surgery for reconstruction of facial skeletal malformations is often achieved by performing LeFort or mandibular osteotomies; therefore, understanding the anatomy of these procedures is beneficial.

D. Craniofacial Bone Structure

Knowledge of basic craniofacial bone structure is important. The facial skeleton comprises three parts: The lower third is the mandible. The middle portion includes the zygomatic arch of the temporal bone, zygomaticomaxillary complex, maxilla, nasal bones, and orbits. Lastly, the superior portion comprises the frontal bone.

E. Temporomandibular Joint Arthroscopy

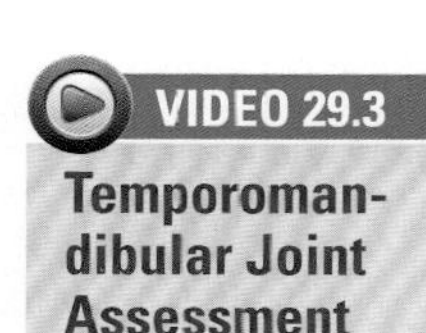

This surgery is indicated when there is displacement of the temporomandibular joint (TMJ) cartilage causing clicking, trismus, fibrosis, or osteoarthritis. Intubation may be oral (if mobility is achieved with GA) or with nasal fiberoptic assistance if the patient is in trismus. Swelling around the surgical site due to irrigation may result in partial or complete airway obstruction.[10,11] Limitation in joint mobility with TMJ arthropathy and/or infection/abscess typically depends on chronicity. The longer it is present, the less likely it will become mobile with GA. This is important to discuss with the oral surgery team prior to induction of anesthesia.

F. Surgery of the Airway

1. Suspension Laryngoscopy and Microlaryngoscopy

These techniques provide direct access and visualization of the airway (ie, no tracheal intubation), while protecting the trachea and maintaining ventilation and oxygenation. These procedures require deep anesthetic levels and muscle relaxation. Total intravenous anesthesia (TIVA) is often the most reasonable choice to avoid uncertainties about volatile anesthetic dosing with an "open" airway. For muscle relaxation, consider rocuronium and reversal with sugammadex. A succinylcholine infusion can be considered for short cases.

Jet ventilation: It provides ventilation without the use of endotracheal intubation for short cases (<30 minutes). Lower pressure (30-50 psi) jet ventilation is used to reduce the risk of barotrauma, which is more likely to occur in children, those with chronic pulmonary disease, and the obese. Stimulation of the larynx may trigger arrhythmias, tachycardia, or hypertension. To block a severe sympathetic response due to stimulation of the larynx, one may administer lidocaine (IV or topical), opiates (eg, remifentanil infusion for faster recovery), and/or beta blockers (**Figure 29.2**).

Laser surgery of the airway: It can be used for microsurgery of the upper airway or trachea. Benefits include coagulation of small vessels, reduced tissue inflammation, and better precision. One serious potential complication

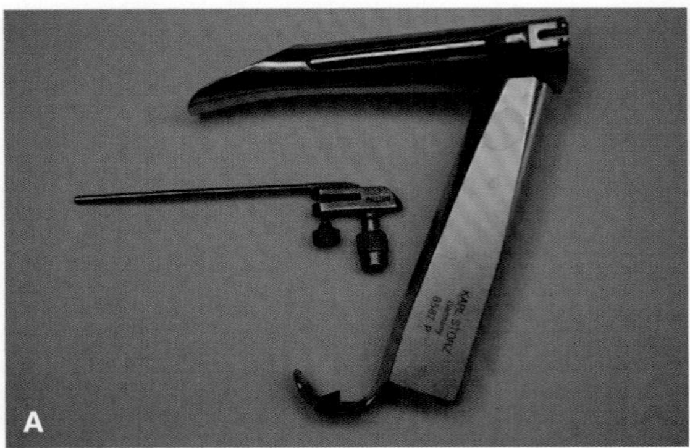

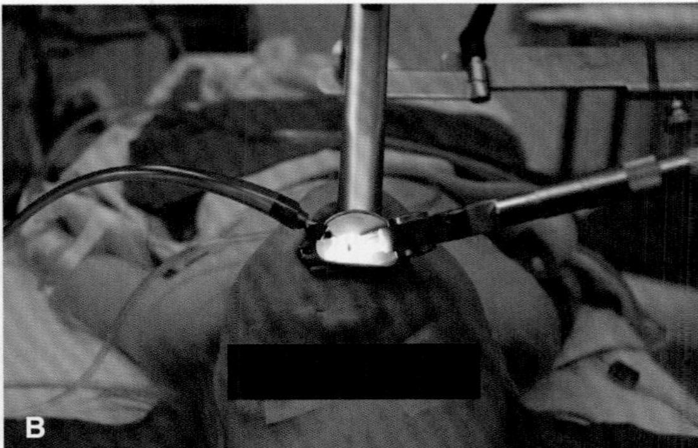

Figure 29.2 The surgical laryngoscope and the jet ventilator needle (A). The surgical view of the laryngoscope positioned in the patient's pharynx and connected to a continuous flow of oxygen through the jet ventilator needle (B).

is airway fire. Usage of fire-resistant, impregnated, or shielded endotracheal tubes, a low FIO_2, and avoidance of nitrous oxide are prudent precautions.[11,12]

2. Bronchoscopy

Bronchoscopy can be flexible or rigid. Flexible bronchoscopy is used to examine the smaller airways. Rigid bronchoscopy is used when there is bleeding of the airway, to perform large airway biopsies, to dilate the airway, or to remove foreign bodies.

Rigid bronchoscopy is performed under GA to prevent airway injury due to coughing, bucking, or straining. Ventilation is administered through a side port of the rigid bronchoscope. The patient may be awakened while being ventilated via mask, laryngeal mask airway (LMA), or endotracheal intubation. Endotracheal intubation may be needed if the patient has received neuromuscular blocking agents or if the protective airway reflexes are compromised.[10,13]

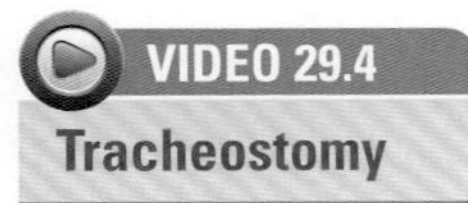

3. Tracheostomy

Tracheostomy is indicated when there is severe upper airway obstruction, loss of protective reflexes, or vocal cord paralysis. In conscious patients with respiratory distress, it is important to perform a physical examination and determine if a tracheostomy should be done with the patient awake or under GA.

G. Infection

Infections of the ear, nose, and throat largely result from by gram-negative bacteria. These may be associated with fever, chills, drooling, and difficulty swallowing and speaking.

1. Peritonsillar/Retropharyngeal Abscess and Ludwig Angina

Occasionally, the abscess must be decompressed under local anesthesia prior to induction. This decreases airway obstruction and the risk of abscess rupture while placing the endotracheal tube. Difficult intubation due to distorted anatomy or trismus may require awake fiberoptic intubation, mask induction with spontaneous breathing, or tracheostomy (**Figure 29.3**).

Ludwig angina is a cellulitis of the submandibular region that displaces the tongue upward and obstructs the airway.

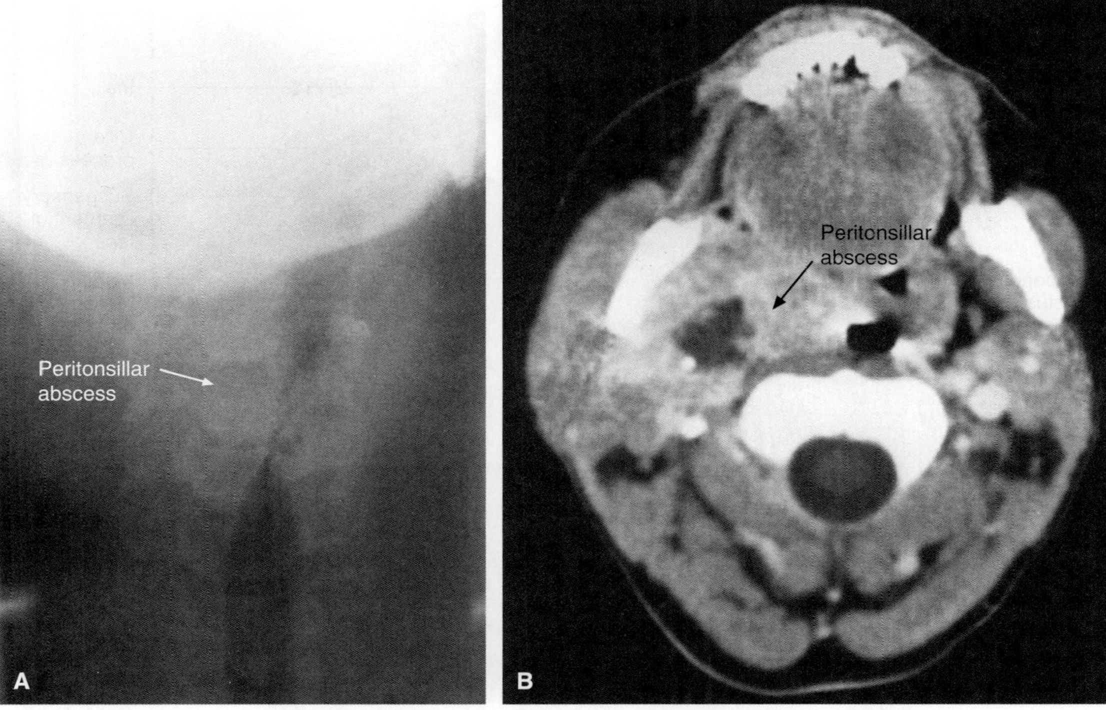

Figure 29.3 Anterior neck radiograph (A, *left*) and computed tomography scan (B, *right*) of a patient with a right peritonsillar abscess. Note displacement of the airway to the left and external compression of the supraglottic airway. (From Ferrari LR, Park RS. Anesthesia for otolaryngologic surgery. In: Barash PG, Cahalan MK, Cullen BF, et al, eds. *Clinical Anesthesia*. 8th ed. Wolters Kluwer; 2018:1357-1372. Figures 48.4 and 48.5.)

H. Neck Dissections and Free Flaps

Patients with head or neck cancer often have a history of heavy smoking and alcohol use with underlying malnutrition and pulmonary and cardiovascular disease. Preparations for potential difficult intubation must be taken due to associated anatomic abnormalities.

A free flap is a transfer of cutaneous and subcutaneous tissue from one part of the body to another. The vascular supply is disconnected during the transfer and reconnected microsurgically. Vasopressors may compromise flap viability and should be avoided.

IV. Extubation

It is essential to engage in closed-loop communication with both the anesthesiology and surgical teams to assure a systematic, step-wise approach to tracheal extubation. All decisions must be individualized for each patient and take into account multiple factors.

ANESTHESIA FOR OPHTHALMIC SURGERY

I. Ocular Anatomy

The eye is formed by the orbit, globe, extraocular muscles, eyelid, and lacrimal system (**Figure 29.4**).

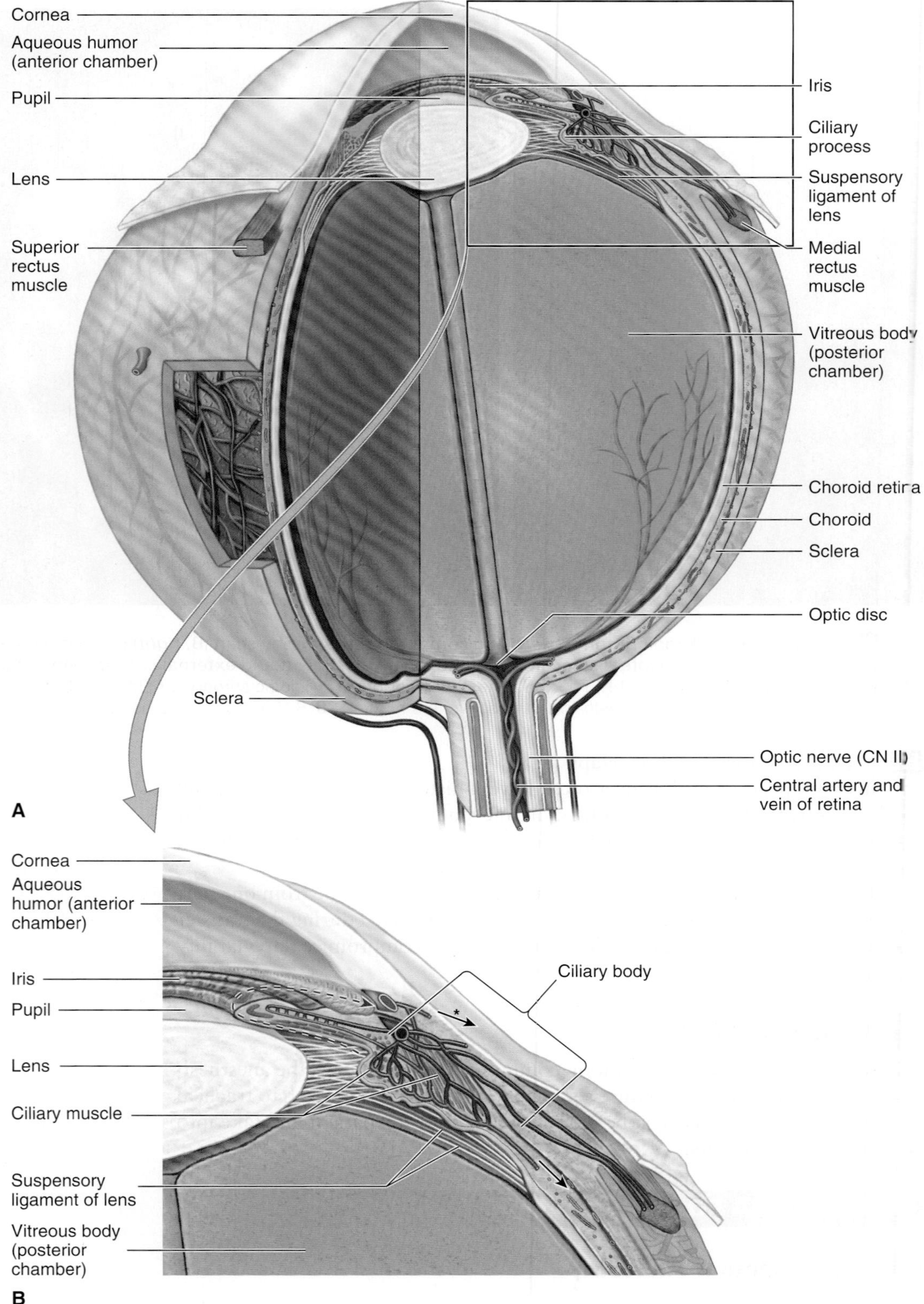

Figure 29.4 A, Gross anatomy of the eye. B, Magnified view of lens and aqueous humor system. (From Moore KL, Agur AMR, Dalley AF. *Clinically Oriented Anatomy*. 7th ed. Wolters Kluwer; 2013.)

The outer fibrous layer forms the sclera, cornea, and corneoscleral junction. The middle layer is formed by the choroid, ciliary body, ciliary processes, and the iris. The choroid contains a dense vascular bed, while the ciliary body controls lens thickness. The pupil is an aperture, the diameter of which is controlled by the sphincter pupillae (parasympathetic innervation) and dilator pupillae (sympathetic innervation). The former constricts the pupil and the latter dilates it.

II. Ocular Physiology

A. Formation and Drainage of Aqueous Humor

Aqueous humor production and drainage are a vital aspect of maintaining normal intraocular pressure (IOP) and vision. Aqueous humor is produced continuously by the ciliary body and secreted behind the iris through the pupil. Stimulation of beta-2 receptors increases the production of aqueous humor; stimulation of alpha-2 receptors decreases such production. Secretion of chloride by the ciliary epithelium leads to an osmotic influx of fluid, a secondary mechanism mediated by carbonic anhydrase.

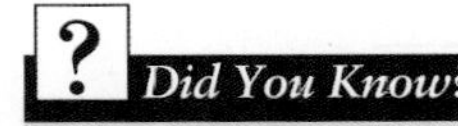

Aqueous humor is produced continuously by the ciliary body and secreted behind the iris through the pupil.

Drainage of aqueous humor occurs primarily through the canal of Schlemm. Aqueous humor can also be reabsorbed via the ciliary muscle. This "uveoscleral" flow is increased by ciliary muscle relaxation and is typically mediated by prostaglandins. Therefore, topical prostaglandin analogues can be used to relieve IOP. Topical beta-blockers can also decrease IOP by reducing aqueous humor production.[14]

B. Maintenance of IOP

Volatile anesthetics and sedatives/hypnotics (with the exception of ketamine) reduce IOP. Opioids may also lower IOP. Nondepolarizing paralytics indirectly reduce IOP by attenuating mechanical reflexes that raise IOP, such as coughing.

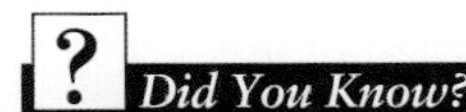

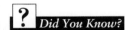

Volatile anesthetics and sedatives or hypnotics (with the exception of ketamine) reduce IOP.

Succinylcholine may cause an elevation in IOP, but it is unclear if this effect has clinical significance. As it is the drug of choice for rapid-onset paralysis, the risks of elevated IOP must be weighed against the risk of not obtaining ideal intubation conditions.[9] Alternatively, rocuronium may be used for rapid-onset paralysis to facilitate tracheal intubation.

To relieve IOP acutely, raise the head and prevent other causes of venous congestion. Under GA, hypocapnia can be used. Additional tactics include the use of muscle relaxants during intubation, the use of an LMA in lieu of intubation, deep extubation, or local anesthetization of the airway. IV sedatives can also rapidly relieve IOP.

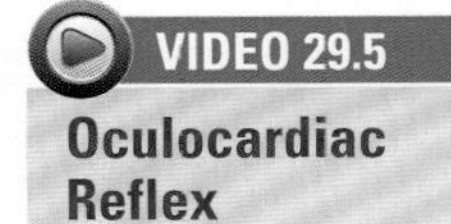

C. Oculocardiac Reflex

Via this reflex, ocular stimulation may trigger hypotension, syncope, bradycardia, and even asystole.

Treatment begins with cessation of any stimuli and ensuring adequate airway and ventilation. If these measures do not succeed, antimuscarinic agents should be administered intravenously. Atropine (20 μg/kg) or glycopyrrolate (15 μg/kg) are both good agents for treatment or prophylaxis. Deepening of the anesthesia, whether local or general, also blunts the reflex, in some instances, leading to a net increase in mean arterial pressure.

III. Glaucoma

Glaucoma is a chronic condition of increased IOP, causing gradual loss of sight. There are two types: open-angle and closed-angle glaucoma. In the setting of either type of glaucoma, additional acute increases in IOP during the perioperative period can put the patient's vision at high risk.

Pupillary constriction moves the iris away from the canal, which lowers the resistance for outflow of aqueous humor. Therefore, muscarinic antagonists or sympathetic alpha-1 agonists, which cause mydriasis, decrease outflow. Conversely, topical cholinergics and acetylcholinesterase inhibitors increase outflow, and so they are indicated as treatment for glaucoma.[15]

> **? Did You Know?**
>
> Echothiophate (phospholine iodide), which is used in the treatment of refractory glaucoma, results in a reduction of pseudocholinesterase activity, causing a longer duration of action for succinylcholine and ester-type local anesthetics.

IV. Anesthetic Implications of Ophthalmic Drugs

Absorption of topical ophthalmic drugs may be sufficient to cause systemic effects. Additionally, some medications that are administered systemically may have significant ophthalmic effects. Constant communication between the anesthesia team and the surgical staff regarding all medications and dosages administered is required to prevent unintended adverse effects.

A. Anticholinesterase Agents

Long-acting topical anticholinesterase agents, such as echothiophate are used in the treatment of refractory glaucoma. They result in a reduction of pseudocholinesterase activity that may last several weeks. In their presence, one can expect a longer duration of action for succinylcholine (prolonged apnea) and ester-type local anesthetics; thus, lower dosages of these medications may be required.

B. Cyclopentolate

Cyclopentolate is used as a mydriatic agent. Concentration-dependent central nervous system (CNS) toxicity occurs with its use. Manifestations of CNS toxicity include dysarthria, disorientation, and psychotic episodes. Seizures have been observed in children. Use should be limited to concentrations below 1%.

C. Epinephrine

Epinephrine (2%) is useful in the treatment of open-angle glaucoma. However, systemic absorption may result in hypertension, headaches, and cardiac dysrhythmias. Dipivefrin is a prodrug of epinephrine that reduces the production of aqueous humor, increases its outflow, and has fewer side effects than epinephrine.

D. Phenylephrine

Phenylephrine decreases capillary congestion and causes mydriasis. Systemic absorption may result in hypertension, headaches, tremors, and bradycardia. In patients with coronary artery disease, it could trigger myocardial ischemia. In small children and the elderly, a solution of 2.5% phenylephrine should be used instead of the usual 10%. To minimize absorption, its use should be limited to the time before incision (to avoid absorption in open venous beds).

E. Topical Beta Blockers

Timolol is a nonselective beta blocker that decreases aqueous humor production. Systemic absorption may cause bradycardia, bronchospasm, congestive heart failure, exacerbation of myasthenia gravis, and postoperative apnea in neonates. Exercise caution when prescribing to patients with preexisting reactive airway diseases, congestive heart failure (CHF), and conduction abnormalities greater than first-degree heart block.

Betaxolol is a newer antiglaucoma beta blocker that is more oculoselective than timolol and has minimal systemic effects. Nonetheless, it may potentiate the effects of systemic beta blockers and is contraindicated in patients with sinus bradycardia, first-degree or higher heart block, CHF, and cardiogenic shock.

F. Intraocular Sulfur Hexafluoride

Sulfur hexafluoride (SF6) is commonly used in retinal detachment repair to replace the volume of vitreous humor lost during surgery. Its low water solubility ensures persistence of the intraocular bubble for several days to weeks.

Nitrous oxide (N_2O) is 34 times more soluble in SF6 than nitrogen; thus, it enters the bubble quicker than nitrogen can exit. This "entrainment" of N_2O causes expansion of the gas bubble, increasing the IOP and potentially compromising the retinal blood flow, especially in the presence of systemic hypotension. N_2O should be discontinued 15 minutes prior to injecting SF6 or any other gas. Abrupt discontinuation of N_2O after injection of SF6 will result in a sharp decrease in the volume of the bubble with a corresponding drop in IOP to below awake levels, possibly jeopardizing the surgical repair. N_2O must be avoided up to 5 days after injection of air, 10 days after the injection of SF6, and 70 days after injection of perfluorocarbons. A Medic Alert bracelet should be considered to prevent this complication, particularly after use of perfluorocarbons.

G. Systemic Drugs

1. Oral Glycerol

Oral glycerol is used to lower the IOP during the treatment of acute glaucoma attacks. Its side effects include hyperglycemia, glycosuria, disorientation, and seizures.

2. Mannitol

Mannitol is used to decrease IOP to enhance surgical exposure (achieve a "soft eye") and occasionally to treat glaucoma. Rapid administration of large doses of mannitol has been associated with renal failure, CHF, fluid overload, electrolyte imbalance, hypertension due to rapid increase in intravascular oncotic pressure, hypotension from the subsequent diuresis, and myocardial ischemia. Allergic reactions have been described as well.

3. Acetazolamide

Acetazolamide, a carbonic anhydrase inhibitor, is used to decrease IOP. Because of its renal tubular effects, acetazolamide can result in the loss of sodium bicarbonate and potassium. Metabolic acidosis and cardiac arrhythmias have been described as well. Acetazolamide should not be used in patients with severe liver or renal dysfunction.[16]

V. Preoperative Evaluation

All patients undergoing ophthalmologic surgery should receive a thorough perioperative evaluation. Timing for the preanesthesia evaluation is based on the invasiveness of the procedure and the general medical condition of the patient.

The components of the preanesthesia evaluation are as follows: full patient history, allergies, medications, anesthetic history (personal and familial), and an anesthesia-focused physical examination. A complete account of all topical and systemic medications is necessary. This includes over-the-counter medications and alternative therapies. Clear instructions should be given to the patient regarding which medications to take and which ones to hold prior to surgery. Special attention should be paid to anticoagulants and antiplatelet medications. Continue warfarin (at least for cataract surgery) due to lack of evidence for a clinically significant increase in the risk of hemorrhage. Dual antiplatelet therapy should be continued in patients with cardiac stents during the perioperative period. Consultation with the patient's cardiologist, primary care physician, and ophthalmologist regarding management of anticoagulants and antiplatelet medications may be necessary. The physical examination must include, at a minimum, general condition and vital signs, airway examination (including range of motion of the cervical spine), and dental, cardiac, and lung examinations.

VI. Anesthetic Techniques

A. Retrobulbar, Peribulbar, and Sub-Tenon Blocks

1. Retrobulbar Block

The patient is placed supine with the eye in a neutral position. A 23 to 25 gauge needle is inserted through the lower lid or conjunctiva at the level of the inferior orbital rim in the inferotemporal quadrant (**Figure 29.5**). The needle is advanced toward the apex of the orbit until loss of resistance is felt (a "pop"). Then 4 to 6 mL of local anesthetic is injected within the muscle cone (four recti muscles and two oblique muscles), obtaining fast and reliable anesthesia and akinesia.

2. Peribulbar Block

The needle is advanced along the inferior orbital floor parallel to the globe, and local anesthetics are injected in the extraconal space, diffusing to adjacent tissue. Greater amounts of local anesthetics are needed in comparison with a retrobulbar block, raising the concern for potential increases in IOP, perforation of the globe, and myotoxicity.

Aspiration before injection is required for both blocks, followed by gentle massage or orbital compression to promote spread of the anesthetic.

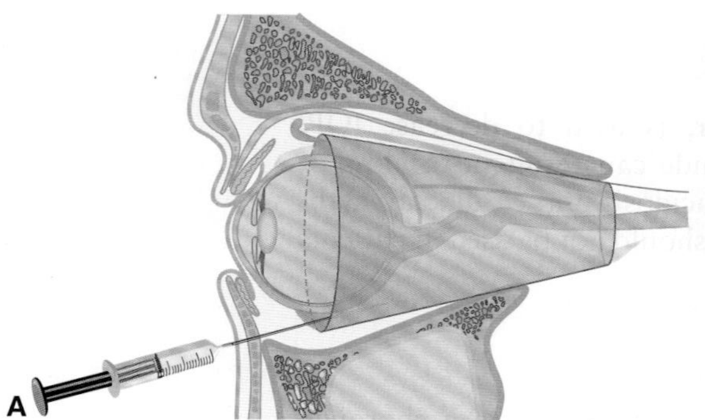

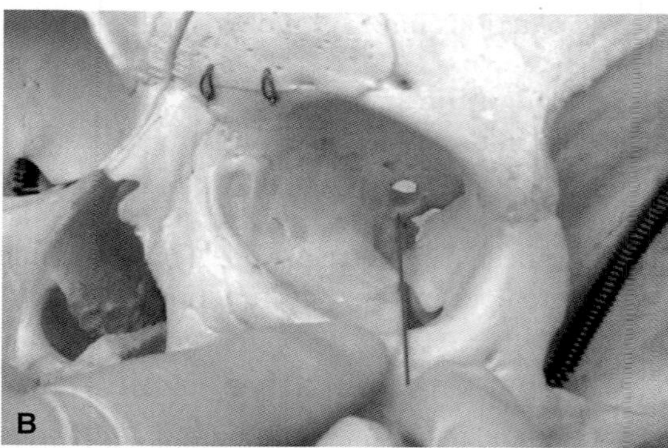

Figure 29.5 **Schematic illustration (A) and skeletal demonstration (B) of proper needle placement for the retrobulbar block.** (From McGoldrick KE, Gayer SI. Anesthesia for ophthalmologic surgery. In: Cahalan MK, Cullen BF; Stock MC, et al, eds. *Clinical Anesthesia*. 8th ed. Wolters Kluwer; 2018:1373-1399, Figures 49.4 and 49.5.)

3. Episcleral (Sub-Tenon) Block

Local anesthetic is injected into the episcleral space (posterior sub-Tenon space). Needle entry is into the fornix at the angle tangential to the globe, between the conjunctival semilunaris fold and globe. Upon entry into the conjunctiva, the needle is shifted medially and advanced posteriorly until a click is felt.[10,16]

Complications of regional eye blocks include optic nerve trauma, brain stem anesthesia (amaurosis, gaze palsy, apnea, dilatation of the contralateral pupil, cardiac arrest), retrobulbar hemorrhage (proptosis of the eye), globe perforation, oculocardiac reflex, seizures, and myocardial depression.

B. Topical Anesthesia

Topical anesthesia includes drops or gels. Local anesthetics include proparacaine (least irritating), lidocaine, bupivacaine, and tetracaine.[10,16] Benefits of topical anesthesia include no risk of hemorrhage, brainstem anesthesia, optic nerve damage, or perforation of the globe. Disadvantages include lack of akinesia and limited use for cataract surgery.

C. Choice of Local Anesthetic, Block Adjuvants, and Adjuncts

The anesthetic approach for ophthalmologic surgery is based on the procedure length and type. Topical anesthesia combines local anesthetics and vasoconstrictors. Vasoconstrictors delay the washout of local anesthetics, prolonging their action.

Adjuvants like clonidine, sodium bicarbonate, morphine sulfate, vecuronium, and hyaluronidase (increased tissue permeability) may also be used to prolong the duration of the blocks.

Increased IOP after administration of local anesthetics can be reduced with the aid of IV osmotic agents or mechanical devices to compress the globe. Mechanical devices may compromise blood flow and result in ischemic optic neuropathy or central retinal artery occlusion.

D. Monitored Anesthesia Care

The goals of this type of sedation exclusively are to provide deep sedation during the administration of regional anesthesia and to otherwise keep the patient comfortable during the remainder of the procedure. The patient should be responsive, cooperative, and able to protect the airway.

E. General Anesthesia for Ophthalmic Surgery

General anesthesia is indicated for procedures that require an immobile surgical field or for patients unable to lie still. Emergence should be smooth, with minimal coughing, bucking, or gagging, in order to minimize elevations in IOP. Patient should be spontaneously breathing, and prophylaxis with opioids or lidocaine to blunt the cough reflex may be administered prior to extubation.[10,16]

VII. Anesthetic Management of Specific Situations

A. Open Eye-Full Stomach

The management of a patient with a lacerated globe and a full stomach requires awareness of the relative risks of each condition. The most controversial issue is how to quickly secure an airway in a patient at risk for aspiration without causing a significant increase in IOP, which could extrude eye contents and cause blindness.

A large dose of an induction agent such as propofol (2 mg/kg) addresses both problems by facilitating conditions for endotracheal intubation while reducing the risk of straining or coughing. Succinylcholine is arguably the most appropriate paralytic for rapid sequence induction in a patient at risk for aspiration; however, it is known to increase IOP 10 to 20 mm Hg, peaking at 2 to 4 minutes and lasting 7 to 10 minutes.[17] There is also anecdotal evidence of succinylcholine causing extrusion of vitreous humor in an open globe,[18] but there is no evidence that succinylcholine causes damage to an intact globe that has elevated IOP, such as in glaucoma.

Alternatively, a high dose of a nondepolarizing agent (eg, rocuronium 2 mg/kg) has been shown to provide paralysis within 60 seconds, 90% of the time. The major drawback is the prolonged paralysis. although the availability of sugammadex addresses the issues of failed airway and unintended neuromuscular block at the end of the procedure.

If GA is contraindicated, local anesthesia should be considered. With an open-globe, penetrating nerve blocks are contraindicated because the pain of injection and the fluid injected may raise IOP. Topical agents are a safer alternative in such situations.

> **? *Did You Know?***
>
> With an open globe, penetrating nerve blocks are contraindicated because the pain of injection and the fluid injected may raise IOP.

Important measures to utilize regardless of the anesthetic type include the following: eliminating any significant increases in IOP, keeping the head elevated, not impairing venous drainage at the neck through the application of cricoid pressure or palpation of the carotid artery, avoiding direct pressure on the globe (eg, face mask), and avoiding painful or intense stimuli of the eye prior to the full onset of the chosen anesthetic.

B. Strabismus Surgery

Strabismus is a persistent misalignment of the visual fields, typically correctable by surgery to counteract the deviation. The surgical repair provides the most benefit when performed before the age of 5 years, at which time the neural pathways involved in vision have neared maturation.[9]

Typically, these repairs are performed under GA due to the immobility required for the work and the pain of the skin and muscle incisions. Endotracheal intubation is preferred to secure the airway due to its proximity to the surgical field and the risk of inadvertent contact.

Acetaminophen may combat the eye irritation felt postoperatively. Fentanyl IV is also an appropriate adjunct.

Strabismus repair has one of the highest rates of PONV of any commonly performed operation, with some studies showing up to 80% in patients who receive no prophylaxis.[19]

Dexamethasone (0.5 mg/kg IV up to 4 mg), ondansetron (0.15 mg/kg IV up to 4 mg), and full replacement of fluid deficits with crystalloids have been shown to reduce the incidence of PONV. Consider gastric emptying with oro-/nasogastric tube while the patient is still deeply anesthetized, in the absence of any contraindications.

C. Intraocular Surgery

The majority of intraocular surgery is performed under local anesthesia rather than GA, the latter having a higher morbidity, higher resource consumption, and longer hospital stay. Various nerve blocks are used to provide surgical analgesia (see previous section) and are also critical for blunting the oculocardiac reflex. Some contraindications to using regional anesthesia for eye surgery include procedures lasting longer than 2 hours, local anesthetic allergy, and the patient's inability to lie supine, be still, or remain awake throughout the surgery. Some surgeons may tolerate a patient who falls into natural sleep, but it carries the risk of sudden movement during REM sleep or upon awakening.

D. Retinal Detachment Surgery

As with other ophthalmic surgeries, the primary concern is choosing GA versus nerve block. For vitreoretinal surgery, a gas bubble is often placed by the surgeon to provide steady pressure that will aid reattachment of the retina to the pigment epithelium. N_2O should be avoided during surgery and, depending on the type of gas installed in the eye, for the next 2 to 12 weeks.[20,21]

VIII. Perioperative Ocular Complications

A. Corneal Abrasion

Corneal abrasions are the most common ophthalmic complications after anesthesia. Decreased tear production and incomplete eyelid closure increase the susceptibility of the cornea to mechanical trauma. Chemical trauma and laser injuries may also occur.

Several risk factors have been correlated with corneal abrasion, including advanced age, high blood loss, Trendelenburg position, prolonged length of stay in the postanesthesia care unit (PACU), and oxygen supplementation during recovery. Sufferers report a foreign body sensation, photophobia, tearing, blurry vision, and pain that tends to increase with blinking. Corneal abrasions heal in 24 to 48 hours and rarely result in long-term sequelae.

Anesthesiologists must evaluate patients who complain of symptoms suggestive of a corneal abrasion. An eye examination usually reveals conjunctival injection with normally reactive pupils. One recommendation is to start ophthalmic antibiotic ointment immediately and continue four times daily for 48 hours. Erythromycin is the first-line therapy, while bacitracin may be used for patients with a contraindication to erythromycin. Patients may require evaluation by an ophthalmologist while in the hospital or shortly after discharge, depending on symptom severity. Topical nonsteroidal anti-inflammatory drugs (NSAIDs) can mask unresolved damage and should not be used because unresolved pain is an important diagnostic sign of injury resolution. The affected eye should not be covered because it has not been shown to improve symptoms. Furthermore, the loss of binocular vision may place the patient at risk for falls or other accidents.

Precautions against corneal abrasions in the OR need to be considered on a case-by-case basis. Taping is the preferred method of eye protection; aggressive application and removal of tape have been associated with corneal abrasion and periocular soft tissue damage. Ointments must be used with care. Both petroleum-based and methylcellulose ointments can result in irritation and allergic reactions and may induce the patient to scratch their eyes.

B. Perioperative Visual Loss

Perioperative visual loss (POVL) is a rare but devastating complication with a prevalence of less than 0.1%. Cardiac and major spine surgery have the highest frequency of POVL. There are two major types of POVL: retinal artery occlusion (RAO) (central and branch) and ischemic optic neuropathy (ION).

1. Retinal Artery Occlusion

Central retinal artery occlusion (CRAO) affects the entire retina and is associated with improper positioning and direct external pressure to the eye. Branch retinal artery occlusion (BRAO) has a segmental deficit distribution and is likely the result of microemboli and/or vasospasm. BRAO is associated with visual loss after cardiac surgery. Lastly, retrobulbar hemorrhage may result in ischemic ocular compartment syndrome.

All types of RAO have poor prognoses and no effective treatment. Therefore, prevention is critical: Prone patients must be positioned using modern foam headrests with cutouts or skull clamp, and goggles must not be used. Positioning and eyes must be checked every 20 minutes. Horseshoe headrests should not be used.

2. Ischemic Optic Neuropathy

The causative factors of ION are poorly understood, but it is known that ION results from disruption of the blood supply to the optic nerve. Anterior ischemic optic neuropathy (AION) is associated with cardiac surgery. Posterior ischemic optic neuropathy (PION) is associated with lengthy spine surgery >6 hours) when performed in the prone position, particularly cases with significant blood loss. There are also case reports of ION being associated with the steep Trendelenburg position during laparoscopic robotic radical prostatectomies.

As with RAO, there is no effective treatment for ION; therefore, prevention is paramount. The Postoperative Visual Loss Study Group recently identified the use of a Wilson frame as an independent significant risk factor; it is the only significant risk factor that is easily controllable.[22] The American Society of Anesthesiologists recommends positioning the head at or higher than the level of the heart and in a neutral position to prevent venous congestion.[23]

Patients deemed to be at high risk for POVL after spinal surgery must be immediately evaluated postoperatively. In the event of positive findings or concerns, an immediate ophthalmology evaluation should occur. The following measures should also be instituted without delay: optimize hemoglobin/hematocrit, hemodynamics, and oxygenation; also, consider an MRI to rule out an intracranial cause.

For further review and interactivities, please see the associated Interactive Video Lectures and "A Closer Look" infographic accessible in the complimentary eBook bundled with this text. Access instructions are located in the inside front cover.

References

1. Groundine SB, Hollinger I, Jones J, DeBuono BA. New York State guidelines on the topical use of phenylephrine in the operating room. *Anesthesiology*. 2000;92:859-864. PMID: 10719965.
2. Bluestone CD, Casselbrant ML, Stool SE, et al, eds. *Pediatric Otolaryngology*. Vol 1. Saunders; 2002.
3. Isaacson G. Tonsillectomy care for the pediatrician. *Pediatrics*. 2012;130(2):324-334. PMID: 22753552.
4. Shi M, Miao S, Gu T, Wang D, Zhang H, Liu J. Dexmedetomidine for the prevention of emergence delirium and postoperative behavioral changes in pediatric patients with sevoflurane anesthesia: a double-blind randomized trial. *Drug Des Devel Ther*. 2019;13:897-905. PMID: 30936683.

5. Jeyakumar A, Brickman TM, Williamson ME, et al. Nonsteroidal anti-inflammatory drugs and postoperative bleeding following adenotonsillectomy in pediatric patients. *Arch Otolaryngol Head Neck Surg*. 2008;134(1):24-27. PMID: 18209131.
6. Perterson J, Losek JD. Post-tonsillectomy hemorrhage and pediatric emergency care. *Clin Pediatr (Phila)*. 2004;43(5):445-448. PMID: 15208749.
7. Steketee KG, Reisdorff EJ. Emergency care for the Posttonsillectomy and Postadenoidectomy hemorrhage. *Am J Emerg Med*. 1995;13(5):518-523. PMID: 7662054.
8. Malone E, Meakin GH. Acute stridor in children. *Contin Educ Anaesth Crit Care Pain*. 2007;7(6):183-186.
9. Coté CJ, Lerman J, Anderson BJ, eds. *A Practice of Anesthesia for Infants and Children*. Elsevier Saunders; 2013.
10. Donlon JV. Anesthesia for eye, ear, nose, and throat surgery. In: Miller RD, Fleisher LA, Johns RA, et al, eds. *Miller's Anesthesia*. 6th ed. Elsiever; 2005:2527-2555.
11. Sasaki K, Watahiki R, Tamura H, Ogura M, Shibuya M. Fluid extravasation of the articular capsule as a complication of temporomandibular joint pumping and perfusion. *Bull Tokyo Dent Coll*. 2002;43:237-242.
12. Mariano ER. Anesthesia for otorhinolaryngology surgery. In: Butterworth JF, Mackey DC, Wasnick JD, ed. *Morgan & Mikhail's Clinical Anesthesiology*. 5th ed. McGraw-Hill; 2013:773-787.
13. Cauley BD, Anesthesia for head and neck surgery. In: Levine WC, Allain RM, Alston TA, et al eds. *Clinical Anesthesia Procedures of the Massachusetts General Hospital*. 8th ed. Lippincott Williams & Wilkins; 2010:409-421.
14. Murgatroyd H, Bembridge J. Intraocular pressure. *Contin Educ Anaesth Crit Care Pain*. 2008;8(3):100-103.
15. Raw D, Mostafa SM. Drugs and the eye. *Br J Anaesth CEPD Reviews*. 2001;1:161-165.
16. McGoldrick KE, Gayer SI. Anesthesia for ophthalmologic surgery. In: Barash PG, Cullen BF, et al, ed. *Clinical Anesthesia*. 7th ed. Lippincott Williams & Wilkins; 2013:1373-1399.
17. Wilson A, Soar J. *Open eye injury with full stomach*. In: *Anaesthesia for Emergency Eye Surgery*. 2000. Issue 11. Article 10: 1-2 pp 1 of 3.
18. Lincoff HA, Breinin GM, DeVoe AG. Effect of succinylcholine on the extraocular muscles. *Am J Ophthalmol*. 1957;44:440-444.
19. Hardy JF, Charest J, Girouard G, Lepage Y. Nausea and vomiting after strabismus surgery in preschool children. *Can Anaesth Soc J*. 1986;33:57-62. PMID: 3948048.
20. Hunnigher A. Anesthesia for retinal detachment. *Br Med J*. 2008;336(7657):1325-1326. PMID: 18556286.
21. Jaffe RA, Samuels SI, Schmiesing CA, et al, eds. *Anesthesiologist's Manual of Surgical Procedures*. 4th ed. LippIncott Williams and Wilkins; 2009.
22. Roth S. Perioperative visual loss: what do we know, what can we do? *Br J Anaesth*. 2009;103(suppl 1):i31-i40. PMID: 20007988.
23. American Society of Anesthesiologists Task Force on Perioperative Visual Loss. Practice Advisory for perioperative visual loss associated with spine surgery: an updated report by the American Society of Anesthesiologists Task Force on Perioperative Visual Loss. *Anesthesiology*. 2012;116:275-285. PMID: 22227790.

INTRAOCULAR PRESSURE AND ANESTHESIA

A CLOSER LOOK

A multitude of factors related to the patient's medical diagnoses, the type of surgical procedure, anesthetic techniques and drugs can have dramatic influences on intraocular pressure (IOP).

Decreased Po_2, increased Pco_2 and PEEP > 15 cm H_2O all ↑ IOP

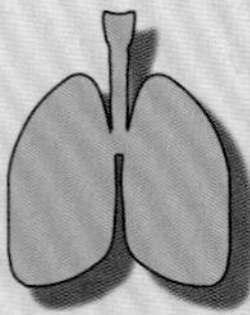

Scopolamine is contraindicated in patients that have a diagnosis of glaucoma

Normal intraocular pressure is

16 mm Hg ± 5 mm Hg

Ocular perfusion pressure (OPP) = MAP - IOP

Thus, safety and integrity of patients' visual function not only requires avoiding excessive increases in IOP, but also ensuring adequate blood pressure.

IOP can ↑ to 100 mm Hg during ocular surgery

Coughing or bucking on an ETT ↑ IOP by about 40 mm Hg

Laparoscopy in head down position ↑ IOP 2-3 X

Laryngoscopy ↑ IOP 2 X, but less so with videolaryngoscopy

Supraglottic airways have minimal effect

Succinylcholine ↑ IOP by about 10 mm Hg

Ketamine may ↑ IOP but this is controversial

Opiates, intravenous anesthetics and volatile anesthetics all ↓ IOP

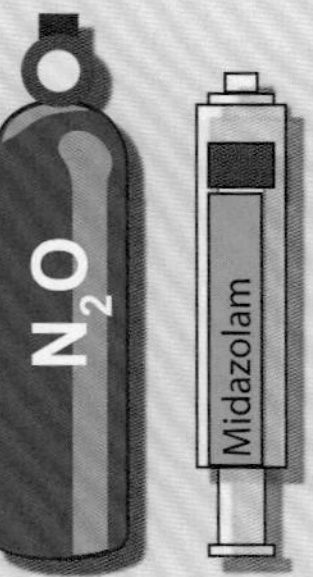

Nitrous oxide and midazolam have no effect on IOP. Be aware if a patient has had an intraocular sulfur hexafluoride (SF_6) injection for retinal detachment surgery, then N_2O is **CONTRAINDICATED**. It can dangerously expand the SF_6 bubble inside the eye!

Infographic by: Naveen Nathan MD

Questions

1. **A 49-year-old, 45 kg woman with a past medical history of hypertension, diabetes mellitus type 2, and chronic sinusitis presents to the ambulatory surgery unit for a functional endoscopic sinus surgery under general anesthesia. Preoperative vital signs: BP 138/78, HR 75, and Spo_2 97% on room air. Five minutes after the surgeon inserted a nose pack impregnated with phenylephrine, her blood pressure reading is 180/111 and the heart rate is 48. What is the appropriate next step for her anesthetic management?**

   A. Deepen the anesthetic, instruct the surgeon to withhold further vasoconstrictors, and wait
   B. Administer intravenous labetalol
   C. Administer intravenous glycopyrrolate
   D. Start a sodium nitroprusside infusion

2. **A four-year-old boy with a past medical history of premature birth at 33 weeks due to maternal cervical incompetence presents to the emergency department with high-pitched breathing sounds, throat pain, and increased respiratory effort. His parents found him crying in his older brother's room but report he had been feeling well earlier in the evening. They administered acetaminophen elixir PO at home before coming to the hospital, hoping to alleviate whatever pain they feared the child may be having. Radiography of the neck, throat, and chest are unremarkable. Vital signs: BP 105/65, HR 105, Spo_2 94%, Temp 98.9°F on room air. What would be the appropriate next step in his management?**

   A. Obtain intravenous access and administer cephalosporins
   B. Consult an otolaryngologist and consider rigid bronchoscopy
   C. Discharge to home after treatment with nebulized albuterol
   D. Continue PO acetaminophen and admit for observation

3. **While taking care of a patient who has been brought to the operating room for acutely elevated intraocular pressure due to intraocular hemorrhage, all of the following strategies may help reduce the risk of loss of vision EXCEPT:**

   A. Elevation of the head of the bed
   B. Induction of general anesthesia with propofol, lidocaine, and rocuronium
   C. Reduction of controlled respiratory rate while the patient is being ventilated with positive pressure
   D. Avoidance of oropharyngeal stimulation if the patient is moderately sedated

4. **Basic safety precautions for laser surgery of the airway include all of the following EXCEPT:**

   A. Low Fio_2.
   B. A supply of saline available next to surgical field.
   C. Use of nitrous oxide-narcotic technique to maintain general anesthesia.
   D. Use of a metallic endotracheal tube.

5. **A 45-year-old man with a history of hypertension, hypercholesterolemia, gout, and obstructive sleep apnea (OSA), who had tonsillectomy/adenoidectomy 7 days ago as treatment for his OSA, presents to the emergency department with active oropharyngeal bleeding. All of the following factors may reduce the risk of morbidity/mortality of this situation EXCEPT:**

   A. Treatment of hypertension with titration of short-acting antihypertensives.
   B. Prenotification of the blood bank prior to arrival in the operating room.
   C. The availability of epinephrine soaked gauze that can be applied by McGill forceps.
   D. Early discharge in the setting of minor bleeding, to avoid iatrogenic sequelae.

Answers

1. A

Phenylephrine has a short duration of action. Mild to moderate hypertension secondary to topical application of vasoconstrictors can be managed expectantly and by deepening of the anesthetic level. Severe hypertension must be treated with direct vasodilators. The use of beta blockers in this scenario is associated with pulmonary edema and cardiac arrest. Glycopyrrolate is not indicated for the treatment of the mild reflex tachycardia in this example.

2. B

This child was found distressed and with acute onset of stridor and was out of sight from a responsible adult. Vital signs and clinical course are not typical of an infectious process. A foreign body in the airway is a highly likely diagnosis. Radiolucent foreign bodies are not visible on x-ray. An otolaryngology consult and consideration for rigid bronchoscopy are necessary. A foreign body in the airway is a life-threatening condition and must be resolved as soon as possible.

3. C

Worsening of elevated intraocular pressure can lead to vision loss. Actions that help prevent further elevation of intraocular pressure include enhancement of venous drainage by elevating the head of the bed and avoidance of coughing and gaging. Intravenous and volatile anesthetics, except ketamine, reduce intraocular pressure. Nondepolarizing muscle relaxants like rocuronium have no effect on intraocular pressure. Hypercapnia and positive pressure ventilation (impairing venous return) can cause elevation of the intraocular pressure.

4. C

Laser surgery of the airway poses a high risk of surgical fire. All fires require the presence of three elements: ignition source, oxidizer, and fuel. To mitigate the risk of a fire, one or more elements of the fire triad must be removed. The risk of fire is lower with an $FIO_2 < 0.3$ and a noncombustible laser-safe endotracheal tube such as a metal tube. Normal saline or water can be used to extinguish a fire and must be readily available in all high-risk cases. Nitrous oxide is an oxidizer and must not be used.

5. D

Posttonsillectomy hemorrhage can be a life-threatening complication. A mean arterial pressure of 65 mm Hg or less minimizes arterial bleeding. Individuals with chronic, poorly controlled hypertension may need higher perfusion pressures. A careful risk-benefit analysis must be conducted prior to determining a safe reduction in blood pressure to aid in controlling hemorrhage. Anesthesiologists must be prepared to administer blood products. Topical vasoconstrictors may be useful in controlling the bleeding. Leaning forward and facing down drains blood away from the airway. It is common for minor bleeding to become severe, so this patient must not be discharged until the hemorrhage is controlled.

30 Anesthesia for Neurosurgery

John F. Bebawy and Antoun Koht

Neuroanesthesia is the practice of anesthesia related to the treatment of real or impending neurologic injury to the ***central nervous system (CNS)*** or ***peripheral nervous system (PNS)***. The CNS encompasses the brain and spinal cord, while the PNS includes all of the peripheral nerves of the body emanating from the spinal cord. As such, neuroanesthesia is the provision of anesthesia and analgesia for a multitude of procedures, including invasive, minimally invasive, and neurointerventional procedures, involving the brain, spinal cord, and peripheral nerves.

I. Neuroanatomy

The adult brain accounts for only 2% of total body weight but 20% of total body oxygen consumption. The different regions of the brain and spinal cord are responsible for distinct functions (**Table 30.1**). Blood flow to the brain is accomplished by two carotid arteries anteriorly (70%) and two vertebral arteries posteriorly (forming the basilar artery) (30%), which subsequently converge to form an anastomotic ring at the base of the skull known as the circle of Willis (**Figure 30.1**). The spinal column is composed of 33 vertebrae (7 cervical, 12 thoracic, 5 lumbar, and 9 fused sacral and coccygeal), with nerve roots leaving the enclosed spinal cord and exiting through corresponding intervertebral foramina. The blood supply to the spinal cord entails one anterior spinal artery and two posterior spinal arteries. The anterior spinal artery originates from radicular arteries branching off the aorta, with the largest one being the artery of Adamkiewicz (usually at L1 or L2). The posterior spinal arteries originate from the posterior cerebral circulation (**Figure 30.2**). The spinal cord itself terminates at L1 or L2 in adults, ending in structures known as the conus medullaris terminus and filum terminale.

II. Neurophysiology

The ***cerebral metabolic rate of oxygen consumption ($CMRO_2$)*** is normally 3 to 3.8 mL/100 g/min in adults. Normal ***cerebral blood flow (CBF)*** is 50 mL/100 g/min at rest, while glucose consumption is approximately 5 mg/100 g/min. The brain is dependent on a continuous supply of oxygen and glucose, with starvation and hypoxic damage resulting after roughly 5 minutes of global ischemia. The results of focal ischemia are less certain.

Cerebral perfusion pressure (CPP) is the difference between mean arterial pressure (MAP) and either ***intracranial pressure (ICP)*** or central venous pressure (CVP), depending on which is higher. Fortunately, even wide swings in

Table 30.1 Functionality of Central Nervous System Structures

Anatomic Location	Structure	Function
Postcentral gyrus	Primary somatosensory cortex	Sensation
Precentral gyrus	Primary motor cortex	Movement
Occipital lobe	Primary visual cortex	Vision
Temporal lobe	Primary auditory cortex	Hearing
Wernicke area (angular gyrus of dominant hemisphere)	Primary language association cortex	Language
Frontal lobe	Primary personality cortex	Personality/intellect
Medial brain	Limbic cortex	Emotion
Medial brain	Hippocampus	Memory
Medial brain	Hypothalamus	Vegetative regulation
Brainstem	Reticular activating system	Consciousness
Brainstem	Vasomotor center	Circulatory/respiratory control
Spinal cord	Dorsal horn (sensory)/ventral horn (motor)	Movement/sensation/reflexes

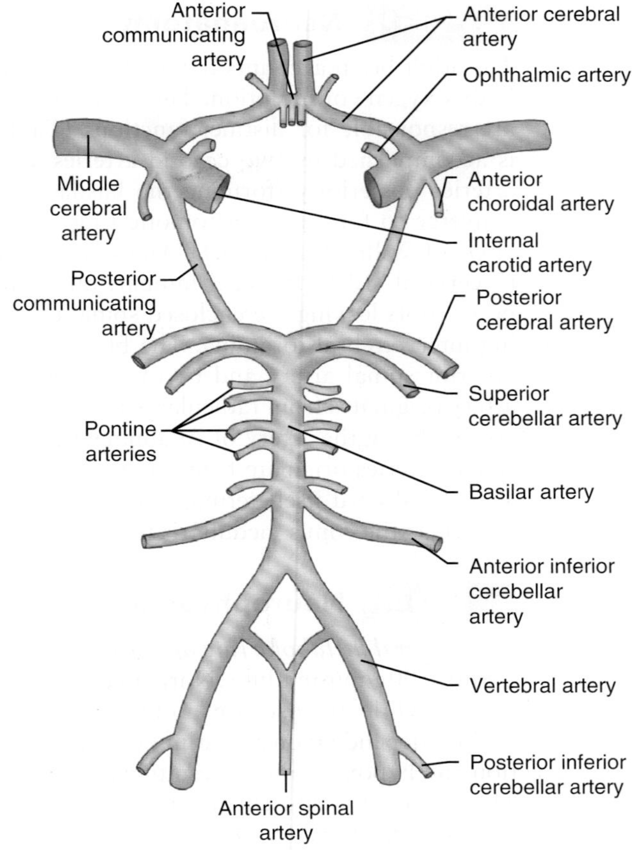

Figure 30.1 The circle of Willis, demonstrating the anterior and posterior blood supply to the brain.

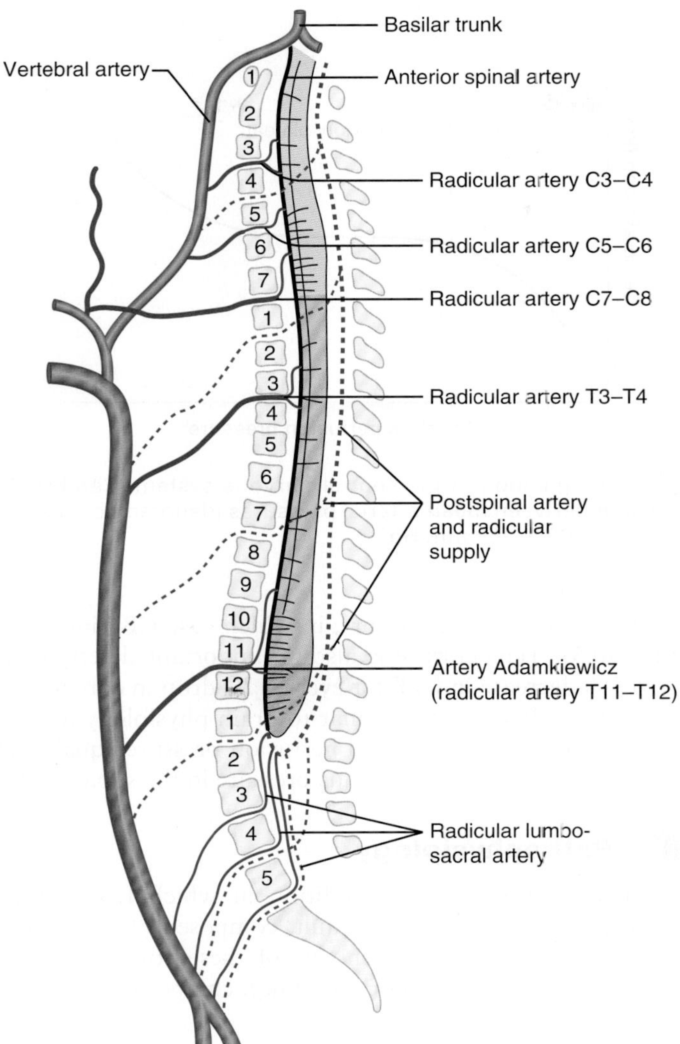

Figure 30.2 The spinal cord blood supply. Note that the cervical spine is served by the posterior circulation emanating from the circle of Willis.

MAP will yield a consistent CBF of 50 mL/100 g/min, thanks to ***autoregulation***, which remains intact between an MAP of approximately 60 to 160 mm Hg (**Figure 30.3**). The autoregulatory curve is shifted rightward in cases of chronic hypertension. Above and below these limits, CBF becomes pressure dependent as cerebral vessels are either maximally vasodilated (lower limit of autoregulation) or vasoconstricted (upper limit of autoregulation).

Besides MAP, other physiologic parameters play an important role in controlling CBF. Arterial carbon dioxide tension ($Paco_2$) is the most important of these variables. CBF is linearly associated with $Paco_2$ between 20 and 80 mm Hg. Hence, hyper- and hypoventilation (either patient-determined and iatrogenic) play critical roles in maintaining, decreasing (with hyperventilation), or increasing (with hypoventilation) CBF (**Figure 30.4**). Oxygen tension in the arterial blood (Pao_2) plays less of a role in controlling CBF unless marked

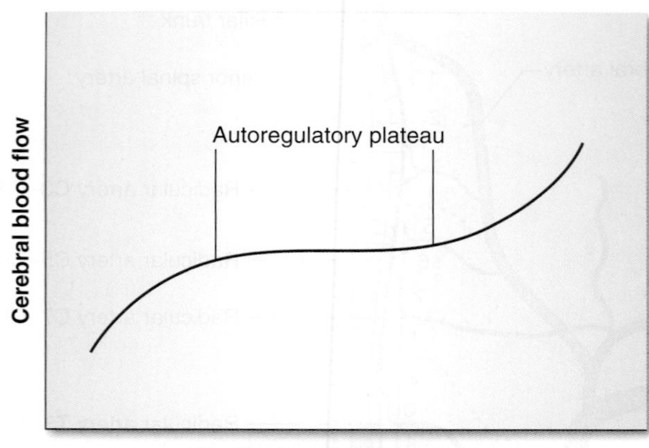

Figure 30.3 Autoregulation in the central nervous system. Cerebral blood flow remains constant between mean arterial pressures (denoted here as cerebral perfusion pressure) of 60 to 160 mm Hg.

hypoxemia ($Pa{O_2}$ <50 mm Hg) occurs, in which case CBF increases dramatically (**Figure 30.5**). Temperature is also an important determinant of CBF, with a 6% to 7% decrease in CBF for every 1 °C drop in core temperature.

Spinal cord physiology is very similar to brain physiology in that autoregulation is maintained and spinal cord perfusion pressure equals MAP minus ICP (or, for spinal cord perfusion, minus pressure in the subarachnoid space).

III. Pathophysiology

VIDEO 30.1 Intracranial Hypertension

Intracranial hypertension is any condition in which ICP is raised above 15 mm Hg. The cranium is a closed vault, composed of brain tissue, blood, and cerebrospinal fluid (CSF). When one of these components enlarges to occupy more space (eg, brain tumor, bleeding), compensation occurs, usually

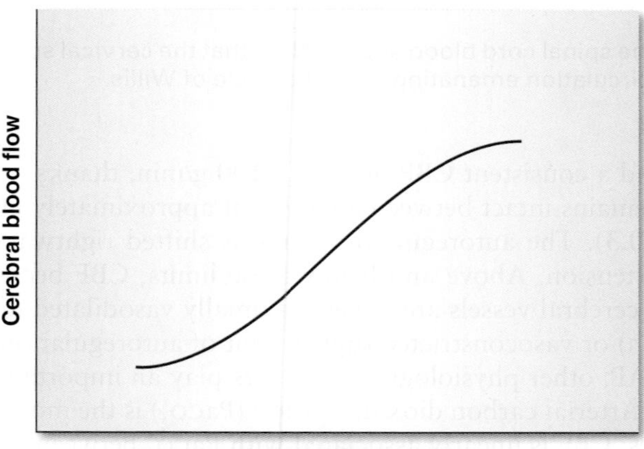

Figure 30.4 Autoregulation in the central nervous system. Cerebral blood flow varies linearly between arterial carbon dioxide partial pressures of 20 to 80 mm Hg.

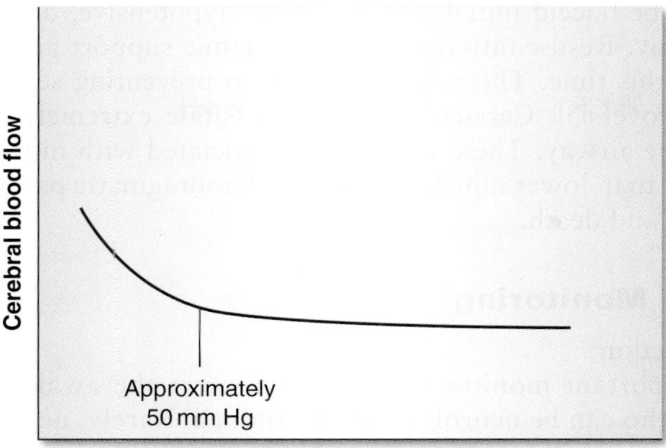

Figure 30.5 Autoregulation in the central nervous system. Cerebral blood flow remains constant above an arterial oxygen partial pressure of 50 mm Hg.

by vasoconstriction and CSF drainage out of the cranium and into the spinal column. ***Intracranial elastance***, however, becomes very limited as ICP reaches a critical point, where sudden, even very small increases in volume can lead to dramatic increases in pressure within the cranium (**Figure 30.6**). The results can be neurologically devastating, with herniation of the brainstem into the foramen magnum and subsequent irreversible damage or even death. Hence, meticulous care in those patients in whom elevated ICP is suspected (eg, avoiding hypoventilation, emergent surgical decompression, or CSF diversion) is critical.

As for the spinal cord, damage can be acute (leading to weakness, loss of sensation, or paralysis) or chronic (causing pain and deformity). ***Acute spinal cord compression***, due to trauma or tumor, is usually a surgical emergency, as time to decompression is correlated with functional outcome.

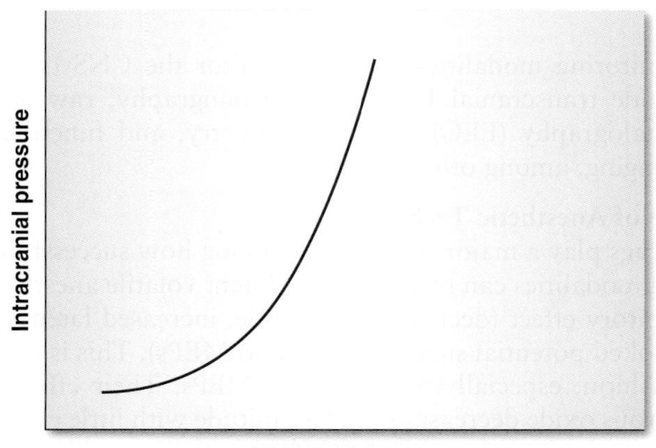

Figure 30.6 The intracranial elastance curve is composed of three sections. (**1**) Intracranial pressure remains low and relatively constant at low volumes until the "elbow" of the curve is reached. (**2**) At this point, small changes in volume lead to moderate changes in pressure. (**3**) When a critical intracranial volume is reached, the pressure increases precipitously.

VIDEO 30.2
Intracranial Compliance Curve

Patients may be flaccid initially and severely hypotensive, due to a relative sympathectomy. Resuscitation and hemodynamic support are mainstays of treatment at this time. The role of steroids in preventing secondary injury is more controversial. Cervical injuries necessitate extremely careful management of the airway. These injuries are associated with more physiologic perturbations than lower injuries, including diaphragmatic paralysis, cardiac disturbances, and death.

IV. Monitoring

A. CNS Function

The most important monitor of CNS function is the awake and responsive patient who can be neurologically examined. Rarely, neurosurgery can be performed with an awake patient. Under general anesthesia, however, other modes of monitoring the CNS are necessary. ***Electrophysiologic (evoked potential) monitoring*** is commonly used in the operating room to assess the functional integrity of the CNS during surgeries that might put CNS structures at risk.[1] The most commonly used modalities of evoked potential monitoring are ***somatosensory-evoked potentials (SSEPs), motor-evoked potentials (MEPs), and electromyography (EMG)***, with brainstem auditory-evoked potentials and visual-evoked potentials being less commonly used.

SSEPs are elicited from a peripheral nerve (eg, median, ulnar, posterior tibial) and usually measured at the level of the subcortex and cortex. This modality is especially useful for monitoring the integrity of the dorsal columns of the spinal cord and the sensory cortex of the brain, where sensory fibers travel. MEPs are produced at the level of the cortex by direct or indirect stimulation and measured as compound muscle action potentials at the muscular level. MEPs are useful for assessing the motor cortex and the anterior spinal cord (corticospinal tracts) during surgeries that may put these structures at risk. EMG is a monitor that continuously assesses distinct nerve or nerve root integrity, either spontaneously or through elicited current, and is sensitive to mechanical and thermal damage to these structures.

Other monitoring modalities used to monitor the CNS (see section that follows) include transcranial Doppler ultrasonography, raw and processed electroencephalography (EEG), cerebral oximetry, and functional magnetic resonance imaging, among others.

B. Influence of Anesthetic Technique

Anesthetic drugs play a major role in determining how successfully these neuromonitoring modalities can be employed. Potent volatile anesthetics have the greatest inhibitory effect (decreased amplitude, increased latency) on obtaining robust evoked potential signals (SSEPs and MEPs). This is done in a dose-dependent fashion, especially as related to MEPs. Their effect on EMG is minimal. Nitrous oxide decreases signal amplitude with little effect on latency. Intravenous anesthetics have much less effect on SSEPs, MEPs, and EMG, but high doses of propofol can depress these signals. Etomidate and ketamine may increase the amplitude of SSEPs, whereas opioids generally have very little effect on evoked potentials. Neuromuscular blocking drugs inhibit MEPs and EMG by directly acting at the neuromuscular junction but often will improve SSEPs by removing myogenic interference.[2]

V. Cerebral Perfusion

A. Processed EEG Monitoring

Processed EEG monitoring is a useful, practical, and increasingly popular technology in the operating room that utilizes proprietary algorithms and methodologies to produce, among other parameters, a unitless index value (based on the raw EEG signal) which reflects the depth of anesthesia. Gamma-aminobutyric acid (GABA) agonists are associated with various changes in the raw EEG pattern, in a typically reliable and dose-dependent fashion, and processed EEG monitors take advantage of these patterns to give an indication of the level of anesthetic depth. Advantages of using a processed EEG monitor include a tailored approach to anesthetic delivery which may produce a more rapid emergence with fewer side effects (ie, may decrease the overall amount of anesthetic administered) and potentially a decrease in the possibility of recall or "awareness" under general anesthesia. Some studies also demonstrated the potential for a decrease in the incidence of postoperative delirium and postoperative cognitive dysfunction (POCD) when using processed EEG. Importantly, the index value generated reflects the EEG activity of the frontal cortices only, over which the monitor lies, and is subject to regional cerebral blood flow and neuronal activity, as well as to contamination from electromyographic (EMG) activity from the overlying scalp.[3]

B. Transcranial Doppler Ultrasonography

Transcranial Doppler ultrasonography (TCD) is a tool used in neurosurgery and neurocritical care by which an ultrasound probe is placed over a "window" (usually the temporal bone) to measure flow velocities of major cerebral vessels (usually the middle cerebral artery). Blood flow velocity is recorded by the ultrasound probe, which emits a high-pitched sound wave. That sound wave bounces off red blood cells and returns to the probe. The speed of the blood in relation to the probe causes a phase shift, with a higher or lower frequency directly correlated to a higher or lower velocity, respectively. Changes in these flow velocities (higher velocities) can indicate narrowing, emboli, or vasospasm of these vessels. Notably, TCD is unable to determine actual CBF; rather, it is primarily a technique for measuring relative changes in CBF over time.[4]

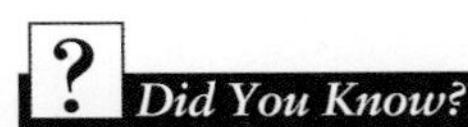

Transcranial Doppler ultrasonography can noninvasively assess changes in cerebral blood flow.

C. ICP Monitoring

ICP monitoring is a useful tool for patients suffering from any cause of dangerously elevated ICP (eg, brain trauma, bleeding, mass). Normal ICP is 5 to 15 mm Hg, and monitoring or treatment is generally initiated when ICP is >20 mm Hg. Waveforms of ICP can be transduced (A, B, and C waves) and may be useful diagnostically over time. ICP monitoring can be accomplished using a variety of devices, all of which currently are invasive. The most commonly used device is an ***external ventricular drain***, which measures ICP by way of a transducer connected via tubing to the ventricle. It is also capable of removing CSF to relieve ICP. Other methods of monitoring ICP include the use of a ***subdural screw*** (usually performed urgently) placed through the skull and dura mater, an epidural sensor placed between the skull and the dura mater, or a tissue sensor placed directly in the brain parenchyma. These methods are incapable of diverting CSF.

D. Cerebral Oxygenation and Metabolism Monitors

Other devices used to monitor the homeostasis of the brain, including its oxygenation and metabolism, are available (often experimental) but may not be commonly used in the clinical setting. Jugular bulb venous oximetry is the most common of these techniques, which involves a fiberoptic catheter placed in a retrograde fashion into the jugular vein. This catheter is capable of measuring the mixed cerebral venous oxygen tension, which is indicative of the brain's oxygen consumption or extraction. Other monitors used to measure ***cerebral metabolism*** include microdialysis catheters, which are multiparameter catheters that can detect focal brain tissue oxygen tension, glucose, pyruvate, lactate, glutamate, and glycerol levels by way of obtaining local perfusate from the brain. These catheters are becoming more popular in neurocritical care units but remain primarily research tools.[5] Lastly, cerebral oximetry has become more prevalent in the clinical setting recently, which involves a noninvasive measurement of regional cerebral blood oxygenation over the frontal cortices bilaterally. Oxygenation is given as a percentage, reflecting the contribution of both arterial (25%) and venous (75%) blood.[6]

VI. Cerebral Protection

? Did You Know?

The brain is particularly susceptible to rapid ischemic injury because of its high oxygen and glucose consumption, inability to store substrate, and inability to dispose of toxic metabolites.

A. Ischemic and Reperfusion

Because of its high oxygen and glucose consumption, inability to store substrate, and inability to dispose of toxic metabolites, the brain is especially susceptible to rapid ischemic injury. With the accumulation of intracellular calcium under these ischemic conditions, neuronal damage quickly occurs and is compounded by the accumulation of lactic acid. Global ischemia, seen in conditions such as cardiac arrest, is responsive to interventions that restore total cerebral perfusion and oxygen-carrying capacity, such as cardiopulmonary resuscitation or red blood cell transfusion. Focal ischemia, on the other hand, is usually due to a regional insult, such as an embolus or intentional or unintentional arterial disruption. Treatment must be focused on restoring perfusion to the region in question. In cases of focal ischemia, a penumbra of salvageable tissue (watershed) usually surrounds the area that is damaged. Efforts must also be directed at "saving" this tissue, which is being supplied to some degree by collateral circulation. Much of the research being performed in ***cerebral protection*** today deals with this concept of "saving the penumbra." Practical methods include augmentation of CPP and reducing brain edema in the acute setting (see section that follows). Another area under heavy study is that of reperfusion and "reperfusion injury," in which reperfusion of previously ischemic brain tissue can actually worsen neurologic outcomes largely due to the production of free radicals derived from oxygen and mediators of inflammation.

B. Hypothermia

Research into the cerebroprotective effects of ***hypothermia*** in humans has been largely disappointing, despite some encouraging animal studies. Theoretically, hypothermia should be extremely protective to the brain and spinal cord, as it lowers the $CMRO_2$ for the CNS to a much greater extent than anesthetics would. Although anesthetics can cause an isoelectric EEG (electrical silence), reducing the brain's metabolic activity by up to 60%, hypothermia can do far more by reducing even the brain's homeostatic (eg, mitochondrial) need for oxygen, which is required for basic neuronal survival. Despite this, mild to moderate reductions in core temperature in the face of cerebral ischemia have not yielded protective results in human studies and have been associated with worsened immunologic and clotting function.[7]

C. Medical Therapy for Cerebral Protection

Similar to hypothermia, medical therapy for ***cerebral protection*** in its application to humans has been difficult to ascertain. Anesthetics, especially barbiturates, have been widely used in an attempt to lessen the burden of ischemia on neurons. Nearly all anesthetics (notable exceptions being ketamine and etomidate in low doses) can lower $CMRO_2$ and theoretically protect the brain. But only barbiturates have been shown in humans to provide some protection from focal (not global) ischemia. No agents have been definitively shown to provide protection from global ischemia. Nimodipine, a calcium channel blocker, is frequently used in the setting of subarachnoid hemorrhage. It may have the benefit in neurologic protection during brain ischemia, although its protective mechanism remains elusive. Within 8 hours of acute spinal cord injury, methylprednisolone (a steroid) has been used to limit the degree of secondary injury due to edema, although controversy still surrounds this technique. Other more experimental agents, such as lidocaine, tirilazad (steroid), magnesium, dexmedetomidine (α_2 agonist), and vitamin E (antioxidant) have been used in various ischemic settings, all with mixed results on neurologic protection and outcomes.

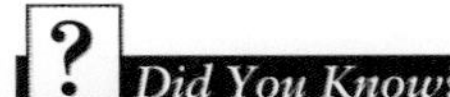

Did You Know?

Glucose is the only substrate that can be aerobically metabolized by the brain under normal conditions.

D. Glucose and Cerebral Ischemia

As mentioned previously, ischemia is rapidly detrimental to the nervous system not only because of oxygen starvation, but also because glucose is the only substrate that can be aerobically metabolized by the brain under normal conditions. Glucose is not stored in the nervous system, so when glucose is absent due to limited or absent cerebral circulation, adenosine triphosphate is no longer available to neurons and cellular injury quickly ensues. Cerebral glucose consumption (5 mg/100 g/min), on a time scale, mimics $CMRO_2$, so hypoxemia and hypoglycemia are roughly equally detrimental to the brain. With cerebral ischemia and hypoglycemia, lactate is metabolized to some extent in the brain, but with much less efficacy than glucose. Hyperglycemia (serum blood glucose >180 mg/dL) in the setting of cerebral ischemia has also been shown to worsen neurologic outcomes, presumably by worsening cerebral acidosis in an anaerobic setting in which glucose is converted to lactic acid.[8]

Did You Know?

The reason cellular injury ensues more quickly in the nervous tissue is because glucose is not stored in the nervous system, so when glucose is absent due to limited or absent cerebral circulation, adenosine triphosphate is no longer available to neurons and cellular injury quickly ensues.

E. A Practical Approach

"True" cerebral protection is hard to achieve or to prove, but practically speaking, certain techniques are commonly used for their possible benefit. Inhaled and intravenous anesthetics are generally "protective," based on their known effect on $CMRO_2$. For operations in which there is planned regional ischemia (eg, temporary clipping of cerebral vessels during aneurysm surgery), propofol given in a large bolus (1-2 mg/kg) followed by a high-dose infusion (150 µg/kg/min) is often used and titrated to induce burst suppression on the EEG ***prior*** to the planned ischemia (ischemic preconditioning). In cardiac or neurologic surgeries in which circulatory arrest is planned (eg, aortic arch repair, giant basilar aneurysm clipping), deep hypothermia (12°-18 °C) has been instituted to "protect" the nervous system with seemingly great success. Another example of practical neurologic protection involves the placement of a lumbar CSF drain prior to thoracoabdominal aortic repair, used to lower CSF pressure and ostensibly maintain spinal cord perfusion when radicular arteries originating from the aorta are at surgical risk.

Did You Know?

Hyperglycemia (serum blood glucose >180 mg/dL) in the setting of cerebral ischemia has also been shown to worsen neurologic outcomes, presumably by worsening cerebral acidosis in an anaerobic setting in which glucose is converted to lactic acid.

VII. Anesthetic Management

A. Preoperative Evaluation

The preoperative evaluation of the neurosurgical patient is of paramount importance in ensuring a safe and successful anesthetic. For patients with intracranial mass lesions, the most important fact to ascertain is the presence and extent of intracranial hypertension, or elevated ICP, and this should be assumed until information proves otherwise. This information can be obtained most readily from the history and physical examination, computed tomography (CT) and magnetic resonance imaging (MRI) scans, and ICP measurements (if available). Patients with elevated ICP may complain of headaches, dizziness, visual or gait disturbances, nausea or vomiting, and seizures. On physical examination, such patients may exhibit abnormalities such as papilledema, loss of strength or sensation, and cranial nerve dysfunction. CT or MRI of the brain are generally most helpful in quantifying the degree of ICP derangement, with slit ventricles and a midline shift >5 mm indicating advanced pathology. Lastly, a careful evaluation of laboratory values may demonstrate electrolyte disturbances, which can be due to pituitary pathology (eg, ***syndrome of inappropriate antidiuretic hormone [SIADH]*** secretion), diuretics, or anticonvulsants being taken by the patient.

> **? *Did You Know?***
>
> CT or MRI of the brain is generally most helpful in quantifying the degree of ICP derangement.

In patients with elevated ICP, sedative or anxiolytic premedication must be carefully titrated or avoided completely. Benzodiazepines and opioids, even in small doses, can depress respiration, leading to elevated $Paco_2$ and subsequent brain herniation. On the other hand, steroids (eg, dexamethasone) and anticonvulsants should be continued preoperatively.

Preoperative evaluation of patients presenting for spine surgery, especially in the acute setting, should focus on (1) the level of injury, (2) the degree of neurologic impairment (complete vs incomplete), (3) the timing of injury (less or more than 8 hours), (4) the complete neurologic examination, (5) current hemodynamic conditions, and (6) the airway examination. Carefully planning endotracheal intubation and subsequent hemodynamic management of these patients is vital. Advanced airway techniques (eg, awake fiberoptic intubation) and critical blood or fluid management with concomitant vasopressor use (eg, during spinal shock) may be required.

> **? *Did You Know?***
>
> ICP can be best controlled during induction of anesthesia by using a generous dose of opioid and intravenous lidocaine (1.5 mg/kg) prior to the induction drug to blunt the sympathetic response to laryngoscopy, while simultaneously ensuring eucapnia.

B. Induction of Anesthesia and Airway Management

Proper induction of anesthesia and airway management are critically important in neuroanesthesia, especially in those patients who have elevated ICP and unsecured aneurysm or cervical spinal cord injury. Elevated ICP demands constant attention during induction and intubation; ICP must be controlled, while CPP must be maintained. To that end, anesthetic induction of patients with elevated ICP should be slow and controlled, with constant attention to the blood pressure throughout the process. In many cases, preinduction arterial catheterization, osmotic diuresis, and CSF drainage are helpful. Patients with elevated ICP should receive a generous dose of opioid and intravenous lidocaine (1.5 mg/kg) prior to the induction drug to blunt the sympathetic response to laryngoscopy, at the same time maintaining normo- to hyperventilation to ensure eucapnia. Following induction and muscle relaxation, hyperventilation by mask should be performed in anticipation of the period of apnea that will accompany the intubation attempt. During intubation, strict control of blood pressure is important, as a rapid increase in arterial blood pressure will worsen ICP, while hypotension and decreased CPP would also be detrimental. In the case of a cervical spinal cord injury, maintenance of MAP is important during induction, while the actual performance of intubation may require more complex techniques (eg, awake fiberoptic intubation, midline stabilization, etc) to ensure that the spinal cord is not further compromised.

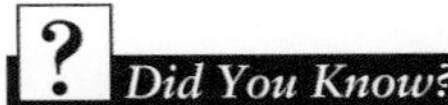

Until the dura is open, strict control of blood pressure and ICP is important, as a rapid increase in arterial blood pressure will worsen ICP, while hypotension will decrease CPP—both of which are detrimental.

C. Maintenance of Anesthesia

The maintenance of anesthesia in neurosurgical patients requires regimens that vary depending on the hemodynamic and monitoring goals for that procedure. Generally speaking, for intracranial surgeries, ICP control is paramount until the dura is opened. To this end, once Mayfield fixation of the head and positioning are safely completed, mannitol (0.5-1.5 g/kg) is administered, as are steroids (eg, dexamethasone 10-20 mg) and, in some cases, a prophylactic anticonvulsant. Anesthetic regimen depends on the ICP and whether neuromonitoring is being employed. For patients with elevated ICP, volatile anesthetics are often limited to 0.5 minimum alveolar concentration (MAC) to minimize the degree of cerebral vasodilation and inhibition of autoregulation that they cause. Half-MAC volatile anesthesia is supplemented with intravenous agents such as propofol or opioid by infusion. This regimen works well in neuromonitoring cases also, where >0.5 MAC of volatile agent may interfere with SSEP and MEP monitoring (MEP is more sensitive than SSEP). Muscle relaxants are generally used, unless they are limited by the MEP monitoring. Nitrous oxide is generally avoided because of its mild vasodilating effects, potential for expanding pneumocephalus, and unfavorable effects on neuromonitoring. Throughout the procedure, CPP must be maintained (often requiring a vasopressor). Because CBF autoregulation is greatly inhibited due to the disease process or the anesthetic, CBF will be directly dependent on MAP (or CPP). In cases of acute spinal cord injury, many of the same principles apply regarding maintenance of anesthesia, as spinal cord perfusion (especially in cervical spine surgery) and the ability to perform neuromonitoring are of great concern.

D. Ventilation Management

Ventilatory management of patients undergoing neurosurgery is also a key consideration. For patients undergoing an intracranial procedure, tidal volume should be maintained at 6 to 8 mL/kg (ie, lung-protective strategy) to minimize potential inflammatory injury to the lungs, with peak pressures kept at <30 cm H_2O. These principles hold especially true for patients with subarachnoid hemorrhage, who may already exhibit acute lung injury or adult respiratory distress syndrome. Positive end-expiratory pressure (PEEP) should be avoided unless needed to improve oxygenation, as it increases intrathoracic pressure and may impede cerebral venous drainage. Positive pressure ventilation is generally used for neurosurgical procedures, as it allows direct control of $Paco_2$. Positive pressure ventilation is especially beneficial during sitting craniotomies, where negative intrathoracic pressure that would occur during a spontaneous breath may contribute to the development of venous air embolism.

E. Fluids and Electrolytes

For many years, fluid maintenance during craniotomy was aimed to keep the patient "dry," so as to minimize the amount of reactive cerebral edema both during the surgery and postoperatively. This strategy is generally no longer considered optimal, as it is now known that the primary goal of fluid management in these cases should be to maintain cerebral perfusion, which is a more important consideration and will actually lessen cerebral edema. Hence, the goal of fluid management should be to keep the patient euvolemic at all times. Isotonic solutions should always be used (eg, 0.9% normal saline), as hypotonic solutions (eg, 0.45% half normal saline) in greater amounts can contribute to cerebral edema. Glucose-containing solutions are avoided, as hyperglycemia is detrimental to cerebral metabolism (see above), and because glucose is quickly metabolized and not osmotically active, leaving hypotonic free water, which can worsen edema.

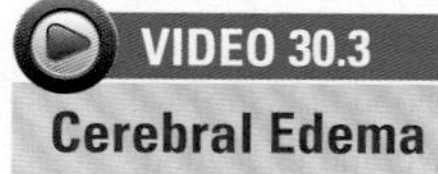

Depending on patient comorbidities and length of the surgery, electrolyte derangements may be common and require close monitoring. Certainly, patients with pre- or intraoperative SIADH or ***diabetes insipidus (DI)*** will require careful monitoring of electrolytes. Hypertonic saline (3%) supplementation (given slowly to prevent central pontine myelinolysis) may also be needed. ***Mannitol***, especially at large doses, can cause mild electrolyte derangements, which are generally short lived (eg, hyponatremia, hyperkalemia). These should be monitored as well. Given in large amounts, 0.9% normal saline can cause hyperchloremic metabolic acidosis, and care should be taken to avoid this.

F. Transfusion Therapy

The transfusion of blood and blood products is often needed during neurosurgical procedures. Preoperatively, coagulation studies should be noted. Anticoagulants should be discontinued in consultation with the physician prescribing anticoagulation. Neurosurgical patients having nonemergency surgery should have a platelet count >100,000/mm^3. Red blood cells that have been typed and crossed should be available for most craniotomies, especially for neurovascular procedures (eg, aneurysm clipping, arteriovenous malformation [AVM] resection) or for resection of tumors that invade the cranial sinuses. Coagulopathies may develop with the release of brain tissue thromboplastin. These should be treated with fresh frozen plasma, platelets, or cryoprecipitate as needed. Complex spine surgery (especially with planned osteotomies or due to tumor) is usually associated with more profound blood loss and transfusion therapy. In these cases, multiple units of blood products should be immediately available and close, repeated monitoring of the hemoglobin level and coagulation studies should be performed.

G. Glucose Management

As discussed previously, glucose management is very important in neurosurgical cases, with the desire to avoid both hypo- and hyperglycemia. Some have advocated for "tight glucose control," in which the range of acceptable serum glucose perioperatively is very narrow (eg, 90-120 mg/dL) and tightly controlled with insulin. Others disagree with such intensive glucose control, arguing that the incidence of hypoglycemia is increased with such a strategy. In any case, most neuroanesthesiologists agree that serum glucose during neurosurgical procedures should be maintained in the 90 to 180 mg/dL range. For hyperglycemia exceeding this range, regular insulin should be readily available and can be given intravenously as a bolus with or without an infusion. In these cases, monitoring of serum glucose must be frequent enough to capture episodes of hypoglycemia. In cases of hypoglycemia, dextrose (eg, dextrose 50% in water) should be administered in 20 to 50 mL doses depending on the degree of hypoglycemia.

H. Emergence

Emergence from anesthesia after neurosurgical procedures requires meticulous attention to maintaining stable hemodynamic and ventilatory parameters, yet ensuring a patient is sufficiently responsive as to allow neurologic examination immediately after the operation. Postcraniotomy hypertension is a well-described, albeit poorly understood, phenomenon, but can certainly be detrimental as it may increase cerebral bleeding from the resection bed and worsen cerebral edema. Careful analgesia (so as not to obtund the patient postoperatively) is helpful in controlling this hypertension, but usually antihypertensive medications are required as well (eg, labetalol, nicardipine). Patients emerging from cerebral AVM resection are particularly vulnerable because the resection bed is more likely to bleed. Patients having undergone posterior fossa surgery, who may also have brainstem compromise, may emerge more slowly and the time to safe extubation may be prolonged. Coughing on emergence should be avoided for all patients because it increases the risk of bleeding and elevation in ICP. A low-dose opioid infusion or intravenous lidocaine may be helpful in this regard. Likewise, postoperative nausea and vomiting should be prophylactically treated in these cases for the same reasons.

> **? Did You Know?**
>
> Postcraniotomy hypertension is detrimental because it may increase cerebral bleeding from the resection bed and worsen cerebral edema.

> **? Did You Know?**
>
> Coughing on emergence should be avoided for all patients because it increases the risk of bleeding and elevation in ICP.

VIII. Common Surgical Procedures

A. Surgery for Tumors

Neurosurgery is commonly performed to remove tumors, both benign and malignant, that emanate from or spread to the CNS or PNS. Common primary tumors include meningiomas, astrocytomas, glioblastomas, schwannomas, and oligodendrogliomas, whereas metastatic tumors may arise from various primary sites (eg, lung, breast, skin). Independent of their histology, the morbidity of brain tumors is associated with their size, rate of growth, and proximity to or invasion of nearby structures. Patients with dangerously elevated ICP preoperatively may require preoperative CSF drainage and intravenous glucocorticoids. Generally speaking, surgery for intracranial tumors can be safely accomplished with the induction and maintenance regimen mentioned above, as well as normo- or hyperventilation and adequate vascular access (usually two peripheral intravenous catheters and an arterial catheter). ICP and CPP are of great concern for these cases. An arterial catheter is very helpful in monitoring CPP closely while also allowing the titration of $Paco_2$ (by revealing its gradient with end-tidal carbon dioxide via arterial blood gas measurement). Usually, patients are extubated in the operating room at the conclusion of the case.

B. Pituitary Surgery

Although elevated ICP is of great importance for supratentorial and infratentorial masses, it is not usually a grave concern in pituitary surgery, as the sellar space usually has room to accommodate most tumors. Pituitary surgery is usually performed endoscopically and transnasally. Anesthetic concerns for pituitary surgery include optic chiasm compression (leading to cranial nerve III compression and classically a bitemporal hemianopsia), acromegaly, electrolyte and fluid disturbances caused by SIADH or DI, and inadvertent surgical trespass into the cavernous sinus or internal carotid artery. Patients with a sellar mass (usually a pituitary adenoma or a craniopharyngioma) may exhibit visual field defects. It is important to differentiate between organic and anesthetic causes of visual problems after surgery. Growth hormone–secreting tumors can commonly cause acromegaly, which is vitally important to the anesthesiologist as airway and hemodynamic management can be much more difficult. Despite an adequate oral opening, acromegalic patients tend to have an abundance of pharyngeal soft tissue and a small glottic opening, which may make mask ventilation and intubation challenging and may require a smaller-sized endotracheal tube and awake fiberoptic intubation. Furthermore, long-standing acromegalics are prone to cardiac rhythm disturbances and cardiomyopathies, and caution with cardiac depressant medications is warranted.

SIADH is common with sellar tumors due to compression of the posterior pituitary and an oversecretion of antidiuretic hormone (ADH), which may lead to intravascular volume overload and hyponatremia. Extracellular body water is usually normal, and edema or hypertension are usually not seen. Treatment of perioperative SIADH involves judicious water restriction, removing the underlying cause (the tumor), and demeclocycline (which is a long-acting inhibitor of ADH, but less helpful in the acute setting). Perioperatively, central DI is also occasionally seen (due to a lack of ADH secretion), the hallmark being a large, dilute urine output. Postoperative DI is usually short lived and can be treated with fluid restriction. Rarely is exogenous desmopressin needed.

Because accidental surgical entry into the cavernous sinus or internal carotid artery is a potential, albeit infrequent, complication of pituitary surgery, two intravenous catheters and an arterial catheter are recommended. Intraoperative hyperventilation is generally not used in pituitary surgery and may make the sellar structures more difficult to access endoscopically. Similarly, a lumbar subarachnoid catheter is sometimes placed before or after pituitary surgery, both to inject small amounts of sterile saline to facilitate surgical exposure and to drain CSF postoperatively to decrease CSF pressure where a dural sealant or fat graft has been used.

C. Cerebral Aneurysm Surgery and Endovascular Treatment

Anesthesia for ***cerebral aneurysm*** clipping requires stable blood pressure so as not to rupture the aneurysm prior to exposure, to maintain CPP, and to have a plan in place in the event of intraoperative rupture. The maintenance regimen should allow neuromonitoring that is used to detect regional ischemia. During exposure of the aneurysm, burst suppression on the EEG is often sought (**Figure 30.7**) to decrease the impending ischemic burden on the brain from temporary occlusion of large cerebral vessels. Additional vasopressor may be required during this time. Prior to direct clipping of the aneurysmal neck, the surgeon may place temporary clips to "soften" the neck and make it more amenable to direct clipping while minimizing the chances of rupture. Alternatively, when temporary clips are anatomically difficult to place, adenosine 0.3 to 0.4 mg/kg may be safely given as a bolus to cause transient circulatory arrest and profound hypotension, allowing safe permanent clip application.[9]

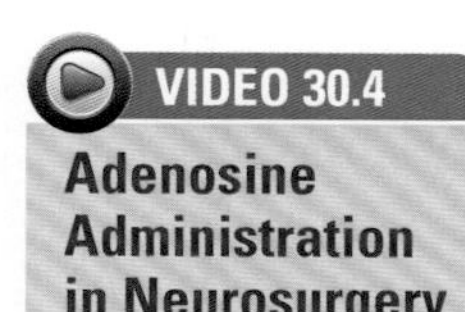

Inadvertent rupture is possible during dissection around the aneurysm. The plan for this must include the availability of blood products and adenosine for rescue. Thus, large bore intravenous access is required for these cases and central venous access is recommended. Arterial catheters are routinely used for aneurysm surgery.

The endovascular treatment of aneurysms involves femoral arterial access and coils deployed to the aneurysmal sac to cause thrombosis and eventual obliteration of the aneurysm. General anesthesia is used and movement should be prevented. An arterial catheter is needed to monitor the blood pressure

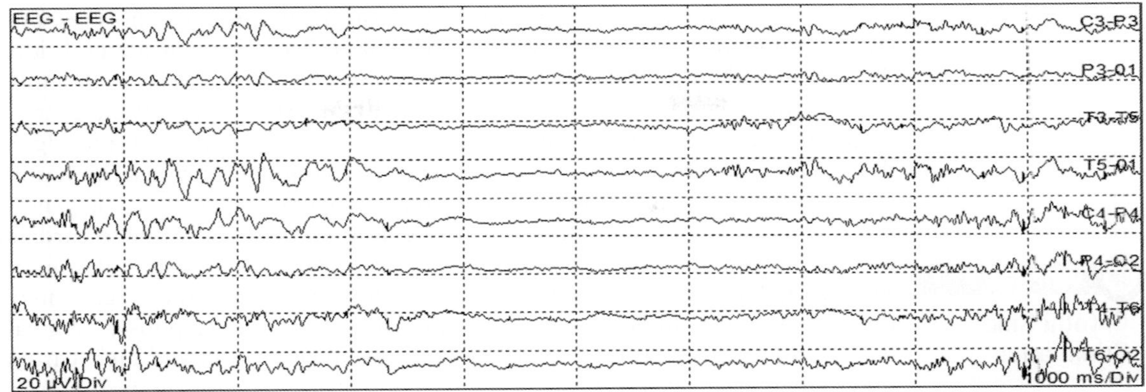

Figure 30.7 Burst-suppression electroencephalogram. Note the "burst" of electrical activity, followed by a period of "suppression," followed again by a "burst."

closely and to obtain blood samples for coagulation measurements at repeated intervals, as heparin is given periodically. The anesthesiologist should communicate very closely with the interventionalist throughout the procedure, as any extravasation of dye into the brain parenchyma may be indicative vascular rupture. Coils may embolize to other parts of the brain. Thus, prompt neurologic examination at the procedure's conclusion is important.

D. Arteriovenous Malformations

Cerebral AVMs are congenital abnormalities in which a plexus of arteries and "arterialized" veins are bunched together and may lead to cerebral hemorrhage, headaches, or seizures, usually between the ages of 10 and 40 years. These lesions may be embolized in the interventional radiology suite (preoperatively or curatively), radiated, or surgically removed. More than in any other intracranial neurosurgical procedure, vascular access is of great importance and a central venous catheter is highly recommended. The greatest risk of AVM resection is bleeding, both intraoperatively and postoperatively, and strict control of blood pressure is required to maintain CPP without worsening blood loss from the resection bed. Blood products should be immediately available, and vasodilators are very often needed, especially at emergence. The phenomenon of normal perfusion pressure breakthrough is a type of autoregulatory inhibition caused by the AVM and affecting the surrounding "normal" brain, in which previously normal cerebral vessels are maximally vasodilated due to long-standing "steal" caused by the AVM. After the AVM has been resected, these "vasoparalyzed" vessels are unable to constrict, leading to cerebral hyperemia, cerebral congestion, headache, and possibly worsened postoperative bleeding. Neuromonitoring is increasingly being used for cerebral AVM resections. Arterial catheterization and careful induction and intubation, as described with cerebral aneurysms, are standard.

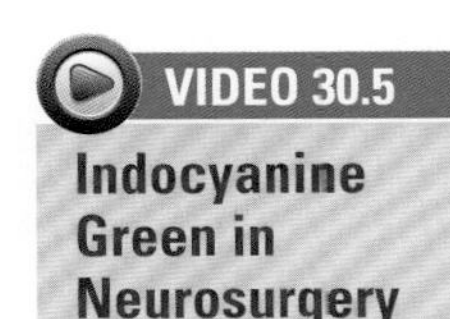

E. Carotid Surgery

Carotid endarterectomy is performed to remove carotid plaque that is ≥70% occlusive. It can be performed either awake (regional technique) or asleep (general anesthesia), with neither technique proven to be superior in terms of neurologic outcome. Awake carotid surgery usually involves a superficial and sometimes deep cervical plexus block, along with low-dose analgesia and

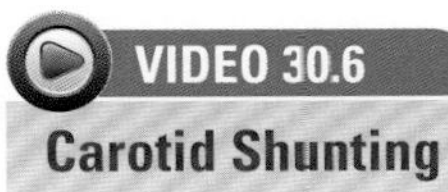

sedation (eg, remifentanil, propofol), while ensuring that the patient is responsive to commands and able to perform manual tasks on the contralateral side. Asleep carotid surgery employs general endotracheal anesthesia. Frequently some form of neuromonitoring is used (eg, EEG, SSEPs, cerebral oximetry), or the measurement of carotid stump pressure is performed (>50 mm Hg is desirable) to ensure adequate CBF during cross-clamping. In either case, arterial blood pressure monitoring is preferred, as operative morbidity is generally due to neurologic complications, while mortality is usually due to cardiac complications, and blood pressure control is critical. During manipulation of the carotid baroreceptor, bradycardia is not uncommon, and the surgeon may infiltrate the carotid sinus with lidocaine to prevent this response. Surgical denervation of the carotid baroreceptor causes hypertension and tachycardia upon emergence, which must be tightly controlled. Because cerebral vessels distal to the carotid have been maximally vasodilated for a long period of time, autoregulation is not intact and a "steal" phenomenon can occur in which cerebral hyperemia and bleeding can potentially occur. Beta-blockers are helpful in this regard. Lastly, the anesthesiologist must be keenly aware of the potential for a postoperative neck hematoma, which may quickly compromise the airway. Immediate intubation, which may be more difficult, and surgical exploration of the wound is required.

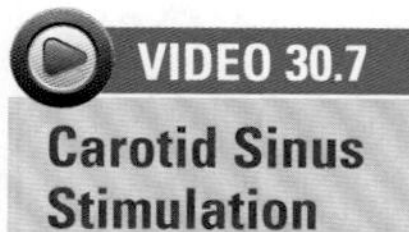

F. Epilepsy Surgery and Awake Craniotomy

Surgery for intractable epilepsy that is not responsive to medical management requires a keen understanding of the pharmacologic effects of both anesthetics and anticonvulsants. Anticonvulsants taken by the patient can induce liver enzymes to a great extent and generally cause a very high metabolism of muscle relaxants and opioids. This leads to a "resistance" to the effects of these drugs and the need for higher dosages. On the other hand, anesthetics have very mixed and variable excitatory and inhibitory effects on seizure activity, and if used improperly can be detrimental to seizure focus mapping. Generally speaking, benzodiazepines should be avoided when electrocorticography (ECoG) is planned. Induction of anesthesia with propofol, muscle relaxant, and opioid is acceptable. During maintenance of anesthesia and prior to ECoG, any anesthetic regimen that allows craniotomy is used, but 30 minutes prior to ECoG initiation, propofol infusion should be stopped and potent volatile anesthetic held to a minimum or stopped as well. To prevent awareness, scopolamine, nitrous oxide, and high-dose opioid infusion can be used with very little adverse effect on ECoG. In any case, the patient should be counseled about the possibility of intraoperative awareness. In some cases, methohexital or etomidate can be used to elicit seizure activity. Once ECoG is complete, a "routine" general anesthetic can be resumed during the resection.

Awake craniotomy has gained popularity in some institutions and is used in cases in which a cranial lesion lies adjacent to either "eloquent," motor, or sensory cortex. The advantage of awake craniotomy lies in its ability to allow speech, motor, or sensory mapping in real time, hence facilitating a subtotal resection of the tumor and avoiding the loss of these functions. The anesthesiologist must be attentive to the patient's analgesic, ventilatory, and emotional needs. Thus, constant communication with the patient is of paramount importance. Generally, an arterial catheter is placed and very light sedation or analgesia (eg, propofol, remifentanil, dexmedetomidine) is used. A selective scalp nerve block may be performed preoperatively, either unilaterally or bilaterally, blocking the six nerves on each side that innervate the scalp and dura mater. The brain itself has no pain or sensory receptors, so only the scalp and dura require anesthesia.

G. Endovascular Therapy for Acute Ischemic Stroke

In cases of cerebrovascular accident (CVA) in which large-vessel occlusion has occurred because of thrombosis, endovascular therapy (ie, mechanical thrombectomy) is sometimes indicated to restore blood flow to the ischemic penumbra and avoid secondary cerebral damage. During this "brain attack," every moment is critical and every effort should be made to hasten the patient to the neurointerventional radiology suite, which may preclude a complete preoperative evaluation. In the setting of hypoxemia or an unprotected airway, general anesthesia with an endotracheal tube is indicated, whereas in a patient with adequate oxygenation and intact airway reflexes, Monitored Anesthesia Care may be preferred. With either anesthetic strategy, meticulous hemodynamic control is paramount, as most randomized, prospective studies have shown that functional neurologic outcome can be influenced by tight blood pressure control rather than by the anesthetic technique used. In this regard, an arterial catheter, placed rapidly or accessed by the proceduralist during groin access, is recommended whenever possible or feasible.

Prior to reperfusion (recanalization), higher systolic blood pressures should be maintained (140-180 mm Hg), which may require vasopressor support, especially in the setting of a greater depth of anesthesia. After recanalization has occurred, the blood pressure can be liberalized to a level of 120 to 140 mm Hg. Close communication with the proceduralist, with a clear consensus on hemodynamic goals, is critical throughout the procedure and into the postprocedure recovery phase.[10] As with other neuroendovascular procedures (eg, aneurysm coiling, AVM embolization), protamine should be immediately available to reverse a heparin effect should arterial perforation occur. Protamine is generally not indicated for routine reversal of heparin in these cases.

IX. Anesthesia and Traumatic Brain Injury

A. Overview of Traumatic Brain Injury

Traumatic brain injury is often associated with other trauma (eg, thoracic, abdominal, and orthopedic injuries) and is a common cause of death and disability in young people. Death following traumatic brain injury is often associated with secondary insults, which emergency and anesthetic management are designed to minimize. Patients presenting with traumatic brain injury are graded according to the ***Glasgow coma scale (GCS)*** on presentation (score of 3-15) and are intubated when GCS is 8 or less, as this corresponds to 35% mortality (**Table 30.2**). Noncontrast CT scan that shows midline shift >5 mm or absent ventricles should also lead to immediate intubation, as ICP is very high in these cases and ventilation must be controlled. ICP monitoring is frequently used in these cases and can be instituted in the emergency department by an external ventricular drain, where mannitol, hyperventilation, and propofol are used to control elevated ICP. Operative management is normally indicated for depressed skull fractures and expanding brain bleeding, including subdural and epidural hematomas.

Table 30.2 Glasgow Coma Scale

	1	2	3	4	5	6
Eye	Does not open	Opens to painful stimulus	Opens to voice	Opens spontaneously	NA	NA
Verbal	Makes no sound	Incomprehensible sound	Inappropriate words	Disoriented, confused	Normal speech	NA
Motor	Makes no movement	Extension to painful stimulus (decerebrate movement)	Flexion to painful stimulus (decorticate movement)	Withdrawal to painful stimulus	Localizes to painful stimulus	Follows commands

NA, not applicable.
Note that the lowest attainable score is 3 and the highest is 15.

B. Anesthetic Management

Patients presenting with traumatic brain injury are assumed to have concomitant cervical spine injury, and the plan for intubation must take this into account. Hypoxemia is common, which may be further exacerbated by pulmonary injury. Induction doses of anesthetics must be tailored so as to avoid worsening systemic hypotension. Succinylcholine is controversial in the face of a closed head injury, as it may raise ICP transiently. But most anesthesiologists would use it to facilitate securing the airway in a rapid and predictable fashion. Nasal intubation is contraindicated if a basilar skull fracture is present or suspected. Once the airway is secured, attention must be paid to hemodynamics, as systolic blood pressure <80 mm Hg is associated with a worse neurologic outcome. Fluid resuscitation and vasopressors are needed to ensure an adequate systemic and cerebral perfusion pressure. Intravascular access should include an arterial catheter and large-bore intravenous cannulae, if not a central venous line. Anesthetic maintenance hinges on a good understanding of ICP management (see above), with intravenous agents and inhalational agents used in balance to avoid excessive cerebral vasodilation. Additional mannitol may be given, but hyperventilation should not continue beyond 2 to 6 hours, as normalization of the pH in the CSF begins to occur and its effect is only to decrease cerebral perfusion. Of note, the release of brain tissue thromboplastin may lead to disseminated intravascular coagulation, and coagulopathy must be aggressively sought and treated. Likewise, neurogenic pulmonary edema may be present, and a "lung-protective strategy" using PEEP and low tidal volumes may be needed to maintain oxygenation. Extubation at the conclusion of surgery depends on the degree of ICP elevation and the severity of injury, with most of these patients being admitted to the neurointensive care unit intubated and sedated.

X. Anesthesia for Spine Trauma and Complex Spine Surgery

A. Spinal Cord Injury

Acute spinal cord injury often necessitates emergency surgery to stabilize the spinal column and prevent secondary injury. Spinal cord injuries, like traumatic brain injuries, often involve young people, and may be due to motor vehicle accidents, falls, violence, or sports-related accidents. Cervical spine injuries are most common, as this is the most mobile part of the spine, followed by thoracic and lumbar injuries. Incomplete tetraplegia (C3-5) is the most common neurologic outcome, followed by complete paraplegia (T1 and below), complete tetraplegia, and incomplete paraplegia. Cervical injuries are the most devastating from a neurologic perspective, as high cervical injuries may impair vital respiratory function (C3-5) necessitating permanent tracheotomy and ventilator support and cardiac accelerator function (T1-5). Following acute spinal cord injury, spinal cord autoregulation is impaired and "spinal shock" may be seen, characterized by flaccid paralysis and decreased spinal cord perfusion, lasting 24 hours. During this time, it is critical to prevent secondary injury by providing aggressive hemodynamic support.

B. Comorbid Injuries

Up to 42% of patients presenting with acute spinal cord injury may also have a concomitant injury. Life-threatening injuries must be addressed, while ensuring that spinal alignment is maintained to avoid adding secondary injury to the spinal cord.

C. Initial Management

Patients presenting with acute spinal cord injury must be immediately evaluated for compromised ventilatory and hemodynamic function. Airway management in cervical spinal injury focuses on maintaining in-line stabilization throughout the intubation process, and may require the use of fiberoptic intubation. In a stable patient, radiographic studies are helpful in assessing the degree of cervical injury and options for intubation. Succinylcholine is safe in the initial 24 hours following spinal cord injury. Extrajunctional nicotinic receptors, which may cause a hyperkalemic response, have not yet fully developed. Fluid or blood product resuscitation and vasopressors or inotropes are often needed to support the blood pressure, which is important both from a systemic standpoint and to prevent secondary injury in the spinal cord due to ischemia and worsening edema due to cellular dysfunction. Arterial blood pressure monitoring and large-bore intravenous access are required. Other strategies to protect the spinal cord, such as corticosteroids, naloxone, or hypothermia, may be instituted at this time, but convincing data for these therapies are lacking. Most anesthesiologists will, however, maintain the mean arterial pressure above 85 mm Hg to ensure adequate spinal cord perfusion (recommended for at least 7 days from the date of injury).

D. Intraoperative Management

Anesthetic choice during maintenance of anesthesia for spinal cord injury should focus on two key considerations: maintaining blood pressure (mean > 85 mm Hg) and allowing for intraoperative neuromonitoring (SSEPs, MEPs, EMG). Complex spine surgery, which often involves multiple level fusions and osteotomies, should also take into account the real possibility of significant (sometimes multiple blood volumes) surgical bleeding and the need for postoperative mechanical ventilation in light of massive transfusion. Adequate intravascular access is vitally important. Measurements of arterial blood gas, coagulation parameters, and hemoglobin levels should be performed frequently. Close communication with the surgeon is important. In noninfectious, nontumor cases, intraoperative cell salvage can be quite helpful in reducing the total amount of allogeneic blood transfused. Other blood-sparing techniques, such as acute normovolemic hemodilution and deliberate hypotension, have largely fallen out of favor, due to the known harmful effects of anemia and hypotension on the neurologic and cardiovascular systems.

E. Complications of Anesthesia for Spine Surgery

Fortunately, complications specifically related to anesthesia for spine surgery are rare, but they are often devastating when they occur. ***Postoperative visual loss (POVL)*** is one such complication, with an incidence of 0.3% after spine surgery.[11] Most cases of POVL are thought to be due to posterior ischemic optic neuropathy, with central retinal artery occlusion and cortical blindness being much less common. Risk factors for POVL (associated but not necessarily causative) include hypotension, anemia, blood loss >1000 mL, surgical duration >6 hours, and the prone position itself which causes increased intraocular pressure. Ophthalmologic consultation should be immediately undertaken if this complication is suspected. Another complication of spine surgery in which anesthetic technique may be implicated is anterior spinal artery syndrome, which is caused by a sustained hypoperfusion of the anterior spinal artery and leads to motor weakness. Finally, deliberate hypotension, hypothermia, and hypovolemia may predispose spine surgery patients to the formation of deep venous thromboses (DVT) and subsequent pulmonary emboli (PE). Lumbar fusion is associated with an incidence of symptomatic DVT of up to 4%, with a 2% incidence of PE. Because prophylaxis with an anticoagulant is often impossible prior to spine surgery (for fear of worsening blood loss and formation of epidural hematoma), an inferior vena cava filter is often placed prior to these surgeries to minimize the chance of developing a significant PE.

For further review, please see the associated Interactive Video Lectures accessible in complimentary eBook bundled with this text. Access instructions are located on the inside front cover.

References

1. Isley MR, Edmonds Jr HL, Stecker M; American Society of Neurophysiological Monitoring. Guidelines for intraoperative neuromonitoring using raw (analog or digital waveforms) and quantitative electroencephalography: a position statement by the American Society of Neurophysiological Monitoring. *J Clin Monit Comput.* 2009;23(6):369-390.
2. Sloan TB, Heyer EJ. Anesthesia for intraoperative neurophysiologic monitoring of the spinal cord. *J Clin Neurophysiol.* 2002;19(5):430-443.
3. Chan MTV, Hedrick TL, Egan TD, et al; Perioperative Quality Initiative (POQI) 6 Workgroup. American society for enhanced recovery and perioperative quality initiative joint consensus statement on the role of neuromonitoring in perioperative outcomes: electroencephalography. *Anesth Analg.* 2020;130(5):1278-1291.
4. Kalanuria A, Nyquist PA, Armonda RA, et al. Use of transcranial Doppler (TCD) ultrasound in the neurocritical care unit. *Neurosurg Clin.* 2013;24(3):441-456.
5. Kitagawa R, Yokobori S, Mazzeo AT, et al. Microdialysis in the neurocritical care unit. *Neurosurg Clin.* 2013;24(3):417-426.
6. Ghosh A, Elwell C, Smith M. Cerebral near-infrared spectroscopy in adults: a work in progress. *Anesth Analg.* 2012;115(6):1373-1383.
7. Todd MM, Hindman BJ, Clarke WR, et al; Intraoperative Hypothermia for Aneurysm Surgery Trial (IHAST) Investigators. Mild intraoperative hypothermia during surgery for intracranial aneurysm. *N Engl J Med.* 2005;352(2):135-145.
8. Pasternak JJ, McGregor DG, Schroeder DR, et al; IHAST Investigators. Hyperglycemia in patients undergoing cerebral aneurysm surgery: its association with long-term gross neurologic and neuropsychological function. *Mayo Clin Proc.* 2008;83(4):406-417.

9. Bebawy JF, Gupta DK, Bendok BR, et al. Adenosine-induced flow arrest to facilitate intracranial aneurysm clip ligation: dose-response data and safety profile. *Anesth Analg.* 2010;110(5):1406-1411.
10. Talke PO, Sharma D, Heyer EJ, Bergese SD, Blackham KA, Stevens RD. Society for neuroscience in anesthesiology and critical care expert consensus statement: anesthetic management of endovascular treatment for acute ischemic stroke*. Endorsed by the society of NeuroInterventional surgery and the neurocritical care society. *J Neurosurg Anesthesiol.* 2014;26(2):95-108.
11. American Society of Anesthesiologists Task Force on Perioperative Visual Loss. Practice advisory for perioperative visual loss associated with spine surgery: an updated report by the American Society of Anesthesiologists Task Force on Perioperative Visual Loss. *Anesthesiology.* 2012;116(2):274-285.

Questions

1. **Cerebral perfusion pressure is calculated as the difference between:**

   A. Cerebral blood flow and cerebral vascular resistance.
   B. Mean arterial pressure and intracranial pressure.
   C. Central venous pressure and intracranial pressure.
   D. Diastolic blood pressure and intracranial pressure.

2. **Autoregulation in the brain within a range of blood pressure is responsible for maintaining:**

   A. Intracranial pressure.
   B. Cerebral perfusion pressure.
   C. Cerebral blood flow.
   D. Cerebrovascular resistance.

3. **Cerebral blood flow is not directly controlled by which of the following physiologic parameters?**

   A. pH
   B. $Paco_2$
   C. MAP (mean arterial pressure)
   D. $CMRO_2$ (cerebral metabolic rate of oxygen consumption)

4. **Cerebral protection for global ischemia in humans is known to occur with which of the following?**

   A. Steroids
   B. Mild hypothermia
   C. Barbiturates
   D. None of the above

5. **Neuromuscular-blocking agents may limit the success of which of the following neuromonitoring modalities?**

   A. Somatosensory-evoked potentials (SSEPs)
   B. Brainstem auditory-evoked potentials (BAEPs)
   C. Visual-evoked potentials (VEPs)
   D. Electromyography (EMG)

Answers

1. B

The cerebral perfusion pressure, the mean blood pressure which exists within the major vessels of the cerebral circulation (ie, the Circle of Willis), is a function of the systemic mean arterial pressure less the pressure exerted "against" these vessels externally, namely the intracranial pressure (or the central venous pressure, which is a postcapillary impediment to forward flow, if that is higher). Cerebral vascular resistance, systolic blood pressure, and diastolic blood pressure exert their effects on cerebral perfusion pressure indirectly, by affecting the mean arterial pressure in the brain, but do not determine the cerebral perfusion pressure in a direct way.

2. C

While many physiologic parameters are tightly regulated by the brain to maintain homeostasis, the term "autoregulation" refers specifically to the neuronal mechanisms which maintain the cerebral blood flow at a constant level throughout a range of blood pressure. Intracranial pressure is kept normal by its own compensatory mechanisms (involving cerebrospinal fluid diversion and shifting of cerebral water content and blood volume). Cerebral perfusion pressure is dependent on mean arterial pressure (see Question 1 above). Cerebrovascular resistance is a dynamic parameter which depends on chemical and pressure-related changes to determine vascular tone within the brain, contributing to the vasodilation and vasoconstriction needed to maintain cerebral blood flow autoregulation with fluctuating blood pressure.

3. A

Carbon dioxide tension, mean arterial pressure, and cerebral metabolic demand all have a direct effect on cerebral blood flow. The extracellular pH, however, does not affect cerebral blood flow directly. It does, however, exert a profound effect in the respiratory centers of the brain (medulla and pons), which is the basis for the ventilatory changes which govern the maintenance of pH homeostasis via acid-base balance.

4. D

While steroids, hypothermia, and anesthetics of various types have shown varying degrees of promise in preclinical and animal models of global ischemic injury, no single agent has been proven definitively to afford global ischemic protection in humans.

5. D

SSEP signals are not diminished by neuromuscular-blocking agents, since they reflect the integrity of the sensory pathways alone, and may in some cases be enhanced by the administration of neuromuscular-blocking agents (because of the removal of EMG artifact). Likewise, BAEPs and VEPs are not affected at all by muscle relaxants, as they do not rely on any motor components. Only EMG can be affected by neuromuscular-blocking agents, as the blocking of neuromuscular transmission at the nicotinic motor end plate can, in varying degrees, abolish the muscular response to nerve stimulation.

31 Obstetrical Anesthesia

Chad T. Dean and Barbara M. Scavone

I. Physiologic Changes of Pregnancy

Pregnancy induces many ***physiologic changes***, most of which are adaptations to support blood flow and oxygen delivery to the fetus.

> **? Did You Know?**
>
> The anemia of pregnancy is caused by a disproportionate increase in plasma volume relative to red cell volume.

A. Hematologic Changes

Blood volume increases by 40% to approximately 100 mL/kg; plasma volume increases by 40% to 50% and red blood cell volume by 20% to 30%, causing a physiologic ***anemia of pregnancy*** (**Table 31.1**). Blood viscosity is decreased, allowing easier flow to the fetus. Normal hemoglobin range during pregnancy is 10.5 to 14 g/dL and is lowest in the second trimester (**Table 31.2**).

Pregnancy is a prothrombotic state, and pregnant patients carry a greater risk of venous thromboembolism. Production of all clotting factors, except factors XI and XIII, increases. Fibrinogen levels significantly increase and are normally >400 mg/dL in the third trimester. A secondary fibrinolysis occurs later in pregnancy, and coagulation changes resemble a state of compensated disseminated intravascular coagulation (DIC). Platelet count may decrease during pregnancy due to dilution as well as increased consumption. Gestational thrombocytopenia is common, occurring in 8% of pregnancies, and is not associated with an increased risk of neuraxial hematoma.

Mild leukocytosis is normal during pregnancy. However, pregnancy is an immunosuppressed state, and pregnant patients do not tolerate the physiologic effects of systemic infection well, and mortality from sepsis is increased. In general, autoimmune diseases improve during pregnancy due to relative immunosuppression.

B. Cardiovascular Changes

Due to increased blood volume, stroke volume, and heart rate, cardiac output increases up to 50% by the end of the first trimester. During labor, cardiac output increases by another 50%, up to 80% over prelabor values immediately postpartum. Cardiovascular changes resolve several days postpartum. Systemic vascular resistance decreases, sometimes causing a mild decrease in blood pressure. Pregnant patients are less responsive to vasopressors and more sensitive to decreases in preload. After 20 weeks' gestation, pregnant patients may experience ***supine hypotension syndrome*** when lying flat, because the

Table 31.1 Summary of Physiologic Changes of Pregnancy at Term

Variable	Change	Amount
Plasma volume	↑	40%-50%
Total blood volume	↑	25%-40%
Hemoglobin	↓	10.5-14 g/dL
Fibrinogen	↑	100%
Serum cholinesterase activity	↓	20%-30%
Systemic vascular resistance	↓	50%
Cardiac output	↑	30%-50%
Systemic blood pressure	↓	Slight
Functional residual capacity	↓	20%-30%
Minute ventilation	↑	50%
Alveolar ventilation	↑	70%
Functional residual capacity	↓	20%
Oxygen consumption	↑	20%-50%
Carbon dioxide production	↑	35%
Arterial carbon dioxide partial pressure	↓	10 mm Hg
Arterial oxygen partial pressure	↑	10 mm Hg
Minimum alveolar concentration	↓	40%

Adapted from Braveman FR, Scavone BM, Blessing ME, Wong CA. Obstetrical anesthesia. In: Barash PG, Cahalan MK, Cullen BF, et al, eds. *Clinical Anesthesia*. 8th ed. Wolters Kluwer; 2018:1144-1177.

Table 31.2 Normal Lab Values in Pregnant Patients

Laboratory Value	Nonpregnant Female	First Trimester	Second Trimester	Third Trimester
Hemoglobin (g/dL)	12-16	11.5-14	9.7-15	10.5-14
Platelets (× 10^9/L)	160-420	180-400	155-420	145-420
WBC (× 10^3/mm^3)	3.5-9	6-14	5.5-15	6-17
Creatinine (mg/dL)	0.5-0.9	0.4-0.7	0.4-0.8	0.4-0.8
Fibrinogen (mg/dL)	230-490	245-500	290-540	400-620
pH	7.38-7.42			7.39-7.45
$Paco_2$ (mm Hg)[a]	38-42			28-32
Bicarbonate (mEq/L)	22-26			18-22
Pao_2 (mm Hg)[a]	90-100			92-107

[a]Blood gas values are arterial.

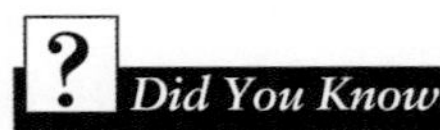

VIDEO 31.1

Left Uterine Displacement

gravid uterus can compress the inferior vena cava and decrease venous return. Therefore, left uterine displacement (LUD) is the preferred position for pregnant patients over 20 weeks' gestation.

Did You Know?

Left uterine displacement should be used for pregnant patients over 20 weeks' gestation to prevent compression of the inferior vena cava by the gravid uterus.

C. Respiratory Changes

Oxygen consumption increases by 20% to 50% and minute ventilation by 50% at term. Minute ventilation increases mainly due to an increase in tidal volume and to a lesser extent respiratory rate. This physiologic hyperventilation decreases arterial partial pressure of carbon dioxide ($Paco_2$) levels to 28 to 32 mm Hg and may cause a slight increase in arterial partial pressure of oxygen (Pao_2) levels. Compensatory metabolic acidosis occurs, bicarbonate levels are normally 18 to 22 mEq/L, and pH only slightly increases (7.45). Vital capacity and closing volume remain the same, but expiratory reserve volume and functional residual capacity decrease, making the pregnant patient quick to desaturate during periods of apnea, in particular in the supine position. A rightward shift in the hemoglobin-oxygen dissociation curve occurs, facilitating oxygen transfer to the fetus.

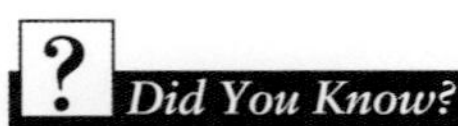

Did You Know?

The normal arterial partial pressure of carbon dioxide ($Paco_2$) during pregnancy is 28 to 32 mm Hg.

D. Airway Changes

Mucosal edema and capillary engorgement occur as pregnancy progresses, and Mallampati class increases at term. The incidence of difficult mask ventilation and laryngoscopy also increases, with difficult or failed intubation occurring in one of 224 pregnant patients versus one of 2500 in the general surgical population.[1] A longer second stage of labor and preeclampsia are both associated with increased ***airway edema***. Proper positioning and preoxygenation assume additional importance during induction of general anesthesia and intubation of pregnant versus nonpregnant patients (**Figure 31.1**).

Did You Know?

The incidence of difficult mask ventilation and laryngoscopy is greater in pregnant patients than in the general surgical population.

E. Gastrointestinal Changes

The gravid uterus causes ***mechanical gastroesophageal sphincter dysfunction***. Progesterone decreases lower esophageal sphincter tone, predisposing pregnant patients to reflux of stomach contents into the oropharynx. In addition, the gravid uterus increases abdominal pressure and, thus, intragastric pressure, furthering risk of reflux of stomach contents. Gastrin secretion by the placenta causes greater acidity of stomach contents. Finally, progesterone slows gastric emptying and gastrointestinal mobility. Pregnant women often have a gastric volume of over 25 mL with pH < 2.5, both of which are associated with aspiration pneumonitis syndrome. Administration of a nonparticulate antacid is the only reliable way to change gastric content pH and possibly reduce the chance of aspiration pneumonitis syndrome should aspiration occur.

F. Neurologic and Musculoskeletal Changes

Minimum alveolar concentration (MAC) decreases by 40% during pregnancy, possibly due to elevated progesterone levels, and returns to baseline by 1 week postpartum. Pregnant women are also more sensitive to neuraxial local anesthetics and require lower doses than nonpregnant patients. Epidural space volume is decreased due to epidural vein engorgement, and cerebrospinal fluid (CSF) pH is decreased. Ligamentous relaxation occurs, and lumbar lordosis is accentuated, raising the intercristal line from L4-5 in nonpregnant patients to L3-4 in pregnant patients.

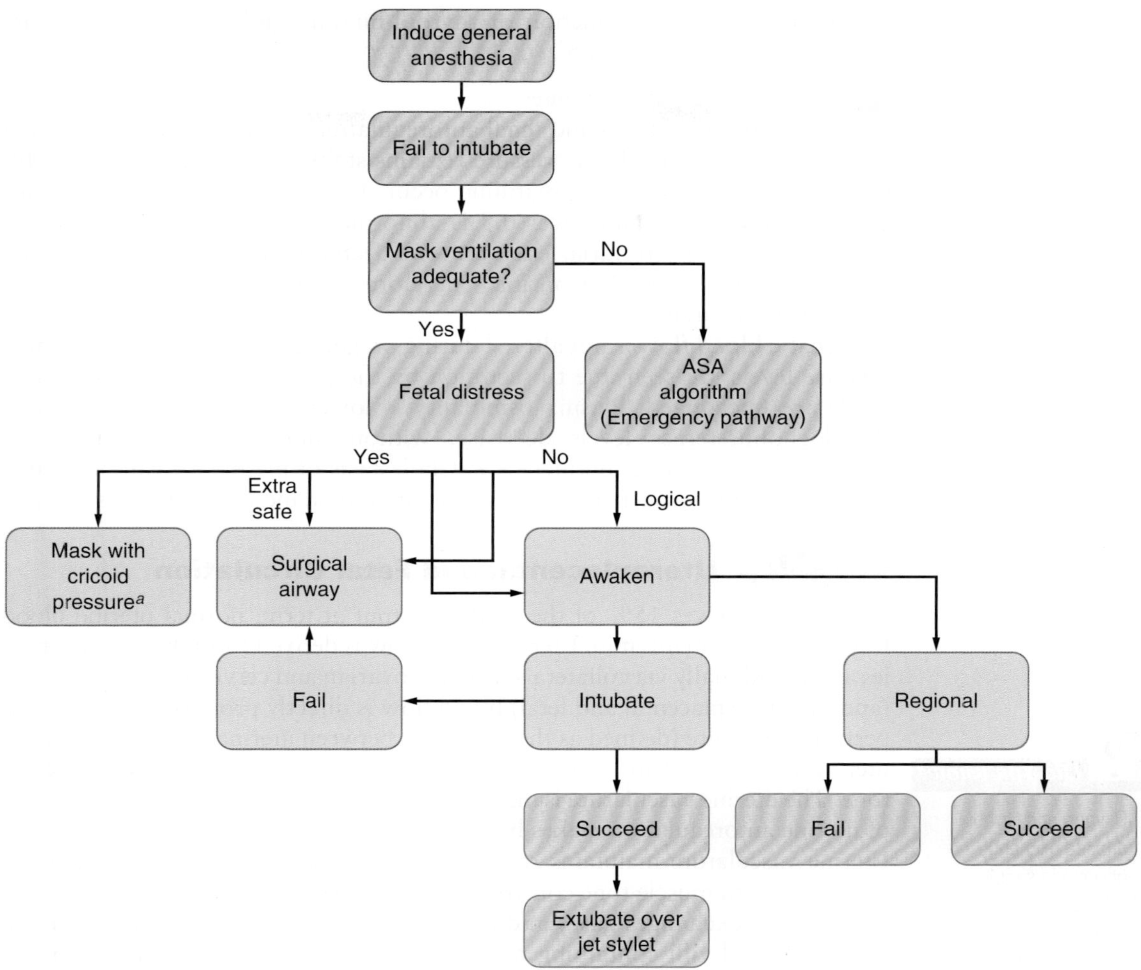

Figure 31.1 Management of the difficult airway in pregnancy with special reference to the presence or absence of fetal distress. When mask ventilation is not possible, the clinician is referred to the American Society of Anesthesiologists algorithm for the emergency airway management. [a]Conventional face mask or laryngeal mask airway. (Reprinted with permission from Kuczkowski KM, Reisner LS, Benumof JL. The difficult airway: risk, prophylaxis, and management. In: Chestnut DH, ed. *Obstetric Anesthesia: Principles and Practice*. 3rd ed. Elsevier-Mosby; 2004:550.)

G. Endocrine Changes

1. Glucose Control

Pregnancy is a diabetogenic state, due to human placental lactogen's anti-insulin effects. Routine screening for gestational diabetes is done via a carbohydrate load between 24 and 26 weeks. Women with gestational or pregestational diabetes are at greater risk for fetal macrosomia and pregnancy complications. Tight glucose control during labor is the standard of care for diabetic women, with goal blood sugar range between 80 and 110 mg/dL in order to avoid neonatal hypoglycemia.

2. Thyroid

Human chorionic gonadotropin is similar in structure to thyroid-stimulating hormone and causes thyroid hormone levels to increase during pregnancy.

Estrogen stimulates production of thyroid-binding globulin, allowing more thyroid hormone to circulate.

H. Renal and Hepatic Changes

Blood flow to the kidneys and renal autoregulation remains unchanged during pregnancy as long as blood pressure remains stable. Increased glomerular filtration rate and decreased creatinine occur due to increases in cardiac output, and serum creatinine over 0.8 is abnormal. Proteinuria is common, as is asymptomatic bacteriuria. Ureteral tone decreases and asymptomatic bacteriuria can lead to pyelonephritis. Therefore, urine is screened for infection during routine prenatal visits.

Hepatic blood flow is not altered during pregnancy. Elevated alkaline phosphatase levels are seen due to secretion by the placenta. Liver transaminase levels are unchanged. Plasma osmolality is lower, leading to tissue edema. Pseudocholinesterase levels decrease, without much clinical significance. Clotting factor production increases. Cholestasis of pregnancy can occur due to the effects of estrogen and causes pruritus and an increased risk of stillbirth.

II. Uteroplacental and Fetal Circulation

The uterus receives 15% of the cardiac output at term; normal uterine blood flow is 700 to 900 mL/min. Uterine blood flow is derived from the uterine arteries and additionally via collaterals from the ovarian and cervical arteries. Uterine (and therefore placental and fetal) blood flow is directly proportional to uterine perfusion pressure (defined as the difference between uterine arterial pressure vs uterine venous pressure), and inversely proportional to uterine artery vascular tone. The uterine vasculature is maximally vasodilated during pregnancy. A lack of uterine autoregulation makes blood flow proportional to perfusion pressure. Uterine vasculature maintains responsiveness to vasoconstrictors. Increases in uterine smooth muscle tone constrict uterine vessels, decreasing flow.

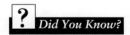

Oxygen and carbon dioxide exchange occurs via simple diffusion; higher maternal Pa_{O_2} favors diffusion to the fetus, and fetal carbon dioxide is higher than maternal carbon dioxide, favoring diffusion back to the mother.

? *Did You Know?*

Most anesthetic drugs cross the placenta, with the exception of paralyzing agents and glycopyrrolate. Heparin and insulin also do not cross the placenta. Most drugs that cross the blood-brain barrier also cross the placenta to the fetus.

The fetus exchanges gases and nutrients with the mother via the placenta. Fetal placental villi containing fetal capillaries are bathed in maternal blood supplied by the spiral arteries, which are branches of the uterine arteries. A normal umbilical cord has three vessels: one vein containing oxygenated blood from the placenta and two arteries carrying deoxygenated blood and waste back to the placenta. A number of mechanisms of transport from mother to fetus and back exist, including simple diffusion (most common, due to fetal or maternal concentration gradient), transcellular transfer, endocytosis, and exocytosis. Oxygen and carbon dioxide exchange occurs via simple diffusion; higher maternal Pa_{O_2} favors diffusion to the fetus, and fetal CO_2 is higher than maternal CO_2, favoring diffusion back to the mother.

Fetal hemoglobin has greater O_2 carrying capacity. The Bohr effect is more profound in the fetus because fetal hemoglobin encounters more hydrogen ions (H^+) in the fetus, which is relatively more acidotic than in the mother, and is more likely to release the O_2 it is carrying to fetal tissues. ***Fetal circulation*** differs from adult circulation in that it bypasses the lungs (**Figure 31.2**).

The majority of maternally administered drugs will reach the fetus via the placenta. The fetal/maternal ratio describes the concentration of drug in the fetal umbilical vein versus maternal serum concentration. Nonionized, nonprotein-bound, lipid-soluble drugs with molecular weights below 600 Da easily cross the placenta. Large, ionized, hydrophilic drugs are less likely to transfer. Most anesthetic drugs cross the placenta, with the exception of paralyzing

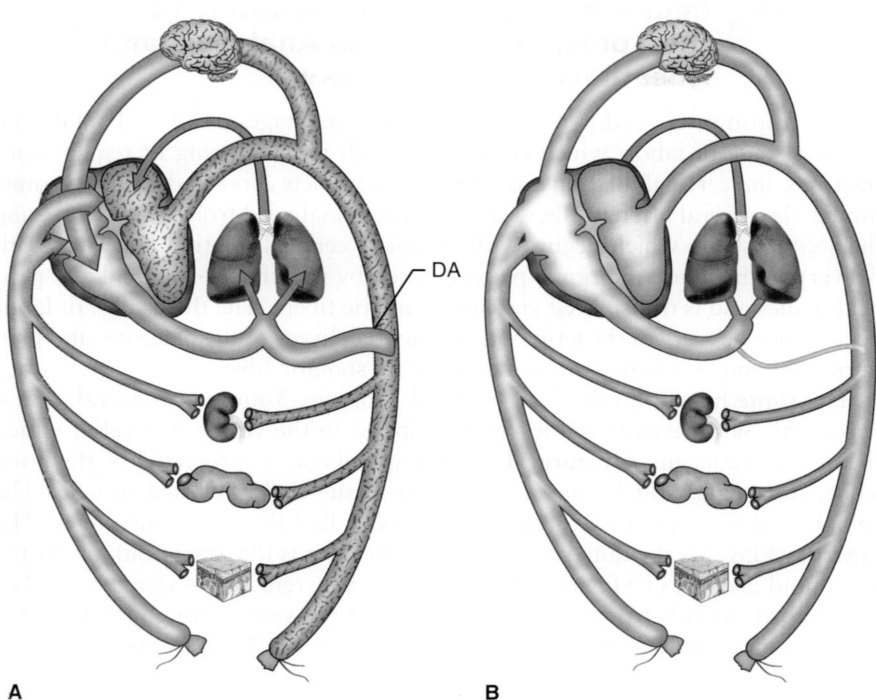

Figure 31.2 A, Schematic representation of the fetal circulation. Oxygenated blood leaves the placenta in the umbilical vein (*vessel without stippling*). Umbilical blood joins blood from the viscera (represented here by the kidney, gut, and skin) in the inferior vena cava. Approximately half of the inferior vena cava flow passes through the foramen ovale to the left atrium, where it mixes with a small amount of pulmonary venous blood. This relatively well-oxygenated blood (*light stippling*) supplies the heart and brain by way of the ascending aorta. The other half of the inferior vena cava stream mixes with superior vena cava blood and enters the right ventricle (blood in the right atrium and ventricle has little oxygen, which is denoted by *heavy stippling*). Because the pulmonary arterioles are constricted, most of the blood in the main pulmonary artery flows through the ductus arteriosus (DA) so the descending aorta's blood has less oxygen (*heavy stippling*) than does blood in the ascending aorta (*light stippling*). B, Schematic representation of the circulation in the normal newborn. After expansion of the lungs and ligation of the umbilical cord, pulmonary blood flow and left atrial and systemic arterial pressures increase. When left atrial pressure exceeds right atrial pressure, the foramen ovale closes so all inferior and superior vena cava blood leaves the right atrium, enters the right ventricle, and is pumped through the pulmonary artery toward the lung. With the increase in systemic arterial pressure and decrease in pulmonary artery pressure, flow through the ductus arteriosus becomes left to right, and the ductus constricts and closes. The course of circulation is the same as in the adult. (Redrawn from Phibbs R . Delivery room management of the newborn. In: Avery GB, ed. *Neonatology, Pathophysiology and Management of the Newborn*. 2nd ed. Philadelphia, PA: JB Lippincott; 1981:184.)

agents and glycopyrrolate. Heparin and insulin also do not cross the placenta. Transient fetal or neonatal depression can be seen after administration of induction agents, anesthetic gases, opioids, and benzodiazepines. The long-term effects of general anesthetic agents on neonatal outcome are unknown. Theoretically, nitrous oxide can interfere with DNA synthesis via oxidation of vitamin B_{12}. However, in animal studies only prolonged (>24 hours) exposure to high-concentration nitrous oxide produces fetal loss.

? Did You Know?

Pain during the first stage of labor, which commences with the beginning of regular contractions and cervical dilation and ends with complete cervical dilation, is transmitted via visceral afferent fibers entering the spinal cord from T10-L1.

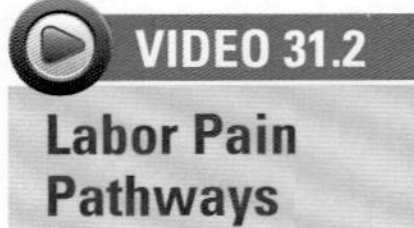

VIDEO 31.2

Labor Pain Pathways

III. Pain Pathways in Labor, Anatomy of the Spine, and Neuraxial Analgesia and Anesthesia

Pain is transmitted via different means in different stages of labor. Pain during the first stage of labor, which commences with the beginning of regular contractions and cervical dilation and ends with complete cervical dilation, is transmitted via visceral afferent fibers entering the spinal cord from T10-L1. During the second stage, which begins with complete cervical dilation and ends with delivery of the fetus, additional pain is caused by stretching of vaginal and perineal tissues and is transmitted via sacral somatic fibers. The third stage of labor begins after delivery of the fetus and ends with delivery of the placenta, and pain during this stage is also transmitted via sacral somatic fibers.

The ***spine*** has 33 levels: 7 cervical, 12 thoracic, 5 lumbar, 5 sacral, and 4 coccygeal. Skin dermatomal levels correspond to the vertebral level at which their nerve roots enter (**Figure 31.3**). The spinal cord is protected by the bony spine, ligaments, and layers of connective tissue and is bathed in CSF. The spinal cord is covered by three membranes, called the spinal meninges. The outermost layer is the dura mater, deep to the dura is the arachnoid, under the arachnoid layer lies CSF, and the pia mater is adherent to the spinal cord. The spinal cord extends from its inception off the brainstem through the foramen magnum and continues to L1 in most adults. About 10% of adults have spinal

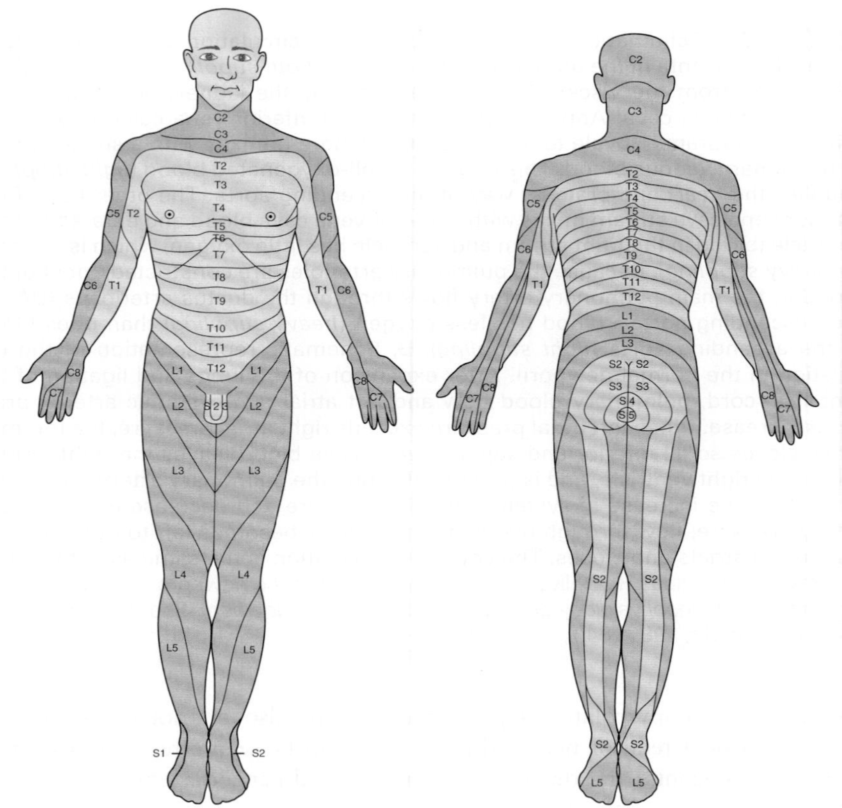

Figure 31.3 **Human sensory dermatomes.** (From Norris MC. Neuraxial anesthesia. In: Barash PG, Cahalan MK, Cullen BF, et al, eds. *Clinical Anesthesia*. 8th ed. Wolters Kluwer; 2018:914-944, Figure 35.9.)

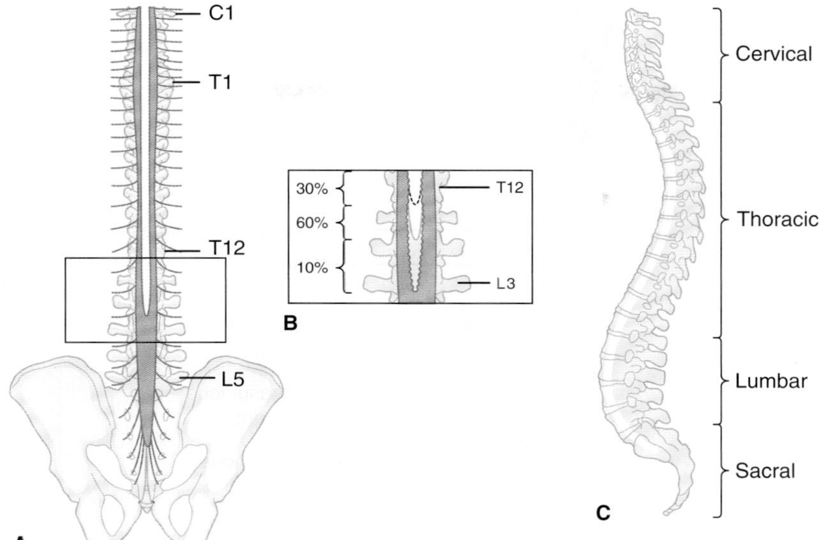

Figure 31.4 Posterior (A) and lateral (C) views of the human spinal column. Note the inset (B), which depicts the variability in vertebral level at which the spinal cord terminates. (From Bernards CM, Hostetter LS. Epidural and spinal anesthesia. In: Barash PG, Cullen BF, Stoelting RK, et al, eds. *Clinical Anesthesia.* 7th ed. Wolters Kluwer Health; 2013:905-933, Figure 34.1.)

cords that terminate lower, at L3. It is therefore prudent to perform neuraxial procedures below this level.

The spinal cord terminates as the cauda equina and the dural sac extends to S2. The epidural space spans from the foramen magnum to the sacral hiatus. It is a potential space and contains nerve roots, fat, valveless veins, lymphatics, and spinal arteries (**Figures 31.4** and **31.5**).

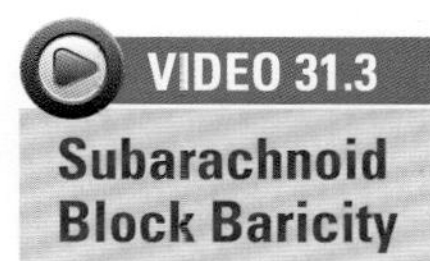

Neuraxially administered local anesthetics cause blockade of sympathetic, sensory, and motor input and, depending on the dose, can provide analgesia or complete anesthesia. Small, myelinated, rapidly firing, active nerve fibers are more sensitive to local anesthetic blockade than larger, unmyelinated fibers. Degree of blockade from highest to lowest after administration of neuraxial local anesthetic is as follows: temperature sensation, vasomotor tone, sensory, and finally motor. Spinal anesthesia occurs via direct action of local anesthetic on the spinal cord, and block level depends on several factors, of which baricity and dose are the most significant.

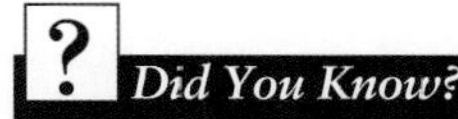

The goal of avoiding excessive motor blockade, while still providing adequate analgesia, is commonly accomplished by administering low-concentration (0.0625%-0.125% bupivacaine), high-volume, patient-controlled epidural anesthesia, with small amounts of opioid in the solutions.

Epidural anesthesia occurs via local anesthetic action on nerve roots and, to a lesser extent, has a direct effect on the spinal cord, via diffusion of local anesthetic into the intrathecal space. Usually 1 to 2 mL of epidural local anesthetic is required per lumbar dermatomal level requiring blockade.

Neuraxial labor analgesia provides excellent pain relief without effects on fetal or labor outcomes, with the exception of slightly increasing the length of the first and second stages of labor and the risk of instrumented vaginal delivery.[2] Avoiding excessive motor blockade, while still providing adequate analgesia, is ideal in labor. This goal is commonly accomplished by administering low-concentration (0.0625%-0.125% bupivacaine) high-volume, patient-controlled epidural anesthesia (PCEA), with small amounts of opioid in the solutions.

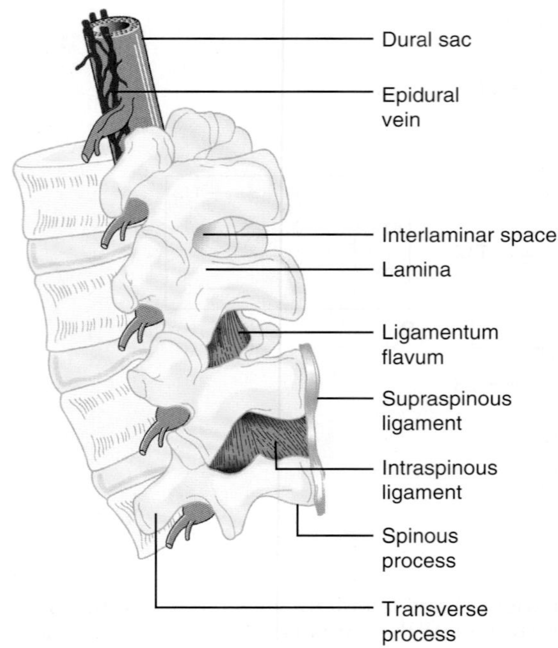

Figure 31.5 Detail of the lumbar spinal column and epidural space. Note that the epidural veins are largely restricted to the anterior and lateral epidural space. (From Bernards CM, Hostetter LS. Epidural and spinal anesthesia. In: Barash PG, Cullen BF, Stoelting RK, et al, eds. *Clinical Anesthesia*. 7th ed. Wolters Kluwer Health; 2013:905-933, Figure 34.2.)

After history, physical examination, and determination that the patient is a candidate for neuraxial anesthesia (**Table 31.3**), preparation for placement of a neuraxial block begins. A functioning intravenous line, resuscitation equipment, and blood pressure and heart rate monitoring are required, as are sterile precautions including hat, mask, hand hygiene, and sterile gloves.

The patient is placed in either the sitting or lateral decubitus position, and the desired lumbar level is identified by palpation of the iliac crests and spinous processes. Most neuraxial catheters for labor are placed between L2-3 and L5-S1. After sterilizing the back with an antiseptic and placing a sterile drape, the anesthesiologist places a skin wheal of local anesthesia at the intended needle placement site. Either a midline or paramedian approach to the epidural space is possible. Midline is more common and easier to perform

Table 31.3 Contraindications to Neuraxial Block
Patient refusal
Severe hypovolemia or shock
Coagulopathy
Condition in which hypotension is physiologically very undesirable (ie, right heart failure, severe aortic stenosis)
Elevated intracranial pressure
Infection at the block site

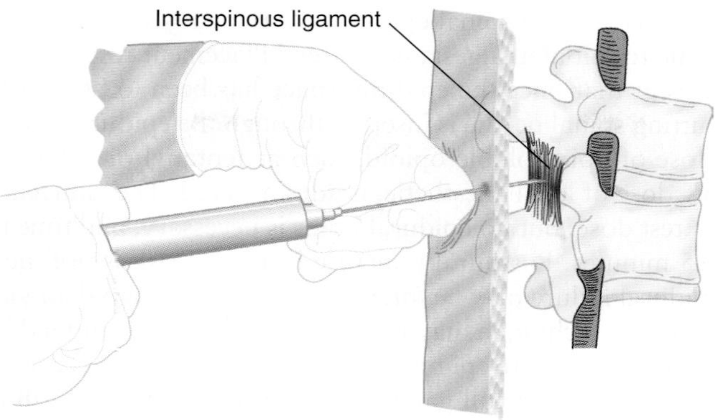

Figure 31.6 Proper hand position when using the loss-of-resistance technique to locate the epidural space. After embedding the needle tip in the ligamentum flavum, a syringe with 2 to 3 mL of saline and an air bubble is attached. The left hand rests securely on the back and the fingers of the left hand grasp the needle firmly. The left hand advances the needle slowly and under control by rotating at the wrist. The fingers of the right hand maintain constant pressure on the syringe plunger but do not aid in advancing the needle. If the needle tip is properly engaged in the ligamentum flavum, it should be possible to compress the air bubble without injecting the saline. As the needle tip enters the epidural space, there will be a sudden loss of resistance and the saline will be suddenly injected. (From Mulroy MF. *Regional Anesthesia: An Illustrated Procedural Guide*. 3rd ed. Wolters Kluwer Health; 2002, Figure 34.8.)

for beginners. Layers traversed by the epidural needle during placement of epidural block include, from superficial to deep, skin, subcutaneous tissue, supraspinous ligament, interspinous ligament, and ligamentum flavum.

The epidural space is a potential space lying deep to the ligamentum flavum. The hollow, large-bore epidural needle with stylet is placed into the superficial ligaments, the stylet is removed, and an air- or saline-filled syringe is attached. The syringe will give tactile resistance when pushed until the ligamentum flavum is traversed, and the epidural space is entered, at which time tactile resistance disappears. Both the thickness of the ligamentum flavum and depth of the epidural space are usually 3 to 5 cm.

Once the space is entered, saline may be injected to confirm loss of resistance, and the depth at which the epidural space was entered is noted (most epidural needles have centimeter markings on them). A soft catheter is then threaded into the space 3 to 5 cm. A test dose of lidocaine mixed with 15 μg of epinephrine is commonly administered via the catheter to ensure that it is not intravascular or intrathecal. Criteria for a positive intravascular test dose include an increase in heart rate by 20 beats per minute or an increase in systolic blood pressure by 15 mm Hg within 45 seconds of administration. The catheter must be removed and replaced at the same or a different interspace if a positive intravascular test occurs. A profound sensory and motor block within 5 minutes after administration of test dose confirms a positive intrathecal. If an intrathecal catheter is accidentally placed, it may be used for labor analgesia with appropriate dosing or it may be removed and replaced at a ***different*** level (**Figure 31.6**).

Epidural activation begins with an initial bolus of dilute local anesthetic mixed with lipid-soluble opioid, such as 0.125% bupivacaine mixed with fentanyl 50 to 100 μg, given in 5-mL increments, for a total of 10 to 20 mL. Time to analgesia is typically 10 to 20 minutes.

Alternatively, combined spinal epidural (CSE) analgesia has gained popularity because time to initial analgesia is shorter.[3] Placement resembles an epidural procedure, except that once the epidural space has been located, a long, small-gauge, noncutting spinal needle is inserted through the epidural needle. Then an intrathecal dose of lipid-soluble opioid, such as fentanyl or sufentanil, with or without a low dose of local anesthetic, is administered. The clinician commonly administers a test dose, but no epidural bolus is necessary, and time to analgesia is typically <5 minutes. Postdural puncture headache risk is not increased, and the risk of epidural failure may be ***lower*** with CSE, although data yield conflicting results.[3,4] A CSE technique may result in increased rates of fetal bradycardia and pruritus. Dural puncture epidural (DPE) is a relatively newer technique. The dura is punctured with a small gauge spinal needle, just as it is during a CSE; however, no medicine is administered into the intrathecal space, and instead, medication is infused through the epidural catheter. This technique produces a marginally faster sensory blockade when compared to epidural alone with less unilateral analgesia and more reliable sacral coverage for the second stage of labor without the potential adverse effects of the CSE technique.[5]

If an intrathecal catheter is placed, the dose is about one-tenth the volume of a typical epidural dose, administered either as a continuous infusion or via intermittent ***provider-administered*** bolus every 1 to 2 hours. The patient's nurse and any subsequent providers must be notified that the catheter is intrathecal, and both the catheter and pump must be clearly labeled so that accidental overdose does not occur.

The use of ultrasound guidance for placement of neuraxial catheters is becoming more common and can be useful in obese patients or for patients with spinal abnormalities. Location of midline, accurate assessment of lumbar level, and measurement of depth of the epidural and intrathecal spaces are all possible via ultrasound.

IV. Anesthesia for Cesarean Delivery

In the United States, 32% of babies are born via cesarean delivery,[6] and recently an increase in the rate of vaginal birth after cesarean delivery has been observed, especially in younger aged women.[7] Most cesarean deliveries are performed under neuraxial anesthesia, via either spinal, epidural, or CSE anesthesia.

Elective cesarean deliveries are performed at term (≥39 weeks), under ***neuraxial*** anesthesia unless there is a contraindication, because the risk to both mother and fetus is lower with neuraxial versus general anesthesia. In preparation for surgery, patients are instructed not to eat solids for 8 hours prior to surgery and not to drink clear fluids for 2 hours prior to surgery. Preoperative labs may include a complete blood count and type and screen. An 18-gauge or larger peripheral intravenous line is placed, and balanced salt solution is administered.

Pfannenstiel skin incision with low transverse uterine incision is the most common type of operative approach. To provide adequate anesthesia for cesarean delivery, blockade must include both incisional or somatic and peritoneal pain fibers up to the celiac plexus. Therefore, a dermatomal block from at least T6 to sacrum is required. Anesthesia care providers commonly employ either spinal or epidural anesthesia to achieve this level.

Spinal bupivacaine (10-12 mg) or lidocaine (60-100 mg) represents viable options for cesarean delivery anesthesia. Intrathecal lidocaine spinal has become less popular due to concern about transient neurologic symptoms. The anesthesiologist commonly administers short-acting and long-acting intrathecal opioids along with the local anesthetic. Typically fentanyl (10-20 µg) or sufentanil (2.5-5 µg) is given. The duration of either is 2 hours, and intraoperative pain, nausea, and vomiting occur less frequently when they are used. Long-acting hydrophilic morphine provides postoperative analgesia.

Hypotension commonly accompanies initiation of spinal anesthesia for cesarean delivery and can be prevented or lessened by placing the patient in 15° to 30° of left uterine displacement and administering a co-load of crystalloid 10 to 20 mL/kg or colloid 5 mL/kg. However, this degree of uterine displacement is difficult to achieve. Administration of crystalloid with prophylactic phenylephrine infusion titrated to maintain baseline blood pressure decreases the incidence of spinal-related hypotension, nausea, vomiting, and results in no significant difference in umbilical cord gas values when compared to LUD.[8] Nausea is common after initiation of spinal anesthesia and may be related to hypotension or to increased vagal tone from sympathectomy.

> **? Did You Know?**
>
> Nausea is common after initiation of spinal anesthesia and may be related to hypotension or to increased vagal tone from sympathectomy.

Epidural anesthesia for cesarean delivery is achieved via 2% lidocaine or 3% chloroprocaine, 15 to 25 mL, incrementally dosed in nonemergency situations. In emergency situations, 3% 2-chloroprocaine 20 mL is preferred because it has the shortest onset time (3-4 minutes) and desirable maternal and fetal safety profiles. Of note, chloroprocaine may decrease the efficacy of opioids and local anesthetics administered subsequently. The addition of sodium bicarbonate will decrease time to blockade by converting more of the local anesthetic to its nonionized form. The dose is typically 1 mEq/10 mL local anesthetic volume. Epinephrine (5 µg/mL) can be added to increase the density and extend the duration of block and to test dose a labor epidural catheter that will be used for cesarean delivery anesthesia. Preservative-free morphine can be given via the epidural catheter for postoperative analgesia, typically after umbilical cord clamping.

General anesthesia for cesarean delivery is generally reserved for emergency cases or when contraindications to neuraxial anesthesia exist. Standard of care requires American Society of Anesthesiologists' (ASA) standard monitors and preoxygenation. Proper positioning and preoxygenation help mitigate the desaturation that occurs, and they assume special importance in pregnant patients who are particularly prone to desaturation after a period of apnea. Administration of a nonparticulate antacid and rapid sequence induction and intubation, with an assistant providing cricoid pressure, are also standard, due to the increased risk of aspiration. The surgeon prepares and drapes the patient's abdomen prior to induction of anesthesia to be ready to perform surgery immediately after endotracheal tube placement is confirmed. Induction was historically with thiopental; however, propofol has replaced thiopental as the induction agent of choice, mainly because of its availability. Succinylcholine (1 mg/kg) given with induction provides muscle relaxation. Once the trachea is intubated, the anesthesiologist notifies the obstetrician and surgery begins.

Temperature monitoring and stomach decompression with an orogastric tube are generally recommended. Oxygen and inhaled anesthetic are administered until delivery of the fetus. Inhaled anesthetic over 1 MAC may decrease uterine tone, so after delivery of the fetus, a nitrous oxygen mixture is started, along with low-concentration inhaled anesthetic. An analgesic, amnestic, and sometimes additional muscle relaxant are given. After delivery of the placenta, an oxytocin infusion is started, and additional uterotonics are given as needed.

A. Postoperative Analgesia

Intrathecal or epidural morphine provides long lasting analgesia and appears to have a ceiling effect around 150 μg (intrathecal) and 3 to 4 mg (epidural).[9,10] Higher doses do not increase analgesia and cause more nausea, respiratory depression, and pruritus. Peak morphine effects occur about 6 hours postadministration and cease by 12 to 18 hours postadministration. Published ASA recommendations call for monitoring of sedation and respiratory rate every hour during the first 12 hours and every 2 hours for the next 12 hours after dosing.[11] Medications to treat side effects include naloxone to treat respiratory depression or sedation, a mixed opiate agonist-antagonist to treat pruritus, and an intravenous antiemetic. Oral analgesics should be ordered, such as acetaminophen and nonsteroidal anti-inflammatory drugs. Additional opiates may be administered if needed, as long as vigilant monitoring takes place. Prophylaxis with an intraoperative dose of antiemetic decreases the incidence of nausea and vomiting associated with neuraxial morphine. Alternatively, the anesthesiologist may leave the epidural catheter in place and administer PCEA with low-concentration local anesthetic and lipid-soluble opioid, typically for 24 hours postdelivery.

For patients who do not receive neuraxial morphine or PCEA, transversus abdominis plane (TAP) blocks improve analgesia by decreasing incisional pain. TAP blocks may be performed immediately postoperatively with ultrasound guidance, typically with 10- to 15-mL long-acting local anesthetic per side.

V. Fetal Assessment and Neonatal Resuscitation

> **? Did You Know?**
>
> Continuous fetal heart rate monitoring is recommended by major obstetric organizations and accompanies almost 90% of US deliveries.

Fetal heart rate (FHR) monitoring during labor attempts to identify fetal hypoxemia or acidosis and avoid resultant fetal neurologic damage or death. FHR monitoring can be intermittent, via auscultation or Doppler, or continuous, via external Doppler or fetal electrocardiogram (ECG). Fetal ECG requires internal monitor placement on the fetal scalp. The mother must be dilated and ruptured for this to occur. Continuous FHR monitoring is recommended by major obstetric organizations and accompanies almost 90% of US deliveries.[12] Despite the emphasis on FHR patterns and neonatal neurologic outcome, cerebral palsy is most often due to an antepartum, not intrapartum, event. Continuous FHR monitoring is associated retrospectively with lower rates of cerebral palsy and death. However, no randomized prospective data are available due to ethical issues. Intermittent versus continuous fetal monitoring has been compared prospectively, and the only difference in outcome is a higher rate of cesarean delivery ***without benefit to the neonate***, and in general a lower risk of neonatal seizures.[13]

> **? Did You Know?**
>
> Fetal heart rate tracing interpretation is very sensitive, but not very specific. Thus, a normal fetal heart rate and variability without decelerations almost always indicates a nonacidotic fetus, but a healthy fetus may have fetal heart rate abnormalities not due to acidosis or distress.

FHR tracing interpretation is very sensitive but not very specific. Therefore, a normal FHR and variability without decelerations almost always indicates a nonacidotic fetus, but a healthy fetus may have FHR abnormalities not caused by acidosis or distress. Fetal tachycardia may be due to hypoxemia, but it may also result from maternal fever or infection or maternally administered drugs (β agonists in particular). Many maternally administered drugs, including magnesium and opioids, may decrease FHR variability (**Figure 31.7**).

The American Congress of Obstetrics and Gynecology (ACOG) classifies FHR tracings into three categories.[10] A Category I tracing is highly predictive of a healthy nonacidotic fetus and must have the following characteristics:

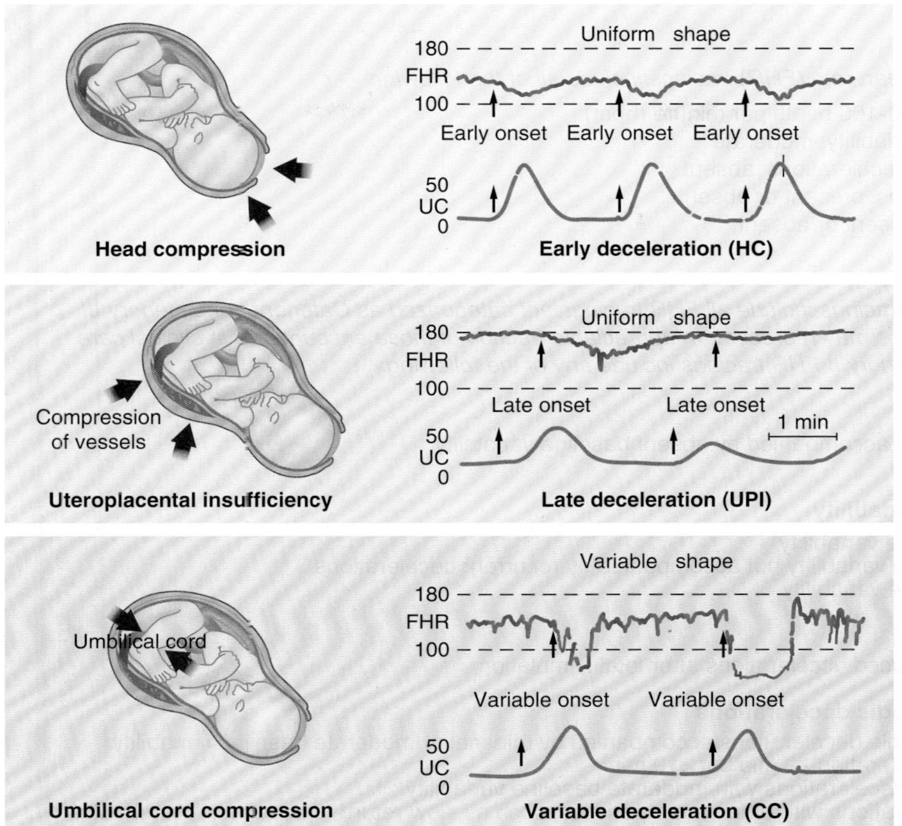

Figure 31.7 Classification and mechanism of fetal heart rate patterns. CC, cord compression; HC, head compression; UPI, uteroplacental insufficiency. (Adapted from Hon EH. *An Introduction to Fetal Heart Rate Monitoring*. Harty Press; 1969:29 and from Braveman FR, Scavone BM, Blessing ME, Wong CA. Obstetrical anesthesia. In: Barash PG, Cahalan MK, Cullen BF, et al, eds. *Clinical Anesthesia*. 8th ed. Wolters Kluwer; 2018:1144-1177, Figure 41.8.)

normal baseline heart rate, normal variability, and no decelerations other than early. A Category III designation is associated with fetal acidosis and has the following characteristics: absent variability ***accompanied by*** late or variable decelerations occurring with >50% of contractions or sinusoidal pattern. Category II includes any tracing not meeting the qualifiers of Category I or III (**Figure 31.8**).

A. Intrauterine Resuscitation

Fetuses with Category III tracings or with prolonged bradycardia require rapid treatment. Treatment of maternal hypotension with lateral positioning, fluid bolus, and vasopressors; administration of high-flow oxygen via face mask; and cessation of uterine contractions with nitroglycerin or terbutaline are primary therapies. If no improvement is seen, immediate delivery is indicated.

Prolonged ***fetal bradycardia*** will lead to emergency cesarean delivery if intrauterine resuscitation measures are ineffective. An existing epidural catheter can be dosed with 20 mL of 3% chloroprocaine, which should provide a surgical level within 3 to 4 minutes. General anesthesia is usually chosen if fetal bradycardia persists in the operating room and no neuraxial catheter is present.

Category I

Category I fetal heart rate (FHR) tracings include all of the following:

- Baseline rate: 110-160 beats per minute (bpm)
- Baseline FHR variability: moderate
- Late or variable decelerations: absent
- Early decelerations: present or absent
- Accelerations: present or absent

Category II

Category II FHR tracings include all FHR tracings not categorized as Category I or Category III. Category II tracings may represent an appreciable fraction of those encountered in clinical care. Examples of Category II FHR tracings include any of the following:

Baseline rate

- Bradycardia not accompanied by absent baseline variability
- Tachycardia

Baseline FHR variability

- Minimal baseline variability
- Absent baseline variability not accompanied by recurrent decelerations
- Marked baseline variability

Accelerations

- Absence of induced accelerations after fetal stimulation

Periodic or episodic decelerations

- Recurrent variable decelerations accompanied by minimal or moderate baseline variability
- Prolonged deceleration ≥2 min but <10 min
- Recurrent late decelerations with moderate baseline variability
- Variable decelerations with other characteristics, such as slow return to baseline, "overshoots," or "shoulders"

Category III

Category III FHR tracings include either:

- Absent baseline FHR variability and any of the following:
  - Recurrent late decelerations
  - Recurrent variable decelerations
  - Bradycardia
- Sinusoidal pattern

Figure 31.8 **Three-tier fetal heart interpretation system.** (From Macones GA, Hankins GD, Spong CY, Hauth J, Moore T. The 2008 National Institute of Child Health and Human Development Workshop on Electronic Fetal Monitoring: Updates on definitions, interpretations, and research guidelines. *Obstet Gynecol.* 2008;112:661, with permission.)

B. Ancillary Fetal Testing

High-risk fetuses or pregnancies sometimes require closer monitoring or additional testing to assess fetal status. A nonstress test (NST) consists of 30 minutes of continuous external FHR monitoring, during which time at least two accelerations of at least 15 beats per minute lasting 15 seconds or more must be seen, indicating a healthy fetus. NSTs are done weekly or daily depending on the diagnosis.

A biophysical profile further assesses fetal status. It has five components each with a maximum of two points, including an NST, measurement of amniotic fluid index, fetal tone, fetal movement, and fetal breathing attempts. Lower scores are indications for admission and continuous monitoring and sometimes delivery.

Table 31.4 Apgar Scores

Sign	0	1	2
Heart rate	Absent	<100 beats/min	>100 beats/min
Respiratory effort	Absent	Slow, irregular	Good, crying
Muscle tone	Limp	Some flexion of extremities	Active motion
Reflex irritability	No response	Grimace	Cough, sneeze, or cry
Color	Pale, blue	Body pink, extremities blue	Completely pink

From Braveman FR, Scavone BM, Blessing ME, Wong CA. Obstetrical anesthesia. In: Barash PG, Cahalan MK, Cullen BF, et al, eds. *Clinical Anesthesia*. 8th ed. Wolters Kluwer; 2018:1144-1177.

Umbilical artery Doppler studies are performed in fetuses with growth restriction or in mothers with hypertension or placental abnormalities to monitor for signs of worsening fetal perfusion (indicated by poor flow in diastole or elevation in placental resistance). The ratio of flow in systole versus diastole is measured, and a score over 3 is concerning. The resistance index is also measured, and a score of >0.6 is indicative of elevated placental resistance. Absent end diastolic flow (AEDF) occurs when flow in diastole stops due to increased placental resistance. Reverse end diastolic flow (REDF) occurs when flow in diastole moves from the placenta to the fetus in the umbilical artery, indicating very elevated placental resistance. REDF is always an indication for delivery. AEDF is an indication for delivery depending on gestational age and other factors. Both are associated with increased fetal morbidity and mortality.

The ***Apgar score*** is a global assessment of neonatal status immediately after birth. The score's intended use is to guide acute intervention, not to provide prognosis. Neonatal breathing, heart rate, reaction to stimulus, tone, and color are each assessed at 1, 5, and sometimes 10 minutes postnatal and given a score of 0 to 2 per category. A score of ≥7 is considered normal. Scores <7 necessitate further intervention (**Table 31.4; Figure 31.9**).

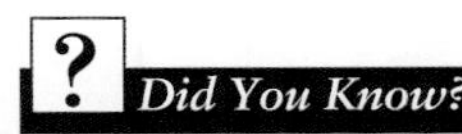

The Apgar score is a global assessment of neonatal status immediately after birth; the score's intended use is to guide acute intervention, not to provide prognosis.

VI. Comorbidities and Obstetric Diseases

A. Pregnancy-Induced Hypertensive Disorders

The pregnancy-induced hypertensive disorders include gestational hypertension, preeclampsia or eclampsia, and hemolysis-elevated liver enzymes with low platelets (HELLP) syndrome. Pregnancy normally causes a slight decrease in blood pressure. Elevated blood pressure in pregnancy is pathologic and associated with fetal and maternal morbidity and mortality. Gestational hypertension is defined as elevated blood pressure occurring after 20 weeks' gestation, without accompanying proteinuria. Preeclampsia is defined by elevated blood pressures after 20 weeks' gestation, accompanied by proteinuria or other organ-system effects. Eclampsia is preeclampsia with seizure.[14] The HELLP syndrome is a variant of severe preeclampsia associated with liver dysfunction and thrombocytopenia.

Preeclampsia can be further categorized as having severe features if any of the following conditions are met: blood pressure elevated over 160 mm Hg systolic or 110 mm Hg diastolic, or end-organ dysfunction, which can manifest as severe headache, vision or cerebral disturbance, pulmonary edema

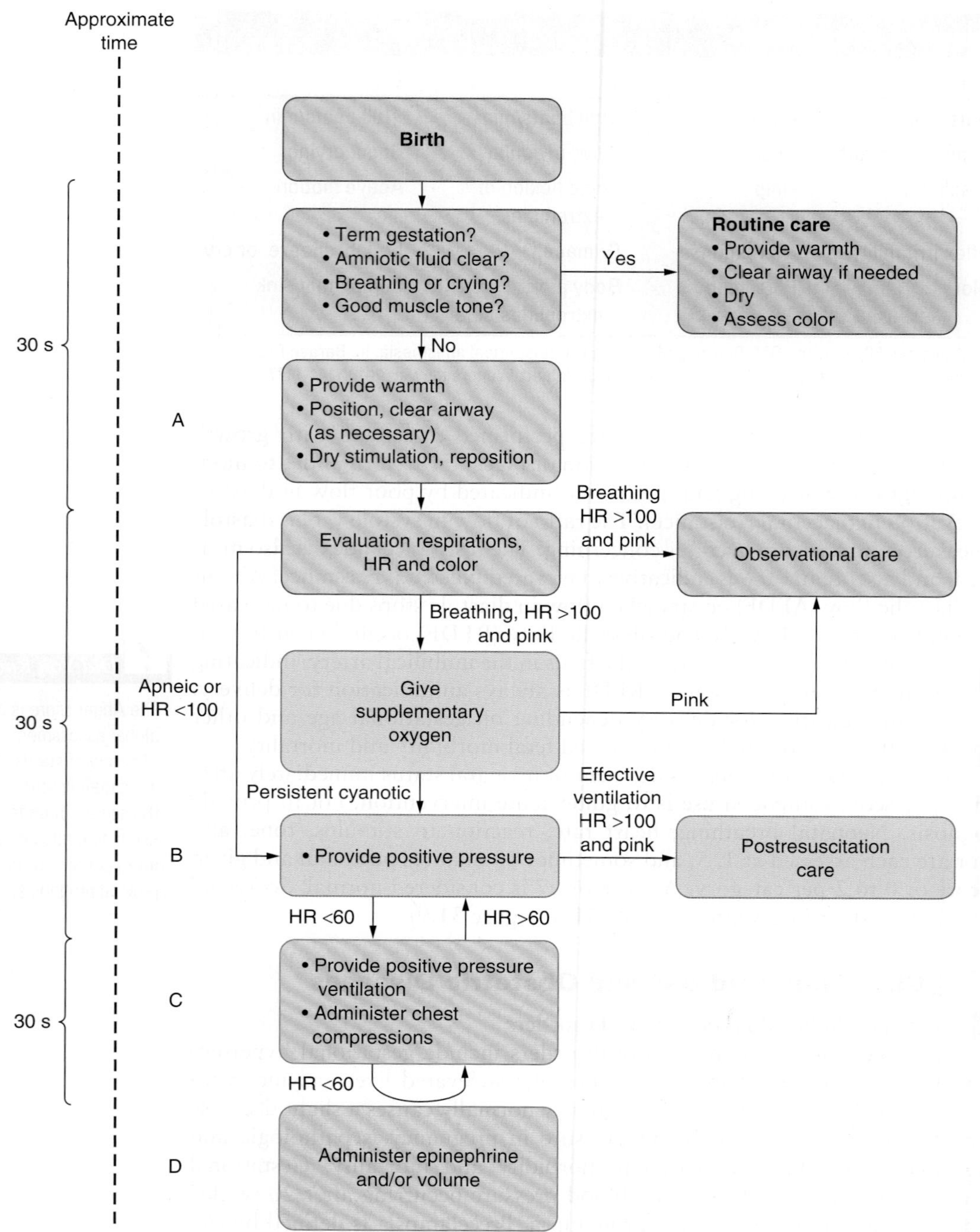

Figure 31.9 **Algorithm for neonatal resuscitation. HR, heart rate.** (From Kattwinkel J, Perlman JM, Aziz K, et al. Special Report–Neonatal Resuscitation; 2010. American Heart Association guidelines for cardiopulmonary resuscitation and emergency cardiovascular care. *Circulation.* 2010;122:S9, with permission.)

or cyanosis, oliguria or renal failure, liver dysfunction, thrombocytopenia (less than 100,000/μL), or severe epigastric pain. Severe proteinuria and fetal growth restriction are no longer used as indicators of severe features but do frequently occur with the disorder.[14]

The etiology of preeclampsia is still being studied, but abnormalities in placental implantation and placental production of thromboxane and prostacyclin may play a role. Poor placental perfusion causes systemic endothelial dysfunction and activation of the renin-angiotensin-aldosterone system, resulting in arteriolar hypertension and edema. Platelet aggregation occurs at sites of endothelial injury, resulting in coagulopathy.

Severe hypertension can cause focal cerebral ischemia, cerebral edema, or hemorrhage, leading to eclampsia or seizures and death or major disability. A recent ACOG Executive Summary recommends immediate control of blood pressure with intravenous antihypertensives to prevent morbidity and mortality.[14] Intravenous labetalol and hydralazine are most commonly used, and direct arterial pressure monitoring may be necessary. Magnesium infusion prevents eclampsia.[15] Magnesium increases the seizure threshold, but has many unwanted side effects. Sedation, decreased reflexes, muscle weakness and potentiation of neuromuscular blockade, and respiratory and cardiovascular depression or arrest are associated with magnesium overdose, which occurs more frequently in patients with renal dysfunction. The practitioner must examine the patient's neurologic status and monitor magnesium levels to prevent overdose. Intravenous calcium is the primary treatment for arrest related to magnesium overdose.

Ultimately, treatment of preeclampsia requires delivery and removal of the placenta. Early preeclampsia without severe features can be managed expectantly with careful maternal and fetal monitoring and antihypertensives to prevent preterm birth. Preeclampsia with severe features usually represents an indication for delivery once the patient is stabilized and steroids have been administered to hasten fetal lung maturity. Neuraxial anesthesia is contraindicated if coagulopathy is present. If general anesthesia is necessary for cesarean delivery, laryngoscopy and intubation may be difficult due to systemic and airway edema, and short-acting intravenous antihypertensives should be used to prevent severe hypertension during airway management.

B. Diabetes Mellitus

Pregnancy is a diabetogenic state, and women can develop gestational diabetes mellitus. Preexisting diabetes often requires insulin therapy. Blood glucose control is very important during pregnancy to avoid fetal central nervous system and cardiovascular malformations and fetal morbidity and mortality. Babies born to diabetic women with poor glucose control have higher rates of macrosomia, shoulder dystocia, respiratory distress, cardiomyopathy, polycythemia and persistent pulmonary hypertension, and term neonatal intensive care unit admission. During labor, tight glucose control, often with an insulin infusion titrated to maintain blood glucose values between 80 and 110 mg/dL, is utilized to help prevent neonatal hypoglycemia.

C. Obesity

The majority of Americans are overweight, obese, or morbidly obese. Many of the physiologic implications of obesity mirror those of pregnancy and the two may combine to produce exaggerated untoward effects. In particular, obese patients have increased cardiac output, increased work of breathing, increased oxygen consumption, decreased lung volumes, and more redundant tissue, making them prone to complications during induction and airway management. Obese parturients exhibit exaggerated aortocaval compression when in the supine position. Obesity worsens obstetric and neonatal outcomes, increasing the rates of dysfunctional labor and cesarean delivery, hypertensive diseases of pregnancy, diabetes, fetal macrosomia, shoulder dystocia, and intrauterine fetal demise. Postoperatively these patients demonstrate increased rates of infection, wound disruption, and thromboembolic disease.

Neuraxial anesthetic techniques are fraught with difficulty, and ultrasound guidance may facilitate block placement. Airway management during administration of general anesthesia should cause concern for failure to ventilate, failure to intubate, and aspiration of gastric contents. The clinician should have a low threshold for awake fiberoptic intubation. Obese parturients should be evaluated soon after admission to the labor and delivery unit, and early neuraxial analgesia is encouraged to decrease the risk of general anesthesia requirement should an emergency cesarean delivery become necessary.

D. Fever and Infection

Pregnancy is an immunosuppressed state, and systemic infection is poorly tolerated. Chorioamnionitis is a common severe infection in pregnant patients that can lead to preterm labor, atony, hemorrhage, and sepsis. Urinary tract infections are also frequent and can lead to ascending infection and pyelonephritis due to poor ureteral valve function in pregnancy. Systemic inflammatory response syndrome and sepsis are treated in the same manner as for nonpregnant patients, but mortality rates are higher in pregnant patients.

Genital ***herpes simplex virus*** (HSV) is a common sexually transmitted disease and is an indication for cesarean delivery if active genital or cervical lesions are present because of the risk of neonatal HSV infection. Primary herpes infection is associated with flu-like symptoms and genital lesions. Neuraxial anesthesia is controversial during primary infection because of the potential risk of seeding the central nervous system with HSV. Many anesthesia practitioners will not administer neuraxial anesthesia until the lesions associated with primary HSV have begun healing and no signs or symptoms of systemic infection are present. Secondary infections are not considered a contraindication to neuraxial techniques. ***Oral HSV*** more commonly recurs in patients who receive neuraxial morphine. The etiology of the recrudescence is unclear and may be related to immunomodulation or to facial pruritus and scratching.

Pregnant patients with human immunodeficiency virus (HIV) are treated with highly active antiretroviral therapy, with the goal viral load being <1000 copies/mL. Vaginal delivery is allowed if viral load is <1000 copies/mL. If viral load is >1000 copies/mL, cesarean delivery helps prevent vertical transmission to the infant. During labor and delivery, the administration of intravenous zidovudine decreases the rate of vertical HIV transmission. Breastfeeding is contraindicated. Neuraxial analgesia and anesthesia are not contraindicated.

E. Epidural Fever

Temperature rises about 0.4° per hour in women with epidural labor analgesia versus those without, even when controlling for other factors such as pain medication and infection.[16] The etiology of this temperature rise is unclear, and the clinical significance of the actual temperature difference is also unclear. Women with epidural-related fever during labor may be incorrectly diagnosed with chorioamnionitis.

F. Bleeding Disorders

von Willebrand disease represents the most common inherited coagulopathy in pregnant women. von Willebrand factor (vWF) is important for normal hemostasis, as it causes adhesion of platelets to injured tissue and serves as a cofactor to factor VIII. Three subtypes of vWF deficiency exist, with deficiencies in either quantitative amount of or qualitative function of vWF. The most common subtype, vWF deficiency type 1, is a result of a decrease in circulating vWF levels. Pregnancy increases circulating levels of vWF and may decrease symptoms or need for treatment. If required, initial therapy for type 1 is with desmopressin (DDAVP), which increases vWF release, doubling to quadrupling the circulating concentrations. Intravenous or intranasal DDAVP begins working in 30 to 60 minutes and lasts for 6 hours. Type 2 has four subcategories and is a result of qualitative abnormalities in vWF causing abnormal function. Subtype 2b is associated with thrombocytopenia and thrombosis if DDAVP is given. Therefore, therapy must include factor VIII concentrate containing vWF (Humate). Fresh frozen plasma (FFP) and cryoprecipitate also contain vWF. However, factor VIII concentrate is recommended if available because of a lower risk of viral disease transmission. Type 3 is a severe, recessive disorder with very low circulating vWF levels and severe bleeding. A hematology consult may guide the therapy.

Acquired coagulopathies associated with hemorrhage commonly occur and are due to dilution or DIC. Dilutional coagulopathy occurs after massive hemorrhage, when resuscitation consists primarily of packed red blood cells (PRBC) without plasma or platelets. Additionally, DIC is associated with placental abruption and amniotic fluid embolism. Therapy for acquired coagulopathy is supportive and includes transfusion of plasma, cryoprecipitate, and platelets.

VII. Emergencies

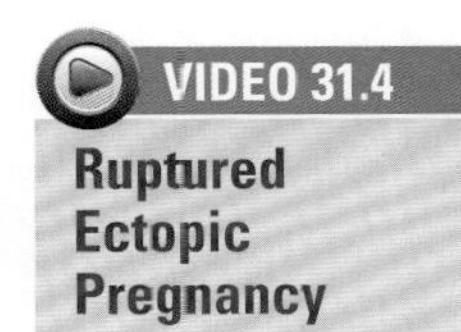

Antepartum hemorrhage occurs due to either acute abnormalities associated with the uterus or placenta (placental abruption or uterine rupture) or abnormal implantation of the placenta (previa).

Placental abruption occurs when a portion of the placenta prematurely separates off its implant site on the uterus. Large abruptions can cause significant blood loss, DIC, and maternal instability, in addition to fetal distress or demise. Risk factors for abruption include advanced age, hypertension, diabetes, smoking, trauma, and cocaine use. Treatment is delivery and fluid and blood product administration. Coagulation should be monitored, including fibrinogen level, as abnormalities may be present contraindicating neuraxial anesthesia.

Uterine rupture occurs most often in women with a history of previous cesarean delivery, in particular with a "classical" vertical uterine scar. Uterine rupture is a surgical emergency and can be associated with severe bleeding. Uterine rupture is less common if a low transverse uterine scar is present, and a vaginal trial of labor (VTOL) may be offered to appropriate patients. A team must be immediately available to provide cesarean delivery for patients undergoing a VTOL.

Placenta previa occurs when the placenta implants either very close to or completely over the cervical os. Vaginal delivery is not possible without maternal and fetal consequences. Placenta previa is associated with maternal hemorrhage and with other abnormalities of placentation such as placenta accreta.

When placenta previa occurs in the setting of five or more cesarean deliveries, the risk of invasive placentation or accreta is at least 75%. Continued bleeding from placenta previa is an indication for emergency cesarean delivery.

Vasa previa occurs when unprotected fetal vessels lie over the cervical os. Any vaginal bleeding may be fetal, and therefore represents an obstetric emergency requiring immediate delivery. Fetal mortality (in an otherwise normal fetus) is higher from vasa previa than any other condition. Therefore, mothers are admitted, and fetuses are continuously monitored until planned early cesarean delivery.

Patients with placenta or vasa previa are more likely to experience postpartum hemorrhage, so blood should be crossmatched and adequate access placed prior to cesarean delivery.

Postpartum hemorrhage (PPH) is the primary cause of maternal death worldwide and a leading contributor to maternal mortality and severe morbidity in the United States. PPH complicates 3% of deliveries[17] and is classically defined as estimated blood loss greater than 500 mL for a vaginal delivery or 1000 mL for a cesarean delivery. However, in clinical practice, these values approximate average blood loss totals. The American College of Obstetricians and Gynecologists revised this definition to also include bleeding associated with signs or symptoms of hypovolemia within 24 hours of delivery regardless of delivery route.[18] The uterine blood flow at term is 700 to 900 mL/min. The uterus normally contracts postpartum, causing mechanical obstruction of bleeding vessels to prevent major maternal hemorrhage. The lack of uterine contraction postdelivery is called ***atony*** and 80% of PPH is due to uterine atony.[17] Risk factors for atony include a history of atony with previous pregnancy, retained placenta, chorioamnionitis, augmented or prolonged labor, uterine relaxants, and an overdistended uterus (macrosomic fetus, polyhydramnios, multiple gestation). Treatment of atony includes bimanual uterine massage, uterotonic drugs, discontinuation of drugs that may impair uterine contraction (inhaled anesthetics), or internal (Bakri balloon) or external (B-Lynch suture) compression of the uterus. Hysterectomy is indicated for severe unresponsive atony.

Medications commonly used for atony include oxytocin, prostaglandins, and methylergonovine (**Table 31.5**).

Abnormalities of placentation represent a major source of massive obstetric hemorrhage. Placenta accreta, increta, and percreta occur when the placenta abnormally adheres to (accreta) or invades (increta) the uterine myometrium or serosa (percreta). Previous cesarean deliveries or uterine surgery are associated with placental implantation abnormalities. Accreta can be diagnosed via ultrasound or magnetic resonance imaging (MRI), although both remain imperfectly sensitive or specific. Planning for cesarean delivery and the possibility of large blood loss is crucial, and adequate large bore intravenous access and type and crossmatched blood products are needed. Safe surgical management of hysterectomy in patients with placenta percreta requires the involvement of subspecialties, including interventional radiology, gynecologic oncology, and general surgery.

Massive blood loss and transfusion can occur in obstetrical patients. Many hospitals have created massive transfusion protocols to facilitate the timely delivery of blood products when needed. High ratios of FFP to PRBC are recommended in the setting of ongoing loss and transfusion. Although the optimal ratio remains controversial, most experts endorse administration of 1:1 or 1:2 FFP to PRBC. One pooled unit of cryoprecipitate and

Table 31.5 Uterotonic Therapy

Drug	Dose	Side Effects
Oxytocin	20-40 U in 1000 mL LR by continuous IV infusion	Hypotension, tachycardia
Ergot alkaloids (Methergine)	0.2 mg IM q2–4h prn	Hypertension, vasoconstriction Coronary vasospasm V/Q mismatch (ventilation perfusion mismatch), elevated pulmonary vascular resistance, and nausea and vomiting
Carboprost (prostaglandin $F_{2\alpha}$/Hemabate)	0.25 mg q15 min × 8 doses, maximum 2 mg	↑ pulmonary vascular resistance Bronchospasm Diarrhea/nausea Fever
Misoprostol	800-1000 mg PR/PV/PO q2h	Fever Nausea
Dinoprostone	20 mg PO q2h	Hypotension Nausea

IM, intramuscular; IV, intravenous; LR, lactated Ringer's; PR/PV/PO, per rectum/per vaginum/per os; prn, as needed.

From Braveman FR, Scavone BM, Blessing ME, Wong CA. Obstetrical anesthesia. In: Barash PG, Cahalan MK, Cullen BF, et al, eds. *Clinical anesthesia*. 8th ed. Wolters Kluwer; 2018:1144-1177.

one pooled unit of platelets should be given for every six PRBCs transfused or based on laboratory values. Experts recommend early identification and aggressive treatment of coagulopathy, and frequent laboratory monitoring can help guide therapy (eg, complete blood cell count, coagulation studies such as prothrombin time and international normalized ratio, partial thromboplastin time, fibrinogen, or thromboelastogram). Obstetric hemorrhage may be accompanied by fibrinolysis. Tranexamic acid use should be considered in PPH early in the course of bleeding unresponsive to uterotonics. Early tranexamic acid was associated with reduced risk of death due to bleeding during PPH without significant adverse effects.[19] Cell saver can be used during massive hemorrhage or for patients who refuse blood transfusion, with the patient's permission.

Amniotic fluid embolism (AFE) occurs when amniotic fluid enters the mother's circulation and causes a severe inflammatory response. AFE often occurs immediately surrounding delivery. Intact survival rate after AFE remains poor. Bronchospasm, acute pulmonary hypertension, circulatory shock, and DIC can all occur with AFE. Treatment is supportive and can include massive transfusion for DIC and resultant hemorrhage. Patients may be placed on extracorporeal membrane oxygenation for support of oxygenation and CO_2 elimination.

A. Cardiopulmonary Arrest

The incidence of peripartum maternal arrest is 1 in 30,000 deliveries.[20] Maternal arrest has many etiologies, including pulmonary or amniotic fluid embolism, drug errors, maternal comorbidities such as preeclampsia, coronary artery disease, severe valvular disease, or complications of general or neuraxial anesthesia. Initial treatment is cardiopulmonary resuscitation (CPR) modified for the pregnant patient, using either manual left uterine displacement, a

Cardiff wedge, or a "human wedge" on the knees of a provider. Other CPR modifications needed for the pregnant state include a slightly higher sternal placement of hands for chest compressions, use of cricoid pressure during bag mask ventilation until the trachea is intubated, and a high index of suspicion for drug errors as the source of the cardiac arrest, in particular magnesium overdose. Use of defibrillation, vasopressors, and inotropes all remain unchanged from adult advanced cardiac life support guidelines. Maternal CPR is almost always suboptimal due to the gravid uterus. If the source of the arrest is unknown or not immediately reversible, cesarean delivery should be performed ***in the labor and delivery room within 5 minutes of arrest.*** To achieve this goal, the team must make the decision to perform a cesarean delivery and make the incision within 4 minutes of arrest. With delivery of the fetus, adequate CPR can be delivered to the mother. Longer arrest-to-delivery intervals are associated with worse neonatal and maternal outcomes.

B. Maternal Mortality

The maternal mortality ratio refers to the number of maternal deaths during a given time period per 100,000 live births. In the United States, the maternal mortality ratio is 17.4 in 100,000. Wide racial and ethnic gaps exist with non-Hispanic black (37.1 in 100,000), non-Hispanic white (14.7), and Hispanic (11.8) women differing largely in terms of maternal mortality.[21] The leading contributors to mortality in the United States are cardiovascular diseases, hemorrhage, venous thromboembolism, infection, hypertensive diseases, cardiomyopathy, mental health diseases, and pregnancy-related conditions such as AFE. Globally, the maternal mortality ratio in low-income nations is 462 per 100,000 live births to as low as 11 per 100,000 in high-income nations.[22] Hemorrhage, sepsis, and pregnancy-induced hypertension are the leading causes of maternal death in undeveloped countries. The anesthesia-related maternal mortality ratio is 1.2 in 1 million; anesthesia is the cause of about 1.5% of maternal deaths in the United States.[23]

VIII. Complications of Neuraxial Anesthesia

A. Postdural Puncture Headache or Epidural Blood Patch

Postdural puncture headache (PDPH) occurs after puncture of the dura, with resultant leakage of CSF. The associated headache is theorized to occur because CSF loss is greater than production, resulting in low CSF volume and pressure. Reflexive cerebral vasodilation then occurs, causing headache. The headache is classically frontal or occipital, may be associated with neck stiffness or pain, increases in severity with sitting position, and is relieved by supine position. It may be accompanied by cranial nerve palsies (abducens palsy is most common), nausea and vomiting, or tinnitus. The majority of PDPHs resolve within 1 week, but some may persist longer. Development of PDPH after dural puncture is higher in young, thin, women with histories of headaches and when larger gauge, cutting needles are used. The risk of headache development in pregnant women after dural puncture with an epidural needle (17-18 gauge) is over 50%.[24]

Treatment of PDPH is either conservative (intravenous fluid and oral caffeine and analgesics) or with epidural blood patch (EBP). During an EBP, the anesthesiologist draws the patient's blood sterilely and injects it into the epidural space, "patching" the dural hole with clot and stopping the CSF leakage. Usually, 15 to 20 mL of blood is administered. Sometimes development of back or neck pain with injection limits the volume of blood that can be used. EBP typically relieves pain immediately, but may need to be repeated if headache recurs as the clot is resorbed. When PDPH does not respond to EBP or is associated with fever or other neurologic abnormalities, further diagnostic testing is indicated to rule out meningitis or intracranial hemorrhage or thrombosis.

B. Local Anesthetic Overdose

Epidural catheters can unintentionally become intravascular during either initial placement or from migration later. If a large dose of intravenous local anesthetic is accidentally given intravenously, systemic toxicity can occur. Neurotoxicity typically manifests before cardiotoxicity and includes changes in mental status, seizures, and obtundation. Cardiovascular effects first become evident as widening of the QRS complex and progress to ventricular tachycardia or ventricular fibrillation and arrest. At the first signs of overdose, local anesthetic should be discontinued, and oxygen and lipid emulsion administered. Lipid emulsion binds free local anesthetic to prevent further blockage of cardiac sodium channels. However, channels that are already affected will not be altered. Therefore, circulatory support, CPR, and even cardiopulmonary bypass may be necessary to rescue, particularly in the case of bupivacaine overdose (**Figure 31.10**).

C. Nerve Damage

Nerve injuries may arise independently of obstetric or anesthetic interventions. They occur at a rate of 0.8% and are thought to be due to fetal head compression of nerves during passage through the pelvis or nerve stretch or compression from patient positioning during labor and delivery. Mean duration of injury is 2 to 3 months. The lateral femoral cutaneous nerve is most often affected and presents with numbness over the lateral thigh, often termed meralgia paresthetica. The femoral nerve is the second most common site of injury, and palsies of this nerve can be sensory, motor, or mixed and occasionally occur bilaterally. Nulliparity, fetal macrosomia, prolonged second stage of labor, instrumented delivery, and prolonged duration of hip hyperflexion are associated with increased rates of injury. Regional labor analgesia was not associated with nerve injury in a large prospective study.[25] Occasionally, root injuries or radiculopathy may present postpartum due to exacerbation of underlying pathologies such as disk herniation. During neuraxial block, a needle or catheter may directly traumatize nerves, resulting in injury. Such an injury is usually preceded by paresthesias during block placement. Persistence of paresthesias or severe pain during a neuraxial technique should prompt withdrawal of the needle or catheter.

Documentation of neurologic examination and preexisting deficits prior to neuraxial procedures is important, and intrinsic nerve injuries due to labor and delivery must be distinguished from those resulting from neuraxial anesthesia. Electromyogram may be helpful in determining the amount of time a deficit has been present.

D. Neuraxial Hematoma or Abscess

Epidural bleeding or abscess can be catastrophic because of pressure exerted on the spinal cord or cauda equina. Neuraxial hematoma is a rare event, but traumatic or difficult placement and coagulopathy or anticoagulant use increase the likelihood of occurrence. The American Society of Regional Anesthesia recommendations for use of anticoagulants and placement of neuraxial anesthesia can be viewed at their website. Motor weakness that persists or worsens

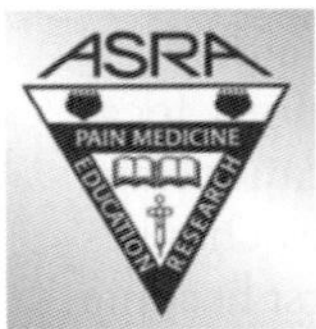

AMERICAN SOCIETY OF
REGIONAL ANESTHESIA AND PAIN MEDICINE

Checklist for Treatment of Local Anesthetic Systemic Toxicity

The Pharmacologic Treatment of Local Anesthetic Systemic Toxicity (LAST) is Different from Other Cardiac Arrest Scenarios

Get Help

Initial Focus

- **Airway management:** ventilate with 100% oxygen
- **Seizure suppersion: benzodiazepines are preferred; AVOID propofol** in patients having signs of cardiovascular instability
- **Alert** the nearest facility having **cardiopulmonary bypass** capability

Management of Cardiac Arrhythmias

- **Basic and Advanced Cardiac Life Support (ACLS)** will require adjustment of medications and perhaps prolonged effort
- **AVOID vasopressin, calcium channel blockers, beta blockers, or local anesthetic**
- **REDUCE individual epinephrine doses to <1 mcg/kg**

Lipid Emulsion (20%) Therapy (values in parenthesis are for 70 kg patient)

- **Bolus 1.5 mL/kg** (lean body mass) intravenously over 1 minute (~100 mL)
- **Continuous infusion 0.25 mL/kg/min** (~18 mL/min; adjust by roller clamp)
- Repeat bolus once or twice for persistent cardiovascular collapse
- Double the infusion rate to 0.5 mL/kg/min if blood pressure remains low
- **Continue infusion** for at least 10 minutes after attaining circulatory stability
- Recommended upper limit: Approximately 10 mL/kg lipid emulsion over the first 30 minutes

Post LAST events at www.lipidrescue.org and report use of lipid to www.lipidregistry.org

Figure 31.10 Checklist for treatment of local anesthetic systemic toxicity. (From Neal JM, Bernards CM, Butterworth JF, et al. ASRA practice advisory on local anesthetic systemic toxicity. *Reg Anesth Pain Med.* 2010;35:152-161, with permission.)

BE PREPARED

- We strongly advise that those using local anesthetics (LA) in doses sufficient to produce local anesthetic systemic toxicity (LAST) establish a plan for managing this complication. Making a *Local Anesthetic Toxicity Kit* and posting instructions for its use are encouraged.

RISK REDUCTION (*BE SENSIBLE*)

- Use the least dose of LA necessary to achieve the desired extent and duration of block.
- Local anesthetic blood levels are influenced by site of injection and dose. Factors that can increase the likelihood of LAST include: advanced age, heart failure, ischemic heart disease, conduction abnormalities, metabolic (e.g., mitochondrial) disease, liver disease, low plasma protein concentration, metabolic or respiratory acidosis, medications that inhibit sodium channels. Patients with severe cardiac dysfunction, particularly very low ejection fraction, are more sensitive to LAST and also more prone to 'stacked' injections (with resulting elevated LA tissue concentrations) due to slowed circulation time.
- Consider using a pharmacologic marker and/or test dose, e.g. epinephrine 5 mcg/mL of LA. Know the expected response, onset, duration, and limitations of "test dose" in identifying intravascular injection.
- Aspirate the syringe prior to *each* injection while observing for blood.
- Inject incrementally, while observing for signs and querying for symptoms of toxicity between each injection.

DETECTION (*BE VIGILANT*)

- Use standard American Society of Anesthesiologists (ASA) monitors.
- Monitor the patient during and after completing injection as clinical toxicity can be delayed up to 30 minutes.
- Communicate frequently with the patient to query for symptoms of toxicity.
- Consider LAST in any patient with altered mental status, neurological symptoms or cardiovascular instability after a regional anesthetic.
- Central nervous system signs (may be subtle or absent)
  - *Excitation* (agitation, confusion, muscle twitching, seizure)
  - *Depression* (drowsiness, obtundation, coma or apnea)
  - *Non-specific* (metallic taste, circumoral numbness, diplopia, tinnitus, dizziness)
- Cardiovascular signs (often the only manifestation of severe LAST)
  - *Initially may be hyperdynamic* (hypertension, tachycardia, ventricular arrhythmias), then
  - *Progressive hypotension*
  - *Conduction block, bradycardia or asystole*
  - *Ventricular arrhythmia* (ventricular tachycardia, Torsades de Pointes, ventricular fibrillation)
- Sedative hypnotic drugs reduce seizure risk but even light sedation may abolish the patient's ability to recognize or report symptoms of rising LA concentrations.

TREATMENT

- Timing of lipid infusion in LAST is controversial. The most conservative approach, waiting until after ACLS has proven unsuccessful, is unreasonable because early treatment can prevent cardiovascular collapse. Infusing lipid at the earliest sign of LAST can result in unnecessary treatment since only a fraction of patients will progress to severe toxicity. The most reasonable approach is to implement lipid therapy on the basis of clinical severity and rate of progression of LAST.
- There is laboratory evidence that epinephrine can impair resuscitation from LAST and reduce the efficacy of lipid rescue. Therefore it is recommended to avoid high doses of epinephrine and use smaller doses, e.g., <1 mcg/kg, for treating hypotension.
- Propofol *should not be used* when there are signs of cardiovascular instability. Propofol is a cardiovascular depressant with lipid content too low to provide benefit. Its use is discouraged when there is a risk of progression to cardiovascular collapse.
- Prolonged monitoring (>12 hours) is recommended after any signs of systemic LA toxicity, since cardiovascular depression due to local anesthetics can persist or recur after treatment.

The ASRA Practice Advisory on Local Anesthetic Toxicity is published in the society's official publication *Regional Anesthesia and Pain Medicine,* and can be downloaded from the journal Web site at www.rapm.org.

Neal JM, Bernards CM, Butterworth JF, Di Gregorio G, Drasner K, Hejtmanck MR, Mulroy MF, Rosenquist RW, Weinberg GL. ASRA practice advisory on local anesthetic systemic toxicity. *Reg Anesth Pain Med* 2010;35:152-161.

Figure 31.10 *(Continued)*

despite discontinuation of local anesthetic is the most common presentation for a neuraxial hematoma. Back pain sometimes accompanies the weakness. Time is important in cases of neuraxial hematoma because neurologic outcomes are worse the longer treatment is delayed. MRI represents the best imaging modality for diagnosis. Neuraxial hematoma necessitates immediate neurosurgical consultation for possible emergent decompression of the clot.

Neuraxial infection may manifest as either meningitis or abscess; both are very uncommon events. Contaminants causing meningitis tend to arise from the nasopharynx of the provider who placed the block. Abscess may be due to the patient's skin flora. Sterile preparation, draping, and use of a surgical mask are standard during placement of neuraxial blocks to prevent iatrogenic infection.

IX. Anesthesia for Nonobstetric Surgery During Pregnancy

Nonobstetric elective surgery during a desired pregnancy is not recommended. Occasionally, emergency conditions warrant surgery during pregnancy, the most common of which are appendicitis or trauma. The safest time to perform surgery during pregnancy is the second trimester because surgery during the first trimester is associated with spontaneous abortion and during the third trimester with preterm labor. Organogenesis occurs early in the first trimester, and it is still unclear what effects anesthetic agents may have on the developing fetus.

Confirmation of fetal heart tones both pre- and postoperatively is recommended. In certain cases, continuous fetal monitoring may be indicated, specifically if the fetus is viable and if staff qualified to perform emergency cesarean delivery are available. Most abdominal surgeries preclude the use of continuous fetal monitoring. Observation postoperatively is generally recommended due to the increased risk of preterm labor.

Regional anesthesia is preferred whenever possible, including for short, uncomplicated open abdominal surgery, such as appendectomy. If not possible (eg, for laparoscopic surgery), general anesthesia should be induced via rapid sequence induction and intubation with cricoid pressure. Patients over 14 weeks' gestation should be positioned in left uterine displacement if feasible. Normotension, maintenance of eucarbia, and adequate oxygenation will provide the fetus and mother with adequate perfusion and oxygenation. Most anesthetic agents, other than the neuromuscular blocking agents, cross the placenta with unknown fetal effects. Neuromuscular blockade reversal agents do cross the placenta, but glycopyrrolate does not. Therefore, the anesthesiologist should reverse blockade with atropine to avoid fetal effects of reversal, including bradycardia.

In summary, providing optimal anesthetic care to pregnant patients requires consideration of the many maternal physiologic changes pregnancy induces, as well as recognition of the effects of anesthesia on both the mother and the fetus. The anesthesiologist is responsible for providing analgesia for labor, but also for guiding the response to complex medical and emergency clinical situations. A thorough knowledge of the medical histories of patients who are admitted to labor and delivery, as well as coordinated multidisciplinary care, is of the utmost importance to ensure optimal outcomes for both mothers and babies.

For further review and interactivities, please see the associated Interactive Video Lectures and "At a Glance" infographic accessible in the complimentary eBook bundled with this text. Access instructions are located in the inside front cover.

References

1. Quinn A, Milne D, Columb M, et al. Failed tracheal intubation in obstetric anaesthesia: 2 yr national case–control study in the UK. *Br J Anaesth*. 2013;110(1):74-80. PMID: 22986421.
2. Sharma S, Alexander J, Messick G, et al. Cesarean delivery: a randomized trial of epidural analgesia versus intravenous meperidine analgesia during labor in nulliparous women. *Anesthesiology*. 2002;96:546-551. PMID: 11873026.
3. Gambling D, Berkowitz J, Farrell T, et al. Randomized controlled comparison of epidural analgesia and combined spinal-epidural analgesia in a private practice setting: pain scores during first and second stages of labor and at delivery. *Anesth Analg*. 2013;116(3):636-643. PMID: 23400985.

4. Pan P, Bogard T, Owen M. Incidence and characteristics of failures in obstetric neuraxial analgesia and anesthesia: a retrospective analysis of 19,259 deliveries. *Int J Obstet Anesth*. 2004;13:227-233. PMID: 15477051.
5. Chau A, Bibbo C, Huang CC, et al. Dural puncture epidural technique improves labor analgesia quality with fewer side effects compared with epidural and combined spinal epidural techniques: a randomized clinical trial. *Anesth Analg*. 2017;124:560-569. PMID: 28067707.
6. Martin JA, Hamilton BE, Osterman MJK, Driscoll AK; National Center for Health Statistics, Centers for Disease Control and Prevention; National Vital Statistics Reports. Births: Final Data for 2018. *Natl Vital Stat Rep*. 2019;68(13):1-47. PMID: 30707672.
7. Osterman MJK. Recent trends in vaginal birth after cesarean delivery: United States, 2016-2018. *NCHS Data Brief*. 2020;(359):1-8. PMID: 32487289.
8. Lee AJ, Landau R, Mattingly JL, et al. Left lateral table tilt for elective cesarean delivery under spinal anesthesia has no effect on neonatal acid-base status. *Anesthesiology*. 2017;127:241-249. PMID: 28598894.
9. Palmer C, Emerson S, Volgoropolous D, et al. Dose-response relationship of intrathecal morphine for postcesarean analgesia. *Anesthesiology*. 1999;90:437-444. PMID: 9952150.
10. Palmer C, Nogami W, Van Maren G, et al. Postcesarean epidural morphine: a dose-response study. *Anesth Analg*. 2000;90:887-891. PMID: 10735794.
11. Horlocker T, Burton A, Connis R, et al. Practice guidelines for the prevention, detection, and management of respiratory depression associated with neuraxial opioid administration: an updated report by the American Society of Anesthesiologists Task Force on Neuraxial Opioids. *Anesthesiology*. 2009;110:218-230. PMID: 19194148.
12. ACOG Practice Bulletin. Intrapartum fetal heart rate monitoring: nomenclature, interpretation, and general management principles. *Obstet Gynecol*. 2009;114(1):192-202. PMID: 19546798.
13. Alfirevic Z, Devane D, Gyte GM. Continuous cardiotocography (CTG) as a form of electronic fetal monitoring (EFM) for fetal assessment during labour. *Cochrane Database Syst Rev*. 2006;3:CD006066. PMID: 16856111.
14. Gestational hypertension and preeclampsia: ACOG Practice Bulletin Summary, Number 222. *Obstet Gynecol*. 2020;135(6):1492-1495. PMID: 32443079.
15. The Eclampsia Trial Collaborative Group. Which anticonvulsant for women with eclampsia? Evidence from the Collaborative Eclampsia Trial. *Lancet*. 1995;345:1455-1463. PMID: 7769899.
16. Segal S. Labor epidural analgesia and maternal fever. *Anesth Analg*. 2010;111:1467-1475. PMID: 20861420.
17. Bateman B, Berman M, Riley L, et al. The epidemioilogy of postpartum hemorrhage in a large, nationwide sample of deliveries. *Anesth Analg*. 2010;110:1368-1373. PMID: 20237047.
18. Committee on Practice Bulletins-Obstetrics. Practice Bulletin No. 183: postpartum hemorrhage. *Obstet Gynecol*. 2011;130(4):e168-e186. PMID: 28937571.
19. Shakur H, Roberts I, Fawole B, et al. The WOMAN Trial (World Maternal Antifibrinolytic Trial). Tranexamic acid for the treatment of postpartum haemorrhage: an international randomised, double blind placebo-controlled trial. *Lancet*. 2017;389:2105-2116. PMID: 20398351.
20. Morris S, Stacey M. Resuscitation in pregnancy. *Br Med J*. 2003;327:1277-1279. PMID: 14644974.
21. National Center for Health Statistics. *National Vital Statistics System*. Centers for Disease Control and Prevention; 2018.
22. World Health Organization. *Trends in Maternal Mortality: 2000 to 2017. Estimates by WHO, UNICEF, UNFPA, World Bank Group and the United Nations Population Division*. World Health Organization; 2019.
23. Hawkins J, Chang J, Palmer S, et al. Anesthesia-related maternal mortality in the United States: 1979–2002. *Obstet Gynecol*. 2011;117:69-74. PMID: 21173646.
24. Choi P, Galinski S, Takeuchi L, et al. PDPH is a common complication of neuraxial blockade in parturients: a meta-analysis of obstetrical studies. *Can J Anesth*. 2003;50(5):460-469. PMID: 12734154.
25. Wong C, Scavone B, Dugan S, et al. Incidence of postpartum lumbosacral spine and lower extremity nerve injuries. *Obstet Gynecol*. 2003;101:279-288. PMID: 12576251.

NEURAXIAL ANESTHESIA FOR CESAREAN SECTION

AT A GLANCE

Approximately one-third of all births in the United States occur through cesarean section. Many c-sections are performed after an unsuccessful attempt at vaginal delivery and the patient may already have a preexisting epidural catheter which can be utilized for surgical anesthesia. In other cases a single shot spinal injection may be used. Below is a comparison of these techniques.

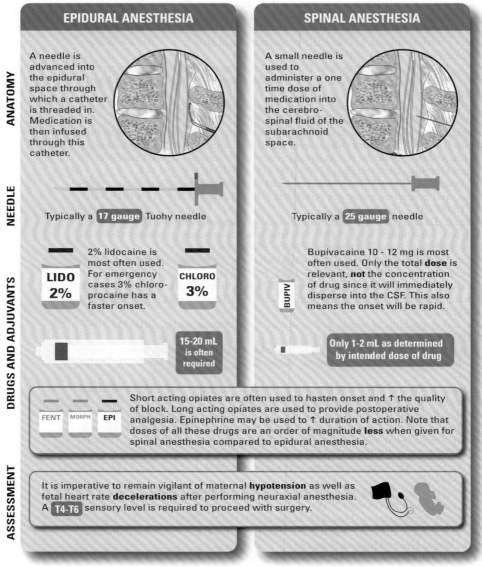

	EPIDURAL ANESTHESIA	SPINAL ANESTHESIA
ANATOMY	A needle is advanced into the epidural space through which a catheter is threaded in. Medication is then infused through this catheter.	A small needle is used to administer a one time dose of medication into the cerebrospinal fluid of the subarachnoid space.
NEEDLE	Typically a 17 gauge Tuohy needle	Typically a 25 gauge needle
DRUGS AND ADJUVANTS	LIDO 2% / CHLORO 3% 2% lidocaine is most often used. For emergency cases 3% chloroprocaine has a faster onset. 15-20 mL is often required	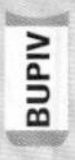 BUPIV Bupivacaine 10 - 12 mg is most often used. Only the total **dose** is relevant, **not** the concentration of drug since it will immediately disperse into the CSF. This also means the onset will be rapid. Only 1-2 mL as determined by intended dose of drug

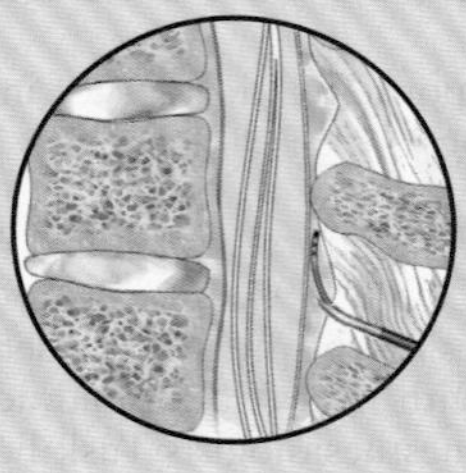

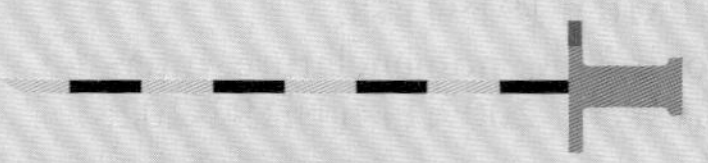

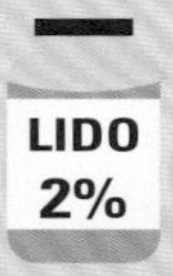

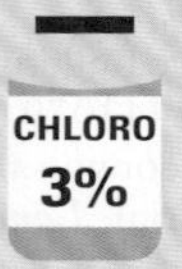

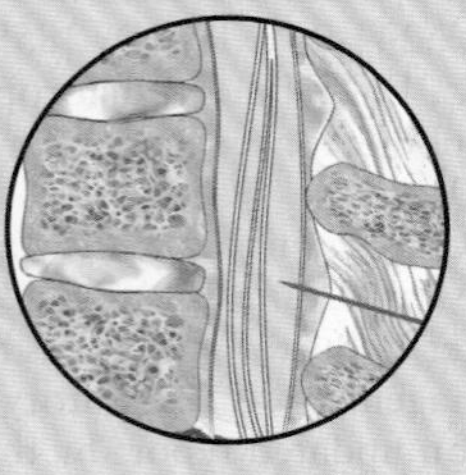

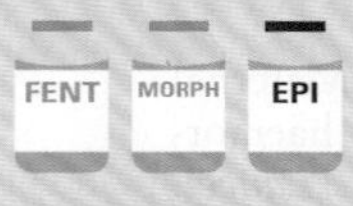

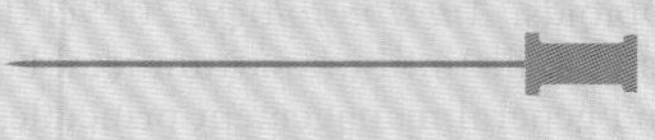

FENT / MORPH / EPI

Short acting opiates are often used to hasten onset and ↑ the quality of block. Long acting opiates are used to provide postoperative analgesia. Epinephrine may be used to ↑ duration of action. Note that doses of all these drugs are an order of magnitude **less** when given for spinal anesthesia compared to epidural anesthesia.

ASSESSMENT

It is imperative to remain vigilant of maternal **hypotension** as well as fetal heart rate **decelerations** after performing neuraxial anesthesia. A T4-T6 sensory level is required to proceed with surgery.

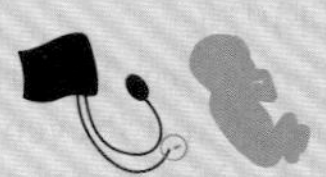

A combined spinal-epidural (CSE) may also be used to take advantage of speed of onset of spinal anesthesia and ability to prolong duration of action with an epidural catheter.

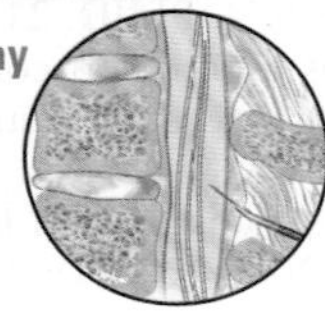

General anesthesia may be indicated if neuraxial anesthesia is contraindicated or in critical emergencies.

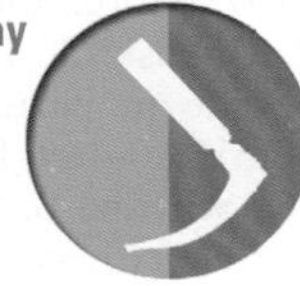

Infographic by: Naveen Nathan MD

Questions

1. **Which of the following arterial blood gas profiles is most consistent with a healthy, term parturient?**

   A. pH 7.40, Pao_2 99 mm Hg, Pco_2 40 mm Hg, HCO_3 24 mEq/L
   B. pH 7.44, Pao_2 103 mm Hg, Pco_2 30 mm Hg, HCO_3 20 mEq/L
   C. pH 7.32, Pao_2 98 mm Hg, Pco_2 44 mm Hg, HCO_3 24 mEq/L
   D. pH 7.40, Pao_2 99 mm Hg, Pco_2 45 mm Hg, HCO_3 26 mEq/L

2. **A 37-year-old parturient with history of moderate persistent asthma requiring frequent steroid use just gave birth to a healthy newborn via cesarean delivery after a failed induction of labor. The obstetrician tells you that they are experiencing uterine atony. Which uterotonic agent is relatively contraindicated in this patient?**

   A. Methylergonovine (IM)
   B. Oxytocin (IV)
   C. 15-Methyl prostaglandin $F_{2\alpha}$ (IM)
   D. Prostaglandin E_2 (buccal)

3. **Which of the following cardiac parameters decreases during pregnancy?**

   A. Systemic vascular resistance
   B. Cardiac output
   C. Stroke volume
   D. Heart rate

4. **During a cesarean delivery under general anesthesia, which anesthetic agent may cause uterine relaxation?**

   A. Nitrous oxide
   B. Volatile anesthetics
   C. Opioids
   D. Propofol

5. **A 25-year-old G1 patient is currently in labor with a well-functioning epidural catheter in place. The patient has a prolonged fetal heart rate deceleration that is not corrected with conservative measures and the decision is made to proceed with an emergent cesarean delivery for fetal well-being. Which of the following local anesthetic combinations will result in the most rapid onset of surgical anesthesia?**

   A. 2% lidocaine with 1:200,000 epinephrine
   B. 2% lidocaine with 1:200,000 epinephrine and sodium bicarbonate
   C. 3% 2-chloroprocaine
   D. 3% 2-chloroprocaine with sodium bicarbonate

Answers

1. B

If a blood gas is obtained on a healthy parturient, you should expect to find a slight respiratory alkalosis with compensatory metabolic acidosis. This is because of the increased minute ventilation observed in pregnancy (increased tidal volume and minimal increase in respiratory rate). You will also observe a slight increase in arterial partial pressure of oxygen. To compensate for this, the kidneys will excrete bicarbonate in the urine creating a compensatory metabolic acidosis. Answer A is a normal blood gas in a healthy, nonparturient. Answer C is consistent with acute respiratory acidosis. Even values of Pco_2 that are considered normal in nonpregnant patient should be concerning for carbon dioxide retention during pregnancy. Answer D is consistent with respiratory acidosis with compensatory metabolic alkalosis.

2. C

Carboprost (15-methyl prostaglandin $F_{2\alpha}$) should be used with caution in patients with poorly controlled asthma, as it may induce bronchospasm. Methylergonovine should be used with caution in patients with poorly controlled hypertension or preeclampsia as it may cause severe hypertension. Oxytocin and misoprostol (prostaglandin E_2) are safe to use in patients.

3. A

Systemic vascular resistance (SVR) decreases about 20% during pregnancy largely due to peripheral vasodilation mediated by an increase in endothelial-related factors. To compensate for this decrease in SVR, there is an increase in cardiac output (by approximately 40%) during pregnancy. This increase in cardiac output is accomplished by both an increase in stroke volume and heart rate.

4. B

Volatile anesthetics, especially when used at levels of 1 MAC or greater, cause uterine relaxation. The other agents (nitrous oxide, opioids, and propofol) do not cause uterine relaxation. Therefore, after delivery of the newborn, volatile anesthetic use should be minimized utilizing a multiagent anesthetic. This can be accomplished by using 0.5 MAC volatile with nitrous or converting to total intravenous anesthesia with propofol infusion. Opioids have no effect on uterine tone and should be used as part of a multimodal approach to treating pain.

5. D

3% 2-chloroprocaine with freshly added sodium bicarbonate will result in the most rapid onset of anesthesia, estimated at about 3 minutes. Despite having a high pK_a (approximately 9), 3% 2-chloroprocaine has the most rapid onset because it is used in high concentrations due to its low systemic toxicity (rapidly metabolized via ester hydrolysis). 2% lidocaine is often utilized for nonurgent cesarean deliveries and results in a surgical level in about 10 minutes. The addition of sodium bicarbonate will hasten the onset of action of both chloroprocaine and lidocaine. Alkalization of the local anesthetic shifts more of the molecules to their nonionized form and therefore the anesthetic passes through the cell membrane more quickly. (Recall that local anesthetics act on the intracellular portion of the cellular sodium channels and therefore must cross into the cell.)

32 Trauma and Burn Anesthesia

Pudkrong Aichholz and Andreas Grabinsky

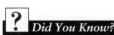

Did You Know?

The primary survey and initial resuscitation of the severely injured patient follow the ABCDE acronym: Airway, Breathing, Circulation, Disability (neurologic function), and Exposure (completely expose and examine the patient so that no injury is missed).

I. Initial Trauma Evaluation and Resuscitation

Traumatic injury is the leading cause of death worldwide, particularly in younger age groups, potentially causing a significant number of life years lost. The treatment of seriously injured patients is time-sensitive and best accomplished by an interdisciplinary team approach, with anesthesia providers being responsible for airway/ventilation management and assisting with vascular access, fluid/blood resuscitation, sedation, and blood pressure control.

Severely injured patients will more likely require fast transport to the operating room for definitive surgical care. Having anesthesia at the bedside in the emergency room (ER) to facilitate such transport is beneficial. In some instances, the direct admission of a trauma patient to the operating room and bypassing the ER may also reduce the time to definitive care.

To facilitate a systematic thinking process and understanding between various specialty providers, the American College of Surgeons' ***Advanced Trauma Life Support (ATLS)*** approach is commonly used to assess and care for injured patients. In short, ATLS management consists of the ***primary survey*** (identification of life-threatening injuries with simultaneous resuscitation), the ***secondary survey*** (comprehensive assessment of all other injuries and associated conditions), and ***definitive care*** (medical, surgical, or critical care). Here, we will focus on the primary survey and resuscitation known by the mnemonic ABCDE.

A. Airway Management With Restriction of Cervical Spine Motion

Assessing and securing the airway is the first step of the primary survey. Rapid assessment is done by asking patients simple questions. Patients who can speak usually have a patent airway and do not immediately require airway management. For more comprehensive assessment, Chapter 20 provides details of airway management in elective and emergent settings.

Standard methods of airway assessment (Tables 20.4-20.6; Figure 20.3) can be limited in the trauma setting by lack of patient cooperation. This makes visual inspection of the face and neck the mainstay of such assessment. A short, fat neck with fewer than three fingerbreadths from the thyroid notch to the jaw tip (ie, thyromental distance) is concerning for a potentially difficult airway. Obvious facial asymmetry further suggests an underlying anatomic abnormality, be it traumatic, congenital, or neoplastic. Limited neck range of motion—whether from preexisting conditions or cervical spine immobilization—further suggests a more challenging airway. The modified LEMON criteria (**Table 32.1**) can be used to predict a potentially difficult airway.

Table 32.1 Modified LEMON Score

	Criteria	Point
L	**Look externally**	
	• Facial trauma	1
	• Beard or mustache	1
	• Large incisors	1
	• Large tongue	1
E	**Evaluate the 3-3-2 rules:**	
	• Interincisor distance <3 fingerbreadths	1
	• Hyoid-mental distance <3 fingerbreadths	1
	• Thyroid-floor of mouth distance <2 fingerbreadths	1
M	**Mallampati score of 3 or 4**: not counted in the modified LEMON total score	-
O	**Obstruction**: Any conditions that cause airway obstruction	1
N	**Neck mobility**: any condition that limit neck mobility including immobilization	1
	Total score	9

The presence of a "full stomach" and high aspiration risk should be assumed for all trauma patients. Thus, rapid sequence intubation (RSI) is generally performed. If possible, secure intravenous (IV) or intraosseous (IO) access and preoxygenation should be ensured before any airway manipulation starts.

Cricoid pressure (CP) is commonly applied as part of the RSI protocol, with the objective of preventing gastric aspiration. However, the evidence supporting CP benefit is controversial and also suggests it may worsen laryngoscopic view.[1] Maintenance of CP during active vomiting risks esophageal injury; therefore, CP is not intended to prevent aspiration in a vomiting patient, but rather to prevent passive reflux of gastric contents into the pharynx. In fact, if a patient begins to vomit, one must release CP, turn the patient on their side (if possible), and suction the emesis.

Until the diagnosis of cervical spinal injury is excluded, the spine should be protected from excessive movement that might result in new or worsening spinal cord injury (SCI). ***Manual in-line stabilization (MILS)*** of the cervical spine is routinely used in emergency airway management of trauma patients at risk for cervical spine and/or cord injury. However, cadaveric studies have shown that MILS does not ensure spine immobility. Rigid adherence to MILS or CP in the context of a poor view of the vocal cords can increase the difficulty and duration of tracheal intubation; therefore, relaxation of MILS or CP must be considered in the context of the overall clinical picture that prioritizes securing the airway.

Mask ventilation and tracheal intubation can both be challenging in trauma patients due to head and neck injuries, recent oral intake that increases aspiration risk, and/or possible lung injury that can negatively impact both oxygenation and ventilation. Adherence to the American Society of Anesthesiologists (ASA) difficult airway algorithm is essential (see Appendix D), including planning and preparation of multiple backup airway management techniques. In patients with severe traumatic injury, however, case cancellation is rarely an option. If the intubation attempt fails, it is indicated to transition rapidly to an emergency surgical airway (cricothyrotomy, tracheostomy), as most trauma patients have limited reserve and will not tolerate prolonged intubation attempts (**Figure 32.1**).

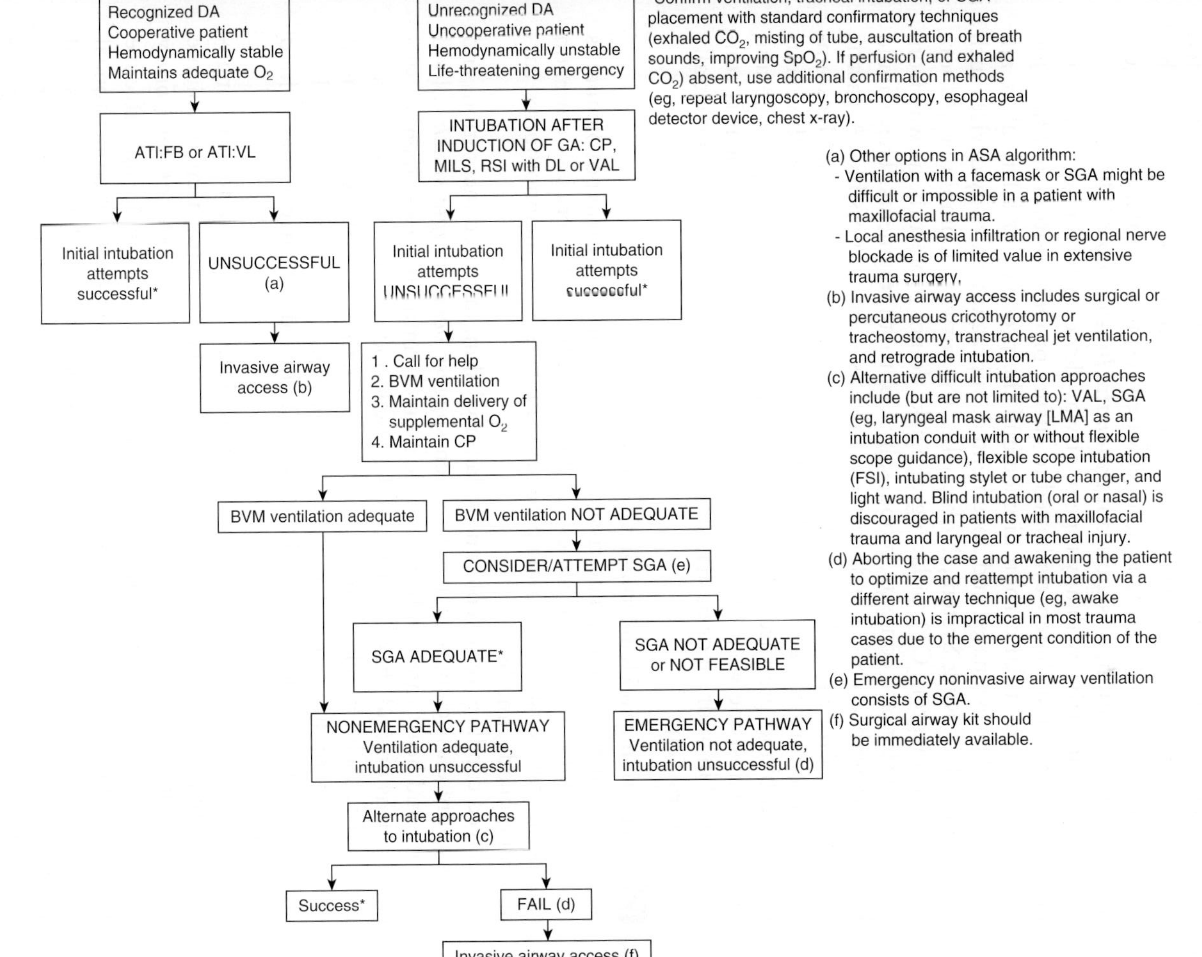

Figure 32.1 American Society of Anesthesiologists Committee on Trauma and Emergency Preparedness airway management algorithm in trauma. ASA, American Society of Anesthesiologists; ATI:FB, awake tracheal intubation using flexible bronchoscopy; ATI:VL, awake tracheal intubation using videolaryngoscopy; BVM, bag-valve-mask; CP, cricoid pressure; DA, difficult airway; DL, direct laryngoscopy; FIS, flexible intubation scope; GA, general anesthesia; MILS, manual in-line stabilization; RSI, rapid sequence intubation; SGA, supraglottic airway; VAL, video-assisted laryngoscopy. (From Hagberg CA, Kaslow O. Difficult airway management algorithm in trauma updated by COTEP. *ASA Monitor.* 2014;78:56-60, Figure 1.)

B. Breathing/Ventilation

Respiratory assessment is a critical component of the primary survey because several pathologies may alter oxygenation and/or ventilation after trauma. Conditions that are life-threatening and often require immediate attention are tension pneumothorax, massive hemothorax, open pneumothorax, and tracheobronchial injuries. Generally, all injured patients should receive supplemental oxygen and monitoring of oxygen saturation with a pulse oximeter. Indications for tracheal intubation include obvious respiratory distress, inability to speak in complete sentences, an elevated respiratory rate, poor oxygenation, poor ventilation, or significant ***traumatic brain injury (TBI)***.

Patients who arrive with any type of airway device placed prior to hospital arrival must be immediately evaluated to ensure proper position and function of the device. End-tidal carbon dioxide and the presence of bilateral breath sounds should be evaluated and documented. Supraglottic airway devices such as the King LT (King System, Noblesville, IN) airway, Combitube (Moore Medical, Farmington, CT), or laryngeal masks do not protect the airway from aspiration of stomach contents, blood, saliva, or tooth fragments. They should be replaced with a cuffed endotracheal tube as soon as possible. A gastric tube should also be placed soon after tracheal intubation to deflate the stomach. This can further mitigate the risk of aspiration and improve both venous return and blood pressure by decreasing both intra-abdominal pressure and pressure against the vena cava. However, nasogastric tube placement is contraindicated in midface or basilar skull fractures, as the tube could potentially enter the cranium.

C. Circulation and Hemorrhage Control

Shock is defined as inadequate tissue perfusion. Blood loss (hypovolemia is the most common cause of shock in trauma patients. Other, less common causes for hypotension in trauma patients include tension pneumothorax, cardiac tamponade, and SCI.

Delayed capillary refill, cold and "clammy" skin, impaired mentation, and oliguria are classic signs that most often suggest ***hemorrhagic shock***. Blood pressure and heart rate can help provide more quantifiable assessment of systemic perfusion and shock. For example, low blood pressure is typically compensated for with an elevated heart rate (see Chapter 3). The Assessment of Blood Consumption score (**Table 32.2**) is a useful tool to determine the likelihood of hemorrhagic shock and the associated need for early massive blood transfusion.

The immediate treatment goals for hemorrhagic shock are to stop ongoing bleeding and restore tissue perfusion by replacing intravascular volume and oxygen carrying capacity (see Chapter 24). Placement of temporary tourniquets on a limb with life-threatening bleeding is a simple and effective hemostasis measure. In cases of significant pelvic trauma and retroperitoneal bleeding, placement of a ***pelvic binder*** can reapproximate pelvic fractures and temporarily limit internal blood loss. Ultimately, the priority is rapid transportation to the operating room or angiography suite for definitive control of internal or external bleeding.

D. Disability (Neurologic Evaluation and Management)

A prompt neurologic evaluation during the primary survey is important for establishing a baseline examination for future treatments. An understanding of the ***Glasgow coma scale*** (GCS) score (see Chapter 30, Table 30.2) is

Table 32.2 Assessment of Blood Consumption Score

Penetrating injury mechanism?	YES/NO
Systolic blood pressure <90 mm Hg?	YES/NO
Heart rate >120 beats per minute?	YES/NO
Positive FAST examination?	YES/NO
If two or more YES answers, then activate massive transfusion protocol.	

FAST, focused assessment with sonography in trauma.

critical to rapidly evaluate and quantify the mental status and motor function of trauma patients. It also guides the need for tracheal intubation in patients with TBI. Of note, the iris contains no nicotinic acetylcholine receptors; therefore, neuromuscular blocking agents do not affect pupil size.

TBI is the leading cause of death in trauma. Any suspicion of TBI should be evaluated with a computed tomography (CT) scan of the head to identify primary injuries (eg, intracranial hematoma) that require immediate surgery or specialized critical care. Throughout the primary survey, however, priority is given to maintaining adequate blood pressure and oxygenation to avoid ***secondary brain injury*** due to neuronal ischemia. In patients with severe TBI defined as GCS of 3 to 8, guidelines from the Brain Trauma Foundation recommend that systolic blood pressure be ≥100 mm Hg for patients 50 to 69 years old or at ≥110 mm Hg for patients 15 to 49 or more than 70 years old. Even transient reductions in blood pressure or oxygen saturation can profoundly affect the mortality of these patients.[2] Perioperative anesthetic management of TBI is discussed in detail in Chapter 30.

> **? Did You Know?**
>
> The 15-point Glasgow coma scale requires cooperative motor responses and verbal skills that are found in older children and adults, but not in younger children or infants; thus, a similar, but modified 15-point pediatric Glasgow coma scale is available and should be used in preverbal children and infants.

In patients who have sustained a ***spinal cord injury (SCI)***, it is important to assess the anatomic level of the neurologic deficit as soon as possible. Sensory level is determined by dermatome level of touch or pain. Motor function is assessed using the American Spinal Injury Association score (see Chapter 26, Table 26.1). Assessment of anal sphincter tone is also an important component of the motor examination.

Methylprednisolone administration, once a standard practice aimed to improve neurologic recovery in SCI patients, was found by recent literature to be associated with negative outcomes such as infection, but with questionable benefit. Thus, the practice is no longer recommended by practice guidelines.[3]

Initial management of suspected SCI includes placement of a rigid cervical collar and strict mobility precautions to minimize spinal motion, particularly in patients with intoxication or TBI when it is challenging to rule out SCI. These patients should remain in a cervical collar until definitive imaging can be performed. Clearance of cervical SCI is only recommended after a negative high-quality C-spine CT scan result[4] and preferably after patient can range the neck without any neurologic deficit.

E. Exposure and Environment Control

The last step of the primary survey is to examine the patient's entire body (including the back) in order to avoid missing any injuries. To evaluate major vascular injury, presence and character of peripheral pulses, as well as skin color and temperature, should be assessed. A cool and poorly perfused limb must be immediately evaluated for possible arterial injury and revascularization. Concurrently, measures to avoid hypothermia should be applied as this can worsen peripheral perfusion and coagulopathy, as well as increase mortality.

After the primary survey is complete, a more detailed history, physical examination, and investigations should be taken to identify any remaining injuries and formulate definitive treatment plans according to urgency of each condition.

F. Interdisciplinary, Team-Based Management

Crew resource management is a concept developed by the aviation industry in which each member of the multidisciplinary team has equal responsibility for passenger safety. For example, any member of a flight crew can alert the pilot in command of a potential hazard. This concept is particularly relevant to trauma, when care is necessarily multidisciplinary and critical events must occur concurrently in a timely fashion. Central to the concept of crew resource management is clear and free communication between all parties, regardless of hierarchy. When several events and therapies must occur simultaneously, it can be valuable to use a checklist to ensure that no critical steps are overlooked.[5] The recommended checklist for trauma and emergency anesthesia is shown in **Figure 32.2**. Assigning predetermined positions to members of the anesthetic resuscitation team is also an effective way to maintain organization in the trauma operating room (**Figure 32.3**).

II. Operative Management: General Considerations

A. Monitoring

Standard ASA monitors are described in Chapter 15. In emergencies, the oxygen saturation monitor can provide reasonably accurate heart rate and oxygen saturation information. A poor quality waveform may also suggest poor peripheral perfusion. An arterial line can provide accurate beat-to-beat measurement of blood pressure and facilitate frequent blood sampling. It can also be used to estimate cardiac output and intravascular volume status (see Chapter 23). Placement of an arterial line, however, should never delay the start of an emergent hemostatic procedure. In severe cases of hemorrhagic shock, the end-tidal CO_2 waveform can be a sensitive indicator for hypoperfusion, as reduced venous return will result in diminished cardiac output and a reduction in end-tidal CO_2. A sudden and significant drop of end-tidal CO_2 in the hypotensive trauma patient is often a sign of imminent cardiovascular collapse.

B. Anesthetic and Adjunct Drugs

Medications should be selected depending on the patient's mental status, injuries, and hemodynamic status. Severely injured patients with hypovolemia are very susceptible to the negative inotropic and vasodilatory effects of anesthetics, particularly certain induction drugs (eg, propofol) and volatile anesthetics. Thus, all anesthetic drugs should be slowly and carefully titrated to avoid cardiovascular collapse in such patients. Unconscious trauma patients may not require much, if any, sedative drugs for tracheal intubation, but will benefit from muscle relaxation to facilitate the intubation. Similarly, hypovolemic yet conscious patients will usually require a significantly reduced dose of anesthetic and benefit from medications such as etomidate or ketamine, which provide better blood pressure stability than propofol. A partial list of commonly used perioperative anesthetic and adjunct drugs, along with specific cautions for use in trauma patients, is provided in **Table 32.3**.

BEFORE PATIENT ARRIVAL

☐ Room temperature 25 °C or higher
☐ Warm IV line
☐ Machine check
☐ Airway equipment
☐ Emergency medications
☐ **BLOOD BANK: "6U O Neg PRBC, 6U AB FFP, 5-6 units of random donor platelets (1 standard adult dose) available"**

PATIENT ARRIVAL

☐ Patient identified for trauma/emergency surgery?
☐ **BLOOD BANK: "Send blood for T&C and initiate MTP now!"**
☐ IV access
☐ Monitors (Sao_2, BP, ECG)
☐ **SURGEON: "PREP & DRAPE!"**
☐ Pre-oxygenation

INDUCTION

☐ Sedative hypnotic (ketamine v. propofol v. etomidate)
☐ Neuromuscular blockade (succinylcholine v. rocuronium)

INTUBATION

☐ **(+) $ETCO_2$ → SURGEON : "GO!"**
☐ Place orogastric tube

ANESTHETIC

☐ (Volatile anesthetic and/or benzodiazepine) + narcotic
☐ Consider TIVA
☐ Insert additional IV access if needed and an arterial line

RESUSCITATION

☐ Send baseline labs
☐ Follow MAP trend
☐ Goal FFP: PRBC controversial, but consider early FFP
☐ Goal urine output 0.5-1 mL/kg/h
☐ Consider tranexamic acid if <3 h after injury; 1 g over 10 min × 1, then 1 g over 8 h
☐ Consider calcium chloride 1 g
☐ Consider hydrocortisone 100 mg
☐ Consider vasopressin 5-10 IU
☐ Administer appropriate antibiotics
☐ Special considerations for TBI (SBP > 90-100 mm Hg, Sao_2 > 90%, Pco_2 35-45 mm Hg)

CLOSING/POST-OP

☐ **ICU: "Do you have a bed?"**
☐ Initiate low lung volume ventilation (TV = 6 mL/kg ideal body weight)

Figure 32.2 **Emergency and trauma anesthesia checklist.** Critical preparation and treatment strategies are shown for each successive step in the emergent, perioperative care of the major trauma victim. AB FFP, type AB fresh frozen plasma; ABG, arterial blood gas, BP, blood pressure; ECG, electrocardiogram; $ETCO_2$, end-tidal carbon dioxide; GCS, Glasgow coma scale; MAP, mean arterial blood pressure; MILS, manual in-line stabilization, MTP, massive transfusion protocol; PRBC, packed red blood cells; RSI, rapid sequence induction, Sao_2, oxygen saturation; SBP, systolic blood pressure; T&C, type and cross; TBI, traumatic brain injury; TIVA, total intravenous anesthesia.

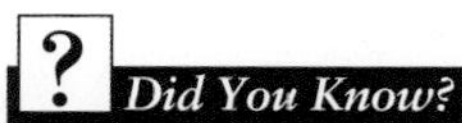

Whereas rapid sequence induction and intubation is generally a two-person procedure, a minimum of three providers are required when performing the procedure in a patient with possible cervical spine injury: one to hold manual in-line neck stabilization, one to provide cricoid pressure, and one to perform tracheal intubation.

C. Induction and Airway Management

Rapid sequence induction (RSI) is the process of intravenous induction of general anesthesia and neuromuscular blockade, after which an endotracheal tube is rapidly placed to secure the airway. This is done with limited positive pressure mask ventilation to minimizing the risk of regurgitation and aspiration of gastric contents (see Chapter 20). RSI is commonly employed in trauma patients. Usually combined with MILS in patients at risk for cervical SCI, it is a safe and

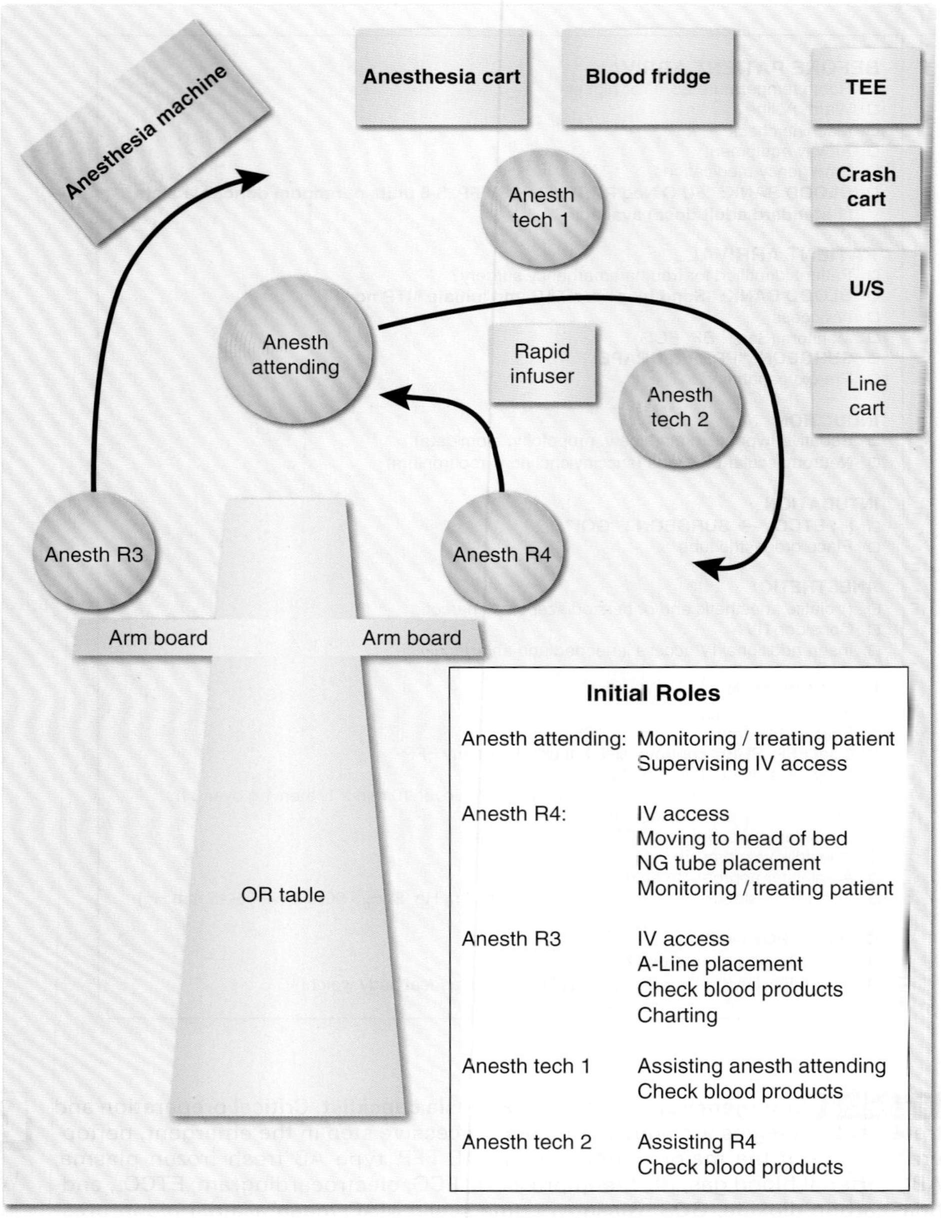

Figure 32.3 **Trauma anesthesia teamwork flow diagram.** The ideal floor plan setup for anesthetic care of the major trauma patient includes assigned spaces for various anesthesia providers, the anesthesia workstation, and critical equipment.

effective method to secure the airway. If a hard cervical collar is in place, the front portion of the collar can be removed, with MILS applied immediately after induction to facilitate mouth opening and laryngeal viewing.

Video laryngoscopy (VL) is increasingly used for emergency airway management. Evidence suggests that VL can improve visualization of the vocal cords and increase the intubation success rate in predicted difficult airway cases (eg, limited mouth opening, higher Mallampati scores). Compared to conventional direct

Table 32.3 Anesthetic and Adjunct Drugs Commonly Used for Trauma Anesthesia and Resuscitation

Medication	Dose	Mechanism of Action	Comments
Sedative/Hypnotics			
Propofol	1.5-2.5 mg/kg	γ-Aminobutyric acid (GABA) agonist	Can reduce systemic vascular resistance (SVR) and blood pressure
Ketamine	1-2 mg/kg	*N*-methyl-D-aspartate (NMDA) antagonist	Maintains airway reflexes and SVR
Etomidate	0.2-0.3 mg/kg	GABA agonist	Single doses for induction can transiently suppress hypothalamic-pituitary-adrenal axis
Neuromuscular Blocking Agents			
Succinylcholine	1 mg/kg	Depolarizing neuromuscular relaxant	Can cause life-threatening hyperkalemia in burns and spinal cord injury after 48 h
Rocuronium	0.6-1.0 mg/kg	Nondepolarizing muscle relaxant	Can be effectively used in rapid sequence induction
Cisatracurium	0.1-0.2 mg/kg	Nondepolarizing muscle relaxant	Eliminated by Hoffman degradation; useful in renal insufficiency/failure
Vecuronium	0.1 mg/kg	Nondepolarizing muscle relaxant	Prolonged duration in hepatic dysfunction
Adjuncts			
Tranexamic acid	1 g over 10 min, then 1 g over 8 h	Synthetic lysine derivative and antifibrinolytic	Improvement in trauma mortality when given within 3 h of injury
Fibrinogen concentrate	50-100 mg/kg	Treat low fibrinogen level (by conventional or viscoelastic testing)	Potential risk of transfusion-transmitted infection
Recombinant factor VII	20-100 μg/kg	Accelerates thrombin formation at site of endothelial injury	Benefits in trauma unclear; potential risk of thrombosis; expensive
Prothrombin complex concentrate (PCC)	25-50 IU/Kg	Reversal anticoagulation from vitamin K antagonist, or direct oral anticoagulant; use with or without fresh frozen plasma (FFP) to replace coagulation factors in bleeding trauma patients	Increases risk of delayed thrombotic complications; expensive
Vasopressin	5-20 IU	Potent vasoconstrictor	Shunts blood to cerebral, cardiac, and pulmonary vascular beds
Calcium chloride	1 g	Facilitates smooth muscle contraction	Used to restore low calcium levels and inotropy during massive transfusion
Hydrocortisone	100 mg	Potent mineralocorticoid	Treats adrenal suppression seen in critical illness

laryngoscopy it also requires less manipulation of the cervical spine. However, it tends to be a slower technique and might not improve the intubation success rate in routine cases.[6] Supraglottic airways (eg, laryngeal mask) provide a blind insertion alternative to tracheal intubation. In the prehospital setting, such devices may be easier to place by providers with limited intubation experience. In the hospital setting, they serve as effective rescue devices in "can't intubate, can't ventilate" scenarios; however, they do not provide reliable protection against aspiration.

D. Hypotension

Hypotension in trauma patients is to be considered of hemorrhagic origin until proven otherwise. While moderate amounts of blood loss can be replaced with crystalloid infusion, more severe blood loss or ongoing hemorrhage will require blood transfusion.

Patients with traumatic injures require adequate intravenous access to allow rapid volume resuscitation. Ideally, severely injured patients should have central venous access with a large-bore sheath introducer (eg, Cordis, Cardinal Health Inc, Dublin, Ohio) or peripheral venous access via a large-bore rapid infusion catheter. Avoiding long IV tubing or tubing extensions ("pig tails") is also recommended, as they will limit the infusion flow rate. For abdominal injuries, IV access is placed preferably in the upper extremities or neck. In case of femoral or iliac vein injury, access in the lower extremity, including femoral line, can cause transfused blood or fluids to flow into the abdomen instead of the central circulation.

Resuscitation is often initiated with warm isotonic crystalloid, such as Plasma-Lyte or lactated Ringer's. Sodium chloride 0.9% should be avoided because of its associated risk of acute kidney injury (see Chapter 23). ATLS currently recommends initiation of 1 L of crystalloid (20 mL/kg for pediatric patients) and early conversion to blood products for unresponsive shock.

Before the bleeding source has been controlled, ***damage control resuscitation (DCR)*** is a useful strategy to reduce blood loss and limit coagulopathy in massively bleeding patients. Aside from early hemorrhage control, DCR focuses on three tenets: permissive hypotension, limiting crystalloid use, and hemostatic resuscitation.

The concept of ***permissive hypotension*** aims to mitigate blood loss by allowing a lower-than-normal blood pressure—just enough to provide vital organ perfusion—until source control of hemorrhage is achieved. In patients without TBI, a target SBP of 80 to 90 mm Hg (MAP 50-60 mm Hg) is generally recommended.[7] Concurrently, crystalloids and colloids are avoided to prevent dilution of coagulation factors, and ***"hemostatic resuscitation"*** is performed with aggressive use of hemostatic blood products combined with packed red blood cells (PRBCs) to prevent and reverse coagulopathy. Early use of PRBCs and empiric administration of fresh frozen plasma (FFP) and platelets before a documented coagulopathy has improved survival of severely injured trauma patients in both the combat environment and the civilian population.[8] The general goal is a ratio of PRBCs to FFP to platelets approaching 1:1:1, or when circumstances permit, a goal-directed transfusion using point-of-care viscoelastic monitoring.

Tranexamic acid (TXA) is a synthetic lysine analogue that inhibits fibrinolysis. Its administration within 3 hours after injury has been shown to reduce mortality in major trauma patients[9] and is increasingly used in this setting.

Hypotension during trauma surgery is most commonly caused by hemorrhage and hypovolemia with compensatory peripheral vasoconstriction, in contrast to hypotension in nontrauma patients that is often caused by vasodilation from anesthetic drugs. Therefore, hypotensive trauma patients should be treated with volume replacement instead of vasopressors. The use of vasopressors (with the possible exception of vasopressin) is associated with increased mortality in trauma resuscitation, and their use should be avoided.[10] However, vasopressors can be used to bridge a short amount of time if blood products are not immediately available for transfusion or to limit excessive crystalloid resuscitation. In case of imminent cardiovascular collapse due to blood loss in a trauma patient, small doses of epinephrine (50-200 μg) can stabilize the blood pressure and allow time for further volume resuscitation. Larger doses of epinephrine might increase the blood pressure significantly, however, and rapidly result in increased blood loss.

E. Hypothermia

The ***"lethal triad" of trauma resuscitation*** consists of hypothermia, coagulopathy, and acidosis. To avoid hypothermia in perioperative trauma care, the operating room should be heated to as warm a temperature as possible, intravenous fluids warmed, and convective warming devices used to maintain a core temperature > 36 °C.

VIDEO 32.1
Hypocapnia

F. Coagulation Abnormalities

Trauma-induced coagulopathy is an endogenous impairment of the coagulation system that occurs early after injury. It is found in at least a quarter of severely injured patient and is associated with at least 2-fold increase in mortality. Thus, accurate assessment of and correction of coagulation status are very important components of trauma resuscitation. Traditionally, blood samples are sent for prothrombin time/international normalized ratio (INR), partial thromboplastin time (PTT), hemoglobin (Hb)/hematocrit, platelet count, and fibrinogen. Low platelet counts, Hb, and fibrinogen are treated with platelets, PRBCs, and cryoprecipitate, respectively. Elevated INR and PTT are treated with FFP. However, these tests are neither timely nor particularly sensitive and specific, thereby limiting their use in acute resuscitation.

Viscoelastic testing, such as ***thromboelastography (TEG)*** and ***rotational thromboelastometry (ROTEM)***, has been increasingly used as a point-of-care test to evaluate various functional aspects of coagulation (**Figures 32.4** and **32.5**) in trauma patients. TEG/ROTEM readout can be divided into three phases, each answering different questions about clot formation. Phase 1 is the preclot formation phase. It shows "how long" it takes for clot formation to start. Prolongation of this phase is treated with FFP or prothrombin complex concentrate. Phase 2 is the clot formation phase, answering "how strong" the clot strength is. This reflects fibrinogen level and platelet mass. A shallow clot angle and amplitude can be treated with platelet, cryoprecipitate, or fibrinogen concentrate transfusion. Lastly, the clot stability phase indicates the status of fibrinolysis. Abnormalities in this phase can be treated with antifibrinolytics such as TXA.

G. Electrolyte and Acid-Base Disturbances

Massive transfusion can cause several metabolic abnormalities. Citrate preservative in both PRBCs and FFP can chelate and decrease the serum calcium level, thereby contributing to hypotension. ***Hypocalcemia*** is associated with increased mortality; therefore ionized calcium levels below 1 mmol/L or persistent hypotension with blood transfusion should be promptly treated with calcium chloride.

Lysis of red blood cells during transfusion can result in ***hyperkalemia***, particularly with older blood products. Hyperkalemia is characterized by peaked T waves on the electrocardiogram. Potassium levels >5 mEq/L should be

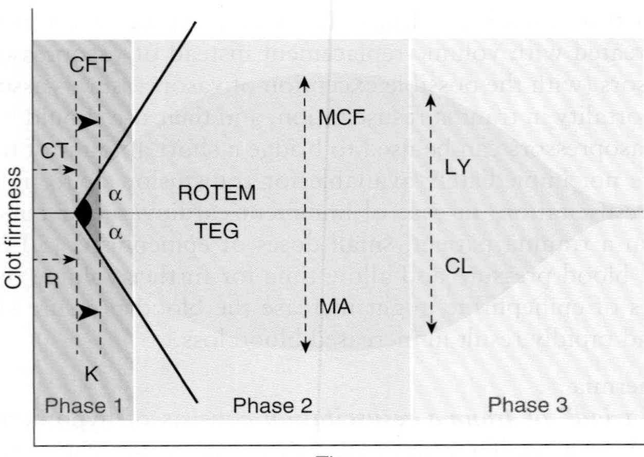

Figure 32.4 Rotational thromboelastometry (ROTEM) and thromboelastography (TEG) tracing and parameters. Three phases of viscoelastic tests shown: phase 1 (preclot formation), phase 2 (clot formation), and phase 3 (stability). α, alpha angle; CFT, clot formation time; CL, clot lysis; CT, clotting time; k, kinetics; LY, clot lysis; MA, maximum amplitude; MCF, maximum clot firmness; R, reaction time.

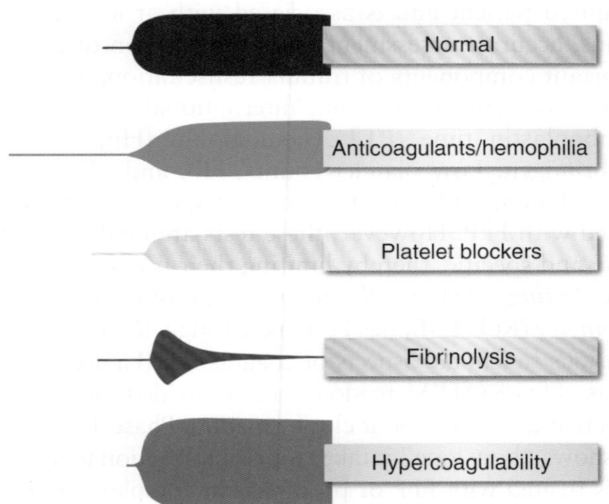

Figure 32.5 Examples of abnormal thromboelastogram tracings. (From da Luz LT, Nascimento B, Rizoli S. Thrombelastography (TEG®): Practical considerations on its clinical use in trauma resuscitation. *Scand J Trauma Resusc Emerg Med.* 2013;21:29, Figure 2)

treated with calcium chloride to stabilize cardiac membrane potentials. Insulin with or without dextrose can also be administered to drive potassium into the cell and lower the serum potassium level; however, blood glucose should be frequently monitored.

III. Anesthetic Management of Specific Injuries

A. Traumatic Brain Injuries or Head Injury

The most important consideration in the anesthetic management of patients with TBI is the prevention of secondary neurologic injury. As noted previously, reductions in blood pressure or oxygenation contribute significantly to mortality and must be avoided in head-injured patients. Perioperative anesthetic management of TBI is discussed in detail in Chapter 30.

B. Spine and Spinal Cord Injury

Clinical presentation of patients with SCI can vary greatly depending on the level and severity of each injury. In addition to spinal immobilization, maintaining mean arterial pressure at 85 to 90 mm Hg is recommended to support spinal perfusion and prevent secondary injury. In high thoracic to cervical SCI cases, ventilation and oxygenation might be compromised (due to diaphragm or intercostal muscle impairment), necessitating airway intervention and ventilatory support. As noted previously, steroids are not indicated in SCI and may worsen patients' outcome. Perioperative management of SCI and spine surgery is discussed in detail in Chapter 26.

C. Soft Tissue Neck Injury

The primary anesthetic consideration with neck injuries is airway management, as the trachea may be involved. Large hematomas outside the airway can cause a midline shift of the trachea. Direct injury to the trachea can create a false passage for the endotracheal tube. Signs of tracheal or laryngeal injury in the trauma patient with neck injury include altered phonation, hoarseness, stridor, and subcutaneous emphysema. As in the management of any traumatized airway, careful preoxygenation and RSI with direct or video laryngoscopy are generally safe. However, if there is significant concern for airway involvement, ***awake tracheal intubation with flexible bronchoscopy*** is indicated.

D. Chest Injury

Chest injuries can involve the heart, lungs, great vessels, and aerodigestive tract. Primary survey evaluation includes assessment of breath sounds and heart tones. Absent or asymmetric breath sounds suggest ***pneumothorax*** or ***hemothorax***, while distant heart tones, especially when accompanied by distended jugular veins, suggest ***cardiac tamponade***. A portable chest x-ray can confirm pneumothorax or hemothorax but should not delay immediate decompression of a ***tension pneumothorax*** if cardiovascular instability is present. Hemothorax and pneumothorax are both treated by placement of a chest tube. If blood >2 L is initially removed or >150 mL/h is drained from the chest tube, then an exploratory thoracotomy is indicated. Surgeons will often require one-lung ventilation in these cases, necessitating placement of a lung isolation device such as a double-lumen endotracheal tube (see Chapter 35). In an emergency, a simple endotracheal tube can be advanced into the right mainstem bronchus to isolate the left lung.

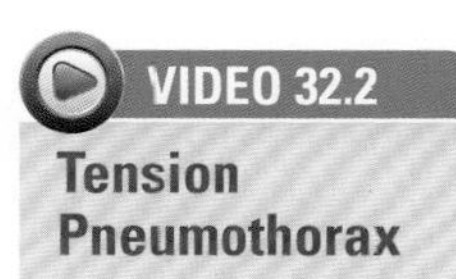

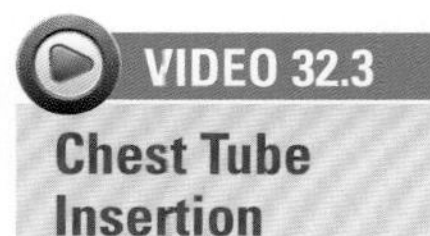

Cardiac tamponade in trauma is a life-threatening condition in which blood fills the pericardium and restricts both venous return and cardiac output. Transthoracic ultrasound is used to quickly evaluate both cardiac function and the presence of pericardial fluid. Tamponade can be relieved by ***pericardiocentesis*** or a ***pericardial window***. Before the procedure, care must be taken to minimize positive intrathoracic pressure (to facilitate venous return) and maintain systemic vascular resistance (eg, phenylephrine) to ensure adequate coronary perfusion.

E. Abdominal and Pelvic Injuries

The ***focused assessment with sonography in trauma (FAST)*** examination evaluates the pericardium, hepatorenal recess (Morison pouch), splenorenal region, and pelvic floor. Hypoechoic signals represent free fluid (blood) and suggest the

? *Did You Know?*

"Damage control surgery" refers to emergent surgical procedures or emergency interventional radiology procedures with the specific limited goals of rapidly identifying and treating life-threatening blood loss or other conditions, but transiently postponing definitive surgical repair until the patient can be medically stabilized.

need for exploratory surgery in blunt trauma settings. In hemodynamically stable patients, an abdominal CT scan identifies intra-abdominal and pelvic injuries with more anatomic specificity. Unstable patients, however, should be taken immediately to the operating room without CT imaging. Major abdominal trauma can include devastating solid organ injury, major vascular injury, and hollow organ contamination. To facilitate surgical exposure, abdominal wall relaxation must be maintained for the duration of the surgery. As noted above, surgeons may perform ***"damage control surgery,"*** with goals of identifying and packing sites of major hemorrhage, control of contamination and temporary abdominal closure, thereby allowing time for resuscitation and correction of hypothermia and coagulopathy. More stable patients are later returned to the operating room for more definitive and lengthy surgical repairs.

Selected abdominopelvic injuries are increasingly being treated in the ***interventional radiology*** setting. A hybrid operating room that includes advanced imaging is often used. These facilities require the same level of anesthesia equipment and staffing as a standard operating room to ensure optimal anesthetic management and resuscitation.

F. Extremity Injuries

Extremity injuries can run the spectrum from simple lacerations and fractures to traumatic amputations. Blood loss from extremity injuries can be surprisingly high (**Table 32.4**) and must be anticipated. Obvious bleeding from an extremity should be promptly controlled, initially with direct pressure and elevation of the extremity. Tourniquets should be considered early in cases of uncontrolled hemorrhage and can be left in situ for 2 to 3 hours, and then released only when the team is fully prepared for surgical intervention.

G. Open Globe Injuries

Important perioperative consideration for open globe injury is avoiding increases in the ***intraocular pressure (IOP)*** that could lead to extruded vitreous and loss of vision. Thus, succinylcholine should be avoided, and rocuronium is used as an alternative neuromuscular blocker for RSI (see Chapter 29).

IV. Burn Injuries

A. Initial Evaluation and Management of Burn Injuries

In addition to stopping the burning process by removing clothing from the burned area, burn-injured patients merit special consideration in the primary trauma survey, given the possibility for airway involvement with thermal injury or smoke inhalation. If the patient was injured in an enclosed space (eg, house fire), has carbonaceous sputum, singed nasal hairs, or other signs suggesting ***inhalation injury***, it is prudent to perform tracheal intubation

Table 32.4 Estimated Internal (Occult) Blood Loss for Closed Fractures in Adults

Pelvic Fracture	2-3 L
Femur fracture	1-2 L
Proximal tibia fracture	0.5-1 L
Humerus fracture	0.5 L

early. Delaying tracheal intubation can allow airway edema to form—particularly after significant fluid resuscitation—and make later airway management extremely difficult. As noted in **Table 32.3**, succinylcholine can cause life-threatening hyperkalemia in burn-injured patients, but not until 48 to 72 hours after injury when upregulation of acetylcholine receptors occurs. Thus, either succinylcholine or rocuronium can be used for RSI in the immediate postinjury setting. Environment control and prevention of hypothermia are also essential due to patient's impaired ability to thermoregulate.

B. Burn Severity Estimation

The magnitude of burn injury should be evaluated by estimation of depth and percentage of total body surface area (%TBSA) involved to guide treatment. Burn depths are characterized as ***superficial*** (eg, sunburn), ***partial thickness***, or ***full thickness***. Full-thickness burns include all layers of the epidermis and dermis and require surgical debridement. The patient's handprint is considered approximately 1% of the total body surface area (TBSA). For larger burns, the most common method to estimate %TBSA is the "Rule of Nines" (**Figure 32.6**). However, this method is less accurate in children and tends to overestimate in obese patients.

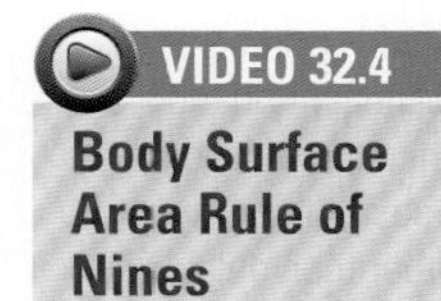

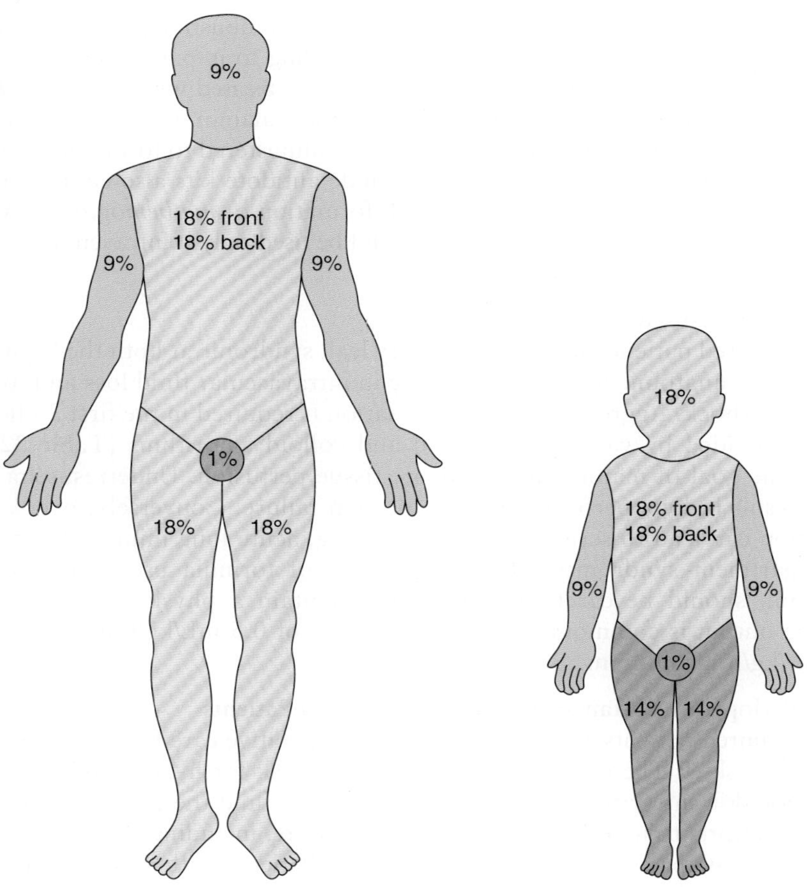

Figure 32.6 **Rule of Nines burn man/child diagram**. The percentage of total body surface area for burn injuries can be estimated from age-specific figures of percentage surface areas for different anatomic regions.

C. Inhalation Injury

In addition to burn severity, inhalation injury is a major prognostic factor for burn victims. Aside from direct thermal and chemical irritation of the upper and lower airway, inhalation of combustion chemical byproducts can cause systemic toxicity. The most common of them are carbon monoxide and cyanide poisoning.

> **? Did You Know?**
>
> Even if respiratory distress is not present upon hospital arrival, patients with significant facial burns or inhalation injury should undergo early tracheal intubation when the procedure is easier to perform, rather than delay until fluid resuscitation and inflammation create a difficult airway due to massive soft tissue edema.

Carbon monoxide (CO) has an affinity for hemoglobin several hundred times higher than that of oxygen. Patients with CO toxicity rarely present with the classic cherry red complexion, and oxygen saturation by pulse oximetry will erroneously appear normal. CO-oximetry is needed in this setting to yield accurate values for both elevated ***carboxyhemoglobin*** and reduced hemoglobin oxygen saturation. CO poisoning interferes with oxygen delivery to peripheral tissues and with cellular respiration, leading to metabolic acidosis. It is also associated with ***central demyelination*** and long-term neurologic sequelae. In cases of suspected CO poisoning, the carboxyhemoglobin level should be determined. Also, high concentration oxygen should be administered immediately as this can create a gradient that displaces CO from hemoglobin. Hyperbaric oxygen therapy can reduce the half-life of CO in the blood even further, but chambers are rarely available and pose logistic issues for other intensive and burn care.

Cyanide toxicity can result from inhalation of combustion products, as well as prolonged use of sodium nitroprusside, leading to impaired cellular respiration and metabolic acidosis. Cyanide toxicity is treated with ***hydroxocobalamin***; it combines with cyanide to form cyanocobalamin, which is eliminated in the urine. ***Sodium thiosulfate*** can also be administered to form thiocyanate, which is eliminated via the kidneys. Cyanide antidote kits also contain ***amyl nitrite***, which can clear cyanide through formation of ***methemoglobin***. Amyl nitrite is a temporizing measure that should be used only if intravenous access or hydroxocobalamin is unavailable.

D. Fluid Resuscitation

Burn-injured patients develop a capillary leak syndrome at both the burn site and distal anatomic locations, resulting in intravascular fluid loss and hypovolemic shock. Aggressive fluid resuscitation is required in the first 24 hours and is guided by various crystalloid and colloid algorithms (**Table 32.5**), with the goal of maintaining adequate tissue perfusion. Underresuscitation can result in hypoperfusion and multiorgan failure. Conversely, overresuscitation can lead to serious complications (eg, acute lung injury, abdominal compartment syndromes). Thus, regardless of formula used, fluid resuscitation should be carefully titrated to maintain a physiologic endpoint. Urine output is commonly used with the goal of 0.5 mL/kg/h in adults and 1 mL/kg/h in children.

E. Perioperative Management of Burn-Injured Patients

Burn-injured patients require specialized perioperative care for several injury-specific risks.[11] These patients are at increased risk for hypothermia because of poor skin integrity and aggressive intravenous fluid therapy. They require special efforts to maintain their body temperature, including elevated operating room temperature and warming devices. Patients with severe inhalation injury may require special ventilation strategies (eg, high-frequency percussive ventilation) and necessitate use of the intensive care unit ventilator in the

Table 32.5 Guidelines for Initial Fluid Resuscitation After Burn Injury

Adults and Children >20 kg
Parkland formula[a]
4.0 mL crystalloid/kg/% burn/first 24 h
Modified Brooke formula[a]
2.0 mL lactated Ringer's/kg per % burn per first 24 h
Children <20 kg
Crystalloid 2-3 mL/kg per % burn per 24 h[a]
Crystalloid with 5% dextrose at maintenance rate
100 mL/kg for the first 10 kg and 50 mL/kg for the next 10 kg for 24 h
Clinical End Points of Burn Resuscitation
Urine output: 0.5-1 mL
Pulse: 80-140 per min (age dependent)
Systolic BP: 60 mm Hg (infants); children 70-90 plus 2 × age in years mm Hg; adults MAP >60 mm Hg
Base deficit: <2

BP, blood pressure; MAP, mean arterial pressure.
[a]50% of calculated volume is given during the first 8 hours, 25% is given during the second 8 hours, and the remaining 25% is given during the third 8 hours.
From Capon LM, Miller SM, Scher C. Trauma and burns. In: Barash PG, Cahalan MK, Cullen BF, et al, eds. *Clinical Anesthesia*. 8th ed. Wolters Kluwer; 2018:1486-1536, Table 53.14.

operating room. Such cases will require total intravenous anesthesia to provide hypnosis and analgesia. If neuromuscular blockade is required, succinylcholine should be avoided after 48 hours following injury, as noted previously. Nondepolarizing muscle relaxants are safe but will have shortened durations of action because of the quantitative and qualitative changes in neuromuscular acetylcholine receptors that occur in the early days following burn injury. Postoperative pain control is a major priority for the burn patient, and multimodal therapy should be considered wherever possible. Patient-controlled analgesia, regional anesthesia, opioids, gabapentin, acetaminophen, and ketamine are all options in the burn patient, and consultation with a pain specialist is often helpful.

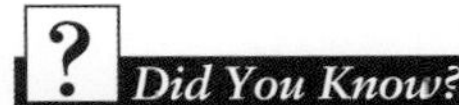

Burn excision and skin grafting procedures are associated with potentially significant blood loss, hypothermia, cardiovascular instability, as well as significant postoperative pain at both the injury and skin donor sites, all of which require comprehensive perioperative planning.

V. Disaster Preparedness

A. Mass Casualties

Any event that overwhelms the medical capacity of a given facility is defined as a ***mass casualty incident***. These events run the spectrum from natural disasters to public transit accidents to warfare. The concept of ***triage*** is used to sort patients who are most likely to benefit from the limited medical resources that are available. Patients who are conscious, able to maintain their airway, and are ambulatory are considered "walking wounded" and are labeled low priority. Patients in cardiac arrest are considered nonsalvageable and are managed expectantly. Conscious or unconscious patients who are in need of emergent surgery to save life, limb, or eyesight are given the highest priority. Less critically ill patients, including those who will survive for at least several hours without surgery, are given medium priority.

Anesthesia departments should have an established ***disaster plan*** to structure procedures and staffing in mass casualty events. This plan should include anesthesia staffing in the triage area or emergency department to coordinate the flow of patients to the operating room and to coordinate anesthesia resources. In the operating room, all cases already undergoing surgery should be finished, while new elective cases should be postponed. The departmental disaster plan should also include a process for mass casualty deactivation and return to the usual activity.

B. Biologic, Chemical, and Nuclear Warfare

The role of the anesthesiologist in a biologic, chemical, or nuclear attack is limited. Any therapy that is undertaken will be of a basic nature. Proper training with chemical or biologic protective gear is necessary to manage patients at any level of care. Proper decontamination is mandatory before patients enter a "clean" environment (eg, the hospital).

In biologic attacks, a healthy immune system and appropriate vaccinations are the main line of defense for care providers. Prompt identification of the involved organism can guide antimicrobial therapy. In chemical attacks, agents are typically dispersed quickly, and protective gear is needed to survive the initial phases of the attack. Similarly, identification of the chemical is mandatory to guide therapy with appropriate antidotes. In nuclear attack, the initial and secondary blasts do the most damage. Nuclear fallout presents a risk of radiation exposure. The only protection against this sort of attack is reinforced shelter and distance from the event. The long-term risk of cancer from radioactive fallout is unclear and often overestimated. Interestingly, the citizens of Hiroshima and Nagasaki experienced lower-than-expected rates of cancer following the nuclear attacks there in 1945. Some groups advocate iodine supplementation in the event of nuclear disasters (ie, nuclear power plant meltdown). However, any protection from radiation exposure that is provided by iodine is limited to the thyroid gland and is not a widely recommended practice.

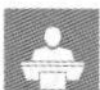

For further review, please see the associated Interactive Video Lectures accessible in complimentary eBook bundled with this text. Access instructions are located on the inside front cover.

References

1. Algie CM, Mahar RK, Tan HB, Wilson G, Mahar PD, Wasiak J. Effectiveness and risks of cricoid pressure during rapid sequence induction for endotracheal intubation. *Cochrane Database Syst Rev*. 2015;(11):CD011656. PMID: 26578526.
2. Chesnut RM, Marshall LF, Klauber MR, et al. The role of secondary brain injury in determining outcome from severe head injury. *J Trauma*. 1993;34(2):216-222. PMID: 8459458.
3. Hurlbert RJ, Hadley MN, Walters BC, et al. Pharmacological therapy for acute spinal cord injury. *Neurosurgery*. 2015;76(suppl 1):S71-S83. PMID: 25692371.
4. Patel MB, Humble SS, Cullinane DC, et al. Cervical spine collar clearance in the obtunded adult blunt trauma patient: a systematic review and practice management guideline from the Eastern Association for the Surgery of Trauma. *J Trauma Acute Care Surg*. 2015;78(2):430. PMID: 25757133.
5. Tobin JM, Grabinsky A, McCunn M, et al. A checklist for trauma and emergency anesthesia. *Anesth Analg*. 2013;117(5):1178-1184. PMID: 24108256.

6. Nouruzi-Sedeh P, Schumann M, Groeben H. Laryngoscopy via Macintosh blade versus GlideScope: success rate and time for endotracheal intubation in untrained medical personnel. *Anesthesiology*. 2009;110(1):32-37. PMID: 19104167.
7. Spahn DR, Bouillon B, Cerny V, et al. The European guideline on management of major bleeding and coagulopathy following trauma. *Crit Care*. 2019;23(1):98. PMID: 30917843.
8. Holcomb JB, Wade CE, Michalek JE, et al. Increased plasma and platelet to red blood cell ratios improves outcome in 466 massively transfused civilian trauma patients. *Ann Surg*. 2008;248(3):447-458. PMID: 18791365.
9. Williams-Johnson J, McDonald A, Strachan GG, Williams E. Effects of tranexamic acid on death, vascular occlusive events, and blood transfusion in trauma patients with significant haemorrhage (CRASH-2): a randomised, placebo-controlled trial. *West Indian Med J*. 2010;59(6):612-624. PMID: 21702233.
10. Plurad DS, Talving P, Lam L, Inaba K, Green D, Demetriades D. Early vasopressor use in critical injury is associated with mortality independent from volume status. *J Trauma*. 2011;71(3):565-572. PMID: 21908995.
11. Kaiser HE, Kim CM, Sharar SR, Olivar HP. Advances in perioperative and critical care of the burn patient: anesthesia management of major thermal burn injuries in adults. *Adv Anesth*. 2013;31(1):137-161.

Questions

1. **Which of the following statements regarding "damage control resuscitation" of the hemodynamically unstable trauma patient is TRUE?**

   A. Crystalloid should be administered as first-line resuscitative fluid to reduce complications from transfusion of blood products.
   B. Blood pressure goals for permissive hypotension are similar in patients with or without traumatic brain injury.
   C. The hemodynamic goal is lower than normal blood pressure that still provides adequate perfusion to vital organs until hemostasis is achieved, after which the blood pressure is normalized.
   D. Any surgical procedures should be postponed until patients are fully resuscitated and the hemodynamic goal is met.

2. **All of the following statements regarding manual in-line stabilization (MILS) during laryngoscopy and tracheal intubation are true EXCEPT:**

   A. MILS must be performed whenever the rigid cervical collar is removed from any trauma patients with potential cervical spine injury.
   B. MILS facilitates direct laryngoscopy and tracheal intubation by improving laryngoscopic view.
   C. During rapid sequence induction, MILS can be relaxed if it hinders intubation.
   D. Patients with cervical spinal cord injury rarely have worsening of their neurologic function when intubation is performed with MILS.

3. **A 65-year-old otherwise healthy woman was rescued from a house fire and arrives shortly at the hospital receiving 10 L/min supplemental oxygen via facemask. She has no apparent burn injuries, but she is lethargic and coughing up carbonaceous sputum. Which of the following laboratory assessments would you NOT EXPECT to observe?**

   A. Pulse oximetry reading of 97%
   B. Carboxyhemoglobin level of 28%
   C. Arterial blood gas with partial pressure of oxygen ($Pa{O_2}$) of 57 mm Hg
   D. CO-oximeter measured arterial oxyhemoglobin saturation of 72%

4. **A 5-year-old, 22 kg boy sustains a 27% total body surface area burn after pulling a pot of boiling water off the stove. What volume of isotonic crystalloid should he receive in the first 8 hours of hospitalization according to the Parkland formula?**

   A. 400 mL
   B. 800 mL
   C. 1200 mL
   D. 1600 mL

5. **When caring for the trauma and burn patients, unintended hyperkalemia can result in all of the following clinical scenarios EXCEPT:**

   A. Administration of four units of 23-day-old red blood cells to a 3-year-old girl with a traumatic leg amputation from a lawn mower accident.
   B. Release of a thigh tourniquet, which was placed in the field 4 hour earlier, in a 29-year-old man with blast injury.
   C. Hemolytic transfusion reaction in a 23-year-old woman who received improperly cross-matched fresh frozen plasma following traumatic brain injury.
   D. Succinylcholine administration to a 44-year-old man with 43% total body surface area burn on day 1 of hospitalization.

Answers

1. C

Hemodynamic goals consist of lower than normal blood pressures aiming to provide just adequate vital organ perfusions until hemostais is achieved, afterwhich the blood pressures are normalized.

2. B

MILS can worsen laryngoscopic view and increase intubation time and failure rate.

3. C

Carbon monoxide poisoning is suspected in victims of inhalation burn injury. Carbon monoxide has very high affinity to bind with hemoglobin thus replacing oxy-hemoglobin. However, this will not effect the partial pressure of oxygen in blood (Pao_2) which should be high with oxygen treatment.

4. C

Calculated by 4 ml of crystalloid per weight in kg per percentage of burn area for 24 hour. Fifty percent of calculated volume given during the first 8 hours.

5. D

Succinylcholine should be avoid after 48 hours of burn injury due to reports of lethal hyperkalemia, but is safe to use in the first 48 hours after burn injury.

33 Neonatal and Pediatric Anesthesia

Jorge A. Gálvez, Rebecca S. Isserman, Ian Yuan, and Alan Jay Schwartz

I. Physiology

A. Cardiovascular System

1. Normal Fetal to Pediatric Cardiovascular Transition

Development of ***normal cardiovascular physiology*** in the pediatric patient depends on the transition from fetal circulation to an adult flow pattern.[1,2] The fetus uses the low vascular resistance placenta as the organ of respiration and therefore does not require pulmonary blood flow. Placental venous blood streams past the liver through the ductus venosus to provide venous inflow to the right atrium and is shunted across the foramen ovale and ductus arteriosus into the left heart and aorta bypassing the right heart flow and the pulmonary circuit (**Figure 33.1**).

During the birthing process, elimination of the low resistance placental circulatory bed results in a rise in the neonate's *systemic vascular resistance*. This is coupled with the decrease in neonatal pulmonary vascular resistance. This reduces and eventually eliminates the blood flow that had been directed away from the lungs through the foramen ovale and ductus arteriosus. The rise in arterial oxygen level when the neonate initiates breathing is essential to maintain blood flow through the alveolar vascular bed.

Although the pulmonary vascular resistance declines at birth, it is not at the normal adult level until the end of the neonatal period. Any factor that can cause a rise in the ***pulmonary vascular resistance*** (eg, hypoxia, hypothermia, respiratory, or metabolic acidosis) can precipitate a reversion to a fetal circulatory pattern, with reopening of the foramen ovale and ductus arteriosus shunting blood away from the neonate's lungs. There are other differences in cardiac function that distinguish the pediatric heart from the adult heart. Most notable is the fact that the young child has a relatively noncompliant heart that depends on rate rather than contractility to boost cardiac output.

2. Common Congenital Cardiac Malformations

Malformations of the cardiac anatomy include many variations in which the ventricular and atrial chambers and the cardiac valves are deformed, causing abnormal blood flow patterns. Viewing congenital heart disease as a physiologic assessment enables the clinician to group the various lesions into three general categories: lesions that cause obstruction to blood flow without

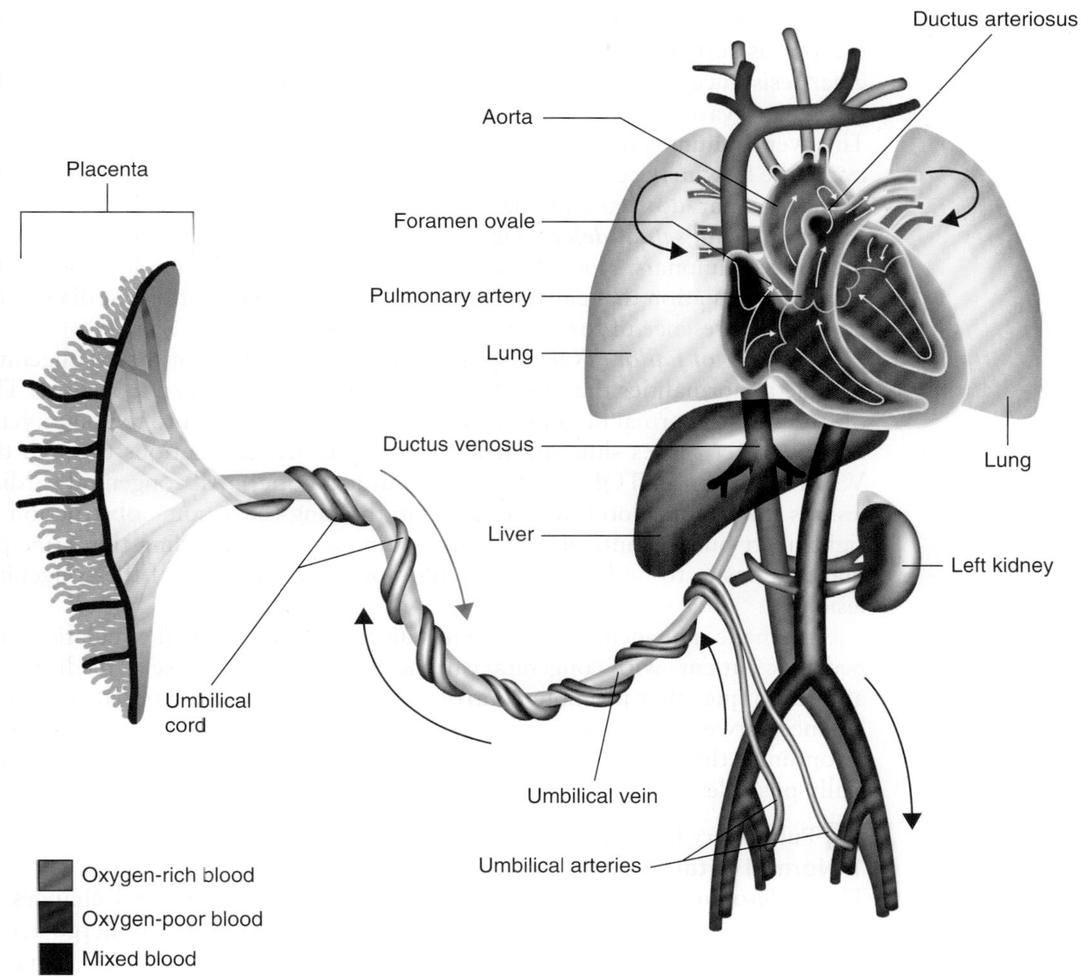

Figure 33.1 Fetal circulation showing direction of blood from the placenta (umbilical artery) that allows blood to bypass the fetal lungs via the foramen ovale and ductus arteriosus.

shunting, lesions that result in an increase in pulmonary blood flow through a shunt pathway, and lesions that result in a decrease in pulmonary blood flow through a shunt pathway.

Congenital aortic stenosis and *coarctation of the aorta* represent examples of non–shunt-obstructing congenital cardiac defects (**Figure 33.2A and B**). The major physiologic impairment is an increase in myocardial workload. Congenital aortic stenosis can be associated with rapid cardiac arrest when the stenotic valve is so narrow that the left ventricle fails to generate sufficient forward cardiac output to supply oxygen to the coronary circulation. A critical difference from adult aortic stenosis is that the pediatric heart does not have sufficient time to adapt and hypertrophy to compensate and overcome the valvular obstruction.

Ventricular septal defect (VSD) is the most common congenital cardiac lesion (**Figure 33.2C**). It results in shunting of blood from the higher pressure left ventricle to the lower pressure right ventricle. As long as the shunt communication is sufficiently large to allow flow through it and the pulmonary vascular resistance is sufficiently low to allow flow from the right ventricle to the pulmonary vascular bed, lesions like VSD will increase pulmonary blood flow. The overall shunt is from left to right. However, at any time during the cardiac cycle, the flow may cease or become right to left, highlighting the distinct possibility for paradoxical embolization from the venous to arterial circulation. When an ***atrial septal defect*** (**Figure 33.2D**) (another example of a lesion that increases pulmonary blood flow) is present, paradoxical embolization to the cerebral circulation that causes a stroke in adult life may be the first diagnostic clue of the presence of the intracardiac communication.

Tetralogy of Fallot (TOF) (**Figure 33.2E**) is an example of those congenital cardiac abnormalities that result in a decrease in pulmonary blood flow. The obstruction to normal blood flow out of the right ventricle into the pulmonary outflow tract causes shunting from the right to left circulations through the VSD that is part of TOF (right to left shunt [cyanotic]). All congenital cardiac lesions that shunt blood flow away from the lungs have some obstruction to right heart outflow into the pulmonary circuit. Understanding this principle makes it easier to understand the physiology and anatomy of the congenital lesions.

Anesthetic management of neonates displaying transitional circulation and pediatric patients with congenital cardiac lesions mandates use of medications and techniques that promote control of pulmonary vascular resistance and a balance between the pulmonary and systemic vascular resistances. The goal is to optimize the ratio of pulmonary to systemic circulation as best as anatomically possible.

B. Pulmonary System

1. Normal Fetal to Pediatric Transition

The ***pulmonary system*** is involved in dramatic developmental changes in the transition from fetal to postnatal physiology.[1,2] The lungs undergo active development throughout the gestational period and childhood. Alveolar development primarily occurs in the third trimester beginning in the saccular stage (24-38 weeks) and peaking in the alveolar stage (36 weeks-8 years).[1] Infants born prematurely benefit from maternal antenatal administration of glucocorticoids, which promote maturation of the fetal lung and surfactant production.

Surfactant is one of the most important factors contributing to adequate gas exchange during the transition to postnatal life. Surfactant is produced by type II endothelial cells, which proliferate during the alveolar stage. It is a mixture of neutral lipids, phospholipids, and specific proteins with an amphipathic nature, which leads to a decrease in surface tension that stabilizes alveoli and provides alveolar inflation while reducing hydrostatic forces that cause pulmonary edema.

During the transition to extrauterine life, the first breaths lead to an increase in pulmonary arterial oxygen (PO_2) and a decrease in partial pressure of carbon dioxide (PCO_2), which stimulates pulmonary vascular dilation, decreases ***pulmonary vascular resistance***, and causes constriction of the ductus arteriosus (**Table 33.1**).

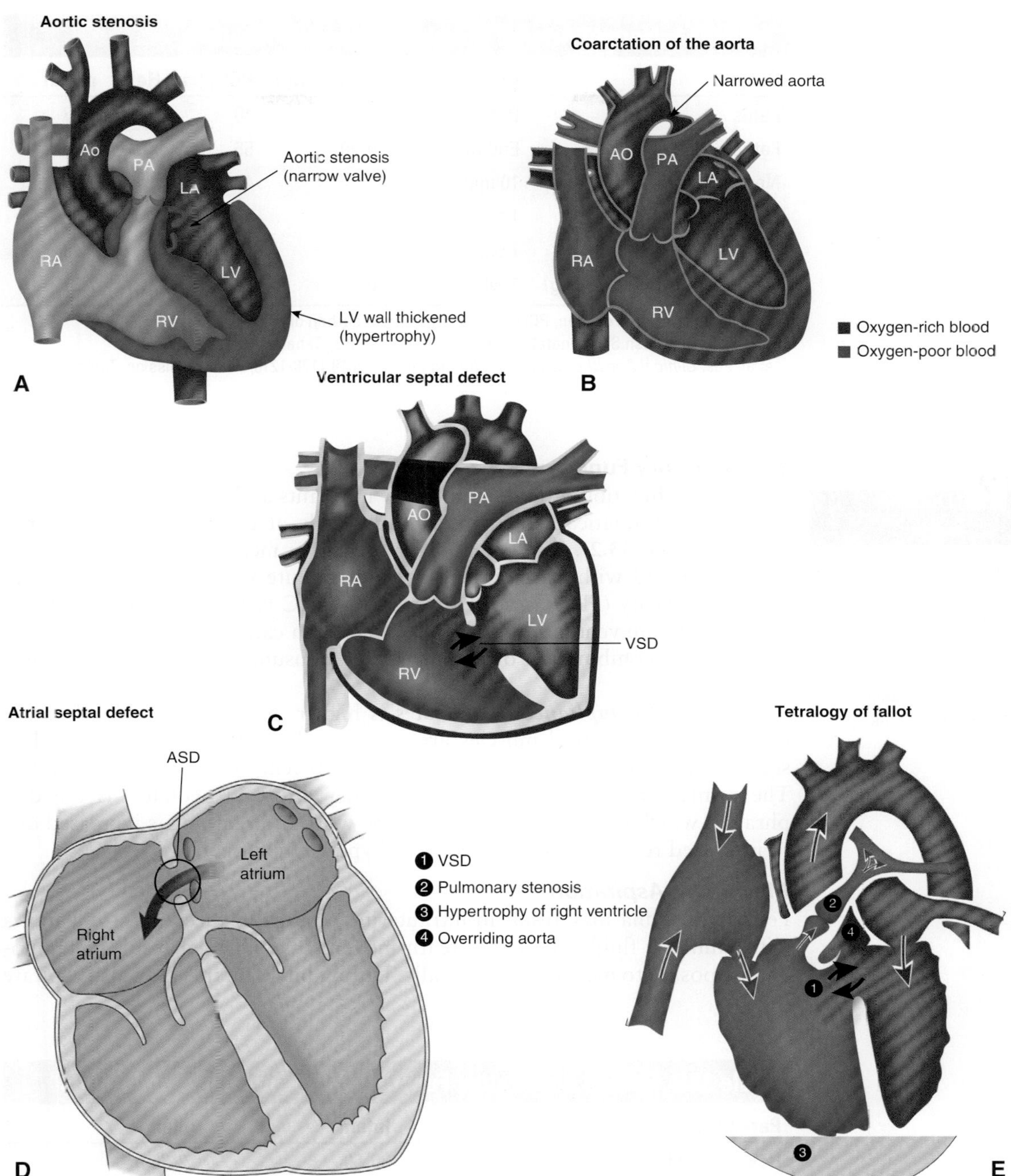

Figure 33.2 A, Aortic stenosis. B, Coarctation of the aorta also can lead to intracardiac shunting. Depending on the location of coarctation in relation to a patent ductus arteriosus, intracardiac shunting can be either right to left (preductal) or left to right (postductal). C, Ventricular septal defect leads to intracardiac shunting. Direction (right to left or left to right) depends on associated cardiac anatomy. D, Atrial septal defect leads to intracardiac shunting. Direction (right to left or left to right) depends on associated cardiac anatomy. E, Tetralogy of Fallot (TOF) consists of four anatomical abnormalities: (1) ventricular septal defect, (2) right ventricular outflow tract obstruction, (3) right ventricular hypertrophy, and (4) overriding aorta. (If an atrioventricular defect is present, the malformation is termed a pentalogy of Fallot.) TOF lesion leads to a right to left intracardiac shunt. ASD, atrial septal defect; AO, aorta; LA, left atrium; LV, left ventricle; PA, pulmonary artery; RA, right atrium; RV, right ventricle; VSD, ventriculoseptal defect.

Table 33.1 Normal Arterial Blood Gas Values in Neonate

Subject	Age	PO_2 (mm Hg)	PCO_2 (mm Hg)	pH (u)
Fetus	Before labor	25	40	7.37
Fetus	End of labor	10-20	55	7.25
Newborn (term)	10 min	50	48	7.20
Newborn (term)	1 h	70	35	7.35
Newborn (term)	1 wk	75	35	7.40
Newborn (preterm, 1500 g)	1 wk	60	38	7.37

PO_2, pulmonary arterial oxygen; PCO_2, partial pressure of carbon dioxide.
From Long JB, Suresh S. Neonatal anesthesia. In: Barash PG, Cahalan MK, Cullen BF, et al, eds. *Clinical Anesthesia.* 8th ed. Wolters Kluwer; 2018:1178-1218, with permission, Table 42.1.

? Did You Know?

Inhalation induction as well as emergence of anesthesia is faster in infants and children as a result of increased minute ventilation relative to adults.

2. Respiratory Function

Respiratory function differs significantly in infants and children. Oxygen consumption is dramatically higher than adult levels, at approximately 7 to 9 mL/kg/min (**Table 33.2**). The demand for oxygen is met with increased minute ventilation and with an increased ratio of minute ventilation to functional residual capacity (FRC) ratio. However, the FRC is relatively low compared with the minute ventilation. Infants and children can rapidly develop hypoxemia from a combination of higher oxygen consumption and lower oxygen reserve.

Chest wall compliance in neonates is higher than that in adults because the ribs and intercostal muscles are not fully developed, which can lead to significant retractions that do not provide efficient effort for gas exchange. The primary mechanism driving respiratory effort in neonates is the diaphragm, which is easily fatigued when the work of breathing is increased due to increased resistance to ventilation or hyperventilation.

Meconium Aspiration

Fetal hypoxemia may result in intrauterine passage of meconium that mixes with amniotic fluid. The fetal breath movements will then result in pulmonary exposure to meconium prenatally. During birth, infants may also aspirate

Table 33.2 Normal Respiratory Function Values in Infants and Adults

Parameter	Infant	Adult
Respiratory frequency	30-50	12-36
Tidal volume (mL/kg)	7	7
Dead space (mL/kg)	2-2.5	2.2
Alveolar ventilation (mL/kg/min)	100-150	60
Functional residual capacity (mL/kg)	27-30	30
Oxygen consumption (mL/kg/min)	7-9	3

From Long JB, Suresh S. Neonatal anesthesia. In: Barash PG, Cahalan MK, Cullen BF, et al, eds. *Clinical Anesthesia.* 8th ed. Wolters Kluwer; 2018:1178-1218, Table 42.2.

Table 33.3 Factors That Impair Vasodilation of the Pulmonary Vascular Tree

Anatomic	Physiologic
Congenital heart syndromes (ie, pulmonary artery hypoplasia)	Hypoxemia
Prematurity with lack of surfactant and bronchoalveolar development	Hypercarbia
Congenital diaphragmatic hernia	Hypothermia
Maternal diabetes	Meconium aspiration
Maternal asthma	Birth asphyxia
	Polycythemia
	Sepsis
	Chronic aspiration (postnatal)

meconium produced during labor. The latter scenario is consistent with thick meconium that can cause a mechanical airway obstruction. Current Pediatric Advanced Life Support recommendations do not support routine suctioning for infants born with meconium-stained amniotic fluid. Meconium aspiration may result in alveolar damage, which results in impaired oxygenation as well as increased pulmonary vascular resistance.

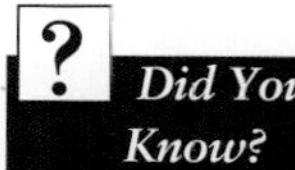

Did You Know?

During resuscitation of a newborn with a very low Apgar score, suctioning may delay other very important therapeutic interventions such as stimulation, assisted ventilation, and chest compressions.

Persistent Pulmonary Hypertension of the Newborn

The pulmonary circulation is highly sensitive to pH and oxygen levels, as well as other mediators such as nitric oxide, adenosine, prostaglandins, and lung inflation.[3] During the newborn period, certain factors can impair vasodilation of the pulmonary vascular tree (**Table 33.3**) and result in elevated pulmonary vascular resistance. Systemic hypotension and cardiac arrhythmias may result, particularly if the right ventricle is not able to compensate and right atrial dilation ensues.

C. Renal System

The kidneys begin to receive increased blood flow after the transition to postnatal circulation. However, the ***glomerular filtration rate (GFR)*** remains lower than adult levels for the first 2 years of life. As a result, infants have impaired ability to retain free water. Therefore, infants are less likely to tolerate prolonged fasting periods, particularly during the first few weeks of life. Their inability to regulate GFR to excrete large amounts of water also leads to an inability to tolerate fluid overload without resulting electrolyte abnormalities. Urine output is initially low, but increases to 1 to 2 mL/kg/h after the first day of life.

D. Hepatic System

The synthetic and metabolic functions of the ***liver*** remain immature in term newborns. The enzymes required for metabolism and drug elimination are present but have not been induced yet.[4] The results are variable, depending on the medication and elimination pathways. Morphine relies on hepatic biotransformation for elimination; therefore, it has a prolonged half-life in neonates. Alternatively, lidocaine does not demonstrate prolonged elimination. Synthetic function is also limited, as exhibited by decreased albumin and vitamin K production, which is one of the medications routinely administered at birth to prevent postpartum hemorrhagic complications such as intraventricular hemorrhage.

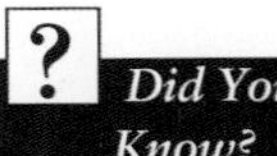

Did You Know?

Neonatal glycogen stores are decreased, especially in preterm infants, thus increasing the risk of hypoglycemia.

E. Central Nervous System

The infant central nervous system (CNS) experiences rapid growth and development from synaptogenesis, pruning, and neuronal myelination.[5] Although neurodegeneration and apoptosis are part of normal neural development, over the past 20 years, there has been concern on anesthetic-induced neurodegeneration.[6,7] This is seen in infant animal models with all commonly used anesthetics and displays a dose-duration dependency.[6,8] Retrospective studies on the effects of anesthesia on the developing human brain showed equivocal result; some showed a very small decrease in performance on neurodevelopmental tests later in life.[9-13] As a result, the U.S. Food and Drug Administration stated that exposure to anesthetic medicines for lengthy or multiple periods may negatively affect neurodevelopment in children aged 3 years or younger, while also recognizing that many surgeries or procedures that require anesthesia should proceed if medically necessary, and that consideration should be given to delaying elective surgery where appropriate.[14] Recently three large prospective studies showed no difference in neurodevelopmental outcomes in human infants exposed to short anesthetics (<1 hour) early in life.[15-18] Most most pediatric surgical procedures are not truly elective, but in light of the recent evidence, it is unlikely that undergoing anesthesia for a short period will affect neurodevelopmental outcomes.

II. Pharmacology

Administration of appropriate doses of anesthetic agents, analgesics, and all medications in the pediatric setting requires consideration of ***pharmacologic differences*** between children and adults.[4] Several variables in pediatric patients affect pharmacokinetics. For most parameters, developmental differences are greatest in neonates and premature infants. For example, total body water comprises 70% to 83% of weight in premature babies and term neonates, whereas it is approximately 60% of weight in infants 6 months through adulthood. Increased total body water translates to larger volumes of distribution of hydrophilic medications, which (assuming similar pharmacodynamics) translates to increased dosing requirements per kilogram of body weight. A selection of pharmacokinetic variables and their influence on drug metabolism are presented in **Table 33.4**. Volatile anesthetic MAC requirements are greatest at approximately 1 month of age.

III. Equipment

The three factors that affect design and choice of ***pediatric breathing circuits*** are excessive resistance to flow, excessive dead space, and decreased heat and humidification. It is for these reasons that a variety of valveless breathing systems have been devised (**Figure 33.3**).[1,2]

Table 33.4 Pharmacokinetic Variables and Their Clinical Influence in Infants and Children

Pharmacokinetic Variable	Physiology	Effect	Clinical Example
Hepatic metabolism	Immature phase 1/phase 2 metabolic pathways in neonates and infants	Decreased metabolism, longer drug half-lives	Phase 1: Amide local anesthetic accumulation with infusion Phase 2: Immature morphine glucuronidation in neonates and early infancy
Renal clearance	Adult glomerular filtration rate not achieved until 6-12 mo	Renally excreted drugs prolonged half-life in infants under 6 mo	Prolonged effect of pancuronium, reduced infusion requirements of other renally excreted drugs (eg, aminocaproic acid)
Total body water	Increased in neonates and infants	Increased volume of distribution for hydrophilic drugs	Increased succinylcholine dose requirement in neonates and infants
Plasma protein content and composition	Reduced α_1-acid glycoprotein and albumin, fetal albumin in neonates	Increased free (unbound) fraction for both acidic and basic drugs	Potentially increased pharmacodynamic effects for a wide variety of drugs

Ayre T-piece has no unidirectional gas flow valve and is effective for the spontaneously breathing patient. It is compact, can provide supplemental oxygen, and is not associated with rebreathing of carbon dioxide. Once neuromuscular relaxants were introduced into anesthesia practice, however, Ayre T-piece became ineffective, as it was difficult to provide the required positive pressure breathing with this device. The Jackson Rees modification of the Ayre T-piece solved this problem while maintaining the valveless system by adding a reservoir

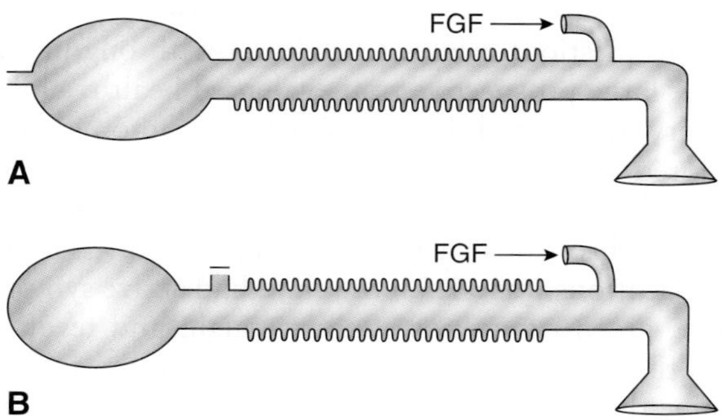

Figure 33.3 **Anesthesia breathing circuits. A, Jackson Rees modification of Ayre T-piece. B, Mapleson D circuit. FGF, fresh gas flow.** (Adapted from Willis BA, Pender JW, Mapleson WW. Rebreathing in a T-piece: volunteer and theoretical studies of the Jackson-Rees modification of Ayre's T-piece during spontaneous respiration. *Br J Anaesth*. 1975; 47:1239, and Ruitort KT, Eisenkraft JB. The anesthesia work station and delivery systems for inhaled anesthetics. In: Barash PG, Cahalan MK, Cullen BF, et al, eds. *Clinical Anesthesia*. 8th ed. Wolters Kluwer; 2018:644-705.)

bag with a variable occlusion pop-off (a variably occluded pigtail on the bag). Although the Jackson Rees modification of the Ayre T-piece solved the need to be able to provide positive pressure breathing, it became apparent that another technical issue had to be solved—the potential for rebreathing carbon dioxide.

Mapleson introduced variations on the Jackson Rees system to address the potential for rebreathing. Mapleson recognized that while rebreathing could occur because this system did not contain unidirectional gas flow valves, the sequential placement of the fresh gas inlet, the pop-off, the reservoir bag, and the connection to the patient can be varied. Depending on whether the patient was breathing spontaneously or was controlled with positive pressure, if the fresh gas flow was sufficient, carbon dioxide rebreathing could be minimized. There are six variations of the Mapleson system, the Mapleson D being commonly used in pediatric patient care. ***The Mapleson D system*** places the fresh gas inlet close to the connection to the patient's airway. The pop-off is farther away from the patient and fresh gas inflow, and the bag is distal to the pop-off. The popularity of the Mapleson D system results from its ability to minimize carbon dioxide rebreathing when controlled ventilation is the ventilatory mode. Rebreathing is also eliminated during spontaneous ventilation when the fresh gas flow is two to three times the patient's minute ventilation.

Modern-day pediatric anesthesia patient care effectively employs the ***circle breathing system***, without undue resistance to the patient when opening the valves. It has the added benefit of conservation of the patient's heat and airway humidity. If concern exists that airway heat and humidity will be lost during ventilation with the anesthesia machine, a heater and humidifier can be incorporated into the circle system.

Recent reports demonstrate that by using the proper-sized ***cuffed endotracheal tube***, the ability to provide positive pressure ventilation was enhanced. There was also less operating room anesthetic gas contamination, better isolation of the airway from gastric contents, and less need for additional laryngoscopies in attempts to select the proper size tube.

IV. Perioperative Management

A. Preoperative Assessment

Children should be evaluated for common coexisting conditions.[1,2] One of the most common questions relates to children with ongoing ***upper respiratory infections***. A large prospective trial evaluated healthy children scheduled for elective surgery. It assessed their respiratory symptoms for nasal drainage (clear or discolored yellow/green) as well as cough (dry or productive and color of sputum), lethargy, and fever for correlation with respiratory complications, including bronchospasm and laryngospasm.[19] The relative risk for respiratory complications was >1.5 if the child had active symptoms, including clear runny nose, green runny nose, moist cough, and fever. A general discussion between the parents, child, surgeon, and anesthesiologist should take place to determine the risk-benefit ratio for every scenario. A thorough preanesthetic discussion with the parents or responsible guardians should include the possibility of admission to the hospital for postoperative management.

The first observation of a child's behavior offers great insight into the developmental stage, as the ***developmental stages*** may not always correlate with a child's age. Children will naturally express anxiety around strangers and may not tolerate a thorough physical examination. ***Neurologic examination*** should focus on the child's activity level and note any anomalies such as contractures, weakness of extremities, or abnormal appearance. The ***cardiovascular examination*** focuses on auscultation of the heart sounds, noting that heart murmurs are common in newborns (patent ductus arteriosus continuous murmur, patent foramen ovale, atrial septal defect, and VSD). The presence of a murmur should warrant further exploration of signs or symptoms of cardiac disease, particularly fainting, discoloration such as blue lips, or failure to thrive. Furthermore, the ***abdominal examination*** may reveal a large or very small liver, which correlates with volume status as well as the ability for the heart to handle preload.

Pulmonary examination focuses on determining the presence of abnormal air movement, including absent breath sounds, wheezing, or coarse breath sounds. It can often be challenging to differentiate coarse lung sounds from transmitted upper airway sounds in the presence of nasal congestion. The abdominal examination evaluates for signs of trauma, distention, or discomfort. Furthermore, umbilical hernias may be appreciated. The extremities should be assessed for range of motion, contractures, or deformities as well as possible sites for intravenous access. There should be a discussion with the patient and guardians regarding the risks and benefits of delivering general versus regional anesthesia to the child. The risks of anesthesia that are specific to pediatrics include, in particular, respiratory depression, particularly in ex-premature infants, respiratory complications, such as bronchospasm and laryngospasm, hypoxia, and aspiration pneumonia.

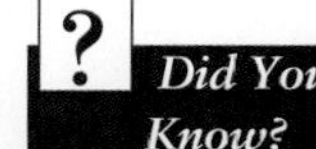

Adolescents may be in a position where they can provide assent to a procedure, but ultimately the legal guardian must provide consent.

B. Fasting Guidelines

The American Society of Anesthesiologists recommends that infants and children fast preoperatively to reduce the risk of pulmonary aspiration; however, fasting times for children are frequently much longer than these guidelines[20,21] (**Table 33.5**). Prolonged fasting in children can increase irritability and lead to adverse physiologic and metabolic effects.[22]

The emphasis in pediatric preoperative fasting has therefore shifted to encouraging drinking, particularly of clear fluids, during the allowable period. Professional societies throughout the world including the European Society for Pediatric Anesthesia have also reduced clear fluid fasting times to 1 hour prior to elective procedures, unless clinically contraindicated.[23]

C. Preoperative Anxiolysis

Children as young as 10 months of age may experience anxiety when transferring to the operating room, with the toddler to preschool range (aged 1-7 years) being the highest risk population. Strategies to mitigate anxiety include premedication, parental presence, and virtual reality techniques.

Oral premedication with a benzodiazepine (eg, midazolam 0.5 mg/kg up to 10 mg) is effective preoperatively due to a rapid onset (5-15 minutes) and a short duration of action.[24] Intranasal or oral dexmedetomidine (1µg/mg) has an onset of 30 to 45 minutes but, with adequate time, can provide excellent separation from parents.[25]

Parental presence during induction of anesthesia eliminates the stress caused by separation. This approach is most effective when parents are calm and adequately prepared as to what to expect.[25]

1. Technology for Anxiety Reduction

Technological advances over the last two decades have had an important impact on the nonpharmacologic strategies available to facilitate anxiolysis in the perioperative setting. Smartphones and tablets can be used to provide

Table 33.5 Preprocedure Fasting Guidelines

Ingested Material	Fasting Time (h)
Clear liquid	2
Breast milk	4
Infant formula	6
Solids/nonhuman milk	6+[a]

[a]Amount and type of food must be considered.

Adapted from American Society of Anesthesiologists Practice guidelines for preoperative fasting and the use of pharmacologic agents to reduce the risk of pulmonary aspiration: an updated report. *Anesthesiology.* 2017;126(3):376-393.

distractions in a number of ways such as playing music, watching a favorite video, playing games, or even interacting with parents via video call during transport and induction of anesthesia. Virtual reality systems are becoming increasingly available and show promise in a variety of pediatric settings including distraction during intravenous line placement and even invasive procedures like upper endoscopies.[26,27]

D. Induction of Anesthesia

Induction of anesthesia represents a stressful event for children (and parents!). Beyond the mandatory goals of maintaining a patent airway and stable hemodynamics, the goals of a pediatric induction also include a smooth separation from the parent (if a parent is not present for induction) and a cooperative child during the process of induction, while establishing and meeting parental expectations during the process. Two of the most commonly used approaches for minimizing the stress of induction (which may be used alone or in combination) are discussed in the sections that follow.[1,2]

1. Inhalation Induction of Anesthesia

In the absence of contraindications, an ***inhaled induction*** of anesthesia has a number of advantages in children. It is painless and it is successful on the first attempt (whereas intravenous cannulation has an inherent failure rate). In the United States, inhalation inductions are performed almost exclusively with sevoflurane, as the availability of halothane is severely limited. In cooperative patients, 50% to 70% nitrous oxide in oxygen may be delivered first (which is odorless), titrating sevoflurane up to 8%. This may allow the child to both tolerate and not remember the less pleasant volatile agent. Because inhaled inductions are performed in children prior to securing vascular access and there is the potential for laryngospasm and bradycardia, succinylcholine (4 mg/kg) and atropine (0.02 mg/kg) should be immediately available for intramuscular administration. Caution is advised for inhalation induction for children with medical conditions (ie, trisomy 21 or Down syndrome) who may develop bradycardia from high sevoflurane concentrations.

2. Intravenous Induction

Intravenous induction is typically preferred in children who have established venous access. For children coming for elective surgery, some centers routinely place an intravenous line for induction of anesthesia. Premedication with a benzodiazepine and application of topical local anesthetic cream can minimize the stress of intravenous line placement.

3. Intramuscular Induction

Occasionally, a patient may not be able to cooperate with any element of preoperative preparation (eg, autistic children) or induction of anesthesia (including taking oral premedication). ***Intramuscular injection*** of ketamine (3-5 mg/kg) may be the best option in these circumstances, but this requires a careful team approach and family preparation to be safe and successful.

E. Pediatric Airway Management

Understanding the anatomical and physiologic differences between adults, infants, and children is necessary to provide safe and successful airway management tailored to the infant or child. In general, these differences and their impact on ***airway management*** are greatest in the neonatal and infant period. Multiple laryngoscopy attempts can lead to an increase in morbidity and mortality in children and, particularly, so for children with known or anticipated difficult airways.[28,29] Passive oxygen delivery during intubation attempts may increase the time before desaturation and provide laryngoscopists with valuable time to secure the airway.[30,31]

Anatomically, an infant has a larger occiput, a larger tongue size relative to the size of the oropharynx, and a more cephalad larynx (**Table 33.6**). The larger occiput may promote airway obstruction and interfere with laryngoscopy when a head pillow is used to achieve the classic sniffing position. Instead, a shoulder roll is often more useful both for promoting a patent airway and for facilitating direct laryngoscopy. Although it was originally postulated that the narrowest portion of the pediatric airway is at the level of the cricoid ring, newer magnetic resonance imaging–based research suggests the glottic opening and the immediate subvocal cord level are the narrowest.[32] Furthermore, the shape of the larynx is cylindrical, as in the adult, so it is important to remember clinically because the endotracheal tube fit (resistance to endotracheal tube passage) must be assessed after it has passed through the vocal cords. Tightly fitting tubes may cause clinical problems such as ***postextubation stridor*** and postextubation croup. A leak pressure of less than 20 to 25 cm H_2O should be targeted to minimize this risk.

> **? Did You Know?**
>
> Infants and young children have a relatively large tongue and a more cephalad larynx effectively shortening the distance in which the oral, pharyngeal, and tracheal axes must be aligned to achieve laryngeal exposure during direct laryngoscopy.

Normal healthy infants have overlap with tidal breathing and closing volumes, and their oxygen consumption rates are nearly three times that of an adult; so under anesthetized conditions, their FRC is reduced (**Table 33.2**). The clinical impact of this is rapid oxyhemoglobin desaturation following brief periods of apnea, resulting in shorter times to perform apneic intubation techniques. Additionally, oxyhemoglobin desaturation will rapidly occur when ventilation is compromised (eg, coughing, airway obstruction). ***Difficult airway management*** in pediatric patients often requires deep sedation or general anesthesia.

1. Anesthetic Conditions for Laryngoscopy and Endotracheal Intubation

Traditionally, intubation of the trachea in children can result in activation of the airway in the form of laryngospasm and/or bronchospasm. Adequate depth of anesthesia prior to laryngoscopy and endotracheal intubation is essential. This can be done with deep sevoflurane anesthesia alone, but it is also often performed with a propofol bolus (eg, 2 mg/kg) or a fast-acting opioid (eg, remifentanil or fentanyl 2 µg/kg) following inhalational induction of anesthesia with sevoflurane. Insufficient depth of anesthesia without neuromuscular blockade may result in coughing, laryngospasm, oxyhemoglobin desaturation, and regurgitation. Garcia-Marcinkiewicz et al report that neuromuscular

Table 33.6 Anatomic Differences Between Infant and Adult Airways

Anatomic Relationship	Pediatric	Adult
Occiput	Large	Normal
Tongue	Large	Normal
Epiglottis	Relatively longer, narrower, and stiffer	Firm
Epiglottis shape	Omega shaped	Flat, broad
Relative larynx location	Cephalad	Caudal
Larynx size/shape	Proportionately smaller/ cylindrical	Cylindrical
Glottic level	C3-C4	C5-C6
Narrowest point	Vocal cords	Vocal cords
Vocal cords	Inclined posterior to anterior	Perpendicular to larynx
Mucosa	More vulnerable to trauma	Less vulnerable to trauma

Data from Lerman J. Pediatric anesthesia. In: Barash PG, Cullen B, Stoelting RK, et al, eds. *Clinical Anesthesia*. 7th ed. Wolters Kluwer/Lippincott Williams & Wilkins; 2013:1216-1256, and Litman RS, Weissend EE, Shibata D, et al. Developmental changes of laryngeal dimensions in unparalyzed, sedated children. *Anesthesiology*. 2003;98:41-45, with permission.

blockade may reduce the risk of airway complications due to laryngospasm in pediatric patients with difficult airway.[33]

Succinylcholine

In the early 1990s, the U.S. Food and Drug Administration applied a black box warning for succinylcholine contraindicating its use for routine airway management. However, in the absence of absolute contraindications (malignant hyperthermia susceptibility, history of burns, etc.), succinylcholine is acceptable in scenarios such as laryngospasm and rapid sequence induction and intubation and may be the preferred agent.

Reversal of Neuromuscular Blockade

Sugammadex is a selective muscle relaxant binding molecule designed for the acute reversal of neuromuscular blockade by rocuronium or vecuronium. It exhibits strong binding to rocuronium, and vecuronium to a lesser degree.[34] It is not effective for reversal of pancuronium or other pharmacological classes of neuromuscular blocking agents such as cisatracurium.[34] Although it was approved for use in the European Union in 2008 and the United States in 2015, the evidence for pediatric use remains sparse, particularly for children younger than 2 years.[35,36] Specific concerns for pediatric care relate to the efficacy of acute reversal of rocuronium, the potential for deposition in bones and growth plates, and the interaction with oral contraceptives for postpubertal girls and adolescents.

2. Direct Laryngoscopy

Traditionally, the ***straight blade (Miller)*** has been used in children, although there is little or no comparative evidence to show that this blade performs better than the ***curved blade (Macintosh)*** (Chapter 20, Figure 20.5). After sweeping the tongue, the blade tip is advanced beyond the vallecula and the epiglottis is directly lifted. Alternatively, the straight blade can be used in the manner of the Macintosh and the epiglottis lifted indirectly with the blade tip in the vallecula.

3. Laryngeal Masks and Supraglottic Airways

Laryngeal mask airways are frequently used in pediatric anesthesia. In general, the indications and contraindications are similar to adults. Laryngeal masks with gastric drain channels as well as laryngeal masks designed to facilitate intubation are available in pediatric sizes.

4. Endotracheal Tube Selection

Historically, ***uncuffed endotracheal tubes*** were recommended in children; however, in the current era, cuffed tubes are in most circumstances superior. The incidence of postintubation stridor is less when properly sized cuffed tubes are used, possibly from the decreased need or frequency of repeated laryngoscopy for tube change when too large a tube is placed initially. ***Cuffed endotracheal tubes*** also offer advantages of improved sealing of the trachea, which decreases operating room pollution, allows for lower fresh gas flows, improves ventilator performance, and may offer greater protection from macroaspiration. Although cuffed tubes can be safely used and often preferred for surgical procedures in neonates and preterm infants, uncuffed tubes are commonly used for long-term ventilation in the neonatal intensive care unit (NICU). When tracheal intubation is performed, the correct tracheal tube size must be chosen. Most commonly, the modified ***Cole formula*** is used for uncuffed endotracheal tubes, where the predicted tube size is 4 plus the age divided by 4. In infants and smaller children, a half-size smaller should be selected when a cuffed tube is used. For example, for a 4-year-old child, one would select a (4 + 4/4 = 5) 5.0 uncuffed endotracheal tube or a (4 + 4/4 − 0.5 = 4.5) 4.5 cuffed endotracheal tube.

5. Tracheal Intubation and Positioning of the Endotracheal Tube

Indications for tracheal intubation in children are largely similar to those for adults. In addition, many anesthesiologists intubate the trachea and control ventilation in neonates and preterm infants in the absence of other traditional indications. Careful attention must be paid to positioning the tracheal tube tip in the midtrachea. Small tube movements may result in endobronchial intubation or inadvertent extubation in infants. Assessing the adequate depth of the endotracheal tube can be performed by deliberately advancing the endotracheal tube into the main stem bronchus while simultaneously auscultating and providing breaths with hand bag ventilation. When the endotracheal tube enters the right or left main stem bronchus, breath sounds will be absent in the opposite side. The tube is then withdrawn by 1 cm in infants and 2 cm in older children to achieve a mid-tracheal position, and breath sounds should be used to confirm both lungs are being ventilated. When a cuffed tube is used, it may be easier and more reliable to position the tube so that the cuff can be palpated by ballottement in the suprasternal notch. This translates to the tip of the tube being in an intrathoracic and midtracheal location.

6. Rapid Sequence Induction and Intubation in Pediatrics

One of the clinical manifestations of the high oxygen consumption rate and reduced FRC of an infant under anesthesia is rapid oxyhemoglobin desaturation following apnea. If a "traditional" ***rapid sequence induction*** is performed, nearly all infants will have an oxyhemoglobin saturation below 90%

after 1 minute of apnea. Therefore, many pediatric anesthesiologists perform a modified rapid sequence induction with gentle positive pressure ventilation in addition to cricoid pressure prior to intubation because oxygen delivery is prioritized over aspiration risk from a risk-benefit standpoint.[24]

V. Temperature Management

Children are at increased risk of ***hypothermia*** under anesthesia; infants and, in particular, premature infants and neonates are at greatest risk. Similar to adults, the primary modes of heat loss are as follows:

1. Radiation
2. Evaporation
3. Convection
4. Conduction

Neonates under anesthesia behave as poikilotherms; their temperature approaches that of their surroundings. Hypothermia can be prevented and normothermia maintained using a combination of strategies tailored to the individual patient. Warming the operating room prior to arrival (convection or radiation), forced air warming (convection), use of a circulating warm water mattress (conduction), heated humidified gases or humidified moisture exchanger (evaporation), and overhead infrared warming lights (radiation) are among the available methods.

VI. Fluid and Blood Management

A. Intravenous Fluid Requirements

Intravenous fluid requirements in fasting children are usually determined using the ***4-2-1 rule***. The hourly infusion rate is calculated as 4 mL/kg for the first 10 kg, plus 2 mL/kg for the second 10 kg, and 1 mL/kg for each additional kilogram. Fasting fluid deficits are calculated based on this formula and the duration the child has been nil per os. These are replaced intraoperatively in a manner similar to adults. The generally accepted guideline is 50% of the deficit replaced in the first hour, followed by 25% of the deficit replaced in each of hours 2 and 3 to complete the entire deficit.

Infants under 6 months of age, and neonates in particular, are at increased risk of hypoglycemia with fasting durations commonly seen in anesthetic practice. Liberalized fasting guidelines (eg, clear liquids until 2 hours prior to surgery) may help prevent hypoglycemia and improve patient comfort.

B. Blood Loss Replacement and Transfusion

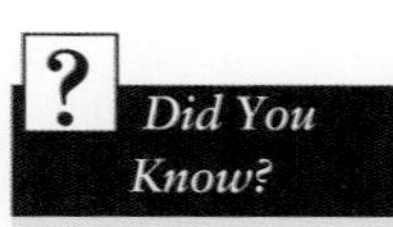

Hypovolemia associated with hemorrhage is the most common cardiovascular cause of perioperative cardiac arrest in children.

Underestimation of blood loss, inadequate preparation (vascular access, blood preparation), and massive hemorrhage are identified as contributors to ***cardiac arrest*** in the pediatric patient.[37,38] Blood loss is replaced with crystalloids (without glucose). Although transfusion thresholds are ultimately tailored to the individual patient and clinical scenario, in most scenarios, red blood cell transfusion is indicated when the hemoglobin is below 7 g/dL and is often indicated sooner depending on the age of the patient and clinical scenario.[37-39] Packed red blood cells (5 mL/kg) can be expected to raise the hemoglobin approximately 1 g/dL. Indications for hemostatic blood component therapy are similar to those for adults. Suggested dosing for blood components are presented in **Table 33.7**.

Table 33.7 Pediatric Blood Component Administration

Component	Dosing Guideline	Comments
PRBCs	5-10 mL/kg	Expected hemoglobin increase of 1-1.5 g/dL for every 5 mL/kg. Infants/small children at risk of hyperkalemia with rapid infusion of PRBCs that have been stored for a prolonged time. Consider fresh/washed PRBCs when anticipated.
FFP	10-15 mL/kg	During massive hemorrhage dilutional coagulopathy of soluble clotting factors develops after >1 blood volume of loss; FFP treatment recommended.
Platelets	10-15 mL/kg	Usually indicated for platelet counts <50,000/μL; higher thresholds may be used for certain procedures (eg, neurosurgery).
Cryoprecipitate	0.1 U/kg	Indicated for fibrinogen levels <80-100 mg/dL.

FFP, fresh frozen plasma; PRBC, packed red blood cells.

C. Regional Anesthesia

There are many useful applications for ***regional anesthetic*** techniques in pediatrics.[40,41] Caudal injections are among the most common procedures performed in pediatric anesthesia. Conversely, there are rare scenarios that may require spinal anesthesia in infants, such as the evaluation of a child for a congenital myopathy that may be associated with malignant hyperthermia. In such cases, a spinal anesthetic provides adequate conditions for a muscle biopsy of the thigh without exposure to triggering agents. Epidural catheters may be threaded to various levels via a caudal approach. Furthermore, peripheral nerve blocks may be helpful for a variety of orthopedic procedures, ranging from osteotomies to arthroscopic procedures for tendon repairs. Ultrasound imaging provides visualization of nerves, anatomic landmarks, and the needle and spread of local anesthetic, which allows for safe and effective administration of regional anesthesia. Other chapters of this book discuss epidural or regional anesthesia blocks.

Prior to administration of caudal anesthesia, informed consent should be obtained from the patient's parent or legal guardian. Physical examination should note the presence of any sacral dimples, which may be associated with occult spina bifida or tethered cord, thus increasing the risk of neurologic complications from the administration of local anesthetics via the caudal approach. The surface landmarks that should be palpated include the sacral cornua as well as the coccyx. The sacral hiatus and sacrococcygeal ligament are located inferior to the cornua. The block can be safely performed with either bupivacaine 0.25% with epinephrine (limit 1 mL/kg) or ropivacaine 0.2% (limit 1 mL/kg).[40] A test dose should consist of epinephrine 5 μg/kg. Criteria for identifying an intravascular injection include an increase in 10 beats per minute in heart rate as positive, recognizing that heart rate changes can be delayed by as much as a minute after administration of the test dose.

VII. Surgical Procedure Considerations

A. Myelomeningocele

Spina bifida refers to a range of congenital anomalies of the CNS. The most common is a myelomeningocele, which involves bulging of the spinal cord into a sac filled with cerebrospinal fluid (CSF; **Figure 33.4**). The incidence of myelomeningocele remains at 3.4 per 10,000 live births. Long-term survivors

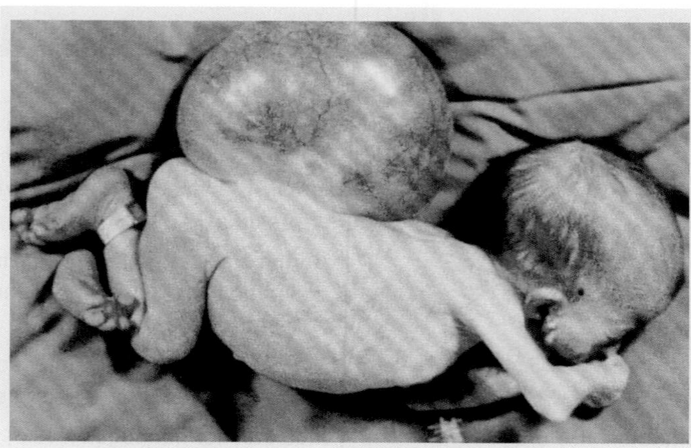

Figure 33.4 Neonate with spina bifida cystica.

with myelomeningocele have neurologic deficits, including bladder and bowel incontinence as well as sensory and motor deficits related to the level of spinal cord involved in the defect. Surgical interventions can be performed in utero or immediately following birth. Fetal interventions show improved motor outcomes and lower need for CSF shunts.[42] Long-term care involves frequent bladder catheterization and potential risk of developing sensitivity to latex products. Latex precautions should be exercised regardless of any history of allergic sensitivity to latex products.

B. Ventriculoperitoneal Shunts

Children may present with ***elevated intracranial pressure*** as a result of various lesions, including anatomic obstruction of CSF flow such as Chiari malformations or tumors. In order to relieve the obstruction of CSF flow, an intraventricular shunt may be placed to redirect flow to a body cavity such as the peritoneal cavity, the pleura, or less commonly an intravascular location such as the right atrium. Patients with existing shunts may present with shunt malfunction or infection and may require emergency surgery to alleviate the shunt malfunction. Preanesthetic evaluation should focus on assessing signs of ***increased intracranial pressure***, such as depressed consciousness, nausea, vomiting, bradycardia, and hypertension. Induction of anesthesia should weigh the potential risk of aspiration with the risk of brain herniation in the setting of elevated intracranial pressure. Surgical approach typically requires access to the head, neck, thorax, and abdomen. Infants and children are particularly prone to hypothermia due to exposure to surgical preparation solution as well as an inability to provide adequate heat source during the procedure. Patient positioning may also result in endobronchial intubation, particularly in small children. Although the risk of hemorrhage is small, it is significant particularly in young children as well as shunt revisions that may involve a vascular component. Patients should be considered for an awake examination after surgery unless the patient's baseline condition is not suitable for extubation and emergence.

C. Craniofacial Surgery

Craniofacial reconstruction is performed for children with premature fusion of cranial sutures during development. Surgical correction is performed to improve appearance as well as to reduce the risk of increased pressure on areas of the developing brain and potential long-term effects on development resulting from inhibited brain growth. Depending on the type and severity of the deformity, it may be corrected in one or more stages typically during the first years of life. Each surgical procedure is associated with variable scalp dissection and cranial osteotomies. Children should be evaluated for associated syndromes (ie, ***Crouzon*** and ***Saethre-Chotzen***), which can be associated with difficult airway as well as difficult intravascular access. Intraoperative management typically includes continuous arterial blood pressure monitoring. To detect ***air embolism***, use of a Doppler monitor is suggested. Central venous access should be considered to assist management in complex procedures, particularly if peripheral vascular access is not adequate (at least two large bore intravenous lines). Despite surgical efforts to minimize hemorrhage, patients typically require transfusion of approximately one circulating blood volume.[43] Preemptive administration of fresh frozen plasma during surgery has been demonstrated to reduce the incidence of postoperative coagulopathy. Surgical complications may include tearing of dural sinuses as well as tearing of the dura during osteotomies.

D. Tonsillectomy

Children presenting for tonsillectomy or adenoidectomy comprise a large amount of all pediatric anesthesiology practices. The indications for the procedures range from recurrent tonsillitis to ***obstructive sleep apnea*** with various levels of symptomatology.[44] Children with Down syndrome, craniofacial anomalies, neuromuscular disorders, sickle cell disease, or mucopolysaccharidoses are at increased risk for postoperative complications from adenotonsillectomy, particularly in terms of postoperative airway obstruction. Airway obstruction can increase the duration of inhalation induction as well as emergence of anesthesia. Furthermore, children with chronic sleep apnea may have increased sensitivity to the respiratory depressant effects of opioids. Airway management is typically performed with an oral Ring-Adair-Elwyn (RAE) endotracheal tube that allows surgical access to the airway for the procedure. During emergence, anesthesiologists should take care to avoid contact with the tonsillar beds by oral airways or suctioning equipment to minimize the risk of hemorrhage. Postsurgical hemorrhage is associated with morbidity and mortality, particularly if there is active hemorrhage during airway management phases such as induction or emergence of anesthesia. Postoperative care ranges from ambulatory surgical care to monitoring in an intensive care unit and is based on the individual comorbidities as well as the postoperative course exhibited by an individual patient. Postoperative nausea and vomiting is a significant risk and should be treated prophylactically with dexamethasone and ondansetron unless otherwise contraindicated (ie, dexamethasone is contraindicated for patients with leukemia due to possibility of tumor lysis syndrome and interference with chemotherapy protocols). Children scheduled for ambulatory tonsillectomy or adenoidectomy should be carefully observed for adequate analgesia and any signs of airway obstruction prior to discharge from the facility.

E. Cleft Lip and Palate

Cleft lip and palate make up the ***most common congenital deformity*** of the head and neck, affecting between 0.5 and 1 child per 1000 births with variation across ethnic groups worldwide (**Figure 33.5**). Maternal exposure to

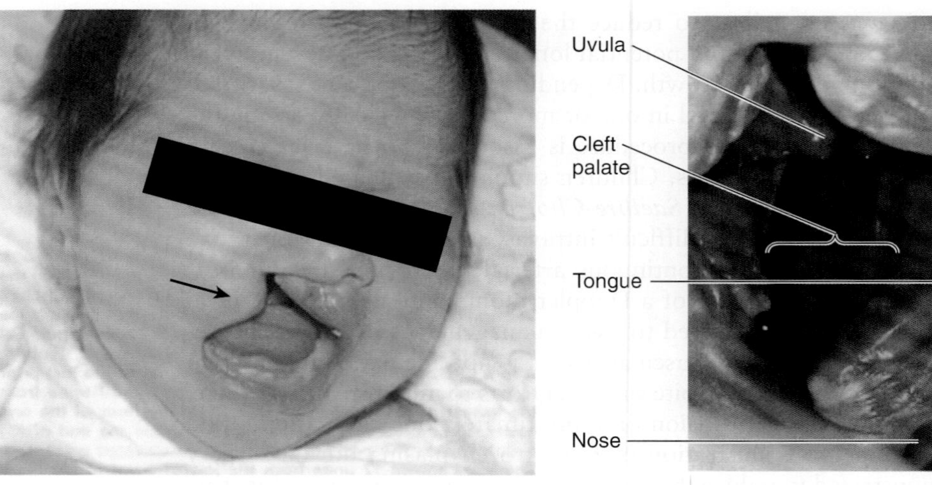

Figure 33.5 A, Unilateral cleft lip (*arrow*). B, Bilateral cleft palate (laryngoscopic view).

phenytoin has been shown to increase the risk of cleft lip, and tobacco use nearly doubles the risk of cleft lip. Various syndromes and genetic disorders may be associated with cleft lip or palate as well and may be a predisposing factor for perioperative airway complications.[45] The anesthetic management plan should recognize these comorbidities. Surgical correction varies based on the type of defect as well as the age of the child and may be performed in one or more stages. Anesthetic management may be highlighted by difficulty with laryngoscopy if either the laryngoscope blade or endotracheal tube is caught in the cleft. Furthermore, positioning of the child during surgery may result in dislodgement of the endotracheal tube or endobronchial intubation. Typically, an oral RAE endotracheal tube is preferred to facilitate surgical access to the airway. Children undergoing repair may be as young as 10 weeks, thus choosing an appropriately sized endotracheal tube is critical. Cuffed oral RAE tubes may not be universally available. As a result, uncuffed endotracheal tubes may result in a large leak or inappropriate depth. When uncuffed tubes are used, large leaks may be managed by inserting a throat pack. Following the repair, children are prone to airway obstruction upon extubation. It is critical that nasopharyngeal airways are avoided unless they are placed by the surgeon at the time of the repair. Postoperative care should focus on maintaining adequate respiration while managing analgesia and hydration.

F. Diaphragmatic Hernia

Diaphragmatic hernias occur as a result of a defect in the diaphragm that results in ***herniation of abdominal contents*** into the thoracic cavity (**Figure 33.6**). There are anatomic variants, including Bochdalek (70%-90%), Morgagni (20%-30%), and central (1%-2%) diaphragmatic hernias.[46,47] This condition usually begins to develop in early gestation during the first trimester. As a result, the affected lung is compressed and not able to develop due to the presence of abdominal organs in the hemithorax. The diagnosis can be made by prenatal diagnostic tests such as ultrasound and magnetic resonance imaging.

Because one lung will be underdeveloped, the patient will have elevated pulmonary vascular resistance as well as limited capacity for gas exchange, which

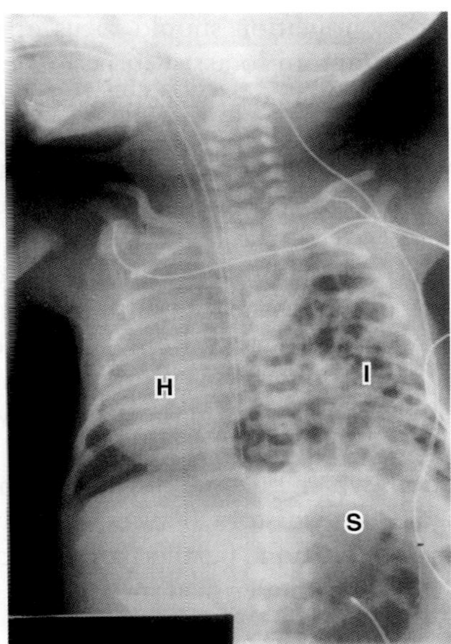

Figure 33.6 Diaphragmatic hernia showing intestine (I) in left thorax. Note position of stomach bubble (S) and shift of heart (H) into right thorax.

can be life-threatening. The prevalence ranges from 1 in 2500 to 4000 and has a 30% to 60% mortality rate. Even after surgical correction, children may develop chronic lung disease as well as pulmonary hypertension. Furthermore, the herniated organs can become distended (ie, stomach distention during mask ventilation or crying), which could result in further impairment of lung mechanics for both lungs. Depending on the severity of the condition, the child may not be able to sustain oxygenation and circulation without assistance. In some cases, the patient may be placed on ***extracorporeal membrane oxygenation (ECMO)*** as a bridge prior to surgical repair.

Considerations for anesthetic management depend on the severity of the case and whether the child can be safely transported from the NICU to the operating room. In some cases, the procedure may be done at the NICU bedside with ECMO. If a patient is not intubated or on ECMO, the anesthesiologist must take care to avoid airway obstruction and ensure ventilation takes place without excessive pressure to avoid overdistention of the stomach and intestines. Distended organs may lead to increased difficulty with ventilation as well as increased difficulty of the surgical procedure. Adequate intravenous access should be ensured with at least two peripheral intravenous lines. The surgical approach may be by laparotomy or thoracotomy. Laparotomy precludes the use of umbilical lines for vascular access. Continuous arterial monitoring is warranted to allow for blood gas monitoring for oxygenation and ventilation as well as for monitoring hemoglobin during the procedure.

G. Anterior Mediastinal Mass

Anterior mediastinal masses range from benign to malignant but may become life threatening due to ***compression of vital structures*** such as the trachea, great vessels, or the heart.[48] The etiology includes lymphoma, thymoma, germ cell tumors, metastatic lesions, bronchogenic masses, or thyroid masses. Preoperative assessment is critical to determine the extent of symptomatology, particularly if there is dyspnea, stridor, or syncope and any postural component. History and examination should focus on identifying any position that exacerbates the symptom to assist in perioperative care. Diagnostic imaging may include plain radiographs, computed tomography scan, and echocardiogram to characterize the mass as well as signs of cardiovascular compromise. Initial management typically involves obtaining a tissue sample to establish a diagnosis prior to initiating treatment such as chemotherapy or radiation to reduce the size of the mass. Induction of general anesthesia may be catastrophic if the mass shifts in position and compresses the airway or cardiovascular structures in the chest, resulting in an inability to ventilate and marked reduction in cardiac output. In high-risk scenarios, the priorities should always be to maintain spontaneous ventilation and to avoid neuromuscular blockade and positive pressure ventilation. In the event that cardiovascular collapse or difficulty with ventilation is encountered, the patient should be placed in a rescue position, which consists of the positions that improved the symptoms based on preoperative history. This may involve the upright sitting, lateral decubitus, or prone position. Furthermore, cardiopulmonary bypass may be required for a patient with a critical mediastinal mass.

H. Tracheoesophageal Fistula or Esophageal Atresia

Tracheoesophageal fistula results when an abnormal connection from the esophagus to the trachea is present due to failed fusion of tracheoesophageal ridges in early embryonal development.[1] This can occur in 1 of 3500 live births and is usually a postnatal diagnosis. Children may present with inability to eat or recurrent aspiration with oxygen requirement. In most cases, a nasogastric or orogastric tube is advanced and is unable to pass to the stomach. The specific diagnosis is usually confirmed by bronchoscopy prior to surgical repair. There are five types of tracheoesophageal fistula (**Figure 33.7**). The most common is a proximal blind esophageal pouch and a distal esophageal segment that communicates with the trachea (approximately 90% of cases), with the other types being less common.

There can be associated conditions, most notably the VATER or VACTERL syndromes (*V*ertebral anomalies, *A*nal atresia, *C*ardiac defects, *T*racheoesophageal fistula and/or *E*sophageal atresia, *R*enal and radial anomalies, and *L*imb defects). Although surgical correction is paramount to allow the child to eat and grow, a complete workup including echocardiogram should be performed to rule out any associated cardiac anomalies.

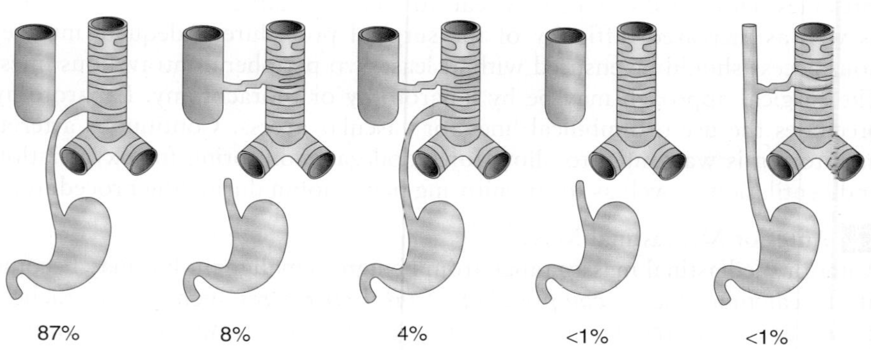

Figure 33.7 Relative frequencies of anatomic variations of esophageal atresia and tracheoesophageal atresia.

Prior to surgical correction, a Replogle tube is typically placed in the esophagus to empty any secretions. The child is not fed, and efforts should be made to soothe the child, as crying may lead to stomach distention, resulting in abdominal compression and respiratory distress. The initial approach typically requires flexible or rigid bronchoscopy to establish the anatomic location of the defect. The surgical approach will be dictated by the location of the defect, ranging from a thoracotomy or laparotomy, and may be completed over multiple stages. Induction of general anesthesia should focus on limiting stomach distention as well as adequate positioning of the endotracheal tube in relation to the fistula. In some cases, the fistula can be large enough to fit the endotracheal tube, and changing the patient's position throughout the procedure may result in "intubation" of the fistula.

I. Pyloric Stenosis

Pyloric stenosis is one of the most common conditions requiring surgical intervention in infants, with an incidence of 2 to 9 per 1000 live births.[1] Infants typically present with an inability to tolerate oral feeding and classic projectile vomiting in the first 3 months of life, resulting in ***hypochloremic, hypokalemic metabolic alkalosis***. If untreated, the condition can be fatal. Initial management consists of adequate resuscitation with intravenous fluids to restore normal circulating blood volume and electrolyte anomalies. The diagnosis may be confirmed with palpation of the thickened pylorus or by ultrasound studies. Anesthetic management should focus on minimizing aspiration of gastric contents.

> **? Did You Know?**
>
> Suctioning the infant's stomach immediately prior to the induction of anesthesia until little or no gastric fluid is retrieved has been successfully applied to reduce the risk of gastric content reflux during induction of anesthesia.

J. Necrotizing Enterocolitis

Necrotizing enterocolitis (NEC) remains a devastating problem affecting preterm infants during the first weeks to months of life.[1] Despite advances in perinatal and neonatal care, the incidence of NEC has not decreased, and its ***morbidity and mortality remain high***. Infants may present with abdominal distention resulting in hemodynamic instability and respiratory failure. Breast milk has been found to offer protection against developing NEC, despite advances in neonatal formula mixtures over the years. Though management strategies have evolved, the common therapies include cessation of gastric feeding, mechanical ventilation, and antibiotic therapy. Infants requiring surgical management are at the highest risk for morbidity and mortality and may not be stable enough to be transported out of the NICU. In such extreme cases, the surgical procedure may be performed at the NICU bedside. Surgical procedures may be complicated by hemorrhage as well as large fluid shifts. Infants may require transfusions in excess of 100 mL/kg and are at risk of transfusion-related complications such as coagulopathy and hyperkalemia.

K. Omphalocele and Gastroschisis

Omphalocele and ***gastroschisis*** are rare abdominal wall defects affecting 2 in 10,000 live births and 3 in 10,000 live births, respectively.[1] Gastroschisis is not associated with an overlying sac and results in exposed intra-abdominal organs. Gastroschisis is not usually associated with other congenital defects. Omphalocele is characterized by herniation of abdominal contents through a defect, although they are protected from the environment by a membrane. Omphalocele is associated with other anomalies including pentalogy of Cantrell, bladder or cloacal exstrophy, trisomy 21 (Down syndrome), or Beckwith-Wiedemann syndrome.[1] Both gastroschisis and omphaloceles require surgical management, which typically involves gradual reduction of the externalized abdominal contents via a mesh or silo. The process can be performed through various procedures to allow for gradual expansion of the abdominal cavity. It can be complicated by abdominal competition and difficulty with ventilation due to increased intrathoracic pressures from a bulging diaphragm.

L. Scoliosis

Children may present for surgical correction of ***scoliosis*** that results from neuromuscular defects with misalignment of the vertebral column or simply as "idiopathic" scoliosis.[2] In severe cases, gross deformities of the chest and abdomen may result in thoracic insufficiency and impair lung development. Furthermore, some patients may suffer neurologic sequelae such as nerve compression, which manifests as weakness, and sensory defects depending on the affected area. Surgical correction of scoliosis in a growing child remains controversial and treatment alternatives vary by surgeon, patient age, and coexisting disease. Surgical options include posterior spine fusion and vertical expandable prosthetic titanium rib. Anesthetic management should be tailored to meet the monitoring needs, as neurophysiologic monitoring may be used to assist and provide safety in the surgical approach. Agents that may affect the quality of motor and somatosensory-evoked potentials should be avoided, including volatile anesthetics, nitrous oxide, and neuromuscular blockade. Total intravenous anesthesia with propofol infusion and opioid infusions such as fentanyl or remifentanil are commonly used. The surgical procedures may be associated with significant hemodynamic derangements, including massive hemorrhage, spinal shock, coagulopathy, and hypothermia. Furthermore, positioning the patient should be done carefully to avoid pressure on the eyes, shoulders, and genitals to minimize position-related complications. Postoperative visual loss is uncommon but devastating and may occur as a result of ischemic optic neuropathy associated with the long duration of surgery. Intraoperative management should place specific emphasis on adequate intravascular access, with consideration for continuous arterial blood pressure monitoring as well as central venous access on a case-by-case basis. Blood conservation strategies such as antifibrinolytic agents, blood salvage techniques, and autologous blood donation may be used based on the resources available. Postoperative pain management may require support from a dedicated team.

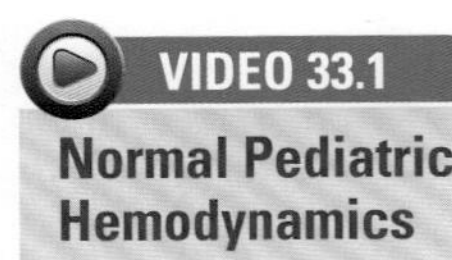
VIDEO 33.1 Normal Pediatric Hemodynamics

VIII. Common Pediatric Perioperative Complications

A. Postoperative Apnea

Infants and neonates born preterm are at increased risk for postoperative apnea following administration of anesthetic and sedative agents.[49] In addition to prematurity, a history of apnea and anemia are risk factors for postoperative apnea. Intravenous caffeine may be administered and is effective in reducing the incidence of apnea, although postoperative admission is still warranted based on postconceptional age. Based on the available data, many institutions admit all former preterm infants until they reach between ***55 and 60 weeks of postconception age***.[50] Postconceptual age is determined by the sum of gestational age and chronological age in weeks. Furthermore, children with obstructive sleep apnea may be especially sensitive to respiratory depression associated with narcotics and general anesthesia.

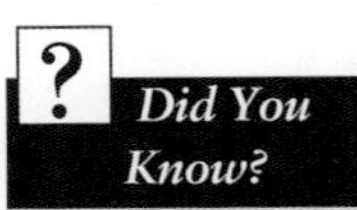
Did You Know?

Children at risk for postoperative apnea should be admitted and observed on a ward with cardiorespiratory monitoring.

B. Laryngospasm

Incidence of ***laryngospasm*** is more common in children than adults. The estimated incidence rate ranges from 1 to 17.4 per 1000 anesthetics.[51] When properly managed, laryngospasm typically results in no significant sequelae. However, it is a significant concern and continues to be a cause of cardiac arrest in children.[37,38] Treatment is with 100% oxygen, positive pressure, and maneuvers to ensure that upper airway obstruction is not present. Laryngospasm not relieved by these maneuvers should be treated with succinylcholine.[49] If there are contraindications to succinylcholine, such as malignant hyperthermia or extensive burn injuries, a nondepolarizing neuromuscular blocking agent may be appropriate. Deepening the anesthetic (eg, with 1-2 mg/kg of propofol) is an option in the early management of laryngospasm. Once desaturation has occurred, rapid neuromuscular blockade (succinylcholine) without delay is the treatment of choice. Secondary complications such as gastric insufflation, regurgitation, and aspiration can occur as a result of the sustained positive upper airway pressure that comprises appropriate management of laryngospasm.

C. Postextubation Stridor

Smaller children and infants are at increased risk for ***postextubation stridor*** due to their smaller diameter tracheas. Symptoms include a barky sounding cough (similar to infectious croup). More severe symptoms include respiratory compromise with retractions and dyspnea. Treatment for mild symptoms includes humidified air or mist. Dexamethasone 0.5 mg/kg up to 10 mg may be administered intravenously. More severe cases are treated with nebulized racemic epinephrine in addition to dexamethasone. Following treatment with racemic epinephrine, patients with improved symptoms should be observed for at least 4 hours to ensure rebound edema does not occur. Recrudescence of symptoms necessitates admission.

D. Emergence Agitation or Delirium

Emergence delirium is characterized by a state of delirium (confusion, lack of orientation to surroundings, agitation) in the immediate postoperative period following emergence from anesthesia.[41] Since the introduction of sevoflurane into clinical practice, the incidence of emergence agitation has surged. Risk factors include young age (2-7 years), sevoflurane use, poor adaptability, and procedures near the face (ear, nose, throat, or ophthalmology). Emergence agitation is a significant concern because agitated children can injure themselves, injure staff, or pull out catheters or drains and require additional staff to safely restrain and protect them. Emergence agitation also upsets parents and creates dissatisfaction. Most strategies have focused on prevention, and a variety of regimens are effective, including maintenance of anesthesia with propofol or intraoperative administration of dexmedetomidine, clonidine, and opioids. Initial management is typically observation and protection of the child from harm. More severe cases or prolonged cases may be managed with benzodiazepines, opioids, or subhypnotic doses of other sedatives.

IX. Outpatient Procedures or Ambulatory Surgery

A. Indications and Contraindications

In general, children presenting for outpatient procedures require being in optimal health and having no ongoing cardiorespiratory processes such as upper respiratory infections.[1,2] Furthermore, the procedure must be amenable to pain control with medications administered by mouth. Although it is not necessary to demonstrate that a child is able to eat prior to discharge, the child should be willing and able to drink fluids and ensure he or she can take the necessary medications as indicated. Additional elements to consider for eligibility for outpatient surgery include the care environment at home as well as the distance to travel home. For example, it may not be prudent to discharge a child from the hospital in the evening if the family has to drive several hours to get home.

There is a clear contraindication to ambulatory surgery in ex-premature infants during the first months of life due to the risk of postoperative apnea. The recommendation applies to premature infants defined as postgestational age of 37 weeks or less. There is an absolute cutoff at 52 weeks of postconceptual age where children must be admitted for overnight observation. Premature infants between 52 and 60 weeks postconceptual age may be observed in the postanesthesia care unit, and the decision to discharge the child can be left to the discretion of the providers caring for the child.

For further review and interactivities, please see the associated Interactive Video Lectures and "A Closer Look" infographic accessible in the complimentary eBook bundled with this text. Access instructions are located in the inside front cover.

References

1. Long JB, Suresh S. Neonatal anesthesia. In: Barash PG, Cahalan MK, Cullen BF, et al, eds. *Clinical Anesthesia*. 8th ed. Wolters Kluwer; 2018:1178-1218.
2. Barash PG, Cullen BF, Stoelting RK, et al. *Clinical Anesthesia*. [eBook Without Multimedia]. 8th ed. Wolters Kluwer; 2018.
3. Healy F, Hanna BD, Zinman R. Clinical practice: the impact of lung disease on the heart and cardiac disease on the lungs. *Eur J Pediatr*. 2010;169(1):1. PMID: 19639339.
4. Alcorn J, McNamara PJ. Pharmacokinetics in the newborn. *Adv Drug Deliv Rev*. 2003;55(5):667-686. PMID: 12706549.
5. Tierney AL, Nelson CA III. Brain development and the role of experience in the early years. *Zero Three*. 2009;30(2):9. PMID: 23894221.
6. Jevtovic-Todorovic V. Exposure of developing brain to general anesthesia: what is the animal evidence? *Anesthesiology*. 2018;128(4):832-839. PMID: 29271804.
7. Lin EP, Lee J-R, Lee CS, Deng M, Loepke AW. Do anesthetics harm the developing human brain? An integrative analysis of animal and human studies. *Neurotoxicol Teratol*. 2017;60:117-128. PMID: 27793659.
8. Jevtovic-Todorovic V, Hartman RE, Izumi Y, et al. Early exposure to common anesthetic agents causes widespread neurodegeneration in the developing rat brain and persistent learning deficits. *J Neurosci*. 2003;23(3):876-882.
9. Vutskits L, Davidson A. Update on developmental anesthesia neurotoxicity. *Current Opin Anesthesiol*. 2017;30(3):337-342.
10. O'Leary JD, Janus M, Duku E, et al. A population-based study evaluating the association between surgery in early life and child development at primary school entry. *Anesthesiology*. 2016;125(2):272-279. PMID: 27433745.
11. Hu D, Flick RP, Zaccariello MJ, et al. Association between exposure of young children to procedures requiring general anesthesia and learning and behavioral outcomes in a population-based birth cohort. *Anesthesiology*. 2017;127(2):227. PMID: 28609302.
12. Glatz P, Sandin RH, Pedersen NL, Bonamy A-K, Eriksson LI, Granath F. Association of anesthesia and surgery during childhood with long-term academic performance. *JAMA Pediatr*. 2017;171(1):e163470. PMID: 27820621.
13. Graham MR, Brownell M, Chateau DG, Dragan RD, Burchill C, Fransoo RR. Neurodevelopmental assessment in kindergarten in children exposed to general anesthesia before the age of 4 years: A retrospective matched cohort study. *Anesthesiology*. 2016;125(4):667-677. PMID: 276655179.

14. United States Food and Drug Administration. *FDA Drug Safety Communication: FDA Approves Label Changes for Use of General Anesthetic and Sedation Drugs in Young Children*. US Food and Drug Administration, Drug Safety Communication; 2017.
15. McCann ME, De Graaff JC, Dorris L, et al. Neurodevelopmental outcome at 5 years of age after general anaesthesia or awake-regional anaesthesia in infancy (GAS): an international, multicentre, randomised, controlled equivalence trial. *Lancet*. 2019;393(10172):664-677. PMID: 30782342.
16. Sun LS, Li G, Miller TL, et al. Association between a single general anesthesia exposure before age 36 months and neurocognitive outcomes in later childhood. *J Am Med Assoc*. 2016;315(21):2312-2320. PMID: 27272582.
17. Vutskits L, Culley DJ. GAS, PANDA, and MASK no evidence of clinical anesthetic neurotoxicity! *Anesthesiology*. 2019;131(4):762-764. PMID: 31246606.
18. Warner DO, Zaccariello MJ, Katusic SK, et al. Neuropsychological and behavioral outcomes after exposure of young children to procedures requiring general anesthesia: the MASK study. *Anesthesiology*. 2018;129(1):89. PMID: 29672337.
19. von Ungern-Sternberg BS, Boda K, Chambers NA, et al. Risk assessment for respiratory complications in paediatric anaesthesia: a prospective cohort study. *Lancet*. 2010;376(9743):773-783. PMID: 20816545.
20. American Society of Anesthesiologists Practice guidelines for preoperative fasting and the use of pharmacologic agents to reduce the risk of pulmonary aspiration: an updated report. *Anesthesiology*. 2017;126(3):376-393. PMID: 28045707.
21. Engelhardt T, Wilson G, Horne L, Weiss M, Schmitz A. Are you hungry? Are you thirsty?–fasting times in elective outpatient pediatric patients. *Pediatr Anesth*. 2011;21(9):964-968. PMID: 21489044.
22. Dennhardt N, Beck C, Huber D, et al. Optimized preoperative fasting times decrease ketone body concentration and stabilize mean arterial blood pressure during induction of anesthesia in children younger than 36 months: a prospective observational cohort study. *Pediatr Anesth*. 2016;26(8):838-843. PMID: 27291355.
23. Thomas M, Morrison C, Newton R, Schindler E. Consensus statement on clear fluids fasting for elective pediatric general anesthesia. *Paediatr Anesth*. 2018;28(5):411-414. PMID: 29700894.
24. Kain ZN, Mayes LC, Wang S-M, Caramico LA, Hofstadter MB. Parental presence during induction of anesthesia versus sedative premedication which intervention is more effective? *Anesthesiology*. 1998;89(5):1147-1156. PMID: 9822003.
25. Malde AD. Dexmedetomidine as premedication in children: status at the beginning of 2017. *Indian J Anaesth*. 2017;61(2):101. PMID: 28250477.
26. Caruso TJ, George A, Menendez M, et al. Virtual reality during pediatric vascular access: a pragmatic, prospective randomized, controlled trial. *Pediatr Anesth*. 2020;30(2):116-123.
27. Nguyen N, Lavery WJ, Capocelli KE, et al. Transnasal endoscopy in unsedated children with eosinophilic esophagitis using virtual reality video goggles. *Clin Gastroenterol Hepatol*. 2019;17(12):2455-2462. PMID: 30708107.
28. Fiadjoe JE, Nishisaki A, Jagannathan N, et al. Airway management complications in children with difficult tracheal intubation from the Pediatric Difficult Intubation (PeDI) registry: a prospective cohort analysis. *Lancet Respir Med*. 2016;4(1):37-48. PMID: 26705976.
29. Galvez JA, Acquah S, Ahumada L, et al. Hypoxemia, bradycardia, and multiple laryngoscopy attempts during anesthetic induction in infants: a single-center, retrospective study. *Anesthesiology*. 2019;131(4):830-839. PMID: 31335549.
30. Humphreys S, Lee-Archer P, Reyne G, Long D, Williams T, Schibler A. Transnasal humidified rapid-insufflation ventilatory exchange (THRIVE) in children: a randomized controlled trial. *Br J Anaesth*. 2017;118(2):232-238. PMID: 28100527.
31. Jagannathan N, Burjek N. Transnasal humidified rapid-insufflation ventilatory exchange (THRIVE) in children: a step forward in apnoeic oxygenation, paradigm-shift in ventilation, or both? *Br J Anaesth*. 2017. 118(2):150-152. PMID: 28100516.
32. Litman RS, Weissend EE, Shibata D, Westesson P-L. Developmental changes of laryngeal dimensions in unparalyzed, sedated children. *Anesthesiology*. 2003;98(1):41-45. PMID: 12502977.
33. Garcia-Marcinkiewicz AG, Adams HD, Gurnaney H, et al. A retrospective analysis of neuromuscular blocking drug use and ventilation technique on complications in the pediatric difficult intubation registry using propensity score matching. *Anesth Analg*. 2019;131:1. PMID: 31567318.

34. Asztalos L, Szabó-Maák Z, Gajdos A, et al. Reversal of vecuronium-induced neuromuscular blockade with low-dose sugammadex at train-of-four count of four. *Anesthesiology*. 2017;127(3):441-449. PMID: 28640017.
35. Tobias JD. Current evidence for the use of sugammadex in children. *Pediatr Anesth*. 2017;27(2):118-125. PMID: 28585399.
36. Won YJ, Lim BG, Lee DK, Kim H, Kong MH, Lee IO. Sugammadex for reversal of rocuronium-induced neuromuscular blockade in pediatric patients: a systematic review and meta-analysis. *Medicine (Baltimore)*. 2016;95(34):e4678. PMID: 27559972.
37. Bhananker SM, Ramamoorthy C, Geiduschek JM, et al. Anesthesia-related cardiac arrest in children: update from the pediatric perioperative cardiac arrest registry. *Anesth Analg*. 2007;105(2):344-350. PMID: 17646488.
38. Christensen RE, Lee AC, Gowen MS, Rettiganti MR, Deshpande JK, Morray JP. Pediatric perioperative cardiac arrest, death in the off hours: a report from wake up safe, the pediatric quality improvement initiative. *Anesth Analg*. 2018;127(2):472-477. PMID: 29677059.
39. Rouette J, Trottier H, Ducruet T, Beaunoyer M, Lacroix J, Tucci M. Red blood cell transfusion threshold in postsurgical pediatric intensive care patients: a randomized clinical trial. *Ann Surg*. 2010;251(3):421-427. PMID: 20118780.
40. Gurnaney H, Kraemer FW, Maxwell L, Muhly WT, Schleelein L, Ganesh A. Ambulatory continuous peripheral nerve blocks in children and adolescents: a longitudinal 8-year single center study. *Anesth Analg*. 2014;118(3):621-627. PMID: 24413546.
41. Voepel-Lewis T, Malviya S, Tait AR. A prospective cohort study of emergence agitation in the pediatric postanesthesia care unit. *Anesth Analg*. 2003;96(6):1625-1630. PMID: 12760985.
42. Adzick NS, Thom EA, Spong CY, et al. A randomized trial of prenatal versus postnatal repair of myelomeningocele. *N Engl J Med*. 2011;364(11):993-1004. PMID: 21306277.
43. Stricker PA, Shaw TL, Desouza DG, et al. Blood loss, replacement, and associated morbidity in infants and children undergoing craniofacial surgery. *Pediatr Anesth*. 2010;20(2):150-159. PMID: 20078812.
44. Roland PS, Rosenfeld RM, Brooks LJ, et al. Clinical practice guideline: polysomnography for sleep-disordered breathing prior to tonsillectomy in children. *Otolaryngol Head Neck Surg*. 2011;145(1 suppl):S1-S15. PMID: 21676944.
45. Jackson O, Basta M, Sonnad S, Stricker P, LaRossa D, Fiadjoe J. Perioperative risk factors for adverse airway events in patients undergoing cleft palate repair. *Cleft Palate Craniofac J*. 2013;50(3):330-336. PMID: 23083121.
46. Canadian Congenital Diaphragmatic Hernia Collaborative, Puligandla PS, Skarsgard ED, Offringa M, et al. Diagnosis and management of congenital diaphragmatic hernia: a clinical practice guideline. *Can Med Assoc J*. 2018;190(4):E103. PMID: 29378870.
47. Mielniczuk M, Kusza K, Brzeziński P, Jakubczyk M, Mielniczuk K, Czerwinska-Szaflarska M. Current management of congenital diaphragmatic hernia. *Anaesthesiol Intensive Ther*. 2012;44(4):259-264. PMID: 22481155.
48. Blank RS, de Souza DG. Anesthetic management of patients with an anterior mediastinal mass: continuing professional development. *Can J Anesth*. 2011;58(9):853. PMID: 21779948.
49. Cote CJ, Zaslavsky A, Downes JJ, et al. Postoperative apnea in former preterm infants after inguinal herniorrhaphy: a combined analysis. *Anesthesiology*. 1995;82(4) 809-822. PMID: 7717551.
50. Davidson AJ, Morton NS, Arnup SJ, et al. Apnea after awake regional and general anesthesia in infants the general anesthesia compared to spinal anesthesia study – comparing apnea and neurodevelopmental outcomes, a randomized controlled trial. *Anesthesiology*. 2015;123(1):38-54. PMID: 26001033.
51. Burgoyne LL, Anghelescu DL. Intervention steps for treating laryngospasm in pediatric patients. *Pediatr Anesth*. 2008;18(4):297-302. PMID: 18315634.

ANESTHESIA AND PREMATURE INFANTS

A CLOSER LOOK

Caring for a neonate can be a daunting effort. The premature infant poses additional challenges that place them at higher risk of perioperative morbidity. In general, premature infants (patients born <37 wk gestation) have immature organ systems. The anesthesia care provider must be cognizant of this during management. Illustrated below are major focus areas during clinical care.

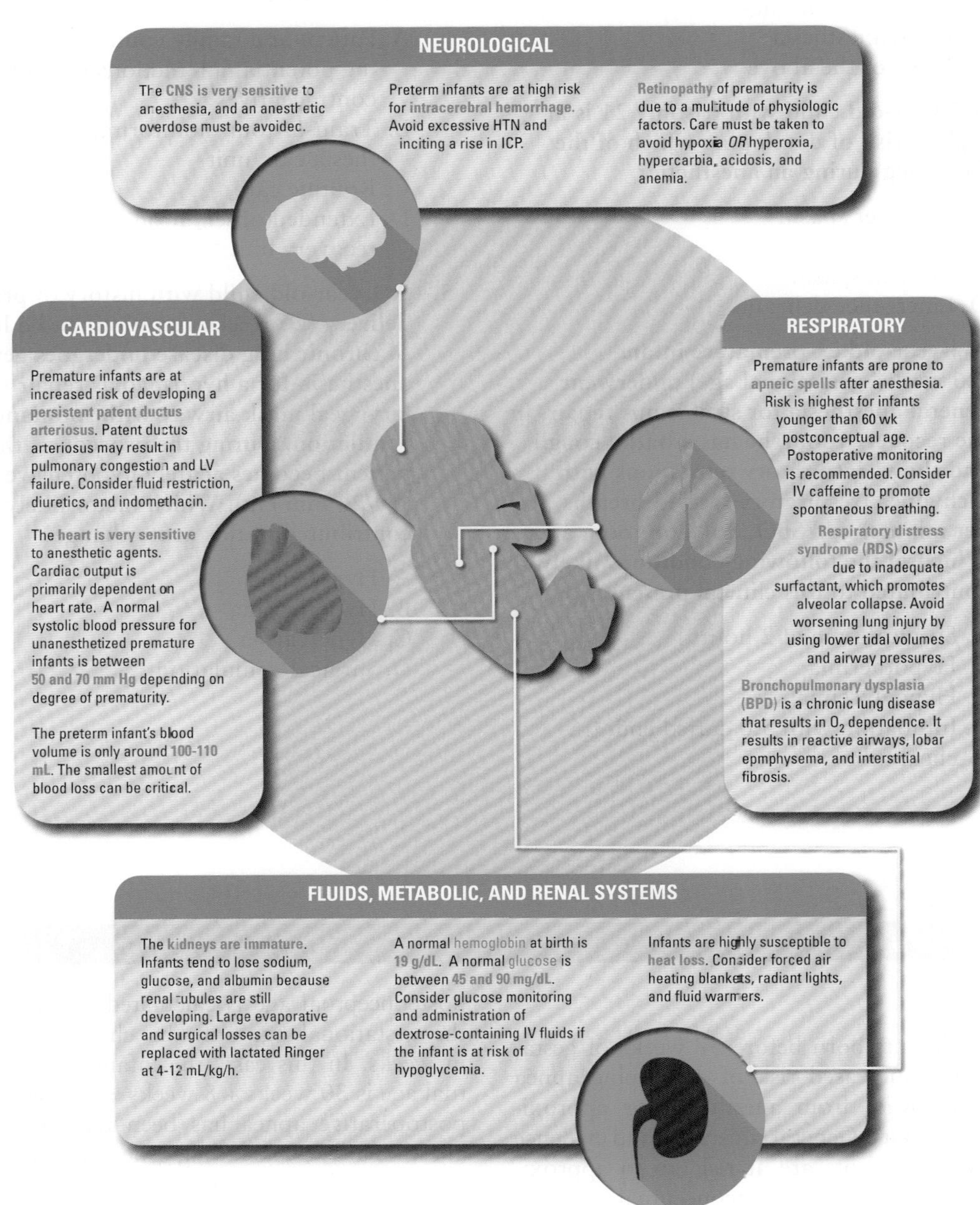

NEUROLOGICAL
The CNS is very sensitive to anesthesia, and an anesthetic overdose must be avoided.
Preterm infants are at high risk for intracerebral hemorrhage. Avoid excessive HTN and inciting a rise in ICP.
Retinopathy of prematurity is due to a multitude of physiologic factors. Care must be taken to avoid hypoxia OR hyperoxia, hypercarbia, acidosis, and anemia.
CARDIOVASCULAR
Premature infants are at increased risk of developing a persistent patent ductus arteriosus. Patent ductus arteriosus may result in pulmonary congestion and LV failure. Consider fluid restriction, diuretics, and indomethacin.
The heart is very sensitive to anesthetic agents. Cardiac output is primarily dependent on heart rate. A normal systolic blood pressure for unanesthetized premature infants is between 50 and 70 mm Hg depending on degree of prematurity.
The preterm infant's blood volume is only around 100-110 mL. The smallest amount of blood loss can be critical.
RESPIRATORY
Premature infants are prone to apneic spells after anesthesia. Risk is highest for infants younger than 60 wk postconceptual age. Postoperative monitoring is recommended. Consider IV caffeine to promote spontaneous breathing.
Respiratory distress syndrome (RDS) occurs due to inadequate surfactant, which promotes alveolar collapse. Avoid worsening lung injury by using lower tidal volumes and airway pressures.
Bronchopulmonary dysplasia (BPD) is a chronic lung disease that results in O2 dependence. It results in reactive airways, lobar epmphysema, and interstitial fibrosis.
FLUIDS, METABOLIC, AND RENAL SYSTEMS
The kidneys are immature. Infants tend to lose sodium, glucose, and albumin because renal tubules are still developing. Large evaporative and surgical losses can be replaced with lactated Ringer at 4-12 mL/kg/h.
A normal hemoglobin at birth is 19 g/dL. A normal glucose is between 45 and 90 mg/dL. Consider glucose monitoring and administration of dextrose-containing IV fluids if the infant is at risk of hypoglycemia.
Infants are highly susceptible to heat loss. Consider forced air heating blankets, radiant lights, and fluid warmers.

Infographic by: Naveen Nathan MD

Questions

1. **A 2-month-old preterm infant born at 30 weeks is now scheduled for repair of bilateral inguinal hernia repair. Which anesthetic plan has the lowest risk of postoperative apnea?**

   A. General anesthesia
   B. Neuraxial anesthesia
   C. Local anesthesia
   D. None of the above

2. **A 7-year-old child with trisomy 21 is at highest risk of developing which of the following during an anesthetic?**

   A. Masseter spasm
   B. Bradycardia
   C. Bronchospasm
   D. Emergence delirium

3. **A 4-year-old ex-premature infant (26 weeks' gestational age) underwent general anesthesia for strabismus repair. In the recovery room, he has a barky cough and shows inspiratory retractions with tachypnea (respiratory rate 45 breaths per minute) and SpO_2 96% on room air. Which of the following conditions likely contributed to this clinical presentation?**

   A. Surgical time of 2 hours
   B. Hypothermia
   C. Hypoglycemia
   D. Intubation with 5.0 cuffed endotracheal tube

4. **A 12-year-old girl undergoes rapid sequence induction with propofol and rocuronium for a laparoscopic appendectomy. She receives sugammadex for acute reversal of neuromuscular blockade. Which of the following considerations should be followed?**

   A. Patient and family counseling regarding potential interactions with oral contraceptives
   B. Train-of-four monitoring in postanesthesia care unit
   C. Routine care
   D. Extended observation in postanesthesia recovery unit

5. **A 1-year-old child with history of preterm delivery (26 weeks gestation) and a history of chronic lung disease undergoes general anesthesia for a hypospadias repair with a laryngeal mask airway with spontaneous ventilation. During the procedure, the patient becomes acutely hypotensive (50/26 mm Hg). Which factor likely contributed to this acute change?**

   A. Hypoxemia
   B. Hypothermia
   C. Hypercarbia
   D. Surgical stimulation

Answers

1. D

Preterm infants born before 37 weeks of gestation are at increased risk of developing apnea during recovery from anesthesia for approximately 24 hours. General consensus and evidence suggest that infants are at risk up to approximately 55 to 60 weeks postconceptual age. The postconceptual age is calculated by the sum of the gestational age and the chronological age in weeks. In this case, the infant's postconceptual age is 30 weeks + 8 weeks = 38 weeks. Late postoperative apnea has been reported for all anesthesia types, including general and neuraxial anesthesia irrespective of opioid use.

2. B

Individuals with trisomy 21, also known as Down syndrome, have a higher prevalence of congenital heart conditions including atrioventricular canal and related defects. Bradycardia is particularly common during inhalational induction with sevoflurane, regardless of the patient's cardiac anatomy. Close monitoring of heart rate and perfusion should be maintained during all phases of induction of anesthesia. Volatile anesthetic concentration should be titrated to maintain adequate anesthesia depth. Bradycardia should be treated promptly by reducing anesthesia dose (ie, decreasing sevoflurane concentration). Administration of atropine or epinephrine may be indicated based on the hemodynamic presentation. Please refer to pediatric bradycardia management algorithms form the American Heart Association.

Patients with trisomy 21 are not at increased risk of masseter spasm or other conditions associated with malignant hyperthermia. Patients with trisomy 21 do not have a higher risk of developing bronchospasm or emergence delirium.

3. D

This patient is experiencing croup secondary to endotracheal intubation. In this case, the endotracheal tube used was likely too large for the patient. The Cole formula (16 + age)/4 – 0.5 = 4.5 for this patient. The 5.0 cuffed endotracheal tube and laryngoscopy likely contributed to airway edema that is resulting in a barky, or croupy, cough. This patient should continue to be monitored for symptom progression. Treatment includes administration of racemic epinephrine via nebulizer. Following treatment, the patient must be observed for a minimum of 4 hours in case the airway edema recurs when the epinephrine wears off.

Hypothermia, hypoglycemia, or prolonged surgical time do not contribute specifically to development of airway edema.

4. A

Sugammadex is a cyclodextrin that selectively binds to rocuronium or vecuronium and reverses acute neuromuscular blockade. It also interacts with steroid compounds including hormonal contraceptives, potentially limiting their efficacy. Postmenstrual girls and their families should be counseled regarding this potential interaction.

Neuromuscular function can be assessed by train-of-four monitoring. However, this technique is painful and not indicated on an awake patient unless they are demonstrating signs of muscle weakness. Postmenarchal patients who receive sugammadex should receive additional counseling; therefore, routine care is not indicated. This patient may not require additional observation in the postanesthesia care unit.

5. C

Preterm infants are at higher risk of pulmonary complications due to underdevelopment of the lower airways and pulmonary vasculature. Acute changes in pulmonary perfusion can be attributed to mild changes in carbon dioxide tension, as could be expected in this procedure. In this case, the patient is breathing spontaneously with a laryngeal mask airway, which could lead to hypercarbia. Severe hypoxemia can result in elevated pulmonary vascular resistance, but these changes are unlikely to occur at normal oxygenation levels. Hypothermia and surgical stimulation are unlikely to contribute to acute hypotension in this scenario. Surgical stimulation may result in tachycardia and hypertension.

34 Anesthesia for the Older Patient

Douglas A. Rooke, G. Alec Rooke, and Itay Bentov

Since 1900, the percentage of Americans aged 65 years and older has more than tripled, from 4.1% in 1900 to 15.2% in 2016. In the coming decades, it is expected that older adults will comprise an even larger fraction of the population (**Figure 34.1**). While our patients may live longer, they are not necessarily healthier, as the burden of chronic diseases increases with age. Furthermore, despite the great variability in how age affects an individual, many age-related physiologic changes (such as changes in body composition and reduction in physiological reserve) are common and inescapable.[1]

As of 2018, the US national health expenditure accounted for almost 18% of the gross domestic product, with 21% ($750.2 billion) of the national health budget spent on Medicare.[2] As impressive as Medicare expenditures may be, federal spending grossly underestimates the total cost of caring for people older than 65 years. One of the challenges for the modern healthcare system is to provide safe yet cost-effective care for this vulnerable population.

> **? *Did You Know?***
>
> In 1935 when social security began, only 6% of the US population was older than 65 years. Now that value is 16%.

Older adults often suffer from multiple comorbidities, are subject to polypharmacy, and have worse outcomes than young adults. Anesthesia providers should be familiar with clinically relevant aspects of aging to provide appropriate clinical practice modifications to have a positive impact on a susceptible patient's outcome during the vulnerable perioperative period.

I. Physiology of Organ Aging

Biological aging is accompanied by changes that lead to a progressive decline in physiological reserve. Despite the body's reparative mechanisms, oxidative stress and other processes result in accumulation of cellular damage and senescence. Systemic conditions that cause inflammation and exhaustion of stem cells in turn result in the development of comorbidities and chronic disease. Age-related reductions in strength and activity lead to loss of muscle mass and function, resulting in frailty and disability. Defining what constitutes "normal aging" is difficult. Longitudinal studies that follow a group of healthy subjects over a long period provide an opportunity to examine age-related changes. Below we will discuss some of the changes that occur in older adults and their respective influence on anesthesia care. The reader is reminded to keep two principles in mind. First, the effect of aging varies considerably from one individual to another. Second, disease processes interact with aging processes to further diminish functional organ reserve.

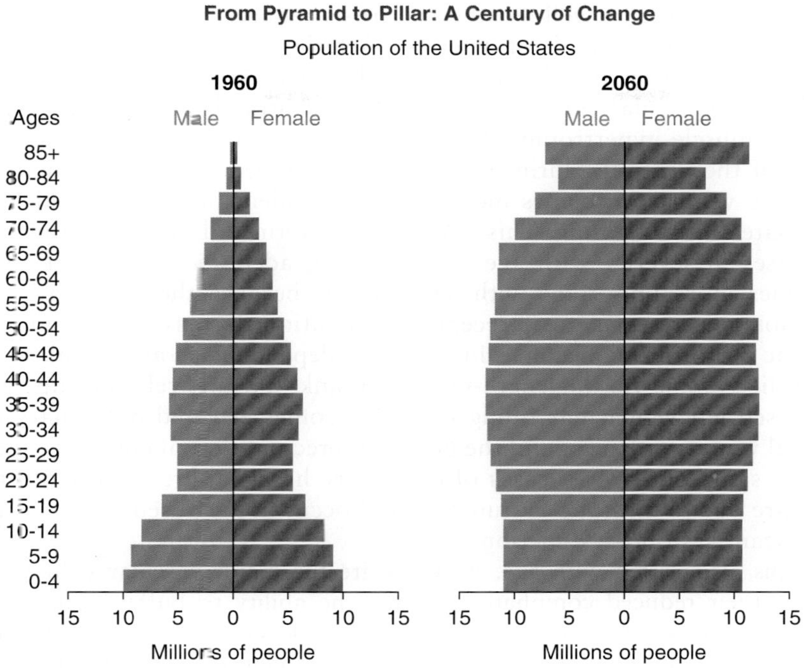

From Pyramid to Pillar: A Century of Change

Population of the United States

1960 — Male / Female; 2060 — Male / Female

Ages: 85+, 80-84, 75-79, 70-74, 65-69, 60-64, 55-59, 50-54, 45-49, 40-44, 35-39, 30-34, 25-29, 20-24, 15-19, 10-14, 5-9, 0-4

15 10 5 0 5 10 15

Millions of people

Figure 34.1 Past and future breakdown of Americans by age group. (Data from the U.S. Census Bureau, 2018.)

A. Cardiovascular Aging

Virtually all components of the cardiovascular system are affected by aging.[3] The major changes include the following: (1) decreased response to β-receptor stimulation; (2) stiffening of the myocardium, arteries, and veins; (3) changes in the autonomic nervous system, specifically, increased sympathetic activity and decreased parasympathetic activity; (4) conduction system changes; and (5) defective ischemic preconditioning. Although mechanisms of aging contribute to the development of atherosclerosis, it is not clear that aging inevitably leads to functional impairment or disease. **Table 34.1** outlines some of the most common cardiac changes and comorbidities associated with aging.

Table 34.1 Age-Related Cardiovascular Changes and Associated Comorbidities

Physiologic Change	Associated Comorbidity
Sinus node dysfunction	Symptomatic bradycardia
Conduction abnormalities	Heart block/dysrhythmia
Atrial enlargement	Atrial fibrillation
Diastolic dysfunction	Heart failure
Arterial stiffening	Systolic hypertension
Venous stiffening	Poor tolerance of hyper- and hypovolemia

Vascular aging as well as atherosclerosis reduces elasticity and lead to progressively less compliant arteries.[4] Arterial stiffening creates a retrograde wave of pressure that returns to the heart during late ejection. The decrease in vascular elasticity increases left ventricular work and leads to cardiac muscle hypertrophy. As hypertrophy progresses, it impairs relaxation of the ventricle during diastole which impedes left ventricular filling. The ventricle becomes increasingly dependent on the atrial kick for adequate diastolic filling. This phenomenon, termed diastolic dysfunction, increases in severity with age. Furthermore, adequate ventricular filling becomes more important with age. This is because the contractile and chronotropic response to β-receptor stimulation decreases with age, and cardiac performance becomes increasingly dependent on an adequate end-diastolic volume via the length-tension (Frank-Starling) relationship. With increased left ventricular filling pressures comes elevated pulmonary and central venous pressures and the potential precipitation of congestive heart failure symptoms. Most cases of congestive heart failure in very old persons are due to diastolic dysfunction and occur in the absence of clinically significant systolic dysfunction.

Veins also stiffen with age. As veins are the major vascular volume reservoir, their reduced compliance impairs the ability to buffer against even modest changes in venous blood volume, as evidenced by the fact that elderly persons are more likely to exhibit postural hypotension compared to young adults.

Rhythm disturbances may develop with age. Fibrosis of the conduction system may lead to conduction blocks. Loss of sinoatrial node cells makes older patients more prone to sick sinus syndrome. The prevalence of atrial fibrillation increases exponentially with age, largely due to atrial enlargement.

B. Pulmonary Aging

Total lung capacity (TLC) and functional residual capacity (FRC) remain relatively constant with age. However, expiratory reserve volume (ERV) decreases and residual volume (RV) increases. These changes are mainly due to loss of connective tissue and elasticity of the lung parenchyma. The lung volume at which the small airways (respiratory bronchioles) begin to close is termed the "closing capacity." In older patients, closing capacity exceeds FRC, resulting in atelectasis at baseline for many elderly patients (**Figure 34.2**).[5]

With aging, the thorax becomes barrel shaped and the chest wall stiffens, which leads to flattening of the diaphragm. There is also age-related loss of muscle mass. With these two effects combined, it is easy to understand why the older patient is more prone to fatigue when challenged by an increase in minute ventilation, and thus more likely to experience respiratory failure. Aging also blunts the ventilatory responses to hypercapnia and hypoxia, especially at night.[6] Aging results in less effective coughing and impaired swallowing and may play a role in the development of postoperative pulmonary complications.

C. Metabolic Changes, Liver, and Kidney Aging

Changes in body composition with age are primarily characterized by a gradual loss of skeletal muscle and an increase in body fat, even if body weight remains stable. Basal metabolic rate declines with age, but it is not clear if changes in body composition lead to a reduction in metabolic rate or if reduction in basal metabolic rate and fat oxidation lead to loss of muscle and accumulation of fat.

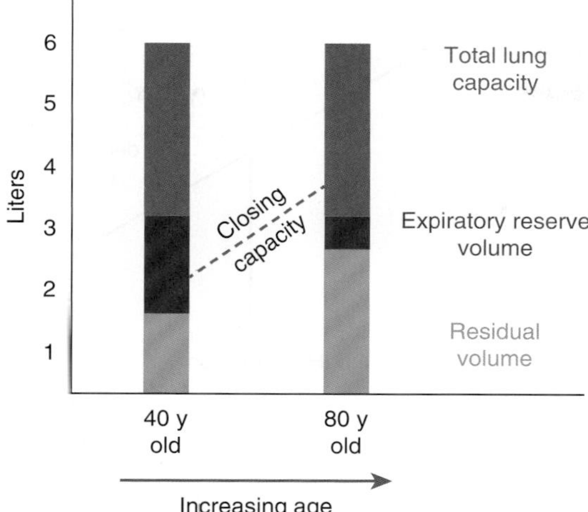

Figure 34.2 Changes in spirometry values with aging. There is virtually no change in total lung capacity. However, expiratory reserve volume decreases and residual volume increases. The sum of these—functional residual capacity—is largely unchanged. Note that closing capacity can exceed functional residual capacity leading to increased atelectasis.

Aging is associated with decreased insulin secretion in response to a glucose load, along with increased insulin resistance, particularly in skeletal muscle. Thus, even healthy elderly patients may require perioperative insulin therapy more often than their younger counterparts. Despite this fact, one should be careful to avoid hypoglycemia when insulin therapy is administered. Insulin is degraded by the liver and kidneys, and in older adults, hypoglycemia is more common and leads to worse outcomes.[7]

Liver mass and its blood flow decreases with age. Consequently, a modest reduction in phase I drug metabolism and bile secretion is expected.[8] However, there is a significant reserve built into the liver, and unless liver function is simultaneously affected by another pathological process, one can generally expect only minor age-related dosing changes for most anesthetic drugs. However, changes in body composition may alter pharmacodynamics and result in markedly increased metabolic half-lives for many drugs, especially benzodiazepines and opioids.

Quite different are the kidneys where significant pharmacokinetic changes occur with age. After about the age of 40 years, glomerular filtration rate (GFR) decreases by about 1 mL/min every year (**Figure 34.3**).[9] Common comorbidities of the elderly such as hypertension and diabetes can greatly accelerate this decrease in GFR. The dosing of many commonly used medications must account for renal impairment once GFR falls below 60 mL/min. Also, as GFR decreases, maintaining fluid and electrolyte hemostasis becomes increasingly difficult.

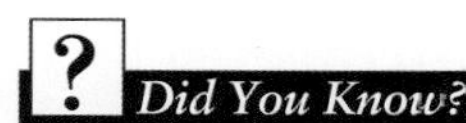

The metabolic half-life of diazepam in a 72-year-old is approximately 3 days.

D. Central Nervous System Aging

As we grow older, there is a loss of brain volume, especially in the frontal cortex. Age-related changes to cerebral vasculature and a higher prevalence of hypertension increase the risk for stroke and ischemia; white matter lesions are often observed on imaging studies. The major effect of brain aging on anesthetic management is an increased sensitivity to many anesthetic agents.

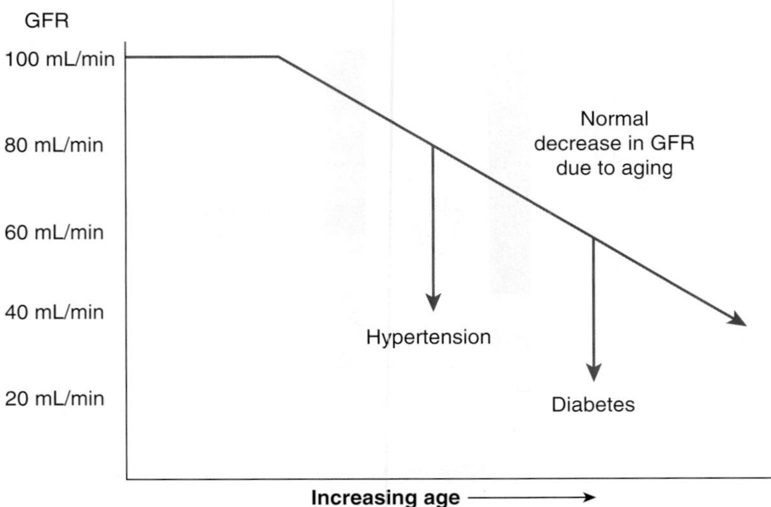

Figure 34.3 At around 40 years of age, glomerular filtration rate (GFR) decreases at a rate of 1 mL/min per year. In addition to this steady decrease, other common comorbid conditions such as hypertension and diabetes can further decrease GFR.

Perhaps the best-known example is the approximately 6% decrease in minimum alveolar concentration (MAC) that occurs per decade after the age of 40 years (**Figure 34.4**). For example, the MAC of sevoflurane for an 80-year-old is 1.4%, whereas it is around 2.1% for a 20-year-old.[10] Age-adjusted MAC should be used for inhalational agents. The brain is also more sensitive to the effects of many intravenous anesthetic agents. The dose of intravenous anesthetics should be reduced and titrated slowly due to longer circulation times. It is much more challenging to manage and quantify the potential interaction

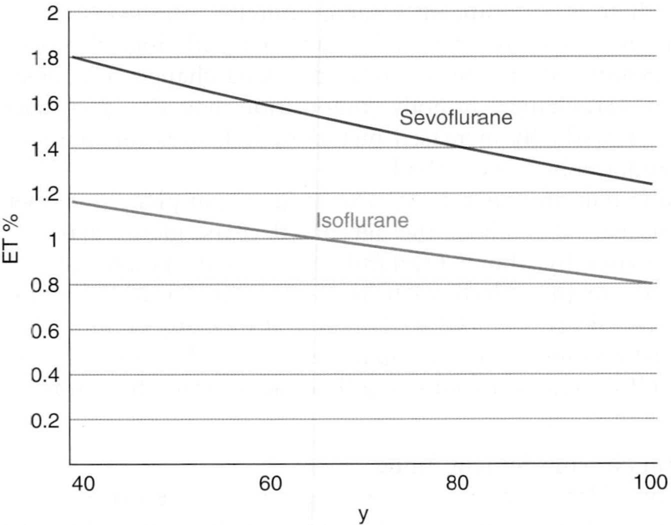

Figure 34.4 Minimum alveolar concentration (MAC) decreases with age for all volatile anesthetics. Illustrated above are the age-associated decreases in MAC for sevoflurane and isoflurane. ET%, end tidal %.

of anesthesia and surgical stress on a brain with reduced reserve. Postoperative neurocognitive disorders (delirium and cognitive decline) are a major challenge for providers and source of fear and anxiety for patients and their families.

II. Conduct of Anesthesia

A. Frailty, Disability, and Comorbidity

Older adults are medically more complex because they suffer from more age-related comorbid conditions (eg, hypertension, diabetes, and heart disease), higher rates of disability (defined as limitations and restrictions of daily activities), and increased incidence of frailty (a state of increased vulnerability that results from decline in reserve and function across multiple physiologic systems). Comorbidity, disability, and frailty are different, yet they often overlap (**Figure 34.5**). Consideration of all three should occur in the assessment of the elderly patient. Disability occurs when patients are unable to perform activities of daily living independently (such as self-feeding, personal hygiene, functional mobility, and dressing). These everyday tasks can be clear markers of a decline in functional status. Frailty or physiologic reserve can account for the patient's ability to recover from a stressor (eg, illness or surgery). When the patient's physiologic limit is reached, the likelihood of functional recovery is low. Frail, older adults may have difficulty recovering from even a medium- or low-risk surgery.

After puberty, there is little increase in the functional capacity of the major organs such as the heart, lungs, liver, and kidneys. Generally, the physiologic reserve plateaus during young adulthood and is followed by a gradual decline starting around the age of 40 years. Around the eighth or ninth decade, a more rapid decline occurs. Frailty occurs when the functional reserve declines to the point at which there is limited resistance to stressors (**Figure 34.6**).

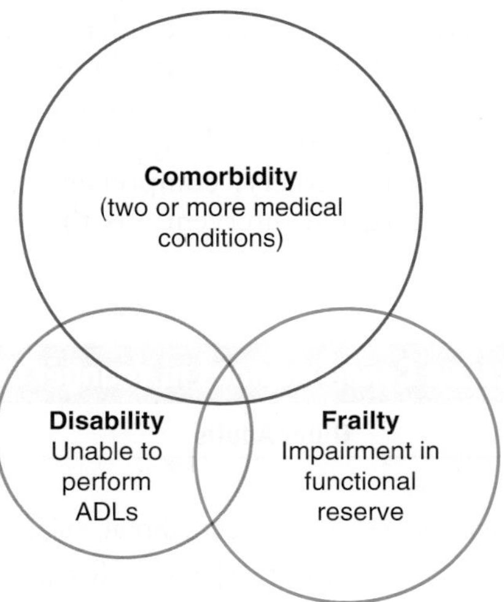

Figure 34.5 Comorbidity is defined as the presence of two or more chronic medical conditions. Disability is defined as the inability of a person to perform many of the activities of daily life (ADLs). Frailty occurs when there is impairment in physical and physiologic functional reserve. Comorbidity, disability, and frailty do not necessarily overlap.

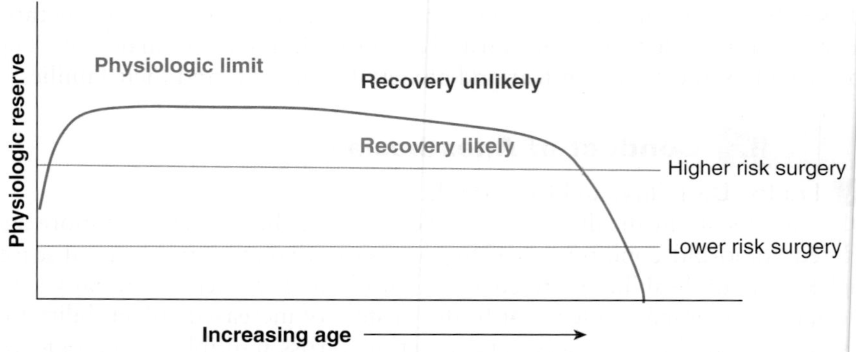

Figure 34.6 Schematic representing the changes in physiologic reserve with age. Recovery becomes less likely the more the stress of surgery exceeds a person's physiologic reserve. Most people retain their physiologic reserve through middle age before it gradually starts to decline. Near the end of life, there is a steeper decline as frailty sets in and patients have little tolerance to physiologic stressors.

B. Preoperative Assessment

Many aspects of preoperative assessment are similar in the young and old. However, additional assessments are often required for older adults (**Table 34.2**). For example, older adults are more likely to be using medications that require adjustment in the perioperative period (eg, anticoagulants, antihyperglycemic medications). Informed consent discussions should include broader considerations, such as goals of care, especially in patients undergoing major procedures.[11] Older adults are more likely to have advanced care directives; it is important to be aware of the patient's long-term care goals and recognize any durable powers of attorney for health care.

> **? Did You Know?**
>
> The elderly often require more preparation for surgery than young adults due to their polypharmacy and poor functional status; their goals for surgery are often different than for younger patients.

Comprehensive geriatric assessment is a framework for integrating clinical evaluation and intervention in vulnerable elderly patients. The assessment generally includes an evaluation physical attributes such as functional status, physical frailty, polypharmacy, and cognition; it also includes an assessment of the patient's social and financial support as well as their individual goals of care. Before elective surgery, comprehensive geriatric assessment may be applied to guide targeted interventions that will lead to improved outcomes.[12,13]

Table 34.2 Preoperative Considerations in Younger Versus Older Adults

Young Adults	Older Adults
Major comorbidities	
Inconveniences and common risks such as sore throat, chipped teeth, etc.	
	Risk of major adverse cardiac event
	Polypharmacy
	Frailty
	Baseline activities of daily living assessment
	Goals of care

C. Polypharmacy

Polypharmacy and drug interactions are common in older adults. The risk of adverse drug reactions increases with the number of medications taken. Up to 30% of ambulatory older adults require medical care for adverse drug events, and upwards of 30% of hospitalizations in the elderly are related to drug effects.[14] It is important for the anesthesia provider to review the patient's medications (especially central nervous system acting agents, anticoagulants and cardiovascular medications) and be prepared for potential interactions with drugs used in the perioperative period.

D. Malnutrition

Reduced appetite and impaired thirst mechanism are common in older adults and can lead to malnutrition and dehydration. Malnutrition screening can help identify those who will benefit from oral nutrition and multinutrient supplements. When malnutrition is identified, oral enteral supplementation should be started before (or soon after) major surgery because it may prevent complications.[15] Prolonged preoperative fasting should be avoided.

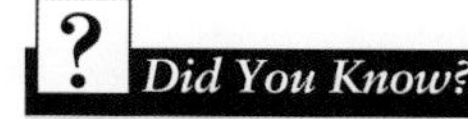

Many medications commonly used in anesthesia are relatively contraindicated for use in the elderly. Care should be taken to find alternative medications when possible.

E. Neurocognitive Decline and Depression

Neurocognitive decline often develops with age and is accompanied by depression. Best practice guidelines recommend that screening for neurocognitive decline and depression (and substance abuse) should be performed in all older adults.[16] Simple screening tests for neurocognitive decline, such as the Mini-Cog, are feasible. However, how best to use the information from these screening tools is not obvious. The Beers list (regularly updated by the American Geriatrics Society) is a list of medications that are typically best avoided in older adults. If an older adult is being prescribed one of these medications (**Table 34.3**), it is reasonable to determine whether changes can be made to decrease the dosing or find alternative medications.

F. Frailty

Frailty assessment can be used to improve preoperative risk stratification and perioperative planning (**Figure 34.7**). While no single definition of frailty has been agreed upon, there are several conceptual frameworks that are used. The "frailty phenotype" encompasses the following indicators: unintentional

Table 34.3 Commonly Used Drugs by Anesthesiologists on the Beers List

Class	Example	Deleterious Effect
Benzodiazepine	Midazolam, diazepam	Cognitive impairment, delayed emergence
Anticholinergic	Atropine, scopolamine	Central anticholinergic effects
First-generation antihistamines	Diphenhydramine	Central anticholinergic effects
Dopamine reuptake inhibitors	Haloperidol, metoclopramide	Extrapyramidal effects
H_2 blockers	Ranitidine	Cognitive impairment
Meperidine		Neurotoxic metabolite

Modified from American Geriatrics Society 2019 Updated AGS Beers Criteria® for potentially inappropriate medication use in older adults. *J Am Geriatr Soc*. 2019;67(4):674-694.

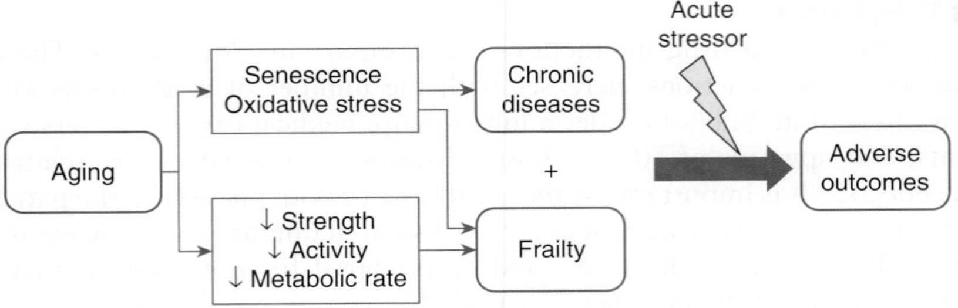

Figure 34.7 Schematic outlining some factors associated with normal aging that put patients at increased risk for adverse outcomes.

weight loss, exhaustion, muscle weakness, slowness while walking, and low levels of activity. Numerous clinical tools have been developed to identify frailty; some are multidimensional and require equipment and time to administer, while others are short and feasible to implement in a preanesthesia clinic.[17] While frailty is associated with increased morbidity, mortality, complications, increased hospital length of stay, and discharge to an institution, different tools are more strongly associated with specific outcomes.[18]

G. Prehabilitation

Once vulnerability is identified preoperatively, it is postulated that a preoperative habilitation program (prehabilitation) designed to increase physical, physiological, metabolic, and psychosocial reserves might be able to improve surgical outcomes.[19] Prehabilitation include a bundle of interventions that have been shown to improve outcomes in the nonsurgical population. These include exercise, education (eg, smoking cessation or psychological preparation), and nutritional support. Although small trials in high-risk surgeries show potential benefits, a major challenge to these programs is low adherence to the prehabilitation protocols.

III. Intraoperative Management

A. Drug Pharmacology and Aging

With increasing age, lean body mass decreases and body fat percentage increases (**Figure 34.8**). Consequently, the volume of distribution for lipid-soluble drugs increases. Also, renal clearance decreases with age. These changes increase the half-lives or the context-sensitive half-times of many drugs.[20] In general, smaller doses are needed in comparison with young adults. In addition, more time should be allowed for the drug to achieve its peak target organ (brain) effect. For example, propofol dosing should probably be decreased by around 50% in older adults and is best titrated to effect.

B. Choice of Anesthetic Technique

Large clinical studies and several meta-analyses have not found an advantage to regional versus general anesthesia in older adults. In a meta-analysis of 21 studies involving patients older than 50 years who underwent major surgery (cardiac and noncardiac) and were cognitively normal at baseline, the incidence of postoperative delirium was not different between those who received general or regional anesthesia.[21] Although regional anesthesia techniques probably provide the most effective analgesia (at least for the duration of the block),

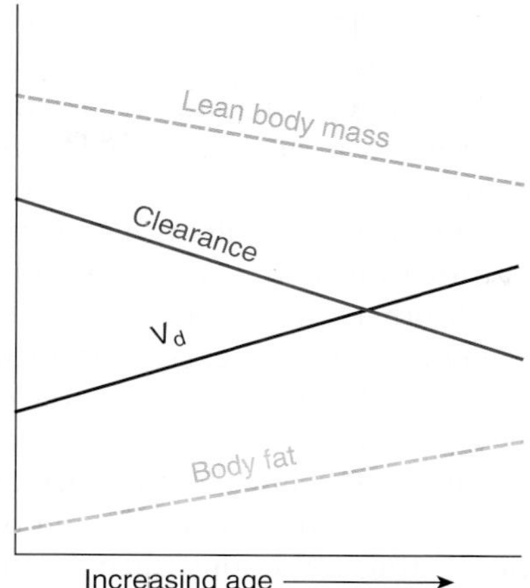

Figure 34.8 With age, lean body mass decreases and body fat percentage increases. Glomerular filtration rate (GFR) decreases with age. Consequently, the context-sensitive half-life of many drugs is increased in the elderly.

most studies suggest that this does not translate into improved long-term outcomes.[22] Hip fractures carry ominous in-hospital and 30-day mortalities (roughly 5%-10%) with high rates of cardiovascular and pulmonary complications and substantial postoperative disability. With an estimated annual incidence of more than 1.5 million cases worldwide, any potential improvement for this vulnerable group would have far-reaching social and economic implications. A retrospective analysis of a large cohort of patients undergoing hip fracture repair found a small difference in length of stay favoring regional over general anesthesia; however, there was no difference in mortality.[23]

C. Blood Pressure Management

Induction of anesthesia in older adults is often accompanied by hypotension, and prolonged hypotension is associated with adverse outcomes.[24] While it is unclear whether the association between hypotension and adverse outcomes is causal, it is hypothesized that avoidance of hypotension may help mitigate risk. Many strategies can be used to minimize hypotension during anesthesia.[25] One strategy focuses on the choice and dose of induction agents (eg, reduction in the propofol dose and use of adjuncts such as opioids, ketamine, or etomidate). Another option is to use vasopressors prophylactically (eg, treat anticipated hypotension with phenylephrine). Intraoperative blood pressure goals in older adults should probably be higher than younger adults due to the high incidence of baseline hypertension, especially in patients with significant arterial disease.[26] However, an excessive hypertensive response to intubation can be harmful to the older heart; thus, care must be taken to dose induction agents adequately. Ultimately, the goal is hemodynamic stability with minimal swings in blood pressure.

D. Fluids and Transfusion Management

Older adults are susceptible to impaired fluid management and electrolyte abnormalities. Ideally, intraoperative fluid and transfusion management strategies should optimize oxygen delivery and organ perfusion. Unfortunately, clinical signs of intravascular volume status are often difficult to evaluate in older persons, and it can be challenging to maintain intraoperative euvolemia.[27]

While small trials have suggested that using various monitoring modalities to guide administration of intravenous fluid and inotropic drugs could improve postoperative outcomes,[28] a large, pragmatic trial did not.[29] A limited subgroup of patients may benefit from advanced hemodynamic monitoring, but how to identify this subgroup has yet to be established.[30]

Transfusion management in older adults is also a matter of debate. Some advocate a liberal transfusion threshold (maintaining a hemoglobin concentration above 9-10 g/dL), while others support a restrictive threshold (above 7-8 g/dL).[31] Proponents of a liberal strategy suggest that anemia is associated with reduced delivery of oxygen to the tissues and poorer outcomes. Proponents of the restrictive strategy suggest that aggressive correction of anemia with red blood cell transfusions is associated with other adverse outcomes (eg, increased risk of infection and fluid overload). The approach chosen must also consider the patient's preexisting conditions, such as cardiovascular disease.

E. Thermoregulation

Age is an independent risk factor for the development of hypothermia during anesthesia. Hypothermia is common not only during general anesthesia, but also during regional anesthesia. Thermoregulatory responses are blunted in the elderly. This is mostly due to altered regulation of skin blood flow, which leads to a reduction in the threshold for thermoregulatory vasoconstriction. Clinical signs such as shivering are reduced or absent in older patients, and rewarming takes significantly longer than in younger adults. Maintenance of normothermia is important, since hypothermia increases the risk for myocardial ischemia, surgical wound infection, coagulopathy, and impaired drug metabolism.[32]

The initial decrease in core temperature during anesthesia results from the redistribution of heat to the periphery. Prewarming in the preoperative area helps minimize this redistribution of core heat. Active warming in the cold environment of the operating room as well as temperature monitoring are advised, especially during long surgeries.

F. Mechanical Ventilation

Postoperative pulmonary complications are common. If positive-pressure ventilation is utilized in the operating room, an important goal is to have lung volume exceed closing capacity during the respiratory cycle to prevent atelectasis. A ventilation strategy of modest tidal volumes (6-8 mL/kg) with individualized positive end-expiratory pressure between 5 and 8 cm H_2O, as well as repeated recruitment maneuvers has been suggested to decrease the incidence of postoperative pulmonary complications. In addition, use of routine monitoring to avoid hyperoxia and monitoring of neuromuscular blockade to minimize the risk of residual paralysis are advised.[33]

G. Delirium Prevention

Multiple studies have investigated the prophylactic use of medications for the prevention of delirium. While small, single-center studies using medications such as ketamine or dexmedetomidine initially showed promise, larger multicenter studies have not replicated these results.[34,35] Similarly, depth of anesthesia monitoring using processed electroencephalogram also has not been found to be beneficial.[36] Single-center studies found evidence of benefit in specific high-risk populations, but a pragmatic trial in which patients undergoing major surgery were randomized to usual care versus electroencephalographic measurement to prevent burst suppression found no difference in the rates of postoperative delirium.[37]

IV. Postoperative Care and Complications

"Failure to rescue" is defined as death after a potentially treatable complication and is an important measure for surgical quality improvement initiatives.[38] Complications are not only more common in older adults, but once they occur, they are significantly more likely to lead to mortality (**Table 34.4**).[39] In addition, there is increasing evidence that anesthetic management may influence long-term outcomes. Older adults are particularly sensitive to the detrimental effects of anesthesia. Anesthesiologists should not only be familiar with tools to identify patients at risk but be familiar with preventive strategies and treatment modalities.

A. Pain Control

The goals of pain management are no different for an older adult than a young adult; however, they are often more difficult to achieve. Accurate assessment of pain is difficult in patients who have cognitive impairment or delirium. In addition, older adults often suffer from chronic pain conditions but tend to underreport their acute pain levels.[40] Inadequate levels of analgesia are associated with numerous adverse outcomes, including sleep deprivation, respiratory impairment, ileus, impaired mobilization, insulin resistance, tachycardia, and hypertension.

Postoperative pain management in older adults is further complicated by an increased incidence of side effects due to polypharmacy and age-related changes in pharmacokinetics. The side effects of opioids (such as changes in mental status, nausea, vomiting, constipation, respiratory depression and increased fall risk) are more common in older adults. Adjunctive medications such as nonsteroidal anti-inflammatory drugs can reduce opioid requirements but often carry their own risks such as renal damage or gastrointestinal toxicity. Appropriate use of regional analgesia can reduce the need for systemic pain relievers.[41]

B. Perioperative Neurocognitive Disorders

One of the most distressing concerns for older patients and their families is the potential for the development of cognitive changes after surgery. In 2018, a nomenclature for the cognitive changes that may develop throughout the perioperative period was developed by expert consensus.[42] Cognitive changes that occur after emergence from anesthesia until expected recovery from anesthesia and surgery (up to 30 days) are referred to as postoperative

Table 34.4 Effect of Age on Selected Perioperative Complications and Mortality

Complication	Complication Rate		Mortality Rate From Complication	
	Age <80 y	Age ≥80 y	Age <80 y	Age ≥80 y
Myocardial infarction	0.4	1.0	37.1	48.0
Cardiac arrest	0.9	2.1	80.0	88.2
Pneumonia	2.3	5.6	19.8	29.2
Cerebrovascular accident	0.3	0.7	26.1	39.3

delirium or delayed cognitive recovery. If cognitive changes persist after the expected recovery period, they are defined as postoperative cognitive decline (POCD) or neurocognitive disorder (postoperative, for the first year). Emergence delirium, which is sometimes observed immediately after anesthesia, likely represents incomplete recovery from anesthetic agents or other conditions such as pain or a full bladder, not a neurocognitive disorder; as such, the condition might more accurately be referred to as emergence excitation.

C. Postoperative Delirium or Delayed Cognitive Recovery

Delirium is a condition of acute and fluctuating disturbance of attention and cognition. Delirium can be accompanied by perceptual disturbances, delusions, or psychomotor agitation. Delirium is associated with an increased length of stay, poorer long-term functional recovery, and increased mortality. Although delirious patients are often detected because of increased activity and agitation, older adults are more likely to present with hypoactive delirium (apathy, slow movement and speech) or a mixed subtype with both hyperactive and hypoactive features. The development of delirium (**Figure 34.9**) is dependent on preexisting vulnerabilities (age, fewer years of education, lower

PREOPERATIVE FACTORS:
Age, baseline low cognitive function (including dementia), depression, frailty, and visual/auditory impairment
Surgical stress
DELIRIUM RISK
Deliriogenic medications
Foreign location
PRESENTATION:
Waxing and waning mental status often hypoactive
OUTCOMES:
Increased hospital length of stay, poor functional and cognitive recovery, and increased mortality

Figure 34.9 Delirium represents a condition of waxing and waning mental status. There are multiple factors that put patients at risk for delirium. Delirium is associated with poor outcomes for patients and increased cost to the healthcare system.

preoperative cognitive function, frailty and functional impairment). Surgery type is also important; for example, in surgeries that require cardiac bypass or emergency orthopedic procedures, the incidence postoperative delirium is as high as 50% to 65%.

Prevention is the best strategy, as delirium can be difficult to treat. Effective preventive methods include frequent reorientation to time and place, good sleep hygiene, quick return of sensory input devices such as glasses and hearing aids, early mobilization (if walking is not possible, sitting in a chair), and adequate oral hydration and feeding. Both uncontrolled pain and excessive use of opioids or sedatives can lead to delirium. Medications with sedative effects (particularly benzodiazepines) should be prescribed cautiously if not avoided altogether. After the onset of delirium, careful use of antipsychotics can be considered.

D. Postoperative Cognitive Decline

Postoperative cognitive decline (POCD) is condition in which a decline in neurocognitive function (especially in memory and executive functions) is diagnosed more than 30 days after surgery or after expected recovery from surgery. In older adults undergoing noncardiac surgery, 26% had a decline in neurocognitive function 1 week after surgery and 10% continue to be affected after 3 months (of note, 3% of matched controls who did not have surgery also had a decline in neurocognitive function after 3 months).[43] These cognitive effects can persist for years and lead to reduced quality of life; they also frequently produce an economic burden on the patient and society. Unlike delirium, POCD can be difficult to diagnose, as its manifestations can be subtle, and detection often requires sophisticated neuropsychological testing.[44] Risk factors include age and reduced preoperative mental capacity; both lower levels of education and lower preoperative neuropsychologic test scores are associated with higher risk of POCD.

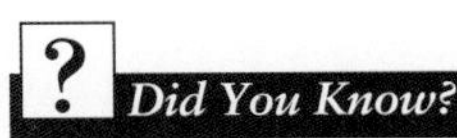

Whether patients who experience postoperative delirium are at increased risk of POCD remains unclear.

Little is known regarding the prevention and treatment of POCD. Trials have examined regional versus general anesthesia and found no differences in POCD risk; other studies are probably underpowered at least in part because of the range of neuropsychological tests used to evaluate cognition and the prolonged follow-up periods that are required.

V. The Future

Innovations in surgical and anesthetic techniques continue to reduce the overall stress to the patient caused by surgery and anesthesia; as such, older and sicker patients are presenting for surgery. Minimizing adverse outcomes involves taking steps throughout the entire perioperative continuum. Preoperatively, vulnerable older adults should be identified, and attempts should be made to improve their baseline status. Intraoperative monitoring of organs with limited reserve may help reduce the potential negative effects of surgery and anesthesia. Comprehensive, interdisciplinary care plans aimed at both preventing and identifying postoperative complications should be employed.

For further review, please see the associated Interactive Video Lectures accessible in complimentary eBook bundled with this text. Access instructions are located on the inside front cover.

References

1. Kennedy BK, Berger SL, Brunet A, et al. Geroscience: linking aging to chronic disease. *Cell.* 2014;159(4):709-713. PMID: 25417146.
2. National Health Expenditure Accounts. In: *NHE Historical and Projections 1960-2028.* Accessed April 3, 2021. https://www.cms.gov/Research-Statistics-Data-and-Systems/Statistics-Trends-and-Reports/NationalHealthExpendData/NationalHealthAccountsProjected
3. Folkow B, Svanborg A. Physiology of cardiovascular aging. *Physiol Rev.* 1993;73:725-764. PMID: 8105498.
4. Rooke GA. Cardiovascular aging and anesthetic implications. *J Cardiothorac Vasc Anesth.* 2003;17(4):512-523. PMID: 12968244.
5. Skloot GS. The effects of aging on lung structure and function. *Clin Geriatr Med.* 2017;33(4):447-457. PMID: 28991643.
6. Peterson DD, Pack AI, Silage DA, Fishman AP. Effects of aging on ventilatory and occlusion pressure responses to hypoxia and hypercapnia. *Am Rev Respir Dis.* 1981;124(4):387-391. PMID: 7294501.
7. Lee SJ. So much insulin, so much hypoglycemia. *JAMA Intern Med.* 2014;174(5):686-688. PMID: 24614940.
8. Schmucker DL. Age-related changes in liver structure and function: implications for disease? *Exp Gerontol.* 2005;40(8):650-659. PMID: 16102930.
9. Mühlberg W, Platt D. Age-dependent changes of the kidneys: pharmacological implications. *Gerontology.* 1999;45(5):243-253.
10. Nickalls RW, Mapleson WW. Age-related iso-MAC charts for isoflurane, sevoflurane and desflurane in man. *Br J Anaesth.* 2003;91(2):170-174. PMID: 12878613.
11. Berger M, Schenning KJ, Brown CH, et al. Best practices for postoperative brain health: recommendations from the Fifth International Perioperative Neurotoxicity Working Group. *Anesth Analg.* 2018;127(6):1406-1413. PMID: 30303868.
12. Eamer G, Taheri A, Chen SS, et al. Comprehensive geriatric assessment for older people admitted to a surgical service. *Cochrane Database Syst Rev.* 2018;1:CD012485. PMID: 29385235.
13. Partridge JS, Harari D, Martin FC, et al. Randomized clinical trial of comprehensive geriatric assessment and optimization in vascular surgery. *Br J Surg.* 2017;104(6):679-687. PMID: 28198997.
14. Budnitz DS, Lovegrove MC, Shehab N, Richards CL. Emergency hospitalizations for adverse drug events in older Americans. *N Engl J Med.* 2011;365(21):2002-2012. PMID: 22111719.
15. Avenell A, Smith TO, Curtain JP, et al. Nutritional supplementation for hip fracture aftercare in older people. *Cochrane Database Syst Rev.* 2016;11:CD001880. PMID: 15846625.
16. Mohanty S, Rosenthal RA, Russell MM, et al. Optimal perioperative management of the geriatric patient: a best practices guideline from the American College of Surgeons NSQIP and the American Geriatrics Society. *J Am Coll Surg.* 2016;222(5):930-947. PMID: 27049783.
17. Bentov I, Kaplan SJ, Pham TN, Reed MJ. Frailty assessment: from clinical to radiological tools. *Br J Anaesth.* 2019;123(1):37-50. PMID: 31056240.
18. Aucoin SD, Hao M, Sohi R, et al. Accuracy and feasibility of clinically applied frailty instruments before surgery: a systematic review and meta-analysis. *Anesthesiology.* 2020;133(1):78-95. PMID: 32243326.
19. Whittle J, Wischmeyer PE, Grocott MPW, Miller TE. Surgical prehabilitation: nutrition and exercise. *Anesthesiol Clin.* 2018;36(4):567-580. PMID: 30390779.
20. Sera LC, McPherson ML. Pharmacokinetics and pharmacodynamic changes associated with aging and implications for drug therapy. *Clin Geriatr Med.* 2012;28(2):273-286. PMID: 22500543.
21. Mason SE, Noel-Storr A, Ritchie CW. The impact of general and regional anesthesia on the incidence of post-operative cognitive dysfunction and post-operative delirium: a systematic review with meta-analysis. *J Alzheimers Dis.* 2010;22 suppl 3:67-79. PMID: 20858956.
22. Hopkins PM. Does regional anaesthesia improve outcome? *Br J Anaesth.* 2015;115(suppl 2):ii26-ii33. PMID: 26658198.

23. Neuman MD, Rosenbaum PR, Ludwig JM, et al. Anesthesia technique, mortality, and length of stay after hip fracture surgery. *J Am Med Assoc.* 2014;311(24):2508-2517. PMID: 25058085.
24. Wesselink EM, Kappen TH, Torn HM, et al. Intraoperative hypotension and the risk of postoperative adverse outcomes: a systematic review. *Br J Anaesth.* 2018;121(4):706-721. PMID: 30236233.
25. Kheterpal S, Avidan MS. "Triple low": murderer, mediator, or mirror. *Anesthesiology.* 2012;116(6):1176-1178. PMID: 22531339.
26. Marx G, Schindler AW, Mosch C, et al. Intravascular volume therapy in adults: guidelines from the Association of the Scientific Medical Societies in Germany. *Eur J Anaesthesiol.* 2016;33(7):488-521. PMID: 27043493.
27. Brown JB, Gestring ML, Forsythe RM, et al. Systolic blood pressure criteria in the National Trauma Triage Protocol for geriatric trauma: 110 is the new 90. *J Trauma Acute Care Surg.* 2015;78(2):352-359. PMID: 25757122.
28. Hamilton MA, Cecconi M, Rhodes A. A systematic review and meta-analysis on the use of preemptive hemodynamic intervention to improve postoperative outcomes in moderate and high-risk surgical patients. *Anesth Analg.* 2011;112(6):1392-1402. PMID: 20966436.
29. Pearse RM, Harrison DA, MacDonald N, et al. Effect of a perioperative, cardiac output-guided hemodynamic therapy algorithm on outcomes following major gastrointestinal surgery: a randomized clinical trial and systematic review. *J Am Med Assoc.* 2014;311(21):2181-2190. PMID: 24842135.
30. Bartha E, Arfwedson C, Imnell A, Kalman S. Towards individualized perioperative, goal- directed haemodynamic algorithms for patients of advanced age: observations during a randomized controlled trial (NCT01141894). *Br J Anaesth.* 2016;116(4):486-492. PMID: 26994228.
31. Brunskill SJ, Millette SL, Shokoohi A, et al. Red blood cell transfusion for people undergoing hip fracture surgery. *Cochrane Database Syst Rev.* 2015;(4):CD009699. PMID: 25897628.
32. Bentov I, Reed MJ. Anesthesia, microcirculation, and wound repair in aging. *Anesthesiology.* 2014;120(3):760-772. PMID: 24195972.
33. Griffiths SV, Conway DH, Sander M, et al. What are the optimum components in a care bundle aimed at reducing post-operative pulmonary complications in high-risk patients? *Periop Med (Lond).* 2018;7:7. PMID: 29692886.
34. Avidan MS, Fritz BA, Maybrier HR, et al. The prevention of delirium and complications associated with surgical treatments (PODCAST) study: protocol for an international multicentre randomised controlled trial. *BMJ Open.* 2014;4(9):e005651. PMID: 25231491.
35. Deiner S, Luo X, Lin H-M, et al. Intraoperative infusion of dexmedetomidine for prevention of postoperative delirium and cognitive dysfunction in elderly patients undergoing major elective noncardiac surgery: a randomized clinical trial. *JAMA Surg.* 2017;152(8):e171505. PMID: 28593326.
36. MacKenzie KK, Britt-Spells AM, Sands LP, Leung JM. Processed electroencephalogram monitoring and postoperative delirium: a systematic review and meta-analysis. *Anesthesiology.* 2018;129(3):417-427. PMID: 29912008.
37. Wildes TS, Mickle AM, Abdallah AB, et al. Effect of electroencephalography-guided anesthetic administration on postoperative delirium among older adults undergoing major surgery: the ENGAGES randomized clinical trial. *J Am Med Assoc.* 2019;321(5):473-483. PMID: 30721296.
38. Ghaferi AA, Birkmeyer JD, Dimick JB. Complications, failure to rescue, and mortality with major inpatient surgery in medicare patients. *Ann Surg.* 2009;250(6):1029-1034. PMID: 19953723.
39. Hamel MB, Henderson WG, Khuri SF, Daley J. Surgical outcomes for patients aged 80 and older: morbidity and mortality from major noncardiac surgery. *J Am Geriatr Soc.* 2005;53(3):424-429. PMID: 15743284.
40. Kaye AD, Baluch A, Scott JT. Pain management in the elderly population: a review. *Ochsner J.* 2010;10(3):179-187. PMID: 21603375.
41. Richardson J, Bresland K. The management of postsurgical pain in the elderly population. *Drugs Aging.* 1998;13(1):17-31. PMID: 9679206.

42. Evered L, Silbert B, Knopman DS, et al. Recommendations for the nomenclature o cognitive change associated with anaesthesia and surgery-2018. *Anesthesiology* 2018;129(5):872-879. PMID: 30325806.
43. Moller J, Cluitmans P, Rasmussen L, et al. Long-term postoperative cognitive dysfunc tion in the elderly ISPOCD1 study. *Lancet*. 1998;351(9106):857-861. PMID: 9525362
44. Cann C, Wilkes AR, Hall JE, Kumar RA. Are we using our brains? Diagnosis of postop erative cognitive dysfunction. *Anaesthesia*. 2010;65(12):1166-1169. PMID: 20964637

Questions

1. **You are seeing an 80-year-old woman in clinic for preanesthetic evaluation. On review of systems, you find that she occasionally has orthopnea symptoms and paroxysmal nocturnal dyspnea and her primary care provider has prescribed a few short courses of furosemide in the past. What is the most likely etiology of her symptoms?**

   A. High-salt diet
   B. Dilated cardiomyopathy
   C. Diastolic dysfunction
   D. Mitral regurgitation

2. **You are called to the recovery room to evaluate an 85-year-old man with an oxygen saturation of 92% on 4 L/min nasal cannula. He is 2.5 hours status post endovascular aortic valve repair with minimal propofol sedation. He is awake and alert although he has been lying supine for quite some time. What is the most likely explanation for this?**

   A. He has elevated P_{CO_2} due to poor ventilation.
   B. There is poor gas exchange due to pulmonary fibrosis.
   C. There was an aspiration event during the procedure.
   D. His pulmonary closing capacity is increased.

3. **After around the age of 40 years, glomerular filtration rate decreases by this amount every year.**

   A. 5 mL/min
   B. 1 mL/min
   C. 0.5 mL/min
   D. It does not change unless the patient has an underlying condition that affects kidney function

4. **What is the expected minimum alveolar concentration (MAC) of sevoflurane in an 80-year-old patient?**

   A. 1.2%
   B. 1.4%
   C. 1.8%
   D. 2.1%

5. **Which of the following are risk factors for the development of postoperative delirium?**

   A. Anticholinergic medications
   B. Frailty
   C. Baseline low cognitive function
   D. All of the above

Answers

1. C

The patient is reporting symptoms and signs of congestive heart failure. All of the above answers can potentially lead to or exacerbate congestive heart failure. In older adults, the most common cause of congestive heart failure is diastolic dysfunction due to cardiac hypertrophy. Ejection fraction is generally preserved.

2. D

The patient likely has a decrease in arterial oxygen partial pressure due to atelectasis. Loss of connective tissue and elasticity with aging lead to an increase in closing capacity and baseline atelectasis. The other answers are possible, however less likely, as the patient has no known history, had minimal sedation, and is awake and alert.

3. B

Glomerular filtration rate decreases by about 1 mL/min per minute each year after the age of 40 years.

4. B

Minimum alveolar concentration for volatile anesthetics decreases with age. The MAC of sevoflurane for a 20-year-old is about 2.1%. By the age of 80 years, the MAC decreases to approximately 1.4%.

5. D

Drugs with central nervous system effects such as anticholinergic medications, frailty, and baseline low cognitive function have all been identified as risk factors for postoperative delirium.

35 Anesthesia for Thoracic Surgery

Katherine Marseu and Peter Slinger

The most common indication for thoracic surgery is malignancy.[1-3] Despite this, a wide variety of pathologies and procedures are commonly encountered when providing anesthetics for patients undergoing thoracic surgery. As a result, there are a number of important preoperative, intraoperative, and postoperative anesthetic considerations for thoracic surgery.

I. Preoperative Assessment

Respiratory and ***cardiac complications*** are the major cause of perioperative morbidity and mortality in the thoracic surgical population. Thus, the preoperative evaluation of these patients focuses on an assessment of respiratory function and the cardiopulmonary interaction. All pulmonary resection patients should have preoperative spirometry to determine postoperative preservation of respiratory function, which has been shown to be proportional to the remaining number of lung subsegments (right upper, middle, and lower lobes = 6, 4, and 12 subsegments, respectively; left upper and lower lobes = 10 subsegments each, for a total of 42 subsegments). The principles discussed in the sections that follow also apply to thoracic surgical patients who are not having lung resections.[1,2]

A. Lung Mechanical Function

A valid single test for postthoracotomy respiratory complications is the ***predicted postoperative (ppo) forced expiratory volume*** in 1 second (ppoFEV_1%), which is calculated as:

$$\text{ppoFEV}_1\% = \text{preoperative FEV}_1\% \times \left(1 - \text{fraction lung tissue removed}\right).$$

For example, a patient with a preoperative FEV_1 of 60% having a right upper lobectomy (6 of 42 lung subsegments) would be expected to have a ppoFEV_1% = 60% × (1 − [6/42]) = 51%. Patients with a ppoFEV_1 >40% are at low risk for postresection respiratory complications, <40% at moderate risk, and <30% are at high risk.[1,2]

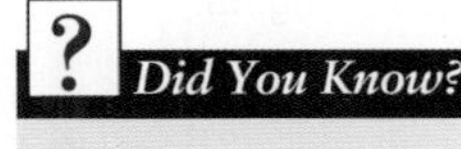

Did You Know?

Patients with a predicted postoperative FEV_1 of >40% are at low risk for postoperative respiratory complications.

B. Lung Parenchymal Function

The most useful test of gas exchange is the ***diffusing capacity*** of the lung for carbon monoxide (DLCO). The preoperative DLCO can be used to calculate a ppo value using the same calculation as for the FEV_1, with similar risk categories: increased risk <40% and high risk <30%.[1-3]

Table 35.1 Summary of Important Values in the Preoperative Respiratory Assessment

Parameter	Value	Risk of Respiratory Complications
ppoFEV_1%	>40%	Low
	<40%	Moderate
	<30%	High
ppoDLCO	<40%	Increased
	<30%	Very high
O_2max	≤15 mL/kg/min	Increased
	≤10 mL/kg/min	Very high

DLCO, diffusing capacity of the lung for carbon monoxide; O_2max, maximal oxygen consumption; ppoFEV_1, predicted postoperative forced expiratory volume in 1 second.

C. Cardiopulmonary Interaction

The most important assessment of respiratory function is an assessment of the ***cardiopulmonary reserve***, and the maximal oxygen consumption (O_2max) is the most useful predictor of outcome. The risk of morbidity and mortality is increased if the preoperative O_2max is ≤15 mL/kg/min and very high if it is ≤10 mL/kg/min. In ambulatory patients, the O_2max can be estimated from the distance in meters that a patient can walk in 6 minutes (6-minute walk test [6MWT]) divided by 30 (ie, 6MWT of 450 m:estimated O_2max = 450/30 = 15 mL/kg/min). The ability to climb five flights of stairs correlates with a O_2max > 20 mL/kg/min and two flights corresponds to a O_2max of 12 mL/kg/min[1-3] (**Table 35.1**).

D. Cardiac Investigations

Patients undergoing thoracic surgery are at risk for cardiac complications, such as myocardial infarction and arrhythmias. Patients should be assessed with the most recent American College of Cardiology and the American Heart Association (ACC/AHA) guidelines for the preoperative assessment of cardiac patients undergoing noncardiac surgery. These guidelines incorporate information based on active cardiac conditions, perioperative cardiac risk factors (**Table 35.2**), and functional capacity, in order to help decide whether patients

Table 35.2 Cardiac Conditions and Risk Factors

Active Cardiac Conditions	Risk Factors as Per the Revised Cardiac Risk Index
Unstable ischemia, recent MI	Ischemic heart disease (stable angina, remote MI)
Decompensated CHF	History of CHF
Significant arrhythmias	History of CVD
Severe valvular disease	Renal insufficiency
Significant pulmonary hypertension	Diabetes mellitus requiring insulin

CHF, congestive heart failure; CVD, cerebrovascular disease; MI, myocardial infarction.

Data from Fleisher LA, Fleischmann KE, Auerbach AD, et al. 2014 ACC/AHA guideline on perioperative cardiovascular evaluation and management of patients undergoing noncardiac surgery: a report of the American College of Cardiology/American Heart Association Task Force on practice guidelines. *Circulation.* 2014;130:2215-2245.

may proceed directly to surgery or should be investigated further, such as with noninvasive stress testing or cardiac catheterization.[1,2,4]

E. Common Pathologies and Comorbidities

Malignancies

The majority of patients presenting for thoracic surgery will have a malignancy, including lung cancers, pleural and mediastinal tumors, and esophageal cancer. These patients should be assessed for the "4-M's" associated with malignancy: ***Mass effects*** (obstructive pneumonia, superior vena cava [SVC] syndrome, etc.), ***Metabolic abnormalities*** (hypercalcemia, Lambert-Eaton syndrome, etc.), ***Metastases*** (brain, bone, liver, and adrenal), and ***Medications*** (adjuvant chemotherapy and radiation).[1,2]

> **? Did You Know?**
>
> The "4-M's" associated with malignancy are: *M*ass effect, *M*etabolic abnormalities, *M*etastases, and *M*edications.

Chronic Obstructive Pulmonary Disease

This is the most common concurrent illness in the thoracic surgical population. Patients should be ***free of exacerbation*** before elective surgery and may have fewer postoperative pulmonary complications when intensive chest physiotherapy is initiated preoperatively. Pulmonary complications are also decreased in thoracic surgical patients who cease smoking for more than 4 weeks before surgery. Patients with chronic obstructive pulmonary disease and limited or unknown exercise tolerance may benefit from an arterial blood gas (ABG) test preoperatively, if the results prove helpful in weaning mechanical ventilation at the conclusion of surgery. Other considerations in chronic obstructive pulmonary disease patients include the presence of bullous disease, pulmonary hypertension with right heart dysfunction, and the risk of dynamic hyperinflation due to gas trapping.[1-3]

II. Intraoperative Management

A. Monitoring

Standard anesthetic monitoring is used in all thoracic surgery cases. An invasive ***arterial line*** is placed for the majority of surgeries. It is useful to measure baseline preoperative ABGs for intraoperative comparison during ***one-lung ventilation (OLV)***, detection of sudden blood pressure changes, and postoperative weaning of mechanical ventilation. A central venous line may be required in some cases for vascular access or for infusion of vasoactive medications. The central venous pressure (CVP) can be a useful intraoperative and postoperative monitor, particularly for cases where fluid management is critical, such as pneumonectomies and esophagectomies. Fluid management for all thoracic procedures should follow either a restricted or a goal-directed protocol. However, recently, concerns about ***acute kidney injury*** have called into question the strategy of fluid restriction in thoracic surgery.[3] No fluids are given for theoretical "third-space" losses. Colloids have not been proven to improve outcome and add considerable expense. Spirometry is particularly useful to monitor breath-by-breath inspired and expired tidal volumes during OLV and may alert the clinician to possible loss of lung isolation, air leaks, and the development of hyperinflation.[1,3]

B. Physiology of OLV

In the majority of thoracic surgery cases, patients transition from being upright, awake, and spontaneously breathing to supine, asleep, and paralyzed. They are then moved from the supine position to the lateral position. Finally,

OLV is initiated, and their chest is opened. Changes in ventilation and perfusion accompany each of these circumstances.

First, functional residual capacity (FRC) is the main factor determining oxygen reserve in patients when they become apneic. Patients will experience a decrease in FRC when in the supine position compared with the upright position. This change will be magnified by the induction of anesthesia and administration of muscle relaxants. When upright, the majority of ventilation and perfusion reach the gravity-dependent portions of the lungs (ie, the bases). With the induction of anesthesia, most of the ventilation now enters the nondependent portions of the lung, increasing ventilation-perfusion (V/Q) mismatch.

Second, in the lateral position, the dependent lung receives more perfusion compared with the nondependent lung. However, the dependent hemidiaphragm is pushed into the thoracic cavity by the abdominal contents, further decreasing FRC and worsening/mismatch.

Third, when the chest is opened, the compliance of the nondependent lung improves relative to the dependent lung, and it is preferentially ventilated, further increasing the/mismatch. However, when OLV is initiated in the dependent lung, it receives the majority of both perfusion and ventilation. There will still be some cardiac output shunted through the collapsed, nondependent lung, but/matching may be improved by hypoxic pulmonary vasoconstriction (HPV) in the nonventilated, nondependent lung (**Figure 35.1**). HPV can be inhibited by many factors, such as extremes of pulmonary artery pressures, hypocapnia, vasodilators, and inhalational agents.[1,3]

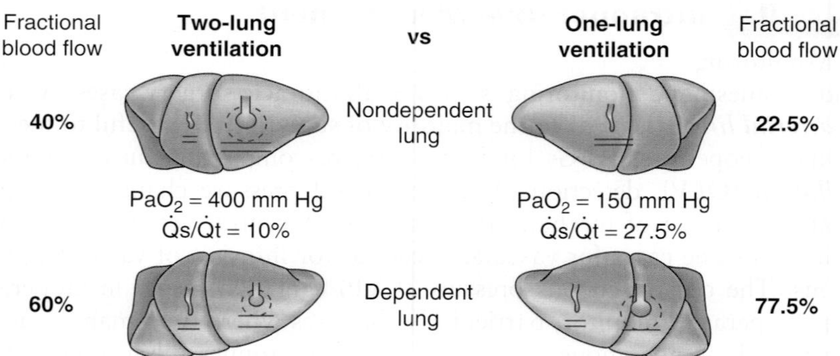

Figure 35.1 Schematic representation of two-lung ventilation versus one-lung ventilation (OLV). Typical values for fractional blood flow to the nondependent and dependent lungs, as well as PaO_2 and Qs/Qt for the two conditions, are shown. The Qs/Qt during two-lung ventilation is assumed to be distributed equally between the two lungs (5% to each lung). The essential difference between two-lung ventilation and OLV is that, during OLV, the nonventilated lung has some blood flow and therefore an obligatory shunt, which is not present during two-lung ventilation. The 35% of total flow perfusing the nondependent lung, which was not shunt flow, was assumed to be able to reduce its blood flow by 50% by hypoxic pulmonary vasoconstriction. The increase in Qs/Qt from two-lung to OLV is assumed to be due solely to the increase in blood flow through the nonventilated, nondependent lung during OLV. PaO_2, partial pressure of oxygen. (Adapted from Benumof JL. *Anesthesia for Thoracic Surgery*. WB Saunders; 1987:112 and Eisenkraft JB, Cohen E, Neustein SM. Anesthesia for thoracic surgery. In: Barash PG, Cahalan MK, Cullen BF, et al, eds. *Clinical Anesthesia*. 8th ed. Wolters Kluwer; 2018:1029-1076, Figure 38.10.)

Table 35.3 Indications for Lung Isolation

High Priority	Intermediate Priority
Prevention of contamination of healthy lung: • Infection • Hemorrhage	Higher indication for surgical exposure: • Thoracic aortic aneurysm repair • Pneumonectomy • Lung volume reduction • Minimally invasive cardiac surgery • Upper lobectomy
Control of distribution of ventilation: • Bronchopleural fistula • Unilateral bullae • Airway disruption	Lower indication for surgical exposure: • Esophageal surgery • Middle and lower lobectomy • Mediastinal mass resection • Bilateral sympathectomies
Unilateral lung lavage	
Video-assisted thoracoscopic surgery	

C. Indications for OLV

High and intermediate priorities for OLV are listed in **Table 35.3**. The highest priorities include prevention of ***contamination*** of the healthy lung by infection or hemorrhage; control of distribution of ventilation in bronchopleural fistula, unilateral bullae, or airway disruption; unilateral lung lavage; and video-assisted thoracoscopic surgery (VATS). Intermediate priorities for OLV include surgical exposure in thoracic aortic aneurysm repair, pneumonectomy, lung volume reduction, minimally invasive cardiac surgery, and upper lobectomy. Lower indications for OLV include surgical exposure in esophageal surgery, middle and lower lobectomy, mediastinal mass resection, and bilateral sympathectomies.[1,3]

D. Methods of Lung Isolation

Lung isolation can be achieved with the use of a ***double-lumen tube (DLT)***, bronchial blocker, or endobronchial intubation with a regular single-lumen tube (SLT) or specialized endobronchial tube. An SLT is rarely used in an endobronchial fashion in adults except in emergent scenarios, as bronchoscopy, suction, or continuous positive airway pressure (CPAP) cannot be applied to the collapsed lung.

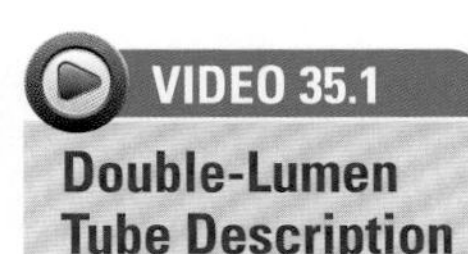

DLTs are the most commonly used method to achieve lung isolation and OLV (**Figure 35.2**). They are available in both left- and right-sided conformations, with the left-sided DLT being the most widely used. Advantages of the DLT include the ability to isolate either lung; apply suction, CPAP, or oxygen insufflation down either lumen; and perform bronchoscopy down either lumen. The DLT is less likely to dislodge than other methods of lung separation, which makes it the ***preferred method*** of isolation in cases of infection or hemorrhage. Disadvantages of the DLT include the fact that it is more challenging to place in a difficult airway, and it will usually need to be exchanged for an SLT if a patient is to remain intubated postoperatively.

A ***bronchial blocker*** placed through an SLT can also be used to achieve lung isolation (**Figure 35.3**). A bronchoscope is used to direct the blocker to the lung or lung segment that is to be collapsed. Several advantages of the blocker include the flexibility for use in an oral or nasotracheal fashion and for

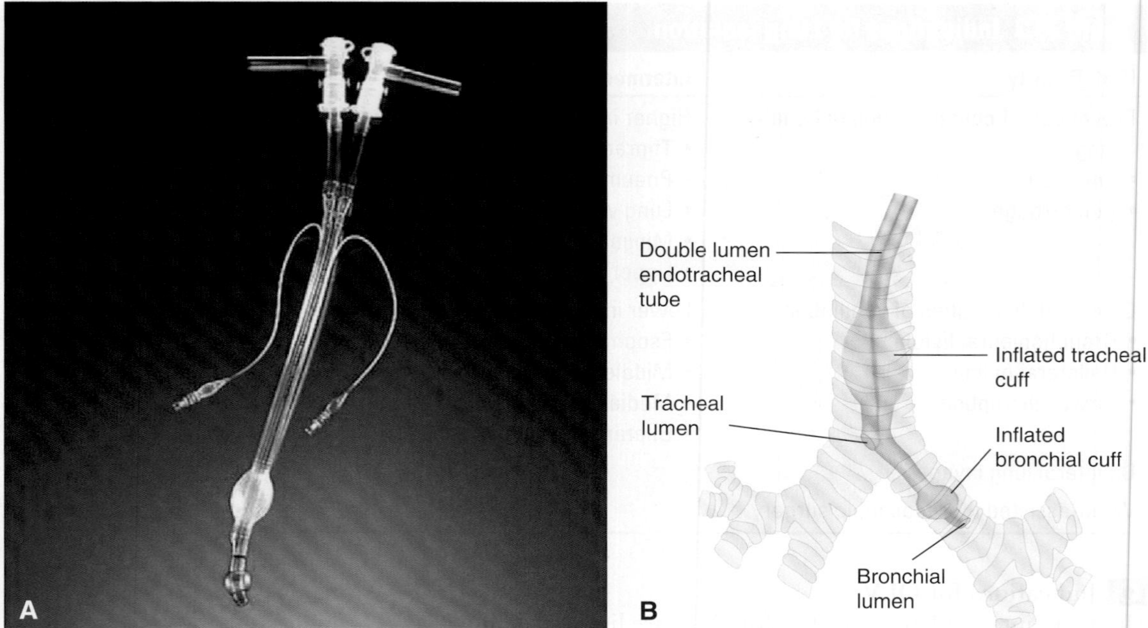

Figure 35.2 A left-sided Robertshaw-type double-lumen tube constructed from polyvinyl chloride (*left*, A). When properly positioned (*right*, B), the distal "bronchial lumen" is placed in the left mainstem bronchus proximal to the left upper lobe orifice, with the "bronchial cuff" inflated just distal to the carina in the left mainstem bronchus. The proximal "tracheal lumen" is positioned above the carina, with the "tracheal cuff" inflated in the mid-trachea. Proper positioning allows for the options of one-lung ventilation on either side (with contralateral lung deflation), as well as two-lung ventilation. (A, Courtesy of Nellcor Puritan Bennett, Inc., Pleasanton, California and B, Redrawn from Hillard EK, Thompson PW. Instruments used in thoracic anesthesia. In: Mushin WW, ed. *Thoracic Anesthesia*. Blackwell Scientific; 1963:315.)

selective lobar blockade. It is particularly useful in scenarios such as a ***difficult airway*** or the need for postoperative ventilation. The main disadvantage of a bronchial blocker is that it can be displaced from changes in patient position or surgical manipulation. This is especially detrimental in a situation where loss of lung separation can lead to contamination from blood or pus.[1,3]

E. Management of OLV

Fraction of Inspired Oxygen

When initiating OLV, a fraction of inspired oxygen (FiO_2) of 1.0 is generally used to prevent hypoxemia. An ABG test may be taken to determine arterial partial pressure of O_2. If this is adequate, the FiO_2 may be titrated down.[3]

Tidal Volume and Respiratory Rate

The current trend in OLV is to use ***lung-protective strategies***. Whether using volume-controlled or pressure-controlled ventilation, tidal volume should be approximately 5 mL/kg. The respiratory rate is then titrated to maintain an acceptable range of end-tidal carbon dioxide (CO_2) or arterial partial pressure of CO_2 (35-40 mm Hg). Peak airway pressures should be maintained at <35 cm H_2O, and preferably <25 cm H_2O.[1,3] In the presence of bullous disease, even lower airway pressures must be considered.

F. Management of Hypoxemia on OLV

Hypoxic pulmonary vasoconstriction can take hours to reach full effect. If hypoxemia develops during OLV, the FiO_2 should be increased to 1.0.

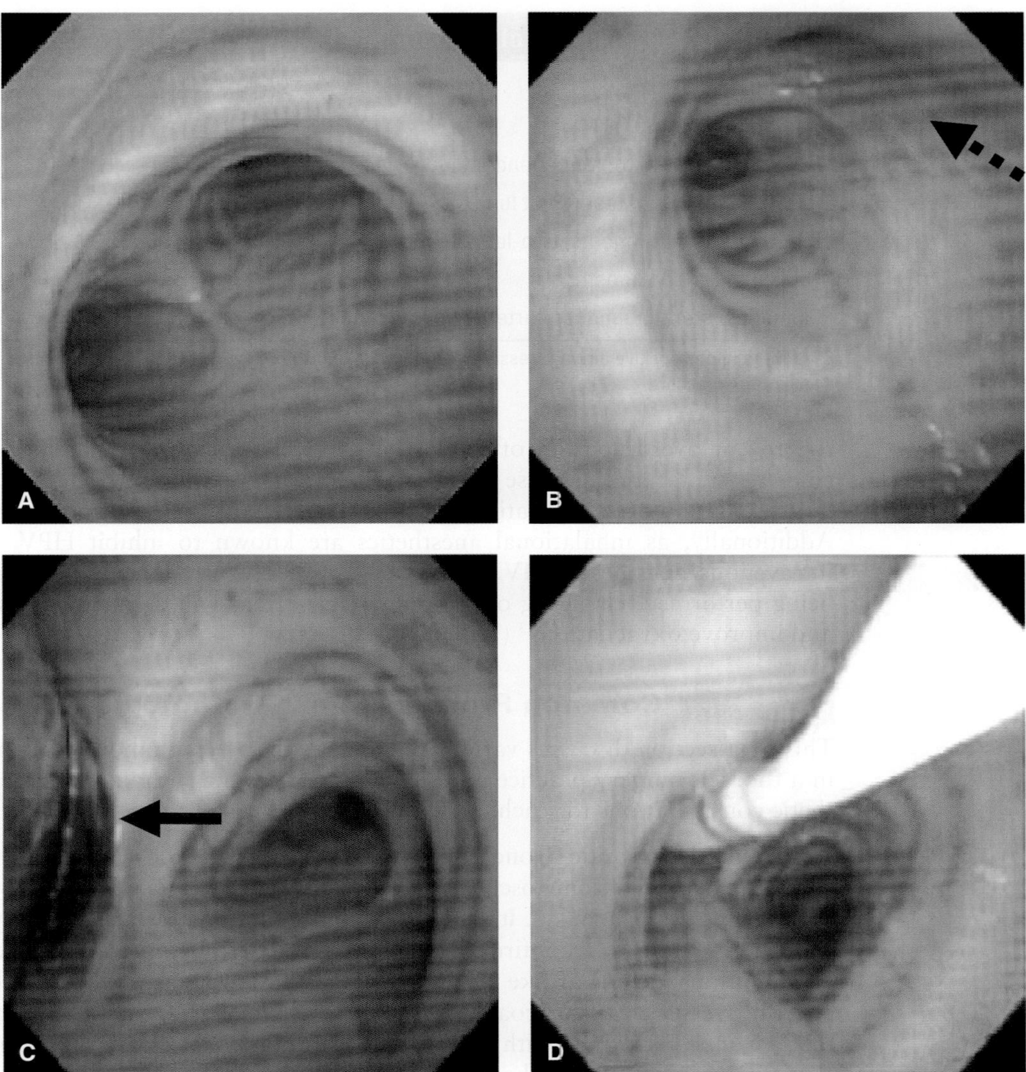

Figure 35.3 A, Bronchoscopic view of the carina through the distal opening of a standard endotracheal tube. Note the C-shaped tracheal rings anteriorly orient the viewer to the left and right mainstem bronchi. B, Bronchoscopic view of the right upper lobe orifice (*dotted arrow*) only 1.5-2.0 cm distal to the carina. This short distance generally prevents the use of right-sided double-lumen tubes. C, Bronchoscopic view of the carina and right mainstem bronchus, demonstrating a properly positioned left-sided double-lumen tube with the blue bronchial cuff (*arrow*) inflated just distal to the carina in the left mainstem bronchus. D, Bronchoscopic view of a bronchial blocker placed through a single-lumen tube and positioned in the left mainstem bronchus to allow one-lung ventilation on the right. (From Eisenkraft JB, Cohen E, Neustein SM. Anesthesia for thoracic surgery. In: Barash PG, Cahalan MK, Cullen BF, et al, eds. *Clinical Anesthesia*. 8th ed. Wolters Kluwer; 2018:1029-1076, Figures 38.12 and 38.13.)

Bronchoscopy should be performed to confirm tube position. The most effective treatment of hypoxemia is to apply 5 to 10 cm H_2O of ***CPAP*** to the nondependent lung. However, as this is the operative lung, CPAP can interfere with the surgical exposure. Thus, the application of positive end-expiratory pressure (PEEP) to the dependent lung may then be useful to increase FRC and / matching. This should be limited to approximately 10 cm H_2O in order

Table 35.4 Management of Hypoxia on One-Lung Ventilation
FiO_2 1.0
Confirm tube position
CPAP 5-10 cm H_2O to nondependent lung
PEEP 10 cm H_2O to dependent lung
Intermittent recruitments, two-lung ventilation
Total intravenous anesthesia
Clamp ipsilateral pulmonary artery in pneumonectomy

CPAP, continuous positive airway pressure; FiO_2, fraction of inspired oxygen; PEEP, positive end-expiratory pressure.

to prevent overdistension of the alveoli, which can elevate pulmonary vascular resistance and increase shunting. ***Recruitment maneuvers*** and intermittent ventilation of the operative lung may be performed if hypoxemia persists. Additionally, as inhalational anesthetics are known to inhibit HPV, total intravenous anesthesia (TIVA) may be considered. If a pneumonectomy is being performed, clamping of the pulmonary artery will eliminate the shunt and improve oxygenation[1,3] (**Table 35.4**).

III. Common Procedures and Pathologies

This next section discusses various procedures that are commonly performed in a thoracic surgery practice and reviews the relevant pathologies and anesthetic considerations for each.

A. Flexible Fiberoptic Bronchoscopy

Flexible fiberoptic bronchoscopy is a diagnostic and therapeutic modality for pathologies of the airways. It is also common to perform bronchoscopy prior to lung resections to reconfirm the diagnosis or determine invasion of the airway. Options include awake with topical anesthesia versus general anesthesia and oral versus nasal approaches. Airway management during general anesthesia can be performed with an endotracheal tube (ETT) or a laryngeal mask airway. ***Intravenous*** anesthesia is preferred if this procedure is going to be prolonged, as volatile agents ***may*** contaminate the operating room.[1,3]

B. Rigid Bronchoscopy

Rigid bronchoscopy is the procedure of choice for dilation of ***tracheal stenosis*** with or without the use of a laser, foreign body removal, and massive hemoptysis. There are four basic methods of ventilation for rigid bronchoscopy: spontaneous ventilation; apneic oxygenation with or without the insufflation of oxygen; positive pressure ventilation (PPV) via the side arm of a ventilating bronchoscope; and jet ventilation with a handheld injector or high-frequency jet ventilator. Rigid bronchoscopy in children is most commonly managed with spontaneous ventilation and a volatile anesthetic. In adults, total intravenous anesthesia (TIVA) and the use of muscle relaxants is more common, with a combination of PPV via the bronchoscope side arm or jet ventilation. Pulse oximetry is vital during rigid bronchoscopy because there is a high risk of desaturation. However, monitoring of end-tidal CO_2 and volatile anesthetics is less useful, because the airway remains essentially open to the atmosphere. Unlike during fiberoptic bronchoscopy via an ETT, with rigid

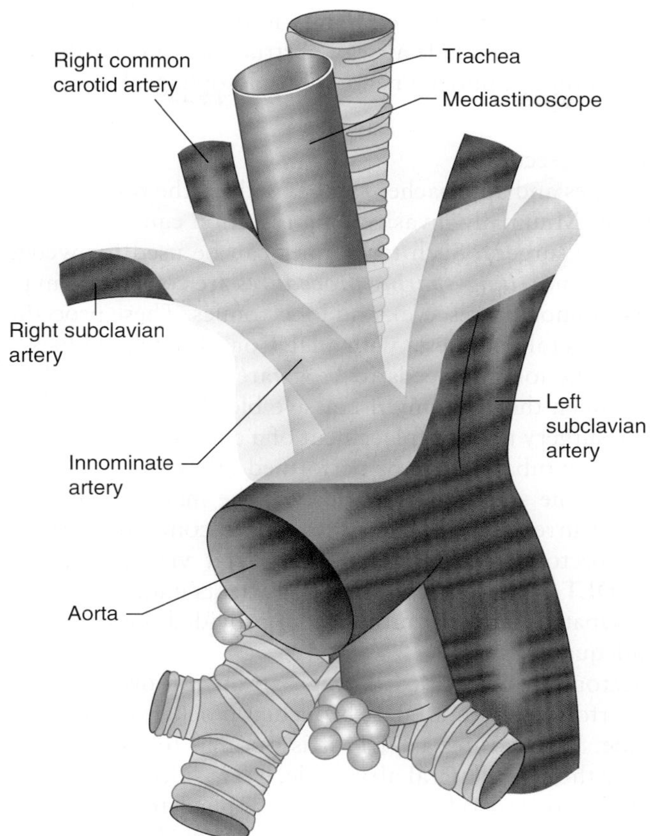

Figure 35.4 **Anatomic relationships during mediastinoscopy. Note the position of the mediastinoscope behind the right innominate artery and aortic arch and anterior to the trachea.** (Adapted from from Carlens E. Mediastinoscopy: a method for inspection and tissue biopsy in the superior mediastinum. *Dis Chest.* 1959;36:343 and Eisenkraft JB, Cohen E, Neustein SM. Anesthesia for thoracic surgery. In: Barash PG, Cahalan MK, Cullen BF, et al, eds. *Clinical Anesthesia.* 8th ed. Wolters Kluwer; 2018:1029-1076, Figure 38.22.)

bronchoscopy, the airway is never completely secure and there is always the potential for aspiration, especially in patients at increased risk. Complications of rigid bronchoscopy include airway perforation, mucosal damage, hemorrhage, postmanipulation airway edema, and potential airway loss at the end of the procedure.[1,3]

C. Mediastinoscopy

Mediastinoscopy is a diagnostic procedure for the evaluation of lymph nodes in the staging of lung cancer and for ***anterior mediastinal masses***. The most common mediastinal procedure is a cervical mediastinoscopy, in which the mediastinoscope is inserted through a small incision in the suprasternal notch and advanced toward the carina (**Figure 35.4**). The majority of these cases require general anesthesia with placement of an SLT. A pulse oximeter or arterial line can be used to monitor perfusion to the right arm, because compression of the innominate artery by the mediastinoscope may occur. The most severe complication of mediastinoscopy is ***major hemorrhage***, which may require emergent sternotomy or thoracotomy. A large-bore intravenous line should be placed in a lower extremity in the event of an SVC tear. Other potential complications include airway obstruction, pneumothorax, paresis of the recurrent laryngeal, phrenic nerve injury, esophageal injury, chylothorax, and air embolism.[1,3,5]

D. Pulmonary Resection

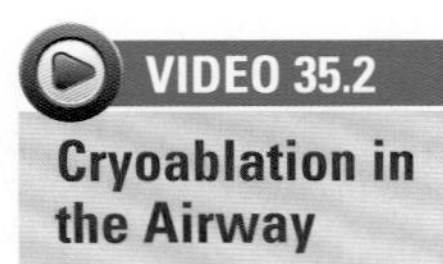

Several techniques and approaches can be used for the resection of pulmonary tissue or tumor. Minimally invasive lung resection can be accomplished with VATS or robotic surgery. Such techniques can be used for wedge resections and segmentectomies (***lung-sparing procedures*** are considered in patients with limited cardiopulmonary reserve), and lobectomies. These procedures are performed under general anesthesia with a DLT or a bronchial blocker to achieve OLV. The anesthesiologist needs to be aware of the potential for emergent conversion to open thoracotomy if massive bleeding ensues. The majority of thoracoscopic surgery requires placement of a chest tube with underwater seal drainage so that extubation can be performed safely.

Lobectomy is the standard operation for the management of lung cancer because local recurrence of the tumor is reduced compared with that of lesser resections. Lobectomy is commonly performed via ***open thoracotomy*** or VATS with a DLT or a bronchial blocker. Patients undergoing lobectomy can usually be extubated in the operating room provided preoperative respiratory function is adequate.

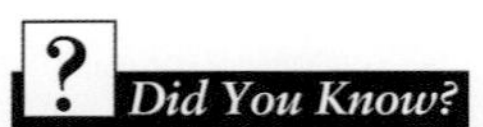

Suction applied to a chest tube placed after pneumonectomy can cause mediastinal shift, resulting in hemodynamic collapse.

Pneumonectomy is performed through an open thoracotomy. Lung isolation can be performed with a DLT, bronchial blocker, or single-lumen endobronchial tube. When using a DLT, it is optimal to use a device that does not interfere with the ipsilateral airway (ie, a left-sided DLT for a right pneumonectomy). Postoperatively, if suction is applied to a chest drain or it is connected to a standard underwater seal system, ***mediastinal shift*** may ensue with hemodynamic collapse. A postoperative chest radiograph is mandatory to assess for mediastinal shift. The mortality rate following pneumonectomy exceeds that for lobectomy because of postoperative cardiac complications and acute lung injury. The risk of complications increases fivefold in patients aged 65 years and older.[1,3,6] The complication of cardiac herniation will be discussed in the last section of this chapter.

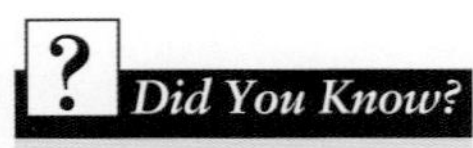

Restrictive fluid strategy for patients undergoing pulmonary and esophageal surgery has become controversial because of a concern about its potential to induce acute kidney injury.

E. Esophageal Surgery

General considerations, which apply to almost all esophageal patients, include an increased risk of ***aspiration*** due to esophageal dysfunction and the possibility of ***malnutrition***. Esophagectomy is a potentially curative treatment for esophageal cancer and for some benign obstructive lesions. It is a major surgical procedure and is associated with high morbidity and mortality rates (10%-15%). There are multiple surgical procedures for esophagectomy that combine three fundamental approaches: transthoracic approach, transhiatal approach, and minimally invasive surgery. Outcomes are improved with early extubation, thoracic epidural analgesia, and vasopressor or inotrope infusions to support blood pressure.[1,3,7]

F. Tracheal Resection

Tracheal resection is indicated in patients who have a tracheal obstruction as a result of a tracheal tumor, trauma (most commonly due to postintubation stenosis), congenital anomalies, vascular lesions, or tracheomalacia. The airways of patients with congenital or acquired tracheal stenosis are unlikely to collapse during induction of anesthesia. However, intratracheal masses may lead to ***airway obstruction*** with induction of anesthesia and should be managed similarly to anterior mediastinal masses (see below). A variety of methods for providing adequate ventilation have been used during tracheal resection, including standard orotracheal intubation; insertion of a sterile SLT into the opened trachea or bronchus distal to the area of resection; high-frequency jet ventilation with a catheter through the stenotic area; high-frequency PPV; and the use of cardiopulmonary bypass (CPB). After the tracheal resection is completed, most patients are kept in a position of neck flexion to reduce tension on the suture line. ***Early extubation*** in these cases is highly desirable. If a patient requires reintubation, it should be performed with a flexible fiberoptic bronchoscope by advancing an SLT under direct vision over the bronchoscope to avoid damage to the repair.[1,3,8]

G. Bronchopleural Fistula

A bronchopleural fistula may be caused by rupture of a lung abscess, bronchus, bulla, cyst, or parenchymal tissue into the pleural space; erosion of a bronchus by carcinoma or chronic inflammatory disease; or stump dehiscence of a bronchial suture line after pulmonary resection. In patients with bullous lung disease, such as emphysema, there is a risk of bulla ***hyperinflation*** and rupture whenever PPV is used. The complications of bulla rupture can be life-threatening due to ***hemodynamic collapse*** from ***tension pneumothorax*** or inadequate ventilation due to a resultant bronchopleural fistula. If bronchial disruption occurs early in postresection patients, it can also be life-threatening. It is possible to redo the thoracotomy and resuture the bronchial stump. Late or chronic postresection disruption is managed with chest tube drainage or with the Clagett procedure, which includes open pleural drainage and the use of a muscle flap to reinforce the bronchial stump.

Concerns for the anesthesiologist in a patient with a bronchopleural fistula include the need for ***lung isolation*** to protect healthy lung regions, the possibility of tension pneumothorax with PPV, and the possibility of inadequate ventilation due to air leak from the fistula. Placement of a chest drain should be considered prior to induction to avoid the possibility of tension pneumothorax with PPV. A DLT is the optimal choice for airway management, as lung isolation should be performed before initiating PPV or repositioning the patient. This is most commonly performed with a modified rapid sequence induction of anesthesia and immediate fiberoptic positioning of the DLT. However, depending on the context, awake intubation maintenance of spontaneous ventilation may be used.[1,3]

H. Bronchiectasis, Lung Abscess, and Empyema

Infectious conditions, including bronchiectasis, lung abscess, and empyema, are indications for thoracic surgery, such as decortication. Anesthetic considerations for these conditions include the need for ***lung isolation*** to protect uninvolved lung regions from soiling by pus. A DLT facilitates suctioning of debris and copious secretions that are present in the trachea-bronchial tree and is less subject to dislodgement during patient movement or surgical manipulation than would be a bronchial blocker. Due to the inflammation, surgery is technically more difficult, and there is a greater risk of massive hemorrhage, particularly during decortication. Some of these patients may present with sepsis at the time of surgery. If the lung has been chronically collapsed, expansion should be done gradually to avoid the development of pulmonary edema upon re-expansion.[1]

I. Mediastinal Masses

Tumors of the anterior mediastinum include thymoma, teratoma, lymphoma, cystic hygroma, bronchogenic cyst, and thyroid tumors. Patients may require anesthesia for biopsy of these masses by mediastinoscopy or VATS, or they may require definitive resection via sternotomy or thoracotomy. Mediastinal masses may cause ***obstruction*** of ***major airways*** or vascular structures. During induction of general anesthesia, airway obstruction is the most common and feared complication. A history of ***supine dyspnea*** or cough should alert the anesthesiologist to the possibility of airway obstruction upon induction. General anesthesia and muscle relaxants will exacerbate extrinsic intrathoracic airway compression due to reduced lung volume and tracheobronchial diameters, bronchial smooth muscle relaxation, and loss of the normal transpleural pressure gradient that dilates the airways during spontaneous inspiration and minimizes the effects of extrinsic intrathoracic airway compression. It is important to note that the point of tracheobronchial compression may be in the distal airway, so it may not be bypassed by an ETT. The other major complication is cardiovascular collapse secondary to compression of the heart or major vessels. Symptoms of supine presyncope suggest vascular compression.

> **? Did You Know?**
>
> In a patient with an anterior mediastinal mass, a history of supine dyspnea or cough may be predictive of airway collapse following induction of general anesthesia.

Patients who are symptomatic or have evidence of airway or cardiovascular involvement on imaging should have diagnostic procedures performed under local or regional anesthesia whenever possible. When general anesthesia is indicated, awake intubation of the trachea is a possibility in some adult patients, if imaging shows an area of noncompressed distal trachea to which the ETT can be advanced before induction. Alternatively, spontaneous ventilation should be maintained with either an inhalation induction or titration of an agent such as ketamine. If muscle relaxants are required, ventilation should first be gradually taken over manually to ensure that PPV is possible and only then can a short-acting muscle relaxant be administered.

Intraoperative life-threatening ***airway compression*** may respond to repositioning of the patient (it must be determined before induction if there is a position that causes less symptoms) or rigid bronchoscopy and ventilation distal to the obstruction (this means that an experienced bronchoscopist and equipment must always be immediately available in the operating room for these cases). Institution of femorofemoral CPB before induction of anesthesia is a possibility in some adult patients. The concept of CPB "standby" during attempted induction of anesthesia should not be considered because there is not enough time after a sudden airway collapse to establish CPB before hypoxic cerebral injury occurs.[1,3,9]

J. Myasthenia Gravis

Myasthenia gravis is an autoimmune disease of the neuromuscular junction, in which affected patients have weakness due to a decreased number of acetylcholine receptors at the motor end plate. Patients may or may not have an associated thymoma. Thymectomy is frequently performed to induce clinical remission, even in the absence of a thymoma. Thymectomy may be performed via full or partial sternotomy or a minimally invasive approach via a transcervical incision or VATS.

Medical treatments for myasthenia gravis include anticholinesterases, such as pyridostigmine, immunosuppressive drugs, such as steroids, and plasmapheresis. On the day of surgery, patients should continue their usual pyridostigmine dosing. Myasthenic patients are unpredictably ***resistant*** to ***succinylcholine*** and extremely ***sensitive*** to ***nondepolarizing blockers***. Ideally, the use of intraoperative neuromuscular relaxation is avoided. Induction of anesthesia with propofol, remifentanil, and topical anesthesia of the airway facilitates intubation without the use of muscle relaxants. Alternatively, inhalational induction with a volatile agent may be performed. Referral for surgery early in the course of the disease, preoperative medical stabilization, and minimally invasive surgical approaches have made the need for postoperative ventilation infrequent.[1,3,10]

IV. Postoperative Management

A. Pain Management

Thoracic epidural analgesia (TEA) has been considered the gold standard for postoperative pain control in patients undergoing thoracotomy. When thoracotomy pain is controlled, the risk of pulmonary complications is decreased. In patients with coronary artery disease, thoracic epidural local anesthetics also seem to reduce myocardial oxygen demand. When there is a contraindication to placement of a thoracic epidural, another excellent choice for analgesia is a paravertebral infusion of local anesthetic via a catheter that may be placed by the anesthesiologist using a landmark or ultrasound-guided technique or directly by the surgeon during an open thoracotomy. This has been shown in a systematic review to be as effective as TEA.[11] Other regional anesthesia options for analgesia in thoracic surgery include intercostal blocks and the more recently described serratus anterior plane block and erector spinae plane block.[12] Additionally, patient-controlled opioid analgesia may be used with multimodal analgesia, such as acetaminophen, gabapentin, and nonsteroidal anti-inflammatories. Postoperative ketamine use is increasing in the thoracic surgical population.[13] Institutions differ in their practices regarding the use of catheter techniques versus intravenous patient-controlled analgesia for minimally invasive thoracic surgeries.[1,3] Optimal analgesia will help contribute to enhanced recovery after thoracic surgery, a movement that has been gaining ground in a variety of surgical specialties.[14]

B. Complications

As mentioned previously, respiratory and cardiac complications account for the majority of morbidity and mortality following thoracic surgery. There are multiple potential complications that can occur in the immediate postoperative period, such as ***torsion*** of a remaining lobe after lobectomy, dehiscence of a bronchial stump, hemorrhage from a major vessel, or cardiac ischemia or arrhythmias. Among these possible complications, two will be discussed in more detail: respiratory failure and cardiac herniation.

Respiratory Failure

Patients with decreased respiratory function preoperatively are at increased risk of postoperative respiratory complications. In addition, age, the presence of coronary artery disease, and the extent of lung resection play major roles in predicting postoperative respiratory failure. Decreased pulmonary complications in high-risk patients are associated with the use of TEA during the perioperative period. Chest physiotherapy, incentive spirometry, and early ambulation are also crucial in order to minimize pulmonary complications after lung resection. For an uncomplicated lung resection, ***early*** extubation is desirable to avoid potential complications that can arise due to ***prolonged*** intubation and mechanical ventilation. Current therapy to treat acute respiratory failure is aimed at supportive measures that provide better oxygenation, treat infection, and provide vital organ support without further damaging the lungs.[1]

Cardiac Herniation

Acute cardiac herniation is an ***infrequent complication of pneumonectomy*** when the pericardium is incompletely closed or the closure breaks down. It usually occurs immediately or within 24 hours after chest surgery and is associated with >50% mortality. When cardiac herniation occurs after a right pneumonectomy, the impairment of venous return to the heart leads to a sudden increase in CVP, tachycardia, profound hypotension, and shock. An acute SVC syndrome ensues due to the torsion of the heart. In contrast, when the cardiac herniation occurs after a left-sided pneumonectomy, there is less cardiac rotation, but the edge of the pericardium compresses the myocardium. This may lead to myocardial ischemia, the development of arrhythmias, and ventricular outflow tract obstruction.

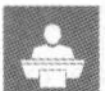

Did You Know?

One of the catastrophic complication of pneumonectomy is cardiac herniation, and it requires immediate surgical treatment to ensure survival.

The differential diagnosis of hemodynamic instability after thoracic surgery should include massive intrathoracic hemorrhage, pulmonary embolism, or mediastinal shift from improper chest drain management. Immediate diagnosis and surgical treatment of cardiac herniation by ***relocation of the heart*** to its anatomic position is key to patient survival. Maneuvers to minimize the cardiovascular effects include positioning the patient in the full lateral position with the ***operated side up***. Vasopressors or inotropes are required to support the circulation while exploration takes place.[1]

For further review and interactivities, please see the associated Interactive Video Lectures and "A Closer Look" infographic accessible in the complimentary eBook bundled with this text. Access instructions are located in the inside front cover.

References

1. Slinger P, Campos J. Anesthesia for thoracic surgery. In: Gropper M, ed. *Miller's Anesthesia*. 9th ed. Elsevier, Inc; 2020:1648-1716.
2. Slinger P, Darling G. Preanesthetic assessment for thoracic surgery. In: Slinger P, ed. *Principles and Practice of Anesthesia for Thoracic Surgery*. Springer; 2011:11-35.
3. Eisenkraft J, Cohen E, Neustein S. Anesthesia for thoracic surgery. In: Barash P, Cullen B, Stoelting R, Cahalan M, Stock M, Ortega R, eds. *Clinical Anesthesia*. 7th ed.. Wolters Kluwer Health/Lippincott Williams and Wilkins; 2013:1030-1075.
4. Fleisher LA, Fleischmann KE, Auerbach AD, et al. 2014 ACC/AHA guideline on perioperative cardiovascular evaluation and management of patients undergoing noncardiac surgery: a report of the American College of Cardiology/American Heart Association Task Force on practice guidelines. *Circulation*. 2014;130:2215-2245. PMID: 25085962.
5. Lohser J, Donington JS, Mitchell JD, Brodsky JB, Raman J, Slinger P. Anesthetic management of major hemorrhage during mediastinoscopy. *J Cardiothorac Vasc Anesth*. 2005;19:678-683. PMID: 16202909.
6. Powell ES, Pearce AC, Cook D, et al. UK pneumonectomy outcome study: a prospective observational study of pneumonectomy outcome. *J Cardiothorac Surg*. 2009;4:41. PMID: 19643006.
7. Buise M, Van Bommel J, Mehra M, Tilanus HW, Van Zundert A, Gommers D. Pulmonary morbidity following esophagectomy is decreased after introduction of a multimodal anesthetic regimen. *Acta Anaesthesiol Belg*. 2008;59:257-261. PMID: 19235524.
8. Pinsonneault C, Fortier J, Donati F. Tracheal resection and reconstruction. *Can J Anaesth*. 1999;46:439-455. PMID: 10349923.

9. Takeda S, Miyoshi S, Omori K, Okumura M, Matsuda H. Surgical rescue for life-threatening hypoxemia caused by a mediastinal tumor. *Ann Thorac Surg*. 1999;68:2324-2326. PMID: 10617025.
10. White MC, Stoddart PA. Anesthesia for thymectomy in children with myasthenia gravis. *Pediatr Anaesth*. 2004;14:625-635. PMID: 15283820.
11. Joshi G, Bonnet F, Shah R, et al. A systematic review of randomized trials evaluating regional techniques for postthoracotomy analgesia. *Anesth Analg*. 2008;107:1026-1040. PMID: 18713924.
12. Jack J, McLellan E, Veryck B, Englesakis MF, Chin KJ. The role of serratus anterior plane and pectoral nerve blocks in cardiac surgery, thoracic surgery and trauma: a qualitative systematic review. *Anaesthesia*. 2020;75(10):1372-1385. PMID: 32062870.
13. Moyse D, Kaye A, Diaz J, Qadri MY, Lindsay D, Pyati S. Perioperative ketamine administration for thoracotomy pain. *Pain Physician*. 2017;20:173-184. PMID: 28339431.
14. Raft J, Richebe P. Anesthesia for thoracic ambulatory surgery. *Curr Opin Anaesthesiol*. 2019;32:735-742. PMID: 31567511.

VENTILATION AND PERFUSION

A CLOSER LOOK

During lung surgery, an often overlooked influence on ventilation and oxygenation is the effect of general anesthesia in the lateral decubitus position. As seen below, the effectiveness of ventilation, as defined by lung compliance ($\Delta V/\Delta P$), changes throughout the lungs and can be well- or poorly matched to perfusion.

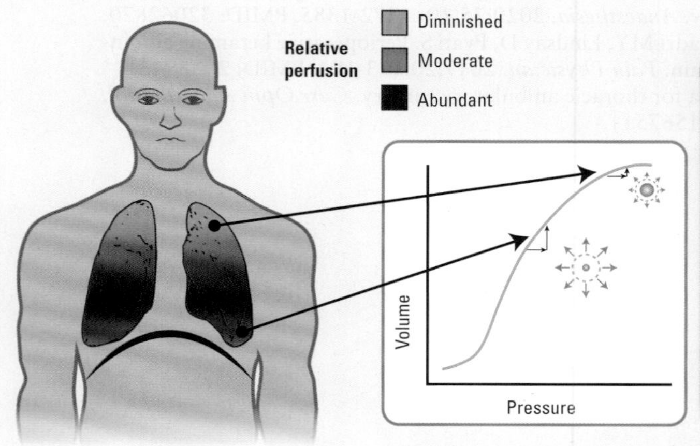

AWAKE, UPRIGHT

Basilar alveoli expand and recoil completely due to their proximate location to the diaphragm. For a given change in respiratory pressure, they produce an effective volume. *Apical* alveoli only participate in minor expasion and recoil. For the same change in pressure, the change in volume is minimal. Ventilation is **well-matched** to perfusion.

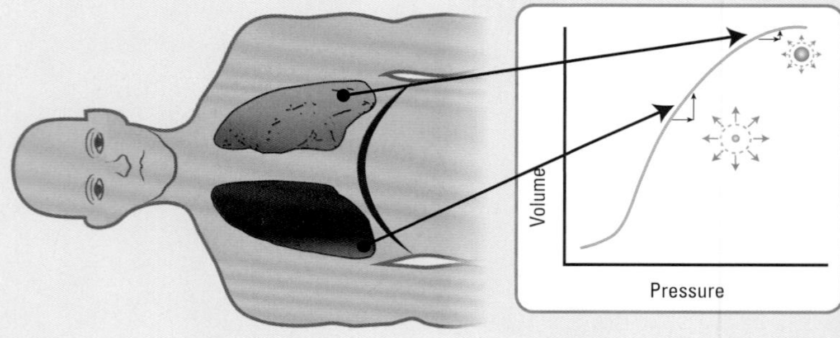

AWAKE, LATERAL

The ventilation pattern in the lateral decubitus position follows that of the upright position only it is transposed to the anatomy. Instead of apical vs. basilar regions of both lungs, ventilation is now *least effective* in the **upper** (nondependent) lung and *most effective* in the **lower** (dependent) lung. Ventilation is still **well-matched** to perfusion.

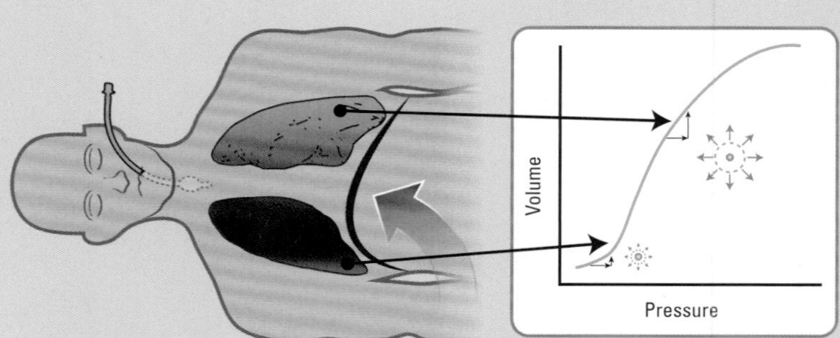

ANESTHETIZED, LATERAL

Under general anesthesia, the diaphragm is *paralyzed* and no longer controls ventilation. This also results in the abdominal contents bearing down on the lower lung causing atelectasis. *Both lungs change to new positions on the compliance curve.* Positive pressure ventilation will deliver tidal volumes preferentially to the *upper lung* which has the least perfusion. **V/Q matching is poor.**

In addition to these changes described, when the chest is opened, the nondependent lung is preferentially ventilated which increases V/Q mismatch. This is counterbalanced when one-lung ventilation of the dependent lung begins. Hypoxic pulmonary vasoconstriction may also occur but is tempered by inhalational agents.

Infographic by: Naveen Nathan MD

Questions

1. **Which is the largest segment of the lung?**

   A. Right lower lobe
   B. Left upper lobe
   C. Left lower lobe
   D. Right middle lobe

2. **Which of the following is NOT a perioperative cardiac risk factor?**

   A. Severe valvular disease
   B. History of cerebrovascular disease
   C. Insulin dependent diabetes mellitus
   D. Renal insufficiency

3. **A patient has a known history of previous difficult intubation. He is now coming for urgent left-sided thoracotomy, lobectomy for cancer, and drainage of empyema. Which is the best option for securing the airway?**

   A. Videolaryngoscopy with the single-lumen tube, then tube exchange over a catheter to a double-lumen tube
   B. Single-lumen tube and bronchial blocker
   C. Endobronchial intubation on the right side
   D. Direct laryngoscopy and left-sided double-lumen tube

4. **Which is the best choice of induction drug for use in a patient with myasthenia gravis (MG):**

   A. Remifentanil
   B. Succinylcholine
   C. Rocuronium
   D. High-dose morphine

5. **Which of the following factors can contribute to increased risk of postoperative respiratory failure in patients following thoracic surgery?**

   A. Presence of coronary artery disease
   B. Use of thoracic epidural analgesia
   C. Early ambulation
   D. Young age

Answers

1. A

A, right lower lobe, is correct because it is made up of 12 subsegments. B, left upper lobe, and C, left lower lobe, are made up of 10 subsegments. D, right middle lobe, is made up of 4 subsegments.

2. A

A, severe valvular disease, is correct because it is considered an active cardiac condition. B, C, and D are incorrect because they are risk factors.

3. A

A, videolaryngoscopy, is the correct answer because it satisfies both problems of the difficult airway and needing secure intraoperative lung isolation for the empyema. B is incorrect because a single-lumen tube will be easier to place in a difficult airway, but the blocker will be prone to dislodgment in the context of the empyema. C is incorrect because endobronchial intubation is easier to place in a difficult airway, will isolate the side with the empyema, but not ideal as will be unable to suction/bronch/apply CPAP etc to the nonventilated side if needed. D is incorrect because direct laryngoscopy will be more difficult in the context of a difficult airway.

4. A

Remifentanil. A is the correct answer because remifentanil will assist with intubation and is short acting. B, succinylcholine, is incorrect because patients with MG may be resistant to succinylcholine. C, rocuronium, is incorrect because patients with MG are very sensitive to nondepolarizing muscle relaxants and they should be avoided if possible or used in very small quantities. D, high does of morphine, is incorrect because it may contribute to postoperative respiratory depression in patients with MG.

5. A

A, presence of coronary artery disease. B, use of thoracic epidural analgesia, is incorrect because a working epidural and adequate analgesia have been shown to decrease the risk of postoperative respiratory complications. C, early ambulation, is incorrect because this has also been shown to decrease the risk of postoperative respiratory complications. D, young age, is incorrect because older age is associated with increased risk of postoperative respiratory failure.

36 Cardiac Anesthesia

Candice R. Montzingo, Sasha Shillcutt, and James P. Lee

Patients with heart disease present unique challenges for the anesthesiologist. This chapter provides an overview of those challenges and the associated physiologic changes and anesthetic management strategies needed to safely provide care to patients undergoing cardiac surgical interventions.

I. Coronary Artery Disease

Coronary artery disease (CAD) is one of the most common causes of death in highly developed nations. It results from the buildup of atherosclerotic lesions in the coronary arteries. Myocardial ischemia is a hallmark of CAD. It is caused by an imbalance between myocardial oxygen supply and demand. The anesthesiologist must understand the determinants of this delicate relation and avoid myocardial injury by minimizing myocardial oxygen demand while optimizing myocardial oxygen delivery.

A. Myocardial Oxygen Demand

Systolic wall tension, contractility, and heart rate are the primary determinants of myocardial oxygen demand. ***Wall tension*** is directly proportional to systolic blood pressure and chamber size (preload) and inversely proportional to wall thickness. Thus, increases in preload increase wall tension exponentially because as chamber size increases, ventricular wall thickness must thin to accommodate the additional volume. Increases in ***heart rate*** are especially deleterious because increases in heart rate increase oxygen demand directly and decrease oxygen delivery indirectly by shortening diastole. The left ventricle (LV) receives its coronary blood flow only during diastole. Thus, increases in wall tension, ***contractility***, and heart rate above normal resting levels must be avoided in patients with CAD.

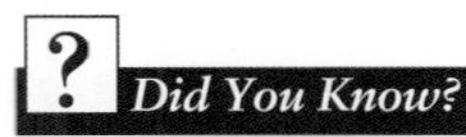

The left ventricle receives its blood flow only during diastole, while the right ventricle is perfused throughout the cardiac cycle.

B. Myocardial Oxygen Supply

The two main factors contributing to myocardial oxygen supply are arterial ***oxygen content*** and ***coronary blood flow***. Recall that arterial oxygen content is represented by the formula:

$$O_2 \text{ content} = (\text{hemoglobin})(1.34)(\% \text{ saturation}) + (0.003)(PO_2).$$

Because hemoglobin levels and blood volume are usually adequately maintained during cardiac surgery, coronary blood flow is the most critical factor

Table 36.1 Treatment of Intraoperative Ischemia

Clinical Manifestation	
Increased demand	
↑ HR	Treat usual reasons, beta-blocker
↑ BP	↑ anesthetic depth
↑ PCWP	Nitroglycerin
Decreased supply	
↓ HR	Atropine, pacing
↓ BP	↓ anesthetic depth, vasoconstrictor
↑ PCWP	Nitroglycerin, inotrope
No changes	Nitroglycerin, calcium channel blockers, ? heparin

↑, increase; ↓, decrease; HR, heart rate; BP, blood pressure; PCWP, pulmonary capillary wedge pressure.

From Skubas NJ, Lichtman AD, Wang CJ, Sharma A, Thomas SJ. Anesthesia for cardiac surgery. In: Barash PG, Cahalan MK, Cullen BF, et al, eds. *Clinical Anesthesia*. 8th ed. Wolters Kluwer; 2018: 1077-1111, Table 39.2.

in maintaining myocardial oxygen supply. Coronary blood flow is directly related to coronary perfusion pressure and inversely related to coronary vascular resistance and heart rate (time for perfusion in diastole). ***Coronary perfusion pressure*** is estimated as the difference between systemic (aortic) diastolic pressure and left ventricular diastolic pressure. In normal hearts, coronary blood flow is autoregulated for systolic blood pressures between 50 and 150 mm Hg. In patients with CAD, the area of the heart most at risk for ischemia is the subendocardium of the LV. The right ventricle (RV) is perfused during the entire cardiac cycle due to its low intracavitary pressure. Thus, low left ventricular diastolic pressure, normal systemic diastolic pressure, and low heart rate improve myocardial oxygen supply.

C. Monitoring for Ischemia

Flat or downsloping ***ST segment*** depression ≥0.1 mV on the electrocardiogram (ECG) is the most reliable ECG sign of myocardial ischemia. However, transesophageal echocardiography (TEE) has been shown to detect myocardial ischemia earlier and more frequently than the ECG and is very often used in cardiac surgery. Pulmonary artery catheters may reveal acute increases in left atrial pressures associated with ischemia-induced stiffening of the LV. However, the pulmonary artery catheter is neither a sensitive nor specific monitor for myocardial ischemia because so many other things influence left atrial pressure during surgery.

D. Treatment of Ischemia

Myocardial ischemia may occur at any time during coronary bypass surgery. The treatment depends largely on the etiology and can be seen in **Table 36.1**. Thorough review of the pharmacologic effects of nitrates, peripheral vasoconstrictors, calcium channel blockers, and beta-blockers can be found in Chapter 13.

II. Valvular Heart Disease

Growing experience with TEE has significantly increased the role of anesthesiologists in the intraoperative evaluation and management of valvular heart disease (VHD). VHD can be classified into two primary lesions: ***regurgitant*** and ***stenotic***. *Regurgitant lesions* lead to volume overload, while *stenotic valve disease* leads to pressure overload. Although disease of the tricuspid and pulmonic valves presents unique challenges to the anesthesiologist, this chapter will focus on the much more common left-sided valvular lesions. Additional information is provided in the 2014 AHA/ACC "Guidelines for the Management of Patients with VHD."[1]

A. Aortic Stenosis

The normal adult aortic valve comprises three equally sized cusps and has an area of 2 to 3.5 cm^2. Aortic stenosis (AS) is the ***most common*** valvular lesion in the heart and can result from congenital or acquired valvular disease. In congenital AS, there is a partial or complete commissural fusion between cusps, resulting in a unicuspid or bicuspid valve. A bicuspid aortic valve is the most commonly occurring congenital heart defect, affecting approximately 1% to 2% of the population. Bicuspid aortic valves are associated with other congenital abnormalities, specifically diseases of the aorta including coarctation and dilatation of the aortic root. Acquired aortic stenosis results from calcific degeneration or, less commonly, rheumatic disease.

VIDEO 36.1
Aortic Stenosis Auscultation

VIDEO 36.2
Aortic Stenosis TEE Clip

Progressive narrowing of the aortic valve leads to an increased transvalvular gradient. This in turn increases the work of the LV and over time results in ***concentric ventricular hypertrophy***. This compensatory response allows the internal diameter of the LV to remain unchanged and preserves systolic function and stroke volume. However, as the LV thickens, its diastolic function declines, causing an increase in the diastolic filling pressure. Patients often remain asymptomatic until the valve area is <1 to 1.2 cm^2, correlating to a peak transvalvular gradient exceeding 50 mm Hg. The classic triad of symptomatic AS is ***angina***, ***syncope***, and ***congestive heart failure*** (dyspnea). The development of any of these is ***ominous***, indicating a life expectancy from 2 to 5 years without valve replacement.

The consequence of elevated intraventricular pressure and concentric hypertrophy is increased myocardial oxygen demand. At the same time, diastolic filling pressure is increased, resulting in a lower coronary perfusion pressure. Thus, patients with severe AS may experience myocardial ischemia and angina in the absence of CAD, especially if the heart rate increases much beyond resting levels (see prior discussion in the section "Myocardial Oxygen Demand"). Maintenance of ***systemic vascular resistance (SVR)*** is critical in patients with AS to ensure adequate aortic diastolic pressure and thus coronary perfusion pressure. Vasoconstrictors such as vasopressin or phenylephrine will increase SVR without increasing myocardial oxygen demand because the increase in systemic blood pressure they cause is not "seen" by the LV due to the stenotic aortic valve.

B. Hypertrophic Cardiomyopathy

Although not a disease of a valve, hypertrophic cardiomyopathy (HCM) can cause an obstructive lesion similar to that of AS. HCM is an uncommon autosomal dominant genetic disorder with highly variable penetrance. It leads to ventricular hypertrophy that occurs in varying patterns, not just involving the interventricular septum. Presenting symptoms are often dyspnea on exertion, poor exercise tolerance, syncope, palpitations, and fatigue. Some patients remain asymptomatic much of their lives and unfortunately are diagnosed after sudden cardiac death.

Approximately one-third of patients with HCM will have hypertrophy of the interventricular septum that leads to ***dynamic obstruction*** of the left ventricular outflow tract. The resulting pressure gradient increases throughout systole, creating obstruction to cardiac output. Any factor decreasing left ventricular size will increase this gradient and further obstruct cardiac output. Examples include increases in heart rate and contractility and decreases in preload and afterload. Therefore, anesthetic management focuses on avoiding tachycardia and maintaining euvolemia and normal systemic vascular resistance. Hypotension in this population is best treated with α-adrenergic agonists and volume. Treatment with inotropic drugs such as ***epinephrine is contraindicated*** and may worsen the dynamic obstruction and hypotension.

VIDEO 36.3
Aortic Insufficiency TEE Clip

C. Aortic Insufficiency

Aortic insufficiency (AI) can be the result of primary valvular disease or in association with aortic root dilatation (Marfan disease, degenerative aortic dilatation, aortic dissection) despite a normal aortic valve. The natural progression of AI varies depending on the pathophysiology and chronicity of the disease.

Acute AI is often the result of traumatic injury to the aortic root or valvular endocarditis. The consequences of ***acute AI*** are immediate and profound volume overload to the LV. Frequently, the LV is not able to maintain forward stroke volume despite compensatory mechanisms, including increased sympathetic tone, leading to tachycardia and increased contractility. Rapid deterioration of left ventricular function develops, leading to dyspnea and eventual cardiovascular collapse. Acute AI often requires urgent or emergent surgical intervention.

Chronic AI results in an increased left ventricular end diastolic volume that over time leads to eccentric hypertrophy (cavity dilatation). The course of chronic AI is gradual, limiting the increase in left ventricular diastolic pressure. It is not typical for patients to develop symptoms associated with AI until decades into the disease process when the LV has significantly dilated and myocardial dysfunction occurs. Once symptomatic, life expectancy diminishes dramatically, with expected survival of only 5 to 10 years.

The anesthetic management of AI focuses on ***preserving forward stroke volume*** and minimizing regurgitant volume by maintaining a relatively rapid heart rate (about 90 beats per minute) and normal to low SVR.

D. Mitral Stenosis

The mitral valve area is typically 4 to 6 cm^2 and is made up of an anterior and posterior leaflet. Mitral stenosis is almost always due to ***rheumatic heart disease*** and is therefore quite rare in the United States and other highly developed nations. It leads to impaired filling of the LV and a resulting decreased stroke volume. Consequently, the ***left atrial pressure*** becomes chronically elevated resulting in left atrial dilatation and increased pulmonary venous pressure. Patients with mitral stenosis are at high risk for developing ***atrial fibrillation*** which may be the presenting sign of the disease. Mitral stenosis patients are often asymptomatic for decades until the mitral valve area has decreased to 1 to 1.5 cm^2 and the heart is faced with an increased demand for systemic stroke volume (exercise, pregnancy, infection). Any high cardiac output state or the onset of atrial fibrillation can cause significant increases in the left atrial and pulmonary arterial pressures, leading to acute ***congestive heart failure***. Chronically elevated left atrial pressures lead to increases in pulmonary

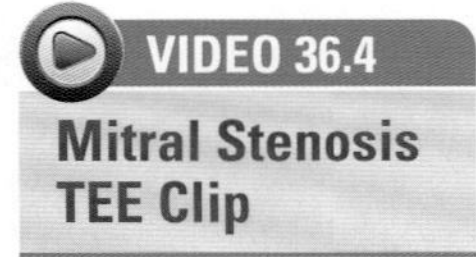

Table 36.2 Hemodynamic Goals in Patients With Valvular Heart Disease

	Aortic Stenosis	Hypertrophic Cardiomyopathy	Aortic Insufficiency	Mitral Stenosis	Mitral Regurgitation
Preload	Full	Full	Increase slightly	Maintain; avoid hypovolemia	Increase slightly
Afterload	Maintain CPP	Increase; treat hypotension aggressively	Decrease to reduce regurgitant fraction	Prevent increase	Decrease
Rate	Avoid bradycardia (decrease CO) and tachycardia (ischemia)	Normal	Increase	Low normal	Increase slightly, avoid bradycardia
Rhythm	Sinus	Sinus is critical	Sinus	Sinus or rate-controlled atrial fibrillation	Sinus or rate-controlled atrial fibrillation

CO, cardiac output; CPP, coronary perfusion pressure.

vascular resistance, pulmonary hypertension, restrictive lung disease, and right heart failure.

Frequently, patients with mitral stenosis have received diuretics preoperatively to control their pulmonary congestion and are relatively hypovolemic. Induction of anesthesia may unmask the ***hypovolemia*** and compromise the transit of blood across the stenotic mitral valve. Thus, adequate fluid administration during anesthesia is crucial, but too much fluid administration can lead to further pulmonary congestion and pulmonary edema. A relatively ***slow heart rate*** (about 60-70 beats per minute) allows ample time for the LV to fill. Tachycardia compromises that filling and may result in severe hypotension. ***SVR*** should be maintained to ensure adequate coronary perfusion pressure, especially to the RV because it is facing increased pulmonary artery pressures.

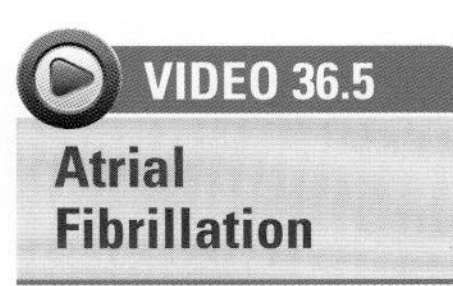

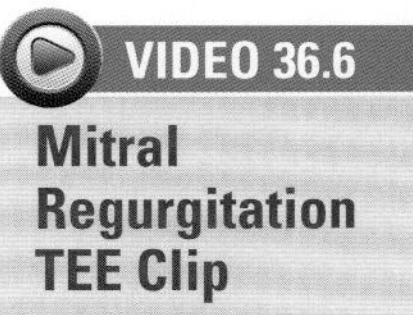

E. Mitral Regurgitation

Mitral regurgitation (MR) results from excessive leaflet motion (prolapse or flail) or restricted leaflet motion (ischemic dilatation, rheumatic heart disease). Similar to AI, MR leads to volume overload. In MR, the stroke volume is made up of blood ejected into the systemic circulation and then regurgitated into the left atrium. The regurgitated blood causes left atrial and ventricular dilatation (eccentric ventricular hypertrophy) and increased ventricular compliance. Unless the MR is due to CAD (eg, ischemic rupture of a papillary muscle), an elevated heart rate (about 90 beats per minute) may be best because it will limit ventricular dilatation. However, the cornerstone in the management of MR is ***reduction of the SVR*** to promote forward ejection of blood and limit regurgitation. In patients with MR and others undergoing valvular heart surgery, TEE has proven beneficial to assess volume status, ventricular function, and, most important, the adequacy of the surgical procedure. **Table 36.2** summarizes the hemodynamic goals in patients with VHD.

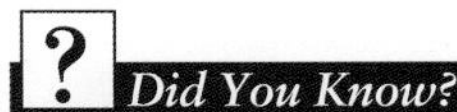

The cornerstone in the management of mitral regurgitation is reduction of the systemic vascular resistance to promote forward ejection of blood and limit regurgitation.

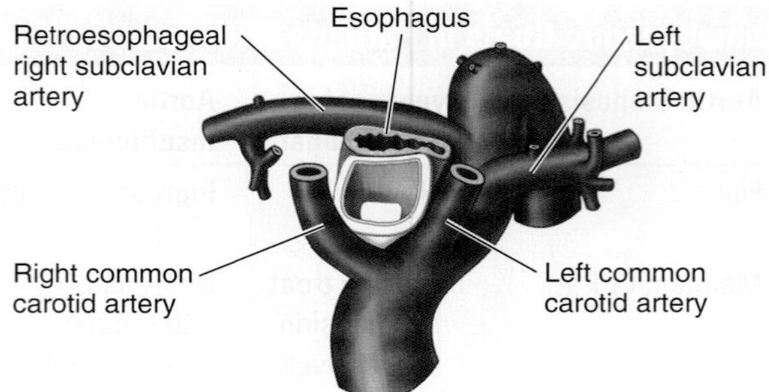

Figure 36.1 Variations and anomalies of branches of aortic arch. **Retroesophageal right subclavian artery.** (From Thorax. In: Moore KL, Agur AMR, Dalley AF. *Clinically Oriented Anatomy.* 8th ed. Wolters Kluwer; 2018:290-403, Figure B4.37.)

III. Aortic Diseases

The aorta is made up of the aortic root, the ascending aorta, the aortic arch, and the descending thoracic aorta, as seen in **Figure 36.1**. Diseases of the aorta can be localized to one segment or multiple segments or involve the entire aorta. Diseases of the aorta may be acquired (traumatic injury, hypertension, occlusive disease, inflammation, infection) or congenital (coarctation, patent ductus arteriosus, connective tissue disorders) and can lead to aortic dissection, aortic aneurysm, intramural hematoma, or aortic transection.

A. Aortic Dissection

Aortic dissection occurs due to a tear in the intimal and medial layers of the aorta, which causes separation of the walls and leads to creation of a ***false lumen***. Blood travels into the false lumen of the media and can travel the length of the vessel. Intimal tears typically originate from an ulcer due to chronic hypertension or connective tissue disorders, such as Marfan syndrome. As the false lumen propagates, thrombus and dissecting layers can cause disruption in perfusion of vital organs due to decreased blood flow to major arteries such as the carotids, subclavian, spinal, or mesenteric arteries.

Type A aortic dissection, which involves the ascending aorta, is a ***surgical emergency*** with a mortality that increases exponentially by the hour. It is often associated with cardiac tamponade, myocardial ischemia (due to dissection of coronary arteries), and acute aortic insufficiency. Symptoms may involve syncope, stroke-like sequelae, and chest pain. ***Type B dissections*** involve the aorta distal to the left subclavian artery and can be ***managed medically*** unless ongoing symptoms (back pain, abdominal pain, or embolic or ischemic phenomenon) persist or end-organ failure develops. Medical therapy focuses on decreasing aortic wall stress and controlling heart rate and blood pressure with beta-blockers and nondihydropyridine calcium channel–blocking agents.[2]

Although contrast-enhanced spiral computed tomography scanning is the gold standard for diagnosis, TEE can be used to confirm the diagnosis in unstable patients where immediate surgery is needed. Also, TEE plays an important role in diagnosing concomitant pathology such as aortic insufficiency, tamponade, and left ventricular failure. However, TEE cannot reliably image the distal ascending aorta and proximal aortic arch. Patients with type A dissection require aortic graft placement and may need aortic valve replacement and reattachment of the coronary arteries or arch vessels, depending on the location of the dissection.

Table 36.3 Acute Aortic Dissection: Hemodynamic Goals

Preload	May be increased if acute AI, increase further in tamponade
Afterload	Decrease with anesthetics, analgesics, arterial dilators (nitroprusside, nicardipine): Keep systolic BP < 100-120 mm Hg
Contractility	May be depressed; titrate myocardial depressants carefully
Rate	Decrease to <60-80 bpm: Use beta-blocker; ensure contractility is adequate
Rhythm	If atrial fibrillation present: Control ventricular response
MVO_2	Compromised if aortic dissection involves coronary vessels
CPB	Alternate site of inflow (arterial) cannulation, deep hypothermic circulatory arrest possible if cerebral vessels are involved

AI, aortic insufficiency; BP, blood pressure; bpm, beats per minute; CPB, cardiopulmonary bypass; MVO_2, myocardial oxygen consumption.

From Skubas NJ, Lichtman AD, Wang CJ, Sharma A, Thomas SJ. Anesthesia for cardiac surgery. In: Barash PG, Cahalan MK, Cullen BF, et al, eds. *Clinical Anesthesia*. 8th ed. Wolters Kluwer; 2018:1077-1111, Table 39.3.

Anesthetic management for aortic dissection involves ***prevention of hypertension***, adequate intravenous access, including central venous access, invasive arterial blood pressure monitoring (usually via the right radial artery), and intraoperative TEE. Hemodynamic goals are listed in **Table 36.3**.

B. Aortic Aneurysm

The aorta is an elastic structure that changes shape with each cardiac contraction. Its normal diameter is 2 to 3 cm. Degenerative diseases, along with age, hypertension, hypercholesterolemia, and atherosclerosis, cause premature loss of its elasticity and are the major cause of aortic aneurysms. Connective tissue diseases such as Marfan syndrome cause cystic medial necrosis, mostly involving the aortic root. Men are more affected than women, and the age of presentation is 50 to 70 years.[3] The majority of people with aortic aneurysms are asymptomatic when diagnosed, unless there is significant aortic insufficiency or mass effect compressing nearby structures such as the trachea or esophagus (eg, hoarseness, cough, dysphagia).

Patients with an aortic ***diameter of 5.5 cm*** or greater should undergo surgical repair. In patients with Marfan syndrome or a bicuspid aortic valve, surgical repair is indicated when the aortic diameter reaches 4.5 cm because in these diseases the rate of aneurysm expansion is faster than in other diseases. Aortic repair with or without coronary implantation and aortic valve replacement may be required in patients with root aneurysms. Involvement of the great vessels may require deep hypothermic circulatory arrest for reconstruction of the aortic arch.

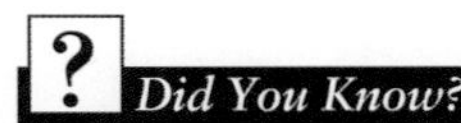

An aortic diameter of >5.5 cm is an indication for surgical repair.

Cerebral protective procedures, such as retrograde or antegrade cerebral perfusion, may also be used to provide hypothermic protective effects on brain tissue, flush toxins, and decrease the cerebral metabolic rate. Cerebral protective effects are controversial and results have been confounding.[4] Left heart bypass, from the left atrium to the femoral artery, can provide retrograde aortic perfusion to aortic branches distal to the repair to perfuse the spine and abdomen.

The anesthetic management for patients with aortic aneurysms is similar to that for patients with aortic dissection. The use of ***spinal fluid drains*** to optimize spinal perfusion pressure during thoracic aortic repair is used in some centers but not others. Intraoperative TEE is recommended to guide hemodynamic management, arterial and venous cannulation, and pre- and postrepair evaluation.

IV. Cardiopulmonary Bypass

The cardiopulmonary bypass (CPB) machine is made up of four basic parts: venous and arterial cannulae to take blood from and back to the heart, a venous reservoir to collect and transiently store the blood drained from the heart, an oxygenator membrane for exchanging carbon dioxide and oxygen, and a pump to propel blood back to the body. The cannula and oxygenator are primed with approximately 800 to 1500 mL of solution that approximates normal plasma osmolarity. When CPB is initiated, this priming volume causes ***sudden hemodilution*** of the patient's circulating blood volume and transient ***hypotension***. Blood is drained from the body via the multiorifice venous cannula that is placed into the right atrium and empties blood from the superior and inferior cavae and right atrium. Venous drainage through this cannula occurs passively by gravity siphon and is dependent on proper cannula position and a drop in height from the heart to the venous reservoir. Once in the venous reservoir, blood travels through a semipermeable membrane oxygenator for carbon dioxide and oxygen exchange. The fraction of inspired oxygen, temperature, the flow rate of the inspired gas, and delivery of volatile agents can all be controlled by the CPB machine. After blood leaves the oxygenator, a roller or centrifugal pump propels the blood via the arterial cannula to the proximal ascending aorta for systemic perfusion. **Figure 36.2** illustrates the basic CPB circuit.

VIDEO 36.7
Extracorporeal Circulation

CPB requires systemic ***anticoagulation***, which is usually accomplished by a single intravenous bolus of 300 U/kg of heparin. Anticoagulation is critical to prevent activation of the clotting cascade and clot formation in the CPB machine due to the exposure of blood to CPB circuitry. Activated clotting times (ACT) are checked to confirm adequate anticoagulation (ACT > 400 seconds) prior to and during CPB.

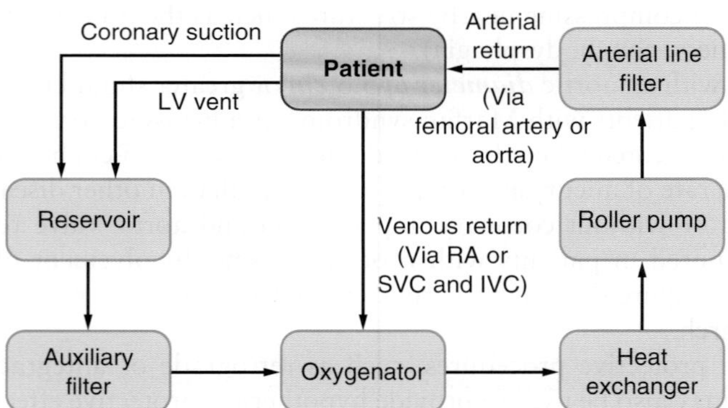

Figure 36.2 The basic circuit for cardiopulmonary bypass. IVC, inferior vena cava LV, left ventricle; RA, right atrium; SVC, superior vena cava. (Adapted from Thomson IR. Technical aspects of cardiopulmonary bypass. In: Thomas SJ, ed. *Manual of Cardiac Anesthesia*. 2nd ed. Churchill Livingstone; 1993:480 and from Skubas NJ, Lichtman AD Wang CJ, Sharma A, Thomas SJ. Anesthesia for cardiac surgery. In: Barash PG, Cahalan MK, Cullen BF, et al, eds. *Clinical Anesthesia*. 8th ed. Wolters Kluwer; 2018:1077-1111 Figure 39.8.)

A. Myocardial Protection

Myocardial protection is accomplished through two mechanisms: (1) the delivery of ***cardioplegia*** solution to arrest, electrically silence, and cool the heart and (2) removal of blood from the heart to minimize wall tension. Cardioplegia solution is a cold or tepid, high-potassium-containing blood solution delivered to the coronaries to decrease myocardial oxygen consumption. It can be delivered antegrade through a cannula placed in the proximal aortic root. However, in the presence of aortic insufficiency, severe coronary stenosis, or valvular surgery, cardioplegia is delivered retrograde by placing a cannula through the right atrium into the coronary sinus. Additional cannulae may be needed to remove any air or blood that collects in the LV from the bronchial circulation or the coronary sinus during CPB. This is critical to prevent dilation of the heart resulting in high wall tension and myocardial ischemia. Surgical blood loss during CPB is returned to the venous reservoir via suction cannulae and a "cardiotomy" reservoir.

V. Preoperative and Intraoperative Management

The preoperative evaluation of the cardiac surgical patient includes the essential elements required for all surgical patients (see Chapter 16). In addition, review of cardiac studies (ECG, echocardiogram, and cardiac catheterization data), laboratory values for hemoglobin, glucose, and renal function, and functional status allow detailed planning of anesthetic management, including the advisability of early extubation after surgery.

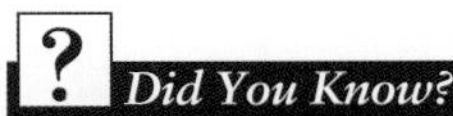

Most current medications should be continued until the time of cardiac surgery, including beta-blockers, antihypertensives, antiarrhythmics, calcium channel blockers, nitrates, statins, and aspirin.

A. Current Drug Therapy

In general, ***most current medications*** should be continued until the time of surgery, including beta-blockers, antihypertensives, antiarrhythmics, calcium channel blockers, nitrates, statins, and aspirin. Insulin administration should be tailored to prevent hyper- or hypoglycemia.

B. Premedication

Anxiolytics may be administered in hemodynamically stable patients with good underlying left ventricular function and respiratory drive. Caution should be used in patients with heart failure, respiratory failure, pulmonary hypertension, or significant obstructive valvular lesions. Benzodiazepines may produce prolonged sedation in elderly patients and prevent early postoperative extubation.

C. Monitoring

Hemodynamic monitoring is discussed in Chapter 15. This section will address techniques specific to the cardiac surgical patient. ***Direct arterial blood pressure monitoring*** is essential. During CPB, noninvasive techniques will not work because blood flow is nonpulsatile. Typically, the radial artery of the nondominant hand is cannulated for this purpose except when this artery will be used for coronary artery bypass grafting. Central venous access is required for infusion of vasoactive drugs and monitoring right atrial pressure. The pulmonary artery catheter or TEE can monitor pulmonary pressures, left ventricular filling pressures, and cardiac output. The use of these techniques is dependent on institutional practice and physician preference and varies widely. A recent study on the practice patterns of cardiac anesthesiologists showed that 67% use TEE in coronary artery bypass surgery, with even higher numbers reported for valve surgery.[5] TEE provides detailed information,

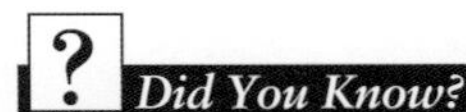

Blood flow during CPB is nonpulsatile, and therefore, blood pressure during CPB cannot be measured with noninvasive techniques.

such as new wall motion abnormalities, valvular abnormalities, guidance of cannula placement, detection of intracardiac air, and prosthetic valve function. Some centers use cerebral oximeters, a noninvasive technique that employs near-infrared spectrophotometry to monitor cerebral perfusion.

D. Selection of Anesthetic Drugs

Outcome studies have not demonstrated the optimal anesthetic agent for patients undergoing cardiac surgery. Commonly, a volatile anesthetic agent and low to moderate doses of a narcotic are used in combination. The volatile agent decreases myocardial oxygen demand by lowering blood pressure and decreasing contractility, decreases the likelihood of awareness during surgery, and possibly provides protection from ischemic injury to the heart via a preconditioning mechanism. The narcotic decreases oxygen demand by lowering the heart rate and provides postoperative analgesia. In addition, the narcotic decreases the required dose of the volatile agent, potentially important in patients with depressed ventricular function. This "balanced" anesthetic is optimal if the goal is to extubate the patient's trachea early after surgery. Nitrous oxide is often avoided because it can increase pulmonary artery pressure and expand air cavities and air emboli. High-dose narcotic and benzodiazepine techniques are rarely practiced today because "***fast-track***" techniques (extubation within 6 hours after surgery) are safe and cost-effective. Narcotics and benzodiazepines, when used concomitantly for induction of anesthesia, can cause hypotension and bradycardia. These effects can be offset with pancuronium but may be worsened by administration of vecuronium or cisatracurium. Etomidate, propofol, and barbiturates have been described as adjunct agents along with narcotics and fast-acting benzodiazepines for induction. Selection of one agent over another depends on the patient's underlying ventricular function and vascular tone. Etomidate is often chosen for induction of anesthesia because of its limited effects on hemodynamics. However, in the rare patient with underlying adrenal insufficiency, it may worsen adrenal dysfunction.

E. Intraoperative Management

In addition to the usual operating room preparations, the cardiac operating room requires significant other preparations for intraoperative patient care: fluid warmers; pressure transducers for central venous, arterial, and pulmonary artery catheters (if used); inotropes, vasodilators, and vasopressor infusions; and pumps for other medication infusions. ***Cross-matched blood*** should be immediately available and checked for correct patient identifiers prior to surgical sternotomy. Even in a prepared environment, placing a hemodynamically unstable patient on emergent CPB takes a minimum 15 to 20 minutes. Preparation and checklists, as found in **Table 36.4**, are key in helping to prevent serious errors.

During the dissection phase of surgery prior to CPB, arrhythmias and hypotension are common, resulting from surgical manipulations near or on the heart, especially in cardiac reoperations. During this time, the anesthesiologist titrates anesthetic depth as needed for the highly variable level of surgical stimulation, performs the baseline TEE examination, and samples arterial blood for determination of blood gas values as well as electrolytes, hemoglobin, and the baseline ACT. ***Sternotomy*** can cause significant sympathetic stimulation that may be prevented by deepening the anesthetic level with narcotics or the volatile agent. Prior to aortic cannulation and initiation of CPB, heparin is

Table 36.4 Anesthetic Preparation for Cardiac Surgery

Anesthesia machine
Routine check
Airway
Nasal cannula for oxygen Ventilation/intubation equipment Suction Difficult airway anticipated? Special equipment Inspired gas humidifier
Circulatory access
Catheters for peripheral and central venous and arterial access Intravenous fluids and infusion tubing and pumps Fluid warmer
Monitors
Standard ASA: ECG leads, blood pressure cuff, pulse oximeter, neuromuscular blockade monitor Temperature: Various probes (nasal, tympanic, bladder, rectal) Transducers (arterial, pulmonary, and central venous pressure) zeroed Cardiac output computer: Proper constant inserted Awareness monitor (BIS) Anticoagulation (ACT) monitor(s) Recorder
Medications
General anesthetic: Hypnotic/induction, amnestic/benzodiazepine, volatile, opioid, muscle relaxant Heparin (predrawn) Cardioactive In syringes: Nitroglycerin/nicardipine, calcium chloride, phenylephrine/ephedrine, epinephrine Infusions: Nitroglycerin, inotrope Antibiotics
Miscellaneous
Pacemaker with battery Defibrillator/cardioverter with external paddles and ECG cables Ultrasound system for central venous line insertion Compatible blood in operating room

ASA, American Society of Anesthesiologists; ECG, electrocardiogram; BIS, bispectral index; ACT, activated clotting time.

From Skubas NJ, Lichtman AD, Wang CJ, Sharma A, Thomas SJ. Anesthesia for cardiac surgery. In: Barash PG, Cahalan MK, Cullen BF, et al, eds. *Clinical Anesthesia*. 8th ed. Wolters Kluwer; 2018:1077-1111, Table 39.12.

administered and an ACT > 400 seconds must be obtained to confirm adequate anticoagulation. During ***aortic cannulation*** and prior to initiation of CPB, the systolic blood pressure should be controlled to no more than 100 mm Hg to minimize the risk of aortic dissection. Once all cannulae are in place and ***adequate anticoagulation*** confirmed, CPB is begun. The patient's head should be examined for any discoloration signaling cannula malposition (plethora may represent venous cannula obstruction or a bright red color may represent aortic cannula malposition), cerebral oximetry monitored (if used), and the surgical field inspected for proper cardiac decompression. Ventilation should stop once CPB machine reaches full flow, which is typically 50 to 60 mL/kg/min.

During CPB, volatile or intravenous anesthetic agents are delivered in the CPB circuit to maintain anesthesia. Muscle relaxants should be continued and mean arterial pressure controlled to a range of 50 to 75 mm Hg by appropriate use of a volatile agent, vasopressor, or vasodilator. Preoperative vasopressor or inotropic support is discontinued during CPB. Blood glucose should be controlled in the 120 to 200 mg/dL range and hematocrit maintained at >20%.

F. Separation From CPB

CPB can be discontinued when surgical hemostasis is adequate, the patient rewarmed to at least 36.5 °C, sinus rhythm restored at a rate between 70 and 100 beats per minute, mechanical ventilation resumed, and metabolic values optimized including pH > 7.36, hematocrit >20%, and serum potassium <6 mEq/L. As the arterial inflow from the CPB machine is decreased, venous drainage from the patient is restricted to allow the heart to generate cardiac output and blood pressure. When these are adequate, CPB is terminated. During this time, blood pressure is monitored closely and TEE is performed to look for intracardiac air, ventricular wall motion abnormalities, and ventricular filling and ejection. Vasoactive and inotropic drugs may be required to obtain adequate hemodynamics and perfusion. Studies have shown risk factors for difficulty in weaning from CPB include age >70 years, left ventricular ejection fraction <20%, female sex, reoperation, emergency operation, and recent myocardial infarction.[7] A checklist prior to discontinuation of CPB is helpful, as provided in **Table 36.5**. Electrical pacing of the heart may be required in the setting of AV nodal dysfunction, which is common after CPB.

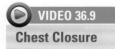

VIDEO 36.8
Protamine Reaction

Once the patient is hemodynamically stable, anticoagulation is reversed by administration of intravenous ***protamine***. Protamine is administered first as a small test dose to detect a possible inflammatory reaction and then, if no adverse effect is noted, given slowly over 5 to 10 minutes (typically 1 mg of protamine is administered for every 100 U of heparin). When one-third of the total protamine dose is administered, the perfusionist is alerted and suction of blood from the surgical into the venous reservoir is terminated to prevent clot formation in the CPB machine. After protamine infusion is complete, an ACT is measured to confirm adequate reversal of anticoagulation and arterial blood sampled to confirm maintenance of appropriate blood gas values, electrolytes, and hemoglobin.

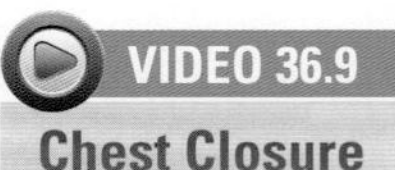

If separation from CPB is difficult, right or left ventricular failure is the likely cause. Ischemia from air embolism, poor myocardial protection, reperfusion injury, and pulmonary hypertension can all cause ventricular dysfunction. Common drug therapy and doses are listed in **Table 36.6**. Patients who require significant inotropic support for ventricular failure may need mechanical support. Placement of an intra-aortic balloon pump should be considered when postbypass ischemia is suspected, whereas severe ventricular dysfunction may require placement of a ventricular assist device until ventricular recovery. Patients who suffer significant pulmonary failure may need oxygenation via extracorporeal membrane oxygenation as a temporary measure.

Table 36.5 Checklist Before Separation From Cardiopulmonary Bypass
Laboratory Values
Hematocrit, ABGs K^+: ? elevated (cardioplegia) Ionized Ca^{2+}
Anesthetic/machine
Lung compliance: Evaluate (hand ventilation) Lungs are expanded, no atelectasis, both are ventilated (manual or mechanical) Vaporizers: Off Alarms: On
Monitors
Normothermia (37 °C nasopharyngeal, 35.5 °C bladder, 35 °C rectal) ECG: Rate, rhythm, ST Transducers rezeroed and leveled Arterial and filling pressures Recorder (if available)
Patient/field
LOOK AT THE HEART! Deaired: Check lead II, TEE Eyeball contractility, size, rhythm LV vent clamped/removed, caval snares released Bleeding: No major sites (grafts, suture lines, LV vent site) Vascular resistance: CPB flow $\propto$ MAP $\div$ Resistance
Support
As needed

ABGs, arterial blood gases; CPB, cardiopulmonary bypass; ECG, electrocardiogram; LV, left ventricle; MAP, mean arterial pressure; TEE, transesophageal echocardiography.

From Skubas NJ, Lichtman AD, Wang CJ, Sharma A, Thomas SJ. Anesthesia for cardiac surgery. In: Barash PG, Cahalan MK, Cullen BF, et al, eds. *Clinical Anesthesia*. 8th ed. Wolters Kluwer; 2018:1077-1111, Table 39.15.

VI. Minimally Invasive Cardiac Surgery

Advances in technology have made minimally invasive cardiac surgical approaches possible in an attempt to avoid complete median sternotomy, aortic cross clamping, and CPB. Decreased time to extubation, decreased length of stay in the intensive care unit, decreased transfusion rates, and decreased incidence of postoperative atrial fibrillation are cited as benefits of minimally invasive cardiac surgery. Although reduction in neurocognitive dysfunction was a primary goal of minimally invasive cardiac surgery, randomized controlled studies have had disappointing results in this area.[8] Minimally invasive cardiac surgery procedures are available for CHD as well as VHD.

However, procedures through small incisions in the chest are technically very challenging. Inexperience with minimally invasive techniques can lead to very significant complications, including inadequate valve repair, paravalvular leaks, and coronary obstruction. Catheter-based percutaneous valve repair and replacement are becoming more common in the United States. These techniques may be best suited for patients who have a history of previous sternotomy or very high perioperative risk of mortality.

VIDEO 36.10
Dobutamine

Table 36.6 Medications Given by Continuous Infusion

Drugs	Usual Initial Dose (mg/kg/min)	Usual Dose Range (mg/kg/min)
Amrinone[a]	2-5	2-20
Dopamine	2-5	2-20
Dobutamine	2-5	2-20
Epinephrine	0.01	0.01-0.1
Isoproterenol[b]	0.05-1	0.1-1
Lidocaine	20	20-50
Milrinone	50 μg/kg (over 3 min)	0.3-0.7
Nitroglycerin	0.5	0.5-5
Nitroprusside	0.5	0.5-5
Norepinephrine	0.1	0.1-1
Phenylephrine	1	1-3
Prostaglandin E_1	0.05-0.1	0.05-0.2
Vasopressin		0.0004

[a]Requires initial bolus of 750 μg/kg over 3 min before start of infusion.
[b]For chronotropic effect following cardiac transplantation, doses of 0.005 to 0.010 μg/kg/min are used.
From Skubas NJ, Lichtman AD, Wang CJ, Sharma A, Thomas SJ. Anesthesia for cardiac surgery. In: Barash PG, Cahalan MK, Cullen BF, et al, eds. *Clinical Anesthesia*. 8th ed. Wolters Kluwer; 2018:1077-1111, Table 39.18.

VII. Postoperative Considerations

Patients in the immediate postoperative period are at high risk for developing life-threatening complications, including respiratory failure, severe hemorrhage, cardiac tamponade, acute coronary graft failure, and prosthetic valve dysfunction (**Table 36.7**).

A. Urgent Reoperations

The incidence of urgent chest exploration after cardiac surgery is between 3% and 5%. The most common reasons are ***persistent bleeding*** and cardiac ***tamponade***. It is critical to distinguish whether persistent bleeding is due to a coagulopathy or inadequate surgical hemostasis. Thromboelastography or coagulation studies, including prothrombin time, activated partial thromboplastin time, fibrinogen level, and platelet count, may confirm a coagulopathy and indicate the optimal treatment. If bleeding persists and coagulopathy is excluded, the patient should return to the operating room for surgical correction of the bleeding.

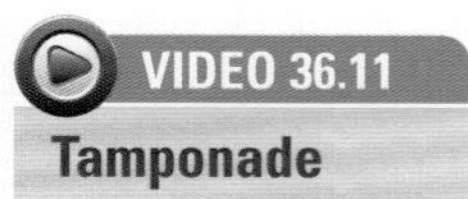

If drainage from the mediastinal chest tubes is not sufficient, cardiac tamponade can result and prompt surgical treatment is imperative. Tamponade must be included in the differential diagnosis of postoperative hypotension or low cardiac output states. It results in the collapse of cardiac chambers due to elevated pressures within the pericardium exceeding the pressures within the heart (particularly the atria). The normal signs and symptoms of tamponade are hypotension, paradoxical pulse, tachycardia, dyspnea, and orthopnea. TEE is an essential tool in making the prompt diagnosis of tamponade and expediting surgical intervention.

Table 36.7 Physiologic Effects of Congenital Cardiac Lesions

Volume overload of the ventricle or atrium resulting in increased pulmonary blood flow
Atrial septal defect (high flow, low pressure)
Ventricular septal defect (high flow, high pressure)
Patent ductus arteriosus (high flow, high pressure)
Endocardial cushion defect (high flow, high pressure)
Cyanosis resulting from obstruction to pulmonary blood flow
Tetralogy of Fallot
Tricuspid atresia
Pulmonary atresia
Pressure overload to the ventricle
Aortic stenosis
Coarctation of the aorta
Pulmonary stenosis
Cyanosis due to a common mixing chamber
Total anomalous venous return
Truncus arteriosus
Double outlet right ventricle
Single ventricle
Cyanosis due to separation of the systemic and pulmonary circulation
Transposition of the great vessels

From Skubas NJ, Lichtman AD, Wang CJ, Sharma A, Thomas SJ. Anesthesia for cardiac surgery. In: Barash PG, Cahalan MK, Cullen BF, et al, eds. *Clinical Anesthesia*. 8th ed. Wolters Kluwer; 2018:1077-1111, Table 39.21.

B. Pain Management

The desire to rapidly awaken and extubate patients following cardiac surgery has driven changes in the pain management. The use of ***shorter-acting narcotics*** (fentanyl and remifentanil) has become a prominent practice along with intrathecal opioids. Studies have confirmed the safety and efficacy of intrathecal opioids to enhance postoperative pain management and facilitate earlier tracheal extubation.[9] ***Dexmedetomidine***, an intravenous α_2-adrenergic agonist, has both sedative and analgesic properties without significant respiratory depression. Dexmedetomidine has been shown in multiple trials to decrease the time to tracheal extubation, and therefore, its use is increasing in postcardiac surgical patients, despite its current high cost.

VIII. Anesthesia for Children With Congenital Heart Disease

Approximately eight children of every 1000 live births have congenital heart disease (CHD). Ventricular septal defect is the most common CHD, and many of these defects will close spontaneously. However, others will require surgical treatment, as will the complex defects such as tetralogy of Fallot, transposition of the great vessels, hypoplastic left heart syndrome, and atrioventricular septal defects. Progress in corrective and palliative surgical techniques for CHD has been enormous in the past 2 decades. Many children with these complex lesions can undergo cardiac surgical procedures and live full and productive

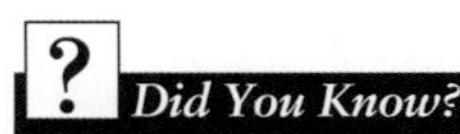

In the United States, there are more adults than children with CHD.

lives. In fact, there are more adults alive today with CHD than children with CHD. Full coverage of anesthesia for CHD is beyond the scope of this chapter and can be found elsewhere.[10]

For further review, please see the associated Interactive Video Lectures accessible in complimentary eBook bundled with this text. Access instructions are located on the inside front cover.

References

1. Nishimura RA, Otto CM, Bonow RO, et al. 2014 AHA/ACC guideline for the management of patients with valvular heart disease. *Circulation*. 2014;129:e521-e643.
2. Hiratzka LF, Bakris GL, Beckman JA, et al. 2010 ACCF/AHA/AATS/ACR/ASA/SCA/SCAI/SIR/STS/SVM guidelines for the diagnosis and management of patients with thoracic aortic disease: executive summary. *Anesth Analg*. 2010;111:279-315.
3. Patel HJ, Deeb GM. Ascending and arch aorta: pathology, natural history and treatment. *Circulation*. 2008;118:188-195.
4. Augoustides JGT, Andritsos M. Innovations in aortic disease: the ascending aorta and aortic arch. *J Cardiothorac Vasc Anesth*. 2010;24:198-207.
5. Dobbs HA, Bennett-Guerrero E, White W, et al. Multinational institutional survey on patterns of intraoperative transesophageal echocardiography use in adult cardiac surgery. *J Cardiothorac Vasc Anesth*. 2014;28:54-63.
6. Hillis LD, Smith PK, Anderson JL, et al. 2011 ACCF/AHA guideline for coronary artery bypass graft surgery. *Circulation*. 2011;124:e652-e735.
7. Denault AY, Deschamps A, Couture P. Intraoperative hemodynamic instability during and after separation from cardiopulmonary bypass. *Semin Cardiothorac Vasc Anesth*. 2010;14:165-182.
8. Cheng DC, Bainbridge D, Martin JE, et al. Does off-pump coronary artery bypass reduce mortality, morbidity, and resource utilization when compared with conventional coronary artery bypass? A meta-analysis of randomized trials. *Anesthesiology*. 2005;102:188.
9. Chaney MA. Intrathecal and epidural anesthesia and analgesia for cardiac surgery. *Anesth Analg*. 2006;102:45-64.
10. Skubas NJ, Lichtman AD, Sharma A, et al. Anesthesia for cardiac surgery. In: Barash PG, Cullen BF, Stoelting RK, et al, eds. *Clinical Anesthesia*. 7th ed. Wolters Kluwer Health/Lippincott Williams & Wilkins; 2013:1076.

Questions

1. **The three primary determinants of myocardial oxygen demand are heart rate, contractility, and:**

   A. Systolic wall tension
   B. Systemic vascular resistance
   C. Preload
   D. Systolic blood pressure
   E. None of the above

2. **The most common valvular heart disease is:**

   A. Mitral stenosis
   B. Mitral regurgitation
   C. Aortic stenosis
   D. Aortic regurgitation
   E. None of the above

3. **Which type of aortic dissection is a surgical emergency?**

   A. Type A
   B. Type B
   C. Type C
   D. Type D
   E. None of the above

4. **Retrograde cardioplegia is delivered by a cannula placed into the:**

   A. Right atrium
   B. Left atrium
   C. Aortic root
   D. Coronary sinus
   E. None of the above

5. **At what activated clotting time is anticoagulation sufficient to initiate cardiopulmonary bypass?**

   A. Greater than 200 seconds
   B. Greater than 300 seconds
   C. Greater than 400 seconds
   D. Greater than 500 seconds
   E. None of the above

6. **The optimal drug for maintenance of anesthesia during cardiac surgery is:**

   A. Fentanyl
   B. Isoflurane
   C. Remifentanil
   D. Propofol
   E. None of the above

Answers

1. A

In its calculation, systolic wall stress incorporates the size of the ventricle (preload) and the systolic blood pressure. Systemic vascular resistance may or may not correlate with myocardial oxygen consumption, but it does not take into account the size of the ventricle or blood pressure.

2. C

Approximately, 1% to 2% of the population in the United States have bicuspid aortic valves, a special risk factor for early development of aortic stenosis.

3. A

Type A dissection involves the ascending aorta. It may cause disruption of blood flow to the coronaries or the arch vessels, or it can rupture into the pericardium, causing cardiac tamponade. The mortality without surgical correction increases exponentially by the hour. Type B dissections can be managed medically in most patients. There are no type C or D dissections.

4. D

The cannula for delivery of retrograde cardioplegia is placed through the right atrium and into the coronary sinus. Cardioplegia solution is infused via this cannula and travels retrograde through the coronary circulation. Antegrade cardioplegia is administered through the aortic root.

5. C

A level >400 seconds prevents activation of the clotting cascade and clot formation in the CPB machine due to the exposure of blood to CPB circuitry.

6. E

Outcome studies have not demonstrated the optimal anesthetic agent for patients undergoing cardiac surgery.

37 Anesthesia for Vascular Surgery

Wendy K. Bernstein, Kyle E. Johnson, and Matthew A. Dabski

I. Vascular Disease: Epidemiologic, Medical, and Surgical Aspects

The incidence of atherosclerosis and vascular disease increases with advancing age. Therefore, it can be expected that there will be higher demand for vascular procedures, especially novel techniques such as angioplasty and endovascular stent placement. In addition, patients undergoing vascular surgery are some of the most complex patients to manage in the perioperative period. This chapter will focus on the principles of that management.

A. Pathophysiology of Atherosclerosis

Atherosclerosis describes a multifactorial ***inflammatory disease*** of the vascular tree. Predisposing risk factors for atherosclerosis include hypertension, dyslipidemia, abdominal obesity, insulin resistance, cigarette smoking, increasing age, family history, pro-inflammatory states, and prothrombotic states. The development of atherosclerosis occurs in two stages: endothelial injury and inflammatory response to injury. The primary injury occurs as low-density lipoprotein and apolipoprotein B–containing lipoproteins invade the vascular endothelium and become pro-inflammatory. As the inflammatory cascade ensues, the subendothelial space is filled with atherogenic lipoproteins and macrophages, which form foam cells. Foam cells form the atheromatous core of a plaque, which becomes necrotic and further enhances the inflammatory process. Disruption of the fibrous cap over a lipid deposit can lead to plaque rupture and ulceration. Vascular disease is not a localized phenomenon, but rather a systemic one affecting multiple organs including the heart with myocardial infarction (MI) and the brain with cerebrovascular accidents (CVAs).

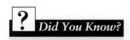

As many as 25% of adults presenting for vascular surgery have severe coronary artery disease.

B. Natural History of Patients With Peripheral Vascular Disease

More than 25 million people in the United States have clinical manifestations of atherosclerotic vascular disease (**Figure 37.1**). For example, 43% of men and 34% of women older than 65 years have >25% carotid stenosis, and stroke remains the leading cause of disability and the third leading cause of death in the United States. Peripheral arterial disease (PAD) can cause claudication and limb ischemia (2% prevalence in aging individuals). Aortic atherosclerotic disease can lead to abdominal aortic aneurysm (AAA), aortic dissection, peripheral atheroembolism, penetrating aortic ulcer, and intramural hematoma. Coronary atherosclerosis that leads to MI is the leading cause of death and disability worldwide.

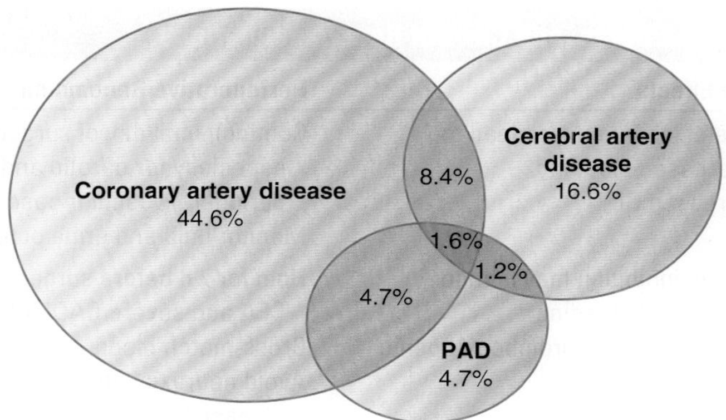

Figure 37.1 Typical overlap in vascular disease affecting different territories. Based on REACH data. PAD, peripheral arterial disease. (Reprinted from: Norgren L, Hiatt WR, Dormandy JA, et al. Inter-society consensus for the management of peripheral arterial disease (TASC II). *J Vasc Surg.* 2007;45(suppl S):S5. Figure A.7, with permission.)

C. Medical Therapy for Atherosclerosis

Management of contributing systemic diseases such as ***hypertension*** (using antihypertensives such as beta blockers), ***hyperlipidemia*** (using statins or other lipid-lowering agents), ***diabetes*** (using oral hypoglycemic agents or insulin therapy), and obesity (through exercise, weight loss, and diet) may significantly retard the progression of atherosclerosis and may reduce perioperative morbidity and mortality after vascular surgery. Treatment with statin drugs reduces progression and may cause regression of atherosclerotic plaques, improve endothelial function, and reduce cardiovascular events. Chronic therapy with aspirin, angiotensin-converting enzyme inhibitors, and especially smoking cessation have all been shown to significantly slow or reverse the progression of atherosclerosis. Most ***medical therapies***, including statins, aspirin, and β blockers, should be continued up to and throughout the perioperative period to reduce the risk of perioperative cardiovascular events (**Table 37.1**).

II. Chronic Medical Problems and Management in Patients Undergoing Vascular Surgery

The patient undergoing vascular surgery likely has systemic vascular disease complicated by medical problems such as coronary artery disease (CAD), systemic hypertension, hyperlipidemia, diabetes, obesity, and tobacco abuse.

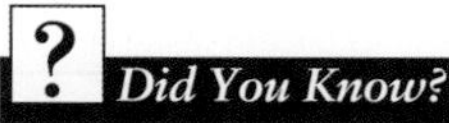

During carotid endarterectomy, emboli from the surgical site are the most common cause of stroke.

A. CAD in Patients With Peripheral Vascular Disease

As many as 25% of patients presenting for vascular surgery have severe CAD. The American Heart Association and others have published guidelines for cardiac evaluation and management prior to noncardiac surgery (**Figure 37.2**).[1]

B. Preoperative Coronary Revascularization

The Coronary Artery Revascularization Prophylaxis trial randomized patients with coronary disease before elective vascular surgery to either coronary revascularization or medical therapy and found no benefit to coronary revascularization if aggressive medical therapy (including beta blockers, aspirin, and statins) was instituted. ***Revascularization*** may therefore be of minimal value in

Table 37.1 Medical Therapy, Side Effects, and Current Recommendations

Medication/Drug Class	Side Effects	Perioperative Recommendations
Aspirin	Platelet inhibition may lead to increased bleeding Decreased GFR	Continue until day of surgery, especially for carotid and peripheral vascular cases. Monitor fluid and urine output.
Clopidogrel	Platelet inhibition may lead to increased bleeding Rare thrombotic thrombocytopenic purpura	Hold for 7 d before surgery except for CEA and severe CAD or DES. Cross-match blood. Avoid neuraxial anesthesia if not held at least 7 d.
HMG CoA reductase inhibitors (statins)	Liver function test abnormalities Rhabdomyolysis	Assess liver function tests. Continue through morning of surgery and continue as soon as possible postoperatively. Check CPK if myalgias.
Beta blockers	Bronchospasm Hypotension Bradycardia, heart block Induction hypotension Cough	Continue through perioperative period.
ACE inhibitors	Induction hypotension Cough	Continue through perioperative period. Consider one-half dose on day of surgery.
Diuretics	Hypovolemia Electrolyte abnormalities	Continue through morning of surgery. Monitor fluid and urine output.
Calcium channel blockers	Perioperative hypotension (especially with amlodipine)	Continue through perioperative period. Consider withholding amlodipine on day of surgery.
Oral hypoglycemics	Hypoglycemia intraoperatively and perioperatively Lactic acidosis with metformin	When feasible, switch to insulin preoperatively. Monitor glucose status intraoperatively and perioperatively.

ACE, angiotensin-converting enzyme; CAD, coronary artery disease; CEA, carotid endarterectomy; CPK, creatine phosphokinase; DES, drug-eluting stents; GFR, glomerular filtration rate; HMG CoA, 3-hydroxy-3-methylglutaryl coenzyme A.

Derived from Morgan GE, Mikhail MS, Murray MJ, eds. *Clinical Anesthesiology*. 4th ed. Lange Medical Books/McGraw-Hill; 2006

preventing coronary events after vascular surgery, except in patients in whom revascularization is indicated for acute coronary syndrome. If a ***coronary stent*** is placed, elective surgery should be delayed: for bare metal stents, a minimum of 30 days of dual antiplatelet therapy (DAPT) with aspirin and a $P2Y_{12}$ inhibitor; and for drug-eluting stents, 6 months (or longer) of DAPT. Aspirin is recommended indefinitely to prevent in-stent thrombosis. In the event that surgery cannot be delayed in patients undergoing DAPT after coronary stent implantation and the procedure requires discontinuation of $P2Y_{12}$ inhibitor therapy, it is recommended to continue aspirin perioperatively and restart the

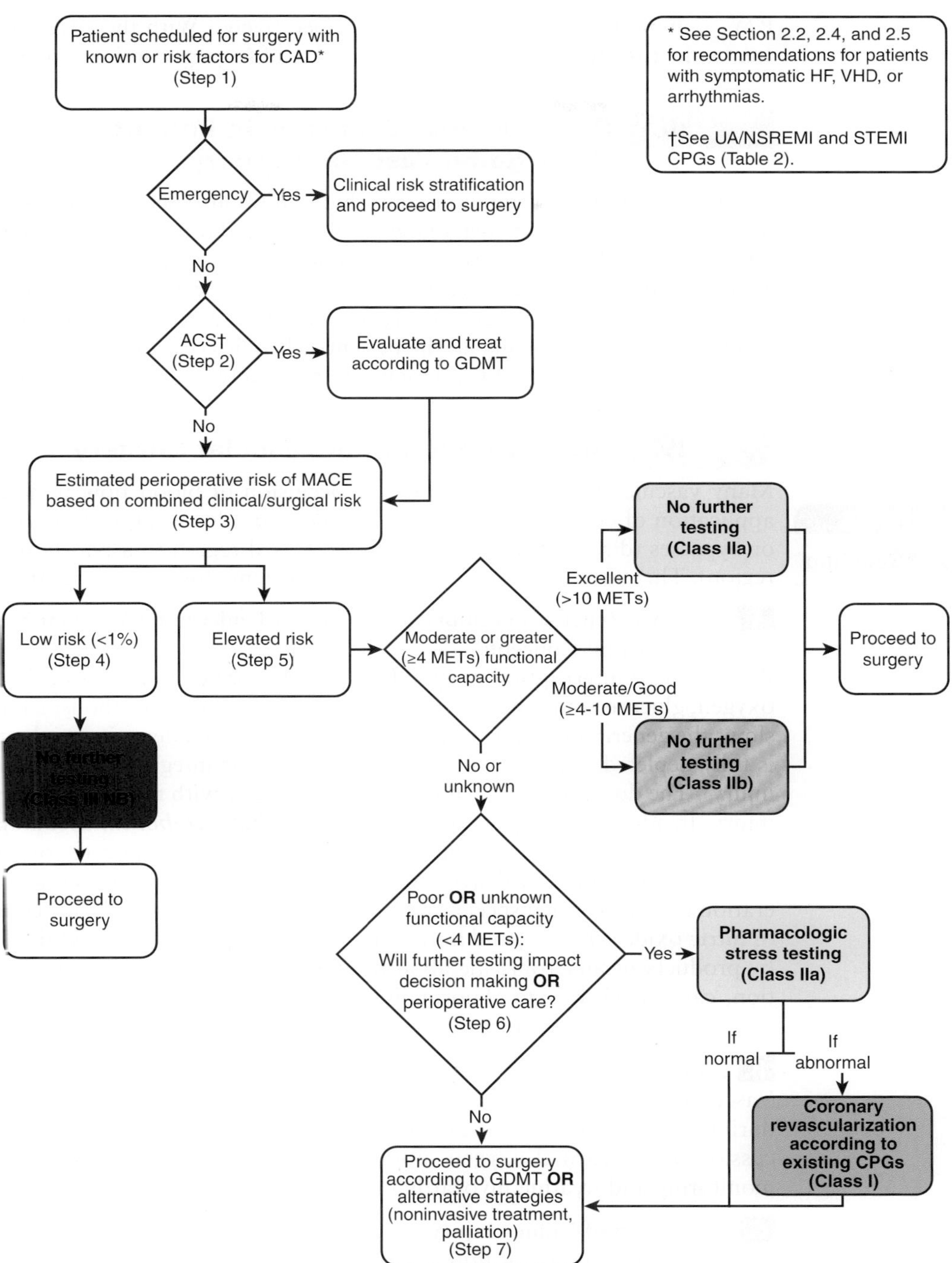

Figure 37.2 Stepwise approach to perioperative cardiac assessment for coronary artery disease. The American College of Cardiology/American Heart Association (ACC/AHA) guideline calls for stepwise cardiac risk assessment involving consideration of the patient's cardiac risk factors, functional capacity, and the planned surgical procedure. ACS, acute coronary syndrome; CAD, coronary artery disease; CPG, Clinical Practice Guidelines; GDMT, guideline-directed medical therapy; MACE, major adverse cardiac event; METs, metabolic equivalents. (From Fleisher LA, Fleischmann KE, Auerbach AD, et al. 2014 ACC/AHA guideline on perioperative cardiovascular evaluation and management of patients undergoing noncardiac surgery: a report of the American College of Cardiology/American Heart Association Task Force on Practice Guidelines. *J Am Col. Cardiol.* 2014;64(22):e77-e137. doi:10.1016/j.jacc.2014.07.944)

$P2Y_{12}$ inhibitor as early as possible postoperatively.[2] With the advent of new stents, the time required for DAPT and delay of surgery continues to evolve.

III. Other Medical Problems in Patients Undergoing Vascular Surgery

In addition to known common comorbid conditions such as CAD, systemic hypertension, hyperlipidemia, diabetes, obesity, and tobacco abuse, the vascular patient may have other undiagnosed conditions including hypercoagulable states, renal insufficiency, heart failure, chronic obstructive pulmonary disease, sleep apnea, and others. If surgery is elective, preoperative management should focus on optimizing all the patient's chronic conditions, a process that cannot be accomplished if the patient presents on the morning of surgery.

IV. Organ Protection in Vascular Surgery

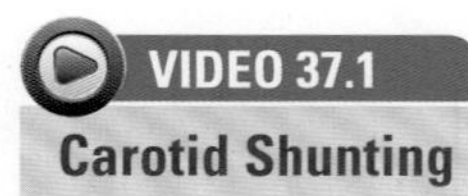

Many vascular procedures involve the occlusion of blood flow through the application of clamps, shunts (providing flow at a lower perfusion pressure), or bypasses (directing flow from a well-perfused region to a poorly perfused region). Therefore, vital organs may suffer ischemia for varying durations.

A. Ischemia-Reperfusion Injury in the Patient Undergoing Vascular Surgery: Fundamental Concepts

Reduction or interruption of blood flow (ischemia) compromises delivery of oxygen, glucose, and other essential nutrients for aerobic metabolism and thus slows the generation of adenosine triphosphate. When adenosine triphosphate is fully depleted, cellular processes fail and cellular integrity is lost (ischemic injury). The duration of ischemia correlates directly with the degree of cellular injury. In addition, toxic metabolites of ***anaerobic metabolism*** accumulate in the low or no-flow regions during the ischemic period. Upon restoration of flow and resumption of delivery of nutrients, further damage occurs via generation of toxic oxygen species, release of cytotoxic amino acids, upregulation of nitric oxide synthase, and initiation of cellular apoptosis. In addition, toxic by-products of anaerobic metabolism are released into the systemic circulation, causing electrolyte abnormalities, labile blood pressures, alterations in systemic vascular resistance, and potentially severe acid-base disequilibrium.

B. Prevention of Myocardial Injury

Vascular surgery can result in dramatic changes in blood pressure, especially during procedures requiring ***aortic clamping***. (See Chapter 36 for further discussion of myocardial oxygen supply and demand as well as techniques for monitoring and treating myocardial ischemia.)

C. Prevention of Kidney Injury

Postoperative ***acute renal failure (ARF)*** results in an increased length of hospital stay, as well as significant morbidity and mortality. Underlying kidney disease, cardiac disease, and especially renal ischemia contribute to its development: suprarenal aortic cross-clamping 15% and infrarenal cross-clamping 5% incidence of ARF. Additional risk factors may include advanced age, hypovolemia, and anemia. Logically, minimizing renal ischemia time and maintaining appropriate hemodynamics are important to preserving renal function. However, currently there is no clinically proven strategy to minimize the risk of postoperative renal insufficiency and ARF.

D. Prevention of Pulmonary Complications

More and more vascular procedures are done via minimally invasive or endovascular techniques for which postoperative pulmonary complications should be minimal. However, for patients who require open surgical procedures, especially aortic procedures, significant pulmonary complications are a real risk due to ***large fluid shifts*** and ***transfusion-related acute lung injury***. In addition, pain from large incisions can compromise respirations and cough. Different centers manage these challenges differently; however, minimizing transfusions and optimizing postoperative analgesia are established ways of improving outcome. After carotid endarterectomy (CEA), the carotid body on the operative side is denervated, and this blunts the ventilatory response to hypoxemia and virtually eliminates this response after bilateral CEA. Postoperative surgical site bleeding after CEA can distort, compress, or occlude the trachea rapidly, necessitating emergent evacuation of the causative hematoma.

> **? Did You Know?**
>
> The most urgent and potentially devastating complication of carotid endarterectomy is clot formation at the surgical site and the associated thromboembolism to the cerebral circulation.

E. Protection of the Central Nervous System and Spinal Cord

In patients undergoing vascular surgery, neurologic injury is most common after CEA (***stroke***) and thoracic aortic procedures ***(paraplegia)***. During CEA, emboli from the surgical site are the usual cause of stroke. However, hypoperfusion of the brain on the operative side can result during carotid clamping if the patient's perfusion via the circle of Willis or the surgical shunt around the site of carotid clamping is inadequate. In thoracic aortic procedures, compromise of the spinal cord vascular supply, especially the artery of Adamkiewicz, is a major risk. For strategies to improve neurologic outcome, please see subsequent chapters on the specific procedures (**Figure 37.3**). Unfortunately, no pharmacologic intervention has proven beneficial.

> **? Did You Know?**
>
> Endovascular repair of aortic aneurysms has evolved into a first-line treatment choice.

V. Carotid Endarterectomy

A. Management of Asymptomatic Carotid Stenosis

Screening asymptomatic patients for carotid stenosis is not recommended because CEA is beneficial for only a very select group of asymptomatic patient and only if the expected risk of CVA is less with CEA than without it.[3]

B. Management of Symptomatic Carotid Stenosis

Symptoms of carotid artery stenosis include sudden unilateral vision loss (amaurosis fugax) and unilateral changes in motor function, dysarthria, and aphasia. These symptoms require ***urgent evaluation*** and treatment to minimize the risk of permanent neurologic damage. If performed expertly, CEA is effective in reducing this risk in symptomatic patients with moderate and high-grade carotid stenosis.

> **? Did You Know?**
>
> Spinal fluid drainage during thoracic aneurysm can be employed to enhance spinal cord perfusion pressure.

C. Preoperative Evaluation and Preparation for Carotid Endarterectomy

The preoperative evaluation of vascular surgical patient includes the essential elements required for all surgical patients (Chapter 16). CEA is defined by the American College of Cardiology/American Heart Association (ACC/AHA) as an intermediate-risk procedure, with the possibility of cardiac death or nonfatal MI being <5%.[1] The ACC/AHA algorithm defines an evidence-based approach to the preoperative evaluation (**Figure 37.2**). If preoperative medical management with ***anticoagulants*** or ***antiplatelet drugs*** does not control symptoms of carotid stenosis, CEA is urgent. Preoperative reduction of hypertension is controversial especially if the carotid stenosis is severe or bilateral. Sudden reduction in blood pressure should be avoided.

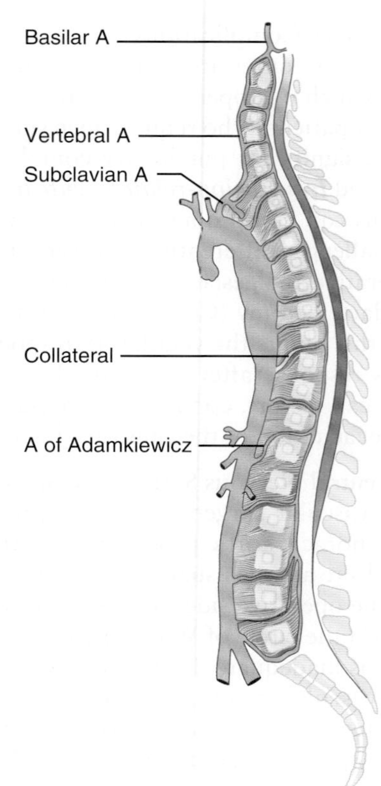

Figure 37.3 The artery of Adamkiewicz usually arises at the T11-T12 level and provides the blood supply to the lower spinal cord. Its variable location and the uncertainty of additional collateral blood supply explain, in part, the unpredictability of paraplegia following descending aortic surgery. (Reprinted from Piccone W, DeLaria GA, Najafi H. Descending thoracic aneurysms. In: Bergan JJ, Yao JST, eds. *Aortic Surgery.* WB Saunders; 1989:249, with permission.)

D. Monitoring and Preserving Neurologic Integrity

Monitoring for cerebral ischemia during CEA is controversial. Some centers advocate providing regional anesthesia and argue that the awake patient can report neurologic changes most reliably. Others advocate general anesthesia to ensure a motionless surgical field, and they rely on continuous electroencephalogram, somatosensory-evoked potentials, transcranial Doppler, or cerebral oximetry. Each method has its limitations and challenges, and neither regional nor general anesthesia has provided better ***neurologic outcomes***. With either technique, if there are signs of cerebral ischemia, blood pressure should be optimized (usually to the patient's normal awake level) or a shunt placed, if not already in use.

E. Anesthetic Management for Elective Surgery

No one anesthetic approach has been proven best for patients undergoing CEA. Both regional and general anesthesia are employed safely.[4] With either approach, the patient must be awake and cooperative at the end of the procedure for ongoing ***neurologic assessment***. Given the very high incidence of CAD and hypertensive heart disease in this patient population, etomidate and esmolol are often used in combination for induction of general anesthesia and abatement of the stimulation of endotracheal intubation. For patients at low risk from the hypotensive effects of propofol, it may be used instead of etomidate to reduce the risk of postoperative nausea and vomiting. General anesthesia can be maintained by intravenous or inhaled anesthetics with the caveat that ***blood pressure*** must be maintained at or near the patient's normal resting level. Isoflurane, sevoflurane, and desflurane reduce cerebral oxygen consumption and provide ischemic preconditioning for the heart and other organs. Despite these potential advantages, they have not been proven to improve outcome, perhaps because the majority of CVAs are caused by ***emboli*** from the surgical site. Regional anesthesia techniques include deep and superficial cervical plexus blocks, as well as cervical epidural anesthesia and local infiltration. In addition to standard American Society of Anesthesiologists (ASA) monitors, continuous direct arterial blood pressure monitoring is highly recommended because blood pressure control is vital during CEA.

F. Carotid Angioplasty With Stenting

Since its clinical introduction over three decades ago, carotid angioplasty with stenting has since emerged as an alternative treatment to CEA. Compared with CEA, carotid stenting is associated with a higher risk of periprocedural stroke and death, especially in older patients. However, long-term data now show that carotid stenting and CEA have similar overall outcomes when comparing risk of stroke, MI, death, and functional status, after 10 years of follow-up.[5]

G. Postoperative Management

The most urgent and potentially devastating complication of CEA is clot formation at the surgical site and the associated ***thromboembolism*** to the cerebral circulation. A new onset neurologic change after surgery requires immediate ultrasound examination of the operative site and reoperation if indicated. Other complications presenting in the early postoperative period include stroke from emboli or hypoperfusion during surgery, severe hyper- and hypotension, myocardial ischemia, cranial and recurrent nerve injuries, and wound hematoma. Control of severe hypertension is vital because if uncontrolled, it is associated with increased mortality and increased cardiac and neurologic complications. Additionally, persistent severe postoperative hypertension increases the risk of cerebral hyperperfusion syndrome, characterized by headaches, seizures, and focal neurologic signs. An ***expanding wound hematoma*** can obstruct the airway, necessitating emergent evacuation of the hematoma before an adequate airway can be reestablished.

VI. Aortic Aneurysms

The management of patients with aortic aneurysms is evolving rapidly with innovative stenting techniques progressively replacing open surgical procedures. However, ***rupture*** of an aortic aneurysm is a ***true surgical emergency*** and one of the greatest anesthetic management challenges.

A. Epidemiology and Pathophysiology of Abdominal Aortic Aneurysms

There are approximately 200,000 AAAs diagnosed annually. Approximately 45,000 of these require surgical repair annually. Risk factors for AAA include male sex, advanced age, smoking, hypertension, low serum high-density lipoprotein cholesterol, high fibrinogen plasma levels, and low platelet count. The annual risk of aneurysmal rupture is directly related to its diameter: 1% for aneurysms measuring <4.0 cm, 2% for aneurysms 4.0 to 4.9 cm, and 20% for aneurysms >5.0 cm. All aneurysms >5.0 cm should be considered for surgical or endovascular repair. Screening is recommended by the U.S. Preventive Services Task Force for men older 65 years with a smoking history.

B. Medical Management Versus Endovascular Repair Versus Open Surgical Repair

Medical management of aortic aneurysms includes smoking cessation and control of hypertension, dyslipidemia, diabetes, and diet. Medical management may slow, but will not halt aneurysm progression completely. For patients with AAAs measuring 4.0 to 5.4 cm, frequent ultrasound monitoring for progression is vital. Since the 1980s, ***endovascular aneurysm repair*** (EVAR) has progressively become the ***dominant*** treatment modality. In this approach, the femoral artery is used to introduce stent graft(s) inside the aneurysm, thereby preventing further enlargement or rupture. Initially, EVAR was used on patients deemed too high risk for an open surgical repair, but now it has evolved into a first-line treatment choice. Nevertheless, EVAR is not without complications, including ***graft leak*** and intraoperative conversion to open repair because of aneurysm rupture, vascular injury, or inability to seal the graft against the wall of the aorta. When compared with open surgical repair, EVAR is associated with shorter recover times and lower 30-day mortality rates (1.4% vs 4.2%). While EVAR offers an early advantage, long-term follow-up data show that overall survival is similar among patients undergoing open and endovascular techniques. However, even with the advent of technologically improved grafts, the rate of reintervention is higher with EVAR, and durability remains a question. Graft costs and reoperation expenses offset other savings, so that ultimately there is no cost benefit to EVAR verses open surgical repair. EVAR is performed using local, regional, or general anesthesia depending on the preferences of the patient and the surgical team.

C. Open Surgical Repair

Open surgical repair of an AAA is performed through either an anterior transperitoneal laparotomy incision or an anterolateral retroperitoneal approach. The surgical exposure for either approach is virtually identical, but the retroperitoneal approach is associated with less fluid shifts, faster return of bowel function, lower pulmonary complications, and shorter intensive care unit stays. After administration of intravenous heparin, the aortic cross-clamp is applied to the supraceliac, suprarenal, or infrarenal aorta, depending on the location of the aneurysm. The higher the *level of cross-clamping*, the greater the stress will be on the left ventricle and the higher the incidence of ischemic injury to the gut, kidney, and spinal cord. Intraoperative blood loss during open AAA repair can be significant, and the extensive retroperitoneal surgical dissection increases fluid requirements (up to 10-12 mL/kg/h). In addition to standard ASA monitors, continuous direct arterial blood pressure monitoring is highly recommended because of the rapid and marked changes in blood pressure during the clamping and unclamping of the aorta. Central venous and pulmonary artery pressure monitoring as well as transesophageal echocardiography are often used depending on the comorbidities of the patient and preferences of the anesthesiologist. General anesthesia or combined general and epidural anesthesia are common approaches. The combined approach has the advantage of providing excellent postoperative analgesia but introduces the risk of epidural hematoma because systemic anticoagulation must be used during surgery.

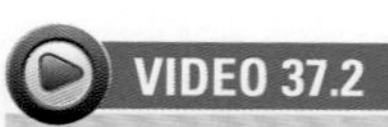

Aortic Cross-Clamping: Blood Volume Redistribution

D. Thoracoabdominal Aneurysm Repair

Thoracoabdominal aortic aneurysm surgery is one of the ***greatest anesthetic management challenges***. Typically, thoracoabdominal aneurysms involve the descending thoracic and abdominal aorta and require an expansive incision extending into these cavities, one-lung ventilation, and the use of partial cardiopulmonary bypass. Selective ("one-lung") ventilation of the contralateral lung is required for optimizing surgical exposure and to prevent the ipsilateral lung from surgical trauma. During thoracic aortic procedures, ***spinal cord ischemia*** may be detected through the use of somatosensory-evoked potential and motor-evoked potentials (**Table 37.2**). To improve spinal cord perfusion pressure, a ***lumbar subarachnoid drain*** can be used to remove cerebrospinal fluid. Partial cardiopulmonary bypass has been used to provide perfusion distal to the operative site. In fact, the incidence of neurologic injury in this setting has been substantially reduced when distal aortic perfusion is combined with drainage of cerebrospinal fluid. Many of the other anesthetic management considerations are the same for thoracoabdominal as noted above for AAA surgery. (See the sections in Chapter 36 on "Aortic Dissection" and "Aortic Aneurysm" and Table 36.2 for a summary of the common hemodynamic goals for all these procedures.)

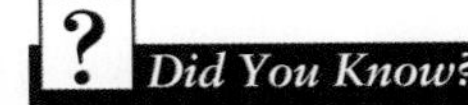

Did You Know?

Approximately 30 to 40 million people in the United States have peripheral arterial disease.

E. Management of Emergency Aortic Surgery

Rupture or leaking of an aortic aneurysm is the most common reason for emergency aortic surgery. Aortic aneurysm rupture has a mortality rate of 85%

Table 37.2 Methods of Spinal Cord Protection During Descending Thoracic Aortic Surgery

Limitation of cross-clamp duration	
Distal circulatory support (partial bypass)	
Reattachment of critical intercostal arteries	
CSF drainage (lumbar drain)	
Hypothermia	Moderate systemic (32°C-34°C) Epidural cooling Circulatory arrest
Maintenance of proximal blood pressure	Pharmacotherapy: Corticosteroids, barbiturates, naloxone, calcium channel blockers, oxygen-free radical scavengers, NMDA antagonists, mannitol, magnesium, vasodilators (adenosine, papaverine, prostacyclin), perfluorocarbons, colchicine Intrathecal: Papaverine, magnesium, tetracaine, perfluorocarbons
Avoidance of postoperative hypotension	
Sequential aortic clamping	
Enhanced monitoring for spinal cord ischemia	Somatosensory-evoked potentials Motor-evoked potentials Hydrogen-saturated saline
Avoidance of hyperglycemia	

CSF, cerebrospinal fluid; NMDA, *N*-methyl-d-aspartate.

Derived from Thomas DM, Hulten EA, Ellis ST, et al. Open versus endovascular repair of abdominal aortic aneurysm in the elective and emergent setting in a pooled population of 37,781 patients: a systematic review and meta-analysis. *ISRN Cardiol.* 2014;2014:149243.

unless surgery is performed immediately, and even then the ***mortality rate is 50%***. If the patient survives emergency surgery, the incidence of renal impairment, pulmonary injury, MI, and spinal cord injury is significantly greater than in elective aortic surgery. Ruptures most commonly occur into the retroperitoneum, and this site allows temporary tamponade of the hemorrhage. About 25% of aneurysms rupture into the peritoneal cavity, and rapid exsanguination occurs. Massive blood loss will occur during this surgery, and, therefore, preparations for blood replacement, including rapid infusion devices, are critical. For this true surgical emergency, both EVAR and open surgical repair are used in different centers depending on the resources and expertise available.[6]

VII. Lower Extremity Revascularization

The incidence of PAD is increasing, especially in the aging population. Roughly 10 million people in the United States have symptomatic PAD, and another 20 to 30 million have asymptomatic PAD. The three indications for elective revascularization procedures include claudication, ischemic rest pain or ulceration, and gangrene. High-risk procedures, including iliofemoral bypass, femoral-femoral bypass, and aortofemoral bypass, reestablish blood flow to an ischemic extremity and relieve debilitating symptoms of claudication. However, advances in minimally invasive percutaneous techniques have made ***endovascular procedures*** the primary modality for revascularization. Regional or local anesthesia with or without sedation is often used for endovascular approaches. The majority of the procedure is not painful. However, tunneling the graft and deployment of the stent can be quite painful and trigger patient movement or hypertension and tachycardia. Heparin is given prior to deployment of grafts or stents, and anticoagulation may be needed in the postoperative period to maintain graft patency.

For further review, please see the associated Interactive Video Lectures accessible in complimentary eBook bundled with this text. Access instructions are located on the inside front cover.

References

1. Fleisher LA, Fleischmann KE, Auerbach AD, et al. 2014 ACC/AHA guideline on perioperative cardiovascular evaluation and management of patients undergoing noncardiac surgery: a report of the American College of Cardiology/American Heart Association Task Force on Practice Guidelines. *J Am Coll Cardiol*. 2014;64(22):e77-e137. doi:10.1016/j.jacc.2014.07.944
2. Levine GN, Bates ER, Bittl JA, et al. 2016 ACC/AHA guideline focused update on duration of dual antiplatelet therapy in patients with coronary artery disease: a report of the American College of Cardiology/American Heart Association Task Force on Clinical Practice Guidelines. *J Am Coll Cardiol*. 2016;68(10):1082-1115. doi:10.1016/j.jacc.2016.03.513
3. Jonas DE, Feltner C, Amick HR, et al. Screening for asymptomatic carotid artery stenosis: a systematic review and meta-analysis for the U.S. Preventive Services Task Force. *Ann Intern Med*. 2014;161(5):336-346. doi:10.7326/M14-0530
4. Malik OS, Brovman EY, Urman RD. The use of regional or local anesthesia for carotid endarterectomies may reduce blood loss and pulmonary complications. *J Cardiothorac Vasc Anesth*. 2019;33(4):935-942. doi:10.1053/j.jvca.2018.08.195
5. Bonati LH, Dobson J, Featherstone RL, et al. Long-term outcomes after stenting versus endarterectomy for treatment of symptomatic carotid stenosis: the International Carotid Stenting Study (ICSS) randomised trial. *Lancet*. 2015;385(9967):529-538. doi:10.1016/S0140-6736(14)61184-3
6. Swerdlow NJ, Wu WW, Schermerhorn ML. Open and endovascular management of aortic aneurysms. *Circ Res*. 2019;124(4):647-661. doi:10.1161/CIRCRESAHA.118.313186

Questions

1. **Atherosclerosis occurs in two stages, the first is endothelial injury and the second is:**

   A. An inflammatory response
   B. A thrombogenic response
   C. A cytotoxic response
   D. An angiogenic response
   E. None of the above

2. **What percentage of men older than 65 years have carotid stenosis?**

   A. Over 20%
   B. Over 30%
   C. Over 40%
   D. Over 50%
   E. None of the above

3. **How long should elective surgery be delayed after placement of a drug-eluting coronary stent?**

   A. 6 weeks
   B. 3 months
   C. 6 months
   D. 12 months
   E. None of the above

4. **The risk of cardiac-related death or nonfatal myocardial infarction after carotid endarterectomy is less than:**

   A. 1%
   B. 2%
   C. 5%
   D. 10%
   E. None of the above

5. **Signs and symptoms of cerebral hyperperfusion syndrome after carotid endarterectomy include headache, seizures, and:**

   A. Focal neurologic deficits
   B. Hypertension
   C. Bradycardia
   D. Apnea
   E. None of the above

6. **At what diameter should an aortic aneurysm be considered for surgical repair?**

   A. Greater than 4 cm
   B. Greater than 4.5 cm
   C. Greater than 5.0 cm
   D. Greater than 5.5 cm
   E. None of the above

Answers

1. A

In response to the injury, an inflammatory cascade ensues, causing the subendothelial space to be filled with atherogenic lipoproteins and macrophages, which form foam cells.

2. C

Forty-three percent of men and 34% of women older than 65 years have >25% carotid stenosis due to atherosclerosis, and stroke remains the leading cause of disability and the third leading cause of death in the United States.

3. D

If a coronary stent is placed, elective surgery should be delayed: for bare metal stents, a minimum of 6 weeks of DAPT; and for drug-eluting stents, 12 months (or longer) of DAPT.

4. C

The American Heart Association defines carotid endarterectomy as an intermediate-risk procedure, with the possibility of cardiac death or nonfatal MI <5%.

5. A

Persistent severe postoperative hypertension increases the risk of cerebral hyperperfusion syndrome, characterized by headaches, seizures, and focal neurologic signs. Although hypertension is very common after carotid endarterectomy, it is not a sign of hyperperfusion syndrome.

6. C

The annual risk of aneurysmal rupture is directly related to its diameter: 1% for aneurysms measuring <4.0 cm, 2% for aneurysms 4.0 to 4.9 cm, and 20% for aneurysms >5.0 cm.

38 Management of Acute and Chronic Pain

Dost Khan, Yogen Girish Asher, and Honorio T. Benzon

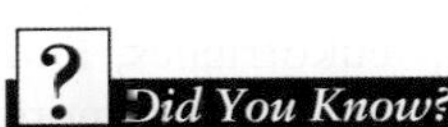

When chronic pain is associated with neuroplastic changes in the central and peripheral nervous systems that may manifest as hypersensitivity, windup, and allodynia, the pain itself becomes a disease state.

Pain is defined by the International Association for the Study of Pain (IASP) as "an unpleasant sensory and emotional experience associated with actual or potential tissue damage, or described in terms of such damage."[1] ***Acute pain*** is a normal physiologic response to injury, disease, or surgery and is usually temporally self-limited. Though unpleasant, pain is protective and serves the purpose of avoiding, stopping, or minimizing tissue damage and should be seen as a symptom of an underlying disease. ***Chronic pain*** is usually defined as pain lasting more than 3 months. It can be due to ongoing disease or tissue injury or can persist after resolution of or in the absence of injury. Chronic pain is associated with neuroplastic changes in the central and peripheral nervous systems that may manifest as hypersensitivity, windup, and allodynia. When these changes occur, the pain itself can be called a disease state.

Nociceptive pain results from transmission of a noxious stimulus through an intact nervous system. Nociceptive pain can be worsened by inflammation, which causes ***hyperalgesia,*** the phenomenon of normally painful stimuli being perceived as more painful than usual. Nociceptive pain can be somatic or visceral. ***Somatic pain*** originates within the skin, superficial tissue, and musculoskeletal system and is typically easy to localize and described as sharp. ***Visceral pain*** is typically vague, diffuse, and achy and may refer to surrounding areas.

In contrast to nociceptive pain, ***neuropathic pain*** results from a lesion in the central or peripheral nervous system. It is often described as electric or lancinating in character. If found in the distribution of a known nerve, it is termed ***neuralgia.*** Neuropathic pain is often associated with altered sensations. ***Paresthesias*** are abnormal, spontaneous, or evoked sensations. ***Dysesthesia*** are unpleasant abnormal sensations. ***Allodynia*** is the perception of pain from a normally nonpainful stimulus (such as light touch). ***Hyperesthesia*** is increased sensitivity to stimulation, and ***hypoesthesia*** is decreased sensation of stimulus.

I. Anatomy, Physiology, and Neurochemistry of Pain

A. Pain Processing

The physiology of pain processing functionally comprises four steps: transduction, transmission, modulation, and perception. These processes are clinically relevant as each provides targets for pain treatment and prevention (**Figure 38.1**). ***Transduction*** is the generation of an action potential from a noxious chemical, mechanical, or thermal stimulus. ***Transmission*** is the propagation of the signal through the afferent pathway from the nociceptor to the sensory cortex. ***Modulation*** is the positive or negative adjustments in the pain signal along the afferent pathway, while ***perception*** is the integration of the pain signal into consciousness.

B. Transduction

Nociceptors are located in the skin, mucosa, muscle, fascia, joint capsules, dura, viscera, and adventitia of blood vessels. Most Aδ and C nociceptors are polymodal (ie, their terminals express transducer channels that are sensitive to multiple stimuli). When they are activated by pressure, chemical, or thermal stimuli, the channels activate voltage-sensitive sodium and calcium channels, starting an action potential. Nociceptors can be activated by bradykinin, serotonin, and protons and sensitized by prostaglandins, leukotrienes, and cytokines. Glutamate, substance P, and nerve growth factor can also promote transduction of a pain signal (**Table 38.1**).

C. Transmission

Pain transmission occurs via a three-neuron afferent pathway, beginning in the periphery (**Figure 38.2**). First-order neuronal cell bodies are located in the dorsal root ganglia with fibers projecting to peripheral tissue where the receptors are located. Fibers enter the spinal cord and travel up or down through

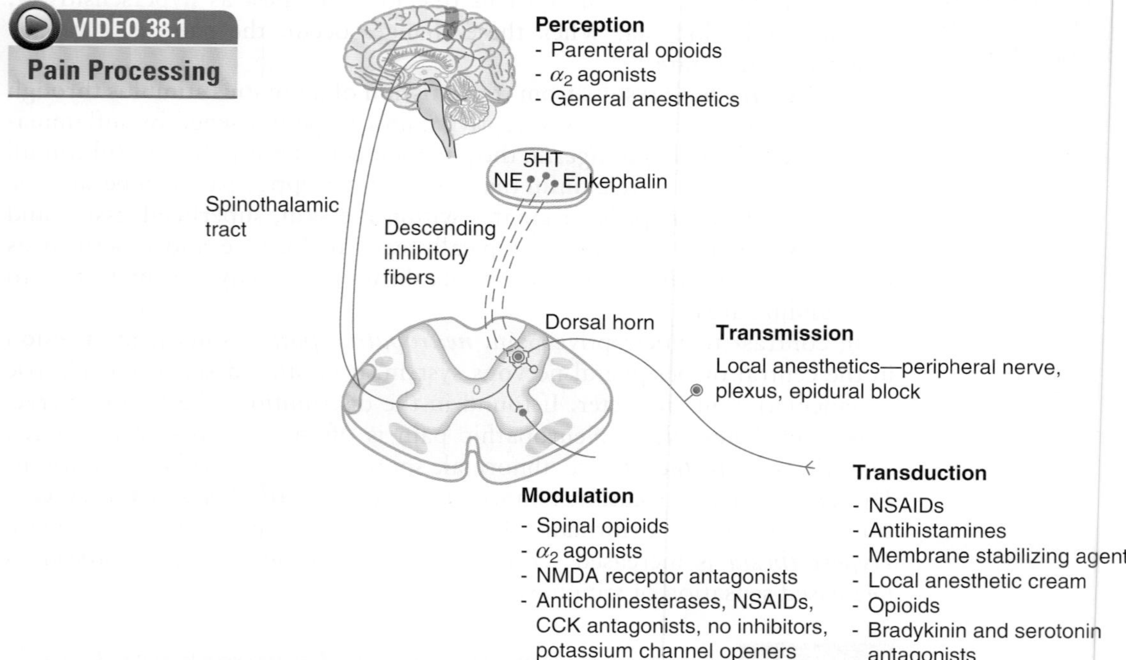

Figure 38.1 The four elements of pain processing: transduction, transmission, modulation, and perception. CCK, cholecystokinin; NMDA, *N*-methyl-D-aspartate; NSAIDs, nonsteroidal anti-inflammatory drugs. (From Macres SM, Moore PG, Fishman SM. Acute pain management. In: Barash PG, Cahalan MK, Cullen BF, et al, eds. *Clinical Anesthesia*. 8th ed. Wolters Kluwer; 2018:1562-1606, Figure 55.6.)

Table 38.1 Classification of Neural Fibers

Fiber Type	Modality	Function	Receptor	Diameter
Aα	Proprioceptive	Muscle tension, length, velocity	Golgi and Ruffini endings, muscle spindle afferents	15-20 μm
Aβ	Mechanosensitive	Touch, motion, pressure, vibration	Meissner, Ruffini, Pacinian corpuscles; Merkel disk	5-15 μm
Aδ	Thermoreceptive	Cold	Free nerve endings	1-5 μm
	Nociceptive	Sharp pain		
C	Thermoreceptive	Warmth	Free nerve endings	<1 μm
	Nociceptive	Burning pain		

Derived from Macres SM, Moore PG, Fishman SM. Acute pain management. In: Barash PG, Cahalan MK, Cullen BF, et al, eds. *Clinical Anesthesia*. 8th ed. Wolters Kluwer; 2018:1562-1606.

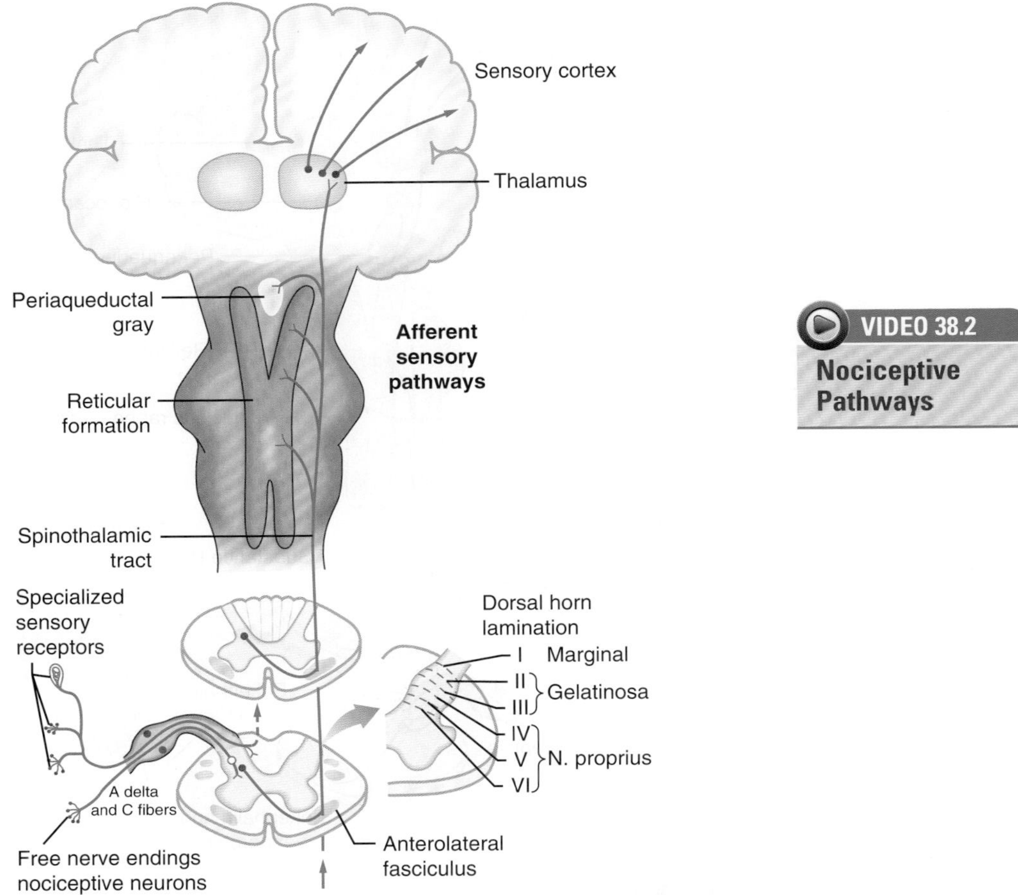

Figure 38.2 The afferent nociceptive pathway. (From Macres SM, Moore PG, Fishman SM. Acute pain management. In: Barash PG, Cahalan MK, Cullen BF, et al, eds. *Clinical Anesthesia*. 8th ed. Wolters Kluwer; 2018:1562-1606, Figure 55.1.)

VIDEO 38.2
Nociceptive Pathways

the posterolateral tract before entering the dorsal horn to synapse on second-order neurons. Second-order neuron cell bodies are located in the dorsal horn and are either nociceptive specific or wide dynamic range. Axons transmitting somatic nociception decussate and ascend via the contralateral spinothalamic tract, while axons transmitting visceral nociception ascend via the ipsilateral dorsal column medial lemniscus. Both synapse on the third-order neurons in the thalamus, the axons of which terminate in the sensory cortex. In the face, the primary afferent neuron has its cell body in the trigeminal ganglion and synapses on the second-order neuron in the medulla in the spinal trigeminal nucleus. From here, the signal is transmitted to the thalamus, as are pain signals from the rest of the body.

D. Modulation

Modulation of the pain response occurs at many levels and can be positive or negative (**Figure 38.3**). Activity between first- and second-order neurons is decreased by feedback from interneurons and descending inhibition from

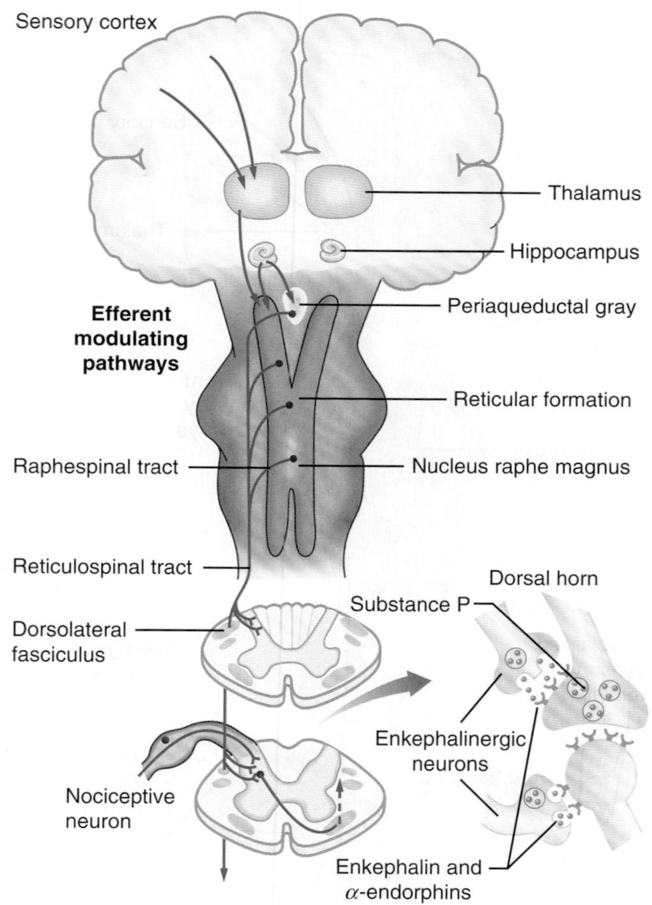

Figure 38.3 **The efferent pathway for modulation of nociception.** (From Macres SM, Moore PG, Fishman SM. Acute pain management. In: Barash PG, Cahalan MK, Cullen BF, et al, eds. *Clinical Anesthesia*. 8th ed. Wolters Kluwer; 2018:1562-1606, Figure 55.2.)

the periaqueductal gray matter, rostral ventromedial medulla, and the dorsolateral pontine tegmentum. Augmentation of pain may occur as part of the transition from acute to chronic pain. Repetitive activation of wide dynamic range neurons by C fibers causes windup. Axonal sprouting causes crosstalk between different fibers, causing nonnoxious stimuli to become painful. In addition, neuromas and axonal sprouting may be associated with upregulation of sodium and downregulation of potassium channels, which cause destabilized cell membranes to become more prone to forming an action potential. Normally Aβ fibers do not produce substance P, but in the presence of tumor necrosis factor-α from injury, Aβ fibers can secrete it. This transition is termed ***phenotypic switch***.

E. Perception

Perception of pain is mediated by multiple structures. The primary and secondary somatosensory cortices are involved with sensory discrimination of pain. The frontal cortex and insula may facilitate learning and memory of pain. The anterior cingulate gyrus is related to emotional significance of pain, while the lentiform nucleus and cerebellum are involved in self-protective reflexes related to pain.

II. Assessment of Pain

Pain is a highly subjective experience and affects many aspects of life. As such, the evaluation of the patient in pain relies primarily on patient-reported information and should include assessment of multiple domains. Because pain is dynamic, it should be reassessed regularly and adjustments to therapy made as appropriate. The location of the pain and where it radiates, if at all, are important. In the postoperative setting, it is still necessary to ask where the pain is located rather than presume the pain is incisional. Patients may have additional pain related to preexisting conditions, positioning or retraction during surgery, and immobility. The onset and temporal pattern as well as exacerbating and ameliorating factors are established. The quality of the pain can help indicate its origin and possible treatment options—sharp incisional pain may respond well to opioids and nerve blocks, but shooting neuropathic pain may respond to an antiepileptic agent.

The intensity of pain should be assessed in multiple contexts. The baseline level of pain is the pain that exists at all times, while breakthrough pain escalates beyond the background intensity. Multiple tools exist to aid in the assessment of pain intensity, all of which are arbitrary, are subjective, and have a high degree of variability between patients. Despite these flaws, they are useful to determine trends in pain control. The numerical rating scale is most commonly used, which asks patients to rate their pain from 0, no pain, to 10, worst pain imaginable. For young children or patients with cognitive impairments, the facial grimace scale allows for a more descriptive approach (**Figure 38.4**).

Because pain impacts many activities, it is important to investigate the patient's functional status including the ability to eat, sleep, ambulate, work, and perform one's activities of daily living. Any side effects from pain therapy should be thoroughly discussed as well. Physical examination is focused on possible etiologies of pain and should include a thorough neurologic and musculoskeletal examination.

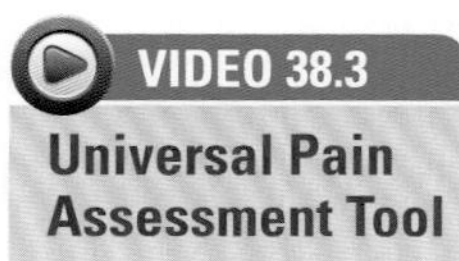

Universal pain assessment tool

This pain assessment tool is intended to help patient care providers assess pain according to individual patient needs. Explain and use 0–10 scale for patient self-assessment. Use the faces or behavioral observations to interpret expressed pain when patient cannot communicate his/her pain intensity.

	0	1	2	3	4	5	6	7	8	9	10
Verbal descriptor scale	No pain		Mild pain		Moderate pain		Moderate pain		Severe pain		Worst pain possible
Wong-Baker facial grimace scale	Alert smiling		No humor serious flat		Furrowed brow pursed lips breath holding		Wrinkled nose raised upper lips rapid breathing		Slow blink open mouth		Eyes closed moaning crying
Activity tolerance scale	No pain		Can be ignored		Interferes with tasks		Interferes with concentration		Interferes with basic needs		Bedrest required

Figure 38.4 **Universal pain assessment tool. Different scales can be used depending on the patient's age and other medical conditions.** (From Macres SM, Moore PG, Fishman SM. Acute pain management. In: Barash PG, Cahalan MK, Cullen BF, et al, eds. *Clinical Anesthesia*. 8th ed. Wolters Kluwer; 2018:1562-1606, Figure 55.12.)

III. Pharmacologic Management of Pain

A. Opioids

Opioids are useful for acute pain and cancer-related pain and can be a component of a chronic pain regimen. In acute pain, short-acting agents are typically used alone. In chronic pain, 80% of the daily dose is given in a basal long-acting medication with the remainder given as a short acting opioid as needed for breakthrough. When assessing patients for opioid management, it is important to inquire about the level of analgesia provided, whether the patient's functional status is improved, the side effects of therapy, and whether the patient displays aberrant behaviors (ie, early refills, lost pills, unscheduled appearance in the clinic).

Opioids bind to the μ, κ, and δ receptors to cause analgesia and side effects, such as pruritus, nausea, constipation, and respiratory depression. Various opioids have different potencies, bioavailabilities, and dosages (**Table 38.2**). For ease of comparison and conversion from one medication to another, they are all compared to the prototypical opioid, morphine. When converting from one opioid to another, it is important to reduce the expected dosage by 25% to 50% to account for incomplete cross-tolerance to the new agent. When treating patients with opioids, precision of terminology is important. ***Tolerance*** is the phenomenon of decreased effect of a given amount of medication. It usually occurs after prolonged administration of the drug. ***Dependence*** is the physiologic condition of withdrawal symptoms when an opioid is discontinued. ***Addiction*** is a disease marked by altered behavior to seek the desired substance despite negative consequences. ***Pseudoaddiction*** is aberrant drug-seeking behavior due to undertreatment of pain.

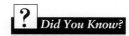

It is important to know the differences between drug tolerance, dependence, addiction, and pseudoaddiction.

Morphine is metabolized by the liver to morphine-6-glucuronide (M6G) and morphine-3-glucuronide (M3G), which are renally excreted. M6G is analgesic due to μ-binding activity and is responsible for respiratory depression, sedation, and nausea. M3G has no μ effect and is associated with hyperalgesia, seizures, and tolerance. Morphine's half-life is 2 hours, but its duration of action is 4 to 5 hours due to its slow elimination from the brain compartment.

Hydromorphone is five times more potent than morphine and is associated with fewer side effects. It is metabolized in the liver to dihydromorphine and

Table 38.2 Opioid Pharmacokinetics and Equianalgesic Dosing

Drug	Onset	Duration	Active Metabolite	Oral Equianalgesic Dose	IV Equianalgesic Dose
Fentanyl	IV: immed IM: 7-8 min	IV: 30-60 min IM 1-2 h Transdermal: 72 h	—	—	100 µg
Hydromorphone	IM: 15 min PO: 30 min	4-5 h	—	6-8 mg	1.5-2 mg
Meperidine	PO: 15 min IM/SQ: 10-15 min IV: immed	2-4 h	Normeperidine	300 mg	100 mg
Methadone	IV: 10-20 min PO: 30-60 min	4 h ($t_{½}$ is 8-59 h)	—	Variable	Variable
Morphine	IM: 10-30 min	4-5 h	Morphine-6-glucuronide	30 mg	10 mg
Oxymorphone	5-10 min	3-6 h	—	10 mg	1 mg
Oxycodone	<60 min	3-4 h	—	20 mg	10-15 mg
Remifentanil	Rapid	5-10 min	—	—	50 µg
Sufentanil	IV: immed Epidural: 10 min	Epidural: 1.7 h	—	—	10-40 µg

IM, intramuscular; immed, immediately; IV, intravenous; PO, oral; SQ, subcutaneous; $t_{½}$, half-life.
Derived from Benzon HT, Hurley RW, Hayek SM, et al. Chronic pain management. In: Barash PG, Cahalan MK, Cullen BF, et al, eds. *Clinical Anesthesia*. 8th ed. Wolters Kluwer; 2018:1607-1631.

dihydroisomorphine, which are active, and hydromorphone-3-glucuronide, which does not cause analgesia but is similar in side effects to M3G. Its onset is 15 minutes when administered intravenously and its duration of action is similar to that of morphine.

Fentanyl is 80 times more potent than morphine and is associated with less histamine release and pruritus. It is more lipophilic than morphine. It is metabolized by the liver and is appropriate for patients with renal failure. It is available as a transdermal patch. Due to gradual absorption of the drug, the patch requires 6 to 8 hours to reach maximum plasma concentrations. The patch provides steady-state analgesia without periods of side effects related to high serum concentrations and periods of pain due to low serum concentrations. After removal of the patch, significant serum levels remain; hence, intramuscular opioid should not be given immediately.

Sufentanil is 1000 times as potent as morphine and is typically used in intraoperative infusions or neuraxially. It has a slightly shorter elimination half-life than fentanyl. Alfentanil is 10 times the potency of morphine and has its peak effect within 2 minutes. It has a very short duration of action, <10 minutes, and is ideal for brief periods of intraoperative stimulation. Remifentanil is approximately 100 times the potency of morphine. Like alfentanil, it is also rapid acting. It is eliminated by plasma cholinesterases, so its terminal half-life is 10 to 20 minutes. Its termination of analgesia is so rapid that it may result in rebound hyperalgesia.

Methadone is a unique opioid because it enhances analgesia by antagonizing the *N*-methyl-D-aspartate (NMDA) receptor and inhibiting serotonin reuptake in addition to its μ effect. It is metabolized in the liver by cytochrome P450 and has many drug interactions. It has a variably long elimination half-life, between 8 and 80 hours, requiring slow titration to avoid accidental overdose. After a single dose, it provides analgesia for 3 to 6 hours, but with prolonged around-the-clock dosing, the duration of analgesia can be 8 to 12 hours. Methadone can cause prolonged QT and torsades de pointes, requiring periodic electrocardiograms.

Meperidine is a short-acting opioid that is metabolized in the liver to normeperidine, which can be neurotoxic and result in seizures, especially in the setting of renal failure or prolonged dosing. It is indicated for short-term use only. Its most common usage is in low doses to treat postoperative rigors.

Oxycodone is activated by conversion to oxymorphone; it is approximately twice as potent as morphine. Both drugs are associated with less pruritus than morphine. Tramadol, hydrocodone, and codeine are considered weak opioids. Tramadol is a μ agonist with monoaminergic properties. It carries low rates of constipation, respiratory failure, and abuse. Codeine is a prodrug that is metabolized to morphine by cytochrome P450 2D6. Reductions in enzymatic activity, as seen in children and certain ethnic groups (whites and Asians), cause decreased analgesia and increased respiratory depression.

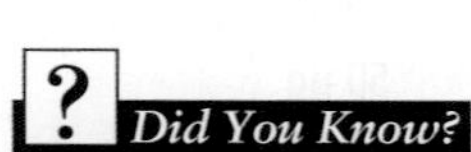

Did You Know?

Acetaminophen is a centrally acting COX inhibitor with minimal peripheral action that causes analgesia and antipyrexia but has no anti-inflammatory effect.

B. Nonsteroidal Anti-inflammatory Drugs

Nonsteroidal anti-inflammatory drugs (NSAIDs) work by inhibiting cyclooxygenase (COX) enzymes, exerting anti-inflammatory, antipyretic, and analgesic effects. COX-1 is present in healthy tissue and serves gastroprotective and hemostatic functions. COX-2 is induced in injury and produces prostaglandins that sensitize peripheral nociceptors to pain and promote hyperalgesia. NSAIDs are effective at reducing postoperative pain and opioid consumption and are commonly used in both acute and chronic pain. Side effects include platelet dysfunction, nephrotoxicity, and gastric ulcers. Acetaminophen is a centrally acting COX inhibitor with minimal peripheral action. It causes analgesia and antipyrexia but has no anti-inflammatory effect.

? *Did You Know?*

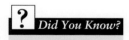

Chronic nerve damage is associated with spontaneous ectopic firing of neurons and anticonvulsants reduce ectopic signals by blocking sodium or calcium channels. Thus, anticonvulsants may be useful in treating neuropathic pain.

C. Anticonvulsants

Chronic nerve damage is associated with spontaneous ectopic firing of neurons and changes in sodium and calcium channel expression. Anticonvulsants reduce ectopic signals by blocking sodium or calcium channels. Gabapentin and pregabalin both block α_2-δ subunit of calcium channels. Both have been shown to be helpful in multiple neuropathic pain syndromes, including postherpetic neuralgia (PHN), diabetic painful neuropathy (DPN), trigeminal neuralgia, human immunodeficiency virus (HIV) neuropathy, spinal cord injury pain, phantom limb pain, and poststroke pain. In acute pain, preoperative gabapentin has been shown to decrease narcotic requirements, improve pain control, and reduce opioid-related side effects. Neither gabapentin nor pregabalin have significant drug-drug interactions. Side effects of both drugs include dizziness, fatigue, peripheral edema, cognitive slowing, and reduced renal function.

D. Antidepressants

Tricyclic antidepressants (TCAs) and serotonin-norepinephrine reuptake inhibitors (SNRIs) exert an independent analgesic effect distinct from their mood stabilizing properties. TCAs affect many pathways, including inhibition of the reuptake of serotonin and adenosine, interaction with α receptors, opioid receptor binding, and blockade of sodium channels, calcium channels, and NMDA receptors. They are effective at treating neuropathic pain, especially PHN and diabetic peripheral neuropathy (DPN), but frequent side effects limit their use. These include sedation, xerostomia, urinary retention, and blurred vision and tend to be more pronounced in the elderly. Nortriptyline and desipramine are better tolerated than amitriptyline.

SNRIs cause pain relief by inhibiting the reuptake of norepinephrine more than serotonin. SNRIs (duloxetine and milnacipran) are effective in DPN and fibromyalgia and are commonly prescribed in other neuropathic pain syndromes because of their minimal side-effect profile compared with TCAs. Selective serotonin reuptake inhibitors (SSRIs) have not been proven to have analgesic properties outside of their beneficial effect on depressive symptoms.

E. *N*-methyl-D-aspartate Antagonists

NMDA receptors provide a nonopioid strategy for pain management and can be helpful in the opioid-dependent patient. NMDA stimulation is thought to play a role in development of chronic pain, opioid-induced hyperalgesia, and windup. Ketamine is the prototypical NMDA antagonist. It has poor oral bioavailability, so it is used in intravenous infusions to reduce opioid requirements. Dosage is limited by side effects, including tachycardia, salivation, and dysphoria.

F. Alpha Adrenergics

Clonidine and dexmedetomidine are both central α_2 agonists. Binding causes reduced norepinephrine output, which causes sedation and analgesia in addition to reduced heart rate and blood pressure without affecting respiratory drive. The half-life of clonidine is 9 to 10 hours. It can be given orally, intravenously, or intrathecally. When given as a transdermal patch, it can be helpful to mitigate adrenergic symptoms of opioid withdrawal. The half-life of dexmedetomidine is 2 hours. Because it is much more selective for α_2 than α_1, as compared with clonidine, intravenous infusion is used for profound sedation with analgesia, with a lower incidence of bradycardia and hypotension.

G. Glucocorticoids

Glucocorticoids, including dexamethasone, inhibit phospholipase A2 to block the production of prostaglandins and leukotrienes and have analgesic and anti-inflammatory effects. They are useful perioperatively to reduce pain and nausea but may be associated with poor wound healing. Bursts of steroids (eg, hydrocortisone, methylprednisolone) can be useful in the management of chronic pain, such as radiculitis, but side effects such as gastric ulcers, osteoporosis, water retention, hypertension, and hyperglycemia limit long-term use.

H. Local Anesthetics

Lidocaine can be delivered in patch form directly to an area of neuropathic pain. The medication is slowly absorbed and blocks sodium channel locally, rather than a systemic effect. It can be helpful in PHN, peripheral neuropathy, osteoarthritis, myofascial pain, and low-back pain. It may require as long as 2 weeks of daily patch use to obtain relief. Intravenous lidocaine infusion can be given for neuropathic pain resistant to other treatments. Dosing is typically 5 mg/kg over 30 minutes. Mexiletine is an orally available local anesthetic with a similar effect to intravenous lidocaine.

I. Topical Agents

Capsaicin's mechanism of action is to stimulate TRPV1 receptors, which then causes reduced nerve fiber density. Substance P may also be depleted. It is available in a low concentration cream, which must be applied three to four times daily for weeks to experience relief. A patch form (8%) is effective in PHN, DPN, and HIV neuropathy when applied. Local anesthetic ointment must be applied for an hour before the patch to mitigate the burning sensation of the patch; relief from one application can last 12 weeks.

IV. Acute Pain

A. Surgical Stress Response and Preventive Analgesia

Postoperative pain occurs by the mechanisms described above. The surgical stress response is the systemic response to the operation, in which cytokines are released with various negative responses. Chemical mediators of the surgical stress response include interleukin-1, interleukin-6, and tumor necrosis factor-α, which promote inflammation. Poorly controlled pain results in increased levels of catecholamine release, which in turn disrupts the neuroendocrine balance. Hormonal changes include increased secretion of cortisol and glucagon paired with decreased secretion of insulin and testosterone. Together these result in a catabolic state with a negative nitrogen balance, hyperglycemia, poor wound healing, muscle wasting, fatigue, and immune compromise. Other negative effects of the surgical stress response are tachycardia, hypertension, increased cardiac work, bronchospasm, splinting, pneumonia, ileus, oliguria, urinary retention, thromboembolism, impaired immunity, weakness, and anxiety. Preventive analgesia is the concept of perioperative strategies for reducing pain-mediated sensitization of the nervous system with the goal of reducing long-term pain. To be effective, preventive analgesia must cover the entire surgical field and be adequate enough to prevent nociception during surgery as well as the entire perioperative period.[2] This period of time is variable for each patient and type of surgical procedure, but typically is less than 30 days.

B. Strategies for Acute Pain Management

Patient-Controlled Analgesia

Intravenous patient-controlled analgesia (IV PCA) has been shown to be a safe alternative to intermittent intravenous boluses of opioids for acute pain, with improved patient satisfaction, decreased nursing requirements, and lower opioid requirements. The general principle is that the patient self-administers incremental boluses of medication at safe intervals, building up the dose until adequate analgesia is achieved. The most common agents for PCA use are morphine, hydromorphone, and fentanyl (**Table 38.3**). Programmable variables include

Table 38.3 Common Dosing Parameters for Patient-Controlled Analgesia in Opiate-Naive Patients

Opioid	Demand Dose	Lockout (min)	Basal Infusion
Fentanyl	20-50 μg	5-10	0-60 μg/h
Hydromorphone	0.2-0.4 mg	6-10	0-0.4 mg/h
Morphine	1-2 mg	6-10	0-2 mg/h

Derived from Macres SM, Moore PG, Fishman SM. Acute pain management. In: Barash PG, Cahalan MK, Cullen BF, et al, eds. *Clinical Anesthesia*. 8th ed. Wolters Kluwer; 2018:1562-1606.

starting bolus, demand dose and interval, basal infusion rate, and 1- or 4-hour limit. The demand dose should be a fraction of the usual therapeutic dose. The dosing interval should be after the medication effect begins and before it starts to wane to allow for cumulative effect. A basal infusion may be employed in a patient on long-term opioid therapy, but should seldom, if ever, be used in the opioid-naïve patient. The 1- and 4-hour limits may be used to control overall dosage, but care must be taken not to restrict it so severely that the patient uses all the allowable boluses in the first portion of the time interval and is without analgesia for the remainder. PCA may result in overdose and respiratory depression. Side effects include nausea, pruritus, and altered mental status. Risk factors include obstructive sleep apnea, congestive heart failure, pulmonary disease, renal or hepatic failure, head injury, and altered mental status.

? *Did You Know?*

The programmable variables when administering IV PCA include starting bolus, demand dose and interval, basal infusion rate, and 1- or 4-hour limit.

Neuraxial and Regional Analgesia

Epidural infusion provides improved pain control with activity, decreased respiratory complications, and decreased postoperative ileus compared with systemic opioids. The placement of the catheter should be chosen to cover the dermatome levels of the surgical incision. Epidural local anesthetic provides somatic analgesia but may cause hypotension and weakness. Epidural opioids provide visceral analgesia but can cause pruritus, respiratory depression, and urinary retention. The combination of opioids and local anesthetic is synergistic and allows for reduced dosage compared with single-agent infusions, minimizing side effects. Clonidine may be a useful adjuvant but could contribute to bradycardia and hypotension. Hypotension usually responds to fluid administration. Pruritus is due to spinal μ binding and is independent of histamine. Therefore, treatment is best accomplished with a low dose of mixed opioid agonist-antagonist, such as nalbuphine. Epidural infusions are usually continuous or continuous with a patient-administered bolus programmed. A relatively new strategy for epidural infusion dosing called programmed intermittent bolus (PIB) can additionally be utilized, which replaces the continuous slow infusion (usually over an hour) with a set bolus at a set time each hour.

Peripheral nerve blocks and continuous catheters are an important component of multimodal pain therapy as well. The discussion of this mode of anesthesia is beyond the scope of this chapter but is well discussed in Chapter 21.

C. Special Cases in Acute Pain

Pediatrics

Acute pain management in children must be tailored to the individual child and family. Assessment of pain is sometimes difficult in younger children, but family and other caregivers can aid in this evaluation. The same techniques can be employed in children as in adults. PCA in older children is safe, as long as no one other than the patient delivers a bolus dose. Epidural infusions and ultrasound-guided peripheral nerve blocks are useful and are commonly placed after induction of anesthesia, rather than awake, as in adults. Caudal injection of local anesthetic is an excellent treatment for postoperative pain for perineal, lower extremity, and lower abdominal cases. Local anesthetic must be dosed appropriately for weight.

The Opioid-Dependent Patient

As a general rule, the perioperative period is not a time to wean opioid usage. Clinical observations show that opioid requirements are approximately doubled from baseline in the postoperative period. The patient's long-acting

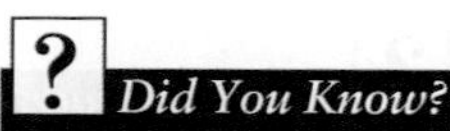

Opioid requirements in the opioid-dependent patient are approximately doubled from baseline in the postoperative period.

opioid should be continued unchanged. If fasting status prohibits dosing of oral medication, the equianalgesic amount should be administered as the baseline infusion in a PCA. The bolus dose should be set 25% to 50% higher than for an opioid-naïve individual. Regional and epidural analgesia is helpful in reducing overall opioid dosage, though care should be taken not to administer opioids through more than one route. To avoid cumulative effect, epidural infusions often consist of local anesthetic only, paired with intravenous opioid PCA. Ketamine, NSAIDs, antiepileptics, acetaminophen, and antidepressants can assist with pain control and limit opioids as well. Medications should be weaned to baseline postoperatively.

Enhanced Recovery After Surgery and Multimodal Analgesia

Many institutions employ enhanced recovery after surgery (ERAS) protocols to facilitate the care of their surgical patients in the preoperative, intraoperative, and postoperative settings. This multidisciplinary approach has been shown to decrease length of stay and reduce postoperative complications by using evidence-based strategies to reduce pain and nausea, minimize fluid shifts, and improve return of postoperative bowel function and ambulation.[3] Minimizing opioid use is crucial to reducing postoperative ileus and other side effects including respiratory depression and nausea, thus multimodal analgesia is often implemented. In addition to regional anesthesia, other techniques such as scheduled anti-inflammatory medications, gabapentinoids, intravenous local anesthetic (lidocaine), and ketamine infusions can be employed. However, much of the evidence for these protocols is in the colorectal literature and increasing number of subspecialty surgeries are beginning to find use for them.[3]

V. Chronic Pain

A. Management of Common Pain Syndromes

Low-back and buttock pain can have a number of possible etiologies, including disk herniation or internal disruption, facet joint syndrome, piriformis syndrome, sacroiliac joint syndrome, myofascial pain, fibromyalgia, as well as vertebral body compression fractures, inflammatory conditions, spinal neoplastic lesions, infections, and rarely vascular malformations.[4]

Low-Back Pain: Radicular Pain Syndromes

When pain radiates in a dermatomal distribution, it is considered ***radicular*** and can be accompanied by weakness, depressed reflexes, numbness, and tingling in the same dermatomal distribution (**Figure 38.5; Table 38.4**). Pain is typically sharp and lancinating. Physical examination often reveals antalgic gait, limited straight leg raise test, diminished or absent reflexes, reduced strength, and decreased sensation in the affected spinal level. Radicular pain is typically the result of irritation or dysfunction of the spinal nerve root in the epidural space, which can be due to mechanical compression of the nerve root and/or a chemical radiculitis from the inflammatogenic cascade of leukotrienes and cytokines released by the injured disk. Spinal imaging can be helpful in diagnosis and should be obtained early in setting of neurological change, history of IV drug use, suspected infection, history of significant trauma, history of cancer, and in the immunosuppressed host.

Treatment of radicular pain syndromes is best managed in a multimodal fashion. NSAID medications, oral steroids, physical therapy (PT), short periods

Table 38.4 Muscle Innervation and Deep Tendon Reflexes by Spinal Level

Spinal Level	Muscle Action	Reflexes
C5	Shoulder abduction	Biceps
C6	Elbow flexion	Brachioradialis
C7	Elbow extension	Triceps
C8	Thumb extension	—
L2	Hip flexion	—
L3	Knee extension	—
L4	Ankle dorsiflexion	Patella
L5	Great toe extension	Medial hamstring
S1	Ankle plantar flexion	Achilles

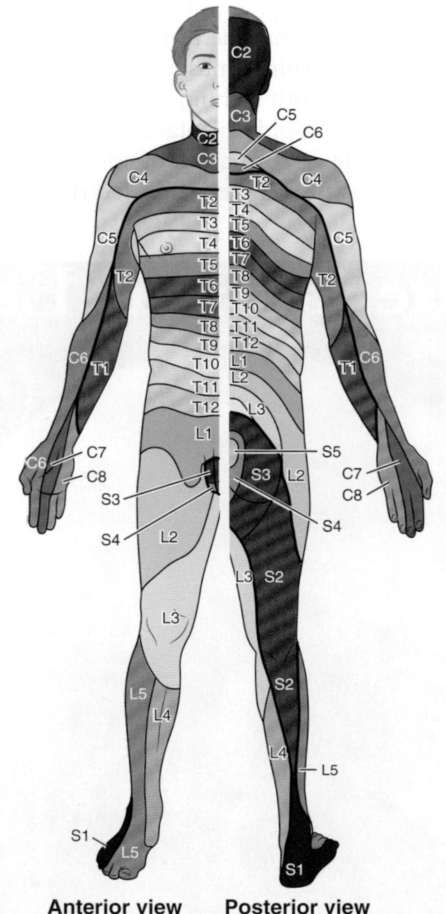

Figure 38.5 **Dermatome map for localization of affected level, planning appropriate epidural placement.** (From Moore KL, Agur AMR, Dalley II AF. *Clinically Oriented Anatomy*. 8th ed. Wolters Kluwer; 2018, Figure 1.36.)

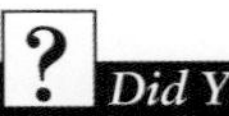

Did You Know?

ESIs are most effective in patients with acute radiculitis and less effective for management of chronic symptoms and nonradicular pain. Surgery does not appear to produce better long-term outcomes for radiculitis than a more conservative approach.

of bed rest, and neuropathic pain medications such as gabapentin or pregabalin can be helpful. If symptoms do not respond to these measures, ***epidural steroid injection (ESI)*** of corticosteroid can reduce inflammation in the epidural space by reducing the activity of phospholipase A2 and blocking nociceptive C-fiber conduction. ESIs have been shown to provide short-term (<3 months) relief of radicular pain. ESIs are most effective in patients with acute radiculitis and less effective for management of chronic symptoms and nonradicular pain. Surgery does not appear to produce better long-term outcomes for radiculitis than a more conservative approach. The natural history of low-back and radicular pain due to a herniated disk is one of gradual improvement with conservative measures. Thus, the use of epidural steroids can minimize the use of systemic medications and their attendant side effects during periods of exacerbation.

ESIs are best performed with fluoroscopy guidance. In the interlaminar approach, a Tuohy epidural needle is advanced through the skin, subcutaneous tissue, supraspinous ligament, interspinous ligament, and finally the ligamentum flavum. A loss of resistance technique to air, or saline, is employed to confirm entry into the dorsal epidural space after traversing the ligamentum flavum. Alternatively, the transforaminal approach may be used, which deposits the steroid more ventrally, closer to the disk-nerve interface. In this technique, the entry point is off midline to the affected side and the needle is directed through skin and paraspinal musculature, traveling medially toward the intervertebral foramen. In both techniques, a small amount of radiopaque contrast is injected to confirm epidural placement, and rule out vascular or intrathecal uptake. Following confirmation of epidural placement, corticosteroid diluted in local anesthetic or saline is injected (**Figure 38.6**).

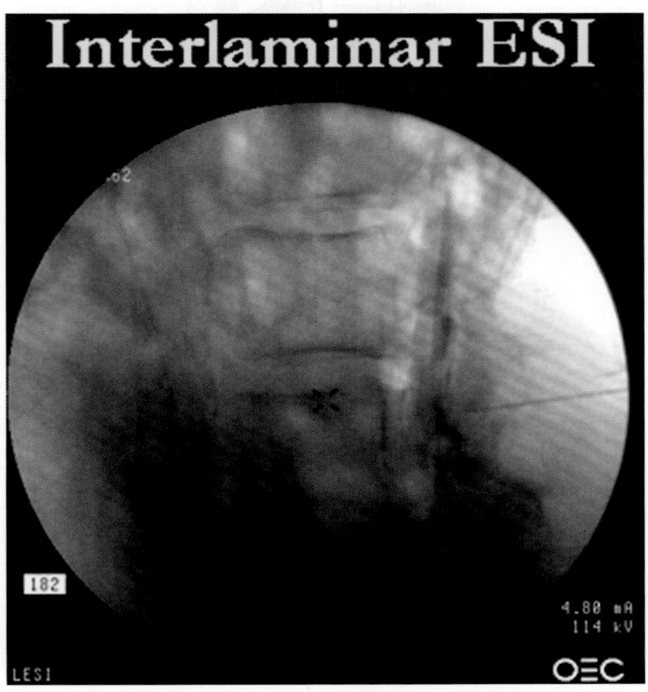

Figure 38.6 Lateral view of an interlaminar approach showing predominant spread of the contrast in the posterior epidural space with minimal spread into the anterior epidural space. ESI, epidural steroid injection.

There are multiple randomized controlled trials investigating the efficacy of ESI with varying results.[5] Most show short-term relief of lumbar radiculopathy symptoms. There are fewer studies of ESIs in cervical radiculopathy, but those also generally show short-term relief of symptoms.[6] There have been comparisons between the transforaminal and interlaminar approaches, which generally favor the transforaminal technique. Comparison of transforaminal to lateral interlaminar (parasagittal) showed better contrast spread in parasagittal injections but with similar efficacy. The short-term relief achieved from ESI can be helpful in returning a patient to function and reducing the toxicity from systemic medications, but it should be used as an adjuvant to multimodal therapy, not a sole treatment.

Complications include damage to the spinal cord or peripheral spinal nerves, epidural hematoma and infection, all of which can cause irreversible neurologic deficit. The incidence of hematoma is reduced by the timely discontinuation of anticoagulant agents per the American Society of Regional Anesthesia (ASRA) guidelines for neuraxial intervention.[7] Penetration of the radicular artery during lumbar transforaminal ESI, or the ascending cervical, deep cervical, or vertebral artery during cervical transforaminal ESI, can result in traumatic shearing, vasospasm, or embolism of steroid, which, in turn, can cause infarction to the brain or spinal cord.

In addition, systemic corticosteroid absorption can cause side effects. Blood pressure and serum glucose levels can be elevated anywhere from 2 days to several weeks after ESI. Exogenous corticosteroids can suppress the hypothalamic-pituitary-adrenal axis, with even a single dose reducing plasma cortisol and corticotropin levels for weeks.

The patient should be reevaluated 2 to 3 weeks after the ESI. If there is no response to a single injection, it can be repeated once, because some patients who did not have relief after one injection have relief after the second. A third injection can be performed if partial relief occurs, but a series of more than three regardless of relief is not advised.

Low-Back Pain: Facet Syndrome

The zygapophyseal joints (facet joints) are paired diarthrodial joints formed by the articulation of the inferior articular process of one vertebra with the superior articular process of the inferior vertebra. Along with the disk, the paired facet joints form the three-joint complex responsible for load bearing and prevent forward displacement and rotatory dislocation of the intervertebral joint. They normally transmit 10% to 15% of the body's weight and are subject to arthritis and increased forces in the presence of spondylolisthesis and disk degeneration. Facetogenic pain is axial and can radiate to the buttock and posterior thigh on the affected side. Physical examination is positive for paraspinal muscle tenderness and pain with ipsilateral rotation during extension. Facet joints are innervated by the medial branches of the dorsal rami, so pain relief from medial branch blocks or facet joint injections can confirm diagnosis. Intra-articular facet joint injections of corticosteroid can produce long-lasting analgesia. If pain relief is transient and there is relief from medial branch blocks, radiofrequency ablation of the medial branches can be performed.[8]

Buttock Pain: Sacroiliac Joint Syndrome

Sacroiliac (SI) joints are paired joints formed by the articulation of the sacrum to the ileum, they are vital load bearing joints with little mobility. Like any joint, the SI joint is subject to arthritis, either intrinsic or secondary to spondyloarthropathies, and vulnerable to any biomechanical abnormalities affecting the lower extremity-pelvis-spine interface. SI joint pain is commonly described near the posterior superior iliac spine (PSIS) and the buttock. It may radiate to the posterior thigh and calf as well as the groin. Physical examination is significant for pain with palpation of the PSIS and stressing of the joint, such as by the FABER (Flexion, Abduction and External Rotation of the hip). Gaenslen, or Yeoman maneuvers. Treatment of SI joint syndrome can include physical therapy, NSAIDs, intra-articular steroid injections, radiofrequency denervation of the L5 medial branch and sacral (S1-S3) lateral branches, and surgical fusion.

Buttock Pain: Piriformis Syndrome

Buttock pain originating from the piriformis occurs from muscular irritation, such as from trauma, infection, or surgery. Pain may radiate to the posterior thigh and calf, indicating irritation of the sciatic nerve by the piriformis muscle. The pain is typically worse with prolonged sitting or moving from sitting to standing. Physical examination reveals pain with *f*lexion, *a*dduction, and *i*nternal *r*otation (FAIR, Lasegue) of the hip, with the patient supine; pain or weakness with resisted abduction with hip flexed (pace), with the patient sitting; and pain with passive internal rotation of an extended thigh (Freiberg sign). Computed tomography (CT) or magnetic resonance imaging may show enlarged piriformis; electromyogram may show signs of neuropathy or myopathy, but the diagnosis is clinical. Treatment includes physical therapy, NSAIDs, and muscle relaxants. Injections of local anesthetic and steroid into the muscle belly can also be helpful. Intramuscular botulinum toxin, or surgical release, can be considered in refractory cases.

Myofascial Pain Syndrome

Trigger points are focal, palpable areas of pain in muscle or fascia. Palpation of these nodules may provoke a twitch response or reproduce radiating pain in a distribution characteristic of the muscle involved. ***Myofascial pain syndrome*** is local, regional, and referred pain that originates from these trigger points. Treatment of myofascial pain syndrome includes massage and stretching, postural training, physical therapy, trigger point injections with local anesthetic or botulinum toxin, and dry needling.

Fibromyalgia

Fibromyalgia is associated with widespread pain, sleep disturbance, fatigue, and cognitive/psychosomatic perturbations. Diagnostic criteria no longer depend upon presence of tender points on physical examination, but place greater emphasis on patient-reported symptoms. Per 2016 revision, the diagnosis of fibromyalgia can be made if all of the following criteria are fulfilled: (1) generalized pain in at least four of five regions (left upper, left lower, right upper, right lower, and axial [jaw, chest, and abdominal pain are not included]), (2) presence of symptoms for at least 3 months, (3) widespread pain index (WPI) ≥ 7 and symptom severity scale (SSS) score ≥ 5 OR WPI of 4 to 6 and SSS score ≥ 9, and (4) diagnosis of fibromyalgia is valid regardless of other diagnoses.[9] Other regional pain syndromes (headaches, irritable bowel syndrome, temporomandibular joint dysfunction, interstitial cystitis) may also be present. Treatment of fibromyalgia is multimodal and should include an exercise program, cognitive behavioral therapy, land- and/or aquatic-based PT, and medications. Opiates are typically not effective, but SNRIs (eg, milnacipran, duloxetine, venlafaxine), pregabalin, gabapentin, and TCAs can be helpful.

Neuropathic Pain Syndromes

Herpes Zoster (HZ) and PHN

PHN is a chronic neuropathic pain following reactivation of latent varicella zoster virus (VZV) infection within neuronal cells. HZ classically manifests as pain and a vesicular eruption within a dermatomal fashion, and most cases will resolve with medication therapy, but 5% to 20% go on to develop PHN. PHN is characterized by chronic allodynia, hyperalgesia, and dysesthesias within the same dermatome as prior HZ rash, and is attributed to immune versus inflammatory damage to neurons during VZV reactivation. Rates of PHN rise steeply after the age of 65 years, such that 20% to 30% of elderly patients with HZ develop PHN. Besides older age, other risk factors include high intensity of pain during acute zoster, severity of zoster rash, and painful prodrome (presence of pain prior to rash onset). In adults VZV reactivation can be prevented by vaccination with the live attenuated shingles vaccine approved for adults >50 years of age. In adults who develop HZ, the likelihood of developing PHN is reduced by prompt administration of antiviral drugs such as acyclovir, famciclovir, and valacyclovir.[10]

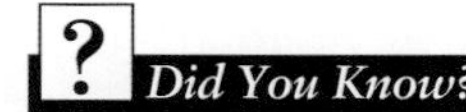

The likelihood of developing PHN is reduced by prompt administration of antiviral drugs. Treatment of PHN is primarily medical, relying on the use of anticonvulsants such as gabapentin and pregabalin, TCAs, and topical lidocaine as first-line treatments.

Opioid analgesics, antidepressants, anticonvulsants, and topical capsaicin can be utilized in conjunction with first-line agents or solely as second-line treatments for refractory disease. Topical medications such as lidocaine patch and capsaicin can also be helpful. The following intervention can be tried if medications are ineffective: subcutaneous injection of botulinum toxin A or triamcinolone, peripheral nerve stimulation, stellate ganglion blockade, paravertebral blocks, and pulsed radiofrequency ablation. If severe pain persists, spinal cord stimulation can be considered. Destruction of the dorsal root ganglion and intrathecal methylprednisolone injection should only be entertained after careful discussion with the patient.

Diabetic Painful Neuropathy

The incidence of DPN increases with age, duration of diabetes, and severity of hyperglycemia. The most common subtypes are distal symmetric polyneuropathy, proximal neuropathy, focal neuropathy, and visceral autonomic neuropathy. It is unknown why some patients experience painful neuropathy and others do not.

Treatments include tight glycemic control and neuropathic medications. The serotonin-norepinephrine reuptake inhibitors (eg, duloxetine, milnacipran) are considered first-line therapy due to their efficacy and favorable side effect profile. Other medications include gabapentin, pregabalin, TCAs, and anticonvulsants. Opioids are considered last-line medications. Spinal cord stimulation has been effective at managing neuropathic symptoms up to 5 years post initiation of treatment.[11,12]

Complex Regional Pain Syndrome

Complex regional pain syndrome (CRPS) is a chronic pain syndrome that can develop after a known nerve injury (type II, formerly causalgia) or in the absence of previous nerve injury (type I, formerly reflex sympathetic dystrophy). It is characterized by sensory, sudomotor, vasomotor, and motor/trophic signs and symptoms.[13] Sensory changes include allodynia, hyperalgesia, hyperesthesia, or spontaneous pain. Sudomotor changes are sweating abnormalities or edema. Vasomotor symptoms are temperature abnormalities or skin color changes. Motor deficiencies include decreased range of motion,

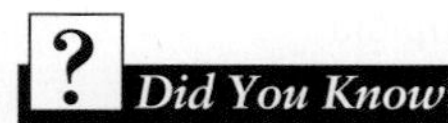

CRPS is diagnosed clinically by meeting specified historical and physical criteria.

Table 38.5 Budapest Criteria for Complex Regional Pain Syndrome

1. Continuing pain, which is disproportionate to any inciting event
2. Must display at least one sign at time of evaluation in two or more of the following categories:
   a. Sensory
   b. Vasomotor
   c. Sudomotor/edema
   d. Motor/trophic
3. Must report at least one symptom in three of the four following categories:
   a. Sensory
   b. Vasomotor
   c. Sudomotor/edema
   d. Motor/trophic
4. There is no other diagnosis that better explains the signs and symptoms

From Harden RN, Bruehl S, Stanton-Hicks M, et al. Proposed new diagnostic criteria for complex regional pain syndrome. *Pain Med.* 2007;8:326-331, with permission.

weakness, tremor, or neglect. Trophic changes are changes in hair or nail growth (**Table 38.5**). Risk factors include female sex, work-related injury, and previous surgery. The diagnosis is one of exclusion, is made clinically utilizing the Budapest criteria, and can be supported by osteopenia on radiographs and metabolic alterations on three-phase bone scan.

Treatment should be multimodal and focus on functional restoration, pain management, and psychological treatment. Physical therapy is useful for desensitization and strengthening. Medications can include gabapentin, pregabalin, duloxetine, TCAs, memantine, opioids, calcitonin, and bisphosphonates. Sympathetic blocks of the upper (stellate) and lower (lumbar paravertebral sympathetic) extremity ganglions with local anesthetic can be effective in the acute phase to reduce allodynia and permit functional restoration. In refractory cases of CRPS spinal cord stimulation (SCS) and/or dorsal root ganglion (DRG) stimulation of the lower extremity can be effective procedural approaches to analgesia.

HIV Neuropathy

Neuropathy in HIV can be viral related or due to nucleoside reverse transcriptase inhibitors used for treatment of the infection. Allodynia and hyperalgesia are most commonly located in the lower extremities and may respond to lamotrigine or gabapentin (**Table 38.6**).

Table 38.6 Recommended Medications for Chronic Pain Conditions

Postherpetic Neuralgia	Diabetic Painful Neuropathy	Spinal Cord Injury	Fibromyalgia	Human Immunodeficiency Virus
Pregabalin	Duloxetine	Pregabalin	Duloxetine	Lamotrigine
Gabapentin	Pregabalin	Gabapentin	Pregabalin	Gabapentin
Opioid	Gabapentin	Lamotrigine	Milnacipran	
Antidepressants	Antidepressants	IV lidocaine	Tramadol	
Tramadol		Mexiletine		
Lidoderm patch				

IV, intravenous.

Derived from Macres SM, Moore PG, Fishman SM. Acute pain management. In: Barash PG, Cahalan MK, Cullen BF, et al, eds. *Clinical Anesthesia*. 8th ed. Wolters Kluwer; 2018:1562-1606.

Phantom Pain

Phantom limb sensation may be experienced by up to 80% of patients with amputated extremities, but phantom pain is significantly less common. The incidence may be reduced by adequate preoperative pain control prior to the amputation. Methods have included epidural infusion and continuous plexus blocks. Treatment includes opioids, gabapentin, NMDA antagonists like ketamine and memantine, and antidepressants. Nonpharmacologic techniques include biofeedback, mirror therapy, transcutaneous electrical nerve stimulation, and spinal cord or peripheral nerve stimulation.

Cancer Pain

Cancer pain is common in up to 90% of patients with advanced disease. It can be somatic pain, which responds well to opioids, NSAIDs, and neural blockade; visceral pain, which responds well to sympathetic blocks; or neuropathic pain, which is best treated with opioids, SNRIs, antiepileptics, and TCAs. Although opioids are the mainstay of treatment for cancer-related pain, management should include a combination of pharmacologic agents, antineoplastic treatment (chemotherapy, radiation), medicinal marijuana, interventional procedures as necessary, and psychological care.[14]

Neurolytic Blocks for Visceral Pain From Cancer

The abdominal organs, with the exception of the descending colon, are innervated by the ***celiac plexus***, which lies on the anterior surface of the aorta at L1. The celiac plexus is made up of sympathetic fibers from the greater, lesser, and least splanchnic nerves, as well as parasympathetic fibers from the vagus nerve. Reduction of pain from the abdominal organs, such as that associated with pancreatic cancer, can be accomplished by the blockade of the splanchnic nerves at the anterior margin of T12 or the retrocrural or anterocrural blockade of the plexus anterior to the L1 vertebral body. Fluoroscopic or CT guidance is mandatory. Alcohol (50%-100%) or phenol (6% aqueous) is used to coagulate the target nerves, allowing for weeks to months of pain relief before the nerves regenerate. Complications can include orthostatic hypotension, transient diarrhea, aortic dissection, back pain, retroperitoneal hematoma, hematuria, pleurisy, hiccups, and paraplegia.

The superior hypogastric plexus, a continuation of the sympathetic chain, innervate the pelvic organs. It is located anterior to the L5-S1 disk space and can be blocked bilaterally or with a single-needle transdiscally.

The perineal area, including the distal rectum, anus, vulva, distal vagina, and distal urethra, are innervated via the ganglion impar, the termination of the sympathetic chain. It is a midline structure located anterior to the sacrococcygeal junction. The transcoccygeal approach is most commonly employed, wherein a needle is placed through the sacrococcygeal ligament until its tip is just anterior to the distal sacrum; care must be taken to avoid rectal puncture.

Interventional Procedures

Minimally Invasive Lumbar Decompression Procedure

The minimally invasive lumbar decompression procedure is indicated to treat spinal stenosis related to ligamentum flavum hypertrophy. An epidural needle is placed and an epidurogram is performed, followed by contouring of the lamina and partial debulking of the hypertrophic ligamentum flavum. This partially decompresses the central canal and alleviates symptoms of back pain and neurogenic claudication attributed to disproportionate ligamentum hypertrophy.

Vertebroplasty and Kyphoplasty

Vertebroplasty and *kyphoplasty* are procedures to treat painful vertebral body compression fractures, usually due to osteoporosis. In both procedures, trocars are inserted percutaneously into the fractured vertebral body, either through the pedicle or extrapedicular approach. In kyphoplasty, a balloon is inflated within the vertebral body fracture to restore height and correct the kyphotic defect. The cavity created after balloon inflation is then filled with cement. In vertebroplasty, the cement is injected directly into the fractured trabeculae without balloon augmentation. In both procedures, the patient remains supine for several hours post intervention to observe neurologic status. Complications can include hematoma, cement leakage into vasculature resulting in pulmonary embolism, and retropulsion of bone fragments or cement into the spinal canal causing neurologic deficit. Long-term sequelae can include return of pain and fracture at an adjacent vertebral level.

Neuromodulation

Spinal cord stimulation involves placement of electrodes within the midline posterior epidural space along the dorsal columns. Electrical stimulation of these tracts can cause paresthesias, masking the sensation of pain. The most commonly postulated theory is modulation of gate control. The stimulator increases the output of larger Aβ fibers responsible for the sensation of touch. These Aβ fibers cause excitation of interneurons in the substantia gelatinosa, which inhibit transmission of signals from smaller pain-mediating C fibers, thereby "closing the gate." The characteristics of electrical pulses and waveforms necessary to form paresthesias can be defined using terminology common to wave theory: frequency, amplitude, and pulse width. By manipulating these parameters, differing electrical waves can be generated and applied to the dorsal columns, thereby enhancing therapeutic options. Early spinal cord stimulator devices provided tonic, constant low-frequency (20-120 Hz) stimulation, to the dorsal columns between the perception (amplitude of stimulation first detected by patient) and discomfort (amplitude where paresthesias became noxious) threshold. Newer therapeutic strategies have been developed focusing on higher frequency and/or burst stimulation. In high-frequency stimulation, up to 10 KHz can be delivered to spinal tracts, resulting in near paresthesia-free stimulation. By altering frequency, different neuronal pathways can be activated, and at 1000 Hz, afferent sensory neuron conduction was altered compared to 50 Hz stimulation. Burst stimulation combines higher frequency stimulation at 500 Hz along with increased pulse width of the pulse waves to create paresthesia-free stimulation. It is theorized this pattern of stimulation is more replicative of endogenous neuronal firing.[15,16] Spinal cord stimulation may help control symptoms and reduce opioid usage in patients with failed back surgery syndrome, neuropathic pain, CRPS, angina, and chronic limb ischemia. Patients should first undergo a psychological screening process to determine appropriateness for therapy and have excellent pain relief from temporary trial leads prior to permanent implantation. Trial leads may be implanted percutaneously in an outpatient clinic and are typically left in 5 to 7 days. Permanent leads may be implanted percutaneously or via laminectomy. The leads exit the epidural space and are tunneled to a battery implanted subcutaneously. Complications of SCS can be stratified into hardware-related issues, such as lead migration, fracture, disconnection, pulse generator pain, implantable pulse generator (IPG) flipping, and charging difficulties; or biologic issues, such as superficial or deep infection, seroma, hematoma, wound dehiscence, or rarely dural puncture and spinal cord/spinal nerve injury.[17]

Focal areas of truncal or lower extremity pain may not be amenable to coverage with traditional SCS, and dorsal root ganglion (DRG) stimulation has emerged as a viable alternative for these refractory pain syndromes. The procedure involves epidural placement of electrodes adjacent to the DRG, within the posterosuperior neuroforamen. The DRG houses the cell bodies of sensory neurons, and stimulation of the DRG is thought to modulate neuronal excitability responsible for neuropathic pain transmission. DRG stimulation has shown efficacy for lower extremity neuropathic pain, CRPS, PHN, and postherniorrhaphy pain. Risks of the procedure are similar to conventional SCS, with higher risk of lead fracture, migration, and unique risks of motor stimulation and possible spinal nerve injury if the neuroforamen is stenotic.[18]

Peripheral nerve stimulation (PNS) is indicated to treat pain originating from a single peripheral nerve. Unlike DRG or conventional SCS, PNS can be utilized anywhere a peripheral nerve can be isolated. Leads are implanted using fluoroscopic or ultrasound guidance to lie adjacent to the painful nerve. The mechanism of peripheral nerve stimulation is thought to involve gate control theory but at the level of the peripheral nerve. Through direct electrical stimulation of larger Aβ fibers within sensory afferents, pain-mediated C-fiber activation is blunted at the level of the spinal interneuron.[19]

Intrathecal Drug Delivery

Intrathecal drug delivery systems, or intrathecal pumps, consist of an intrathecal catheter tunneled under the skin to an internalized pump and drug reservoir. Infused medications may include opioids, bupivacaine, and clonidine. Ziconotide is used for neuropathic pain, and baclofen is indicated for spasticity. The most common opioids used are morphine, hydromorphone, and fentanyl. Intrathecal opioids are indicated in malignant pain when oral and transdermal opioids have failed to provide adequate relief despite appropriate dosing or when side effects limit upward titration of opioids. Medications are placed in the spinal fluid, bypassing the blood-brain barrier and allowing for much lower effective doses and an improved side effect profile. Side effects can include respiratory depression, headache, pruritus, peripheral edema, intrathecal catheter granuloma formation, and hormone disruption. Intrathecal catheter granuloma formation involves the development of an inflammatory mass near the catheter tip, attributed to alterations of cerebrospinal fluid dynamics, and this can cause direct compression of spinal cord contents prompting surgical intervention. Duration of intrathecal therapy is a known risk factor for granuloma formation; other possible risk factors include previous history of spinal surgery, spinal cord injury, and a higher association with hydromorphone infusions.[20,21]

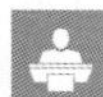

For further review, please see the associated Interactive Video Lectures accessible in complimentary eBook bundled with this text. Access instructions are located on the inside front cover.

References

1. Merksey H, Bogduk N. *A current list with definitions and notes on usage*. In: *Classification of Chronic Pain*. 2nd ed. IASP Press; 1994. Accessed May 7, 2020. www.iasp-pain.org/Education/Content.aspx?ItemNumber=1698

2. Macres SM, Moore PG, Fishman SM. Acute pain management. In: Barash PG, Cullen BF, Stoelting RK, et al, eds. *Clinical Anesthesia*. 8th ed. Wolters Kluwer; 2017:1562-1606.
3. Ljungqvist O, Scott M, Fearon KC. Enhanced recovery after surgery: a review. *JAMA Surg*. 2017;152(3):292-298. doi:10.1001/jamasurg.2016.4952. PMID: 28097305.
4. Benzon HT, Hurley RW, Hayek SM. Chronic pain management. In: Barash PG, Cullen BF, Stoelting RK, et al, eds. *Clinical Anesthesia*. 8th ed. Wolters Kluwer; 2017:1607-1631.
5. Benyamin RM, Manchikanti L, Parr AT, et al. The effectiveness of lumbar interlaminar epidural injections in managing chronic low back and lower extremity pain. *Pain Physician*. 2012;15(4):E363-E404. PMID: 22828691.
6. Cohen SP, Hooten WM. Advances in the diagnosis and management of neck pain. *Br Med J*. 2017;358:j3221. doi:10.1136/bmj.j3221. PMID: 28807894.
7. Narouze S, Benzon HT, Provenzano D, et al. Interventional spine and pain procedures in patients on antiplatelet and anticoagulant medications (second edition): guidelines from the American society of regional anesthesia and pain medicine, the European society of regional anaesthesia and pain therapy, the American academy of pain medicine, the International neuromodulation society, the North American neuromodulation society, and the world institute of pain. *Reg Anesth Pain Med*. 2018;43(3):225-262. doi:10.1097/AAP.0000000000000700. PMID: 29278603.
8. Lord SM, Barnsley L, Wallis BJ, et al. Percutaneous radio-frequency neurotomy for chronic cervical zygapophyseal-joint pain. *N Engl J Med*. 1996;23:1721-1726. doi:10.1056/NEJM199612053352302. PMID:8929263.
9. Wolfe F, Clauw DJ, Fitzcharles MA, et al. 2016 Revisions to the 2010/2011 fibromyalgia diagnostic criteria. *Semin Arthritis Rheum*. 2016;46(3):319-329. doi:10.1016/j.semarthrit.2016.08.012. PMID: 27916278.
10. Mallick-Searle T, Snodgrass B, Brant JM. Postherpetic neuralgia: epidemiology, pathophysiology, and pain management pharmacology. *J Multidiscip Healthc*. 2016;9:447-454. doi:10.2147/JMDH.S106340. PMID: 27703368.
11. Beek M, Geurts JW, Slangen R, et al. Severity of neuropathy is associated with long-term spinal cord stimulation outcome in painful diabetic peripheral neuropathy: five-year follow-up of a prospective two-center clinical trial. *Diabetes Care*. 2018;41(1):32-38. doi:10.2337/dc17-0983. PMID: 29109298.
12. Hurley RW, Henriquez OH, Wu CL. Neuropathic pain syndromes. In: Benzon HT, ed. *Raj's Practical Management of Pain*. 5th ed. Mosby Elsevier; 2014:346-361.
13. Harden RN, Bruehl S, Stanton-Hicks M, et al. Proposed new diagnostic criteria for complex regional pain syndrome. *Pain Med*. 2007;8:326-331. doi:10.1111/j.1526--4637.2006.00169.x . PMID: 17610454.
14. Scarborough BM, Smith CB. Optimal pain management for patients with cancer in the modern era. *CA Cancer J Clin*. 2018;68(3):182-196. doi:10.3322/caac.21453. PMID: 29603142.
15. Miller JP, Eldabe S, Buchser E, et al. Parameters of spinal cord stimulation and their role in electrical charge delivery: a review. *Neuromodulation*. 2016;19(4):373-384. doi:10.1111/ner.12438. PMID: 27150431.
16. Morales A, Yong RJ, Kaye AD, et al. Spinal cord stimulation: comparing traditional low-frequency tonic waveforms to novel high frequency and burst stimulation for the treatment of chronic low back pain. *Curr Pain Headache Rep*. 2019;23(4):25. doi:10.1007/s11916-019-0763-3. PMID: 30868285.
17. Eldabe S, Buchser E, Duarte RV. Complications of spinal cord stimulation and peripheral nerve stimulation techniques: a review of the literature. *Pain Med*. 2016;17(2):325-336. doi:10.1093/pm/pnv025. PMID: 26814260.
18. Harrison C, Epton S, Bojanic S, et al. The efficacy and safety of dorsal root ganglion stimulation as a treatment for neuropathic pain: a literature review. *Neuromodulation*. 2018;21(3):225-233. doi:10.1111/ner.12685. PMID: 28960653.
19. Deer TR, Jain S, Hunter C, et al. Neurostimulation for intractable chronic pain. *Brain Sci*. 2019;9(2):2. doi:10.3390/brainsci9020023. PMID: 30682776.
20. Narouze SN, Casanova J, Souzdalnitski D. Patients with a history of spine surgery or spinal injury may have a higher chance of intrathecal catheter granuloma formation. *Pain Pract*. 2014;14(1):57-63. doi:10.1111/papr.12024. PMID: 23360382.
21. Veizi IE, Hayek SM, Hanes M, Galica R, Katta S, Yaksh T. Primary hydromorphone-related intrathecal catheter tip granulomas: is there a role for dose and concentration? *Neuromodulation*. 2016;19(7):760-769. doi:10.1111/ner.12481. PMID: 27505059.

Questions

1. **If an epidural catheter is placed to provide analgesia for a major abdominal surgery, how do you decide the optimal thoracic interspace to place it?**

   A. There is no difference as all interspaces are equianalgesic.
   B. The placement of the catheter should be chosen to cover the dermatome levels of the surgical incision.
   C. A lumbar catheter should be placed so you can also offer an intrathecal dose.
   D. None of the above.

2. **Which are essential components of an ERAS (enhanced recovery after surgery) protocol?**

   A. A multidisciplinary team that can access the patient before, during, and after the surgery
   B. Applying strategies to minimize fluid shifts that will improve postoperative bowel function and ambulation
   C. Reducing opioid use in order to decrease side effects like respiratory depression and nausea
   D. All of the above

3. **A 45-year-old male patient with history of prostate cancer status post radical prostatectomy presents to the pain clinic for evaluation of worsening low-back pain and new-onset radicular leg pain. Pain is associated with worsening bladder incontinence, which he attributes to his previous urologic surgery. On sensory examination, he has reduced perineal sensation, absent deep tendon reflexes in his lower extremities, altered gait, and weakness of his right extensor hallucis longus with a foot drop. Which of the following is the next best step?**

   A. Referral for physical therapy
   B. Trial of nonsteroidal anti-inflammatory drugs (NSAIDs)
   C. Urgent lumbar spine MRI and spine surgical consultation
   D. Lumbar epidural steroid injection to target right the L5 nerve root

4. **You receive a palliative medicine request for celiac plexus block for a 60-year-old woman with stage IV pancreatic adenocarcinoma. Her tumor has metastasized to the colon causing a malignant bowel obstruction. Despite surgical palliation, her bowel obstruction persists, and her abdominal pain remains severe despite high-dose intravenous opioids. You identify mild thrombocytopenia with platelets 122,000 and normal coagulation parameters, though she is on prophylactic enoxaparin. She has a history of pruritus to iodinated contrast. Which of the following is an absolute contraindication to celiac plexus blockade?**

   A. Relative thrombocytopenia
   B. Malignant bowel obstruction
   C. Hypersensitivity reaction to contrast
   D. Enoxaparin administration

5. **A 28-year-old male patient with cerebral palsy presents to the emergency room with altered mental status, hyperthermia, rigidity, and increased spasticity. His caregiver states he recently missed his intrathecal pump medication refill and the low volume alarm has been beeping for days. Which of the following medications is he most likely withdrawing from?**

   A. Baclofen
   B. Ziconotide
   C. Clonidine
   D. Bupivacaine

Answers

1. B

The epidural catheter should be placed at the vertebral level that innervates the painful area(s).

2. D

ERAS incorporates all the above components for ideal results.

3. C

The worsening bladder incontinence and new-onset radicular leg pain may indicate spine metastases and need to be ruled out.

4. B

Celiac plexus blockade is contraindicated in setting of malignant bowel obstruction because unopposed parasympathetic activity will promote peristaltic activity against a fixed obstruction. Choice A is incorrect because platelets, though low, remain above the 100k threshold for intervention. Choice C is incorrect because her hypersensitivity is mild, and so anaphylaxis to contrast would be an absolute contraindication. Choice D is incorrect because enoxaparin can be held, per American Society of Regional Anesthesia (ASRA) guidelines, prior to spinal intervention.

5. A

Intrathecal baclofen withdrawal associated with increased spasticity, hyperthermia, altered mental status, and labile blood pressure. Prompt resumption of baclofen therapy, whether it be oral, intravenous, or intrathecally administered could be lifesaving. Choice B is incorrect because there have been no reported cases of ziconotide withdrawal. Choice C, clonidine, is incorrect because intrathecal clonidine withdrawal can cause severe hypertension, tachycardia, and agitation. Choice D is incorrect because local anesthetic cessation would lead to gradual return of motor and sensory function, with abolition of hypotension.

39 Nonoperating Room Anesthesia and Special Procedures

Karen J. Souter and Najma Mehter

Nonoperating room anesthesia (NORA) refers to anesthesia services that are provided outside of traditional surgical operating rooms and labor and delivery areas. These locations include, but are not limited to, radiology departments, endoscopy suites, magnetic resonance imaging (MRI), computed tomography (CT) scanners, cardiac catheterization laboratories (CCL) and electrophysiology laboratories (EPL). NORA cases account for over 30%[1] of the procedural work of hospitals, and increasingly, patients or the proceduralists require or request anesthesia or sedation to facilitate these procedures. This chapter will discuss the care of patients requiring anesthesia or sedation for procedures in NORA locations. Anesthesia for surgical procedures performed in offices and ambulatory surgery centers is addressed in Chapter 25, and anesthesia and analgesia provided for labor and delivery is discussed in Chapter 31.

I. The Three-Step Approach to NORA

NORA covers a diverse spectrum of patients, procedures, and locations, and a systematic approach is recommended. The simple ***three-step paradigm***—the ***patient,*** the ***procedure,*** and the ***environment***—may be a useful mnemonic for NORA (**Figure 39.1**).

A. The Patient

Patients may require sedation or anesthesia to tolerate NOR procedures for a number of reasons (**Table 39.1**). Children often require sedation or anesthesia for diagnostic and therapeutic procedures. Patients with significant comorbidities or surgical disease may be too ill to tolerate a major operative procedure, whereas a palliative, less invasive NOR procedure may be possible. All patients presenting for NORA require a thorough ***preanesthesia assessment***[2] and the development of a sound anesthetic plan with appropriate levels of monitoring.

B. The Procedure

Common NOR procedures for which the patient may require anesthesia or sedation are listed in (**Table 39.2**). The anesthesiologist must understand all the details of the NOR procedure, specifically the position the patient will be in, how painful the procedure will be, how long it will take, and any special requirements (such as use of contrast media or the need to wake the patient up halfway through). ***Preoperative communication*** with the proceduralist is essential and must include discussion of contingency plans for emergencies and complications.

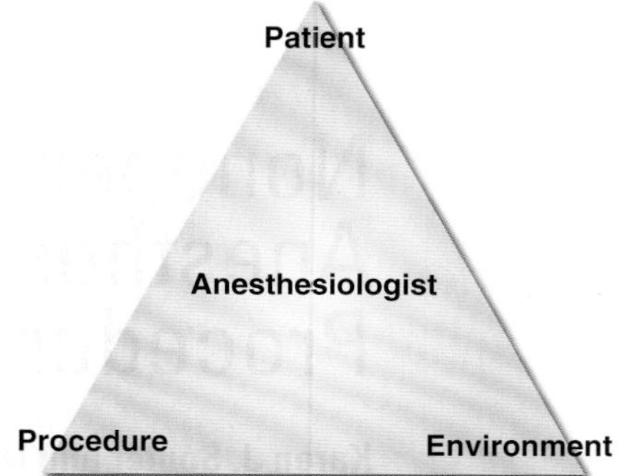

Figure 39.1 A simple three-step paradigm for nonoperating room anesthesia.

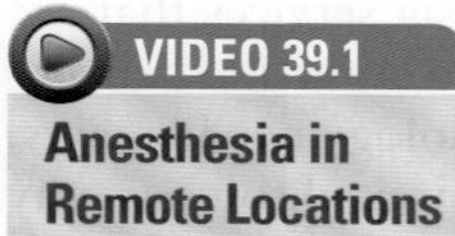

C. The Environment

Unlike in operating rooms, the conditions under which NORA services are delivered may vary greatly in terms of the space, equipment, and staff available. A number of factors contribute to NORA sites being unfamiliar and less optimal environments for anesthesia providers (**Figure 39.2**):

1. These locations were often designed before or without considering whether anesthesia would be needed for patients undergoing care. Access to the patient by the anesthesia provider is often limited by diagnostic and therapeutic equipment such as CT and MRI scanners, fluoroscopes, or endoscopy towers.
2. Hazards unique to specific locations exist such as radiation in fluoroscopy and CT and the magnetic field in MRI.
3. Proceduralists and ancillary staff may be unfamiliar with the requirements for safe anesthesia care and how to assist anesthesia providers when a difficulty is encountered.
4. Away from the operating room, immediate help from anesthesia colleagues in case of emergency may not be readily available.

The American Society of Anesthesiologists (ASA) has developed ***guidelines*** for NORA.[3] Prior to the anesthetic, the presence and proper functioning of all equipment needed for safe patient care must be established; this is described in **Table 39.3**.

The location of immediately available resuscitation equipment should be noted and protocols developed with the local staff for dealing with

Table 39.1 Patient Factors Requiring Sedation or Anesthesia for Nonoperating Room Procedures

- Claustrophobia, anxiety, and panic disorders
- Cerebral palsy, developmental delay, and learning difficulties
- Seizure disorders, movement disorders, and muscular contractures
- Pain related to the procedure or the positioning or unrelated pain
- Acute trauma with unstable cardiovascular, respiratory, or neurologic function
- Increased intracranial pressure
- Significant comorbidity and patient frailty (American Society of Anesthesiologists grades III and IV)
- Child's age, especially children <10 y old

Table 39.2 Common Nonoperating Room Anesthesia Procedures

Radiologic imaging	Computed tomography Magnetic resonance imaging Positron emission tomography
Diagnostic and therapeutic interventional radiology	Various vascular imaging, stenting, and embolization procedures Radiofrequency ablation Transjugular intrahepatic portosystemic shunt
Diagnostic and therapeutic interventional neuroradiology	Occlusive ("closing") procedures Embolization of cerebral aneurysm/arteriovenous malformations/highly vascular tumors (eg, meningiomas) Opening procedures Angioplasty/stenting/thrombolysis in stroke or cerebral vasospasm
Radiotherapy	Radiation therapy Intraoperative radiotherapy Diagnostic and therapeutic interventional cardiology
Cardiac catheterization laboratory	Diagnostic cardiac catheterization/percutaneous coronary interventions/balloon mitral valvuloplasty (usually without anesthesiologist) Interventional techniques for structural heart disease—transcatheter aortic valve replacement (TAVR)/left atrial appendage closure/mitral clip repair (with anesthesiology) Placement of left ventricular cardiac assist devices for hemodynamic support
Electrophysiology laboratory	Electrophysiology studies and arrhythmia ablations Implantation of biventricular pacing systems and cardioverter-defibrillators
Other cardiac-related procedures	Cardioversion and transesophageal echocardiography
Diagnostic and therapeutic interventional gastroenterology	Upper gastroenterology endoscopy Esophageal dilatation or stenting Percutaneous endoscopic gastrostomy tube placement Endoscopic retrograde cholangiopancreatography Colonoscopy Liver biopsy
Psychiatry	Electroconvulsive therapy
Dentistry	Dental extractions Restorative dentistry

emergencies, including cardiopulmonary resuscitation and the management of anaphylaxis.

II. Standards of Care for NORA

Many NOR procedures are performed under ***sedation*** or ***monitored anesthesia care***. Anesthesia care may be thought of as a continuum, with a gradual transition from the awake state, through progressively deepening sedation to general anesthesia (**Table 39.4**).[4]

As sedation deepens, progressive blunting of the airway reflexes, with the potential for airway obstruction, together with depression of spontaneous ventilation can ensue. The individual responsiveness of patients to different

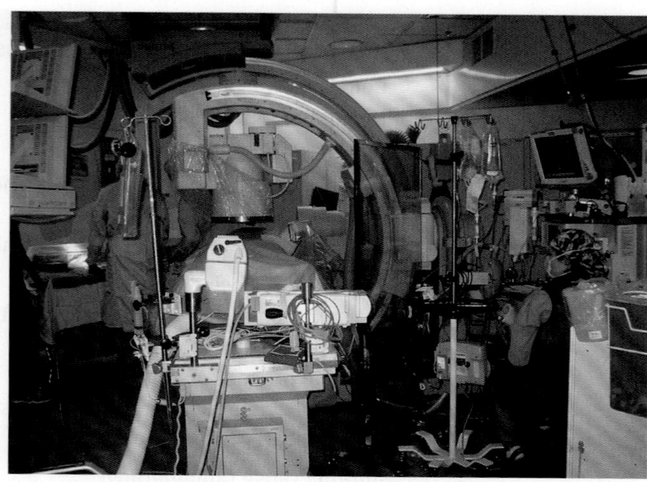

Figure 39.2 A radiology suite showing a C-arm and the high density of equipment that may separate the anesthesiologist from the patient.

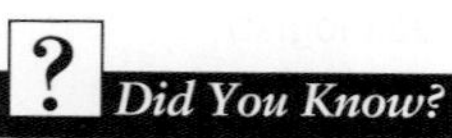

Did You Know?

The same standards for operating rooms should be applied to patients being cared for in all nonoperating room sites.

sedative agents varies, as do the levels of stimulation during the course of a procedure. Consequently, during the course of an NOR procedure under sedation, the patient may drift to a deeper level than is intended, resulting in airway and respiratory depression. It is, therefore, essential that the person providing sedation be properly trained to care for a patient who drifts to a deeper level of sedation than the level originally intended.

At the conclusion of the NOR procedure, the patient should be transported by a member of the anesthesia team to a recovery area that is equipped to the same standards as for all postoperative patients.

III. Adverse Events

?

Did You Know?

More than 80% of surgical patients with obstructive sleep apnea are unaware that they have that disease prior to undergoing surgery.

Significant adverse events in NORA are rare; however, malpractice closed claims analysis[5] demonstrate that while claims for NORA were less frequent than for OR anesthesia, NORA had a higher proportion of claims for death than operating room settings. NORA claims were most frequently seen in cardiology and radiology locations. NORA complications were more likely to occur during monitored anesthesia care and be related to inadequate oxygenation and ventilation. Furthermore, aspiration pneumonitis occurred in a higher proportion of NORA malpractice claims than it did in the operating room.

IV. Environmental Considerations for NORA

A. X-rays and Fluoroscopy

Fluoroscopy (C-arm) is widely used in many NOR locations, including interventional radiology, cardiac catheterization, electrophysiological procedures, and in the gastroenterology suite. The C-arm moves back and forth around the patient during the procedure, requiring large amounts of space, limiting access to the patient, and serving as a means of dislodging intravenous lines and endotracheal tubes (**Figure 39.2**).

B. Computed Tomography

The CT procedure is painless, and most adults do not require sedation or anesthesia. For children or adults with neurologic or psychological disorders,

Table 39.3 American Society of Anesthesiologists' Standards for Nonoperating Room Anesthesia Locations

1. Oxygen-reliable source and full backup equivalent to E-cylinder
2. Reliable and adequate suction that meets operating room standards
3. Scavenging system if inhalational agents are administered
4. Anesthetic equipment
   Backup self-inflating bag capable of delivering at least 90% oxygen by positive-pressure ventilation
   Adequate anesthetic drugs and supplies
   Anesthesia machine with equivalent function to those in the operating rooms and maintained to the same standards
   Adequate monitoring equipment to allow adherence to the ASA standards for basic monitoring
5. Electrical outlets
   Sufficient for anesthesia machine and monitors
   Isolated electrical power or ground fault circuit interrupters if "wet location"
6. Adequate illumination of patient, anesthesia machine, and monitoring equipment
   Battery-operated backup light source
7. Sufficient space for
   Personnel and equipment
   Easy and expeditious access to patient, anesthesia machine, and monitoring equipment
8. Resuscitation equipment immediately available
   Defibrillator/emergency drugs/cardiopulmonary resuscitation equipment
9. Adequately trained staff to support the anesthesiologist and a reliable means of two-way communication
10. All building and safety codes and facility standards should be observed
11. Postanesthesia care facilities:
    Adequately trained staff to provide postanesthesia care
    Appropriate equipment to allow safe transport to main postanesthesia care unit

ASA, American Society of Anesthesiologists.
From *Statement on Nonoperating Room Anesthetizing Locations. Committee of Origin: Standards and Practice Parameters.* Approved by the ASA House of Delegates on October 19, 1994, last amended on October 16, 2013, and reaffirmed October 17, 2018. https://www.asahq.org/standards-and-guidelines/statement-on-nonoperating-room-anesthetizing-locations

sedation or anesthesia may be required. CT scanning may be employed to facilitate invasive and painful procedures such as abscess localization and drainage and ablation of tumors. Patients with acute thoracic, abdominal, and cerebral trauma often require urgent imaging to facilitate diagnosis. These patients may develop hemorrhagic shock, increased intracranial pressure (ICP), depression of consciousness, and cardiac arrest while in the CT scanner.

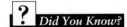

Always secure the airway and resuscitate hemodynamically unstable patients before they undergo CT or any other form of emergency diagnostic imaging!

Hazards of Ionizing Radiation

The effects of ***ionizing radiation*** on biologic tissues are classified as deterministic (severity of tissue damage is dose dependent, such as in cataract or infertility) and stochastic (probability of occurrence is dose related, such as in cancer or genetic effect).[6] Protective measures to reduce patient exposure to radiation should always be taken. Staff exposure to radiation can be minimized by

1. Limiting the time of exposure to radiation
2. Increasing the distance from the source of radiation
3. Using protective shielding (lead aprons, thyroid shields, and leaded eyeglasses)
4. Using dosimeters

Table 39.4 Definition of General Anesthesia and Levels of Sedation or Analgesia

Vital Sign	Minimal Sedation (Anxiolysis)	Moderate Sedation (Conscious Sedation)	Deep Sedation	General Anesthesia
Responsiveness	Normal response to verbal stimulation	Purposeful response to verbal or tactile stimulation	Purposeful response after repeated or painful stimulation	Unarousable, even with painful stimulus
Airway	Unaffected	No intervention required	Intervention may be required	Intervention often required
Spontaneous ventilation	Unaffected	Adequate	May be inadequate	Frequently inadequate
Cardiovascular function	Unaffected	Usually maintained	Usually maintained	May be impaired

From American Society of Anesthesiologists Task Force on Sedation and Analgesia by Non-Anesthesiologists. Practice guidelines for sedation and analgesia by non-anesthesiologists. *Anesthesiology.* 2002;96:1004-1017.

Did You Know?

The intensity of the radiation is inversely proportional to the *square* of the distance from the source (the inverse square law).

C. Magnetic Resonance Imaging

MRI, like CT, is painless and does not require sedation or anesthesia. However, the scanning sequences are considerably longer than for CT, so a scan of ≥30 minutes for younger children as well as adults with neurologic or psychological disorders, including claustrophobia, often requires sedation or anesthesia.[7]

Hazards of MRI

MRI is devoid of the risks related to ionizing radiation. However, magnetizable or ferromagnetic materials and electronic devices represent potential hazards to the patient and staff. For example, cardiac pacemakers may malfunction, intracerebral aneurysm clips may move, and transdermal medication patches may cause burns. Before entering the vicinity of the magnet, patients and staff need to complete a rigorous safety checklist. Ferromagnetic equipment such as intravenous poles, gas cylinders, laryngoscopes, and pens become potentially lethal projectiles if brought too close to the magnetic field. Patient monitors, ventilators, and electrical infusion pumps may malfunction in proximity to the scanner, and magnet-safe technology should be used. In the case of an emergency, resuscitation attempts should take place outside the scanner because equipment such as laryngoscopes and cardiac defibrillators cannot be taken close to the magnet.

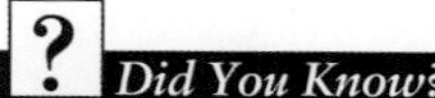

Thirty percent of adult patients experience some degree of anxiety during MRI scanning.

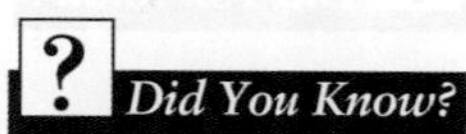

MRI field strength is measured in the units Gauss (G) and Tesla (T). 1 T = 10,000 G. The Earth's magnetic field is approximately 0.3 to 0.7 G, whereas the standard MRI generates a field of 1.5 to 3 T!

D. Intravenous Contrast Agents

Intravenous contrast agents are commonly used in CT and MRI scans to highlight organs, vessels, and tumors. Adverse reactions to contrast agents may occur and can be divided into renal adverse reactions and hypersensitivity reactions.

Renal Adverse Reactions

Contrast agents are eliminated via the kidneys, and patients with preexisting chronic renal disease, diabetes mellitus, dehydration, advanced age, and concomitant use of nephrotoxic drugs (eg, nonsteroidal anti-inflammatory drugs) are at risk of developing contrast-induced nephropathy. Preventative measures against contrast-induced nephropathy include adequate hydration, maintaining a good urine output, and using sodium bicarbonate infusions to improve elimination of the contrast agent. Gadolinium-containing contrast agents used in MRI scans may cause nephrogenic systemic fibrosis in patients with renal insufficiency.

Hypersensitivity Reactions

Hypersensitivity reactions to contrast media are divided into immediate (<1 hour) and non-immediate (>1 hour) reactions. The clinical manifestations of various hypersensitivity reactions to contrast media are outlined in **Table 39.5**. Treatment of moderate and severe immediate hypersensitivity reactions is identical to that of anaphylaxis.

V. Specific Nonoperating Room Procedures

A. Diagnostic and Interventional Radiology

Angiography

Angiography causes minimal discomfort and may be performed under local anesthesia with or without light sedation. Lengthy procedures and patients with recent cerebral vascular accidents, depressed levels of consciousness, or raised ICP may necessitate anesthesia with airway protection (tracheal intubation).

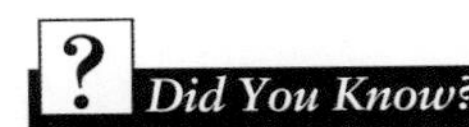

During interventional procedures, the anesthesiologist may be exposed to as much if not more radiation than the interventional radiologist.

Interventional Neuroradiology

Endovascular embolization may be used to treat cerebral aneurysms, arteriovenous malformations, and certain vascular tumors such as meningiomas. The endovascular treatment of acute ischemic stroke is becoming increasingly important with anesthesiologists assuming a vital role in the intraprocedural care of these patients.[8] General anesthesia and conscious sedation are both suitable techniques for interventional neuroradiology depending on the complexity of the procedure, the need for blood pressure manipulation, and the requirement for neurologic assessment during the procedure.

Table 39.5 Clinical Manifestations of Immediate and Nonimmediate Hypersensitivity Reactions to Radiocontrast Agents

Immediate Reactions	Nonimmediate Reactions
Pruritus	*Pruritus*
Urticaria	*Exanthema (mostly macular or maculopapular drug eruption)*
Angioedema/facial edema	Urticaria, angioedema
Abdominal pain, nausea, diarrhea	Erythema multiforme minor
Rhinitis (sneezing, rhinorrhea)	Fixed drug eruption
Hoarseness, cough	Stevens-Johnson syndrome
Dyspnea (bronchospasm, laryngeal edema)	Toxic epidermal necrolysis
Respiratory arrest	Graft-versus-host reaction
Hypotension, cardiovascular shock	Drug-related eosinophilia with systemic symptoms
Cardiac arrest	Symmetrical drug-related intertriginous and flexural exanthema
	Vasculitis

Note: Most frequent reactions are in italics.

Radiofrequency Ablation

CT-guided percutaneous radiofrequency ablation (RFA) is carried out for treatment of primary and metastatic tumors in solid organs. One-lung ventilation and high-frequency jet ventilation may be used in patients for RFA of liver tumors to minimize motion associated with diaphragm excursions from standard ventilation.

Transjugular Intrahepatic Portosystemic Shunt

A transjugular intrahepatic portosystemic shunt (TIPS) procedure is carried out using fluoroscopy and is performed to help alleviate portal hypertension in patients with advanced cirrhosis. The procedure may be performed under sedation or general anesthesia. Patients presenting for a TIPS procedure, in general, have significant hepatic dysfunction and require careful preoperative assessment and intraoperative management.

B. Radiation Therapy

External beam radiation is a common treatment for children with malignancies (**Table 39.6**).[9] The doses of radiation used are very high, and all personnel must leave the room during the treatment. An interfaced system of closed-circuit television, telemetric microphones, and standard monitoring is used to allow close observation of the patient during the procedure. Complete absence of movement is crucial during radiation therapy and general anesthesia or deep sedation techniques, with propofol the anesthetic of choice during these procedures.

C. Interventional Cardiology

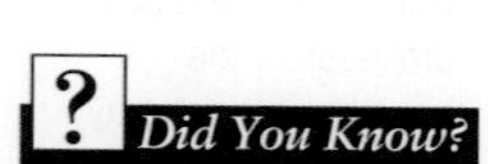

Transcatheter aortic valve implantation or replacement allows replacement of the aortic valve percutaneously in the CCL. High-risk patients who are too sick for open-heart surgery may be treated successfully.

Diagnostic and therapeutic interventional procedures are carried out in the *CCL* and *EPL*. These procedures are outlined in **Table 39.2**. Light or moderate sedation is commonly used under supervision of the cardiologist. However, general anesthesia is increasingly required for more lengthy and complex procedures, especially structural heart procedures.[10]

Electrophysiologic studies (EPS) and ablation of abnormal conduction pathways are performed for the treatment of dysrhythmias caused by aberrant conduction pathways. EPS are lengthy and can cause discomfort, especially when intraoperative dysrhythmias are provoked by the procedure and then terminated using overdrive pacing, or if unsuccessful, by external cardioversion. Anesthetic agents including volatile agents and muscle relaxants may interfere with ablation procedures; thus, communication with the proceduralists is of great importance in planning anesthesia for these procedures.[11] The ability to move the patient rapidly to the operating room and the availability of cardiopulmonary bypass are essential backups for CCL and EPL procedures.

Table 39.6 Common Radiosensitive Tumors in Children
Primary CNS tumor: neuroblastoma, medulloblastoma
Acute leukemia: CNS leukemia
Ocular tumors: retinoblastoma
Intra-abdominal tumors: Wilms tumor
Rhabdomyosarcoma
Other tumors: Langerhans cell histiocytosis

CNS, central nervous system.

D. Cardioversion

Transthoracic cardioversion is commonly used electively to treat dysrhythmias, especially atrial fibrillation and atrial flutter. Cardioversion takes a few seconds; however, it is distressing and painful. Therefore, deep sedation is used except in life-threatening situations. A small bolus of intravenous induction agent such as propofol or etomidate is usually sufficient for the procedure.

E. Nonoperating Room Pediatric Cardiac Procedures

Cardiac catheterization is performed in children with congenital heart disease for both hemodynamic assessment and interventional procedures. These children are often very sick and may present with cyanosis, dyspnea, congestive heart failure, and intracardiac shunts. In patients with a patent ductus arteriosus, high oxygen tension can lead to premature closure, and prostaglandin infusions are often used to maintain duct patency.

> **? Did You Know?**
>
> Pay meticulous attention to preventing air bubbles entering intravenous lines shunts in children with right-to-left shunts because they may cross to the arterial circulation, causing stroke or cardiac arrest.

F. Gastroenterology

Procedures commonly performed in the gastrointestinal endoscopy suite are outlined in **Table 39.2**. The majority of these procedures may be performed with light sedation (commonly fentanyl and midazolam or propofol infusion) without the involvement of an anesthesiologist.

Gastroenterologists, however, universally agree that patients in ASA classes III and IV who are undergoing complex procedures or have histories of adverse or inadequate responses to light or moderate sedation require the care of an anesthesiologist.[12]

The patient's condition, the position of the patient, and the specific procedure determine the anesthetic technique to be used. Local anesthetic may be sprayed into the oropharynx to facilitate passage of the endoscope, although this may abolish the gag reflex and increase the risk of aspiration. High-flow nasal oxygenation (HFNO) is a newer oxygenation technique that may be used in sedated patients. Under general anesthesia, patients usually require tracheal intubation to protect the proximal airway, which is shared with the endoscope during the procedure, although laryngeal mask airways have also been used.

G. Electroconvulsive Therapy

Electroconvulsive therapy (ECT) has been used in the management of severe depression, mania, and affective disorders. Patients typically undergo a series of regular treatments (three times a week for 6-12 treatments, followed by weekly or monthly maintenance). The procedures are usually performed in the postanesthesia care unit, where there is close access to anesthesia support service. Alternatively, they may be performed in the psychiatric unit where anesthesia services are not so readily available. ECT is distressing and possibly dangerous because generalized convulsions may result in limb injuries and significant cardiovascular reactions may occur. Light general anesthesia with muscle relaxation, usually provided with the short-acting muscle relaxant succinylcholine, is used to mitigate the unpleasant effects of a generalized seizure. The anesthesiologist should be aware of the patient's medication regimes because drug interactions between anesthetic agents and psychotropic medications, particularly monoamine oxidase inhibitors, may occur. Skillful airway management using bag and mask ventilation is usually sufficient to maintain oxygenation during anesthesia for ECT.

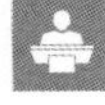

For further review and interactivities, please see the associated Interactive Video Lectures and "A Closer Look" infographic accessible in the complimentary eBook bundled with this text. Access instructions are located in the inside front cover.

References

1. Nagrebetsky A, Gabriel RA, Dutton RP, Urman RD. Growth of nonoperating room anesthesia care in the United States: a contemporary trends analysis. *Anesth Analg*. 2017;124:1261-1267. PMID: 27918331.
2. Chang B, Urman RD. Non-operating room anesthesia: the principles of patient assessment and preparation. *Anesthesiol Clin*. 2016;34:223-240. PMID: 26927750.
3. American Society of Anesthesiologists Committee on Standards and Practice Parameters. *Statement on Nonoperating Room Anesthetizing Locations*. 2018. Accessed March 12, 2020. https://www.asahq.org/standards-and-guidelines/statement-on-nonoperating-room-anesthetizing-locations
4. American Society of Anesthesiologists Task Force on Sedation and Analgesia by Non-Anesthesiologists. Practice guidelines for sedation and analgesia by non-anesthesiologists. *Anesthesiology*. 2002;96:1004-1017. PMID: 11964611.
5. Woodward ZG, Urman RD, Domino KB. Safety of non-operating room anesthesia: a closed claims update. *Anesthesiol Clin*. 2017;35(4):569-658. PMID: 29101947.
6. Miller DL, Vañó E, Bartal G, et al. Occupational radiation protection in interventional radiology: a joint guideline of the Cardiovascular and Interventional Radiology Society of Europe and the Society of interventional Radiology. *Cardiovasc Intervent Radiol*. 2010;33:230-239. PMID: 20020300.
7. Deen J, Vandevivere Y, Van de Putte P. Challenges in the anesthetic management of ambulatory patients in the MRI suites. *Curr Opin Anesthesiol*. 2017;30:670-675. PMID: 28817401.
8. Rasmussen LK, Simonsen CZ, Rasmussen M. Anesthesia practice for endovascular therapy of acute ischemic stroke in Europe. *Curr Opin Anaesthesiol*. 2019;32:523-530. PMID: 31045592.
9. McFadyen GJ, Pelly N, Orr RJ. Sedation and anesthesia for the pediatric patient undergoing radiotherapy. *Curr Opin Anaesthesiol*. 2011;24:433-438. PMID: 21602675
10. Fiorilli PN, Anwaruddin S, Zhou E, Shah R. Catheterization laboratory. Structural heart disease, devices, and transcatheter aortic valve replacement. *Anesthesiol Clin*. 2017;35:627-639. PMID: 29101953.
11. Mandel JE, Stevenson WG, Frankel DS. Anesthesia in the electrophysiology laboratory. *Anesthesiol Clin*. 2017;35:641-654. PMID: 29101954.
12. Kuzhively J, Pandit JJ. Anesthesia and airway management for gastrointestinal endoscopic procedures outside the operating room. *Curr Opin Anaesthesiol*. 2019;32:517-522. PMID: 31082826.

HYPERSENSITIVITY REACTIONS

A CLOSER LOOK

In many nonoperating room anesthesia (NORA) cases, intravenous contrast agents are used. Patients can have a severe allergic response to these drugs. Prompt recognition and treatment is critical.

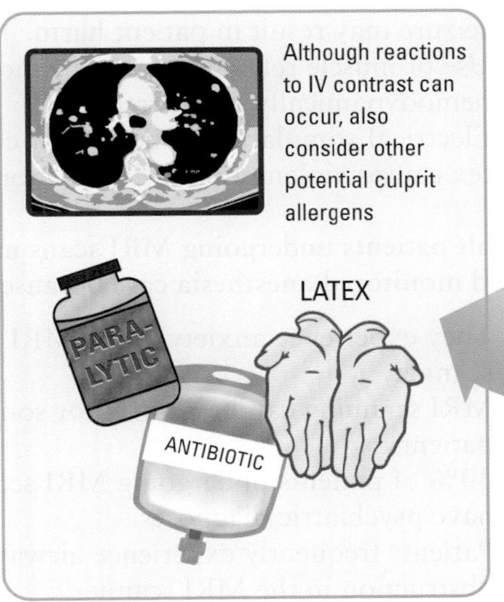

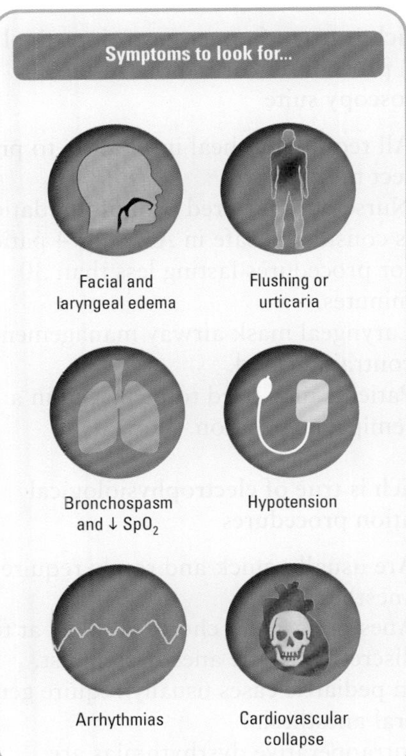

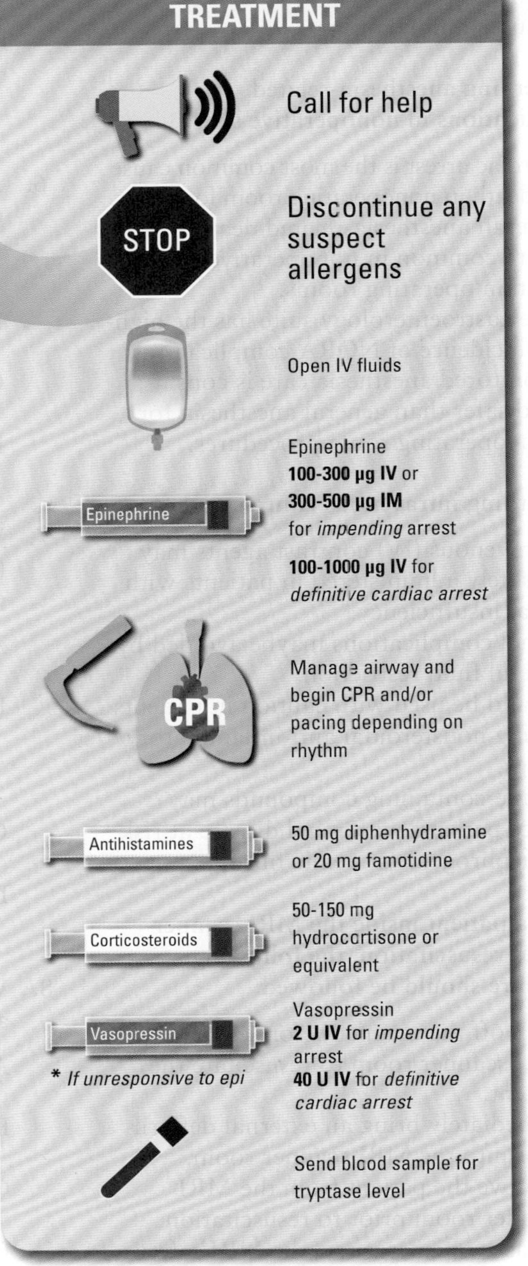

Although reactions to IV contrast can occur, also consider other potential culprit allergens

Symptoms to look for...
Facial and laryngeal edema
Flushing or urticaria
Bronchospasm and ↓ SpO_2

TREATMENT
Call for help
STOP
Discontinue any suspect allergens
Open IV fluids
Epinephrine
Epinephrine
100-300 μg IV or
300-500 μg IM
for *impending* arrest
100-1000 μg IV for *definitive cardiac arrest*
CPR
Manage airway and begin CPR and/or pacing depending on rhythm
Antihistamines
50 mg diphenhydramine or 20 mg famotidine
Corticosteroids
50-150 mg hydrocortisone or equivalent
Vasopressin
* *If unresponsive to epi*
Vasopressin
2 U IV for *impending* arrest
40 U IV for *definitive cardiac arrest*
Send blood sample for tryptase level

Infographic by: Naveen Nathan MD

Questions

1. **What are the most common complications associated with NORA?**

 A. Airway obstruction and respiratory depression
 B. Tachycardia and hypertension
 C. Pain and agitation
 D. Nausea and vomiting

2. **Concerning anesthesia-related complications in nonoperative sites:**

 A. Cardiac arrest is the most common cause of death in nonoperating room locations.
 B. Overall anesthesia-related death is more common in nonoperative sites than in operating rooms.
 C. The gastroenterology suite has the highest incidence of NORA complications.
 D. Monitored anesthesia care is considered safer than general anesthesia for non–operating room procedures.

3. **Concerning intravenous contrast agents:**

 A. Intravenous (IV) contrast agents may be safely administered in patients with renal insufficiency.
 B. Renal complications maybe avoided by careful fluid restriction.
 C. Should be used with caution in patients taking nonsteroidal anti-inflammatory drugs.
 D. Iodine-containing compounds may place patients with renal disease at risk of nephrogenic systemic fibrosis.

4. **When a patient inside the MRI scanner requires resuscitation, the following procedure should be followed:**

 A. Turn off the magnet before entering the MRI scanner room to resuscitate the patient.
 B. Immediately bring an external defibrillator into the MRI scanner room.
 C. Remove the patient from the MRI scanner room prior to resuscitation.
 D. In cases of emergency, the MRI safety checklist may be overlooked prior to entering the MRI scanner room.

5. **Anesthesia for ECT requires the administration of a muscle relaxant because:**

 A. It is imperative to intubate the trachea.
 B. Muscle movements caused by the seizure may result in patient harm.
 C. Use of muscle relaxants creates a more hemodynamically stable treatment.
 D. Electrical stimulation of the motor cortex causes violent muscle contraction.

6. **Adult patients undergoing MRI scans may need monitored anesthesia care because:**

 A. They experience anxiety in the MRI scanner.
 B. MRI scanning can be painful for some patients.
 C. 30% of patients undergoing MRI scans have psychiatric diagnoses.
 D. Patients frequently experience airway obstruction in the MRI scanner.

7. **Which is true of upper gastrointestinal (GI) procedures carried out in the endoscopy suite**

 A. All require tracheal intubation to protect the airway.
 B. Nurse-administered propofol sedation is considered safe in ASA3 or 4 patients for procedures lasting less than 30 minutes.
 C. Laryngeal mask airway management is contraindicated.
 D. Patients may need to be placed in a semiprone position.

8. **Which is true of electrophysiological ablation procedures**

 A. Are usually quick and rarely require anesthesia.
 B. Anesthetic agent choice is solely at the discretion of the anesthesiologist.
 C. In pediatric cases usually require general anesthesia.
 D. Intraoperative dysrhythmias are uncommon.

Answers

1. A

Complications related to NORA are more likely to involve monitored anesthesia care related to inadequate oxygenation and ventilation.

2. B

Significant adverse events in NORA are rare; however, malpractice closed claims analysis5 demonstrate that while claims for NORA were less frequent than for OR anesthesia, NORA had a higher proportion of claims for death than operating room settings.

3. C

Contrast agents are eliminated via the kidneys, and patients with preexisting chronic renal disease, diabetes mellitus, dehydration, advanced age, and concomitant use of nephrotoxic drugs (eg, nonsteroidal anti-inflammatory drugs) are at risk of developing contrast-induced nephropathy.

4. C

Emergency resuscitation attempts should take place outside the MRI scanner because equipment such as laryngoscopes and cardiac defibrillators cannot be taken close to the magnet.

5. B

ECT is distressing and possibly dangerous because generalized convulsions may result in limb injuries. Light general anesthesia with muscle relaxation, usually provided with the short-acting muscle relaxant succinylcholine, is used to mitigate the unpleasant effects of a generalized seizure.

6. A

Scanning sequences are considerably longer for MRI than they are for CT, so a scan of ≥30 minutes for younger children as well as adults with neurologic or psychological disorders, including claustrophobia, often requires sedation or anesthesia.7

7. D

Tracheal intubation is not always required for upper and lower GI procedures. For sicker patients, a trained anesthesia provider is preferable. A laryngeal mask airway may be an alternative airway technique in GI procedures. Patients may be positioned in the semiprone position for GI procedures.

8. C

Electrophysiological procedures performed for the treatment of dysrhythmias are lengthy and can cause discomfort, especially when intraoperative dysrhythmias are provoked by the procedure and then terminated using overdrive pacing, or by external cardioversion. Anesthetic agents including volatile agents and muscle relaxants may interfere with ablation procedures; thus, communication with the proceduralist is of great importance in planning anesthesia for these procedures. In pediatric patients, general anesthesia is preferred.

40 Postoperative Recovery

Louisa J. Palmer and Matthew Grunert

I. Introduction and Postoperative Workflow

It is an American Society of Anesthesiology (ASA) standard that all patients should receive appropriate postanesthesia management following general, regional, or monitored anesthesia care.[1] This management will most commonly be provided in the postoperative care unit (PACU) except on the occasion that either the anesthesiologist responsible for the patient's intraoperative care documents that the patient meets criteria to bypass the PACU and go straight to a regular inpatient floor, or the patient meets criteria for admission to the intensive care unit (ICU). Criteria for direct ICU admission from the operating room include, but are not limited to:

- Ongoing needs for mechanical ventilation.
- High risk of airway obstruction or compromise.
- Dependence on vasoactive medications to support blood pressure and cardiac output.
- Requirement for invasive or frequent neurologic monitoring.
- Need for acute renal replacement therapy.
- Risk for significant ongoing bleeding or coagulopathy requiring resuscitation.

The majority of postoperative patients will end up being managed in the PACU postoperatively. The goal of the PACU is to allow a patient time to recover physiologically from anesthesia and surgery to the point where they are safe to transition either to a regular inpatient floor or back to their home. The PACU provides a closely monitored setting in which acute postoperative conditions can be identified and managed, as described in the following sections. ASA standards help to guide quality care of the PACU patient (**Table 40.1**).

Before leaving the PACU for transfer either to an inpatient unit or home, all patients must be evaluated to assess that they have recovered from the acute effects of anesthesia. Criteria for discharge may vary between institutions and may have modifications dependent on the type of anesthesia administered and the destination of discharge. Generally, criteria will include assessment that the patient has returned to baseline neurologic status with pain at an acceptable level, the ability to maintain a patent airway and stable oxygenation, hemodynamic measurements within acceptable parameters, and no evidence of significant ongoing hypovolemia or bleeding. Additional or modified criteria may

Table 40.1 ASA Standards for Postoperative Care

	ASA Standard
Transport	• Member of the anesthesia team with detailed knowledge of patient's condition present • Appropriate monitoring and support provided
Hand-off	• Verbal report from anesthesia provider to RN • Report should include preoperative comorbidities, allergies, intraoperative course, potential postoperative issues • Initial evaluation by PACU RN • Anesthesia provider remains until PACU RN accepts responsibility
Reevaluation/Monitoring	• Continual evaluation and documentation of patient's condition • Should include oxygenation, ventilation, hemodynamics, fluid balance, level of consciousness and temperature • Responsible physician present to manage complications and provide advanced life support if needed
Discharge from PACU	• Patients may be discharged from the PACU once departmentally approved discharge criteria are met • Discharge criteria may vary depending on the type of anesthesia performed and whether the patient is being discharged to an inpatient setting versus back to the community

PACU, postoperative care unit.

be applied if the patient has undergone neuraxial anesthesia or a peripheral nerve block. If the patient is going to be discharged home, they will need to receive a written summary with instructions, future relevant appointments and prescriptions. Extended recovery units, where patients may be kept overnight for observation but are discharged within 24 hours have also become increasingly common and are an option for PACU discharge at many facilities.

II. Postoperative Pain Management

Uncontrolled postoperative pain can lead to excessive catecholamine release, hypertension, myocardial ischemia, splinting and impaired respiratory mechanics, and worsened patient experience. For these reasons, it is important to identify and treat postoperative pain appropriately in the PACU.[2] Different methods for quantifying postoperative pain include verbal rating scales, numerical rating scales, visual analogue scales, and the Wong Baker faces scale. While traditionally managed with primarily IV opioids, enhanced recovery after surgery (ERAS) protocols and the growing opioid epidemic have emphasized the need for multimodal approaches. These include several classes of adjunctive analgesic medications (**Table 40.2**) as well as regional anesthesia.

ERAS protocols are multimodal care pathways that are implemented in the perioperative period that lead to earlier postoperative recovery, shorter

Table 40.2 Multimodal Pain Medications

	Medications	Advantages	Risks/Side Effects
Opioids	Fentanyl Dilaudid Morphine Oxycodone Tramadol	Potent analgesics, IV forms with rapid onset	Respiratory depression, somnolence, nausea, pruritus, impaired bowel function, urinary retention
Gabapentinoids	Gabapentin Pregabalin	Particularly effective for neuropathic pain	Respiratory depression, dizziness, visual disturbance, depressed mental status
NSAIDs	Ketorolac Ibuprofen Naproxen	Strong anti-inflammatory properties, decreases opioid consumption	AKI, postoperative bleeding, GI bleed, dyspepsia, MI, stroke
COX-2 Inhibitors	Celecoxib	Strong anti-inflammatory, lower bleeding risk	MI, stroke, AKI
Acetaminophen	Acetaminophen	Excellent side effect profile	Risk of hepatic injury
NMDA-Receptor Antagonists	Ketamine	Potent analgesic, may reduce acute opioid tolerance	Hallucinations, anxiety, excessive salivation, potential increase in ICP

AKI, acute kidney injury; GI, gastrointestinal; ICP, intracranial pressure; MI, myocardial infarction; NMDA, N-methyl-D-aspartate; NSAIDs, nonsteroidal anti-inflammatory drugs.

hospital length of stay, and improved patient outcomes.[3,4] While these protocols were initially validated in colorectal surgeries, their scope of implementation has subsequently expanded to include many other types of surgeries, and this trend will likely continue. ERAS protocols encompass the entire perioperative period, and it is important that care of patients in the PACU be consistent with the goals of these protocols when appropriate.

A primary component of ERAS pathways is a multimodal approach to analgesia, geared primarily toward reducing the use of opioids, particularly long-acting ones. Preoperatively, patients may receive several analgesic medications that are intended to improve pain control while also minimizing the use of opioids. These medications include acetaminophen, neuropathic medications like gabapentin or pregabalin, and nonsteroidal anti-inflammatory drugs (NSAIDs) or selective COX-2 inhibitors (**Figure 40.1**). It is important to be aware of the preoperative or intraoperative administration of these medications while taking care of patients in the PACU in order to maintain the appropriate dosing schedules and to avoid potential toxicities related to administration of multiple medications from one class. Additionally, neuropathic

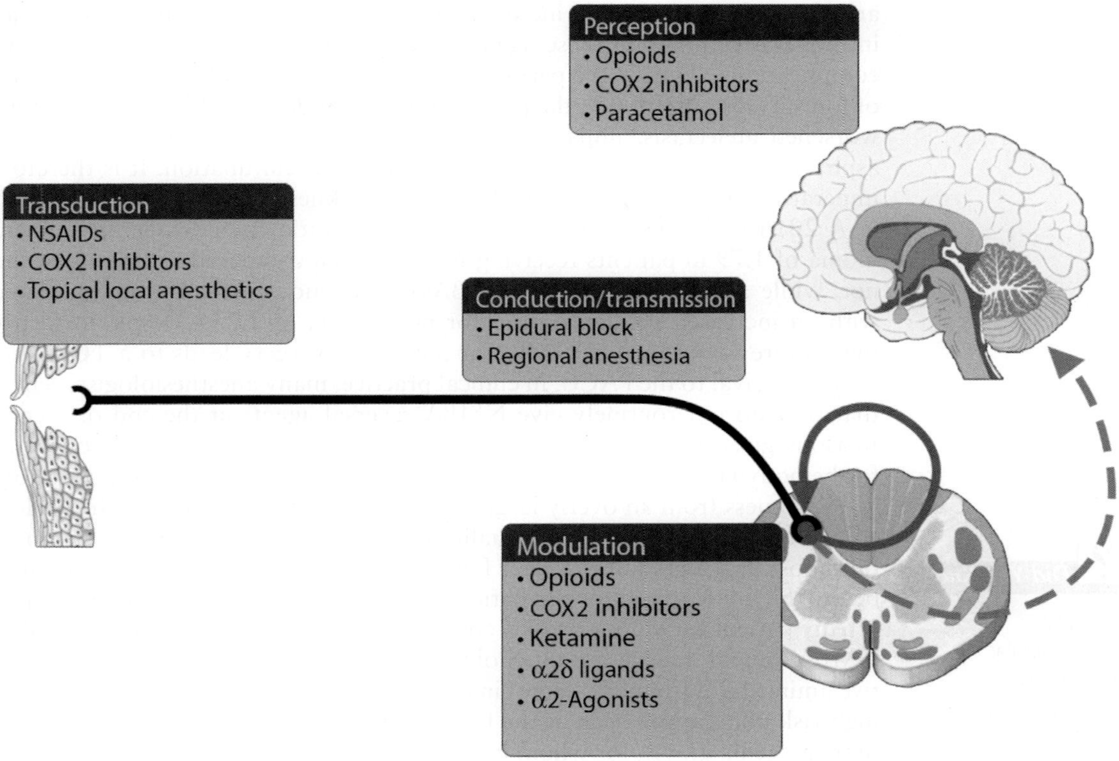

Figure 40.1 Schematic showing neuroanatomical targets for adjunctive pain medications. COX2, cyclooxygenase-2; NSAIDs, nonsteroidal anti-inflammatory drugs. (Redrawn from Schug SA. Multimodal drug therapies for postoperative pain control in adults. In: Carr DB, ed. *Pain After Surgery.* 1st ed. Wolters Kluwer; 2019:249-258.)

medications like gabapentin and pregabalin have been linked to somnolence and respiratory depression, especially when combined with other central nervous system (CNS) depressant medications, which are inevitably present in the perioperative setting. It is important to keep these medications in mind when evaluating patients that are slow to arouse or showing signs of depressed respiratory drive.

The use of regional anesthesia, when feasible, is an equally important component of pain management in ERAS protocols, as these techniques also minimize opioid use. Interventions in the PACU may include optimizing existing epidural or nerve block catheters for patients that had them placed pre- or intraoperatively. Patients with unexpectedly high analgesic requirements may benefit from postoperative nerve blocks or continuous nerve block catheter placement when appropriate. With the expanded use of long-acting liposomal bupivacaine, it is important to determine which patients can safely receive additional doses of local anesthetics without significant risk for local anesthetic systemic toxicity.

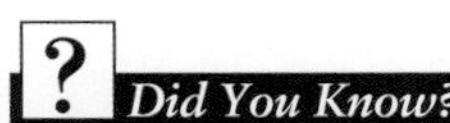

ERAS pathways promote a multimodal approach to analgesia with emphasis toward reducing opioid use.

III. Postoperative Weakness

A. Generalized Weakness

Many procedures performed in the operating room require patients to undergo muscle relaxation with neuromuscular blocking agents (NMBA). Residual weakness from the use of these agents has historically been associated in anesthesia literature with increased morbidity and mortality, with higher intraoperative doses of these agents linked to a higher risk of postoperative complications.[5] During the period between extubation and recovery of a train of four (TOF) ratio of 0.9, the patient is at risk of decreased respiratory effort, worsened atelectasis, impaired protective airway reflexes, increased risk of aspiration events, increased risk of hypoxia, and reintubation. It is therefore imperative to monitor for signs of residual weakness in the PACU.

A 2016 study revealed a relative incidence ratio for postoperative pneumonia of 1.79 in patients receiving NMBA when compared to those that did not, while a failure to reverse NMBAs at the end of a case was associated with an increased incidence ratio for pneumonia of 2.25.[6] Despite evidence that failure to antagonize NMBA at the end of surgery leads to a TOF ratio <0.7 on arrival to the PACU, in clinical practice, many anesthesiologists report that they do not routinely give NMBA reversal agents at the end of a case. Reasons given for avoiding anticholinesterase medications include concerns for hemodynamic changes, postoperative nausea and vomiting, and paradoxical weakness from an overly large dose of neostigmine, as well as the finding of "no fade" with the use of a qualitative twitch monitor. It should be noted that most providers fail to detect fade once the TOF ratio is above 0.4—well below the 0.9 required for the patient to avoid postoperative complications.

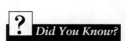

Residual neuromuscular blockade is an underappreciated phenomenon in PACU and is associated with increased risk of postoperative pneumonia.

Any patient for whom there is concern for incomplete or absent reversal of NMBA should receive an anticholinesterase agent or sugammadex (a selective aminosteroid-binding agent) in the PACU. This is especially important for high-risk populations such as the frail and elderly, and patients with a history of myasthenia gravis, for whom it is necessary to identify the last dose of their home anticholinesterase agent and make sure that it is administered on schedule. There are some data to support the notion that these high-risk populations should preferentially be reversed with sugammadex if they have received an intraoperative aminosteroid NMBA.

B. Focal Weakness

The PACU is where patients may first exhibit signs of having sustained an intraoperative positioning injury. The most common of these is injury to the ulnar nerve, followed in prevalence by injury to the peroneal nerve. Signs and symptoms should be carefully evaluated and documented. Most such injuries will improve with time, but follow-up with a neurologist should be considered. Persistent lower extremity weakness following spinal surgery or neuraxial anesthesia needs to be evaluated with an MRI in order to rule out the presence of an epidural hematoma.

Certain procedures such as carotid endarterectomy and intraoperative events such as severe hypertension or hypotension can put patients at increased risk for hemorrhagic, ischemic, or embolic stroke. This diagnosis should be considered in patients with new focal postoperative neurologic deficits, aphasia, or with other unexplained neurologic changes while in PACU. Rapid recognition and notification of appropriate services is essential to provide timely management and intervention.

IV. Altered Mental State

Multiple conditions can lead to postoperative changes in mental state. Those most commonly encountered in the PACU include residual anesthetic opioid side effect, hypoxia, hypercapnia, and hypoglycemia. The patient with significantly depressed mental status should be assessed for airway patency and respiratory function, and consideration should be given to reversal agents such as naloxone and flumazenil. A fingerstick glucose should be checked with initial assessment, and further workup such as electrolytes and arterial blood gas (ABG) should be considered.

On the other end of the spectrum, confusion and agitation are also commonly encountered in the PACU, especially in the pediatric and geriatric populations. Antipsychotics and dexmedetomidine may be considered for management of extreme cases once other etiologies have been ruled out such as pain, full bladder, or respiratory distress.

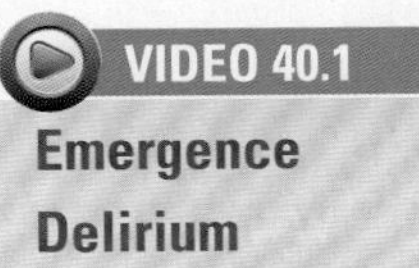

V. Hypoxia

There are several potential causes of hypoxia in the postoperative patient. The most common cause of V/Q mismatch in the PACU is atelectasis. Factors predisposing to atelectasis include obesity, prolonged supine or Trendelenburg intraoperative positioning, increased intra-abdominal pressure, lack of cough or deep breathing under anesthesia, and postoperative splinting due to pain. This can be exacerbated by increased O_2 demand in the setting of pain, shivering, and agitation. For this reason, most postoperative patients will continue to require supplemental oxygen in the postoperative period until they regain their functional residual capacity (FRC) with mobilization and good pulmonary toilet. It is important to be aware that supplemental O_2, while frequently useful, may mask hypoventilation caused by residual anesthesia or sedative medications.

Less common etiologies to keep in mind for the hypoxic postoperative patient include airway compromise, pulmonary edema (from volume overload, negative pressure, or re-expansion) pulmonary embolus, aspiration pneumonitis, or mucous plugging. Pneumothoraces may occur after breast, neck, or thoracic surgery or potentially from abdominal surgery involving compromise of the diaphragm.

Workup of the hypoxic postoperative patient should include initial assessment of level of consciousness, airway patency, adequacy of respiratory effort, and breath sounds. Persistent or profound hypoxia should be further assessed with chest x-ray (CXR) and ABG analysis. Point of care ultrasound is now frequently used to help identify signs of pneumothorax, pulmonary edema, or consolidation. In the setting of pulmonary edema or profound atelectasis, continuous positive airway pressure (CPAP) may be used to potentially avoid reintubation for hypoxia[7] (**Figure 40.2**).

> ? *Did You Know?*
>
> The most common cause of hypoxia in PACU is atelectasis that develops intraoperatively.

A. Airway Compromise

Postanesthesia patients are at high risk for airway obstruction. Signs of potential airway compromise and obstruction include stridor, increased work of breathing, apneic episodes, or neck swelling. Patients at particular risk are those with known or suspected obstructive sleep apnea (OSA) and patients who have had procedures on the neck and upper airway.

Patients recovering from thyroid, parathyroid, and carotid surgery are at risk of developing localized neck hematomas that may distort airway anatomy leading to respiratory compromise. Surgical teams should be notified and rapid hematoma expansion may necessitate reopening of the incision at bedside. Intubation in this scenario may be very difficult or impossible due to altered anatomy, and efforts should be made to maintain

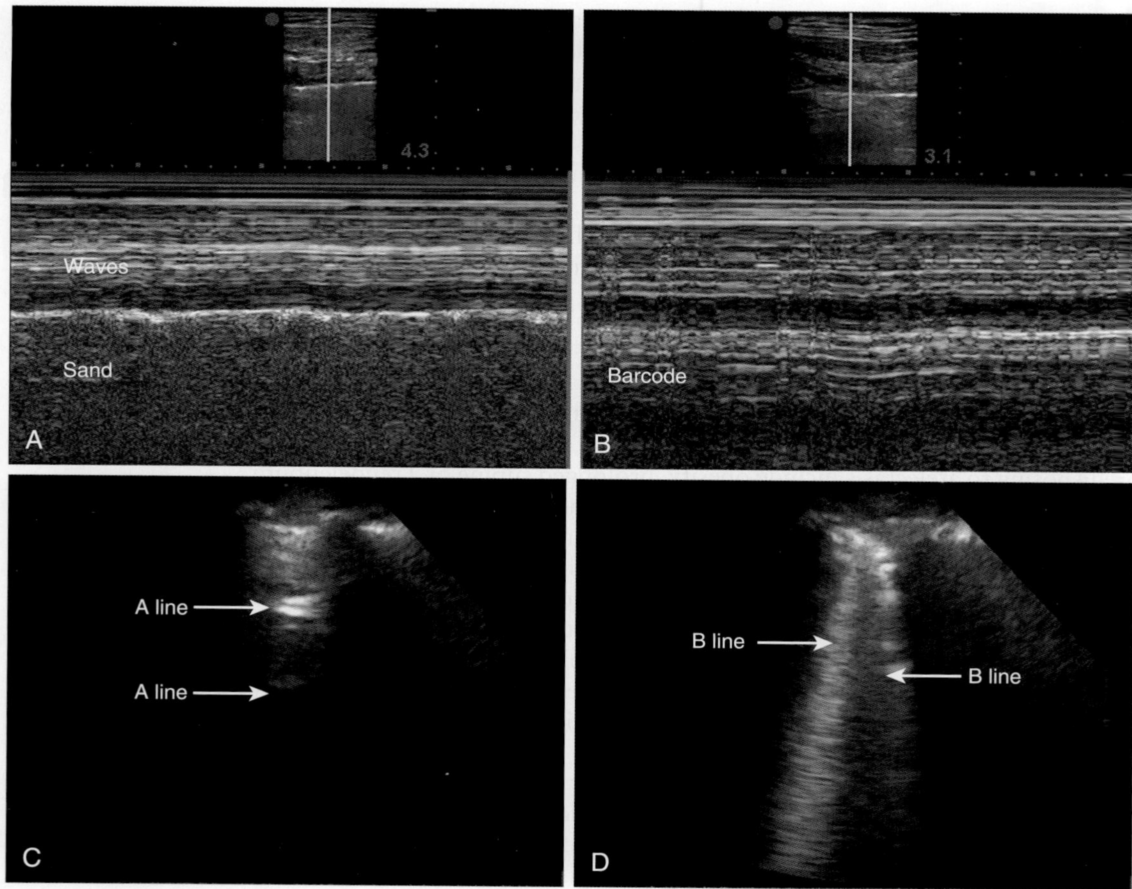

Figure 40.2 Lung ultrasound findings in the postoperative care unit (PACU). A, The "seashore sign M mode is placed across the pleura. With normal lung, there are horizontal "waves" above the pleura and speckled "sand" below. B, In the presence of a pneumothorax when M mode is placed across, the pleura the waves persist below the pleura to create a "barcode" sign. C, With two-dimensional (2D) ultrasound, horizontal A lines are reverberation artifacts of the pleura and represent normally aerated lung. D, In a patient with pulmonary edema, the increased density of the lung causes 2D echo to show vertical B lines.

spontaneous respiration during any intubation attempt. In the absence of obvious neck hematoma, vocal cord injury, edema, or spasm may be the cause of symptoms. Racemic epinephrine and steroids may help if airway edema is thought to be the cause, and ENT evaluation should be considered. Airway compromise can also be the result of postsurgical oropharyngeal bleeding after procedures such as tonsillectomy, and these patients require close monitoring.

VI. Obstructive Sleep Apnea

Patients with OSA can make up a significant portion of patients in the PACU. They are at an elevated risk of apneic episodes and airway obstruction in the postoperative period. Severe hypoxia can result from the combination of airway obstruction and decreased FRC. These patients need to be identified early, either through preoperative testing or using a high-sensitivity scoring system to identify at-risk patients[8] (**Table 40.3**).

Table 40.3 Identifying Patients at Risk of Obstructive Sleep Apnea

Physical Characteristics	BMI > 35 kg/m^2
	Presence of large tonsils
	Craniofacial malformations
	Large neck circumference
	Male
Clinical Symptoms	Loud/frequent snoring
	Observed apnea events while sleeping
	Awakens frequently from sleep
	Frequent daytime somnolence
	Easily falls asleep when not stimulated (eg, on sofa watching TV)

BMI, body mass index.

Adapted from American Society of Anesthesiologists Task Force on Perioperative Management of Patients With Obstructive Sleep Apnea. Practice Guidelines for the perioperative management of patients with obstructive sleep apnea: an updated report by the American Society of Anesthesiologists Task Force on Perioperative Management of patients with obstructive sleep apnea. *Anesthesiology*. 2014;120(2):268-286.

Analgesic regimens should be carefully planned in these patients as the use of sedatives and opioids increases the risk of respiratory depression and airway obstruction. Regional techniques and adjunct medications should be used to minimize opioid requirements. If a patient controlled analgesia is prescribed for pain, a background infusion should be avoided. It is reasonable to use supplemental O_2 in these patients postoperatively to support oxygenation, but it should be kept in mind that this could potentially increase the length of apneic episodes and disguise hypoventilation. All postoperative patients with OSA should be monitored with continuous pulse oximetry, and this should continue after transfer out of the PACU on the floor. Strong consideration should be given to initiating CPAP for any patient who has evidence of persistent hypoxemia or obstruction without surgical contraindication. OSA patients who use home CPAP should be encouraged to bring their machine to the hospital on the day of surgery so they can use it in the postoperative period. Other simple maneuvers to minimize hypoxia and airway obstruction include positioning in a nonsupine position such as sitting or on their sides.

The decision to discharge a patient with OSA home after surgery requires careful consideration. Patients should not be discharged home until they are no longer felt to be at increased risk of postoperative respiratory depression, and this may require a longer PACU stay than their non-OSA counterparts. Before discharge, patients should be able to maintain oxygen saturations without supplemental O_2 in an unstimulating environment. On discharge, they should be instructed to be compliant with their home CPAP (if used) for naps and overnight. They should also be given advice on the use of adjunct, simple pain medications, and advised to minimize any opioid use. Day surgery patients with OSA who are hypoxic in the PACU or score as high risk should be admitted to the hospital for observation (**Table 40.4**).

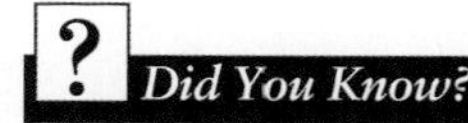

High-risk OSA patients should be considered for overnight observation instead of being routinely discharged home from PACU.

VII. Hypoventilation

While hypoxia is easily recognized on PACU monitors, hypoventilation frequently goes unrecognized and, as mentioned above, may be masked by the routine administration of supplemental O_2 given to postoperative patients.

Table 40.4 Postoperative Risk Stratification for Patients With OSA

		Level of Postoperative Risk
Severity of OSA	Mild	Low
	Moderate	Medium
	Severe	High
Type of surgery/anesthetic	Surgery done purely under local anesthetic	Low
	Low-risk surgery under sedation or general anesthesia	Medium
	Major surgery/airway surgery under general anesthesia	High
Pain medication requirements	No opioids required	Low
	Low-dose/low-frequency opioids	Medium
	High-dose opioids/neuraxial opioids	High

OSA, obstructive sleep apnea.

Adapted from American Society of Anesthesiologists Task Force on Perioperative Management of Patients With Obstructive Sleep Apnea. Practice Guidelines for the perioperative management of patients with obstructive sleep apnea: an updated report by the American Society of Anesthesiologists Task Force on Perioperative Management of patients with obstructive sleep apnea. *Anesthesiology*. 2014;120(2):268-286

Common causes of hypoventilation include sedation from anesthetics and opioids, weakness caused by residual NMB, and splinting from inadequately treated pain. Hypercapnia with respiratory acidosis may lead to either increased agitation or somnolence and should be suspected in both of these scenarios. Patients with a history of asthma or chronic obstructive pulmonary disease (COPD) are prone to exacerbations in the postoperative period which may manifest as respiratory distress with expiratory wheezing. If left untreated, this may progress to significantly impaired air movement with subsequent hypercarbia and hypoxia.

Reversing sedation, improving pain control, bronchodilator therapy, and bilevel positive airway pressure can all be considered for treatment of postoperative hypoventilation depending on the suspected etiology.[7] Refractory hypoventilation resulting in hypoxia may necessitate reintubation and ICU transfer.

VIII. Postoperative Hypertension

Hypertension is commonly encountered in the immediate postoperative period, and while no specific blood pressure cutoff has been established, postoperative hypertension is independently associated with complications after noncardiac surgery. Among the most common causes of hypertension in PACU are inadequately managed pain, nausea, anxiety, bladder distension, hypercarbia, emergence delirium, and perioperative holding of antihypertensive medications. Postoperative hypertension puts patients at risk for myocardial ischemia, stroke, bleeding, and elevated intracranial pressure (ICP) and intraocular pressure. Specific surgical populations are at particularly increased risk of complications and may require more aggressive blood pressure management. These include intracranial procedures, ocular surgery, carotid surgery, and other surgeries involving arterial anastomoses. Typical goals for blood pressure management in the PACU involve maintaining pressure within 20% of baseline. Initial management should involve verification of blood pressure readings and confirmation of appropriate blood pressure cuff size or arterial line transducer placement. After assessment, treatment should address the cause of hypertension. Once all secondary causes of hypertension have been ruled out or treated, titrated doses of labetalol or hydralazine may be appropriate to treat presumed primary hypertension. Patients requiring particularly tight blood pressure control may benefit from continuous infusions of nitroglycerine, nicardipine, or esmolol, and these patients will likely require ICU or step-down admission after PACU discharge. Day surgery patients that require management of postoperative hypertension may benefit from a dose of any home antihypertensive they may have held preoperatively.

IX. Postoperative Hypotension

Postoperative hypotension is common and often transient due to residual vasoplegia and decreased sympathetic tone from anesthetic agents. However, the concern with prolonged or profound hypotension is reduced tissue perfusion leading to supply-demand imbalance and end-organ ischemic injury like acute kidney injury and myocardial ischemia.

Causes of hypotension can be divided into preload, cardiac/obstructive and afterload. Preload etiologies include intravascular hypovolemia from dehydration, third-spacing, or ongoing surgical bleeding. Cardiac or obstructive causes of hypotension include left heart failure, right heart failure, tension pneumothorax, cardiac tamponade, and large pulmonary embolus. The most common postoperative cause of hypotension, as mentioned, is vasoplegia from residual anesthetic leading to significant afterload reduction. This can also lead to peripheral pooling of blood and a resultant decrease in preload.

Workup should include a focused physical examination and evaluation of symptoms and signs such as light-headedness, chest pain, shortness of breath, oliguria, tachycardia or bradycardia, cardiac arrhythmias, and hypoxia. Depending on the severity and suspected etiology, a 12 lead electrocardiogram (ECG), cardiac enzymes, electrolytes, ABG, complete blood count, and CXR can be obtained. The patient's response to a fluid challenge may help to differentiate the etiology of their hypotension.

Increasingly, point of care ultrasound is being used to provide additional information to the clinical examination to aid rapid diagnosis and management of postoperative hypotension.[9,10] A bedside focused cardiac ultrasound examination can rapidly identify if the left ventricle has depressed function or is hyperdynamic, if there are regional wall motion abnormalities, right heart dysfunction, or if there is a pericardial effusion that may be causing tamponade physiology. A small, collapsed inferior vena cava (IVC) correlates with low right atrial pressure and may indicate hypovolemia. Lung ultrasound can be used to diagnose a pneumothorax that may be causing tamponade physiology or pulmonary edema and pleural effusions that may suggest decompensated heart failure. Abdominal ultrasound may identify intraperitoneal free fluid and could suggest ongoing postoperative surgical bleeding in the context of abdominal surgery (**Figure 40.3**).

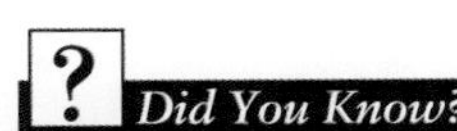

A bedside focused cardiac ultrasound is a useful tool in differentiating various causes of postoperative hypotension.

X. Postoperative Nausea and Vomiting

Postoperative nausea and vomiting (PONV) is an unfortunate but common complaint from patients emerging from anesthesia. PONV can cause significant distress, can negatively impact a patient's postoperative recovery, and

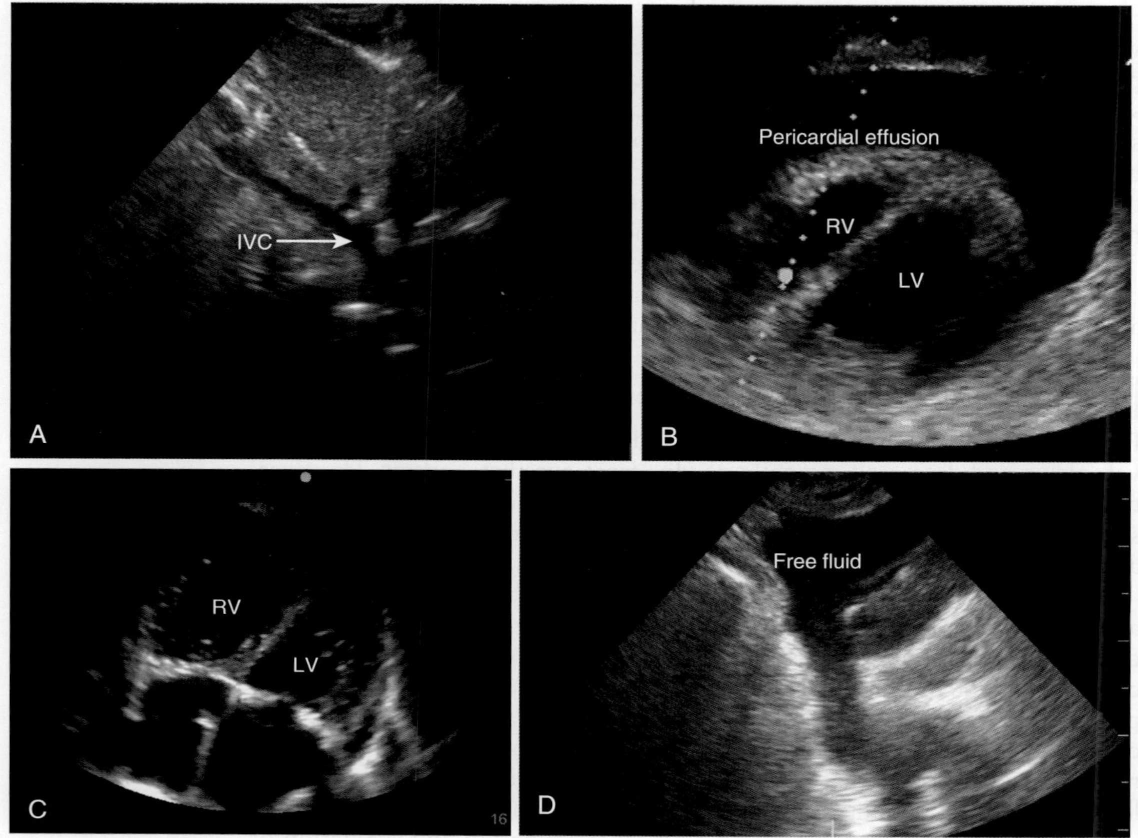

Figure 40.3 Point of care ultrasound (PoCUS) findings in the unstable postoperative care unit (PACU) patient. A, Small, collapsed inferior vena cava (IVC) suggests a low right atrial pressure and would be consistent with hypovolemia in a hypotensive postoperative patient. B, Large pericardial effusion is seen surrounding the heart. C, Severely dilated right ventricle is larger than the left ventricle in a patient with acute car pulmonale. D, Hypoechoic free fluid in the pelvis of a postoperative patient with significant postoperative intra-abdominal bleeding.

is often more poorly tolerated than postoperative pain. In addition, retching caused by PONV can put strain on surgical incision sites and, in worse-case scenarios, can lead to abdominal wound dehiscence or development of a neck hematoma around a neck incision.

The best treatment strategy is prevention with multi-modal antiemetics administered prior to emergence in high-risk patients. Common antiemetic medications include antiserotonergics (ondansetron), antidopaminergics (metoclopramide/haloperidol), antimuscarinics (scopolamine), antihistamines (diphenhydramine), antipsychotics (phenothiazines such as prochlorperazine and promethazine), and dexamethasone. Benzodiazepines and propofol may also have antiemetic properties. Any of the above medications may be used to treat PONV in the PACU, once serious causes of PONV such as hypotension, hypoglycemia, and raised ICP have been ruled out, although it is important to keep the side effect profiles of each in mind. For example, many antiemetics such as ondansetron, metoclopramide, haloperidol, and the phenothiazines can cause QTc prolongation and should be avoided in those patients with a prolonged QTc or those who are already taking QTc prolonging drugs; antidopaminergic agents can cause extrapyramidal side effects and should be avoided or used with caution in the elderly and those with Parkinson disease; dexamethasone can lead to hyperglycemia in diabetic patients; benzodiazepines and scopolamine can lead to confusion and should be avoided in the elderly.

XI. Fluid Management

Perioperative fluid management depends largely on patient and surgical specifics. It is also a central component of ERAS pathways that affects anesthetic management both intraoperatively and in the immediate postoperative period.[11] While pathway specifics may vary depending on patient characteristics, type of surgery, and institutional preference, the goal of fluid management is always to maintain euvolemia. This may involve a zero-balance fluid regimen (also called a restrictive approach) for some low-risk surgeries in low-risk patients or goal-directed fluid therapy in more extensive surgeries and for higher risk patients. In either case, it is important for the PACU physician to be aware of patients that are on ERAS pathways and to adhere to the fluid management goals specific to these patients, as studies have demonstrated that fluid management on the day of surgery is an independent predictor of postoperative complications. Many patients will be transitioned to early enteral feeding and have maintenance IV fluids discontinued in PACU. Other patients will be continued on restrictive maintenance IV fluids and may need titrated boluses for oliguria or hypotension. Some ERAS protocols emphasize volume resuscitation with colloid over crystalloid solutions in order to maximize intravascular volume while minimizing overall volume administration. While some studies suggest that this approach does lead to less volume administered, data showing improved clinical outcomes are inconsistent, and there is not currently a strong consensus favoring one type of fluid over another.

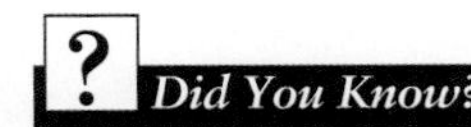

ERAS fluid management aims to maintain euvolemia throughout the perioperative period and may involve a zero-balance or goal-directed fluid therapy approach.

XII. Electrolyte Abnormalities

Electrolyte derangements are common in the postoperative period, and early manifestations of these abnormalities may become apparent in the PACU. Changes in serum sodium, potassium, and calcium are among the most common electrolyte abnormalities encountered.

A. Hyponatremia

In the postoperative period, low serum sodium concentration is most commonly the result of syndrome of inappropriate antidiuretic hormone secretion (SIADH) or significant fluid resuscitation with hypotonic solutions such as lactated ringers (LR) (sodium concentration of 130 mEq/L). Additionally, pseudohyponatremia due to very high blood glucose or triglyceride levels should be ruled out. Mild hyponatremia will typically resolve with time or potentially through diuresis in the hypervolemic patient. Although rare, moderate to severe hyponatremia can result from transurethral resection of prostate (TURP) syndrome, where significant amounts of irrigation fluid are absorbed when under pressure in a closed body cavity. Severe hyponatremia (<120 mEq/L) can lead to life-threatening symptoms including impaired consciousness and seizures and should be corrected with hypertonic saline in a controlled manner to avoid central pontine myelinolysis.

B. Hypernatremia

While less common than hyponatremia in the postoperative period, hypernatremia may result from aggressive diuresis with diuretics like furosemide or osmotic agents like mannitol. Additionally, patients with subarachnoid hemorrhage or traumatic brain injury or those undergoing surgery involving the pituitary gland may be at risk for diabetes insipidus postoperatively. The resultant hypernatremia can be treated with free water repletion and administration of desmopressin.

C. Hyperkalemia

Postoperative hyperkalemia may be the result of perioperative tissue necrosis, reperfusion of ischemic tissue, massive transfusion, hemolytic reactions, significant acidosis, inappropriate succinylcholine administration, or malignant hyperthermia. Patients with significant renal disease will be at increased risk of hyperkalemia due to decreased excretion. Initial workup should include an ECG to look for concerning abnormalities like peaked T waves or QRS widening. Management may include shifting potassium intracellularly with agents like insulin, beta-agonists, or bicarbonate or eliminating potassium in the urine or from the GI tract with agents such as loop diuretics or potassium-binding agents. Severe hyperkalemia may necessitate hemodialysis. In the setting of ECG changes, calcium should be considered to stabilize cardiac myocyte membranes, as these patients are at risk for malignant ventricular arrhythmias.

D. Hypokalemia

A drop in potassium levels may be the result of medication administration (ie, insulin, beta agonists, furosemide), aggressive fluid resuscitation without potassium repletion, or acute alkalosis that shifts potassium intracellularly. Significant hypokalemia may lead to QTc prolongation and predispose patients to malignant arrhythmias including torsades de pointes and atrial fibrillation with rapid ventricular response. IV potassium should be administered either peripherally or through a central venous catheter until levels are normalized.

E. Hypocalcemia

Calcium levels may drop intraoperatively or postoperatively due to calcium chelation with administration of albumin or citrate in blood products. Thyroid or parathyroid surgery may also result in postoperative hypoparathyroidism and subsequent hypocalcemia, although this typically develops after PACU discharge. Hyperventilation from pain or anxiety may result in an acute drop in ionized calcium. Symptoms of acute hypocalcemia typically include perioral numbness, paresthesias, and muscle cramps, and these can progress to severe muscle spasms, laryngospasm, or even seizures. Cardiovascular manifestations may include hypotension due to impaired cardiac contractility and QTc prolongation. Treatment involves correcting ionized calcium levels with IV administration of calcium chloride or alternatively calcium gluconate.

XIII. Postoperative Acid/Base Disturbances

ABG samples are frequently sent for analysis on unstable patients in the PACU. The information provided can help elucidate the etiology and severity of physiologic perturbations. The most common acid-base disorder postoperatively is acute respiratory acidosis due to the respiratory depressant effects of residual anesthetic and analgesic medications. It is present when the pH is <7.4 with a $Paco_2$ > 40 mm Hg. Symptoms can include headache, confusion, agitation, and somnolence. Severe acidosis is present with a pH of <7.25, and consideration should be given to reintubation to reestablish appropriate ventilation. As a ballpark figure, each increase in $Paco_2$ of 10 mm Hg acutely should lead to a 0.08 decrease in pH.

If the pH is higher than would be estimated by the rise in $Paco_2$, there is likely a chronic component of respiratory acidosis. If the pH is lower than would be estimated, then a metabolic acidosis is also present.

Metabolic acidosis can be classified into gap or nongap depending on whether an anion gap is present. The most likely cause of a postoperative nongap metabolic acidosis may be excessive chloride administration in normal saline, but may also result from loss of bicarbonate in the urine from renal tubular acidosis or the GI tract such as with a high-output fistula. When an anion gap is present, it suggests that the body is producing too much acid or the kidneys have a reduced ability to excrete acid. The most common causes postoperatively include lactic acidosis from decreased tissue perfusion, diabetic ketoacidosis, starvation ketoacidosis, and uremia from renal failure. If the pH is <7.2, sodium bicarbonate administration may be required to increase the pH enough for vasopressors to work and to prevent electrolyte disturbances such as hyperkalemia. However, the definitive management for metabolic acidosis with an anion gap is to treat the cause by restoring circulation, administering insulin or dextrose, or initiating renal replacement therapy.

XIV. Postoperative Glycemic Control

A. Hyperglycemia

Management of diabetes can be particularly challenging in the perioperative period due to the significant stress response associated with surgery and anesthesia, perioperative holding of diabetic medications, and patients' NPO status. Even patients without diabetes may be prone to hyperglycemia postoperatively due to a significant neuroendocrine stress response or administration of steroids or sympathomimetic medications. Postoperatively, significant hyperglycemia can put patients at risk for electrolyte disturbances, osmotic diuresis, fluid shifts, and surgical site infection. Goals of glycemic management typically involved keeping blood glucose below 180 mg/dL while being cautious to avoid hypoglycemia. This can be accomplished with administration of IV or SQ regular insulin. Patients with type I diabetes are at risk of developing diabetic ketoacidosis perioperatively, and therefore, it is preferable for them to continue their basal insulin dosing with close monitoring for hypoglycemia for and treatment with IV dextrose.

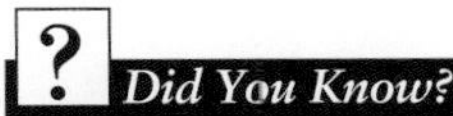

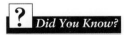

While significant hyperglycemia should be treated in PACU, overly aggressive correction should be avoided, as residual anesthetics can mask the symptoms of hypoglycemia

B. Hypoglycemia

Patients taking oral diabetic medications or insulin as well as malnourished patients are at risk of postoperative hypoglycemia due to their NPO status. Signs and symptoms of hypoglycemia may be difficult to identify in PACU patients with residual anesthetic in their system. However, it is important to have a high suspicion and rapidly recognize hypoglycemia as it may be life-threatening when severe enough. Profound hypoglycemia (<40 mg/dL) can predispose patients to arrhythmias, cardiac events, or cognitive impairment. Rapid administration of IV dextrose (usually a bolus of D50) followed by infusion of a dextrose-containing crystalloid solution is typically sufficient to correct hypoglycemia.

XV. Hypothermia and Hyperthermia

Intraoperatively, many patients are at risk for hypothermia largely due to impaired thermoregulation due to anesthetic medications, cold operating rooms, cold resuscitation fluids, and significant surgical exposure. Forced air warmers and other convection devices reduce this risk, but hypothermia is still a common problem in the PACU. Hypothermia is associated with significant risks, including increased bleeding, infection, myocardial ischemia, altered drug metabolism, longer PACU stays, and decreased patient comfort and satisfaction. Shivering significantly increases oxygen consumption and CO_2 production, leading to increased work of breathing and increasing the risk of respiratory failure. Hypothermia should be aggressively corrected with warming blankets and raising ambient temperature when possible. Meperidine can be used to treat shivering, although patients should be monitored for sedation and respiratory depression.

Conversely, hyperthermia in PACU patients may be the result of overly aggressive intraoperative warming, infection or systemic inflammatory response related to surgery, transfusion reactions, or drug reactions. Less common but highly concerning reactions like malignant hyperthermia or neuroleptic malignant syndrome may also occur. Patients should be thoroughly evaluated as treatment depends largely on determining the underlying cause.

XVI. Incidental Trauma

A. Corneal Abrasion

Corneal abrasion is commonly caused by drying or inadvertent eye contact and can occur intraoperatively, on emergence, during transport, or in the PACU. Abrasion causes tearing, decreased visual acuity, pain, and photophobia, but usually heals without scarring within 72 hours. Topical antibiotics should be applied until symptoms resolve. It is important to be alert for visual impairment in patients who have prolonged surgical procedures in the prone position as they have a one in a thousand chance of developing vision loss in the postoperative period. This is most commonly due to ischemic optic neuropathy, and while the etiology of this condition is unclear, anemia, hypotension, and venous congestion are thought to play the major roles in its development

B. Oral Trauma

Oral trauma can be caused by laryngoscopy, surgical instrumentation, rigid airways, or inadvertent biting. Lip, tongue, or gum abrasions may be treated with icing and topical analgesia as necessary; however, penetrating soft tissue injury may require antibiotics. If dentition is damaged by airway manipulation or jaw clenching, a dental consult should be obtained and foreign body aspiration should be ruled out. Sore throat, dryness, and hoarseness occur in up to 50% of patients after laryngoscopy and can be managed with humidification of oxygen administration while in PACU and topical analgesia if needed. Intubation can also cause temporomandibular joint dysfunction, hypoglossal, lingual or recurrent laryngeal nerve damage, vocal cord evulsion, or tracheoesophageal perforation.

C. Postdural Puncture Headache

Postdural puncture headache can occur after subarachnoid anesthesia, dural puncture during epidural placement, intraoperative dural puncture, or following any procedure involving loss of cerebrospinal fluid. The headache can be debilitating and should be treated with aggressive hydration, analgesia, and caffeine. If the symptoms are particularly severe or persistent, an epidural blood patch can be considered.

D. Soft Tissue Injury

Muscle pain, aching, or stiffness may reflect lack of motion or muscle stretch associated with positioning during surgery, particularly if the procedure is prolonged. Excessive joint extension can lead to backache, joint pain, and even joint instability. Soft tissue ischemia and necrosis can occur at pressure points, especially during surgery in the lateral or prone position, with long duration of surgery, or in patients with a high body mass index (BMI). It is notable that a significant proportion of patients following bariatric surgery (26.5% reported in one study) experience raised serum creatinine kinase to the levels associated with rhabdomyolysis.[12] Entrapment of ears, genitalia, and skin folds can cause also cause necrosis whereas prolonged scalp pressure may cause localized alopecia. Extravasation of intravenous medications can result in local irritation, neuropathy or compartment syndrome. Thermal, electrical, or chemical burns from cautery equipment and surgical prep solutions may also occur. In the event of significant tissue injury or a suspected compartment syndrome, urgent surgical consultation is indicated.

For further review and interactivities, please see the associated Interactive Video Lectures and "A Closer Look" infographic accessible in the complimentary eBook bundled with this text. Access instructions are located in the inside front cover.

References

1. Apfelbaum JL, Silverstein JH, Chung FF, et al. Practice guidelines for postanesthetic care: an updated report by the American Society of Anesthesiologists Task Force on Postanesthetic Care. *Anesthesiology*. 2013;118(2):291-307. doi:10.1097/ALN.0b013e31827773e9. PMID: 23364567.
2. American Society of Anesthesiologists Task Force on Acute Pain Management. Practice guidelines for acute pain management in the perioperative setting: an updated report by the American Society of Anesthesiologists Task Force on Acute Pain Management. *Anesthesiology*. 2012;116(2):248-273. doi:10.1097/ALN.0b013e31823c1030. PMID: 22227789.
3. Ljungqvist O, Scott M, Fearon KC. Enhanced recovery after surgery: a review. *JAMA Surg*. 2017;152(3):292-298. doi:10.1001/jamasurg.2016.4952. PMID: 28097305.
4. Gustafsson UO, Scott MJ, Hubner M, et al. Guidelines for perioperative care in elective colorectal surgery. Enhanced Recovery After Surgery (ERAS) society recommendations: 2018. *World J Surg*. 2019;43(3):659-695. doi:10.1007/s00268-018-4844-y. PMID: 30426190.
5. Murphy GS, Kopman AF. "To reverse or not to reverse?": the answer is clear! *Anesthesiology*. 2016;125(4):611-614. doi:10.1097/ALN.0000000000001280
6. Bulka CM, Terekhov MA, Martin BJ, Dmochowski RR, Hayes RM, Ehrenfeld JM. Nondepolarizing neuromuscular blocking agents, reversal, and risk of postoperative pneumonia. *Anesthesiology*. 2016;125(4):647-655. doi:10.1097/ALN.0000000000001279. PMID: 27496656.
7. Keenan SP, Sinuff T, Burns KE, et al. Clinical practice guidelines for the use of noninvasive positive-pressure ventilation and noninvasive continuous positive airway pressure in the acute care setting. *Can Med Assoc J*. 2011;183(3):E195-E214. doi:10.1503/cmaj.100071. PMID: 21324867.
8. American Society of Anesthesiologists Task Force on Perioperative Management of Patients With Obstructive Sleep Apnea. Practice guidelines for the perioperative management of patients with obstructive sleep apnea: an updated report by the American Society of Anesthesiologists Task Force on Perioperative Management of patients with obstructive sleep apnea. *Anesthesiology*. 2014;120(2):268-286. doi:10.1097/ALN.0000000000000053. PMID: 24346178.
9. Mahmood F, Matyal R, Skubas N, et al. Perioperative ultrasound training in anesthesiology: a call to action. *Anesth Analg*. 2016;122(6):1794-1804. doi:10.1213/ANE.0000000000001134. PMID: 27195630.
10. Zimmerman JM, Coker BJ. The nuts and bolts of performing focused cardiovascular ultrasound (FoCUS). *Anesth Analg*. 2017;124(3):753-760. doi:10.1213/ANE.0000000000001861. PMID: 28207445.
11. Zhu AC, Agarwala A, Bao X. Perioperative fluid management in the Enhanced Recovery After Surgery (ERAS) pathway. *Clin Colon Rectal Surg*. 2019;32:114-120. doi:10.1055/s-0038-1676476. PMID: 30833860.
12. Khurana RN, Baudendistel TE, Morgan EF, Rabkin RA, Elkin RB, Aalami OO. Postoperative rhabdomyolysis following laparoscopic gastric bypass in the morbidly obese. *Arch Surg*. 2004;139(1):73-76. doi:10.1001/archsurg.139.1.73. PMID: 14718280.

OSA AND POSTOPERATIVE RECOVERY

A CLOSER LOOK

Patients with a history of obstructive sleep apnea (OSA) are at high risk for airway obstruction after anesthesia which can result in significant hypoventilation and respiratory acidosis. This can often times be masked with the use of supplemental oxygen.

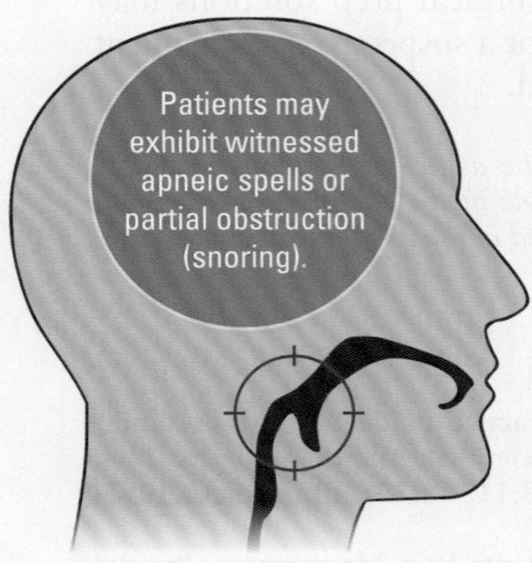

Patients may exhibit witnessed apneic spells or partial obstruction (snoring).

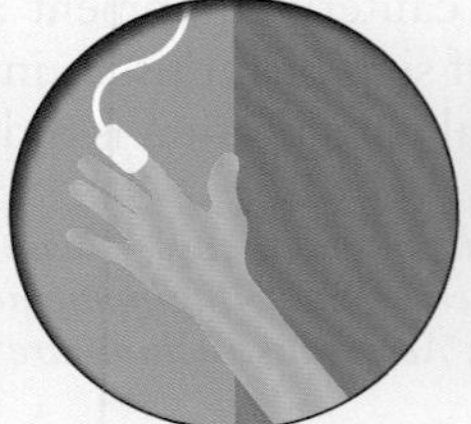

Low SpO_2 or increasing FiO_2 needs

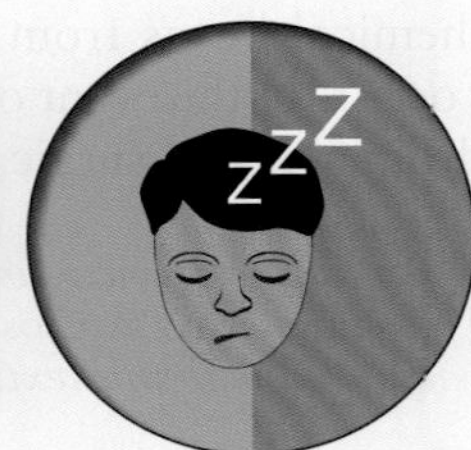

Decreased arousability

In addition, other clinical observations may include...

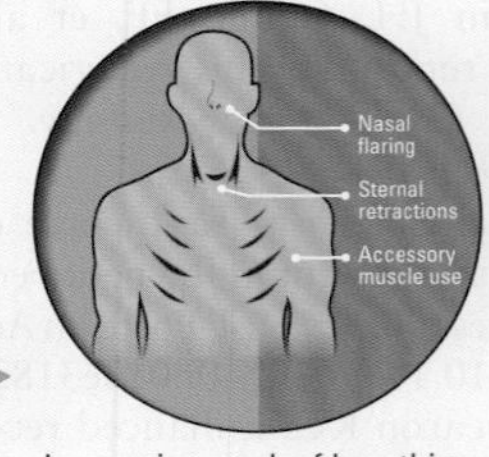

Increasing work of breathing

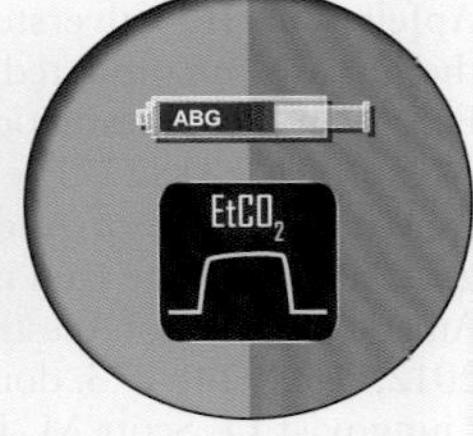

Rising $EtCO_2$ or respiratory acidosis on blood gas

Immediate actions to take...

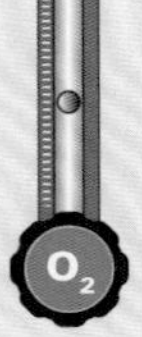

↑ FiO_2

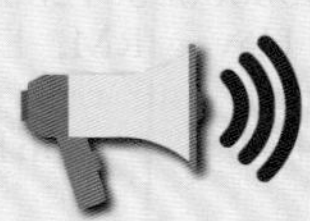

Call for help

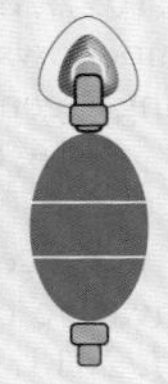

Noninvasive ventilation (eg, CPAP)

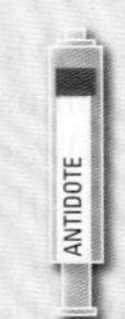

Consider reversing pharmacologic causes with naloxone or sugammadex

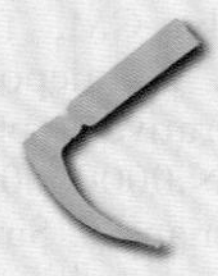

Assess need for reintubation

Intraoperative strategies to reduce risk

Avoid use of long-acting sedatives and anesthetics

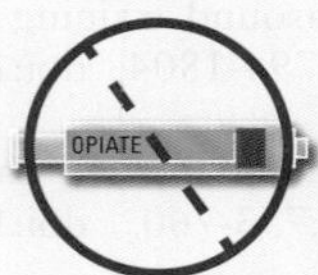

Minimize opioids if possible

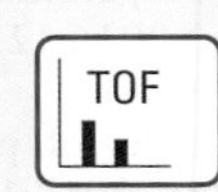

Use quantitative neuromuscular monitoring

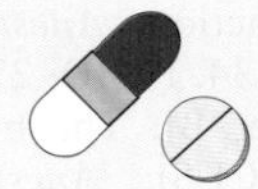

Employ multimodal anesthesia and analgesia

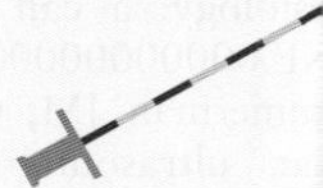

Consider regional anesthesia if feasible

Infographic by: Naveen Nathan MD

Questions

1. **A 36-year-old woman was admitted to PACU 30 minutes ago after a hysteroscopic myomectomy. She is still slow to wake up and appears weak. Labs demonstrate a sodium of 114 mEq/L. What is the most likely cause of her hyponatremia?**

   A. SIADH
   B. Diabetes Insipidus
   C. TURP syndrome
   D. Resuscitation with LR
   E. Acute kidney injury

2. **A 52 year old man is in PACU after a total thyroidectomy. Over the last 20 minutes, the right side of his incision and has become progressively more swollen. He is now starting to develop stridor, although his breathing remains non-labored and his Spo_2 is 95% on RA. What is the most appropriate next step in caring for this patient?**

   A. Intubate immediately
   B. Administer nebulized racemic epinephrine
   C. Call the surgical team emergently to the bedside
   D. Place an laryngeal mask airway (LMA)
   E. Administer nebulized albuterol

3. **A 73-year-old woman is recovering after a laparoscopic partial colectomy and is on an ERAS pathway. She remains somnolent with a slow respiratory rate and has had intermittent apneic episodes that have responded to gentle stimulation by the bedside nurse. She received no long-acting opioids during her surgery and had TAP blocks placed for pain control. Which ERAS medication is likely responsible for her depressed respiratory status?**

   A. Celecoxib
   B. Gabapentin
   C. Acetaminophen
   D. Scopolamine
   E. Famotidine

4. **A 42-year-old man is in the PACU after an uncomplicated cystoscopy under sedation. He has a BMI of 45 kg/m^2, a thick neck and his preop assessment notes that he confirmed frequent night time awakenings and that he feels that he needs to take several naps during the day. In the PACU he has complained of some discomfort that appears to be associated with bladder spasms. His oxygen saturations read 98% on 4 L nasal cannula. The PACU RN is asking for the patient to be signed out so that he can go home. The best next step would be to:**

   A. Sign the patient out and advise him to follow up with his PCP to arrange a sleep study.
   B. Initiate CPAP in the PACU due to his ongoing oxygen requirement.
   C. Admit to an inpatient floor with continuous pulse oximetry.
   D. Ask the PACU RN if the patient has had any observed apneic or hypoxic episodes in the PACU and if not allow the patient to go home with advice to avoid postoperative opioid use.
   E. Observe in the PACU for an extended period of time.

5. **A 72 year old female with chronic myeloid leukemia, coronary artery disease and ejection fraction 45% on preoperative echo is admitted to the PACU following an exploratory laparotomy and splenectomy. On sign out the anesthesia resident notes to the PACU RN that he gave 1 L crystalloid and 250 mL 5% albumin for the case, estimated blood loss was 200 and remarks that the surgical team seemed to have a hard time due to the size of the spleen. You are called over an hour after arrival due to profound hypotension, tachycardia, low urine output and**

patient complaints of abdominal pain and light-headedness. The first thing you do is:

A. Assess the patient, lay them flat, administer fluid bolus and small dose of vasopressor.
B. Assess the patient and use bedside ultrasound to aid your diagnosis before initiating management.
C. Assess the patient, place an arterial line and send a full set of blood work including ABG and lactate.
D. Ask the patient about chest pain, obtain 12 lead EKG, CXR and give a dose of furosemide.
E. Call the surgical team to tell them to take the patient straight back to the operating room.

Answers

1. C

This patient has developed TURP syndrome. While it is rare, use of hypotonic irrigation fluids in a hysteroscopic procedure can lead to significant absorption accompanied by a rapid fall in serum sodium. SIADH or aggressive resuscitation with LR are common causes of postoperative hyponatremia, but would not lead to such severe hyponatremia. Acute kidney injury can lead to hyponatremia, but it is very unlikely to lead to such acute hyponatremia. Diabetes insipidus would cause hypernatremia.

2. C

This patient has an expanding neck hematoma and is developing signs of airway compromise. Fast action must be taken to avoid loss of his airway. While intubation is likely warranted in this case, it is important to have someone available to rapidly open the incision at the bedside if intubation is not possible. Nebulized racemic epinephrine or albuterol will not alleviate the upper airway obstruction caused by a neck hematoma. Placing an LMA would not be appropriate in this case unless needed in a difficult airway algorithm.

3. B

Gabapentinoids have been shown to increase the risk of postoperative respiratory depression, particularly when taken in conjunction with opioids or other CNS depressant medications. Patients should be monitored closely, particularly elderly patients or those with COPD, and dose adjustment should be considered preoperatively in these populations. Celecoxib, acetaminophen, and famotidine are not likely to cause depressed mental status or respiratory depression. While scopolamine can lead to somnolence, particularly in elderly patients, it has not been linked to respiratory depression.

4. E

This patient meets criteria for OSA and therefore should be assessed carefully before discharge to home. He has undergone a minor surgery under sedation, has no ongoing pain that is severe enough to warrant opioid use and therefore is low to moderate risk of postoperative complications. This patient should be able to discharge home with instructions to follow up with his PCP to arrange a sleep study and with advice to use simple analgesics and avoid opioids. There is no report of apneic or hypoxic episodes for this patient that would warrant inpatient admission and potentially CPAP, but he is still receiving supplemental oxygen via nasal cannula. The supplemental oxygen should be weaned off and the patient observed to maintain his saturations before being signed off to go home.

5. A

This patient is hypotensive and has evidence of poor end-organ perfusion. The most likely diagnosis given the scenario is hypovolemia from postoperative bleeding or third-spacing. Attempts to stabilize this patient and obtain more information should be made before heading back to the OR. A bedside ultrasound exam could help identify an underfilled LV and free fluid (blood) in the abdomen expeditiously, and an arterial line and blood work will be certainly be helpful, but again attempts to stabilize the patient should be initiated first. Given the patient's history there is a chance that this presentation could represent an acute coronary syndrome or heart failure. These should be thoroughly investigated if the patient does not respond as expected to initial interventions.

41 Complications of Anesthesia

James E. Szalados

In 1932, William Osler, perhaps the greatest of contemporary physicians, remarked that "errors in judgment must occur in the practice of an art which consists largely of balancing probabilities." The practice of medicine applies as much art as science to the treatment of diverse and unique individuals. The 20th century witnessed a transformation of medicine from a largely humanistic art into a technologically driven enterprise accounting for 1/8th of the US gross domestic product. Anesthesiology and Critical Care are practiced in a highly complex clinical arena where critical decisions are often made in the context of patients presenting with superimposed acute and/or chronic illness. Thus, the clinical context is one of variable physiologic reserve, acute pathophysiology, and interventions often based on relatively sparse data. Thus, despite regular advances in the state of medical knowledge and technology, the risk of complications cannot be completely eliminated.

I. Risks and Complications

A. Mortality and Major Morbidity Related to Anesthesia

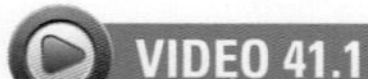

Rates of Selected Anesthetic Complications

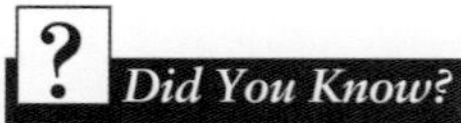

The estimated anesthesia-specific mortality risk has steadily declined from approximately 1 in 1000 in the 1940s to 1 in 10,000 in the 1970s to 1 in 100,000 in the 2000s.

With the advent of specialty training and certification, advances in pharmacology and technology, and improved perioperative medical care, the mortality risk attributed to anesthesia has declined from about 1/1000 anesthesia procedures in the 1940s to 1 in 100,000 in the early 2000s. A study in 2009 reported a rate of anesthesia-related mortality to be 8.2/million hospital surgical discharges.[1] The reliability of these statistics, especially as they relate to causation, is undermined by the lack of a centralized data repository the indirect sources of the data (eg, incident reports and diagnostic codes) the multifactorial and interdisciplinary management of such cases, and the postoperative time period. All available data show that anesthesia-related mortality is directly related to the patient's age (higher at both extremes of age) and their preoperative physical status.

Quantification of the risk of morbidity related to anesthesia is also difficult to quantify because these data are also subject to limitations in reporting and disclosure. Haller et al estimate that more than 1/10 patients will have an intraoperative incident and 1/1000 will suffer an actual injury such as dental damage, an inadvertent dural perforation, peripheral nerve injury, or significant pain.[2] Some morbidity such as venous thromboembolism, myocardial infarction, intraoperative fires and burns, or catheter-related bloodstream infections can be predicted and managed; some morbidity such as aspiration, previously unknown allergies, nerve injuries, or awareness might be mitigated; however, some morbidity such as stroke can neither be well predicted or mitigated.

In addition, data continue to show a large variation between the practice patterns of anesthesia providers and the surgical team which may be as important to outcome as perioperative risk scores.[3] Advances in technology and medical science do not readily translate into their ubiquitous adoption into practice.[4] Potential impediments to the adoption of new technology and even "best practices" include ongoing controversies regarding outcome benefits, costs associated with training and technology acquisition, perceived lack of "need," and culture. Indeed, Cheng et al argue that "we need to respect that we cannot (and should not) 'do it all,' especially if the new techniques or technologies will achieve only marginal benefits at best and at greater risk and cost compared with the existing status quo."[5] Not all presumably "new and improved" interventions are supported by solid scientific evidence. In a strict legal sense, variations in practice are reasonable if they represent sound medical judgment and conform to the standard of care.

II. Risk Management and Patient Safety

A. Ethics

Ethics is a branch of philosophy dedicated to the study of values and customs of groups. In a contemporary context, ethics relates to discourse regarding, and the clinical application of, precepts such as right and wrong, good and evil, and norms for interactions between individuals. Since it is inevitable that disagreements will arise when individual preferences form the basis for healthcare and end-of-life decisions, ethics provides a framework within which clinicians reconcile differing beliefs and values. Thus, ethics provides an accepted structural framework through which dialogue facilitates discourse, and problem-solving in highly complex clinical dilemmas for which there are usually no clear cut answers, and for which decisions are frequently subject to retrospective scrutiny. The importance of such analysis and open dialogue is important in our increasingly diverse society since individual ethical and moral values differ. Ethics provides the theoretical foundation, the structure, and the context, with which healthcare providers can approach discussions with patients, families, and among each other regarding deeply personal topics, such as do-not-resuscitate orders, medical futility, withdrawal of life support, terminal sedation, research design and research subject protections, placebo therapy, triage and rationing, access to healthcare, patient-centered healthcare, apologies in the clinical setting, and the meaning of brain death. "Empathy" implies an understanding of the emotional state of the patient, whereas sympathy merely describes the provider's own response to the situation of patient. The concept of "dignity" represents a generally accepted right of humanness. Dignity in humans involves an expectation of personal respect or preservation of self-esteem; it is a fundamental starting point for any discussion of clinical ethics. Within a society characterized by diversity, open and honest, but structured, dialogue facilitates the equal weighing of differing points of view, without prejudging or arbitrarily imposing one's own personal values.

Although ethics is widely believed to represent a branch of legal doctrine, it applies equally to all professions. Nonetheless, laws apply to interactions between individuals and between individuals and society. Lawyers are trained to simultaneously manage opposing points of view and are trained to develop arguments on behalf of the client whom they are representing at the time. In the United States, laws are derived from the shared ethical and moral principles inherent in the Constitution. Laws, like ethical concepts, form the structure and context, within which lawyers argue the merits of their clients' cases. The important relationship of professions with society suggests that professional values must be congruent with the societal values in which the professionals practice. Ethical decisions made in the medical context are subject to public review; that review most frequently occurs in a judicial or quasi-judicial context; for that reason, clinical ethics decisions must be as unbiased, carefully reasoned, well-documented, and as transparent as possible.

Aristotle distinguished "basic wisdom" (***sophia***), the ability to think about the nature of the world and discern inherent universal truths, in contrast to "practical wisdom" (***phronesis***), the capacity to consider the appropriate action needed in order to bring about changes with the intent of improving the quality of life. Thus, practical wisdom implied an ability to perceive relationships among people. Therefore, in the context of ethics, one could argue that if human dignity is the final denominator, the ethical process must harmonize scientific facts and individual choices. The goal of communication in medicine is the formation of a "therapeutic alliance" which facilitates shared decision-making. Many so-called ethical conflicts in clinical practice can be traced to a lack of effective communication.[6]

Medical malpractice litigation is very closely linked to the perceptions of patients and families regarding honest communication, team cohesiveness, disclosure of adverse events, and, therefore, their subjective impressions regarding the quality of care. Litigation is more likely to result when there is a significant discrepancy between a patient's or family's expectations and perceptions regarding the care that was rendered. In the absence of true medical negligence, patients and families are most likely to remember the respect, care, and attentiveness ("ethical behavior") they encountered during the time of the patient's healthcare encounter.

Ethical codes or "codes of conduct" are largely a set of aspirational values, which are the ethical guiding principles for professions. The Oath of Hippocrates and the American Medical Association's Principles of Medical Ethics represent such professional documents. The Principles of Medical Ethics apply equally to each and every member of the healthcare team.

The principle of "beneficence" stands for the precept that each healthcare practitioner should knowingly strive to always act in the best interest of each individual patient (***salus aegroti suprema lex***). Thus, healthcare decisions should reflect the highest level of care for each patient, without regard to personal gain, societal interests, or the interests of family. Beneficence also refers to the "fiduciary duty" of providers, as professionals, to act in their patients' best interests, as agents on their patients' behalf.

The principle of "nonmaleficence" is embodied in the concept of primum non nocere—"first, do no harm." Harm may be variably interpreted and includes either willful omission or commission of an act which inflicts emotional or psychological distress, pain and suffering, or physical injury. Nonmaleficence is also inherent in the fiduciary duty that is owed by providers to their patients. Nonmaleficence can become legally operative within the context of palliative sedation when the prescription may facilitate a peaceful and pain-free, albeit more expedient, death in which case the ethically and legally operative issue is that of intent. Medical interventions have inherent risks that cannot be eliminated no matter how much care and attention is rendered. Where a therapeutic intervention is prescribed with the intent of "doing good" and an unavoidable but recognized harm may ensue, this is known as the "double effect." Double effect recognizes the detrimental effect of a treatment, such as respiratory depression caused by the administration of opiates for palliative sedation is well-recognized but intends that the desired effect is not respiratory depression, but rather relief from suffering. Thus, palliative sedation is ethically acceptable whereas euthanasia and assisted suicide are not; the process is similar but the intent is dichotomous.

The principle of "autonomy" addresses the patient's right to choose (***voluntas aegroti suprema lex***) and to make informed, uncoerced, voluntary decisions. Autonomy refers to each individual's right to self-determination. American culture has placed great importance on and has had a great respect for the principle of individual autonomy, a notion embodied in the Declaration of Independence, the United States Constitution, and the Bill of Rights. The principle of autonomy is exemplified in the obligation to obtain informed consent and also with the right to refuse medical care. Today there is increased awareness of the need to articulate one's need for life-sustaining treatment before one has lost decision-making capacity or the ability to articulate one's wishes. This has resulted in more widespread adoption of living wills, advance directives, and healthcare proxy designations. The principle of autonomy requires healthcare surrogates (proxies) to use "substituted judgment" in decision-making whereby the surrogate decides for the patient in accordance with what the patient would have done.

The principle of "justice" is bifurcated into distribution and retribution. Distributive justice is an ideal that concerns the hope that all are treated equally and with clear transparency with respect to access to and distribution of limited healthcare resources. Retributive justice addresses retrospective retaliation as punishment, or prospective warnings of imminent punishment as a deterrent to certain actions. In some ways, justice represents the antithesis of the principle of autonomy because where autonomy dictates that a patient's interests are determinative, the principle of distributive justice dictates that the provider must consider the fair allocation of resources without discrimination. Triage in emergencies and in critical care settings represents application of the principle of distributive justice. Retributive justice is largely reserved for disciplinary and legal review.

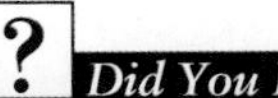

Did You Know?

As a result of several high-profile cases (Nancy Cruzan, Terri Schiavo), the US Supreme Court has judged that competent persons have a constitutionally protected liberty interest to refuse medical treatment, spurring more widespread discussion and adoption of living wills, advance directives, and healthcare proxy designations.

The principle of "paternalism" refers to the instinct for professionals to unilaterally make decisions on behalf of others who are incapable of doing so. Paternalism represents a value-based ethics in which the provider was universally perceived as competent, altruistic, and sincere; the provider's decision was universally accepted since it was widely perceived to be grounded in a fiduciary duty which in turn stemmed from extensive knowledge, training, and experience which was far beyond the understanding of a typical layperson. In its extreme form, the paternalistic provider ignores the wishes and needs of the patient and is not reconcilable with the precept of autonomy. Less obtrusively, paternalism is also manifested when the provider subconsciously withholds crucial information in the belief that bad news, such as a terminal diagnoses or a poor prognosis, might inflict undue emotional distress. Paternalistic decision-making is no longer acceptable in modern medicine.

B. Medical Errors and Patient Safety

The topics of medical error and patient safety attained national prominence in 2000 when the Institute of Medicine (IOM) published "*To Err is Human: Building a Safer Health System*" in which it purported that medical errors accounted for at least 98,000 inpatient deaths annually or at least 270 deaths daily.[7] Medical error can be defined as a mistake, inadvertent occurrence or unintended event in healthcare delivery which may, or may not, result in patient injury. The IOM defines patient safety as "freedom from accidental injury."

Anesthesiology has a long history of leadership in quality and safety and was the first specialty to adopt a national standard for safety improvements. In the mid-20th century, coincident with the blossoming of formal training in anesthesia and establishment of board certification, studies reported that a significant number of anesthetic deaths could be attributed to anesthetic mismanagement. The majority of errors in anesthetic care could be attributed to preventable human error whereas a minority were deemed due to other factors such as faulty equipment, inexperience, poor communication among personnel, haste, and distraction. If one excludes errors due to intentional violation of rules, most errors by providers can be traced to error-prone systems. As an example, the anesthesiologist who administers the wrong medication because its packaging has been changed. Many errors are unrecognized, such as "near misses." Although they may be pervasive, they may remain undiscovered with high potential for future repetition. In general, the more complex the system, the greater the potential for error. Complex systems share common characteristics: high-level technical requirements, the need for quick reaction times, 24 hours per day operations, fatigue, production pressure which frequently involve trade-offs between personnel, and multidisciplinary team coordination.

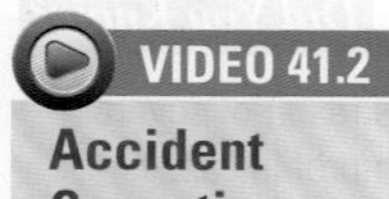

The medical model for team coordination has its origins in the aviation industry which developed the "crew resource management" (CRM) paradigm in 1978; this later evolved onto a clinical multimodality model of patient safety. (**Table 41.1**). CRM fosters an organizational culture which encourages each team member to respectfully question authority while preserving authority and chain of command. CRM encompasses knowledge, skills, and attitudes including communications, situational awareness, problem-solving, decision-making, and teamwork. CRM is a team management system which makes optimum use of all available resources including equipment, procedures, and people in order to promote safety and enhance operational efficiency. The CRM model has now permeated healthcare in the form of a "safety culture" which universally establishes safety as an organizational priority by fostering teamwork, patient involvement, transparency, and accountability. CRM has become an integral part of anesthesiology simulator training. A successful safety culture is characterized by

Table 41.1 The Structure of Crew Resource Management

Communication: Leadership and team management
Workload management: Mission planning, stress management, and workload distribution
Decision-making: Integration and proceduralization (standard operating procedures)
Conflict resolution
Leadership
Team management
Stress management

leadership vision and commitment, shared core values and goals, consistency, nonpunitive responses to adverse events and errors, and promotion of safety through continuous education and training.

The importance of teamwork is further exemplified by the high-reliability organization (HRO). An HRO is one that has succeeded in avoiding catastrophes despite a high level of risk and complexity.[8] Classical examples of HROs include nuclear power plants, air traffic control systems, and naval aircraft carriers. HROs are characterized by five common practices: (1) sensitivity to operations; (2) reluctance to accept "simple" explanations for problems; (3) a preoccupation with failure; (4) emphasis on expertise; and (5) resilience. Healthcare organizations have recently moved to adopt the HRO mindset, but some experts caution that the methodology through which HROs generate and maintain high levels of safety may not be directly applied to healthcare. Rather, they recommend incremental changes which healthcare systems could use to progress toward high reliability: (1) leadership's commitment to achieving zero patient harm; (2) a fully functional culture of safety throughout the organization; and (3) the widespread deployment of highly effective process improvement tools.[9]

Multiple healthcare agencies promote patient safety and reduction of medical error. In 1986, the Anesthesia Patient Safety Foundation was formed and became the first-ever foundation dedicated to patient safety. It was the model for the National Patient Safety Foundation. The Agency for Healthcare Research and Quality (AHRQ) is the federal agency charged with promotion of patient safety in healthcare. The AHRQ also coordinates the Patient Safety Task Force which is a collaboration of agencies with regulatory and data collection responsibilities including the Centers for Disease Control and Prevention (CDC) and its National Electronic Disease Surveillance System, the Centers for Medicare and Medicaid Services (CMS) and state Quality improvement organizations, and the Food and Drug Administration (FDA). Finally, The Joint Commission uses evidence of an institutional commitment to patient safety as an accreditation criterion.

The Institute of Medicine has defined 10 recommendations for improving both quality of care and patient safety: (1) care based on continuous healing relationships; (2) customization based on patient needs and values; (3) establishment of the patient as the source of control; (4) shared knowledge and the free flow of information; (5) evidence-based decision-making; (6) safety as a priority; (7) transparency; (8) anticipation of needs; (9) continuous reduction of waste; and (10) cooperation among clinicians.[10]

C. Informed Consent

A separate and distinct documentation of informed consent for anesthesia and for anesthesia-related procedures is widely held to be the standard. Each patient's right to refuse a proposed intervention; to place limits, restrictions, or conditions on treatment; or to disregard the advice of a provider altogether are all corollaries of the informed consent doctrine. Providers should understand and respect the fact that what may be consented to may also be refused. Documentation of "refusal to consent" is equally important as the documentation of informed consent to treatment.

The doctrine of informed consent is premised on the ethical principle of autonomy which obliges providers to respect patients' right to bodily self-determination and therefore share medical decision-making authority with patients. The cornerstone of valid informed consent is effective communication—a two-way dialogue. There are two distinct legal standards which are applied to the informed consent process: the reasonable provider standard or the reasonable patient standard.

The reasonable patient standard is more commonly applied, is consistent with a respect for patient autonomy, and requires disclosure of that relevant information which a typical and reasonable patient would want to know in order to make an informed decision. The process of informed consent requires disclosure and discussion of all material risks, benefits, and alternatives to proposed therapeutic or investigational interventions.

All disclosure standards require that information and choices be presented comprehensively and in clear terms, with a concomitant explanation of the meaning of the terms, potential short-term and long-term implications of each option, discussions regarding the option to change the plan of care at a later time, the implications of such withdrawal, and reassurance that such decisions will be respected. The dialogue, including an opportunity for patients to ask questions and receive honest answers regarding the proposed treatment, should occur in an atmosphere devoid of any sense of duress or coercion in order for the consent to be truly valid.

Finally, after all disclosures have been made, the options considered, and the accord reached, the signed form within the record will represent the formal documentation of the process. Consent is therefore somewhat analogous to a contract which requires truthful disclosure, consideration, and acceptance and which then subsequently outlines expectations but also imposes duties and obligations on the parties. Similar to contracts, there are potential legal challenges regarding the validity of the consent/contract; such challenges include fraudulent facts or pretenses, duress, lack of capacity, or impaired judgment. A legally competent patient is one who is legally able to make decisions on his or her own behalf. Unemancipated minors, the mentally challenged, or the permanently disabled are possible examples of patients who may lack competency for autonomous decision-making, and therefore, family or court-appointed guardians will make decisions on their behalf. The term "capacity" refers to an impairment in decision-making which is more situational in context, such as use of medications that impair judgment and reasoning; metabolic disturbances; or mental states such as depression, mania, psychosis, and delirium or confusion.

The majority of states have statutory requirements regarding informed consent, where failure to comply with statutory requirements for informed consent can put the provider at risk for a charge of professional misconduct. Medicare conditions of participation and The Joint Commission also separately mandate informed consent. If a course of medical care is litigated for any reason, the lack of documented informed consent can compromise the legal defensibility of that case. A patient can also bring an action against a provider in civil court based on lack of consent premised either as negligent nondisclosure or medical battery. Because battery is not considered to be medical malpractice, providers may not be covered under their medical liability insurance policies for cases alleging battery.

The doctrine of "implied consent" can sometimes address the relatively common clinical situation where the provider could reasonably infer that a patient would have consented to the treatment. Implied consent is essentially a matter of the provider's reasonable interpretation of the overall patient's conduct to be consistent with an intention to authorize a procedure, even though express consent to treatment is lacking. Implied consent should be reserved for emergency care and situations where informed consent from a patient or surrogate is either very impracticable or impossible.

In the instance where a previously competent patient, or a patient with capacity, has clearly expressed their directives, these directives remain binding even after the patient loses competence or capacity. For example, in the case of an adult Jehovah's Witness patient who expressly refuses blood transfusion, with a directive clearly documented in the record, most courts have held the family cannot overrule the patient's decision after he or she loses capacity.

D. Importance of the Medical Record

The medical record is a document which serves medical, legal, and business purposes; it is an ongoing record of treatment which is used to record and communicate the circumstances of patient care to other providers, to substantiate and justify the medical reasoning involved in reaching a diagnosis and determining a plan of care, and to support a claim for reimbursement. The medical record is legally the work product of the healthcare team (**Table 41.2**). There are two aspects of medical records: the physical chart and the information contained in them. The patient has two types of legal rights to his or her medical information: a right of possession and a right of confidentiality. The physical chart is the property of the medical provider who is the legal custodian of the chart and assumes responsibility for its integrity, whereas the information contained within the medical record is legally the property of the patient.

With widespread adoption of the electronic medical record (EMR), there are new risks for providers and institutions. The risk for breach of confidentiality is enhanced with EMRs mainly because (1) unprotected (lost or unencrypted) portable devices can store and access data remotely; (2) the potential for unauthorized access to repositories of records through "hacking"' is substantial; and (3) electronic data transmission can disseminate confidential data faster and further than was possible with photocopy or fax technologies in the past. Many doctrines, laws, regulations, and policies address the confidentiality of medical information; the most widely recognized of which are the Health Insurance Portability and Accountability Act of 1996 (HIPAA) and the Health Information Technology for Economic and Clinical Health Act of 2009 (HiTECH) which address the privacy of personally identifiable health information, and security concerns associated with the electronic transmission of health information and penalties for violations for unauthorized disclosures, respectively. HiTECH has also mandated providers and health systems to provide patients with unfettered access to their EMR records.

The metadata embedded within EMRs provide details regarding the records and images accessed for review, the time and duration of document review

Table 41.2 Purposes of the Medical Record
Written documentation of the healthcare encounter
Basis for longitudinal comparisons of a patient's clinical course over time
Communication and continuity of care among the healthcare team
Basis for coding and billing claims in support of reimbursement for services
Utilization review
Peer review and quality of care evaluations
Collection of research data

and record entry, and changes made. Thus, a detailed log of the exact data and documentation reviewed by a clinician during a patient's evaluation can be retrospectively reconstructed in the event of a lawsuit. Late entries may sometimes be necessary; however, late entries after a bad outcome will be challenged as self-serving and defensive. Templates, checkboxes, and pull-down menus should be reviewed for inaccurate default entries. Typographical errors and word-recognition transcription errors are common: on one hand, errors can be reflective of inattention to detail; on the other hand, some errors are inevitable in the clinical production environment and the mind will frequently autocorrect for recently dictated errors. Nonetheless, a clear and organized narrative will still best reflect the clinician's thought process, differential diagnosis, and clinical judgment and represents a defensible clinical work-product. Providers must be cognizant that when they "copy" and "paste" information from one patient encounter to another they are acknowledging that everything was entirely the same in both visits. Also, they must be cognizant that signing prepopulated checklists, such as parts of a physical examination, legally implies that every checked item on that list has, indeed, been undertaken.

E. Responding to an Adverse Event

A serious adverse perioperative event, especially one which results in severe disability or death to an otherwise healthy patient during elective surgery, can have tremendous psychological impact on the anesthesia care team. Since such events are likely to be rare occurrences during a single practice career, the Anesthesia Patient Safety Foundation has developed an Adverse Event Protocol (AEP) to facilitate an effective, efficient, and coordinated response to a perioperative incident.[11] The AEP represents a "standard operating procedure" whereby the response to an incident is a standardized reasonable best practice, obviating the need to improvise or reinvent protocols for each individual circumstance. The AEP can be divided into a series of components: (1) communication and coordination which is designated to an incident commander who assumes administrative direction and control over the event and coordinates the involvement of consultants and the notification of departmental leadership, administrators, and family members; (2) preservation of evidence which is designed to sequester drugs and equipment to subsequently rule out contamination or malfunction in such a way as to provide credibly unspoiled evidence for later review; (3) debriefing and documentation support which promotes clear, complete, factual, and objective memorialization of the events for the medical record; and (4) subsequent peer review. The verbal, written, and behavioral responses of involved providers after a perioperative incident have potentially enormous legal ramifications: (1) statements made to peers and support staff are discoverable and may be later admitted into evidence against the provider unless they occur in a protected setting; (2) written documentation which is not objective can later be scrutinized and found to be misleading or self-serving; and (3) "cleaning up" the workstation may either result in loss of important evidence (ie, turning off monitors and machines can wipe temporary electronic memory) or be construed as intentional spoliation (intentional loss or destruction) of evidence. A well-designed AEP is communicated to all members of the anesthesia care team before any incident occurs; has been sanctioned by providers, administrators, and legal counsel; and is protocolized and automatically triggered.

The formal discussion of the circumstances surrounding an adverse event has come to be known as "disclosure." The term "disclosure" is most frequently used in the context of a disclosure of a medical error; however, disclosure of the circumstances relating to an adverse event which results in patient harm frequently occurs before it is clear that a medical error did in fact occur. Transparency and truthfulness is widely recognized as an ethical tenet and therefore a professional responsibility of providers. The American Medical Association Code of Ethics, the National Quality Forum, the National Patient Safety Foundation, and The Joint Commission have each either endorsed or have issued statement mandating disclosure. Specifically, The Joint Commission accreditation standards require providers to inform patients about "unanticipated outcomes." However, it is widely recognized that identification and scrutiny of error with implementation of a corrective feedback loop ("root cause analysis" or "RCA") is a critical mechanism to enhance patient safety; the dissemination of specific data regarding an adverse event or medical error has administrative and legal implications to both providers and institutions.

Numerous, but not well-controlled, studies have suggested that patients are more likely to seek legal counsel to explore their legal rights and to bring suit in the absence of a formal explanation or apology, presumably because of an innate sense of suspicion and a need to reach closure. The legal quandary with respect to disclosure meetings is that potentially self-implicating statements made during such meetings can be later discovered by plaintiff attorneys and admitted into evidence. Medicolegal liability from disclosure can be increased in the following ways: (1) Disclosure may inevitably put patients and families on notice that an undesirable outcome or injury was the result of a mishap or medical error and not a consequence of the disease process or other unavoidable complication of treatment. (2) Medical malpractice insurance policies frequently contain a "cooperation" or "duty to cooperate" clause which requires the insured to cooperate with the insurer's best efforts to defend against a claim. A common stipulation within such a clause maintains that an admission of liability to an injured party may nullify the policy coverage for the event. (3) Legal evidentiary rules categorize an admission of guilt is considered to be a "statement against one's own interest" and are excepted from rules regarding hearsay rules.

There is currently an expanding national interest in so-called Communication and Resolution Program (CRP) approaches to the management of an unexpected complication of medical care (ie, medical error). CRPs call for institutions to promote a culture of nonpunitive reporting of adverse events, thorough investigation of adverse events, proactive and honest explanation of what happened to patients and families, use of this experience to improve patient safety and prevent the recurrence of such incidents, and, when appropriate, an apology and offer of fair compensation to the patient or family. In 2016, the federal Agency for Healthcare Research and Quality published a "toolkit" (CANDOR) of best practices for instituting CRP.[12] Early results show that application of CRP in cases of medical error results in greater patient satisfaction and reduced litigation.

With the intent of facilitating truthful communication between providers and patients, some states have enacted "apology statutes" which are "safe harbors" designed to protect providers who apologize to patients for medical errors. Under an "apology statute," expressions of apology are excluded from discoverable evidence in the event of a malpractice claim. Apology statutes permit "offers of expressions of grief" and are primarily intended to encourage open communication through informal conversations between the patient/

family and the healthcare provider. There are two forms of apology statutes: (1) sympathy statutes which protect providers' expressions of sympathy, regret, and condolences; and (2) admission of fault statutes which, in addition, protect admissions of fault and error. Of the states which have enacted apology statutes, most have adopted the sympathy statute only; moreover, 14 states at present have not enacted any form of apology statute. In general, although it is sound practice for medical staff to adhere to regulatory and administrative policies and procedures mandating disclosure of medical errors, it is equally important that the circumstances surrounding the discussion are carefully controlled to the extent possible. Legal advice should be sought before a disclosure policy is implemented, and legal opinion should be obtained prior to a formal disclosure meeting.

? *Did You Know?*

Apology statutes vary by state and are of two types: sympathy statutes, which protect physicians' expressions of sympathy, regret, and condolences, and admission of fault statutes, which protect physicians' admissions of fault or error.

F. National Practitioner Data Bank

The National Practitioner Data Bank (NPDB) was created in 1990 and represents a federal data repository to collect and maintain quality-related information about healthcare providers (**Table 41.3**). The NPDB serves as a central data clearinghouse which collects and releases information related to the professional conduct and competence of physicians, nurses, dentists, and other healthcare practitioners. The intent of the NPDB is to support professional peer review by requiring hospitals, state licensing boards, professional societies, and other healthcare entities to report adverse actions against providers and also to query the databank as part of the credentialing and privileging process. The NPDB contains information about healthcare practitioners' malpractice history, adverse licensure actions, restrictions on professional membership, and negative privileging actions by hospitals. It is important to realize that uncontested adverse actions such as settlements before judgment in malpractice litigation, uncontested denials for medical staff credentialing, and resignations from medical staff while a peer review investigation is ongoing are all reportable to the NPDB.

G. Advance Directives

An advance directive is a statement of instruction (usually, but not always in written form) which, when written, is anticipated to potentially take effect at some point in the future. The purpose of an advance directive is to make one's wishes known to others, in the event that one later loses the ability to communicate, so that one's wishes can be known and respected.

Table 41.3 Examples of Events Reportable to the National Practitioner Databank
Medical malpractice payments
Healthcare-related civil or criminal actions
Adverse licensure actions
Revocation, reprimand, censure, suspension, probation, voluntary surrender
Adverse clinical privileging actions
Adverse professional society membership actions
Drug Enforcement Administration actions
Exclusions from Federal- or State-funded healthcare programs
Private accreditation organization actions
Other due-process adjudications pertinent to healthcare

Advance directives represent a practical application of the ethical principle respecting autonomous decision-making. Examples of advance directives include living wills and healthcare proxies, durable powers of attorney, general do-not-resuscitate requests, or the specific documentation of preferences for interventions such as prolonged mechanical ventilation, artificial nutrition and hydration, or dialysis in the event of severe incapacitating injury.

A "living will" is a common form of advance directive which defines a patient's expectations from providers and the healthcare system; it almost always delineates specific or general parameters for the initiation, continuation, or termination of various levels of life-sustaining medical treatment. Living wills can be prepared by either the patient alone or, more often, in consultation with either his or her provider and/or attorney. A principal practical limitation of living wills is that very few such documents are of sufficient specificity so as to unequivocally define a patient's wishes for all contingencies. Thus, most living wills are practically little more than a general guide to patients' wishes. Thus, even when a living will is available, the patient's surrogate decision-makers are still tasked with the interpretation of the patient's wishes in that specific circumstance.

A healthcare proxy is a surrogate decision-maker who is specifically and legally appointed by the patient, by way of a written designation, for the purpose of making healthcare decisions on his or her behalf. The healthcare proxy need not be a relative, and therefore, a healthcare proxy supersedes statutorily defined surrogacy hierarchies. The proxy or surrogate is merely conveying indirectly the wishes and directions of the patient and should not engage in unilateral decision-making. In the absence of a previously designated healthcare proxy, providers should consult their state laws regarding "statutes of surrogacy" which define the hierarchy of decision-makers who can speak on a patient's.

A "power of attorney" is a legal document empowering another with authority of agency or the authority to act in one's place. Powers of attorney can be specific to financial, administrative, or healthcare matters or may be more general and even unrestricted. Simple powers of attorney are in effect only as long as the patient also has capacity to make decisions and become void when a patient loses decision-making capacity. On the other hand, a "durable power of attorney" is a more powerful document which retains its effect even after a patient loses decision-making capacity. Again, even durable powers of attorney may be restricted in scope and may not necessarily extend to healthcare decisions.

Advance directives also include orders regarding preferences for resuscitation. "Do Not Resuscitate" (DNR) or "Do Not Attempt Resuscitation" (DNAR) orders represent provider orders which are based upon the completion of a standardized form which outlines a patient's resuscitation preferences. The DNR form is similar to the living will, but it is more specific and is frequently a legal form designed and regulated by individual state statutes. While the living will is usually broad and somewhat aspirational, the DNR form is subject to little or no discretion for interpretation. DNR forms closely resemble a "refusal to consent" to treatment since they specify a limitation of medical care. The general legal and ethical considerations that apply to the informed consent process also apply to end-of-life discussions and the DNR order—for a DNR to be legally valid, it must be obtained after full disclosure in a competent patient with capacity and without duress or coercion. Patients who have lost the capacity to understand the implications of their decisions, or those that are suicidal or clinically depressed, are not typically viewed as being in a position to consent to or refuse treatment.

III. Quality Improvement and Patient Safety

A. Structure, Process, and Outcome: The Building Blocks of Safety

The Donabedian model[13] is a conceptual framework for evaluating quality and designing quality of care improvements using three categories of analysis: structure, process, and outcome. The term "structure" describes the factors which impact the context in which care occurs (such as the hospital, staff, training, equipment, and administration); "process" relates to the normative behaviors, relationships, and interactions (such as preventive care, patient education, choice of diagnostic or therapeutic interventions) throughout healthcare delivery; and finally, "outcome" refers to the results obtained and the effect of healthcare encounters on patients or populations (mortality, health status, patient satisfaction, or health-related quality of life). The Donabedian framework can be used to modify structures and processes within a healthcare delivery unit and to evaluate the effects of changes on specified external indicators of quality; however, the model itself does not contain an implicit definition of quality or value. Lohr has defined "quality healthcare" to be "the degree to which health services for individuals and populations increase the likelihood of desired health outcomes and are consistent with current professional knowledge."[14]

The Donabedian model is relevant to discussions of patient safety and quality of care for two reasons: (1) patient safety is related to structure and process, and quality describes outcomes and the manner in which they are achieved; (2) legislators, regulators, healthcare administrators, and payors uniformly require and rely upon this framework. The model describes how regulators, policymakers, and stakeholders analyze the healthcare system and therefore every health system's licensure, regulatory compliance, and condition of participation requirements. It is commonly believed that the majority of medical errors result from faulty systems and processes.

Deming developed the ***Total Quality Management*** (TQM) model which promoted an organizational approach to quality which stressed the importance of teamwork, defined processes, systems thinking, and change programs intended to create an environment supportive of quality improvement. In a similar fashion, ***Continuous Quality Improvement*** (CQI) is a doctrine based in the principle that a potential opportunity exists for improvement in every process, and therefore, objective data are necessary to analyze and improve processes. The "***PDSA cycle***" implements four steps (1) a "Plan" for a change, (2) a "Do" action which carries out that plan, (3) a "Study" of the results, and (4) an "Act" or lasting quality improvement initiative. The ***Six Sigma*** model consists of 5 elements (define, measure, analyze, improve, and control) which represent a quality improvement framework for developing incremental improvement. ***Root cause analysis*** (RCA) is a retrospective rather than prospective model of quality improvement. RCA is a widely used two-step process—thorough examination of adverse outcomes (eg, interviews, document review) and development of plans to strengthen or develop safety systems.

B. Difficulty of Outcome Measurement in Anesthesia

Quality of care is difficult if not impossible to define and measure clinically. The first clinical quality indicators, or ***generic quality screens***, relied on the identification of specific adverse outcomes and subsequent analysis through individual case review to identify potential quality of care issues. Subsequently, The Joint Commission developed a series of anesthesia-related quality indicators by which organizational performance could be continuously monitored and evaluated. This national ***Indicator Measurement System*** evaluated two categories of performance: (1) sentinel event indicators (unexpected occurrences involving death or serious physical injury) and (2) rate-based indicators (trends in a particular type of process or outcome of care). Unfortunately, the validation of anesthetic clinical indicators is largely limited to expert opinion, because at this time, there is insufficient evidence to demonstrate that compliance with evidence-based best practice will systematically and universally result in better patient outcome.[15] For example, compliance with perioperative beta-blockade was initially instituted as a national quality indicator after data suggested that institution of perioperative beta-blockade reduced the incidence of myocardial infarction in high-risk patients undergoing noncardiac surgery. Subsequently, additional data validated the effect of beta-blockade on myocardial infarction rate, but also demonstrated that the risk of death and blindness were increased in noncardiac surgery patients receiving perioperative beta-blockade.

Outcome measurement in anesthesiology is also complicated by the lack of standardized and consensus definitions across systems and countries. For example, perioperative anesthesia-related mortality can be measured by three different indicators: death within 48 hours of a procedure involving anesthesia, death rate associated with procedures involving anesthesia, or deaths within 30 days of surgery. Death as an outcome measure, similar to other perioperative morbidity measures, is dependent on the patient's medical status or severity of illness; institutionally the cumulative medical complexity of patients is reflected in the case-mix index. Although the ***ASA Physical Status Classification System*** is related to perioperative risk, the system is largely subjective and definitions are based on relative severity of disease which result in inconsistent categorization. The complexity of clinical care systems is such that multiple variables are involved in every outcome. Thus, anesthesia-specific outcomes, or outcomes specifically attributable to anesthesia care, remain elusive. It is difficult to attribute causality for the outcome to either a specific surgical, anesthetic, or medical intervention as opposed to the totality of the medical care. The ability of the anesthesiologist in a brief perioperative timeframe to optimize the patient before surgery and to follow the outcomes postoperatively is limited. In addition, it is not possible to accurately predict which of many common but low-morbidity anesthesia outcomes are of highest importance to a particular surgical patient. For example, the specific choice of opiate for the management of postoperative pain may impair the perceived quality of care for a postoperative patient who considers nausea more important than the intensity of pain.

Thus, with respect to the Donabedian model, practical quality improvements based on connections between process and outcomes requires large sample populations, adjustments by case mix, and long-term follow-up; and the meaningful impact of specific interventions on relatively low-frequency adverse outcomes is largely lost in the complexity of the individual patient and multiple healthcare interventions.

C. Regulatory Requirements for Quality Improvement

The Flexner Report established standards for modern medical education and provided an impetus for the development of state departments of public health which were later charged with the supervision of healthcare institutions. In the 1950s, The Joint Commission on Accreditation of Hospitals (JCAH), now referred to simply as The Joint Commission, established an accreditation process for hospitals which became a compulsory standard for facilities seeking state licensure and Medicare participation.

State licensure is a statutory condition of participation for hospitals, while accreditation is a voluntary means of meeting the conditions for participation. Regulatory oversight for healthcare quality occurs at many levels ranging from professional licensure; conditions of participation; training, certification, and accreditation; mandatory reporting; and pay for performance. Compliance with regulatory mandates has made healthcare the most regulated of industries in the United States.

The Federal Health Reform legislation of 2010, the Affordable Care Act (ACA), mandates "value-based purchasing" and assigns bonuses or penalties to providers and hospitals which employ care coordination and safety interventions, which prevent nosocomial infections and unnecessary hospital readmissions, and participate in public reporting of hospital and provider quality performance. Curve-2 Metrics or "Metrics for the Second Curve of Health Care" refers to the transition from the volume-based first curve to the value-based second curve and requires (1) the alignment of hospitals, providers, and other clinical providers across the continuum of care; (2) the adoption of evidence-based practices to improve quality and patient safety; (3) the improvement of efficiency through productivity and financial management; and (4) the development of integrated information systems. Elements of Curve-2 Metrics applicable to anesthesiologists will include measures such as the effective management and measurement of care transitions, the management of utilization variation, the reduction of preventable complications and mortality, and expense per episode of care.

IV. Professional Liability

A. Professionalism and Licensure

Anesthesiologists, legally, are considered professionals. As such, they must have met specific standards of education and training. These standards of practice and ethics are codified in codes of conduct specific to medicine and the specialty. All physicians owe a fiduciary duty to their patients.

Epstein and Hundert[16] define "professionalism" as a "habitual and judicious use of communication, knowledge, technical skills, clinical reasoning, emotions, values, and reflection in daily practice for the benefit of the individual and community being served." An international panel of medical societies defined three fundamental principles of professionalism: (1) the primacy of patient welfare, which addresses altruism, trust, and patient interest; (2) patient autonomy addressing the importance of honesty with patients and the need to empower patients in medical decision-making; and (3) social justice addressing providers' societal contract and distributive justice in consideration of the finite nature of healthcare resources (**Table 41.4**). Specific to anesthesiology, Tetzlaff has defined the essentials of professionalism to include the following: (1) accountability; (2) humanism; (3) personal well-being; and (4)

Table 41.4 Commitments Inherent to Professionalism

Professional competence
Honesty
Patient confidentiality
Appropriate relations with patients
Improving quality of care
Improving access to care
Just distribution of finite resources
Scientific knowledge
Maintaining trust by managing conflicts of interest
Professional responsibilities

ethics.[17] More practically, the three pillars of clinical excellence for anesthesiologists have been defined as availability, affability, and ability.

B. The Adversarial System of Justice

The adversarial system refers to a common law legal system whereby advocates represent their parties' positions before an impartial person or group of people, usually a judge or jury, who attempt to determine the truth of the matters alleged. The aggrieved patient who initiates the lawsuit is the ***plaintiff*** who seeks a legal remedy from the court. If the plaintiff is successful, the court will enter judgment for the plaintiff and issue a court order for damages with the intention of making the plaintiff whole in compensation for having been wronged. The party against whom the complaint is directed is the ***defendant***. In litigation, cases are identified by citing the plaintiff first; thus, a lawsuit is cited as "Plaintiff v. Defendant." In a civil lawsuit, the burden of proof rests with the plaintiff who must establish the requisite elements of his or her case by a "preponderance of evidence" that all the alleged facts have been presented and are more likely than not to be true.

The party who initiates the lawsuit (plaintiff) must file the claim within a specified period of time, a statutorily defined and state-specific time period known as the "statute of limitations." A lawsuit is formally commenced when the plaintiff's attorney files a complaint with the court and the clerk of the court issues a summons. A civil lawsuit in United States is initiated by filing a summons, claim form, or complaint; documents which are collectively referred to as the pleadings. Pleadings describe in detail the alleged wrongs committed by the defendant and include a demand for relief. The legal action is initiated by service of legal process by physical delivery of the pleadings to the defendant. The pleadings are then filed with the court which has jurisdiction over the parties together with an affidavit verifying that they have served on the defendant in accordance with the rules of legal procedure.

Typically, service of the summons is made on the defendant-provider, not on the insurer, and it is important that the provider notify the insurance carrier immediately because the defendant has only a limited period of time during which to answer the complaint. If the answer is not filed by the provider's defense counsel within the statutory time limits, the plaintiff can obtain a default judgment against the defendant-provider, forfeiting the right to contest the matter in court.

If the action is not dismissed, then both parties will begin a process of ***discovery***. Discovery relates to the opportunity of each party to obtain relevant information and documents from the parties to the lawsuit. Discovery may include interrogatories, depositions of key parties, support staff, and families; chart reviews; expert reviews; determination of relevant supporting materials. Interrogatories refer to written questions served on parties; depositions represent formal oral sworn testimony obtained under oath and transcribed by a court reporter.

All states have trial courts where civil disputes are filed and litigated, and there is usually a system of appeals courts, with final judicial authority resting in the state court of final appeal. If the malpractice claim involves the federal government acting through a federally funded clinic or a Veteran's Administration Facility, then the action is filed in a federal district court. Federal courts will also hear malpractice claims when there is complete diversity of state citizenship such as when the parties are domiciled in different states or if a "federal question" is at issue, such as a violation of a fundamental constitutional right during the alleged negligent conduct. The place where the case is filed is usually guided by place where the incident occurred, or the residence of the parties involved, and is known as the ***venue***.

At various times during the litigation process, the parties might choose to settle, attempt alternative dispute resolution such as mediation or arbitration, proffer motions for either summary judgment or dismissal, or voluntarily discontinue the action. Settlement prior to trial is generally encouraged by the courts in the interests of judicial efficiency. Medical malpractice cases frequently settle out-of-court since there are many potential advantages of doing so: (1) juries are unpredictable; (2) the negative consequences and publicity of a guilty verdict are lessened; (3) defense attorney, expert witness, and court costs are potentially lessened; and (4) the precedential impact of the verdict to future similar cases is eliminated. If the matter proceeds to trial, the court will set a trial date on the "docket," or trial calendar. The defense strategy is often a complex interplay between the facts of the case, the credibility of the witnesses, the opinions of experts, and the personalities of the parties. A party generally has the right to appeal a judgment to at least one higher court, which has the power to affirm, reverse, or modify the judgment of the trial court.

> **? *Did You Know?***
>
> In medical malpractice cases, physicians are generally not liable for negligence for errors in judgment but can be liable for care that falls outside recognized standards of good medical practice, defined as care that a reasonably competent and skilled healthcare professional, with similar training, would provide under similar circumstances.

C. Elements of Medical Malpractice, Res Ipsa, and Malpractice Insurance

Since medicine involves decision-making of high complexity, in circumstances where not all the relevant information is available, and often during times of extreme urgency, medicine is an area of professional practice wherein the risk of adverse outcomes, and therefore of litigation, is high. Nonetheless, providers must understand that a bad outcome does not equate with medical malpractice. A provider is generally not liable for errors in judgment; rather, liability can only legitimately be inferred where the treatment rendered clearly falls outside recognized standards of good medical practice. In order to prove medical malpractice, the plaintiff must show that the provider deviated from the standard of care relevant to the specific treatment setting in question. The ***standard of care*** is further defined as that care which a reasonably competent and skilled healthcare professional, with a similar training, would have provided under similar circumstances.

Medical malpractice is a specific type of negligence within a group of legal causes of action known as civil torts governed by the laws of state-specific civil statutes. To be found liable under any specific cause of action, the trial court will require that the plaintiff demonstrate each legal element of that particular cause of action. The legal elements of the civil tort of medical negligence are (1) the existence of a duty; (2) a breach of that duty; (3) proof that the breach of duty was the actual and proximate cause of the adverse outcome; and (4) demonstration that ascertainable damages resulted as a cause of that breach. Medical malpractice usually involves issues that are beyond the usual understanding of laypersons; therefore, the courts require that the elements of malpractice including standard of care, breach, and proximate cause must be proved through expert testimony.

Duty is created by the provider-patient relationship and requires that the provider adhere to that degree of skill and learning ordinarily possessed and employed by other members of the same profession, who are in good standing, and are engaged in the same type of practice or specialty. In practice, however, the norms of generally accepted medical practice, which form the basis for a definition of a relevant standard of care, can be difficult to define because the medical literature is replete with controversy and new advances, and there is great variation between patients. Therefore, both plaintiff and defendant will each introduce expert opinion testimony regarding the applicable standard of care. In order to prove that the defendant-provider committed a breach of duty, the plaintiff must demonstrate that the defendant did not act in accordance with the applicable standard of care.

The plaintiff must prove causation by showing of a reasonably close "causal connection" between the alleged negligent act (or omission) and the resulting injury. The malpractice must be shown to be a "cause in fact" ("actual cause") of the plaintiff's injury. However, in addition, the alleged act of malpractice must be shown to also be the proximate cause ("legal cause") of the plaintiff's injury. The concept of legal causation can be difficult for providers to comprehend because it does not refer to a strict scientific causation. Legal causation considers both "causation in fact" and "foreseeability." Causation in fact is defined using the "but for" test which requires a showing that "but for" the act or failure to act, the complication or injury would not have occurred. "Foreseeability" requires that the patient's injuries be a reasonably foreseeable result of the defendant-provider's actions.

The term "damages" attempts to quantify the actual ascertainable injuries suffered by the plaintiff. The term "damages" is broad and encompasses a range of financial, physical, and emotional injuries. The intent of awarding compensatory damages in a tort action is to "make the plaintiff whole again" which, in most medically related injuries, is an obvious legal fiction but nonetheless the best attempt at compensation. Damages can be special (eg, costs of further care, lost wages), general (noneconomic injuries such as loss of companionship, grief, pain and suffering), or punitive (if the alleged conduct can be shown to be willful, reckless, fraudulent, grossly negligent, or malicious.)

In the event that the elements of medical negligence cannot be proven, or the case is relatively straight-forward, a theory of medical liability can also be premised in the doctrine of "res ipsa loquitur" which literally translates as "the facts speak for themselves." The specific elements of a "res ipsa" claim vary by state; however, in general, a case may be submitted to the jury on the theory of res ipsa only when the plaintiff can establish that (1) the event is one which ordinarily does not occur in the absence of negligence; (2) the event was caused by an agency or instrumentality within the exclusive control of the defendant; and (3) the event cannot have been due to any voluntary action or contribution on the part of the plaintiff.[12] Examples of res ipsa claims include retained instruments, positioning injuries, and intraoperative burns. The legal effect of res ipsa loquitur is to create a prima facie case ("valid on its face") of negligence and does not usually require expert testimony.

Medical malpractice insurance indemnity policies provide insurance coverage for claims arising out of alleged malpractice. The malpractice carrier has two principal obligations to the insured: the duty to defend and the duty to indemnify. In order to provide a legal defense, an insurance carrier will typically retain knowledgeable and experienced defense counsel and pay the legal fees on behalf of the defendant-provider. The duty to indemnify requires the carrier to pay the amount of a settlement or judgment on a covered claim within the set policy limits. There are two general types of medical malpractice insurance policies: ***Occurrence policies*** which cover incidents which occur not only during the period when the policy is in effect but also if it is reported following expiration or discontinuance of that policy. ***Claims-made*** policies only cover occurrences where both the event and the claim occur during the life of the policy. Since the average malpractice claim is made 1 to 2 years following an incident, a provider may no longer be covered under the policy when a claim is made. Therefore, claims-made policies usually require that the provider purchase either "nose" or "tail" coverage in order to maintain coverage during job or insurer-to-insurer transitions.

For further review, please see the associated Interactive Video Lectures accessible in complimentary eBook bundled with this text. Access instructions are located on the inside front cover.

References

1. Li G, Warner M, Lang BH, Huang L, Sun LS. Epidemiology of anesthesia-related mortality in the United States, 1999-2005. *Anesthesiology*. 2009;110(4):759-765. PMID: 19322941.
2. Haller G, Laroche T, Clergue F. Morbidity in anaesthesia: today and tomorrow. *Best Pract Res Clin Anaesthesiol*. 2011;25(2):123-132. PMID: 21550538.
3. Mazzocco K, Petitti DB, Fong KT, et al. Surgical team behaviors and patient outcomes. *Am J Surg*. 2009;197(5):678-685. PMID: 18789425.
4. Boet S, Etherington N, Nicola D, et al. Anesthesia interventions that alter perioperative mortality: a scoping review. *Syst Rev*. 2018;7(1):218. PMID: 30497505.
5. Cheng D, Martin J. Evidence-based practice and health technology assessment: a call for anesthesiologists to engage in knowledge translation. *Can J Anaesth*. 2011;58(4):354-363. PMID: 21264556.
6. Szalados JE. Morality, ethics, and the law: an overview of the foundations of contemporary clinical ethical analysis. In: Szalados JE, ed. *Ethics and Law for Neurosciences Clinicians: Foundations and Evolving Challenges*. Rutgers University Press; 2019.
7. Institute of Medicine. *To Err Is Human: Building a Safer Health System*. National Academy Press; 1999.
8. Sutcliffe KM. High reliability organizations (HROs). *Best Pract Res Clin Anaesthesiol*. 2011;25(2):133-144. PMID: 21550539.
9. Chassin MR, Loeb JM. High-reliability health care: getting there from here. *Milbank Q*. 2013;91(3):459-490. PMID: 24028696.
10. Institute of Medicine. *Crossing the Quality Chasm: A New Health System for the 21st Century*. National Academy Press; 2001.
11. Cooper JB, Cullen DJ, Eichhorn JH, Philip JH, Holzman RS. Administrative guidelines for response to an adverse anesthesia event. The risk management committee of the Harvard Medical School's department of anaesthesia. *J Clin Anesth*. 1993;5(1):79-84. PMID: 8442975.
12. Agency for Healthcare Research and Quality. *Communication and Optimal Resolution (CANDOR) Toolkit*. 2016. Accessed September 8, 2020. http://www.ahrq.gov/professionals/quality-patient-safety/patient-safety-resources/resources/candor/introduction.html
13. Donabedian A. The role of outcomes in quality assessment and assurance. *Qual Rev Bull*. 1992;18:356-360. PMID: 1465293.
14. Lohr KN, Schroeder SA. A strategy for quality assurance in Medicare. *N Engl J Med*. 1990;322:1161-1171. PMID: 2406600.
15. Haller G, Stoelwinder J, Myles PS McNeil JM. Quality and safety indicators in anesthesia: a systematic review. *Anesthesiology*. 2009;110(5):1158-1175. PMID: 19352148
16. Epstein RM, Hundert EM. Defining and assessing professional competence. *J Am Med Assoc*. 2002;287(2):226-235. PMID: 11779266.
17. Tetzlaff JE. Anesthesiology. Professionalism in anesthesiology: "what is it?" or "i know it when I see it". *Anesthesiology*. 2009;110(4):700-702. PMID: 19276965.

Questions

1. **Which of the following is a formal principle of medical ethics?**

   A. Patient autonomy
   B. Beneficence
   C. Nonmaleficence
   D. All of the above

2. **Which of the following is an example of the medical ethical principle of "justice"?**

   A. An anesthesiologist decides on a perioperative care plan based on careful review of the patient's medical history, without discussion with the otherwise mentally competent and communicative patient.
   B. An anesthesiologist working in a mass casualty incident triages patients to settings of emergent care, delayed care, or expectant care.
   C. An anesthesiologist provides the highest level of care, without regard to personal gain or societal interests.
   D. The concept of primum non nocere (first, do no harm).

3. **A healthy 2-month-old, former preterm boy is undergoing an elective inguinal hernia repair under general anesthesia. The "crew resource management" paradigm for perioperative care team coordination includes all of the following examples EXCEPT:**

   A. A preoperative "time-out" takes place for all members of the team to review the surgical safety checklist.
   B. Prior to administering a local anesthetic field block, the surgeon, nursing staff, and anesthesiologist review and agree on the correct drug and dose for the child.
   C. When the surgeon and anesthesiologist disagree on the maximum local anesthetic dose for the child, the procedure is briefly halted to consult with the hospital pharmacy.
   D. On her first day in her anesthesiology clerkship, the medical student assisting the anesthesiologist notices a large volume of air in the intravenous tubing, but refrains from telling the anesthesiologist due to her insecurity.

4. **A healthy, mentally competent, 55-year-old married father of three teenage children is about to undergo an elective open repair of an iliac artery pseudoaneurysm. The patient is a Jehovah's Witness who has noted in writing on both his hospital admission form and his surgical consent form that he will not accept any type of blood product under any condition. The anesthesiologist should:**

   A. Contact hospital risk management to obtain a court order to transfuse blood products, should unexpected life-threatening bleeding occur intraoperatively.
   B. Discuss the issue with the patient to confirm his wishes (even if doing so might put his life in danger) and to discuss potential alternative treatments (eg, intraoperative blood salvage and return).
   C. Arrange for intraoperative blood salvage (eg, cell-saver) to be used without informing the patient.
   D. Refuse to participate in the procedure.

5. **The National Practitioner Data Bank collects and releases information related to the professional conduct and competence of physicians and other healthcare providers, including which of the following?**

   A. Negative privileging actions by a hospital
   B. Previous malpractice claims, irrespective of settlement
   C. Adverse licensure actions by state authorities
   D. All of the above

6. **Which of the following is an example of an advance directive?**

   A. Living will
   B. Do-not-resuscitate (DNR) order
   C. Durable power of attorney
   D. All of the above

7. **Medical malpractice is a type of negligence that is argued in civil court, as opposed to criminal court. Related to the initiation, location, and appeals process for such proceedings, all of the following are true EXCEPT:**

   A. Civil lawsuits are initiated by postal mailing of a summons, claim form, or complaint document to the defendant physician's malpractice insurer.
   B. Civil malpractice disputes are generally filed in state trial courts and final judicial authority generally rests in the state court of appeals.
   C. Civil malpractice disputes can be filed in federal courts only in specific instances where federal issues are involved.
   D. Once a defendant physician receives a proper summons, the defendant has only a limited time to respond to the complaint (ie, statutory time limit).

8. **Regarding medical malpractice insurance indemnity policies, which of the following is TRUE?**

   A. Defendant physicians generally must retain their own defense counsel.
   B. Occurrence policies only cover occurrences where both the event and the claim occur during the life of the policy.
   C. Claims-made policies usually require the physician to purchase a "tail" policy to maintain malpractice coverage for incidents that occurred during the life of the policy but the malpractice claim was filed after the policy ended.
   D. Insurance carriers are not required to pay the amount of a settlement or judgment, even if the amount is within set policy limits.

9. **A 75-year-old mentally competent woman with no living relatives is scheduled to undergo hip replacement surgery and has granted legal and documented "simple power of attorney" to her otherwise unrelated and mentally competent housemate. Is the following statement true or false? "While under general anesthesia, the housemate may make healthcare decisions on behalf of the patient."**

   A. True
   B. False

10. **The Donabedian model, root cause analysis, the PDSA cycle, and the Six Sigma model are all examples of which of the following?**

    A. Adverse event reporting systems
    B. Strategies to document "meaningful use" of electronic health records
    C. Paradigms for decision-making in medical ethics
    D. Quality improvement models

Answers

1. D

The four formal principles of medical ethics are patient autonomy, beneficence, nonmaleficence, and justice, and they provide a structure for case discussions and application to medical ethics decision-making.

2. B

The medical ethical principle of justice has components of distribution and retribution. Distributive justice addresses aspects of providing access to equitable and transparent care within the confines of limited healthcare resources (eg, triage). Retributive justice addresses retaliation or punishment for certain actions and is largely applicable to disciplinary and legal reviews. Making unilateral decisions on behalf of patients without their input is a form of paternalism. Providing the highest level of care typifies the ethical principle of beneficence, whereas primum non nocere typifies that of nonmaleficence.

3. D

As shown in **Table 41.1**, the general structure of the crew resource management paradigm in the operating room is focused on team communication and leadership, workload management, structured decision-making, and stress management. One key tenet is that any team member—regardless of their position in the chain of command—is free and encouraged to respectfully question issues related to patient safety.

4. B

When clearly documented in the medical record, the directive of a mentally competent, adult Jehovah's Witness to not receive intraoperative blood products is binding, even after the patient loses competence or capacity under general anesthesia. The anesthesiologist should explicitly confirm these directives prior to surgery and then agree to follow the directives. If the anesthesiologist has personal or religious objections to carrying out such directives, he or she should arrange for a colleague to provide such care.

5. D

The purpose of the National Practitioner Data Bank is to support professional peer review by requiring hospitals (patient care privileges), state licensing boards (licensure actions), professional societies (restrictions on membership), and other healthcare entities (malpractice claims) to report such adverse actions. Such data can then be released (under strict control) for future physician credentialing and privileging purposes.

6. D

Examples of advance directives include living wills and healthcare proxies, durable powers of attorney, general do-not-resuscitate requests, or the specific documentation of preferences for interventions such as prolonged mechanical ventilation, artificial nutrition and hydration, or dialysis in the event of severe incapacitating injury.

7. A

All states have trial courts where civil disputes such as medical malpractice are filed and litigated, up to and including the appeals process. However, when there is diversity of state citizenship among parties, if a federal question (eg, violation of a constitutional right) is at stake, or if care occurred in a federally funded healthcare facility, the disputes (and possible appeals) will be litigated in federal court. Medical malpractice lawsuits are initiated by physical delivery of the summons, claim form, or complaint to the defendant physician, who must then immediately inform his or her insurance carrier due to the limited time to respond to the complaint (ie, statutory time limit).

8. C

To meet their dual obligations to defend and to indemnify, insurance carriers (not the defendant physician) will typically retain experienced defense council and also pay the amount of a settlement or judgment on a covered claim (within set policy limits). Occurrence policies cover events even if the claim is filed after discontinuation or expiration of the policy. In contrast, claims-made policies only cover events that both occur and are claimed during the life of the policy; thus, a "tail" policy is generally required for such policies.

9. B

Simple power of attorney is in effect only as long as the patient also has the capacity to make decisions but becomes void when a patient loses that capacity. In contrast, a durable power of attorney retains its effect after the patient loses decision-making capacity. Thus, only someone with legal and documented durable power of attorney specifically for healthcare decisions can make such decisions on behalf of the patient while the patient is under general anesthesia.

10. D

The models and strategies noted above can all be used for quality improvement purposes by providing structures to link clinical outcomes with quality of care improvements. Key factors in each approach can include data collection, error identification, clinical outcomes, patient satisfaction, process measures, and analysis.

42 Critical Care Medicine

Matthew R. Hallman and Vanessa M. Cervantes

? *Did You Know?*

Critical care medicine and the development of intensive care units were initiated in response to the increased incidence of respiratory failure observed during the US polio epidemic of the 1940s, with the first critical care medicine training program established by a University of Pittsburgh anesthesiologist, Dr Peter Safar.

The practice of critical care medicine (CCM) and development of intensive care units (ICUs) date to at least the 1940s and perhaps earlier. Advances in surgical interventions along with increased incidences of respiratory failure due to polio epidemics led to an increased demand for physicians specializing in the care of critically ill patients, especially patients with respiratory failure. To meet this demand, the first CCM training program was established by Peter Safar, an anesthesiologist at the University of Pittsburgh, in the 1960s, but it was not until 1986 that the first CCM board certification examination was administered by the American Board of Anesthesiology. As of 2019, approximately 2600 anesthesiologists had completed the CCM certification process. However, <10% of practicing intensivists are anesthesiologists, and the majority of intensivists in the United States continue to be pulmonary physicians. Physicians of other specialties including surgery, pediatrics, emergency medicine, and neurology also pursue training in critical care medicine. Fortunately for those interested in this specialty, the future need for intensivists is expected to be much greater than the supply.

The scope of CCM is vast, covering nearly every aspect of illness and injury and drawing upon knowledge from nearly every medical and surgical specialty. It is also a specialty that continues to undergo tremendous change. New technologies, equipment, and medications along with increased understanding of diseases and pathophysiology allow for the treatment of increasingly ill patients. More recently, as the economics of healthcare delivery have received increased attention, the focus on delivering evidence-based, cost-effective care has also increased. Because the ICU is one of the most resource-intensive areas of modern hospitals, care of patients in the ICU has been identified as an obvious target for increased efficiency.

Although the entire spectrum of critical care is beyond the scope of this chapter, widely applicable aspects of contemporary critical care are reviewed here. The first part of the chapter addresses processes of care that are applicable to most ICU settings, including both medical and surgical ICUs. The second part of the chapter provides an overview of the management for some commonly encountered diagnoses. The entire chapter focuses on evidence-based practices that may improve both patient outcomes and healthcare system performance in the perioperative setting.

I. Processes of Care

A. Staffing

Advances in medical and surgical therapeutics have increased the complexity of care for an aging and increasingly ill population. It has become clear that providing the best care for such a population requires a knowledge base and skill set that are highly specialized and that involving intensivists in the care of critically ill patients is desirable. Compared with low-intensity staffing models, ***high-intensity staffing*** models (ie, an intensivist-led team or mandatory consultation of an intensivist) are associated with lower hospital and ICU mortality as well as shorter hospital and ICU lengths of stay.[1]

Patient outcomes appear to be further improved by the addition of ***multidisciplinary*** providers to intensivist-led teams. Examples include pharmacist participation in daily rounds, as well as the inclusion of nurses, dieticians, and respiratory therapists. These practices significantly reduce costs and medication-related adverse events and are also associated with decreased patient mortality.[2]

B. Checklists

Despite the improvement in communication and information transfer that occurs with multidisciplinary teams, high stress and a massive volume of information in the ICU environment can lead to errors. Checklists have been widely implemented on ICU rounds as cognitive aids that serve as daily reminders to evaluate a limited number of interventions, preventative measures, bundles, and processes of care that can improve outcomes. Their implementation is associated with decreased mortality and ICU length of stay, and their cost is negligible.[3] Considering the potential benefits and the minimal economic investment required for checklist implementation, their use is strongly recommended. In fact, many of the care processes discussed in this chapter commonly appear on checklists and should be considered for every patient, every day. Suggested content for consideration and inclusion in a daily ICU checklist is listed in **Table 42.1**. Content might be added or removed based on local ICU considerations.

C. Resource Management

In 2014, the Critical Care Societies Collaborative released a list of "Five Things Physicians and Patients Should Question" in critical care as part of the Choosing Wisely campaign. The campaign is designed to reduce unnecessary interventions that lack cost-effectiveness and has been supported by many medical specialties. At the top of the list is a recommendation to not order diagnostic studies (chest x-rays, blood gases, blood chemistries and counts, and electrocardiograms) at regular intervals (eg, daily) unless there is a clear indication. Compared with the practice of ordering tests only to answer clinical questions or when doing so will directly affect management, the routine ordering of tests increases costs, does not benefit patients, and may in fact harm them. This and other efforts to minimize unnecessary interventions recognize both the financial impact medical practice decisions have

Table 42.1 Suggested Daily Intensive Care Unit Checklist

- Spontaneous awakening trial
- Spontaneous breathing trial
- Nutrition/diet ordered
- Glucose control adequate
- Deep vein thrombosis prophylaxis initiated
- Unnecessary laboratory tests and imaging discontinued
- Antibiotics discontinued
- Foley catheter removed
- Central venous catheter and arterial line removed

on individual patients and the healthcare system overall. These efforts also emphasize the physician's role in providing not just effective care, but efficient care.

? *Did You Know?*

Once commonplace in intensive care units, the routine, scheduled performance of diagnostic tests (eg, daily chest x-ray) is no longer indicated due to increased costs, questionable clinical benefit, and possible patient harm.

D. Analgesia and Sedation

Pain

Pain is defined as "an unpleasant sensory and emotional experience associated with actual or potential tissue damage, or described in terms of such damage[4]" and is experienced differently by each individual. Agitation and delirium are additional conditions often closely linked with pain in the critically ill population. Both the patient's underlying medical conditions and the assessments and interventions that occur as part of ICU care can contribute to the development of pain, agitation, and delirium (PAD). ***An effective PAD management program should be tailored to each individual patient and involve steps to prevent, detect, quantify, treat, and reassess PAD.***

Opioids are the primary modality of treating moderate to severe pain in critically ill adults. However, they have undesirable side effects including nausea, constipation, respiratory depression, immunosuppression, and alteration of mental status. When titrated to similar end points, there is not one opioid medication that has been shown to be superior to others. In order to reduce opioid-related side effects, nonopioid analgesics such as acetaminophen, nonsteroidal anti-inflammatory drugs, local anesthetics, ketamine, alpha-2 agonists, and γ-aminobutyric acid analogues may be used in conjunction with opioids. In the case of mild pain, acetaminophen or nonsteroidal anti-inflammatory drugs may replace opioids altogether. Regional anesthesia techniques may also be helpful in managing a variety of types of pain including extremity injuries, incisional pain on the torso, and rib fractures. Neuropathic pain, commonly related to diabetes and vascular disease, can be just as debilitating as nonneuropathic pain and therefore deserves equal attention. Although all these medications can play a role in the management of neuropathic pain, the γ-aminobutyric acid analogues, such as gabapentin, pregabalin, and carbamazepine, are recommended as first-line agents.[5] Nonpharmacologic interventions that may also help reduce pain include massage therapy, music, ice packs, and relaxation techniques.

In all instances, before and after assessments of pain severity should be made to guide further analgesic administration. A number of validated assessment instruments exist including the Numeric Rating Scale, Faces Pain Thermometer, Behavioral Pain Scale, and the Critical Care Pain Observation Tool. Family members may be involved in the pain assessment process in certain situations when a patient is unable to self-report. It is important to note that vital signs alone should not be used to assess pain but may be a clue (ie, pain-induced sympathetic nervous system activation) to further investigate whether pain is present.

Agitation and Delirium

A variety of factors may contribute to the development of agitation and delirium including pain, hypotension, hypoxemia, hypoglycemia, alcohol and other drug intoxication or withdrawal, sleep cycle alteration, light, noise, and mechanical ventilation. These contributing factors should be sought out and aggressively corrected. Similar to pain treatment, treating agitation and delirium effectively requires patient assessment followed by an intervention, with a subsequent reassessment to determine the effectiveness of the intervention. There are multiple validated agitation and delirium assessment tools, including the Richmond Agitation Sedation Score and the Sedation-Agitation Scale for agitation and the Confusion Assessment Method for the ICU and ICU Delirium Screening Checklist for delirium. All patients should have daily screening with one of these tools. When agitation and delirium are detected, it is especially important to differentiate pain from other etiologies as appropriate treatment of pain may eliminate the need for additional sedatives. Efforts should also be made in all patients to minimize sleep interruption and to maintain a normal sleep-wake cycle. Opening the window shades, turning on lights, and engaging the patient with cognitive stimulation and mobilization during the day, while turning off lights, minimizing noise, and minimizing procedures at night all help to achieve this goal. It is also important to minimize sensory impairments by providing patients with their glasses or hearing aids whenever possible.

When pharmacologic intervention is necessary, the goal is to use the smallest amount of sedative possible. Although deeper states of sedation may make patient care easier, minimal sedation is associated with improved outcomes including reduced duration of mechanical ventilation and shorter ICU stays. Pharmacologic treatment of agitation commonly involves benzodiazepines, propofol, antipsychotics, and dexmedetomidine. Although all these agents are potentially useful for agitation treatment, benzodiazepines are associated with increased delirium and should be minimized unless alcohol withdrawal is suspected. Regardless of the agent used, unless there is a specific contraindication to stopping sedation, all patients should have a daily ***spontaneous awakening trial (SAT)***.

II. Ventilator Liberation and Spontaneous Breathing Trials

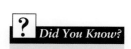

For mechanically ventilated patients in the intensive care unit who are recovering respiratory function, a spontaneous breathing trial (reduced ventilator support while the trachea is still intubated) is often coupled with a spontaneous awakening trial (reduced administration of sedative medications) to determine the likelihood of successful tracheal extubation.

Liberation (sometimes called weaning) from mechanical ventilation is a process that requires, at a minimum, adequate oxygenation and ventilation without mechanical assistance. However, safe removal of the endotracheal tube requires patients to meet additional criteria including the ability to manage secretions and protect their airway from aspiration and obstruction.

Both objective and subjective parameters should be examined in order to determine a patient's suitability for liberation from mechanical ventilation. **Table 42.2** lists commonly used criteria for extubation. The objective criteria require the patient to undergo a ***spontaneous breathing trial (SBT)***. The SBT is a 30- to 120-minute trial of breathing with little or no assistance from the ventilator. It may be performed with a variety of techniques including T-piece trials, pressure support ventilation trials, and continuous positive airway pressure trials. No single technique is superior to another, though pressure augmentation of 5 to 8 cm H_2O during the SBT is recommended for patients ventilated more than 24 hours.[6] An SBT should be performed daily on all patients who qualify. Typically this includes mechanically ventilated patients requiring <60% fraction of inspired oxygen (FIO_2) and positive end-expiratory pressure (PEEP) < 8 cm H_2O. When combined with a protocolized daily SAT, the daily SBT has been shown to shorten the duration of mechanical ventilation and may improve mortality.

Table 42.2 Criteria for Extubation

Subjective Criteria
• Indication for intubation is resolved • Adequate airway reflexes to handle secretions and avoid upper airway obstruction • No signs of increased work of breathing (eg, nasal flairing, accessory muscle use, sternal retractions, diaphoresis)
Objective Criteria (based on spontaneous breathing trial performance)
• Hemodynamic stability: Heart rate and blood pressure change <20% from baseline • Adequate oxygenation: $Sao_2 > 90\%$, $Pao_2 > 60$ mm Hg, $Pao_2/Fio_2 > 150$ • PEEP < 8 cm H_2O and $Fio_2 < 0.5$ • Adequate ventilation: $Paco_2 < 60$ mm Hg, pH > 7.25 • Rapid shallow breathing index (RR/Vt) < 105 • Negative inspiratory force >30 cm H_2O • Vital capacity >10 mL/kg

Fio_2, fraction of inspired oxygen; $Paco_2$, arterial partial pressure of carbon dioxide; Pao_2, arterial partial pressure of oxygen; PEEP, positive end-expiratory pressure; RR/Vt, respiratory rate/tidal volume; Sao_2, arterial oxygen saturation.

These criteria are only guidelines. Decisions regarding extubation should be made on an individual basis.

III. Important Considerations in the Critically Ill Patient

A. Venous Thromboembolism

Deep venous thrombosis (DVT) and venous thromboembolism (VTE) are common problems in critically ill patients. The incidence may be as high as 30% for DVTs and 5% for pulmonary embolism (PE) depending on the population. The pathologist Rudolph Virchow was the first to describe the combination of three factors that predispose patients to venous thrombosis. The triad of hypercoagulability, venous stasis, and vascular endothelial damage bare his name, and almost all ICU patients have at least one of these risk factors. A simple scoring system for VTE risk stratification is shown in **Table 42.3**. Determining VTE risk is important in that it helps in choosing prophylactic therapy and in determining the level of suspicion for VTE in individual patients.[7] ***The clinical decision of which patients to treat prophylactically and how to treat them always balances the risk of VTE with the risks of VTE prophylaxis***, including heparin-induced thrombocytopenia and bleeding. It is generally agreed that high-risk patients without contraindications should receive prophylaxis with low-molecular-weight heparin (LMWH). Patients with low to moderate risk should receive either low-dose unfractionated heparin (UFH) or LMWH. Patients with contraindications to LMWH or UFH may receive prophylaxis with mechanical devices (serial compression devices) and, in some cases, inferior vena cava (IVC) filters. But IVC filters should be reserved for the setting of high VTE risk and ongoing contraindications to anticoagulation. There is no evidence to support the routine preventive placement of IVC filters in the critically ill, including those with traumatic injuries. UFH and LMWH do not need to be routinely held prior to most surgical procedures (unless regional anesthesia is under consideration), but decisions regarding perioperative anticoagulation should be made in conjunction with the surgical team.

Table 42.3 Caprini Risk Assessment Model for Venous Thromboembolism

1 Point	2 Points	3 Points	5 Points
Age 41-60 y	Age 61-74 y	Age > 75 y	Stroke < 1 mo
Minor surgery	Arthroscopic surgery	Personal history of VTE	Elective lower extremity arthroplasty
Body mass index > 25 kg/m^2	Major open surgery > 45 min	Family history of VTE	Hip, pelvis, or leg fracture
Swollen legs	Laparoscopic surgery > 45 min	Any thrombophilia	Acute spinal cord injury < 1 mo
Varicose veins	Bed rest > 72 h	Elevated serum homocysteine	Multiple trauma < 1 mo
Pregnant or postpartum < 1 mo	Immobilizing plaster cast	Heparin-induced thrombocytopenia	
History of miscarriage	Central venous access		
Oral contraceptives or hormone replacement therapy		High Risk: ≥5 points Intermediate Risk: 3-4 points Low Risk: 1-2 points Very Low Risk: 0 points	
Sepsis < 1 mo			
Serious lung disease < 1 mo			
Abnormal pulmonary function			
Acute myocardial infarction			
Congestive heart failure < 1 mo			
History of inflammatory bowel disease			
Medical patient on bed rest			

VTE, venous thromboembolism.

Adapted from Pollak AW, McBane II RD. Succinct review of the new VTE prevention and management guidelines. *Mayo Clin Proc.* 2014;89:394-408.

Although routine DVT screening studies are not recommended, asymptomatic DVTs are common. Thus, VTE should be considered in patients with nonspecific findings such as tachycardia, tachypnea, fever, asymmetric extremity edema, and gas exchange abnormalities. ***Compression Doppler ultrasonography*** is the most commonly used test for diagnosis of DVT. It has a good positive and negative predictive value. However, regularly scheduled screening compression Doppler ultrasonography is not generally recommended. The Wells criteria and D-dimer levels, tests commonly used in the outpatient setting, have little role in critically ill patients due to their lack of specificity.

The mainstay of treatment for VTE in the critically ill patient is heparin, which should be started prior to confirmatory studies if clinical suspicion is high. The advantage of UFH over LMWH in the ICU population is its titratability and rapid reversibility, which may be desirable in patients at high risk for bleeding and in those with renal insufficiency. In patients with PE and hemodynamic instability, chemical thrombolytic therapy or mechanical thrombectomy should be considered (if not contraindicated). Although the data supporting thrombolytic therapy for treatment of PE are limited, patients with massive PE or shock are likely to benefit.

B. Nutrition

Critical illness can lead to hypermetabolic states and an early risk of malnutrition. Poor nutritional status is associated with increased mortality and morbidity among critically ill patients. Therefore, appropriate nutrition is an important aspect of critical care, and adequate nutritional support should be considered a standard of care. The American Society for Parenteral and Enteral Nutrition regularly publishes and updates evidence-based guidelines for best nutritional practices.[8] The most recent guidelines recommend the following practices in the ICU setting:

- For patients suspected to be incapable of adequate volitional intake, nutritional risk based on the Nutritional Risk Screening 2002 or NUTRIC scores should be determined to identify who would benefit most from early enteral feeding. Nutrition should be initiated in the first 24 to 48 hours after ICU admission. In patients unable to take a volitional oral diet, a feeding tube should be placed.
- Caloric needs for most patients can be predicted with a simple formula based on ideal body weight (25-30 kcal/kg/d). Proteins should represent 15% to 20% of this (1.2-2 g/kg/d). In the obese patient (body mass index >30), permissive underfeeding at a level 60% to 70% of ideal body weight–predicted needs is acceptable.
- Enteral feeds should not be held for residual volumes >500 mL unless there is other evidence of feeding intolerance. In the event of gastric feeding intolerance or high aspiration risk, postpyloric positioning of the feeding tube and prokinetic agents (eg, metoclopramide, erythromycin) should be considered.
- Enteral feeds should be halted in settings of escalating vasopressor use, though may be considered in patients on stable low doses of vasopressors.
- Total parenteral nutrition should not be used unless enteral nutrition is anticipated to be inadequate for at least 7 days, as parenteral nutrition is associated with increased infectious complications.

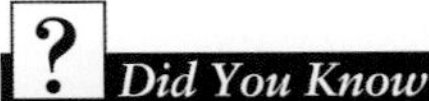

Vigilant glucose control is required in the intensive care unit to minimize morbidity associated with both hyperglycemia and hypoglycemia, although the most appropriate serum glucose range in this setting remains controversial.

C. Glucose Control

Hyperglycemia is common in critically ill patients. It can occur in both diabetics and nondiabetics. It results from both a primary increase in glucose production as well as insulin resistance due to inflammatory and hormonal mediators that are released in response to injury. It can be exacerbated by therapeutic interventions, including corticosteroids and total parenteral nutrition. Hyperglycemia is associated with increased risks of infection as well as poorer outcomes in patients with stroke, traumatic brain injury, and myocardial infarction.

Considering the association of hyperglycemia with negative outcomes, it is not surprising that efforts to improve outcomes by treating hyperglycemia have been made. Although targeting serum glucose levels of 80 to 110 mg/dL (commonly called tight control) was advocated in the past, more recent evidence suggests that this level of control is associated with significant ***hypoglycemia*** and possibly increased mortality.[9] Current serum glucose targets are somewhat variable, but 140 to 180 mg/dL is acceptable in most patients. As insulin delivery and glucose monitoring systems improve, it may become possible to safely target levels less than 140 mg/dL.

D. Stress Ulcer Prophylaxis

Gastric mucosal breakdown with resulting gastritis and ulceration (stress ulceration) is common in critically ill patients, but significant bleeding from the ulcerations is uncommon. Significant bleeding occurs in <4% of high-risk patients (those with a coagulopathy, >48 hours of mechanical ventilation, prior history of GI ulceration, sepsis, or traumatic brain, spinal cord, or burn injury) and in <1% of patients without these risk factors. Despite this being a relatively uncommon event, the mortality from significant bleeding (requiring blood transfusion or resulting in hemodynamic instability) is >45% and has resulted in the common use of pharmacologic agents including H_2 receptor antagonists, proton-pump inhibitors, and cytoprotective agents such as sucralfate for stress ulcer prophylaxis (SUP). These medications are not benign and are associated with increased costs, drug interactions, and adverse drug reactions. In addition, due to changes in the pH of gastric contents, H_2 receptor antagonists and proton-pump inhibitors may be associated with increased rates of pneumonia and *Clostridium difficile* infection. Considering this, routine SUP in critically ill patients is not recommended. Furthermore, enteral feeding may be a safe and more effective strategy for SUP than pharmacologic agents. Among high-risk patients, pharmacologic SUP may be considered, but no agent has been shown to be clearly superior to the others.

E. Transfusion Therapy

Anemia is common in critical illness. Most patients admitted to the ICU are anemic at some point during their hospital stay, and many will receive a blood transfusion. Although both anemia and blood transfusions are associated with mortality, it is important to note this does not imply cause and effect and may simply reflect the severity of illness. Anemia in critical illness has many causes, including blood loss from the primary injury or illness, iatrogenic blood loss due to daily blood sampling, nutritional deficiencies, and marrow suppression.

Transfusion thresholds are a source of ongoing debate. Historically, a hemoglobin (Hb) concentration of 10 g/dL was advocated. This was based on the assumption that critically ill patients have reduced physiologic reserve and require this level for adequate tissue oxygen delivery. However, red blood cell transfusion carries a risk of infection, transfusion-related acute lung injury, transfusion-associated circulatory overload, transfusion-related immunomodulation, microchimerism, and more (see Chapter 24). The undesired effects of transfusion may explain why a large, randomized, prospective trial of transfusion requirements in critical illness failed to show a mortality difference when a restrictive transfusion threshold (Hb < 7 g/dL) was compared with a more conventional threshold of <10 g/dL.[10] These data strongly suggest that routine transfusion of critically ill patients is not necessary and may be harmful unless the Hb concentration is below 7 g/dL. Based largely on the results of this trial, most critical care guidelines now suggest a transfusion threshold of 7 g/dL unless there is evidence of ongoing blood loss, acute myocardial infarction, unstable angina, or possibly acute neurologic injury.

IV. Common Diagnoses in the ICU

A. Nosocomial Infections

Nosocomial infections are a major source of morbidity and mortality in the critically ill, but many of them are preventable with relatively simple interventions. There are four types of infection that are relatively unique to inpatient and ICU care that should be considered when signs suggestive of infection arise. They are ventilator-associated pneumonia (VAP), central line–associated bloodstream infection (CLABSI), catheter-associated urinary tract infection (UTI), and *C. difficile* infection (CDI).

Ventilator-Associated Pneumonia

The risk of developing VAP increases with the duration of mechanical ventilation. This underscores the importance of any intervention that can reduce the duration of mechanical ventilation such as SATs, SBTs, and sedation minimization. The exact definition and diagnostic criteria for VAP are controversial, but most agree that radiologic evidence of pneumonia, fever, leukocytosis, increasing sputum production, and quantitative culture results all may support the diagnosis. VAP is typically classified as early-onset (occurring within the first 48-72 hours of intubation or ventilation) or late-onset (occurring thereafter). Antibiotic-sensitive bacteria including *Haemophilus influenzae, Streptococcus pneumonia,* and methicillin-sensitive *Staphylococcus aureus* are often the causal organisms. In contrast, late-onset VAP is associated with more antibiotic-resistant organisms, including methicillin-resistant *Staphylococcus aureus* (MRSA), *Pseudomonas aeruginosa,* and *Acinetobacter.*

A number of simple and low-cost interventions may reduce the incidence of VAP, including strict handwashing between patients, positioning the patient with at least 30° of head elevation, avoiding inappropriate use of gastric stress ulcer prophylaxis, using closed tracheal suction systems, and the use of chlorhexidine for daily oral decontamination. These practices should be rigorously applied in all ICUs.

Once VAP has developed, early detection and appropriate treatment are essential to reducing morbidity and mortality. As noted previously, the diagnostic criteria for VAP are controversial. However, an invasive diagnostic strategy is likely more accurate than traditional clinical criteria to diagnose VAP and is recommended whenever possible. Invasive strategies typically involve collection of bronchial-alveolar specimens using lavage or protected brushes and then quantitating bacterial growth in the laboratory.

Because delayed treatment of VAP is associated with increased mortality, treatment should not be delayed pending diagnostic evaluation. Treatment should be started after culture specimens are sent if the clinical suspicion of VAP is high. Antibiotics can then be narrowed in spectrum or discontinued depending on the results from quantitative cultures after 48–72 hours. This approach of de-escalating therapy is designed to both ensure adequate initial antibiotic treatment and also to avoid development of antibiotic resistance. In general, antibiotic treatment for early-onset VAP can be relatively narrow in spectrum and limited to a single agent. Late-onset VAP requires broader spectrum antibiotics covering resistant gram-negative organisms and MRSA. **Table 42.4** lists common antibiotic selections for a variety of common infections. However, antibiotic selection should always consider local patterns of

Table 42.4 Suggested Empiric Antibiotic Regimens for Common Intensive Care Unit Infections

Ventilator-Associated Pneumonia	
Early (<72 h of intubation and hospital admission)	Ceftriaxone PLUS azithromycin Consider adding vancomycin or linezolid if known history of MRSA
Late (>72 h of intubation or hospital admission)	Vancomycin OR linezolid AND cefepime Consider adding ciprofloxacin if high incidence of MDR GNRs
Bloodstream	Vancomycin OR linezolid AND cefepime
Urinary Tract	
Noncatheter-associated	Ceftriaxone
Catheter-associated	Ceftazidime ADD vancomycin if GPCs on Gram stain CONSIDER meropenem instead of ceftazidime if concerned for MDR GNRs or ESBLs
Clostridium difficile diarrhea	Vancomycin (oral dosing) IF shock, megacolon, or ileus, then ADD intravenous metronidazole
Meningitis	
Nonsurgical	Dexamethasone AND ceftriaxone AND vancomycin AND ampicillin AND acyclovir
Postsurgical	Cefepime AND metronidazole AND vancomycin
Intra-abdominal	
Community acquired	Ceftriaxone AND metronidazole
Hospital acquired	Vancomycin AND either piperacillin-tazobactam OR meropenem
Sepsis, site unknown	Vancomycin AND meropenem Consider adding ciprofloxacin if concern for MDR GNRs or ESBLs

ESBL, extended spectrum beta-lactamase; GNR, gram-negative rods; GPC, gram-positive cocci; MDR, multidrug resistant; MRSA, methicillin-resistant *Staphylococcus aureus*.
Antibiotic regimens should be narrowed once culture results are available.

infection and hospital-specific antibiograms. Optimal therapy duration is not clear, but 8 days is typically sufficient unless multidrug-resistant organisms are present. In that case, 14 days or longer may be appropriate.

Central Line–Associated Bloodstream Infections

The Centers for Disease Control and Prevention has a complex but strict definition for central line–associated bloodstream infection (CLABSI). The specific criteria have changed over time and are important for epidemiologic and payment reasons but are less important clinically. Conceptually, CLABSIs are infections arising from the placement or use of a central venous catheter. They have received a great deal of attention due to their common occurrence, high financial costs associated with treating these infections, significant mortality, and, most important, preventable nature. The Centers for Disease Control and Prevention's recommendations for practices that minimize such catheter-associated infectious risk are summarized in **Table 42.5**.

Table 42.5 Best Practices for Central Venous Catheter Placement
Subclavian and internal jugular veins are preferred over femoral veins
Prep skin with chlorhexidine (if chlorhexidine allergy, 70% alcohol or tincture of iodine are acceptable alternatives)
Full barrier precautions (full body sterile drape)
Strict aseptic technique (handwashing, sterile gloves and gown, mask, and surgical cap)
Use ultrasound guidance to minimize the number of needle passes
Choose a catheter with the minimum number of lumens possible for the clinical situation
Use a chlorhexidine-impregnated sponge and sterile, transparent semipermeable dressing
Inspect the catheter site daily for signs of infection
Do not routinely replace catheters unless medically indicated[a]
Remove catheters as soon as possible

[a] When adherence to aseptic technique cannot be maintained (eg, catheters placed emergently), the catheter should be replaced with aseptic technique as soon as possible.

CLABSIs are commonly caused by a number of bacteria including *Staphylococcus epidermidis* and *S. aureus,* enteric gram-negative bacteria, *P. aeruginosa* and *Acinetobacter,* and occasionally *Enterococcal* species. Although coagulase-negative staphylococci are commonly isolated from blood cultures, they are in most cases contaminants. When catheter-related bacteremia is suspected, blood cultures should be tested from the catheter and peripheral sites, and consideration should be given to catheter removal. If infection is confirmed, the catheter should be removed promptly and replaced if necessary. As with other infections, prompt initiation of antibiotics may be lifesaving. High clinical suspicion of infection should trigger the initiation of broad-spectrum antibiotic coverage. **Table 42.4** lists the common antibiotic regimens for CLABSI treatment.

Catheter-Associated UTI

UTIs are the second most common source of ICU infection. Because the incidence of catheter-associated UTI (CAUTI) increases with the duration of bladder catheterization, the necessity of an indwelling catheter should be reviewed daily and it should be removed as soon as possible. Other strategies to minimize the risk of CAUTIs include adherence to aseptic technique during placement, using bladder scans to minimize unnecessary catheter insertion, and maintaining the drainage bag below the level of the bladder. The responsible organisms are similar to those causing other nosocomial infections, including *Staphylococcal* species, *Enterococcus* species, enteric gram-negative bacteria, and non–lactose-fermenting gram-negative bacteria such as *Pseudomonas.* Once the diagnosis of a CAUTI has been made, it is reasonable to remove and replace the catheter (if still indicated) in an effort to reduce the microbiologic burden while also starting antibiotics. Recommended antibiotic treatment for UTIs is presented in Table 41.4.

Clostridium difficile Diarrhea

CDI has surpassed MRSA as the most common hospital-acquired infection. Pharmacologic risk factors for CDI include the use of antibiotics, antineoplastic agents, corticosteroids, and proton-pump inhibitors. Although clindamycin, third-generation cephalosporins, and ampicillin are the most commonly implicated antibiotics, nearly all antibiotics, including metronidazole and vancomycin, may increase the risk. Other significant risk factors include prior CDI, chronic dialysis, gastrointestinal surgery, recent hospitalization, and postpyloric feeding. Diarrhea is the most common symptom, but it is not always present. Fever, abdominal pain, constipation, and leukocytosis (commonly with white blood cell counts >20,000/mm^3) should prompt consideration of the diagnosis, which can be further confirmed by a number of laboratory methods. It should be noted, however, that all currently available laboratory tests are imperfect, and considerable debate exists as to which is the best. Once the diagnosis is confirmed, the treatments outlined in Table 41.4 can be initiated.

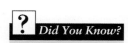

With adoption in 2012 of the Berlin definition of acute respiratory distress syndrome (ARDS), the previous distinction between acute lung injury and ARDS has been replaced by the classification of ARDS into mild, moderate, or severe based on the degree of hypoxemia.

V. Acute Lung Injury and Acute Respiratory Distress Syndrome

Acute respiratory distress syndrome (ARDS) occurs commonly in the ICU. It is characterized by the acute onset of hypoxemic respiratory failure, diffuse alveolar damage, noncardiogenic edema, reduced thoracic compliance, and both increased dead space and shunt. ARDS can occur as a result of direct injury to the lung (eg, aspiration or pneumonia) or in association with extrapulmonary infection (eg, sepsis), injury (eg, multiple trauma or burns), or toxicity from other therapies (eg, transfusion-related acute lung injury or hematopoietic stem cell transplantation).

The definition of ARDS has changed over time. In 2012, a new consensus conference proposed the Berlin definition, which eliminates the distinction between acute lung injury and ARDS, and instead categorizes ARDS as mild, moderate, or severe based on the degree of hypoxemia.[11] The classification system is summarized in **Table 42.6**.

Although ARDS appears to be a diffuse process by chest x-ray, computed tomography imaging and histopathologic specimens demonstrate heterogeneity with severely damaged areas of lung existing next to normal appearing areas. Treatment of ARDS is largely supportive and consists mainly of attempting to preserve the uninjured lung while treating the underlying cause of ARDS.

A. Lung-Protective Ventilation

Lung-protective ventilation (LPV) describes a mechanical ventilation strategy that restricts tidal volumes (Vt) to ≤6 mL/kg and targets a static (plateau) airway pressure of ≤30 cm H_2O. Because minute ventilation can be maintained by increasing the respiratory rate only so far, it is commonly inadequate to eliminate all carbon dioxide that is produced. This results in a state of hypercapnea and respiratory acidosis called ***permissive hypercapnea.*** LPV is the only intervention that has been shown to significantly reduce mortality in patients with ARDS compared with conventional ventilator strategies that rely on Vt > 6 mL/kg.

LPV strategies would result in substantial atelectasis and increased shunt if a reduction in Vt were the only intervention. In order to maintain a

Table 42.6 The Berlin Definition of the Acute Respiratory Distress Syndrome

Timing	Within 1 wk of a known clinical insult or new or worsening respiratory symptoms
Chest imaging[a]	Bilateral opacities not fully explained by effusions, lobar/lung collapse, or nodules
Origin of edema	Not fully explained by cardiac failure or fluid overload. Need objective assessment (eg, echocardiography) if no risk factor present
Oxygenation	
Mild:	200 mm Hg < Pao_2/Fio_2 ≤ 300 mm Hg; PEEP or CPAP ≥ 5 cm H_2O
Moderate:	100 mm Hg < Pao_2/Fio_2 ≤ 200 mm Hg; PEEP ≥ 5 cm H_2O
Severe:	Pao_2/Fio_2 ≤ 100 mm Hg with PEEP ≥ 5 cm H_2O

CPAP, continuous positive airway pressure; Fio_2, fraction of inspired oxygen; Pao_2, arterial partial pressure of oxygen; PEEP, positive end-expiratory pressure.

[a] Chest radiography or computed tomography scan.

Adapted from Force ADT, Ranieri VM, Rubenfeld GD, et al. Acute respiratory distress syndrome: The Berlin definition. *J Am Med Assoc*. 2012;307:2526-2533.

nonatelectatic and open lung, low Vt is typically bundled with higher levels of PEEP. The optimal balance between PEEP and Fio_2 continues to be debated. Alternative approaches to ***open lung ventilation*** include the use of intermittent high-level end-expiratory pressure or sigh breaths, pressure-controlled ventilation, inverse ratio ventilation (prolonged inspiratory time), prone positioning, and high-frequency ventilation, which have all been used successfully.

B. Rescue Techniques

In instances when oxygenation is severely impaired, prone positioning, inhaled vasodilators, neuromuscular blockade, and extracorporeal life support (also known as extracorporeal membrane oxygenation, or ECMO) may be used. Of these techniques, prone positioning and venovenous ECMO have shown mortality benefit in moderate to severe ARDS.[12] Inhaled nitric oxide and inhaled prostacyclins variably and transiently improve oxygenation in ARDS by improving blood flow to ventilated alveoli, but they do not have a proven mortality benefit. Neuromuscular blocking drugs have also not been shown to reliably improve outcomes. Other therapies for ARDS that do not have strong evidence in support of their efficacy include inhaled beta-agonists, albumin infusions, and systemic steroids.

C. Sepsis and Septic Shock

The physiologic response to systemic infections known as sepsis can manifest in varying degrees of severity, and efforts to define this condition have evolved greatly over the years. Earlier definitions, such as the systemic inflammatory response syndrome (SIRS) criteria, focused primarily on vital sign and laboratory abnormalities that were nonspecific for sepsis and have since been abandoned. In 2016, a joint task force at the 45th Critical Care Congress changed the definition of sepsis to "life-threatening organ dysfunction caused by a dysregulated host response to infection.[13]" Septic shock is a severe form of sepsis that results in a distributive shock and is characterized by low systemic

Table 42.7 Management of Severe Sepsis and Septic Shock

- Early recognition of sepsis or septic shock
- Obtain cultures prior to starting antibiotics, but do not delay antibiotics
- Administer empiric, broad-spectrum antibiotics within 1 h of diagnosis
- Control the source of infection if appropriate (ie, surgical intervention if appropriate)
- Initial resuscitation of at least 30 mL/kg with crystalloid fluids for sepsis-induced hypoperfusion
- Use norepinephrine as the first-line vasopressor for a target mean arterial pressure of ≥65 mm Hg
- Consider adding vasopressin as an adjunct to catecholamines
- Consider dobutamine if hypoperfusion persists despite fluid resuscitation and vasopressor support
- Consider stress-dose steroid therapy if blood pressure is poorly responsive to fluid and vasopressors
- Target a hemoglobin of ≥7 g/dL in the absence of myocardial ischemia, severe hypoxemia, or acute hemorrhage

Adapted from Rhodes A, Evans LE, Alhazzani W, et al. Surviving sepsis campaign. International guidelines for management of sepsis and septic shock: 2016. *Intensive Care Med.* 2017;43(3):304-377.

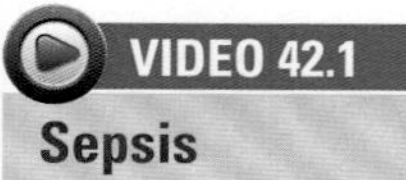

vascular resistance, hypotension, and regional blood flow redistribution, resulting in tissue hypoperfusion and increased mortality compared to sepsis alone. Because survival from sepsis depends heavily on early intervention, the most recent guidelines recommend hospitals implement sepsis screening programs to facilitate prompt recognition of this disease.[14]

Clinical management of sepsis is summarized in **Table 42.7**. The mainstay of early treatment is prompt and appropriate antibiotic administration, intravascular fluid resuscitation using crystalloids, vasopressors if hypotension persists after adequate fluid resuscitation, and inotropes if low cardiac output is suspected.

Fluid Resuscitation

Sepsis commonly causes a state of systemic vasodilation that results in a low effective circulating volume. Restoration of an effective circulating volume may be achieved by increasing absolute intravascular volume with fluid resuscitation or by increasing vascular tone with vasopressors. A wide variety of fluids including blood products, albumin, synthetic colloid solutions, and many different crystalloid solutions have been extensively studied (see Chapter 23). Albumin has generally proven no more effective than crystalloid solutions, and synthetic colloids are associated with increased harm. Older guidelines have advocated that red blood cell transfusion be used as a way to increase oxygen delivery, but newer data suggest that targeting a Hb of 7 g/dL, the same as in most critically ill patients, is appropriate. ***Crystalloids remain the preferred resuscitation fluid in most septic patients.***

Vasopressors

A number of vasopressors, including phenylephrine, norepinephrine, epinephrine, dopamine, and vasopressin, have been evaluated for systemic vascular resistance augmentation in sepsis. Norepinephrine is the recommended first-line agent owing to evidence of improved outcomes and reduced side effects.

Epinephrine may be considered an alternative agent, but it is associated with increased arrhythmias. There is evidence that endogenous vasopressin production is suppressed in sepsis, and this provides the theoretical basis for considering the addition of vasopressin to norepinephrine. However, this has not been shown to improve outcomes. Dopamine and phenylephrine are generally not recommended.

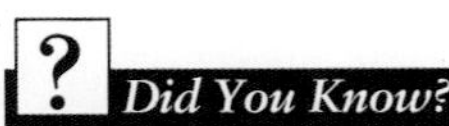

Of the various vasopressors used to augment systemic vascular resistance in the setting of septic shock, norepinephrine is the first-line agent owing to evidence of improved outcomes and reduced side effects.

Inotropes

Myocardial depression is a common phenomenon in patients with septic shock and may result in inadequate cardiac output and oxygen delivery. Once adequate intravascular volume and systemic vascular resistance have been achieved by the administration of fluid therapy and vasopressors, dobutamine or epinephrine may be used to augment cardiac output. Because pulmonary artery catheters are no longer recommended for the routine management of septic patients, central venous oxyhemoglobin saturation of ≥70% or serum lactate clearance may be used as a surrogate marker for adequate cardiac output and oxygen delivery. This may help guide decisions about the addition of inotropes. Both agents may precipitate arrhythmias.

Antibiotics

Identifying the source of the infection, attaining source control, and initiating appropriate antibiotic therapy early are at least as important as providing hemodynamic support in sepsis. Appropriate cultures should always be obtained before antimicrobial therapy is initiated and may include blood, sputum, urine, cerebrospinal fluid, and wounds and other fluid cultures (eg, pleural fluid or ascites). Empiric antibiotic therapy should be started within 1 hour of recognition of sepsis (see **Table 42.4** for antibiotic recommendations). After antibiotic susceptibility testing is available, narrowing the spectrum of antimicrobial treatment is appropriate.

Corticosteroids

The use of stress-dose steroids (eg, hydrocortisone 200-300 mg/d) in sepsis is controversial. Current guidelines recommend they be considered as an adjunct in patients with septic shock who remain hypotensive despite adequate volume resuscitation and vasopressor therapy. Cosyntropin stimulation testing prior to steroid initiation is not recommended. Steroids may also be considered in patients with recent steroid use.

VI. ICU-Acquired Weakness

ICU-acquired weakness (ICUAW) is an increasingly recognized entity that can greatly impede weaning from mechanical ventilation and lengthen the recovery process. It is thought to be due to three primary mechanisms: polyneuropathy, myopathy, and muscle atrophy. Critical illness polyneuropathy is a peripheral nerve disease manifested as symmetric sensory, motor, and autonomic nerve dysfunction. Patients demonstrate reduced compound motor action potentials (CMAPs) and sensory nerve action potentials (SNAPs) with histologic evidence of axonal degeneration late in the disease course. Direct muscle stimulation may demonstrate preserved CMAP amplitudes, indicating no myopathic component. Critical illness myopathy is instead characterized as muscle weakness with retained sensory nerve function. Electrophysiologic studies will demonstrate low-amplitude CMAPs with either direct muscle or nerve stimulation. Histologic studies show atrophy with muscle necrosis. These conditions likely overlap with each other and can present simultaneously. Proposed mechanisms for these conditions include acquired channelopathies, inexcitability of neuromuscular membranes, catabolic state leading to muscle wasting, atrophy from immobilization, and hyperglycemia-induced mitochondrial dysfunction.[15]

Identification of patients with ICUAW is challenging as nerve conduction studies are both resource and labor intensive and clinical diagnoses depends on the patient's ability to be alert and follow commands. The most consistent risk factor for development of ICUAW is severity of illness; however, other factors such as poor premorbid health and exposure to toxic therapies or conditions such as corticosteroids, aminoglycosides, neuromuscular blockers, immobilization, and hyperglycemia have also been implicated. Early mobilization of patients receiving mechanical ventilation has been shown to be safe and feasible and is associated with reduced ICU length of stay and increased functional scores at hospital discharge.[16]

Post–Intensive Care Syndrome

As ICU mortality decreases, survivors of critical illness are found to have ongoing cognitive and physical impairments that can continue for years. The term "post–intensive care syndrome" (PICS) applies to both survivors of critical illness and their family and refers to their decline in physical, cognitive, and mental health after a patient is released from the intensive care unit. Up to 6 out of 10 survivors of critical illness have been found to have at least one PICS problem after 1 year follow-up,[17] with depression being associated with increased mortality in the first 2 years following ICU discharge.[18] No association for the development of PICS has been found for age, sex, disease severity, or ICU length of stay; however, higher premorbid frailty scores and fewer years of education were found to be independent predictors of PICS.[17] These findings point to the importance of understanding social determinants of health, and further research is needed to identify whether targeted therapies in the ICU can reduce the incidence of this syndrome.

For further review and interactivities, please see the associated Interactive Video Lectures and "At a Glance" infographic accessible in the complimentary eBook bundled with this text. Access instructions are located in the inside front cover.

References

1. Wilcox ME, Chong CA, Niven DJ, et al. Do intensivist staffing patterns influence hospital mortality following ICU admission? A systematic review and meta-analyses. *Crit Care Med.* 2013;41:2253-2274.
2. Lane D, Ferri M, Lemaire J, et al. A systematic review of evidence-informed practices for patient care rounds in the ICU. *Crit Care Med.* 2013;41:2015-2029.
3. Hales BM, Pronovost PJ. The checklist—a tool for error management and performance improvement. *J Crit Care.* 2006;21:231-235.
4. Loeser JD, Treede RD. The kyoto protocol of IASP basic pain terminology. *Pain.* 2008;137(3):473-477.
5. Devlin JW, Skrobik Y, Gélinas C, et al. Clinical practice guidelines for the prevention and management of pain, agitation/sedation, delirium, immobility, and sleep disruption in adult patients in the ICU. *Crit Care Med.* 2018;46(9):e825-e873.

6. Ouellette DR, Patel S, Girard TD, et al. Liberation from mechanical ventilation in critically ill adults: an official American College of Chest Physicians/American Thoracic Society Clinical Practice Guideline. Inspiratory pressure augmentation during spontaneous breathing trials, protocols minimizing sedation, and noninvasive ventilation immediately after extubation. *Chest*. 2017;151(1):166-180.
7. Guyatt GH, Akl EA, Crowther M, et al. Executive summary: antithrombotic therapy and prevention of thrombosis, 9th ed. American College of Chest Physicians Evidence-Based Clinical Practice Guidelines. *Chest*. 2012;141:7S-47S.
8. Taylor BE, McClave SA, Martindale RG, et al. Guidelines for the provision and assessment of nutrition support therapy in the adult critically ill patient: society of critical care medicine (SCCM) and American society for parenteral and enteral nutrition (A.S.P.E.N.). *Crit Care Med*. 2016;44(2):390-438.
9. Kansagara D, Fu R, Freeman M, et al. Intensive insulin therapy in hospitalized patients: a systematic review. *Ann Intern Med*. 2011;154:268-282.
10. Hebert PC, Wells G, Blajchman MA, et al. A multicenter, randomized, controlled clinical trial of transfusion requirements in critical care. Transfusion Requirements in Critical Care Investigators, Canadian Critical Care Trials Group. *N Engl J Med*. 1999;340:409-417.
11. Force ADT, Ranieri VM, Rubenfeld GD, et al. Acute respiratory distress syndrome: the Berlin definition. *J Am Med Assoc*. 2012;307:2526-2533.
12. Aoyama H, Uchida K, Aoyama K, et al. Assessment of therapeutic interventions and lung protective ventilation in patients with moderate to severe acute respiratory distress syndrome: a systematic review and network meta-analysis. *JAMA Netw Open*. 2019;2(7):e198116.
13. Singer M, Deutschman CS, Seymour CW, et al. The third international consensus definitions for sepsis and septic shock (Sepsis-3). *J Am Med Assoc*. 2016;315(8):801-810.
14. Rhodes A, Evans LE, Alhazzani W, et al. Surviving sepsis campaign. International guidelines for management of sepsis and septic shock: 2016. *Intensive Care Med*. 2017;43(3):304-377.
15. Jolley SE, Bunnell AE, Hough CL. ICU-acquired weakness. *Chest*. 2016;150(5):1129-1140.
16. Kress JP, Hall JB. ICU-acquired weakness and recovery from critical illness. *N Engl J Med*. 2014;370:1626-1635.
17. Marra A, Pandharipande PP, Girard TD, et al. Co-occurrence of post-intensive care syndrome problems among 406 survivors of critical illness. *Crit Care Med*. 2018;46(9):1393-1401.
18. Hatch R, Young D, Barber V, et al. Anxiety, depression and post traumatic stress disorder after critical illness: a UK-wide prospective cohort study. *Crit Care*. 2018;22(1):310.

EXTUBATION CRITERIA

AT A GLANCE

Extubating a patient who has suffered critical illness should be conducted with careful attention to factors that could potentially require reintubation. Both subjective and objective criteria shown below can guide the decision to extubate.

SUBJECTIVE CRITERIA

Indication for intubation is resolved

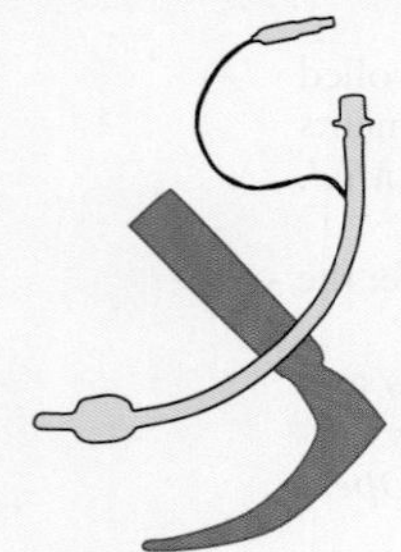

Adequate upper airway reflexes (cough, gag, and swallow) and upper airway muscle tone

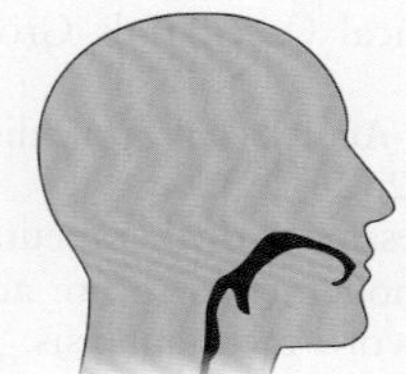

No signs of increased work of breathing

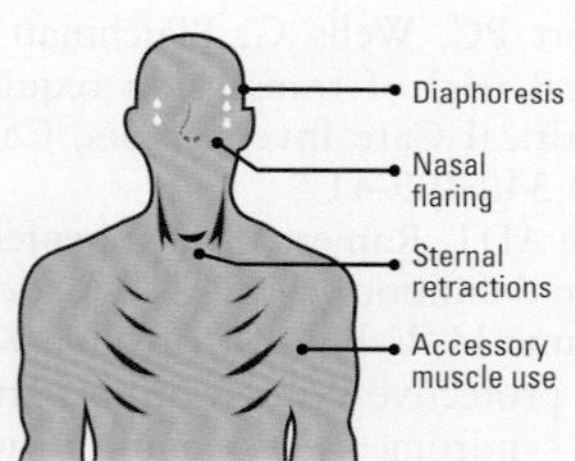

OBJECTIVE CRITERIA

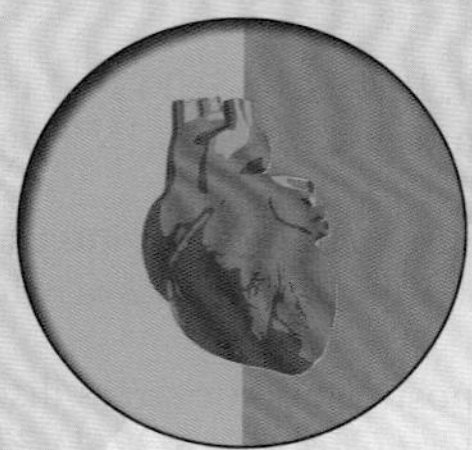

Hemodynamic stability

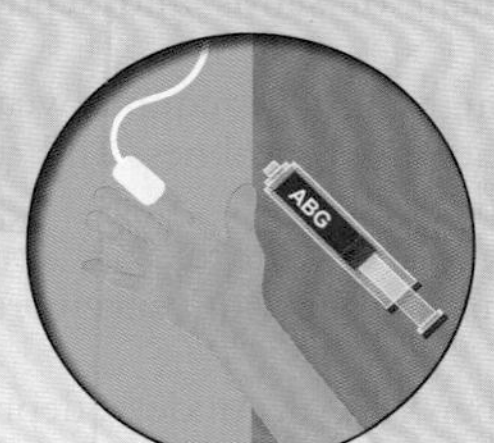

Sao_2 > 90%, Pao_2 > 60 mmHg, Pao_2/Fio_2 >150

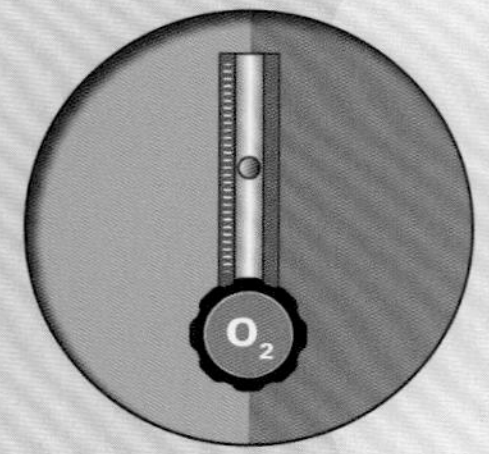

Fio_2 < 0.5, PEEP < 8 cm H_2O

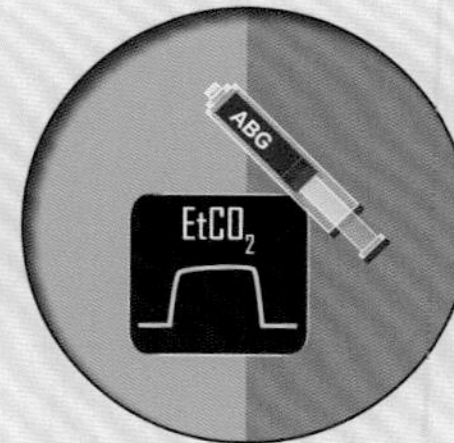

$Paco_2$ < 60 mm Hg, pH > 7.25

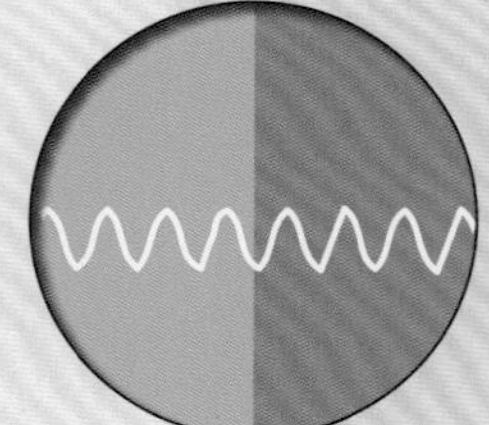

Rapid shallow breathing index (RR/Vt) < 105

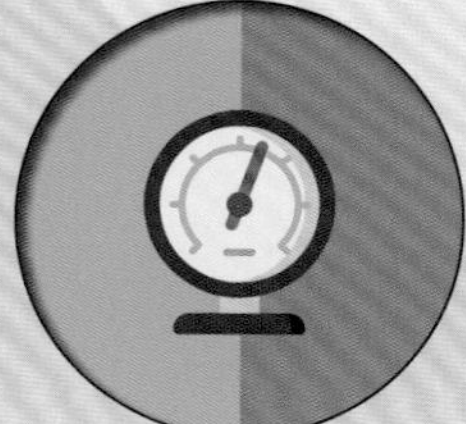

Negative inspiratory force of at least –30 cm H_2O

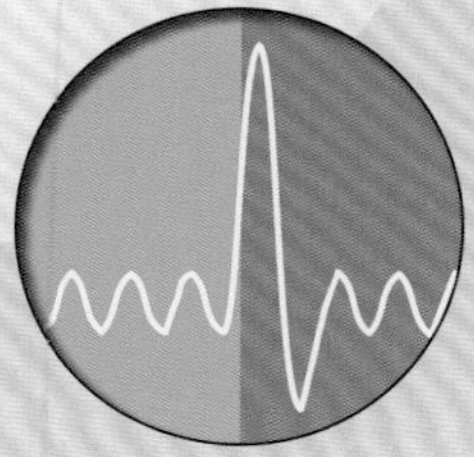

Vital capacity > 10 mL/kg

Infographic by: Naveen Nathan MD

Questions

1. **An 87-year-old woman with multiple acute rib fractures is having difficulty taking deep breaths. She complains of severe pain and is somnolent on examination. What is the MOST appropriate pharmacological intervention?**

    A. Intravenous morphine
    B. Epidural bupivacaine
    C. Intravenous lorazepam
    D. Oral gabapentin

2. **Which of the following is MOST consistent with the acute respiratory distress syndrome (ARDS)?**

    A. Causative insult occurred within 4 days of respiratory failure
    B. Concomitant development of acute kidney injury
    C. Bilateral pleural effusions on chest x-ray
    D. Reduced left ventricular function on echocardiogram

3. **Early use of which of the following interventions is MOST likely to improve mortality in moderate to severe ARDS?**

    A. Inhaled prostacyclin
    B. Neuromuscular blockade
    C. Inhaled nitric oxide
    D. Prone positioning

4. **A 30-year-old, intubated, and mechanically ventilated woman is recovering from sepsis. She repeatedly fails her spontaneous breathing trials due to tachypnea and low tidal volumes. Electrophysiologic studies demonstrate low-amplitude compound motor action potentials (CMAPs). What is the MOST likely factor contributing to the patient's condition?**

    A. Elevated blood glucose concentration
    B. Prolonged sedation with propofol
    C. Obesity
    D. Fatigue from physical therapy

5. **A 50-year-old woman is admitted to the ICU with a ruptured appendix and the following vital signs: P 115/min, BP 75/50, R 28/min, and Spo_2 94% on ambient air. She is confused. What is the MOST appropriate intervention?**

    A. Administer meropenem.
    B. Initiate a neosynephrine infusion.
    C. Obtain a central venous oxygen saturation.
    D. Administer hydrocortisone.

Answers

1. B

Adequate pain control is important for patients with rib fractures to be able to clear their secretions and mobilize to prevent secondary complications such as pneumonia and atelectasis. While opioids are the mainstay of treating severe pain in the ICU, they have undesirable side effects including somnolence, delirium, and respiratory depression. Neuraxial analgesia with local anesthetics such as bupivacaine effectively treat rib fracture pain while avoiding the side effects of systemic opioids. Benzodiazepines including lorazepam are sedative medications that do not have analgesic properties. Gabapentin may play a role in treating neuropathic pain but is limited if any utility in treating nonneuropathic pain such as from rib fractures.

2. A

According to the Berlin definition, ARDS is an acute hypoxemic respiratory failure that develops within 1 week of a known clinical insult and is not fully explained by fluid overload or cardiac failure. Reduced left ventricular function and pleural effusions suggest cardiogenic and intravascular volume–related etiologies of respiratory failure, respectively. Additional end-organ dysfunction such as acute kidney injury is not part of the ARDS definition, although multiple organ dysfunction is common in patients with ARDS.

3. D

Inhaled prostacyclin, neuromuscular blockade, and inhaled nitric oxide may improve oxygenation but have not been shown to consistently improve mortality in patients with moderate to severe ARDS. Prone positioning and venovenous ECMO have been associated with decreased mortality in patients with moderate to severe ARDS.

4. A

The patient likely suffers from ICU-acquired weakness, and she may have both a polyneuropathy and myopathy component. Proposed mechanisms for this condition include hyperglycemia-induced mitochondrial dysfunction, muscle wasting from underfeeding, and neuromuscular toxicity from aminoglycosides, steroids, and neuromuscular blocking drugs, among others. Early and aggressive physical therapy is both potentially preventative and the treatment for ICU-acquired weakness.

5. A

This patient is in septic shock. Her confusion represents end-organ dysfunction in the setting of hypotension caused by an infection. The mainstay of treatment is early and appropriate source control and antibiotics. Fluid resuscitation with crystalloids is the initial intervention to treat hypotension. If hypotension persists, vasopressors and/or inotropes may be added. Central venous oxygen saturation may be used to help guide resuscitation. Steroids are only indicated if hypotension persists following adequate fluid resuscitation and vasoactive support.

43 Anesthesia for Urologic Surgery

Ashleigh Menhadji

As the population of the United States continues to age, urologic procedures remain some of the most frequently performed surgeries in operating rooms around the country. Although some procedures are becoming less common secondary to increasing specialization within the field, they still present with important anesthetic considerations that will be discussed further in this chapter.

I. Transurethral Procedures

A. Cystoscopy and Ureteroscopy

Both cystoscopy and ureteroscopy are considered endoscopic procedures. Cystoscopy allows the surgeon to visualize and treat the lower urinary tract including the urethra and bladder while ureteroscopy allows for examination and treatment of the upper urinary tract including the ureters and kidneys. Cystoscopy is generally less stimulating than ureteroscopy and as such affords more options for anesthesia including local, conscious sedation, regional or general techniques. The choice of anesthetic is governed both by patient related (eg, highly anxious or severe pulmonary disease) and procedural factors (eg, invasiveness and duration). Ureteroscopy, on the other hand, often requires general or regional anesthesia as exploration into the ureters and kidney is generally more stimulating.

B. Resection of Bladder Tumors

Bladder cancer is the sixth most common malignancy in the United States and second most common urologic malignancy. Greater than 90% of these cancers are either urothelial or transitional cell carcinoma.[1] Bladder cancer typically presents as painless hematuria. Initial evaluation consists of cystoscopy and renal function tests +/− bladder cytology depending on risk factors and suspicion. Transurethral resection of the bladder tumor or TURBT is performed for those with abnormal cytology. TURBT can be performed under either regional or general anesthesia. It should be noted that for an inferolaterally located bladder tumor, obturator nerve stimulation may occur with regional anesthesia. The obturator nerve is derived from L3/L4 with some contribution from L2. Surgical stimulation of the obturator nerve can result in potential rapid adductor muscle contraction resulting in injury to the surgeon or bladder perforation, a well-known risk of this procedure. This mechanical stimulation occurs distal to the site of local anesthetic blockade during spinal anesthesia. For this reason, general anesthesia with muscle relaxation or regional anesthesia with supplemental direct obturator nerve blockade is preferred. In an awake patient with regional anesthesia, bladder perforation can be signaled by sudden intense abdominal pain as well as nausea, vomiting, sweating, and abdominal rigidity. If extravasation of the irrigating fluid is suspected, the operation should be stopped as soon as possible as the accumulation of large amounts of irrigating fluid in the intraperitoneal cavity can be life-threatening. Most of these cases will require an open laparotomy in order to repair the bladder perforation and drain the collection. Small perforations, however, usually do not cause significant hemodynamic changes and can be managed conservatively with drains and diuretics.

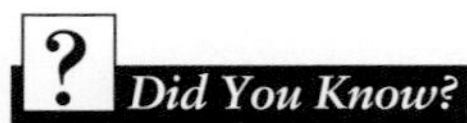

Bladder perforation with extravasation of the irrigating fluid is a well-known risk of transurethral bladder resection.

C. Resection of the Prostate

Benign prostatic hyperplasia (BPH) is one of the most common diseases in aging men with a prevalence between 8% and 80% between the ages of 40 and 90 years. It can lead to lower urinary tract symptoms which can cause urinary retention and necessitates the need for surgical therapy in a large number of aging men. Symptomatic BPH can be treated medically or surgically. The most common surgical procedure performed is a transurethral resection of the prostate (TURP) in which pieces of prostatic tissue that protrude into the urethra and disrupt the flow of urine are removed by a resectoscope to create patency. Continuous irrigation of the bladder and urethra provides a visible field for the surgeon and allows all dissected tissue and blood to be removed.[2] The prostatic capsule is preserved in these cases.

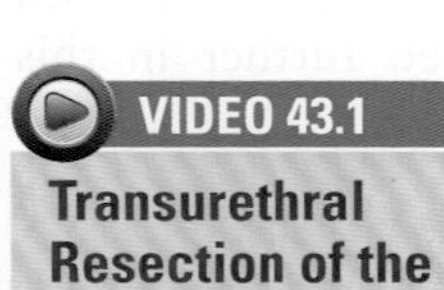

1. Transurethral Resection of the Prostate

Classic monopolar TURP procedures can result in the absorption of large volumes (>2000 mL) of irrigating solution into the plexus of venous sinuses. This excessive fluid absorption results in a constellation of symptoms known as TURP syndrome. Symptoms may include headaches, confusion, nausea/vomiting, dyspnea, anxiety, arrhythmias, hyper-/hypotension, and seizures.[3,4] The symptoms that arise depend on the type of irrigating fluid, as shown in **Table 43.1**. Given the risk of absorption, the ideal irrigating fluid should be isotonic, nonhemolytic, nontoxic when absorbed, nonelectrolytic, not metabolized, clear, and rapidly excreted. Most irrigation solutions, however, are hypo-osmolar and acidic. Common solutions like normal saline and lactated Ringer solution are not routinely used, because although isotonic, they contain electrolytes which can conduct electrical current when a monopolar electrical resectoscope is used. Given that most fluids used are hypo-osmolar, they can cause a dilutional hyponatremia resulting in severe neurological symptoms if sodium values fall below 120 mEq/L. Acute severe hyponatremia can be fatal, so early recognition and treatment, including stopping the offending irrigant is key; see **Table 43.2** for signs and symptoms and **Table 43.3** for a summary of treatments.

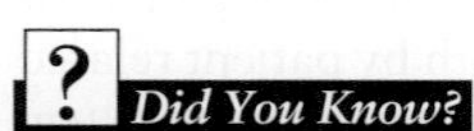

Most irrigating solutions are hypo-osmolar and acidic. Transient blindness is associated with glycine irrigation, hyperglycemia is associated with sorbitol, and volume overload is associated with the use of mannitol.

The amount of fluid absorbed is dependent on the number and size of venous sinuses opened, duration of surgery, experience of the surgeon, and hydrostatic pressure (determined by height above the surgical table of the irrigation solution bag). During resection, irrigating fluid is absorbed at a rate of 10 to 30 mL/min with the majority occurring in the first 30 minutes of the procedure. The volume of fluid absorbed can be estimated with the following formula:

$$\text{Volume Absorbed} = \frac{\text{Preoperative Serum Na}^{+}}{\text{Postoperative Serum Na}^{+}} \times \text{ECF} - \text{ECF}$$

Table 43.1 Properties of Commonly Used Irrigating Solution During Transurethral Resection of Prostate Procedure

Solution	Osmolality (mOsm/kg)	Advantage	Disadvantage
Distilled water	0	Improved visibility	Hemolysis Hemoglobinemia Hemoglobinuria Renal failure Hyponatremia
Glycine (1.5%)	200	Less likelihood of TURP syndrome	Transient blindness Hyperammonemia Hyperoxaluria
Sorbitol (3.3%)	165	Same as glycine	Hyperglycemia, Lactic acidosis (possible) Osmotic diuresis
Mannitol (5%)	275	Isomolar Not metabolized	Osmotic dieresis Acute volume overload

TURP, transurethral resection of prostate.

Table 43.2 Signs and Symptoms Associated With Acute Changes in Serum Na^+ Levels

Serum Na^+ (mEq/L)	Central Nervous System Changes	Electrocardiogram Changes
120	Confusion, restlessness	Possible widening of QRS complex
115	Somnolence, nausea	Widened QRS complex, elevated ST segment
110	Seizure, coma	Ventricular tachycardia or fibrillation

Table 43.3 Treatment of Transurethral Resection of Prostate Syndrome

Ensure oxygenation, ventilation, and circulatory support
Notify surgeon to terminate procedure as soon as possible
Consider insertion of invasive monitors if cardiovascular instability occurs
Send blood to laboratory for electrolytes, creatinine, glucose, and arterial blood gases
Obtain 12-lead electrocardiogram
Treat mild symptoms (serum Na^+ concentration >120 mEq/L) with fluid restriction and loop diuretic (furosemide)
Treat severe symptoms (if serum Na^+ <120 mEq/L) with 3% sodium chloride intravenously at a rate <100 mL/h
The rate at which serum sodium is increased should not exceed 12 mEq/L in a 24-h period to avoid pontine myelinolysis
Discontinue 3% sodium chloride when serum Na^+ >120 mEq/L

? Did You Know?

Absorption of large volumes of irrigating solution leads to intravascular volume overload, hyponatremia, and hypo-osmolality.

where ECF is extracellular fluid volume and Na^+ is the sodium ion.

To mitigate absorption, it is recommended that resections conclude in less than an hour, and limits are placed on irrigating solution bag height to curtail hydrostatic pressure.

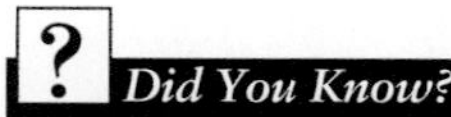

Absorption of the irrigating fluid during TURP is directly related to the number and size of opened venous sinuses, duration of resection, and the height of the bag of irrigating solution above the surgical table.

2. Bleeding and Coagulopathy

Factors affecting blood loss during TURP include duration of surgery, size and vascularity of the prostate, the number of venous sinuses opened during the resection, and presence of infection. Given that blood is mixed with the irrigation fluid, blood loss can be challenging to asses and may necessitate serial hematocrit values and intravascular volume assessment to determine if transfusion is necessary. Significant bleeding after TURP is rare and occurs in less than 1% of cases. Most cases of abnormal bleeding after TURP are likely a result of disseminated intravascular coagulopathy.

? Did You Know?

Disseminated intravascular coagulopathy is the likely etiology of abnormal bleeding after TURP.

3. Bladder Perforation

Bladder perforation during TURP has an incidence of approximately 1%. Signs and symptoms of perforation vary depending on the consciousness of the patient and the dermatomal level of the regional anesthetic. An awake patient under regional anesthesia may experience nausea, vomiting, sweating, and upper or lower abdominal pain depending on location of perforation. Patients may also have referred pain to the shoulder. Under general anesthesia, sudden hyper- or hypotension may occur along with bradycardia.

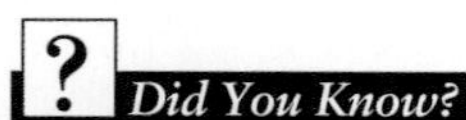

The urologist may suspect perforation by noting the irregular return of irrigating fluid.

4. Transient Bacteremia and Septicemia

Bacteremia as a result of TURP is fairly common, usually asymptomatic and easily treated with commonly used antibiotic combinations that are effective against gram-positive and gram-negative bacteria. Higher rates of bacteremia are associated with recent antibiotic use and presence of an indwelling urinary catheter. Septicemia may occur in some of these patients (approximately 7%), presenting as chills, fever, and tachycardia and can quickly worsen to include bradycardia, hypotension, and cardiovascular collapse. Mortality rates from septicemia range from 25% to 75% and therefore should be aggressively treated with antibiotics and critical care support.

5. Hypothermia

There are many causes of hypothermia during surgery such as circulatory redistribution following general anesthesia and evaporative heat loss from an open surgical field. Heat loss during TURP may also result from irrigation and absorption of room temperature irrigating fluid. Warmed fluids have been shown to minimize this risk.

6. Positioning Complications

Injury to common peroneal, sciatic, and femoral nerves can occur as a result of improper padding or positioning. TURP is most commonly performed in the lithotomy position with slight Trendelenburg.

7. Anesthetic Techniques

TURP can be performed under general or regional anesthesia (spinal or epidural). Classically, regional has been the technique of choice as patients can remain awake allowing for detection of early signs of bladder perforation or

TURP syndrome. For adequate coverage of bladder distention and sacral segments, spinal anesthesia to a T10 sensory level is preferred. Epidural anesthesia may inadequately block discomfort in the sacral segments. General anesthesia with either an endotracheal tube or a supraglottic airway is a very reasonable alternative.

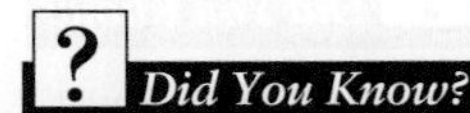

Regional anesthesia has been the anesthetic technique of choice for TURP as the conscious patient can alert the clinicians to the early signs of TURP syndrome or bladder perforation.

8. Morbidity and Mortality After TURP

Most complications after TURP are minor, but more serious complications including severe blood loss, capsule perforations, pulmonary thromboembolism, myocardial infarction, urosepsis, TURP syndrome, and even death have been reported in the literature. Complications are increased unsurprisingly, with increased patient age, comorbidities, and longer surgical times.

9. The Future of TURP

Less invasive surgical treatments have evolved over time and provide options for patients at higher risk of complications following the traditional TURP including the elderly and those with significant comorbidities. Many patients who would have endured classic monopolar TURP are currently treated with bipolar TURP, a common technique characterized by a much lower incidence of complications. Other less invasive options include balloon dilatation, prostatic stents, transurethral incision of the prostate, and laser prostatectomy. These procedures may be done on an outpatient basis, as they are associated with minimal blood loss and less risk of TURP syndrome.[5]

II. Extracorporeal Shock Wave Lithotripsy

In the United States, 12% of the population will experience renal calculi in their lifetimes. The optimal therapy is based on the size of the stone (<4.0 mm usually pass spontaneously), location in the urinary tract, and stone composition. Extracorporeal shock wave lithotripsy (ESWL) can be used for disintegration of urinary stones in the kidney and upper part of the ureters. It has the advantages of being minimally invasive, performed on an outpatient basis, and associated with minimal perioperative morbidity.

The original, first-generation lithotripter required the patient to be placed in a hydraulically supported gantry chair and immersed in a water bath—the so called most expensive bathtub in the world.[6] Modern lithotripters do not require water immersion, simplifying the procedure and eliminating the many adverse effects and difficulties of water immersion. The lithotripter is positioned to contact the patient's flank posteriorly. Shock waves are then applied that traverse the skin and deep tissue targeting the culprit stone. As a result, most *ESWL* procedures can be done on an outpatient basis and rarely require deep sedation or general anesthesia.

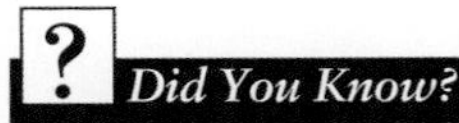

Most ESWL can be done on an outpatient basis and rarely require deep sedation or general anesthesia.

There are several known absolute and relative contraindications for lithotripsy. Absolute contraindications include pregnancy, untreated urosepsis or urinary tract infections, uncorrected coagulopathy, and ureteral obstruction distal to the stone. Some relative contraindications include uncontrolled hypertension, abdominal aortic aneurysms, obesity, renal insufficiency, and pacemakers. Patients with a pacemaker or internal cardiac defibrillator can safely undergo lithotripsy provided the pacemaker is set to the asynchronous mode (if the patient's normal heart rate is pacemaker dependent) and the defibrillator is turned off during the procedure. Renal parenchymal damage is

? Did You Know?

Pregnancy, uncorrected coagulopathy, and obstruction distal to the renal calculi are contraindications to lithotripsy.

believed to be responsible for the hematuria that occurs in nearly all patients, whereas subcapsular hematoma is seen in only 0.5% of patients after lithotripsy. A decrease in postoperative hematocrit should arouse suspicion of a large perinephric hematoma. Up to 10% of patients have significant urinary tract colic, occasionally requiring hospitalization and opioid analgesics. Shock wave lithotripsy can cause damage to adjacent tissues such as the lungs and pancreas. Despite the wide array of potential complications, mortality after ESWL is extremely low.

III. Percutaneous Renal Procedures

Percutaneous nephrostomy (PCN) is a procedure that uses ultrasound guidance to percutaneously puncture the renal pelvis, creating a nephrostomy tract. PCN is used to diagnose and treat a wide variety of urologic problems, including relief of renal obstruction, stone removal, biopsy of tumors, and ureteral stent placement.

Nephroscopy involves passing an endoscope through the nephrostomy tract to examine the kidney. For this procedure, the patient is placed in the oblique prone position and provided local anesthesia and intravenous sedation. Percutaneous nephrolithotomy, a procedure to remove renal calculi too large to be treated with lithotripsy, is one of the most common urologic endosurgical procedures. Anesthesia (general or regional) is required for dilatation of the nephrostomy tract.

Although percutaneous surgical techniques are considerably less invasive than open surgical procedures, a variety of complications can occur depending on location and size of the tract and surgical time. During insertion of the nephrostomy tube, trauma to adjacent structures such as the spleen, liver, and colon can result in acute blood loss necessitating an emergency open surgical procedure. Lung and pleural injury may occur during nephrostomy tract placement when access is created above the 12th rib or when the kidney lies in a more cephalad position than normal. In order to improve the surgical field for the surgeon during nephroscopy, continuous irrigation of fluid through the endoscope is necessary. Extravasation of irrigation fluid into the retroperitoneal, intraperitoneal, intravascular, or pleural spaces is possible and can result in electrolyte abnormalities, fluid overload, hypothermia, and anemia.

IV. Laser Surgery in Urology

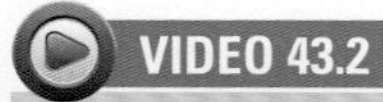

Laser Retrograde Ureteral Lithotripsy

Numerous urologic problems have been treated effectively by laser therapy, such as condyloma acuminatum of the external genitalia, ureteral stricture or bladder neck contracture, interstitial cystitis, BPH, ureteral calculi, and superficial carcinoma of the penis, bladder, ureter, and renal pelvis. Minimal blood loss, decreased postoperative pain, and tissue denaturation are major advantages of laser surgery over traditional surgical approaches. Laser lithotripsy is used for ureteral stones that are low in the ureter and not amenable to ESWL. The stones absorb the laser beam, resulting in their disintegration. Ideally, general anesthesia with paralysis should be maintained to avoid patient movement. If regional anesthesia is chosen, a spinal level of T8 to T10 is required. Because lasers are an integral part of urologic surgery, understanding the indications and limitations of each type of laser is essential (**Table 43.4**).

Table 43.4 Lasers Used for Urologic Surgery

Type of Laser	Characteristics	Uses
Carbon dioxide (CO_2)	Intense heat with vaporization, minimal tissue penetration	Cutaneous lesions of the external genitalia
Argon	Selectively absorbed by hemoglobin and melanin	Coagulation of bleeding sites in the bladder
Pulsed dye	Generates a pulsed output	Destruction of ureteral calculi
Nd-YAG laser (most versatile and widely used)	Can be used in water or urine without loss of effectiveness, deep tissue penetration	Lesions of the penis, urethra, bladder, ureters, and kidneys
KTP-532 laser (double the frequency of Nd-YAG laser)	Better cutting effect, less deep tissue penetration	Urethral strictures and bladder neck contractures

Nd-YAG, neodymium-doped yttrium aluminum garnet.

Protective goggles with appropriate filtering lenses are available for each type of laser to minimize eye damage. The laser equipment should not be activated until all operating room personnel and the patient are wearing the appropriate goggles. All operating room personnel involved in carbon dioxide (CO_2) laser procedures for condyloma acuminatum should wear protective masks that prevent inhalation of the plume (smoke) from the vaporization of tissue. This smoke may contain active human papillomavirus. In addition, the laser plume should be removed from the operating room with a smoke evacuation system.

V. Urologic Laparoscopy

Urologic laparoscopy procedures have gained wide acceptance because they are minimally invasive, more surgically precise, and provide better preservation of periprostatic vascular, muscular, and neural structures. They are also less painful postoperatively and less costly than open surgical procedures. Laparoscopic procedures performed in urology include diagnostic procedures for evaluating undescended testis, orchiopexy, varicocelectomy, bladder suspension, pelvic lymphadenectomy, nephrectomy, adrenalectomy, prostatectomy, and cystectomy. Many structures in the genitourinary system are extraperitoneal (ie, pelvic lymph nodes, bladder, ureters, adrenal glands, kidneys), and urologists use extraperitoneal insufflation during laparoscopic surgery on these organs. CO_2 absorption is greater with extraperitoneal compared with intraperitoneal insufflation. Therefore, general anesthesia with controlled ventilation is the method of choice to maintain normocarbia. Extraperitoneal insufflation results in subcutaneous emphysema that may extend all the way up to the head and neck. Please refer to Chapter 27 for a detailed discussion of the physiologic impact and potential complications of laparoscopy.

VI. Radical Cancer Surgery

Radical surgical procedures are performed to treat prostate, bladder, or kidney cancer. Robotic surgeries are gaining popularity for radical cancer operations.[7] They are often lengthy procedures, requiring a steep

Trendelenburg position to facilitate surgical access to the pelvis. As a result of this positioning, the lower extremities have decreased perfusion while the brain experiences increased mean arterial pressure and decreased venous drainage. Lung compliance and functional residual capacity are decreased, resulting in increased ventilation-perfusion mismatching. Pulmonary congestion and edema have been reported as have increased intracranial pressure and intraocular pressure. Other complications that result from the positioning include ischemic muscle damage in the lower extremities and pelvis and lower extremity and upper extremity nerve injuries. When the operative site in the pelvis is above the heart, the patient is at risk for venous air embolism. In addition to all of these concerns, radical cancer surgery poses a substantial risk for extensive blood loss and the need for transfusion.

? Did You Know?

Radical surgical procedures are associated with extensive blood loss, complications related to positioning, and venous air embolism.

A. Radical Prostatectomy

Prostate cancer is the second leading cause of male cancer-related deaths in the United States with surgery being the treatment of choice for localized prostate disease.[7] Radical prostatectomy can be performed by a perineal, retropubic, or laparoscopic surgical approach. During radical perineal or retropubic prostatectomy, general or regional (epidural or spinal) anesthesia may be used. If regional anesthesia is used, a sensory block of T6-8 is adequate. During the laparoscopic surgical approach, general anesthesia is the technique of choice for the reasons noted above (duration of surgery and steep Trendelenburg positioning). Robotic-assisted radical prostatectomy is associated with better visualization and better surgical dissection, decreased blood loss, less scaring and postoperative pain, shorter hospital stay, and faster return to daily activity.

? Did You Know?

During radical procedures, the anesthesiologist should identify the chemotherapeutic agents used, be aware of the side effects of these drugs, and should be prepared for significant intraoperative hemorrhage.

B. Radical Cystectomy

Radical cystectomy involves en bloc removal of the bladder, prostate, seminal vesicles, and proximal urethra in men, while in women, it is necessary to remove the bladder, urethra, and anterior vaginal wall, as well as to perform a total hysterectomy and bilateral salpingo-oophorectomy. A pelvic lymph node dissection is also routinely included. At completion of the procedure, a urinary diversion is performed, most commonly as an ileal or colon conduit. Significant intraoperative hemorrhage can occur during radical cystectomy. The extent and duration of this surgery mandate general anesthesia. Patients with bladder cancer may have been treated with chemotherapy before their procedure. The anesthesiologist should be aware of prior use of any chemotherapeutic agent so any possible drug toxicity can be elucidated. In particular, doxorubicin has cardiotoxic effects, methotrexate may cause hepatic toxicity, and both cisplatin and methotrexate are associated with neurotoxicity and renal dysfunction.

? Did You Know?

In 5% to 10% of right-sided renal cell carcinomas, the tumor extends into the renal vein, the inferior vena cava, and the right atrium, and thus, transesophageal echocardiography (TEE) is of crucial value.

C. Radical Nephrectomy

Radical or partial nephrectomy is the treatment of choice for renal cell carcinoma.[8] It involves en bloc removal of the kidney and surrounding fascia, the ipsilateral adrenal gland, and the upper ureter. In 5% to 10% of right-sided renal cell carcinomas, the tumor extends into the renal vein, the inferior vena cava, and the right atrium. To operate on these patients safely, the extent of the lesion must be defined preoperatively. If there is tumor extension into the vena cava or right atrium, cardiopulmonary bypass is often required to safely resect it.

Transesophageal echocardiography may be of value in confirming complete removal of the tumor or identifying intraoperative embolization of the tumor and the need to emergently institute cardiopulmonary bypass. Nephrectomy may be performed through a lumbar, transabdominal, or thoracoabdominal incision. If a lumbar approach is used, the patient is placed in the flexed lateral decubitus position with the operative side up and the mechanical kidney support elevated beneath the 12th rib. This mechanical kidney support has been associated with hypotension due to decreased venous return, nerve damage, decreased thoracic compliance, and pulmonary atelectasis. General anesthesia is used because of positioning. Other complications of surgery include pneumothorax if the thoracic cavity is inadvertently entered or venous air embolism if the positioning places the operative site above the heart.

? *Did You Know?*

Hypotension during radical nephrectomy can be multifactorial; mechanical effect, pneumothorax, air embolism, and bleeding.

D. Radical Surgery for Testicular Cancer

All intratesticular masses are considered cancerous until proven otherwise. Radical orchiectomy is performed for both definitive diagnosis and as the initial step of most treatment regimens. Either regional or general anesthesia can be used for this procedure.

Again, the anesthesiologist should identify the chemotherapeutic agents used and be aware of the side effects of these drugs. One commonly used chemotherapeutic agent is bleomycin, an antitumor antibiotic used against germ cell tumors of the testis. Bleomycin use is associated with pulmonary toxicity and postoperative respiratory failure usually within 3 to 10 days after surgery. Risk factors for postoperative respiratory distress include preoperative evidence of pulmonary injury, recent exposure to bleomycin (within 1-2 months), a total dose of bleomycin >450 mg, or a creatinine clearance of <35 mL/min. A retrospective study found that intravenous fluid management, including blood transfusion, was the most significant factor affecting postoperative pulmonary morbidity and clinical outcomes. The authors recommend that intravenous fluid administration consist primarily of colloid and be limited to the minimum volume necessary to maintain hemodynamic stability and adequate renal output.

For further review, please see the associated Interactive Video Lectures accessible in complimentary eBook bundled with this text. Access instructions are located on the inside front cover.

References

1. DeGeorge KC, Holt HR, Hodges SC. Bladder cancer: diagnosis and treatment. *Am Fam Physician*. 2017;96(8):507-514. www.aafp.org/afp. PMID: 29094888.
2. Lim KB. Epidemiology of clinical benign prostatic hyperplasia. *Asian J Urol*. 2017;4(3):148-151. PMID: 29264223.
3. Jensen V. The TURP syndrome. *Can J Anaesth*. 1991;38(1):90-96. PMID: 1989745.
4. Demirel I, Ozer AB, Bayar MK, Erhan OL. TURP syndrome and severe hyponatremia under general anaesthesia. *BMJ Case Rep*. 2012;2012:bcr-2012-006899. doi:10.1136/bcr-2012-006899. PMID: 23166168
5. Strope SA, Yang L, Nepple KG, et al. Population based comparative effectiveness of transurethral resection of the prostate and laser therapy for benign prostatic hyperplasia. *J Urol*. 2012;187(4):1341-1345. PMID: 22341267.
6. Knoll T, Alken P. Looking back at 50 years of stone therapy. *Aktuelle Urol*. 2019;50(2):157-165. doi:10.1055/a-0828-9936. PMID: 30818400.
7. Mikhail D, Sarcona J, Mekhail M, Richstone L. Urologic robotic surgery. *Surg Clin North Am*. 2020;100(2):361-378. doi:10.1016/j.suc.2019.12.003. PMID: 32169184.
8. Cohen HT, McGovern FJ. Renal-cell carcinoma. *N Engl J Med*. 2005;353(23):2477-2490. PMID: 16339096.

Questions

1. **For resection of bladder tumors performed under regional anesthesia it is recommended that which additional nerve block also be performed to avoid inadvertent bladder perforation?**

   A. Femoral nerve
   B. Obturator nerve
   C. Hypogastric nerve
   D. Pudendal nerve
   E. Ilioinguinal nerve

2. **A 74-year-old man with a past medical history significant for diabetes, hypertension, and hyperlipidemia presents to the OR for transurethral resection of the prostate (TURP) under regional anesthesia. During the procedure, he starts to complain of decreased ability to see. What irrigating solution was most likely used?**

   A. Distilled water
   B. Glycine
   C. Sorbitol
   D. Mannitol
   E. Normal saline

3. **All of the following are ways to help mitigate absorption of irrigating fluid during TURP except:**

   A. Keeping the surgical time short.
   B. Limiting the number of venous sinuses opened.
   C. Raising the bag of irrigating fluid high above the surgical table.
   D. All of the above.

4. **Extracorporeal shock wave lithotripsy can safely be performed on which of the following patients?**

   A. A 28-year-old G1P0 at 32 weeks with an otherwise uncomplicated pregnancy who presents with a 5-mm upper ureteral stone
   B. A 78-year-old woman with a 6-mm kidney stone on aspirin and Plavix for placement of drug-eluting stent 2 months ago but no other significant past medical history
   C. A 63-year-old man with an 8-mm upper ureteral stone and history of implanted defibrillator for cardiomyopathy
   D. An otherwise healthy 24-year-old man who presents with a 5-mm kidney stone and untreated urinary tract infection
   E. None of the above

5. **Which chemotherapeutic agent is incorrectly matched to its side effect?**

   A. Doxorubicin—cardiotoxic effects
   B. Methotrexate—neurotoxicity and renal injury
   C. Bleomycin—pulmonary toxicity
   D. Cisplatin—hepatic toxicity

Answers

1. B

Stimulation of the obturator nerve by the lateral bladder wall during a TURBT can cause adductor contraction of the leg resulting in a jerk reflex that increases risk of bladder perforation.

2. B

All of the solutions other than normal saline are the commonly used irrigating solutions during TURP. Glycine, however, is the only one that has a known complication of leading to transient blindness.

3. C

Raising the irrigating solution bag greater than 30 cm above the operating room table can increase the hydrostatic pressure driving fluid into the prostatic veins and sinuses and increase systemic absorption.

4. C

Absolute contraindications for ESWL include pregnancy, anticoagulation, and untreated urinary tract infections or urosepsis. Implanted pacemakers/defibrillators are relative contraindications only, and patients can still safely undergo the procedure as long as the pacemaker function is turned to asynchronous mode for those who are pacer dependent and the defibrillator is turned off during the procedure

5. D

Cisplatin is associated with neurotoxicity and renal injury like methotrexate but not hepatic toxicity. Methotrexate is also associated with hepatic toxicity.

44 Electrical Safety and Fire

Theodora Valovska and Christopher W. Connor

The physics and engineering principles involved in electrical supply and electrical safety are very well established, though they may not be intuitively obvious. Firstly, this is a matter of unfamiliarity—as clinicians and as citizens of developed countries, we usually presume that the electrical supply will be present and equipment will be working safely on a daily basis, without giving much thought to its source or configuration. In the setting of prolonged power failures, or if we had to make do with dilapidated or broken equipment, we might find ourselves at a loss.

Secondly, the terminology of electrical engineering is commonly misused by laypeople leading to imprecise and incorrect usage. For instance, the simple word "ground," "grounded," or "grounding" might take on multiple different meanings in an operating room (OR) setting:

1. The physical surface of the Earth
2. The voltage ascribed, by convention, to the Earth: 0 V
3. Describing an electrical plug or socket that has three pins
4. The green electrical wire, the ground lead, found within electrical power cables
5. The adhesive pad that forms the dispersive return electrode for an electrosurgical unit
6. The act of connecting a patient to some form of electrical apparatus such as the electrosurgical unit. ("Is the patient grounded?")
7. A state of failure of the OR's isolated electrical power system, in which the system "becomes grounded"

In the setting of, for example, a shoulder arthroscopy in an ambulatory surgery center, in which arthroscopic video cameras, instruments, and electrosurgery are being used, this wordage can become important. Suppose a large puddle of joint irrigation solution has accumulated on the floor, spreading among cables, between the feet of the surgeon and anesthesiologist. Who is safe in this situation? Or, if while on bypass in a major cardiac case in the middle of the night, the electrical safety monitors in the room begin to alarm loudly—what is the next step to ensure patient safety? In order to respond confidently and appropriately, it is necessary to understand the principles of intraoperative electrical safety and fire management.

I. Principles of Electricity

A. Introduction

Electrical current is measured in amperes with the symbol I. When an electrical potential exists, current will flow through an electrically conductive substance, which is known as a conductor. The electrical potential is measured in volts, symbolized by E.

This concept can be highlighted by considering a person standing on solid ground while touching a live electrical wire. The ground is considered to be at 0 V, and the wire is a live domestic electrical wire at 120 V. The person would receive an electrical shock due to the difference in voltage between the wire and the ground. However, if the same individual were standing on a metal plate that had a matching voltage of 120 V while touching the same wire, no shock would be delivered because there would be no difference in voltages.

It is the difference in electrical potential (called the potential difference) that generates the current and the delivery of energy, not the absolute voltage. Imagine two patients falling from their beds. Patient A is on the sixth floor of the hospital, and his bed is 20 m above ground level. Patient B is on the third floor, and his bed is 10 m above ground level. Of course, it is not their absolute height in the building (ie, absolute voltage) that matters, but instead, the height of the fall from their beds to the floor of their rooms (ie, potential difference).

Conductors have a property called resistance (R, measured in ohms), which is defined as the tendency to resist the flow of a current for a given potential difference. Potential difference, current, and resistance are related by Ohm law:

$$E = I \times R \text{ or equivalently } I = \frac{E}{R}$$

The electrical resistance of the human body is not constant. It is strongly dependent on the wetness of the skin. Wet skin can generate a resistance of approximately 1000 Ω, whereas dry skin can generate a resistance of up to 100,000 Ω.

B. Direct and Alternating Current

The current flow in a circuit may be either direct current (DC) or alternating current (AC). This depends on whether the direction in which the electrical current flows in the circuit remains the same (DC), or alternates back and forth (AC). Batteries produce a direct current. The positive terminal of the battery remains at a constant higher electrical potential relative to the negative terminal of the battery until the battery is exhausted. Therefore, the current always flows from the positive to the negative terminal.

The electrical current obtained from the mains power supply is alternating current. The potential difference of the live conductor oscillates around the neutral conductor. It is possible to convert AC to DC using a simple circuit called a ***rectifier***, and AC voltages are specified in terms of the equivalent DC voltage that would make the same amount of electrical power available. The mains power supply in the United States, which is nominally 120 V, has a live conductor whose potential difference oscillates sinusoidally between ±170 V relative to the neutral conductor sixty times each second.

C. Capacitors and Inductors, Reactance and Impedance

Capacitors and inductors are both devices capable of storing electrical energy.[1] A capacitor consists of two electrical plates, separated by an insulating material called the ***dielectric***. As a DC voltage is applied to the capacitor, positive

> **? Did You Know?**
> It is possible for electricity to be transmitted from one circuit to another without direct contact. This is an important part of the isolation transformer in use in most ORs.

charge begins to accumulate on one plate of the capacitor, while negative charge begins to build up on the opposite plate. Eventually, a sufficient charge accumulates such that an equilibrium state is produced, in which no further current can flow. The capacitor can be rapidly discharged from this state, producing a pulse of current through the desired part of the circuit—this is similar to how a camera flash operates. Once the capacitor is fully charged, however, no additional electrical current can flow onto it, and its resistance to DC becomes effectively infinite.

An inductor consists of a coil of wire wrapped in a spiral fashion around a ferromagnetic core. As electrical current passes through the coil of wire, an equal and opposing magnetic field is created in the core, and an opposing electrical voltage occurs in the coil. In this regard, an inductor is similar to a simple electromagnet. However, once the current to the inductor is interrupted, the magnetic field in the core collapses, inducing a strong, opposing voltage spike in the electrical coil. Thus, these devices can not only store charge but can also cause electrical and magnetic fields that exist beyond the physical boundaries of the device itself.

When alternating current is applied to a capacitor, the voltage on the plates of the capacitor switches polarity as the AC voltage cycles. This causes electrical charge, in the form of electrical current, to flow on and off the plates of the capacitor. Therefore, even though there is no direct electrical connection between the two plates of the capacitor, and even though the effective electrical resistance to DC is infinite, the act of repeatedly charging and discharging the capacitor allows alternating current to be able to flow through it. This "resistance" to alternating current is called ***reactance***; it is a property of both capacitors and inductors and is dependent on the frequency of the alternating current. The simple and familiar expression of Ohm law above, in which resistance is expressed as R, is only true for direct current. In order to model alternating current at different frequencies, a quantity called ***impedance*** becomes important. Impedance represents a combination of both resistance and reactance.

More precisely, impedance is a complex number whose real component is the electrical resistance and whose imaginary component is the reactance. From a practical standpoint, the existence of reactance makes it possible to design circuits that only allow electrical signals at certain frequencies to pass through them. This is the basis of graphic equalizers for music. It is also the basis for medical signal filters for electrocardiograms (ECGs) that filter and amplify only those frequencies associated with cardiac conduction and reject signals at frequencies that are associated with interference.

By carefully arranging capacitors and inductors, it is possible to design circuits that can receive and respond to external electromagnetic signals, and to design circuits that optimally radiate electromagnetic energy out into the environment. Such circuits form the basis of radios and broadcast towers. However, these properties can also exist in an unwanted form in electrical devices. The proximity of electrical conductors within the power cord of a device or between the windings of an electric motor and its metal case can cause ***stray capacitance or parasitic capacitance***. In turn, these produce the phenomena of ***electrical interference*** and ***leakage current***.

II. Electrical Shock Hazards

A. Alternating and Direct Currents

Electrical current causes the stimulation of nerves and can stimulate direct muscle contraction; this leads to the possibility of therapeutic uses but also the

Table 44.1 Physical Effects of Exposure to a 60 Hz Electric Current for One Second

Electrical Current		Physical Effect
Macroshock (to body via skin contact)		
1 mA	(0.001 A)	Threshold of perception
5 mA	(0.005 A)	Maximum harmless current
10-20 mA	(0.01-0.02 A)	Maximum current before sustained muscle contraction prevents voluntary release of the conductor ("let-go threshold")
50 mA	(0.05 A)	Pain; risk of mechanical injury from muscle contractions
100-300 mA	(0.1-0.3 A)	Threshold for ventricular fibrillation; respiration drive is preserved
6000 mA	(6A)	Sustained myocardial contraction, followed by resumption of heart rhythm. Temporary respiratory paralysis. Burns at areas of high current density
Microshock (to heart via wire or conducting cannula)		
10 μA	(0.01 mA)	Maximum recommended 60 Hz leakage current
100 μA	(0.1 mA)	Ventricular fibrillation

risk of injury or death. Direct current is generally considered to be safer than alternating current; the amount of direct current necessary to induce ventricular fibrillation is around three times higher than the amount of alternating current required to produce the same effect. **Table 44.1** summarizes the physical effects that are experienced from exposure to different thresholds of 60 Hz alternating current as is encountered in the standard US "mains" electricity supply.

The perception of the safety of direct current is reinforced by daily experience of "mains" alternating current being more powerful and dangerous than the relatively small amounts of direct current that are produced from standard batteries. However, a large direct current source such as an automobile battery or marine battery should not be considered harmless—the direct current discharge that can be produced between the terminals can cause significant burns and musculoskeletal injury.

B. Source of Shocks

Whenever a difference in electrical potential exists, current will flow through a suitable conductor placed between those electrical potentials. Consequently, there is always a risk of electrical shock whenever an external source of electricity is touched. The severity of the physical effect of the shock depends upon both the magnitude of the electrical current and the duration of time for which that current is applied. At lower current levels, the electrical shock is first felt as a sensory tingling sensation, rising to pain with increased levels of current. Greater levels of current are able to stimulate contraction of muscles directly, and beyond a certain current level, it becomes impossible to release the contraction of these muscles voluntarily. Beyond this "let-go" threshold, it may no longer be possible for a victim to break contact with the source of electrical shock, further sustaining the electrical exposure.[2] Further escalations in current can cause the onset of ventricular fibrillation as the electrical shock interferes with cardiac conduction and causes direct paralysis of the respiratory muscles. The flow of electrical current through the body also generates heat and can destroy tissue through direct thermal injury. The risk of burning is greatest at the points where the electrical current is entering or leaving the body, as the concentration of electrical current (the ***current density***) is greatest there.

C. Grounding

When electrical current flows through a person, causing a shock, the shock is usually flowing from some other electrical potential to ground. The body of the person is usually either in direct contact with the ground, or electrically connected to the ground via a conductor such as an item of metal furniture. Since an electrical shock can only occur when there is a difference in electrical potential, the aim of electrical safety is to minimize that potential difference so that the magnitude of that electrical shock to ground is made as small as possible. One approach, as seen in small battery-powered devices, is to minimize the total electrical voltage used by the device to such an extent that even the maximum possible shock current that could be generated by it is harmless. However, for devices that require significant electrical power, electrical safety must be achieved by more active means, and in this case, "grounding" refers to the various steps that we can take to reduce the magnitude of the possible electrical shock.

The simplest of these is illustrated in **Figure 44.1**. On the right, a malfunctioning device is shown: it has developed a fault in which a conductor connected to the "hot" or "live" wire of the electrical supply has broken and is now in contact with the casing of the device. Touching the case poses an immediate risk of electric shock because it is possible for this live voltage to flow through the body to ground. However, as a safety precaution, the device also contains a "ground" or "earth" wire which is connected to ground voltage and also to the casing of the device. The electrical current from the case

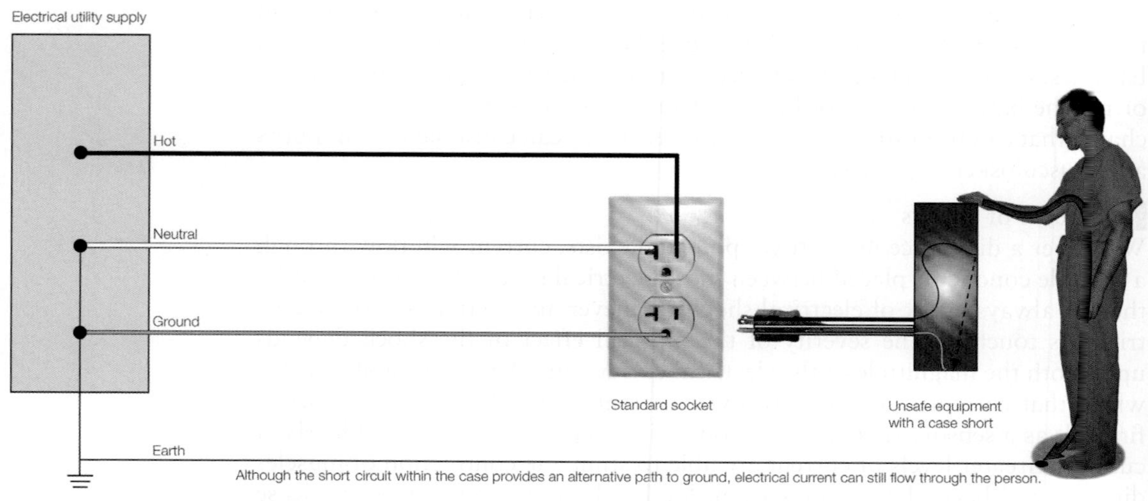

Figure 44.1 Unsafe equipment operating on a standard power supply.

fault is, therefore, able to flow to ground either through the body of the person touching the device, or through the ground wire. Since the electrical resistance of the ground wire is much lower than the resistance of the body, most of the electrical current will preferentially travel to ground through the ground wire, reducing but not eliminating the magnitude of the electrical shock current passing through the person. However, if the ground wire were to break, or if the device were connected instead to a two-pin electrical socket without a ground pin, then the protection afforded by the ground wire would be entirely lost and the person touching the case would be exposed to the full magnitude of the electrical shock current.

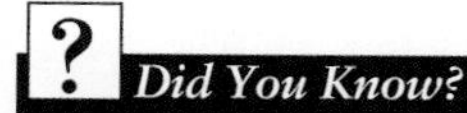

Did You Know?

Use of a three-pin to two-pin "cheater" plug will enable a device to operate, but it will disable the protection afforded by the device's internal ground wire.

III. Electrical Power and Isolation

A. Grounded Power Systems and the Ground Fault Circuit Interrupter

The electrical power supply illustrated in both **Figures 44.1** and **44.2** is referred to as a "grounded power system." It is given this name because the potential of the neutral wire is fixed at the same potential as the ground wire, which in turn is fixed at the same potential as the actual ground (ie, the physical surface of the Earth).

As shown in **Figure 44.1**, although a ground wire within a malfunctioning device can reduce the amount of electric shock current flowing through a person touching that device, it cannot eliminate that shock current entirely. In the scenario shown in **Figure 44.1**, the device will continue to pose an ongoing risk of electrical shock. Furthermore, this risk of shock will likely not be discovered until someone touches the device and experiences a shock. The grounded power system shown in **Figure 44.1** represents the standard for domestic electrical wiring, but it is inadequately safe for the OR.[3]

Figure 44.2 demonstrates a refinement of this electrical system, making use of a device called a ground fault circuit interrupter (GFCI). A GFCI is an electrical device that monitors the ground wire to detect whether any current is flowing in that wire. GFCIs are available as individual units that can be plugged into normal electrical sockets, or alternatively, electrical sockets can

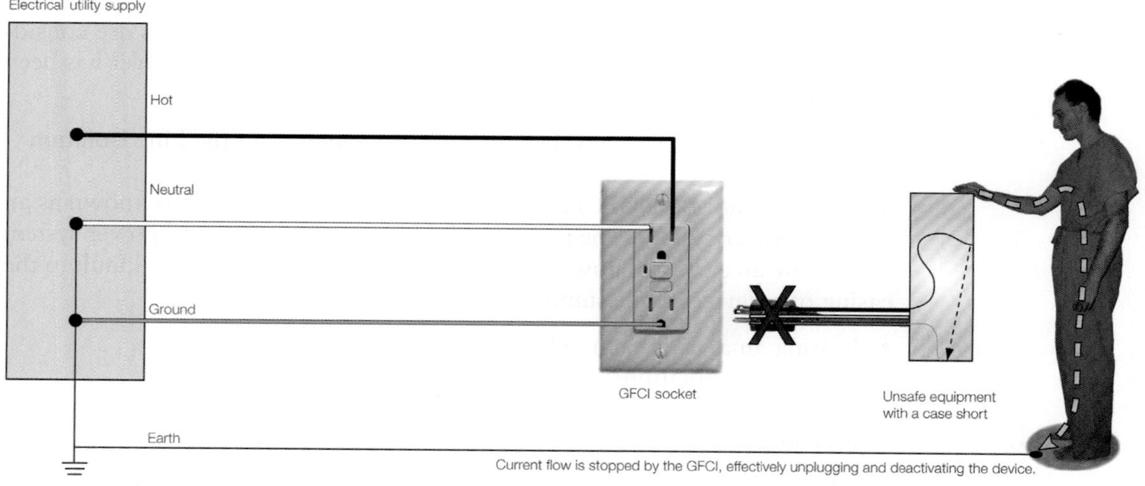

Figure 44.2 Unsafe equipment operating on a power supply with ground fault circuit interrupter (GFCI) protection.

be purchased and installed such that the GFCI circuitry is contained within the socket itself. **Figure 44.2** shows this latter type of installation.

Under normal operating conditions, no electrical current should be flowing in the ground wire. However, if there is an electrical fault that makes the casing of the device electrically live, then some of that fault current will be carried away in the ground wire. The GFCI detects that anomalous current flow, and in response, the GFCI automatically interrupts the electrical supply to the device, deactivating the electrical socket and producing the same effect as if the malfunctioning device were suddenly unplugged. The GFCI also displays a warning light on the socket (shown red in **Figure 44.2**), indicating that the safety provisions of the GFCI have been triggered and that power output from the socket has been disabled. The malfunctioning device is rendered electrically safe, in that it no longer has any electrical power flowing to it, but it is also rendered inactive.

In many regard, this is a significant improvement over the preceding scenario in **Figure 44.1**. A warning light on the GFCI indicates that an electrical fault has occurred. As soon as the fault occurs, the device is automatically rendered safe. If a person subsequently touches the device, no shock can occur. These outcomes are desirable, and hence, GFCIs are commonly used in domestic settings that are at higher risk for electrical shock, such as electrical outlets in bathrooms, in kitchens, and outdoors. However, there are some notable drawbacks. Firstly, once the GFCI is triggered, electrical power to the device is immediately interrupted. This may be dangerous if the device itself is necessary for life support: suddenly interrupting power to a cardiac bypass machine or a ventilator is immediately hazardous to the patient.

Secondly, the GFCI can only work if the ground wire is intact. If the ground wire is broken or the ground wire is not connected to the GFCI because of an intervening two-pin plug, the GFCI can never detect current flow on the ground wire. Its safety features are then made ineffective.

Thirdly, the GFCI relies on an active mechanical circuit breaker to interrupt electrical power to the device. If this mechanical circuit breaker were itself to fail or jam, then theoretically the GFCI might be unable to interrupt the electrical power to the device. For these reasons, GFCIs are not approved for electrical safety in all ORs. GFCIs may be installed for electrical safety only if the OR is certified as a dry location.[4] Since 2012, all new ORs are considered wet locations by default unless a specific risk assessment waiver has been performed.[5]

B. Isolated Power Systems, Isolation Transformers, and the Line Isolation Monitor

The limitations of the GFCI can be overcome by creating what is known as an ***isolated power system***. The purpose of the design of an isolated power system is to create an electrical power supply that can tolerate an electrical fault to the casing of a device, while simultaneously:

- Raising an alarm that an electrical fault has occurred.
- Allowing the malfunctioning device to continue to operate.
- Preventing a risk of shock from the malfunctioning device to a person touching it.

Figure 44.3 illustrates an electrical fault occurring in an isolated power system. The two important new components in this diagram are the isolation transformer and the line isolation monitor (LIM).

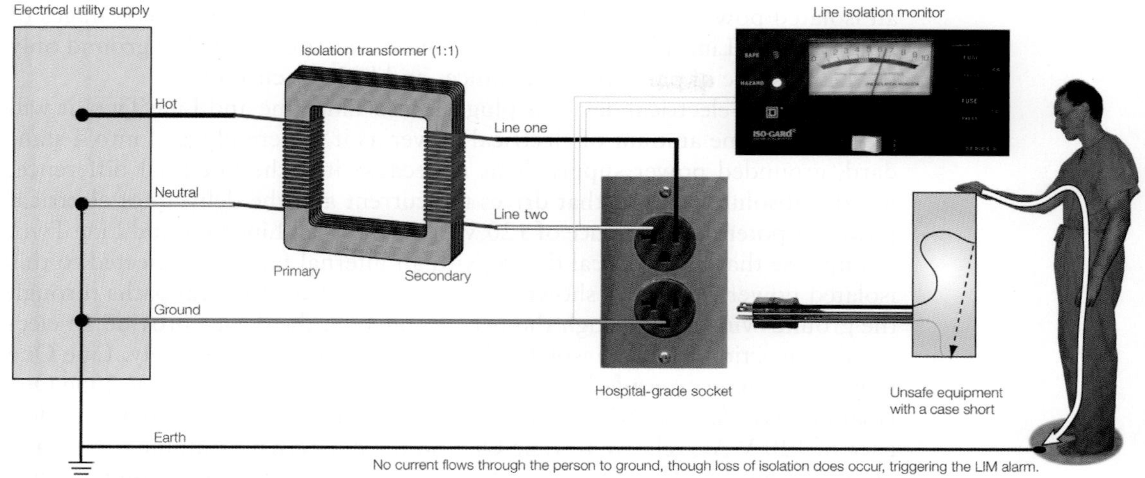

Figure 44.3 Unsafe equipment operating on an isolated power supply. LIM, line isolation monitor.

An isolation transformer allows electrical power to be transmitted from one circuit to another without the existence of a direct electrical connection between them. In **Figure 44.3**, the standard grounded electrical power supply is connected to the primary coil of the isolation transformer. The primary coil consists of a single wire, wrapped in a spiral fashion around a ferromagnetic core. The current flowing in this wire causes a magnetic field to be created in the core, in the manner described earlier for an inductor. However, in this case, the ferromagnetic core is shaped like a loop (a square in this case), and the magnetic field is trapped within the body of this loop. A secondary coil is wrapped around the opposite side of the core. The magnetic field generated by the current in the primary coil circulates around within this ferromagnetic loop. As the magnetic field passes through the windings of the secondary coil, it induces an electrical current causing power to be transmitted from the primary to the secondary. In an isolation transformer, the number of windings in the primary and secondary coil are the same, so that the current flowing in the primary and secondary coil are the same. The purpose of an isolation transformer, therefore, is to convert electrical power into a magnetic field and then immediately convert it back again into electrical power. Although this may initially appear redundant, it produces two important effects:

1. An electrical fault on one side of the transformer cannot spread over to the other side because the two coils of the transformer are physically separated and linked only by a magnetic field.
2. The isolation transformer transmits only the potential difference across the primary coil, not the absolute voltage. A potential difference of 120 V AC exists between the hot and neutral wires attached to the primary coil. The hot wire is at 120 V AC and the neutral wire is fixed at ground. The outputs from the secondary coil are called Line One and Line Two. Only a potential of 120 V AC exists between them. The absolute voltages of Line One and Line Two are unknown. They are now isolated.

In a grounded power system, the voltage of the neutral wire is at 0 V, because it is directly coupled to the ground wire which is also fixed at 0 V. In an isolated power system, this is no longer true, and the absolute voltages of Line One and Line Two are uncertain. These lines are coupled to ground only by the presence of parasitic capacitances and leakage currents.

If a normal electrical device is plugged into Line One and Line Two, it will receive the same amount of electrical power as if it were plugged into a standard, grounded power supply. This is because it is the potential difference, not the absolute voltage, that drives the current and the delivery of electrical power. A potential difference of 120 V exists between Line One and Line Two.

Suppose that an electrical device with an internal fault is connected to this isolated power supply, as shown in **Figure 44.3**. The electrical paths through the ground wire and through the person touching the device provide an electrical connection from the isolated Line One to ground. Effectively, Line One now has ***become grounded***, and its voltage has become fixed at 0 V. Line One is said to have ***lost isolation***. Line Two will continue to have a potential difference of 120 V AC relative to Line One, so the device will continue to operate. However, because Line One has taken on the same voltage as ground, no current can flow through the person to the ground because there is no potential difference. No electrical shock is produced.

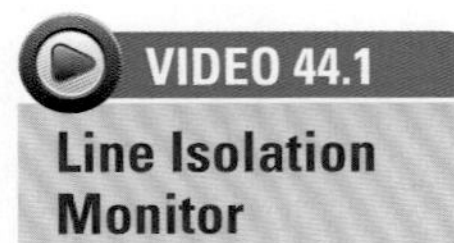

The LIM monitors the electrical potentials and leakage currents that exist between Line One and Line Two and ground. The line isolation monitor is designed to alarm when the isolation of the electrical power system has degraded to the extent that an electrical shock of greater than 5 mA could be produced with the next electrical fault. As shown in **Table 44.1**, a shock current of 5 mA applied to the body is considered to be the threshold below which no physical harm can result. **Figure 44.3** shows that the LIM has detected a loss of isolation and has triggered a hazard alarm.

In summary, in an isolated power system, neither Line One nor Line Two are the hot or neutral wires. However, if a fault occurs such that Line One is brought into contact with a grounded object or person, then Line One will immediately become the neutral wire, having lost isolation and having become grounded. Line Two will in turn become the equivalent of the hot wire. No shock will occur and all equipment will continue to receive electrical power. An isolated power system can therefore accommodate one single electrical fault without producing a shock and without having to shut down potentially life-sustaining medical devices. Of course, once a fault has occurred and the isolated power system has become grounded, then it is only as safe as the standard, grounded power system as shown in **Figures 44.1** and **44.2**.

? *Did You Know?*

If the LIM alarms, all equipment plugged into that circuit will remain operative. However, if the faulty device causing the alarm is not identified and removed, the LIM will no longer provide protection against shock if a second defective piece of equipment is plugged into the circuit.

If a LIM begins to alarm during a surgical case, the anesthesiologist should try to identify which device in the OR is faulty. The anesthesiologist should unplug electrical devices in turn until the alarm stops, thus identifying the device that contains the electrical fault. Once the offending device is disconnected and quarantined, the other devices can be progressively reconnected. If the source of the fault cannot be identified, or if the fault lies within an essential piece of equipment that cannot be disconnected, then it is acceptable to complete the surgical procedure with vigilance; the margin of safety provided by the isolated power system has been lost, and particularly, careful attention must be paid to the arrangement of electrical devices around the patient. It is an absolute contraindication to begin a surgical case in an OR with a known electrical fault.

IV. Microshock

Table 44.1 shows that a current threshold between 100 and 300 mA is required to induce ventricular fibrillation with a 60 Hz AC electrical shock. However, these results are calibrated for electrical current applied to the body. Electrical current applied directly to the heart can induce ventricular fibrillation with currents as low as 100 μA (0.1 mA), known as ***microshock***. The patient can be placed at risk for microshock by any conductive medium that is in contact with the myocardium that also extends outside the body. For example, temporary pacemaker wires or a pulmonary artery (PA) catheter containing a conductive electrolyte solution can lead to microshocks. Since the LIM does not usually alarm until there is a possible shock current of at least 5 mA, the use of an isolated power system and LIM does not necessarily protect against the risk of microshock. The anesthesiologist must remember that a risk of microshock to the myocardium exists whenever devices are manipulated. These devices should not be handled while the anesthesiologist is simultaneously in physical contact with any other piece of electrical apparatus.[6]

V. Electrosurgery

The use of electrosurgery in clinical practice was pioneered in 1926 through a collaboration between neurosurgeon Harvey Cushing and physicist William Bovie.[7] Electrosurgery is different from electrocautery. Electrocautery is the process of using electricity (commonly DC current) to generate heat and then applying that heat to tissue to cauterize it. In electrocautery, the electricity is simply a convenient form of energy to convert to heat at the surgical site.

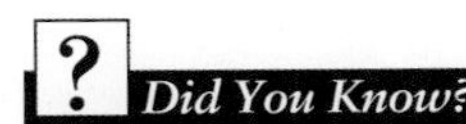

A large dispersive electrode ("grounding pad") is not required for bipolar electrosurgical instruments. The current in one electrode is returned to the adjacent electrode and does not pass elsewhere in the body.

Instead, electrosurgery makes use of alternating current at very high frequencies, on the order of 300 to 500 kHz, generated by an electrosurgical unit (ESU). These frequencies are sufficiently high that they are close to the radio frequencies (RF) used to transmit medium-wave AM radio. Electrosurgery is therefore sometimes referred to as RF electrosurgery in order to further distinguish it from simple cautery. The power output from an ESU operating in "cut" mode exceeds the power required simply to burn or desiccate tissue—it is sufficient to convert the water within the tissue into vapor, effectively exploding the tissue itself. The use of a fine-pointed surgical electrode produces a region of very high current density around the tip and creates precisely controllable surgical tissue dissection.

When using electrosurgery, an electrical current has been introduced into the body. Therefore, the path this current travels through the body and to return to the ESU must be in a manner such that no other surgical effects occur outside of the desired region. Many electrosurgical tools have two electrodes, referred to as ***bipolar instruments***—the current is introduced to tissue through one electrode at the tip of the instrument, and a second electrode nearby receives the return current. This design is appropriate for instruments such as laparoscopic scissors, in which the two blades of the scissors act as the two electrodes. The current transmitted to or through neighboring anatomical structures is very small.

Alternatively, an electrosurgical device may consist of only one electrode—described as ***monopolar***; these devices require a separate electrical return path from the patient to the ESU.[8] This return path is created by sticking a large electrically conductive pad to a substantial part of the body such as the patient's thigh. This pad is often referred to as a ***grounding pad***, but that description is unfortunately misleading. The pad does not ground the patient to earth potential because the patient and the electrosurgical device are electrically isolated by an isolated power system. The purpose of the pad is to act as an electrode to receive the electrosurgical current. The current is retrieved over a large tissue area so that the tissue current density is low. Otherwise, the tissue under the pad might be accidently burned. The grounding pad should therefore, more correctly, be called a ***dispersive electrode***. If the dispersive electrode is improperly applied so that it only contacts the patient's skin in a few small locations, the return current will be concentrated at these points, the current density will be high, and accidental burns may result. It is therefore important that the dispersive electrode is applied smoothly and is not wrinkled. Patients should also be strongly encouraged to remove metal jewelry. For example, a metal wedding ring may come to rest against a metal part of the OR table and form an electrically conductive path back to the dispersive electrode. The wedding ring would then effectively act as an unintended return electrode and could create a circumferential burn to the finger. Metal jewelry that cannot be removed can be covered with tape to provide a layer of electrical insulation.

The frequency of the electrosurgical current is so high that it does not cause depolarization of nerves or muscle fibers. Nerves and muscles possess a property called ***chronaxy***, defined as the shortest duration of electrical impulse necessary to elicit a response. Since the frequency of the AC current produced by an ESU is at several hundred kilohertz, the duration of one oscillation of the electrosurgical current is far shorter than the chronaxy of these tissues. The electrosurgical current can pass through the body without triggering ventricular fibrillation—unlike an electrical shock from equivalent mains power supply current at 60 Hz.

Special care must be taken with patients who have an automatic implantable cardioverter defibrillator (AICD). The AICD continuously monitors the electrical activity of the patient's heart, and it may misinterpret the high-frequency electrical interference from the electrosurgical current as being an episode of ventricular fibrillation requiring a defibrillation shock. Therefore, the AICD must be inhibited from administering this shock during surgery. The AICD can either be reprogrammed pre- and post-surgery, or it can be temporarily inhibited by placing a large magnet on the patient's chest over the AICD insertion site. The AICD detects the presence of this magnetic field, and then the defibrillator action of the AICD is inhibited while the magnet remains in place. Many AICDs emit an audible warning tone that can be heard clearly through the patient's skin when the magnet is placed.

VI. Fire Safety

Although considered a rare event in the OR, OR fires present a steady danger to both patients and staff and are more common than expected. There are about 600 reported OR fires per year,[9] and 90% of these are started secondary to electrocautery.[9,10] The fire triad—oxidizer, ignition, fuel—is commonly known, but recommendations on how to manage OR fires are strictly based on case reports, with no data driven management plan available.

Igniting a fire requires the presence of each element of the "fire triad" —a source of ignition, a fuel to burn, and an oxidizer.[11] The most common sources of ignition are ESUs[9]; these are usually under the control of the surgical team. Multiple types of ESUs exist and deliver energy using various energy types, like thermal energy versus radiofrequency energy.[12] The most common types are the monopolar, the bipolar, and ultrasound.

Ignition can occur via the device itself or human tissue heating to a point where a fire is possible. For example, even though ultrasonic devices do not transfer heat directly to tissue, they can raise tissue temperature to over 200 °C,[12] increasing the risk of fire. Monopolar and bipolar devices both rely on direct heat transfer, but an advantage exists with a bipolar device. The development of a spark is minimized with a bipolar device, as the electrical field is maintained between the two tips of the instrument.[12] With a monopolar ESU, the electrical field is created between the tip of the device and tissue, creating a larger gap for spark formation and an increased risk of fire.[12] Regardless of the type of ESU, however, the risk of fire exists whenever tissue and heat are involved.

Fires related to nonelectrocautery devices were less common than fires caused by ESUs.[10] A closed claim analysis by Mehta et al looked at claims regarding OR fires from the years 1985 to 2009 and showed that out of 103 OR fire claims, only 10 cases were related to non-ESU devices (nine related to lasers and one related to a defibrillator pad).

Typical sources of fuel are drapes, dressings, or gauzes, which may additionally have become soaked in alcohol-based prep solutions or petroleum jelly. These materials are usually under the control of the scrub and circulating nurses. Although dry materials such as sponges, paper gowns, and gauze intuitively seem to possess a higher fire fuel risk,[12] even wet pledgets present in a surgical airway may become combustible.[13] It is also important to note that most drapes used in an OR are actually designed to be water resistant. Thus, if they do serve as fire fuel, extinguishing the fire might be difficult as the entire drape would have to be submerged in water in order to effectively extinguish it.[12]

Although alcohol-based prep solutions might be expected to be a common culprit in OR fires, less than a fifth (14%, $n = 11$) of all ESU fires were related to alcohol-based prep solutions or volatile compounds.[10] Fires are more likely to be fueled by the burning of plastic airway equipment such as nasal cannulas with nose prongs and endotracheal tubes.[10] This remains true even when using reinforced endotracheal tubes, which are ET tubes that are considered laser safe, as they are wrapped in specialized metal. However, the tip of the tube is metal free and can easily serve as fuel if the laser crosses its path. Close to half of all airway fires occurred with ET tubes serving as a fuel source,[12] as ET cuff damage allows oxygen to come into the surgical field.[13]

Closed airway systems, defined as systems that include an endotracheal or laryngeal mask airway are considered less of a fire source than open airway systems using a face mask or nasal cannula.[12] However, a fire risk still exists with closed breathing systems. Inadvertent cuff perforations can occur with reinforced endotracheal tubes; this can serve as strong fire accelerant as oxygen is introduced into the surgical field via the broken cuff.[13] ESU-related fires occurred more commonly during administration of monitored anesthesia care/regional anesthesia, where an open breathing circuit was used. Slightly more than half of these cases had supplemental oxygen delivered to the patient via nasal cannula, and a third were via face mask.[10]

Oxygen is the most common oxidizer in OR fires,[10] with nitrous oxide a close second. These gases are usually under the control of the anesthesiology team and become an essential factor to control especially when an open breathing system is used. Mehta et al showed that 85% of OR fires were related to an open delivery system. Thus, maintaining the lower percentage of inspired oxygen (FIO_2) while keeping the patient saturating becomes important. Even with closed airway systems, however, oxygen can spread into the OR environment via a break in the ET tube, the cuff, or the inspiratory/expiratory limbs of the system.

In a mechanical model looking at fire hazards during laser airway surgery, Roy et al showed that using 40% and 100% of FIO_2 created a long, sustained flame and immediate fire. Even at 29% FIO_2, a small flame was noted. Use of room air did not cause a fire. Multiple sources recommend use of room air or an FIO_2 of less than 30% to avoid fires[12] and, if a greater percentage of oxygen is needed, to convert to a closed breathing system with an endotracheal tube. It is important to note that although titrating the oxygen down decreases the amount of oxygen delivered, there is often a lag between the delivered oxygen and the expired oxygen. Thus, although less oxygen is delivered, the patient might still be exhaling a high concentration of O_2,[12] increasing fire risk. The anesthesiologist should not be lulled into a false sense of security even when delivering lower amounts of inspired oxygen.

Surgical drape tenting also creates an environment around the surgical field that might have a higher concentration of oxygen compared to the FIO_2 delivered to the patient, especially when open breathing systems are used. Although air in the OR is typically exchanged over 20 times, if a patient is draped so that oxygen becomes trapped between the patient and the site, the risk of fire would increase as that area would contain a higher concentration of oxygen.[12]

> **? *Did You Know?***
>
> Although modern inhaled anesthetics are considered nonexplosive or nonflammable, disastrous fires can still occur because both oxygen and nitrous oxide support combustion. Caution must be exercised when these gases come in contact with a source of ignition (eg, laser, ESU) and fuel (eg, paper drapes, prep solution, endotracheal tube).

While the anesthesiologist must always be aware of the potential risk of an intraoperative fire, some procedures present a clearly foreseeable risk.[14]

- During a tracheostomy, the opening of the trachea can potentially release a high concentration of oxygen into the surgical field; this, combined with the presence of gauze and electrosurgical instruments, creates an imminent risk of fire.
- The surgical site prep solution for procedures on the upper chest or neck (eg, port-a-cath placement) may tend to pool or accumulate within the folds of the surgical drapes, producing a potent fuel source. These procedures are commonly performed under monitored anesthesia care (MAC), and oxygen from the face mask can accumulate underneath the drapes. The use of an electrocautery device on the surgical side of the drape can then be sufficient to ignite the drapes over the patient's head. The sudden flash fire, combined with melting of the plastic of the face mask, can produce disfiguring head and facial burn injuries within only a few seconds.[15]
- Laser laryngoscopic surgery typically involves the use of laser surgical tools in close proximity to an airway that has been secured with an endotracheal tube. Appropriate "laser-safe" endotracheal tubes should be used during this type of surgery, but a risk of igniting the endotracheal tube itself is always present.[13] In the event of the endotracheal tube catching fire, the patient must be immediately extubated. Simultaneously, the endotracheal tube should be disconnected from the anesthesia circuit, the surgical field should be quenched with a sterile solution, and any remaining burning material must be removed from the airway. The primary goal is to terminate thermal injury in the shortest possible time. Once the airway fire is extinguished, the patient can be mask ventilated, the airway can be

examined by laryngoscopy or bronchoscopy, and an airway can be secured with a new endotracheal tube.

The OR environment contains ample equipment and materials to fulfill the three parts of the required triad for the outbreak of an OR fire. Unfortunately, because each part of the triad is under the control of a different nursing, surgical, or anesthesia team, deficiencies in team communication can easily lead to OR fires.

For further review, please see the associated Interactive Video Lectures accessible in complimentary eBook bundled with this text. Access instructions are located on the inside front cover.

References

1. Horowitz P, Hill W. *The Art of Electronics*. 2nd ed. Cambridge University Press; 1989:xxiii, 1125. Update to Horowitz 2015.
2. Cadick J, Cadick J. *Electrical Safety Handbook*. 4th ed. McGraw-Hill; 2012.
3. Chambers JJ, Saha AK. Electrocution during anaesthesia. *Anaesthesia*. 1979;34(2):173-175. PMID: 443513.
4. Wills JH, Ehrenwerth J, Rogers D. Electrical injury to a nurse due to conductive fluid in an operating room designated as a dry location. *Anesth Analg*. 2010;110(6):1647-1649. PMID: 19933528.
5. National Fire Protection Association (NFPA). *NFPA 99: Health Care Facilities Code*. National Fire Protection Association; 2018.
6. Baas LS, Beery TA, Hickey CS. Care and safety of pacemaker electrodes in intensive care and telemetry nursing units. *Am J Crit Care*. 1997;6(4):302-311. PMID: 9215428.
7. O'Connor JL, Bloom DA. William T. Bovie and electrosurgery. *Surgery*. 1996;119(4):390-396. PMID: 8644002.
8. Brill AI, Feste JR, Hamilton TL, et al. Patient safety during laparoscopic monopolar electrosurgery – Principles and guidelines. Consortium on Electrosurgical Safety during Laparoscopy. *J Soc Laparoendosc Surg*. 1998;2(3):221-225. PMID: 9876743.
9. Jones SB, Jones DB, Schwaitzberg S. Only you can prevent OR fires. *Ann Surg*. 2014;260(2):218-219. PMID: 25350649.
10. Mehta SP, Bhananker SM, Posner KL, Domino KB. Operating room fires: a closed claims analysis. *Anesthesiology*. 2013;118(5):1133-1139. PMID: 23422795.
11. Culp WC Jr, Kimbrough BA, Luna S, Maguddayao AJ. Mitigating operating room fires: development of a carbon dioxide fire prevention device. *Anesth Analg*. 2014;118(4):772-775. PMID: 24651231.
12. Jones TS, Black IH, Robinson TN, Jones EL. Operating room fires. *Anesthesiology*. 2019;130(3):492-501. PMID: 30664060.
13. Roy S, Smith LP. Surgical fires in laser laryngeal surgery: are we safe enough? *Otolaryngol Head Neck Surg*. 2015;152(1):67-72. PMID: 25344591.
14. Kaye AD, Kolinsky D, Urman RD. Management of a fire in the operating room. *J Anesth*. 2014;28(2):279-287. PMID: 23989633.
15. Culp WC Jr, Kimbrough BA, Luna S. Flammability of surgical drapes and materials in varying concentrations of oxygen. *Anesthesiology*. 2013;119(4):770-776. PMID: 23872933.

Questions

1. **All of the following are characteristics of common "household" electricity EXCEPT:**

   A. The electrical potential is nominally 120 V.
   B. The current oscillates at 60 Hz.
   C. Current always flows from the positive (black) wire to the neutral (white) wire.
   D. The potential difference between the "hot" and neutral conductor oscillates sinusoidally between ±170 V.

2. **In a hospital operating room, the MOST efficacious way to reduce the possibility of harmful shock to personnel is to:**

   A. Use a system that transmits power from one circuit to another without a direct electrical connection between them.
   B. Install GFCI devices at all electrical outlets.
   C. Use only equipment that has a three-pin (conductor) plug.
   D. Only use items of equipment that have been serviced and checked for the absence of leakage current.

3. **All of the following statements regarding a GFCI device are true, EXCEPT:**

   A. It senses current flow in the ground wire of any device plugged into it.
   B. If triggered, it will disconnect ("unplug") all devices plugged into it.
   C. If triggered, a red light will come on, but it will not sound an alarm.
   D. It will remain operative if a two-pin adapter is inserted between a three-pin plug and the outlet.

4. **All of the following statements regarding electrical power supplied to an OR by an isolation transformer in conjunction with a line isolation monitor (LIM) are true EXCEPT:**

   A. Electrical power is delivered by induction of a magnetic field across two separated wire coils.
   B. Under normal operation, the output of the isolation transformer is through two wire leads, one at 120 V and the other at 0 V (ground).
   C. Electrical power will continue to be provided at the outlet if a malfunctioning piece of equipment is plugged in.
   D. If a person touches a malfunctioning piece of equipment plugged into a properly functioning isolation circuit, some current will flow through the person but no shock will be perceived.

5. **If the LIM alarms, the most appropriate next action for the anesthesiologist is to:**

   A. Convert to manual ventilation and prepare to administer intravenous anesthesia.
   B. Have the LIM alarm reset, but be prepared to have all electrical equipment checked at the end of the case.
   C. Recommend the surgical procedure be rapidly aborted and have someone unplug all nonessential pieces of equipment.
   D. Have someone sequentially unplug single pieces of equipment until the LIM alarm stops and the offending device is discovered.

6. **Which of the following statements is TRUE?**

   A. A dispersive pad applied to the patient is required for both mono- and bipolar electrosurgical instruments.
   B. Use of electrosurgical devices is contraindicated when patients have an implanted cardioverter defibrillator (AICD).
   C. The current frequency of the electrosurgical unit is so high that if passed through the heart, ventricular fibrillation is unlikely.
   D. The dispersive plate is grounded so that the patient does not receive a shock.

7. **All of the following scenarios represent a significant risk for fire associated with use of an electrosurgical device EXCEPT:**
   A. Tracheostomy during anesthesia with isoflurane, 70% nitrous oxide, and 30% oxygen.
   B. Laparoscopy during which the pneumoperitoneum is achieved with carbon dioxide.
   C. Laser surgery for laryngeal papilloma with general anesthesia achieved via a standard endotracheal tube.
   D. Facial plastic surgery performed during conscious sedation with 100% oxygen administered via plastic face mask under the drapes.

Answers

1. C

Typical "household" electrical supply is AC. The potential difference of the live conductor oscillates in a sinusoidal manner at ±170 V around the neutral conductor, but is nominally 120 V. The current therefore changes direction at a rate of 60 Hz (cycles per second).

2. A

No system is absolutely foolproof, but the best system is one that employs an isolation transformer that allows power to be supplied to the OR, without the need for a direct wire connection. The system is even more foolproof when combined with a line isolation monitor.

3. D

A GFCI senses current flow in the ground wire of equipment plugged into it. Eliminating the ground connection by use of a two-pin adapter renders the GFCI inoperative. If the equipment malfunctions (eg, metal casing becomes "live"), the GFCI will cut off power to the outlet and a red light will appear. All items of equipment plugged into outlets controlled by the GFCI will also be turned off. No alarm will sound.

4. B

The isolation transformer "isolates" the electrical power in the OR by inducing a magnetic field across two physically separated wire coils. The output from the secondary coil has a potential difference of 120 V but neither lead is grounded (at 0 V). If a person touches a malfunctioning piece of equipment, one wire from the outlet becomes grounded, the LIM will alarm, power will continue to the equipment, and the person will not receive a shock.

5. D

If the LIM alarms, it is not an emergency. Electrical power will continue to be supplied, but the safety feature of the isolation circuit has been bypassed. Each electrical device should sequentially be unplugged until the alarm stops. The faulty piece of equipment must then be removed or replaced. If it is an essential piece of equipment, it is acceptable to continue and complete the surgical procedure.

6. C

A dispersive electrode is only required for monopolar electrosurgical instruments. The current frequency of an ESU is very high and can safely pass through the heart without risk of fibrillation. The dispersive plate, although commonly referred to as a "ground" plate, is not connected to ground. It is safe to use an ESU when patients have an AICD, but a magnet must be placed over it or the AICD must be reprogrammed prior to surgery to prevent the AICD from misinterpreting the ESU as ventricular fibrillation.

7. B

Carbon dioxide does not support combustion so that use of an ESU intraperitoneally is safe. Nitrous oxide supports combustion so it should not be administered if the ESU is to be used at the time of tracheal incision. Oxygen should be diluted with air or nitrogen. Only "laser-safe" endotracheal tubes may be used during laser surgery in proximity to the airway. Oxygen administered via a plastic face mask can contribute to a devastating fire in the event that it is exposed to an ESU or ignited drapes. Administer only enough oxygen to keep the oxygen saturation as measured by pulse oximetry at a safe level.

45 Wellness Principles and Resources for Anesthesiologists

Amy E. Vinson and Robert S. Holzman

In dealing with those who are undergoing great suffering, if you feel "burnout" setting in, if you feel demoralized and exhausted, it is best, for the sake of everyone, to withdraw and restore yourself. The point is to have a long-term perspective.

—Dalai Lama

I. Wellness and the Anesthesiologist

Wellness is personal; therefore, a single definition is elusive. Of diverse cultural and spiritual backgrounds, anesthesiologists operate in a high-stress environment physically, mentally, and emotionally. They are colleagues at different life stages, and therefore, "wellness" means something entirely different to each. Compare the 29-year-old residency graduate in her second year of marriage, starting a family, and paying down medical school debt while learning how to become an autonomous physician and teacher, with the 63-year-old seasoned practitioner celebrating her first grandchild while contemplating retirement, her own health, and the illness or death of a parent. Here the commonality of wellness is defined as the collective thought processes, behaviors, values, and attitudes that lead to increased resilience, decreased burnout, an enhanced sense of well-being, and improved job and life satisfaction. Given that wellness is a multivariate, complex, and personal state of being, it is not the purpose of this chapter to provide a formulaic guide to wellness, but rather, a summary of wellness issues specific to the anesthesiologist, the practice of anesthesiology, and to leaders within anesthesiology-related organizations.

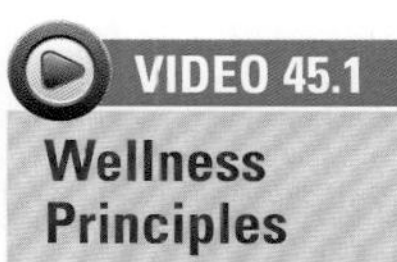

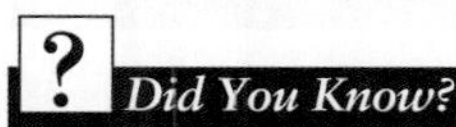

Wellness is a complex and personal state of being, defined by the collective thought processes, values, and attitudes that lead to increased resilience, decreased burnout, and an enhanced sense of well-being, including job and life satisfaction.

Several organizations have identified wellness as a group of competencies to be achieved during training. The Royal College of Physicians and Surgeons of Canada lists "Demonstrate a commitment to physician health and sustainable practice" as the third competency of professionalism in their 2015 framework.[1] The American Board of Anesthesiology, as part of its Milestones project, designated the "Responsibility to maintain personal emotional, physical, and mental health" as a required component of professionalism in the certification process.

Although a definition of wellness remains nebulous, the concept of burnout is well established. The "burnout syndrome" gained attention in the 1970s and 1980s, when Maslach et al[2] developed and marketed the "Maslach Burnout Inventory" (MBI). They defined ***burnout*** as "a syndrome of emotional exhaustion and cynicism that occurs frequently among individuals who do 'people work' of some kind." The MBI characterizes burnout based on three major psychological characteristics: ***emotional exhaustion, depersonalization***, and a ***low sense of personal accomplishment***. The MBI has since become the gold standard in quantifying burnout.

In 1999, in response to a growing body of literature concerning higher rates of suicide, substance abuse, and depression among anesthesiologists, Jackson contemplated the role of stress, closely examining aspects such as personality type, physical implications of stress, life cycle changes, sex stress differences, self-esteem, and workplace stress abatement.[3] He defined stress as the "nonspecific adaptive response of the body to any change, demand, pressure, challenge, threat, or trauma" and related this to the particular stressors encountered within the practice of anesthesiology. Jackson offered that a humanistic approach to medical education, coupled with the teaching of stress management techniques, could improve the overall professional and personal lives of anesthesiologists. Following this, a body of literature has reported the epidemiology and impact of burnout in the larger community of physicians (**Table 45.1**).

> **?** *Did You Know?*
>
> In one large national study, physicians reported higher burnout rates than the average high school graduate, whereas those with nonmedical graduate degrees reported lower burnout rates than the average high school graduate.

The 2020 Medscape Lifestyle Report, based on the surveyed responses of over 150,000 physicians, reported a nationwide burnout rate of 42% (anesthesiologists 41%). Generation X physicians (born between mid-1960s and early 1980s) reported a 10% higher rate of burnout, and female physicians (all specialties averaged) were more likely to experience burnout than their male colleagues (48% compared to 37%). A recent investigation revealed 44.7% of non-Hispanic White physicians, 41.7% of non-Hispanic Asian physicians, 38.5% of non-Hispanic Black physicians, and 37.4% of Hispanic/Latinx physicians report burnout.[4] Anesthesiologists ranked 7 of 23 medical specialties in burnout among physicians. Of all respondents, 38% screened positive for depression and 6% reported suicidal ideations within the past 12 months.

Table 45.1 Physician Burnout: Causes, Consequences, and Epidemiology

Study	Methods and Focus	Findings
Shanafelt TD, Balch CM, Bechamps G, et al. Burnout and medical errors among American surgeons. *Ann Surg.* 2010;251:995-1000.	Survey of 7905 ACS members. MBI, QOL, and depression screens	• 32% response rate. • 8.9% reporting a major medical error in past 3 mo, with 70% citing individual, not systems, errors.
Dyrbye LN, Massie FS, Eacker A, et al. Relationship between burnout and professional conduct and attitudes among US medical students. *J Am Med Assoc.* 2010;304:1173-1180.	Survey of medical students at seven US medical schools. MBI, PRIME-MD depression screen, QOL survey	• 61% response rate. • 52.8% incidence of burnout. • Unprofessional behavior more common among students with burnout. • Burnout associated with lower rates of altruistic views.

Table 45.1 Physician Burnout: Causes, Consequences, and Epidemiology (*Continued*)

Study	Methods and Focus	Findings
Balch CM, Shanafelt TD, Sloan JA, et al. Distress and career satisfaction among 14 surgical specialties, comparing academic and private practice settings. *Ann Surg.* 2011;254:558-568.	14 surgical specialties from ACS data—demographics, career satisfaction, distress parameters	• Academic surgeons less likely to experience burnout, depression, or suicidal ideation and more likely to have career satisfaction. • Academic burnout associations: Negative (older children, pediatric surgery, cardiothoracic surgery, male); positive (trauma surgery, nights on call, hours worked). • Private practice burnout associations: Negative (older children, physician spouse, older age); positive (urologic surgery, 31%-50% nonclinical time, incentive-based pay, nights on call, hours worked).
Shanafelt TD, Boone S, Tan L, et al. Burnout and satisfaction with work-life balance among US physicians relative to the general US population. *Arch Intern Med.* 2012;172:1377-1385.	Survey of 27,276 US physicians from AMA Physician Masterfile, compared with probability-based sample of the general US population. MBI	• 26.7% response rate. • 45.8% with at least one symptom of burnout. • More common in physicians than in the average high school graduate. • Burnout most common in emergency medicine and general internal medicine (anesthesiology was seventh of 23 specialties listed).
West, CP, Dyrbye, LN, Sinsky, C, et al. Resilience and burnout among physicians and the general US working population. *JAMA Netw Open.* 2020;3(7):e209385. doi:10.1001/jamanetworkopen.2020.9385	Survey of 5445 physicians and a probability-based sample of 5198 individuals in the US working population.	• 17.9% response rate. • Mean resilience scores 3.8% higher in physicians. • Physicians without burnout had higher resilience scores. • 29% of physicians with the highest resilience scores still reported burnout.

(*continued*)

Table 45.1 Physician Burnout: Causes, Consequences, and Epidemiology (*Continued*)

Study	Methods and Focus	Findings
Marshall A, Dyrbye L, Shanafelt T, et al. Disparities in burnout and satisfaction with work–life integration in U.S. physicians by gender and practice setting. *Acad Med.* 2020;95:1435-1443.	30,456 physicians were invited to participate; 5445 (17.9%) completed the survey	• Female physicians reported a higher but not statistically significant prevalence of burnout than male physicians in both Academic and Private Practice.
Dyrbye L, Burke S, Hardeman R, et al. Association of clinical specialty with symptoms of burnout and career choice regret among us resident physicians. *J Am Med Assoc.* 2018;320(11):1114-1130.	Of 4696 resident physicians, 3588 (76.4%) completed the questionnaire during the second year of residency.	• 45.2% reported symptoms of burnout. • Career choice regret was reported by 14.1%. • Characteristics associated with higher risk of symptoms of burnout included female sex, risk difference, and higher levels of anxiety during medical school. • A high level of empathy during medical school was associated with a lower risk of symptoms of burnout during residency.
West CP, Dyrbye LN, Sinsky C, et al. Resilience and burnout among physicians and the general US working population. *JAMA Netw Open.* 2020;3(7):e209385. doi:10.1001/jamanetworkopen.2020.9385		• Higher rates of resilience in physicians than the general population. • Concomitant high resilience with high burnout in many physicians. • Myth that resilience training is the antidote to burnout dispelled.

ACS, American College of Surgeons; AMA, American Medical Association; MBI, Maslach Burnout Inventory; PRIME-MD, Primary Care Evaluation of Mental Disorders; QOL, quality of life.

II. Special Circumstances

Some stressors are so vital they require intervention to continue practice. This has resulted in various legislative efforts, as described in the sections that follow.

A. Americans With Disabilities Act

The ***Americans with Disabilities Act (ADA)*** is "an Act to establish a clear and comprehensive prohibition of discrimination on the basis of disability" that was signed into law by George H. W. Bush in 1990. This was followed in 2008 by the ***ADA Amendments Act (ADAAA)***, which broadened the protections offered in the original bill. In order to be protected by the ADA, a person must demonstrate a disability to qualify for protection and then request reasonable accommodation. A major focus of the ADAAA was to clarify the meaning of disability and broaden its definition to include any impairment that "substantially limits" a "major life activity." Although patients' safety must take primary focus, there will occasionally be physicians who have physical or mental limitations, including visual and auditory impairments. Often, reasonable accommodations can be made to enable the anesthesiologist to perform in an acceptable manner. When this is possible, the patient is protected by the ADA. Controversy is introduced, however, when there is a question of whether the proposed accommodations are reasonable or when patient safety appears to be compromised. Further questions—and controversies—arise at the local level with regard to credentialing and privileges and at the indemnification level with liability insurance underwriting. These cases are rare and are generally dealt with on a case-by-case basis.

B. Family and Medical Leave Act

The ***Family and Medical Leave Act*** of 1993 was a federal attempt at protecting work-life balance by ensuring covered employees are job protected, albeit unpaid, and granted leave during times of family need, such as an illness in the family, military leave, personal illness or recovery, pregnancy, or adoption. Certain stipulations (eg, who is considered a covered employee, including employment of 12 months prior to leave) are made, but most employed physicians and trainees fall within this category. Many employers also provide paid leave for various periods of time and circumstances. Controversies persist regarding the relatively higher use by women for maternity leave, although the use of paternity leave does appear to be increasing.

III. Considerations for the Physician

A. The Impaired Physician

The current body of literature relating to physician impairment, with few exceptions, focuses on impairment from substance use disorders. However, it must be noted that factors other than substance use may impair professional performance. These include other forms of addiction (eg, gambling, sex, food), psychiatric conditions (eg, anxiety, depression, obsessive-compulsive disorder), and medical conditions or treatments leading to fatigue or altered mental status (eg, obstructive sleep apnea, seizure disorder, prescribed narcotics).

Anesthesiologists have, for years, been considered at high risk for ***substance use disorder (SUD)***. However, until recently, strong data did not exist to support this assertion or its consequences. In 2013, Warner et al reported on the prevalence of SUD in those entering accredited anesthesiology residencies between 1975 and 2009.[5] Although their primary objective was to define the ***incidence*** of SUD during training, they also reported on the types of substances abused, episodes of relapse, and consequences, including death attributed to SUD. The most commonly abused substances were opioids, with intravenous fentanyl being the most common. Other commonly abused substances were alcohol, anesthetics or hypnotics, marijuana, and cocaine, with many abusing multiple substances. In a follow-up study, Warner et al reported the percentage of anesthesiologists expected to develop SUD within 30 years after completion of training was 1.6%. The most common substances used were opioids (55%), alcohol (40%), and anesthetics/hypnotics (20%). A substantial proportion of anesthesiologists who develop SUD after the completion of training die of this condition, and the risk of relapse is high in those who survive.[6]

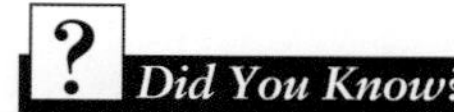

For anesthesiologists who developed a substance use disorder (SUD) during their training, the subsequent risk of death from relapse and SUD-related causes is reported to be 11%—an occupational hazard rate higher than being a firefighter and only slightly lower than being a police officer.

In response to the growing requirements by the Joint Commission, most states now offer specialized support programs for physicians struggling with SUD. These programs vary in their relationship with their respective state medical boards. Anesthesiologists can easily find a local program by doing an online search for "physician health program" in their state. Alternatively, one can simply visit the Federation of State Physician Health Programs (http://www.fsphp.org) and select the appropriate state or access aggregated information links via the American Society of Anesthesiologists Wellness website (https://www.asahq.org/in-the-spotlight/wellness-resources).

B. The Aging Physician

Since 1975, the number of practicing physicians older than 65 years in the United States has increased by more than 374%, and in 2015, 23% of practicing physicians were 65 years or older. With time, physicians gain experience; attain knowledge, judgment, and wisdom; and advance within the field, passing skills on to trainees and shaping the practice environment. While research shows that between the ages of 40 and 75 years the mean cognitive ability declines by more than 20%, there is substantial variability from one person to another, indicating that while some older physicians are profoundly impaired, others retain their ability and skills. There is no set retirement age for physicians, and this question is arising more frequently as many physicians choose to delay retirement in uncertain economic times. In November 2015, the American Medical Association (AMA) Council on Medical Education issued a report on "Competency and the Aging Physician" that called for "guidelines/standards for monitoring and assessing both their own and their colleagues' competency," and in 2016, the American College of Surgeons (ACS) released a "statement on the aging surgeon." Both the AMA and ACS proposals rely on voluntary action by physicians.[7] In 2012, relatively few departments had specific policies for older anesthesiologists. With the publication of findings that same year that found a higher frequency of litigation and a greater severity of injury in patients treated by anesthesiologists in the 65 years and older group,[8] promulgation of further research as well as proposals for neurocognitive and competency testing are evolving in both specialty societies and among regulatory agencies. More frequent ongoing professional performance evaluations have been recommended by the Joint Commission to address competency. As institutions implement such evaluations, they will hopefully become more valid and sensitive to instances of true cognitive decline.

IV. Providing Support

At some point in the anesthesiologist's career, an extraordinarily stressful event will be encountered that will require additional assistance with either processing or navigating the situation. It is unfortunate that not everyone faced with these situations seeks or accepts such assistance. Two specific situations arise during the careers of many anesthesiologists: adverse clinical events and malpractice litigation (see Chapter 41).

A. After an Adverse Event

"War stories" of perioperative catastrophes are occasionally shared in the anesthesia lounge, but until recently, the prevalence and impact of these events was not fully described. In 2012, a survey study was sent to 1200 members of the ASA. Gazoni et al[9] reported on this survey and found that, with a 56%

response rate, 84% of respondents had experienced at least one unexpected perioperative catastrophe. Of these, 19% reported never having fully recovered from the event, nearly all (88%) required some time to recover emotionally, and 67% felt the care they were delivering over the subsequent 4 hours was compromised. Despite this, only 7% were given any time off to recover.

The COVID-19 crisis offered a uniquely stressful milieu for anesthesiologists and critical care specialists to expand individuals' responses to adverse events and to consider front-line healthcare workers as a class with similar values, tasks, and responsibilities. Fleisher et al identified multifactorial stressors within their department as well as its individuals in the context of larger social systems such as the family, the influence of the media, and availability of personal protective equipment (PPE). They also found a significant interaction between trait anxiety of individuals and a culture of anxiety: clinicians who scored lower in trait anxiety showed a greater increase in anxiety related to the culture of anxiety of those around them.[10]

Already moving in this direction prior to the COVID crisis, many hospitals, universities, malpractice providers, and other organizations began to offer structured support following adverse events. These come in the form of peer support, formal counseling, debriefing, and even mandatory time away from clinical practice. It is wise to become familiar with the support resources available in one's practice environment in the event that such assistance is someday required following an adverse clinical event.

B. During or After a Malpractice Claim

Despite the historical role of anesthesiologists in improving patient safety, anesthesiologists can still find themselves named in a malpractice claim. A recent study of malpractice claims for a national carrier demonstrated anesthesiologists to have an annual risk of malpractice claims and payment similar to that of other medical specialists.[11] This can be one of the most stressful events in a physician's life, with distress arising from the uncertainty of outcomes, the prolonged nature of many lawsuits, and the sense of isolation that can occur when advised to not discuss the case with others. Although physicians' ego, financial security, and career are seemingly at risk during the litigation process, they also must repeatedly relive a potentially traumatizing adverse clinical event, adding to the psychological impact of the experience. Many malpractice carriers offer support and assistance during the difficult process of a medical malpractice lawsuit.

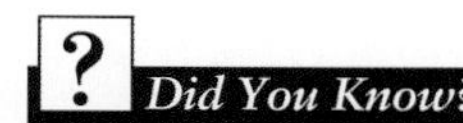

Although fitness, nutrition, proper rest, fiscal responsibility, and work-life balance are all important components of wellness, mindfulness-based stress reduction—an intentional, enhanced, and nonjudgmental awareness of one's environment and an inclination for living in the present moment—is most strongly linked to physician well-being.

V. Promoting Wellness

Although many suggest that personal well-being is an individual responsibility, recent data highlighting rates of burnout, SUD, and SUD-related death underscore the obligation of the profession in promoting well-being for its members. Moreover, as wellness principles become integrated into training and practice, there will likely be an inevitable extension into the concept of personal well-being as a "duty owed" to patients.

The components of wellness are varied, but certain approaches to decrease stress or increase resilience have been well validated and studied. Although fitness, nutrition, proper rest, fiscal responsibility, and work-life balance are all important components of wellness, none have been as solidly linked to improved physician well-being as ***mindfulness-based stress reduction (MBSR)***. Mindfulness carries many different definitions, all of which express the concept of an intentional, enhanced, and nonjudgmental awareness of one's environment and an inclination for living in the present moment. Rooted in Buddhist philosophy, the incorporation of mindfulness in contemporary medical practice has been led by the work of Jon Kabat-Zinn. Decreases in chronic pain and anxiety, and improved wound healing have been reported, with some recent studies demonstrating changes in brain architecture and gene expression as well as improvements in perceived levels of stress. Many medical schools are also starting to integrate MBSR as well as the concept of mindful practice into their curricula. These curricula, while varied, seek to prevent compassion fatigue and burnout, increase physician engagement and self-awareness, and decrease overall stress levels.[12]

Beyond the personal responsibility, however, is the impact of more systemic and external factors on physician well-being. In fact, the COVID-19 pandemic offers an incomparable opportunity to examine the delicate wellness balance between healthcare organizations and the individuals who comprise them; ultimately, the crucible of wellness care for the organization and its patients will be reflected in how the organization took care of its workers. Even prior to COVID-19, many national organizations, such as the National Academies of Medicine, were heavily engaged in addressing well-being at a higher organizational and policy level, representing the future direction of wellness interventions.[13]

VI. Conclusions

In order to provide sustained care, a person must have a degree of well-being. Given the data accumulating on anesthesiologist burnout, depression, suicidality, SUD, and SUD-related death, there should be substantial concern that common, as well as unique, problems exist within the specialty of anesthesiology. Fortunately, research and a body of literature are emerging on recognition and interventions focused on decreasing burnout and improving physician well-being.

For further review, please see the associated Interactive Video Lectures accessible in complimentary eBook bundled with this text. Access instructions are located on the inside front cover.

References

1. Frank J, Snell L, Sherbino J. *CanMEDS 2015 Physician Competency Framework*. Royal College of Physicians and Surgeons of Canada; 2015.
2. Maslach C, Jackson S. *Maslach Burnout Inventory*. 2nd ed. Consulting Psychologists Press; 1986.
3. Jackson S. The role of stress in anaesthetists' health and well-being. *Acta Anaesthesiol Scand*. 1999;43(6).
4. Garcia L, Shanafelt T, West C, et al. Burnout, depression, career satisfaction, and Work-life integration by physician race/ethnicity. *JAMA Netw Open*. 2020;3(8):e2012762. doi:10.1001/jamanetworkopen.2020.12762
5. Warner D, Berge K, Sun H, Harman A, Hanson A, Schroeder D. Substance use disorder among anesthesiology residents 1975-2009. *J Am Med Assoc*. 2013;310(21):2289-2296.
6. Warner D, Berge K, Sun H, Harman A, Wang T. Substance use disorder in physicians after completion of training in anesthesiology in the United States from 1977 to 2013. *Anesthesiology*. 2020;133(2):342-3497.
7. Dellinger E, Pellegrini C, Gallagher T. The aging physician and the medical profession: a review. *JAMA Surg*. 2017;152(10):967-971.
8. Tessler M, Shrier I, Steele R. Association between anesthesiologist age and litigation. *Anesthesiology*. 2012;115(3):574-579.
9. Gazoni F, Durieux M, Wells L. Life after death: the aftermath of perioperative catastrophes. *Anesth Analg*. 2008;107:591-600.
10. Fleisher L, Sweenet R, Clapp J, Barsade S. Managing anxiety in anesthesiology and intensive care providers during the COVID-19 pandemic; an analysis of the psychosocial response of a front-line department. *NEJM Catalyst* 2020. doi:10.1056/CAT.20.0270
11. Jena A, Seabury S, Lakdawalla D, Chandra A. Malpractice risk according to physician specialty. *N Engl J Med*. 2011;365(7):629-636.
12. Dobkin P, Hutchinson T. Teaching mindfulness in medical school: where are we now and where are we going? *Med Educ*. 2013;47(8):768-779.
13. National Academies of Sciences Engineering and Medicine. *Taking Action against Clinician Burnout: A Systems Approach to Professional Well-Being*. National Academy of Medicine; 2019.

Questions

1. **All of the following are major symptoms of burnout as described in the Maslach Burnout Inventory EXCEPT:**

   A. Low sense of personal accomplishment.
   B. Frustration.
   C. Emotional exhaustion.
   D. Depersonalization.

2. **The significance of the Americans with Disabilities Amendments Act (ADAAA, 2008) beyond the Americans with Disabilities Act (ADA, 1990) is that:**

   A. a person must demonstrate a disability and then request reasonable accommodation.
   B. it clarified the meaning of disability to include any impairment that substantially limits a major life activity.
   C. it takes practitioners' disability needs into account as a priority over patient safety.
   D. it resolved that disputes about patient safety and practitioner accommodation should be settled in court.

3. **Which of the following assessment tools has a high positive predictive value for detecting clinical impairments associated with aging?**

   A. Continuing Medical Education (CME) performance
   B. Neurocognitive testing
   C. Maintenance of Certification in Anesthesiology (MOCA) programs
   D. None of the above

4. **The percentage of anesthesiologists expected to develop substance use disorder within 30 years following completion of training is:**

   A. 1.6%.
   B. 5.4%.
   C. 8%.
   D. 10%.

5. **During their career, anesthesiologists can experience a perioperative catastrophe (such as a patient's unanticipated injury or death) associated with their care. All of the following are characteristic of these outcomes EXCEPT:**

   A. These complications are rare.
   B. Of anesthesiologists who experience such an event, approximately 20% report never having fully recovered emotionally from the event.
   C. The majority of anesthesiologists who experience such an event feel that the care they deliver immediately following the event can be compromised.
   D. Providing immediate care to both the harmed patient and the involved anesthesiologist is a recommended practice.

Answers

1. B

The MBI is considered the gold standard for assessing burnout and assesses three psychological characteristics. Frustration is not a component of the tool.

2. B

The 2008 amendment to the 1990 Americans with Disabilities Act (ADA) served to define and clarify the meaning of disability and broaden its definition to "include any impairment that substantially limits a major life activity." Although patients' safety takes primary focus, the amendment recognizes that there will occasionally be physicians who have physical or mental limitations, including visual and auditory impairments, and reasonable accommodations can be made to enable the anesthesiologist to perform in an acceptable manner. If a question arises of whether the proposed accommodations are reasonable, or if patient safety appears to be compromised, they are adjudicated locally on a case-by-case basis with regard to credentialing, practice privileges, and liability coverage.

3. D

Neither CME or MOCA performance have been clearly linked to improved knowledge retention or patient care, and neurocognitive testing has both low positive predictive value and high potential for psychological stress from false-positive results.

4. A

Warner et al (2020) found the cumulative percentage of anesthesiologists expected to develop substance use disorder within 30 years of graduation (Kaplan-Meier estimate) equaled 1.6% (95% CI, 1.4%-1.7%)

5. A

Gazoni et al (2008) reported that 84% of anesthesiologists had experienced at least one unexpected perioperative catastrophe, and of these, 19% reported never having fully recovered from the event. About 88% required some time to recover emotionally, and 67% felt that the care they were delivering over the subsequent 4 hours was compromised. Only 7% were given any time off to recover. Experts believe that the best practice following unanticipated patient harm is to provide immediate emotional support not only to the patient and his/her family, but to the involved practitioners as well.

IV Appendices

A Formulas

Hemodynamic Formulas
Respiratory Formulas
Lung Volumes and Capacities

Hemodynamic Formulas

Hemodynamic Variables: Calculations and Normal Values		
Variable	**Calculation**	**Normal Values**
Cardiac index (CI)	CO/BSA	2.5-4.0 L/min/m^2
Stroke volume (SV)	CO × 1000/HR	60-90 mL/beat
Stroke index (SI)	SV/BSA	40-60 mL/beat/m^2
Mean arterial pressure (MAP)	Diastolic pressure +⅓ pulse pressure	80-120 mm Hg
Systemic vascular resistance (SVR)	$\frac{MAP - \overline{CVP}}{CO} \times 79.9$	1200-1500 dyne-cm-s^{-5}
Pulmonary vascular resistance (PVR)	$\frac{\overline{PAP} - \overline{PCWP}}{CO} \times 79.9$	100-300 dyne-cm-s^{-5}
Right ventricular stroke work index (RVSWI)	$0.0136\ (\overline{PAP} - \overline{CVP}) \times SI$	5-9 g-m/beat/m^2
Left ventricular stroke work index (LWSWI)	$0.0136\ (MAP - \overline{PCWP}) \times SI$	45-60 g-m/beat/m^2

BSA, body surface area; CO, cardiac output; $\overline{CVP}$, mean central venous pressure; HR, heart rate; MAP, mean arterial blood pressure; $\overline{PAP}$, mean pulmonary artery pressure; $\overline{PCWP}$, mean pulmonary capillary wedge pressure.

Respiratory Formulas

	Normal Values (70 kg)
Alveolar oxygen tension $PAO_2 = (PB - 47)\ FIO_2 - PACO_2$	110 mm Hg ($FIO_2 = 0.21$)
Alveolar-arterial oxygen gradient $Aao_2 = PAO_2 - Pao_2$	<10 mm Hg ($FIO_2 = 0.21$)
Arterial-to-alveolar oxygen ratio, a/A ratio	>0.75
Arterial oxygen content $Cao_2 = (Sao_2)(Hb \times 1.34) + Pao_2\,(0.0031)$	21 mL/100 mL
Mixed venous oxygen content $C\dot{v}o_2 = (S\dot{v}o_2)(Hb \times 1.34) + P\overline{v}o_2\,(0.0031)$	15 mL/100 mL
Arterial-venous oxygen content difference $avo_2 = Cao_2 - C\overline{v}o_2$	4-6 mL/100 mL
Intrapulmonary shunt $\dot{Q}S/\dot{Q}T = (Cco_2 - Cao_2)/(Cco_2 - C\dot{v}o_2)$ $Cco_2 = (Hb \times 1.34) + (PAO_2 \times 0.0031)$	<5%
Physiologic dead space $\dot{V}D/\dot{V}T = (Paco_2 - PECO_2)/Paco_2$	0.33
Oxygen consumption $\dot{V}o_2 = CO(Cao_2 - C\dot{v}o_2)$	240 mL/min
Oxygen transport $O_2T = CO\,(Cao_2)$	1000 mL/min

Cao_2, arterial oxygen content; Cco_2, pulmonary capillary oxygen content; CO, cardiac output; $C\dot{v}o_2$, mixed venous oxygen content; FIO_2, fraction inspired oxygen; o_2, oxygen consumption (minute); O_2T, oxygen transport; $PACO_2$, alveolar carbon dioxide tension; $Paco_2$, arterial carbon dioxide tension PAO_2, alveolar oxygen tension; Pao_2, arterial oxygen tension; P_B, barometric pressure; $PECO_2$, expired carbon dioxide tension; $\dot{Q}S/\dot{Q}T$, intrapulmonary shunt; VD, dead space gas volume; VT, tidal volume.

Lung Volumes and Capacities

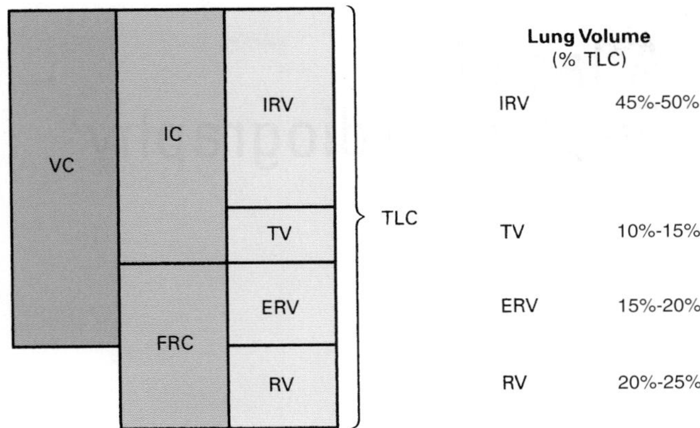

		Normal Values (70 kg)
Vital capacity	VC	4800 mL
Inspiratory capacity	IC	3800 mL
Functional residual capacity	FRC	2400 mL
Inspiratory reserve volume	IRV	3500 mL
Tidal volume	TV	1500 mL
Expiratory reserve volume	ERV	1200 mL
Residual volume	RV	1200 mL
Total lung capacity	TLC	6000 mL

B Atlas of Electrocardiography[1]

Lead Placement

	Electrode	
	Positive	**Negative**
Bipolar Leads		
I	LA	RA
II	LL	RA
III	LL	LA
Augmented Unipolar		
aVR	RA	LA, LL
aVL	LA	RA, LL
aVF	LL	RA, LA
Precordial		
V_1	4 ICS–RSB	
V_2	4 ICS–LSB	
V_3	Midway between V_2 and V_4	
V_4	5 ICS–MCL	
V_5	5 ICS–AAL	
V_6	5 ICS–MAL	

[1]Sections and images of this Appendix were developed, in part, for both Barash PG, Cullen BF, Stoelting RK, et al, eds. *Clinical Anesthesia*. 7th ed. Wolters Kluwer Health/Lippincott Williams & Wilkins; 2013, and Kaplan JA, Reich DL, Savino JS, eds. *Kaplan's Cardiac Anesthesia: The Echo Era*. Elsevier; 2011.

Abbrev.	**Meaning**
LA	Left arm
RA	Right arm
LL	Left leg
ICS	Intercostal space
RSB	Right sternal border
LSB	Left sternal border
MCL	Midclavicular line
AAL	Interaxillary line
MAL	Midaxillary line

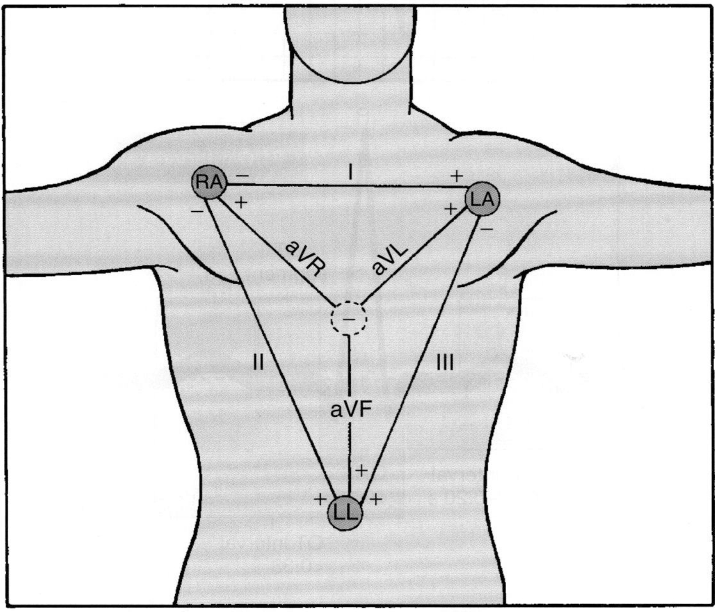

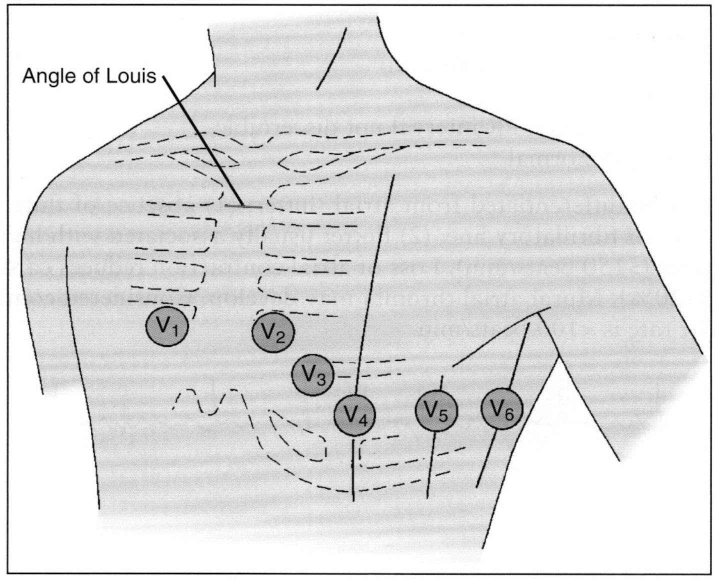

The Normal Electrocardiogram—Cardiac Cycle
The normal electrocardiogram is composed of waves (P, QRS, T, and U) and intervals (PR, QRS, ST, and QT).

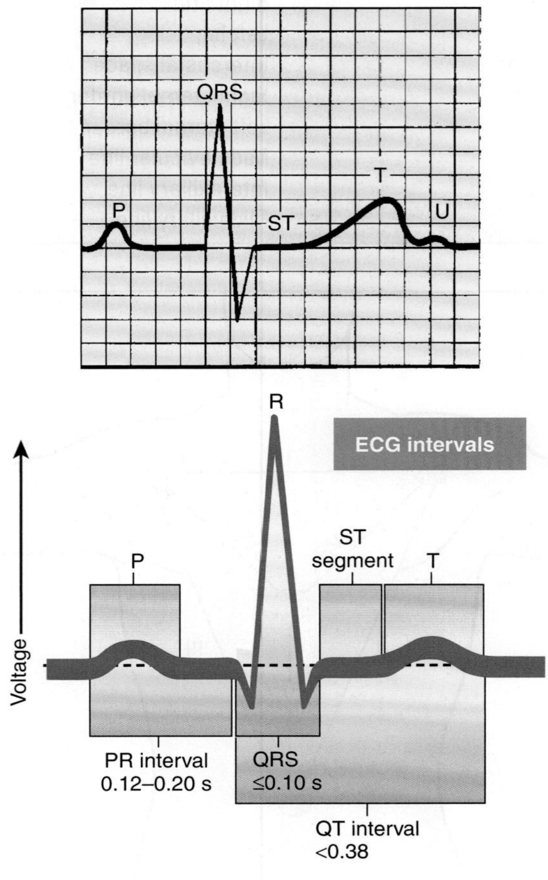

Atrial Fibrillation
Rate: Variable (~150-200 beats/min)
Rhythm: Irregular
PR interval: No P wave; PR interval not discernible
QT interval: QRS normal

Note: Must be differentiated from atrial flutter: (1) absence of flutter waves and presence of fibrillatory line; (2) flutter usually associated with higher ventricular rates (>150 beats/min). Loss of atrial contraction reduces cardiac output (10%-20%). Mural atrial thrombi may develop. Considered controlled if ventricular rate is <100 beats/min.

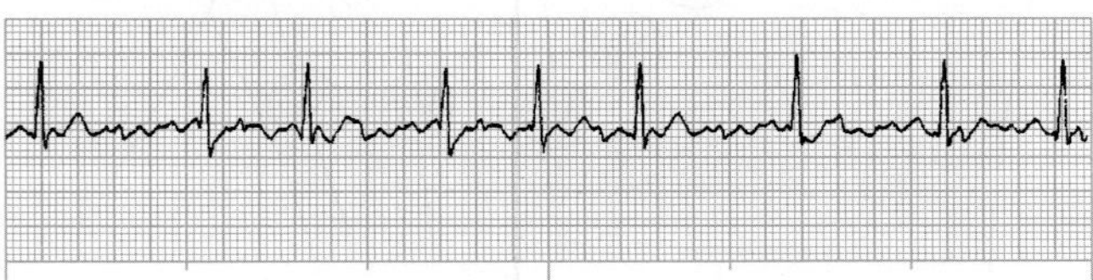

Atrial Flutter
Rate: Rapid, atrial usually regular (250-350 beats/min); ventricular usually regular (<100 beats/min)
Rhythm: Atrial and ventricular regular
PR interval: Flutter (F) waves are saw-toothed. PR interval cannot be measured.
QT interval: QRS usually normal; ST-segment and T waves are not identifiable.

Note: Vagal maneuvers will slow ventricular response, simplifying recognition of the F waves.

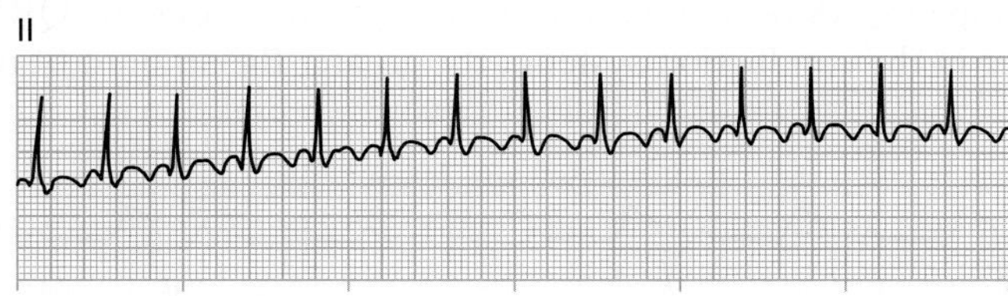

Atrioventricular Block (First Degree)
Rate: 60 to 100 beats/min
Rhythm: Regular
PR interval: Prolonged (>0.20 seconds) and constant
QT interval: Normal

Note: Usually clinically insignificant; may be early harbinger of drug toxicity.

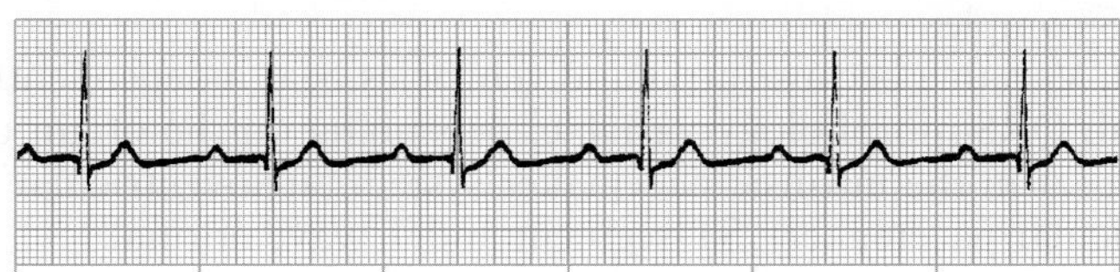

Atrioventricular Block (Second Degree), Mobitz Type I/Wenckebach Block
Rate: 60 to 100 beats/min
Rhythm: Atrial regular; ventricular irregular
PR interval: P wave normal; PR interval progressively lengthens with each cycle until QRS complex is dropped (dropped beat). PR interval following dropped beat is shorter than normal.
QT interval: QRS complex normal but dropped periodically.

Note: Commonly seen in trained athletes and with drug toxicity.

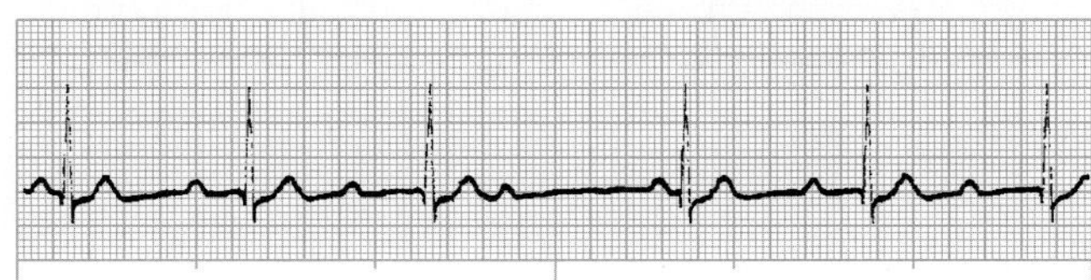

Atrioventricular Block (Second Degree), Mobitz Type II

Rate: <100 beats/min

Rhythm: Atrial regular; ventricular regular or irregular

PR interval: P waves normal but some are not followed by QRS complex.

QT interval: Normal but may have widened QRS complex if block is at level of bundle branch. ST-segment and T wave may be abnormal, depending on location of block.

Note: In contrast to Mobitz type I block, the PR and RR intervals are constant and the dropped QRS occurs without warning. The wider the QRS complex (block lower in the conduction system), the greater the amount of myocardial damage.

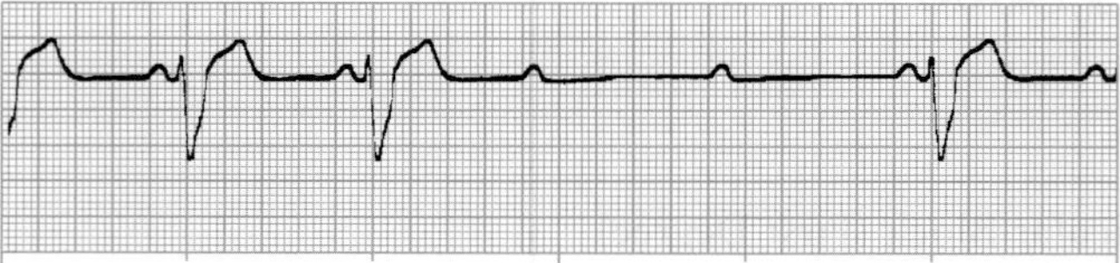

Atrioventricular Block (Third Degree), Complete Heart Block

Rate: <45 beats/min

Rhythm: Atrial regular; ventricular regular; no relationship between P wave and QRS complex

PR interval: Variable because atria and ventricles beat independently.

QT interval: QRS morphology variable, depending on the origin of the ventricular beat in the intrinsic pacemaker system (atrioventricular junctional vs ventricular pacemaker). ST-segment and T wave normal.

Note: AV block represents complete failure of conduction from atria to ventricles (no P wave is conducted to the ventricle). The atrial rate is faster than ventricular rate. P waves have no relationship to QRS complexes (eg, they are electrically disconnected). In contrast, with AV dissociation, the P wave is conducted through the AV node and the atrial and ventricular rates are similar. Immediate treatment with atropine or isoproterenol is required if cardiac output is reduced. Consideration should be given to insertion of a pacemaker. Seen as a complication of mitral valve replacement.

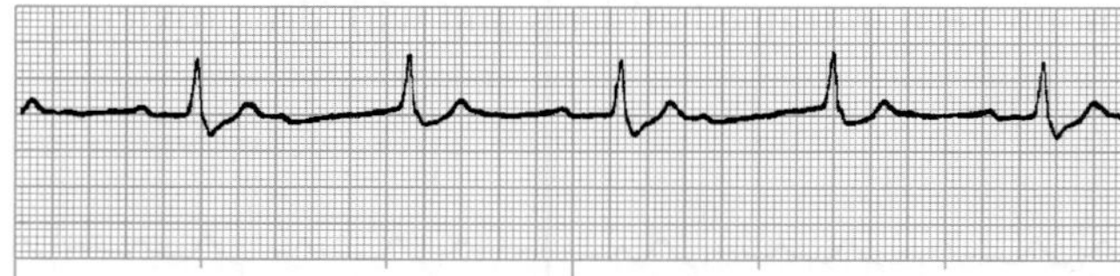

Bundle-Branch Block—Left (LBBB)
Rate: <100 beats/min
Rhythm: Regular
PR interval: Normal
QT interval: Complete LBBB (QRS >0.12 seconds); incomplete LBBB (QRS = 0.10-0.12 seconds); lead V_1 negative RS complex; I, aVL, V_6 wide R wave without Q or S component. ST-segment and T wave direction opposite direction of the R wave.

Note: LBBB does not occur in healthy patients and usually indicates serious heart disease with a poor prognosis. In patients with LBBB, insertion of a pulmonary artery catheter may lead to complete heart block.

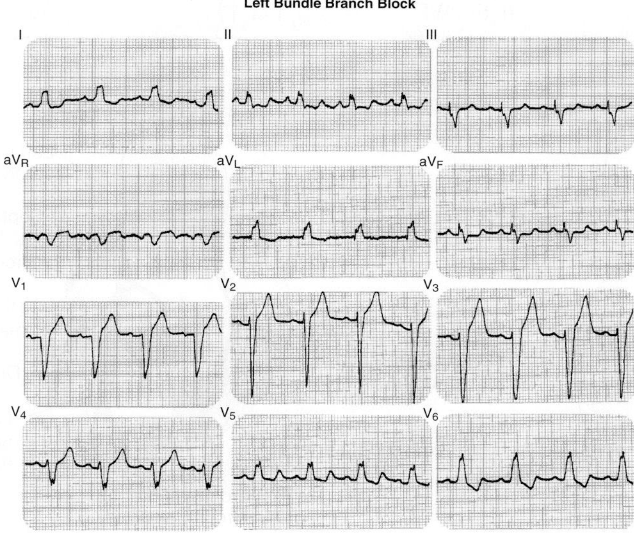

Bundle-Branch Block—Right (RBBB)
Rate: <100 beats/min
Rhythm: Regular
PR interval: Normal
QT interval: Complete RBBB (QRS >0.12 seconds); incomplete RBBB (QRS = 0.10-0.12 seconds). Varying patterns of QRS complex; rSR (V_1); RS, wide R with M pattern. ST-segment and T wave opposite direction of the R wave.

Note: In the presence of RBBB, Q waves may be seen with a myocardial infarction.

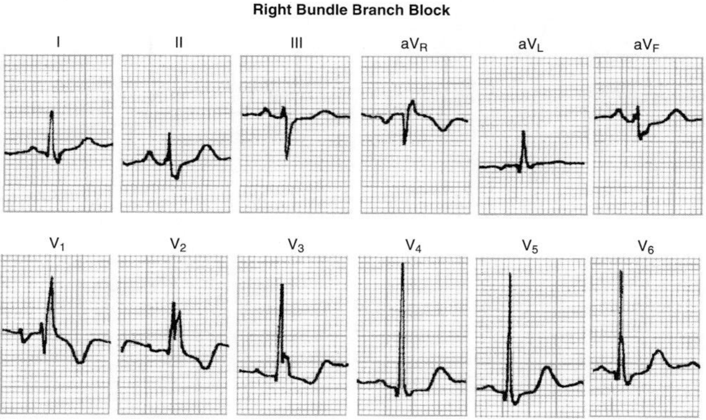

Coronary Artery Disease

Transmural Myocardial Infarction (TMI)

Q waves seen on ECG, useful in confirming diagnosis, are associated with poorer prognosis and more significant hemodynamic impairment. Arrhythmias frequently complicate course. Small Q waves may be normal variant. For myocardial infarction (MI), Q waves >0.04 seconds or depth exceed one-third of R wave. For inferior wall MI, differentiate from RVH by axis deviation.

Myocardial Infarction

Anatomic Site	Leads	ECG Changes	Coronary Artery
Inferior	II, III, AVF	Q, ↑ST, ↑T	Right

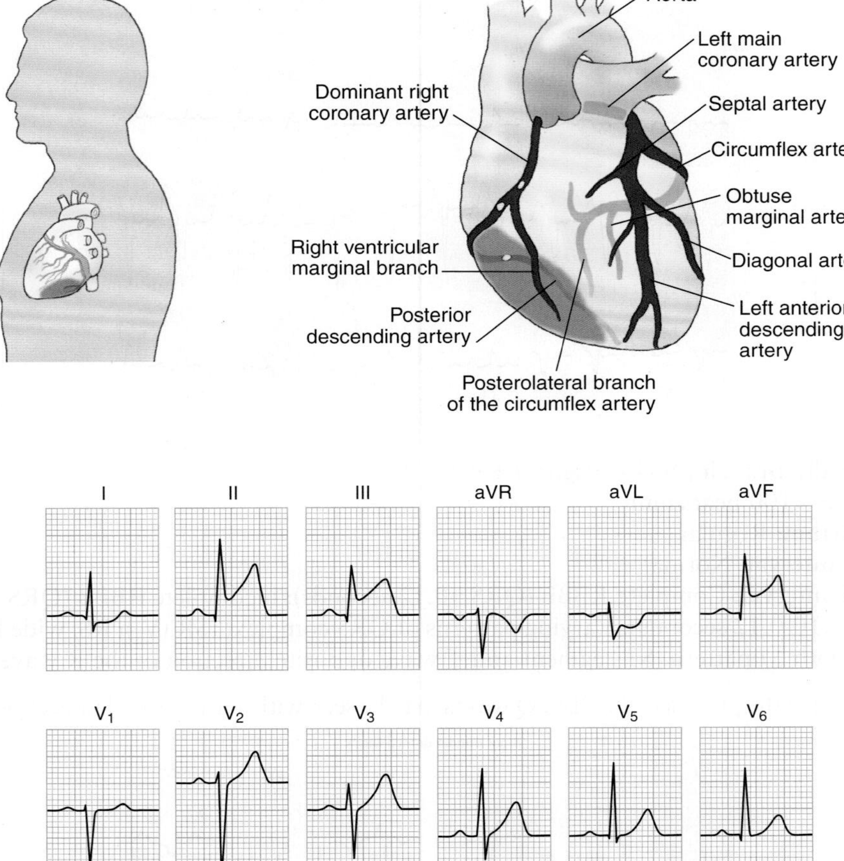

Myocardial Infarction

Anatomic Site	Leads	ECG Changes	Coronary Artery
Posterior	V_1–V_2	↑R, ↓ST, ↓T	Left circumflex

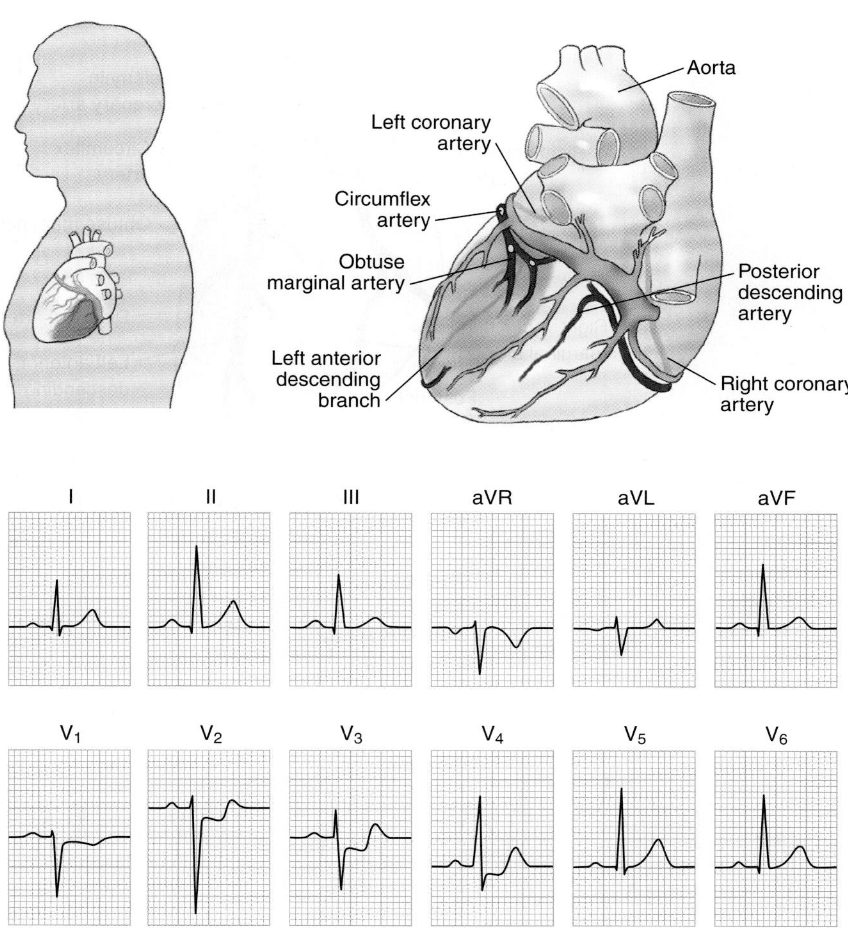

Myocardial Infarction			
Anatomic Site	**Leads**	**ECG Changes**	**Coronary Artery**
Lateral	I, aVL, V_5–V_6	Q, ↑ST, ↑T	Left circumflex

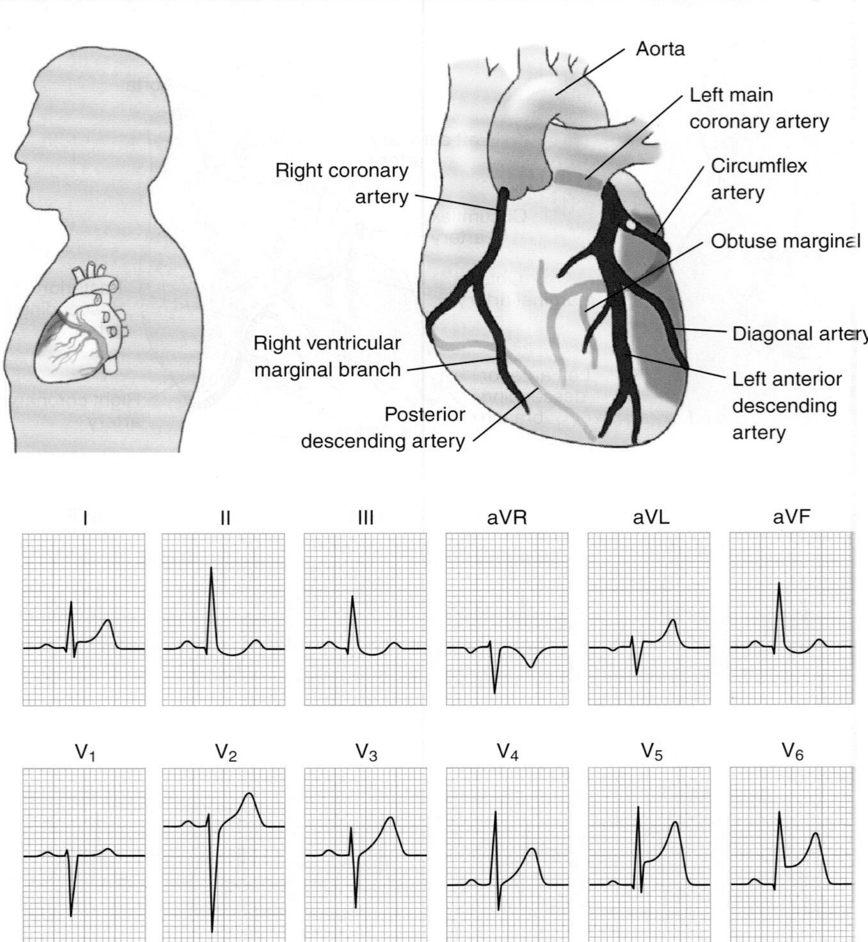

Myocardial Infarction

Anatomic Site	Leads	ECG Changes	Coronary Artery
Anterior	I, aVL, V_1–V_4	Q, ↑ST, ↑T	Left anterior descending

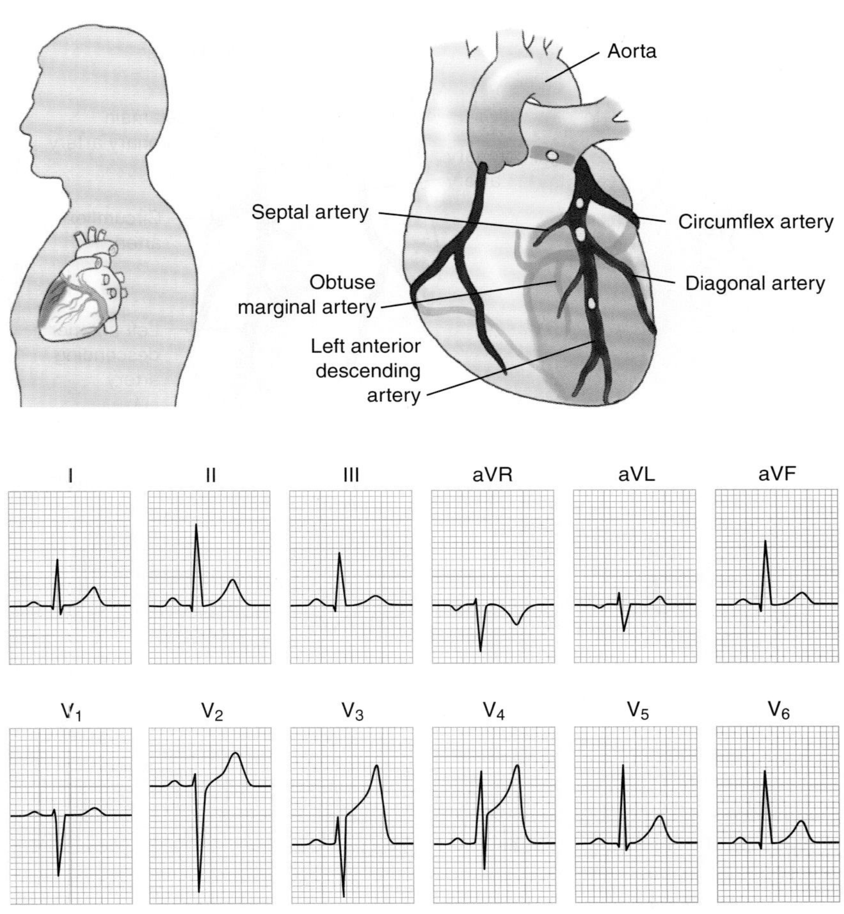

Myocardial Infarction

Anatomic Site	Leads	ECG Changes	Coronary Artery
Anteroseptal	V_1–V_4	Q, ↑ST, ↑T	Left anterior descending

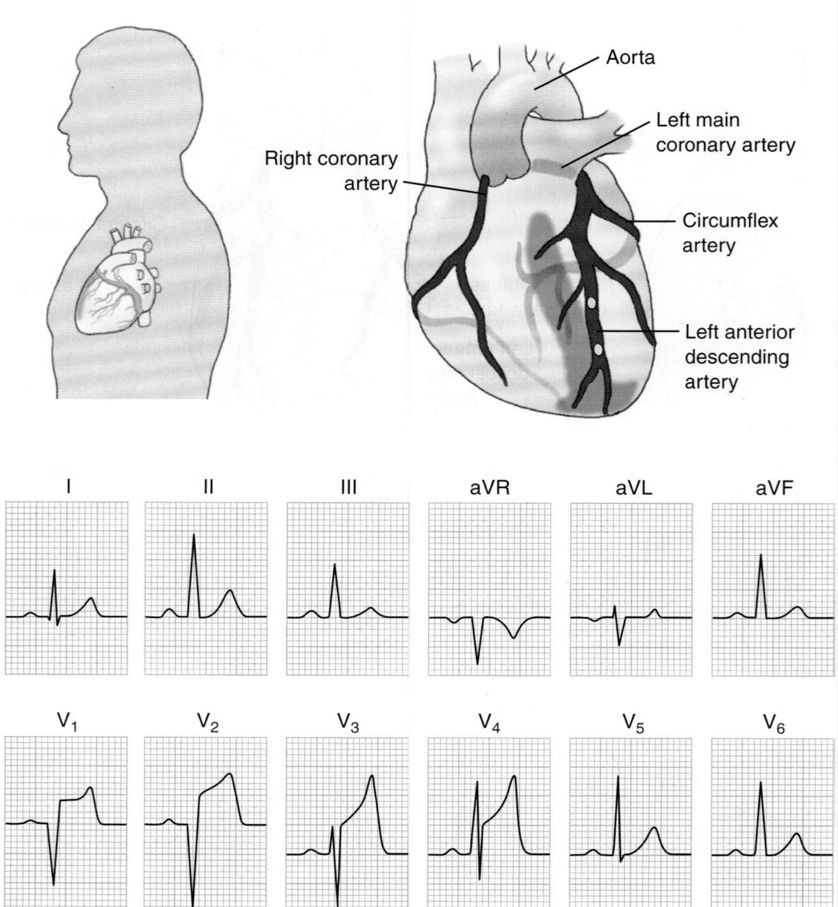

Subendocardial Myocardial Infarction (SEMI)

Persistent ST-segment depression and/or T-wave inversion in the absence of Q wave. Usually requires additional laboratory data (eg, isoenzymes) to confirm diagnosis. Anatomic site of coronary lesion is similar to that of TMI electrocardiographically.

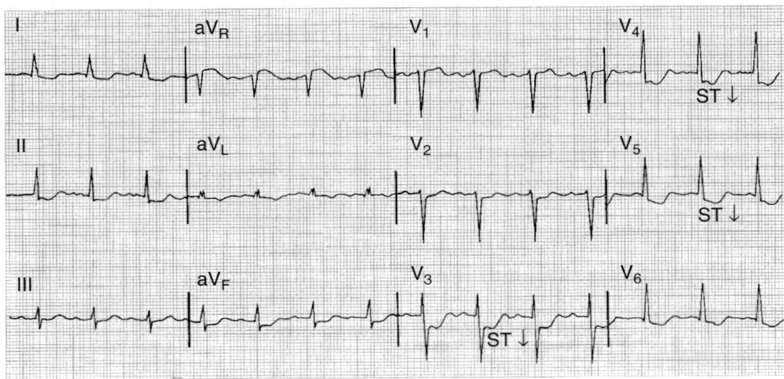

Myocardial Ischemia

Rate: Variable

Rhythm: Usually regular but may show atrial and/or ventricular arrhythmias.

PR interval: Normal

QT interval: ST-segment depressed; J-point depression; T-wave inversion; conduction disturbances. (A) TP and PR intervals are baseline for ST-segment deviation. (B) ST-segment elevation. (C) ST-segment depression.

Note: Intraoperative ischemia usually is seen in the presence of "normal" vital signs (eg, ±20% of preinduction values).

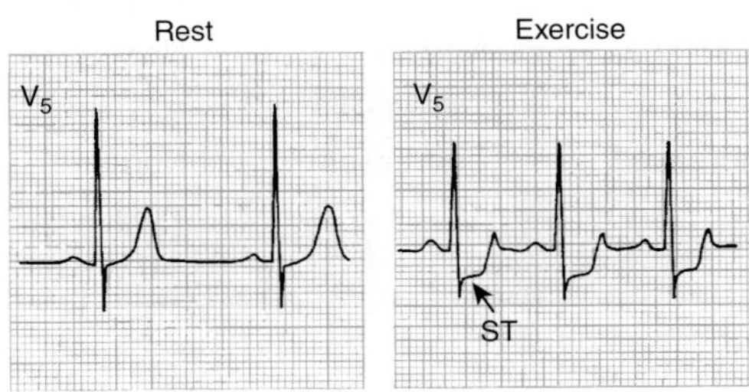

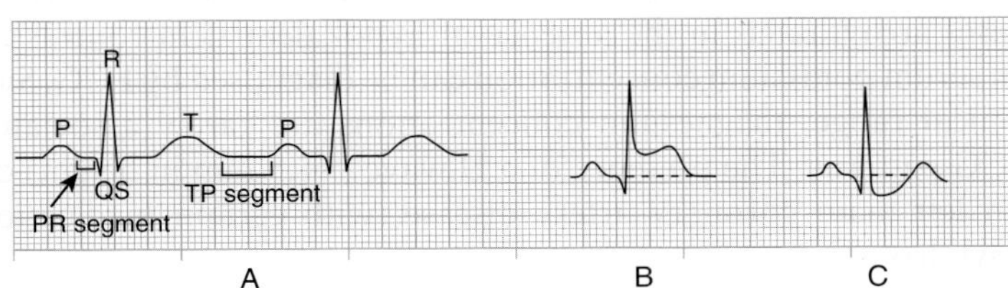

Digitalis Effect
Rate: <100 beats/min
Rhythm: Regular
PR interval: Normal or prolonged
QT interval: ST-segment sloping (digitalis effect)

Note: Digitalis toxicity can be the cause of many common arrhythmias (eg, premature ventricular contractions, second-degree heart block). Verapamil, quinidine, and amiodarone cause an increase in serum digitalis concentration.

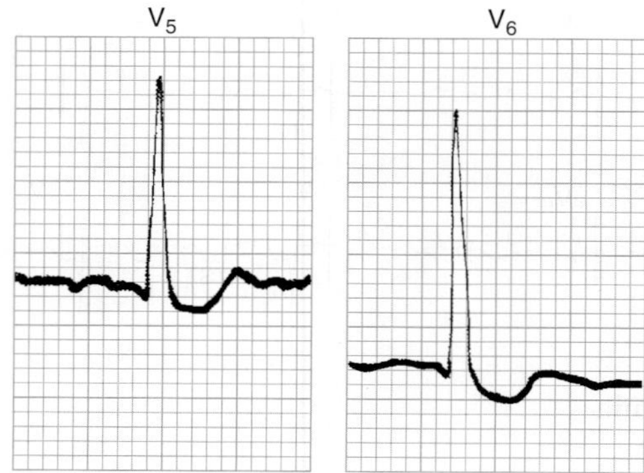

Electrolyte Disturbances

	↓Ca^{2+}	↑Ca^{2+}	↓K^+	↑H^+
Rate	<100 beats/min	<100 beats/min	<100 beats/min	<100 beats/min
Rhythm	Regular	Regular	Regular	Regular
PR interval	Normal	Normal/increased	Normal	Normal
QT interval	Increased	Decreased	Normal	Increased
Other			T wave flat U wave	T wave peaked

Note: ECG changes usually do not correlate with serum calcium. Hypocalcemia rarely causes arrhythmias in the absence of hypokalemia. In contrast, abnormalities in serum potassium concentration can be diagnosed by ECG. Similarly, in the clinical range, magnesium concentrations are rarely associated with unique ECG patterns. The presence of a U wave (>1.5 mm in height) can also be seen in left main coronary artery disease, with certain medications and long-QT syndrome.

Calcium

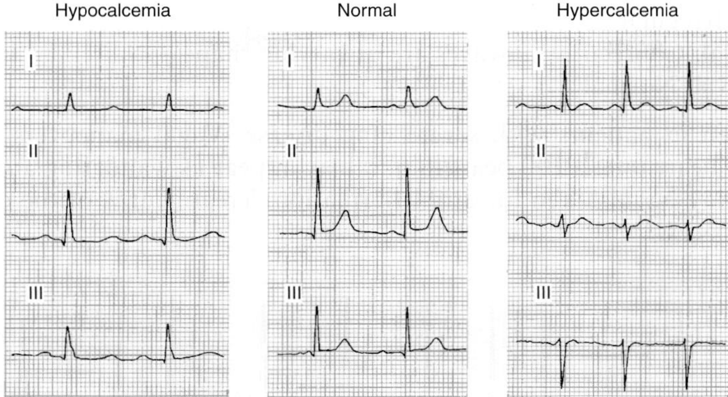

Potassium

Hypokalemia (K^+ = 1.9 mEq/L)

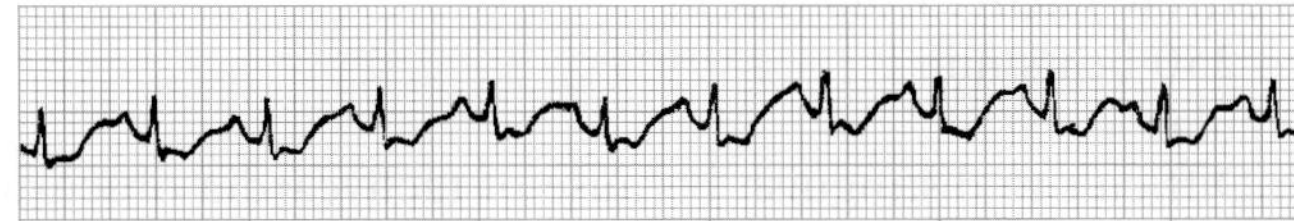

Hyperkalemia (K^+ = 7.9 mEq/L)

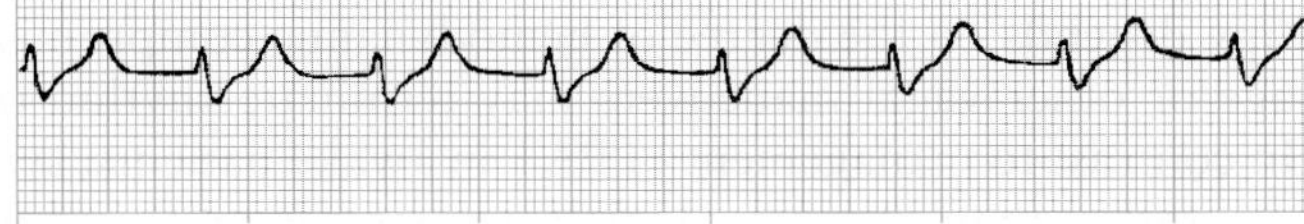

Hypothermia

Rate: <60 beats/min
Rhythm: Sinus
PR interval: Prolonged
QT interval: Prolonged

Note: Seen at temperatures below 33 °C with ST-segment elevation (J point or Osborn wave). Tremor due to shivering or Parkinson disease may interfere with ECG interpretation and may be confused with atrial flutter. May represent normal variant of early ventricular repolarization. (*Arrow* indicates J point or Osborn waves.)

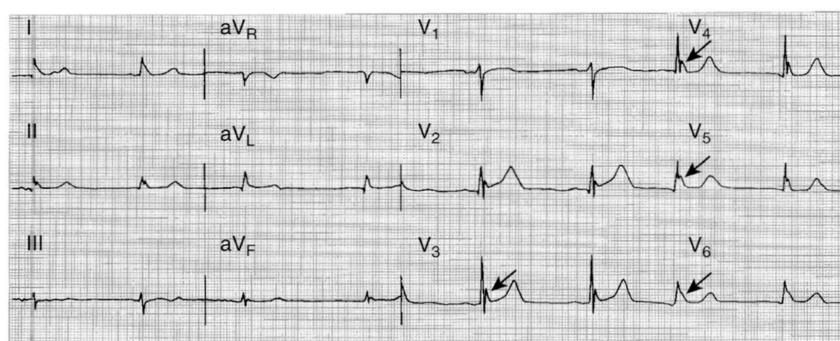

Multifocal Atrial Tachycardia
Rate: 100 to 200 beats/min
Rhythm: Irregular
PR interval: Consecutive P waves are of varying shape.
QT interval: Normal

Note: Seen in patients with severe lung disease. Vagal maneuvers have no effect. At heart rates <100 beats/min, it may appear as wandering atrial pacemaker. May be mistaken for atrial fibrillation. Treatment is of the causative disease process.

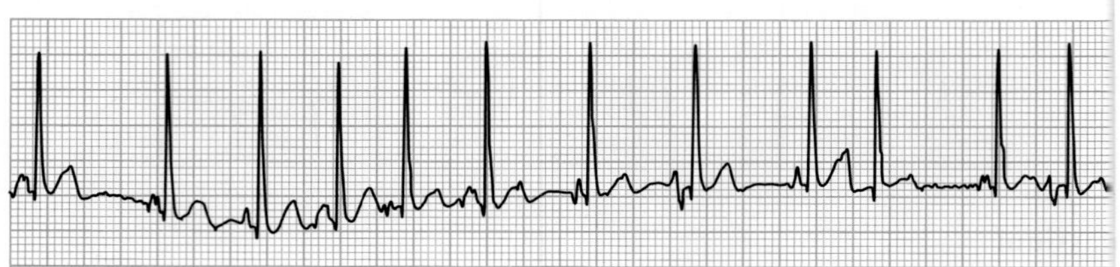

Paroxysmal Atrial Tachycardia (PAT)
Rate: 150 to 250 beats/min
Rhythm: Regular
PR interval: Difficult to distinguish because of tachycardia obscuring P wave. P wave may precede, be included in, or follow QRS complex.
QT interval: Normal, but ST-segment and T wave may be difficult to distinguish.

Note: Therapy depends on the degree of hemodynamic compromise. Carotid sinus massage or other vagal maneuvers may terminate rhythm or decrease heart rate. In contrast to management of PAT in awake patients, synchronized cardioversion, rather than pharmacologic treatment, is preferred in hemodynamically unstable anesthetized patients.

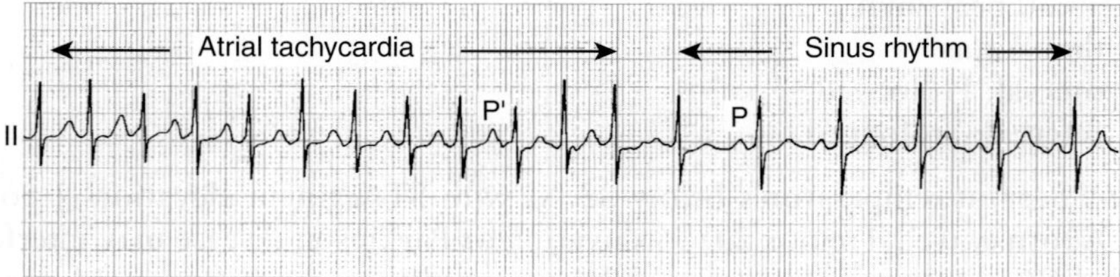

Pericarditis
Rate: Variable
Rhythm: Variable
PR interval: Normal
QT interval: Diffuse ST and T-wave changes with no Q wave and seen in more leads than a myocardial infarction.

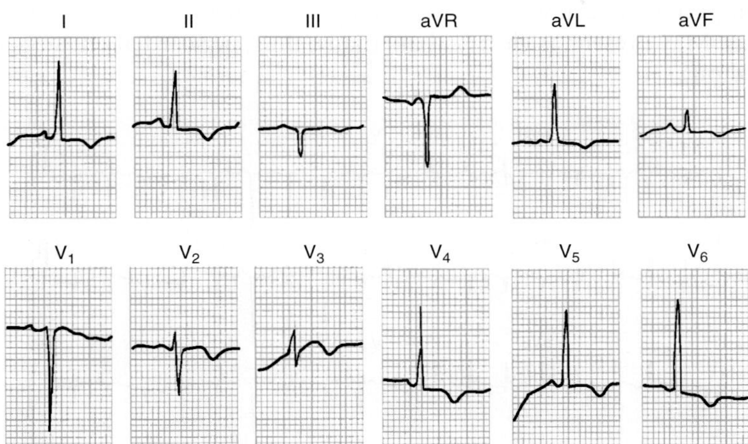

Pericardial Tamponade
Rate: Variable
Rhythm: Variable
PR interval: Low-voltage P wave
QT interval: Seen as electrical alternans with low-voltage complexes and varying amplitude of P, QRS, and T waves with each heartbeat.

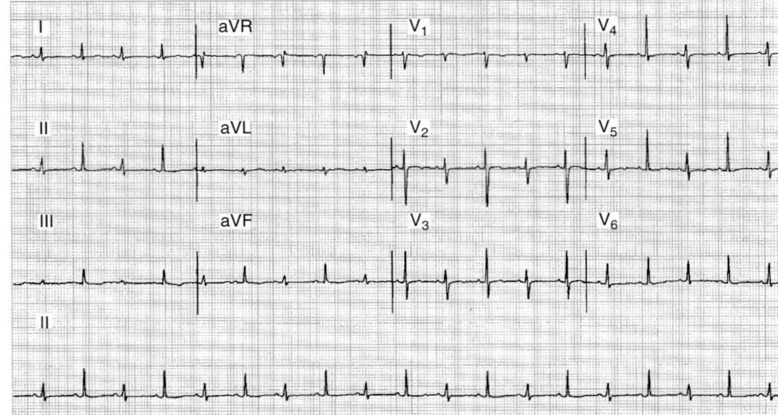

Pneumothorax
Rate: Variable
Rhythm: Variable
PR interval: Normal
QT interval: Normal

Note: Common ECG abnormalities include right-axis deviation, decreased QRS amplitude, and inverted T waves V_1–V_6. Differentiate from pulmonary embolus. May present as electrical alternans; thus, pericardial effusion should be ruled out.

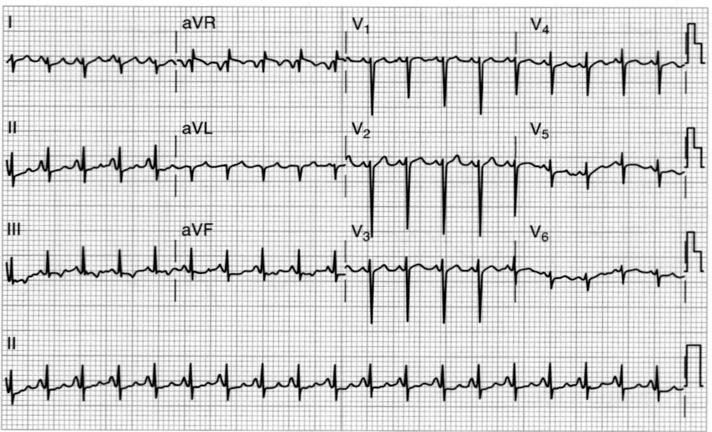

Premature Atrial Contraction (PAC)
Rate: <100 beats/min
Rhythm: Irregular
PR interval: P waves may be lost in preceding T waves. PR interval is variable.
QT interval: QRS normal configuration; ST-segment and T wave normal.

Note: Nonconducted PAC appearance similar to that of sinus arrest; T waves with PAC may be distorted by inclusion of P wave in the T wave.

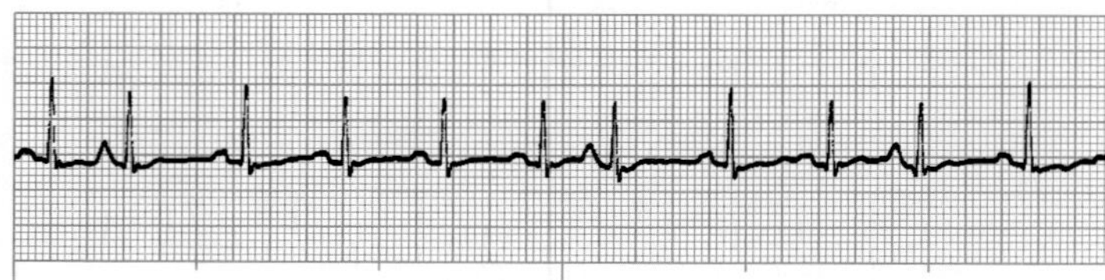

Premature Ventricular Contraction (PVC)
Rate: Usually <100 beats/min
Rhythm: Irregular
PR interval: P wave and PR interval absent; retrograde conduction of P wave can be seen.
QT interval: Wide QRS (>0.12 seconds); ST-segment cannot be evaluated (eg, ischemia); T wave opposite direction of QRS with compensatory pause. Fourth and eighth beats are PVCs.

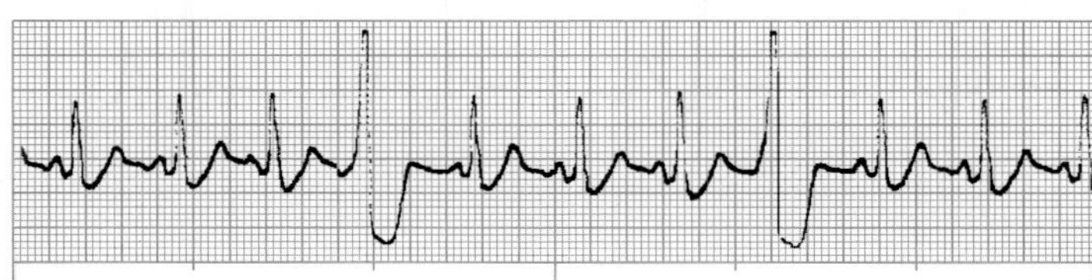

Pulmonary Embolus
Rate: >100 beats/min
Rhythm: Sinus
PR interval: P-pulmonale waveform
QT interval: Q waves in leads III and aVF

Note: Classic ECG signs S1Q3T3 with T-wave inversion also seen in V_1–V_4 and RV strain (ST depression V_1–V_4). May present with atrial fibrillation or flutter.

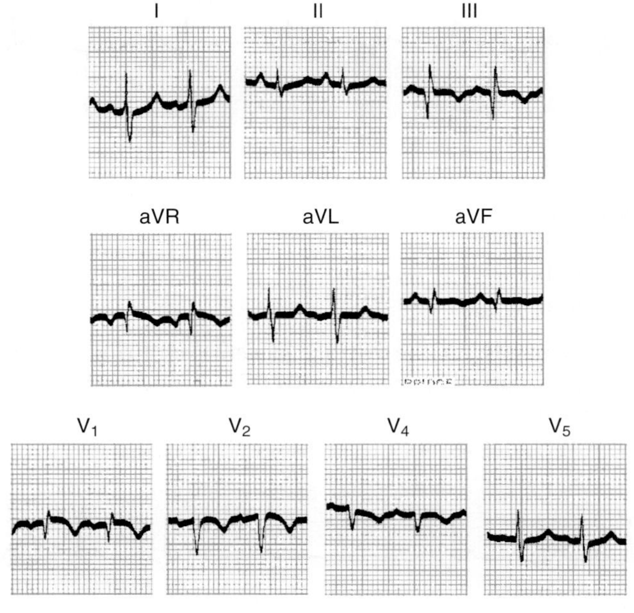

Sinus Bradycardia
Rate: <60 beats/min
Rhythm: Sinus
PR interval: Normal
QT interval: Normal

Note: Seen in trained athletes as normal variant.

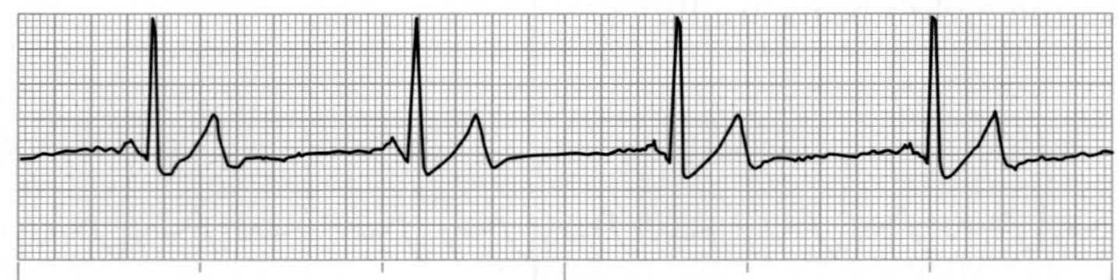

Sinus Arrhythmia
Rate: 60 to 100 beats/min
Rhythm: Sinus
PR interval: Normal
QT interval: R-R interval variable

Note: Heart rate increases with inhalation and decreases with exhalation +10% to 20% (respiratory). Nonrespiratory sinus arrhythmia seen in elderly with heart disease. Also seen with increased intracranial pressure.

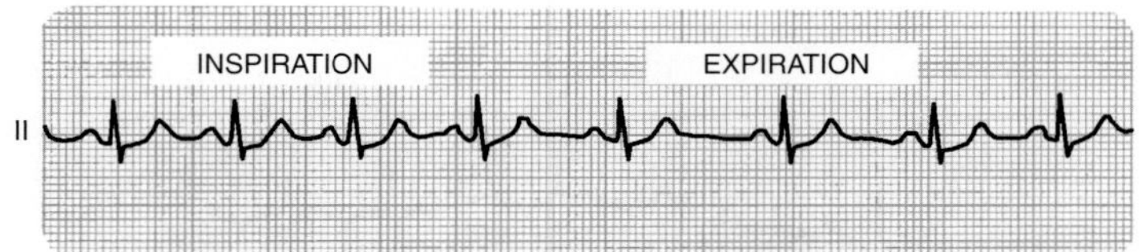

Sinus Arrest
Rate: <60 beats/min
Rhythm: Varies
PR interval: Variable
QT interval: Variable

Note: Rhythm depends on the cardiac pacemaker firing in the absence of sinoatrial stimulus (atrial pacemaker 60-75 beats/min; junctional 40-60 beats/min; ventricular 30-45 beats/min). Junctional rhythm most common. Occasional P waves may be seen (retrograde P wave).

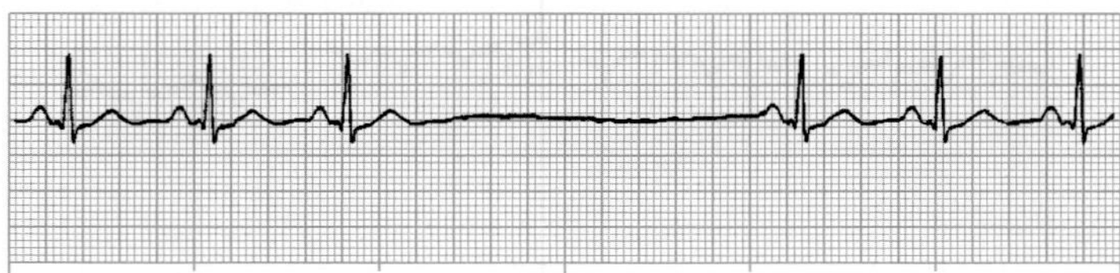

Sinus Tachycardia
Rate: 100 to 160 beats/min
Rhythm: Regular
PR interval: Normal; P wave may be difficult to see.
QT interval: Normal

Note: Should be differentiated from paroxysmal atrial tachycardia (PAT). With PAT, carotid massage terminates arrhythmia. Sinus tachycardia may respond to vagal maneuvers but reappears as soon as vagal stimulus is removed.

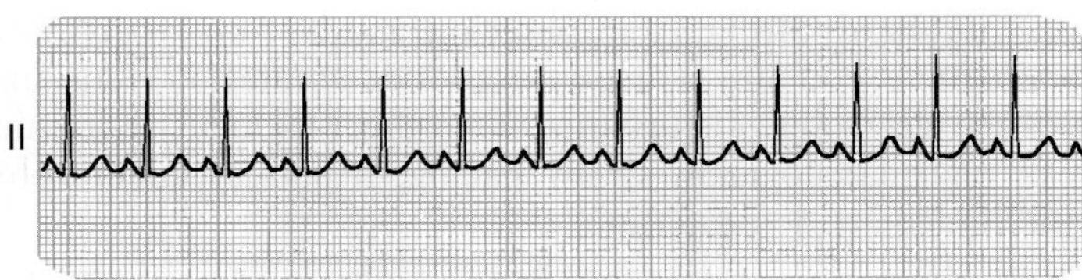

Subarachnoid Hemorrhage
Rate: <60 beats/min
Rhythm: Sinus
PR interval: Normal
QT interval: T-wave inversion is deep and wide. Prominent U waves are seen. Sinus arrhythmias are observed. Q waves may be seen and may mimic acute coronary syndrome.

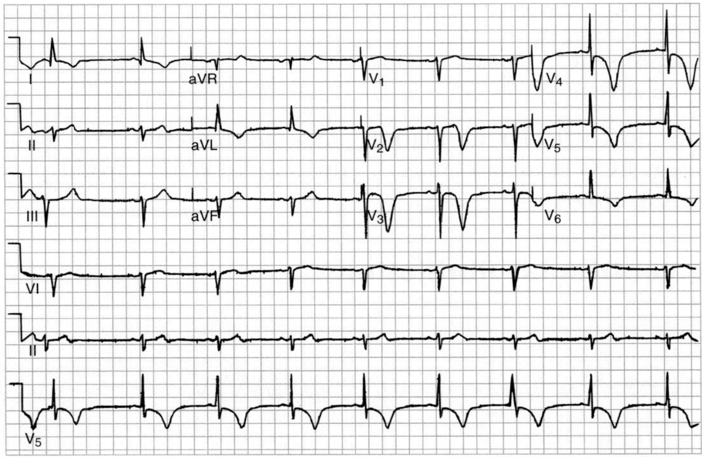

Torsades DE Pointes
Rate: 150 to 250 beats/min
Rhythm: No atrial component seen; ventricular rhythm regular or irregular.
PR interval: P wave buried in QRS complex
QT interval: QRS complexes usually wide and with phasic variation twisting around a central axis (a few complexes point upward, then a few point downward). ST-segments and T waves difficult to discern.

Note: Type of ventricular tachycardia associated with prolonged QT interval. Seen with electrolyte disturbances (eg, hypokalemia, hypocalcemia, and hypomagnesemia) and bradycardia. Administering standard antiarrhythmics (lidocaine, procainamide, etc) may worsen torsades de pointes. Prevention includes treatment of the electrolyte disturbance. Treatment includes shortening of the QT interval, pharmacologically or by pacing; unstable polymorphic VT is treated with immediate defibrillation.

Torsades de Pointes: Sustained

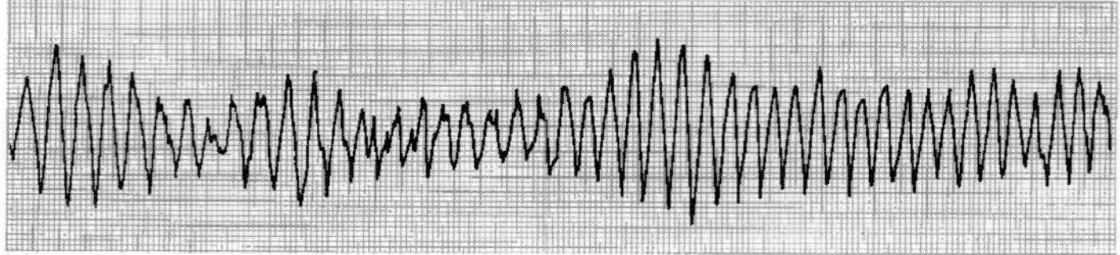

Ventricular Fibrillation
Rate: Absent
Rhythm: None
PR interval: Absent
QT interval: Absent

Note: "pseudoventricular fibrillation" may be the result of a monitor malfunction (eg, ECG lead disconnect). Always check for carotid pulse before instituting therapy.

Coarse ventricular fibrillation

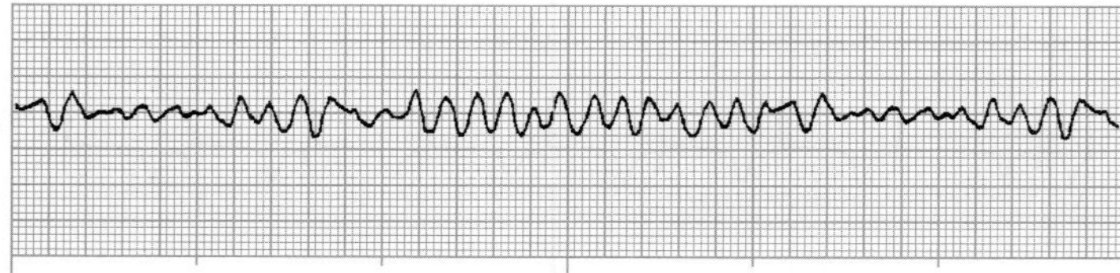

Fine Ventricular Fibrillation

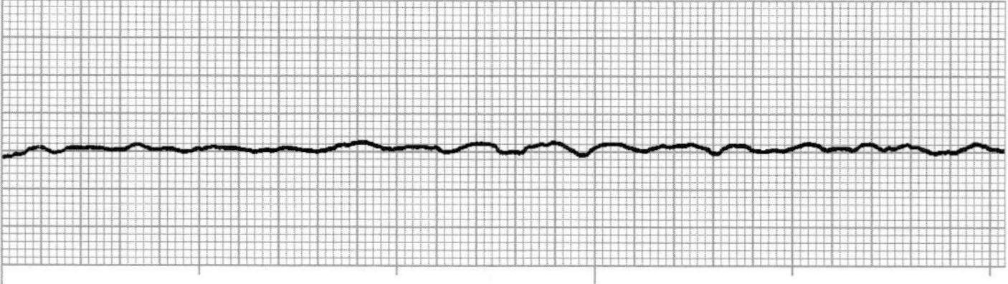

Ventricular Tachycardia
Rate: 100 to 250 beats/min
Rhythm: No atrial component seen; ventricular rhythm irregular or regular.
PR interval: Absent; retrograde P wave may be seen in QRS complex.
QT interval: Wide, bizarre QRS complex. ST-segment and T wave difficult to determine.

Note: In the presence of hemodynamic compromise, VT with a pulse is treated with immediate synchronized cardioversion, whereas VT without a pulse is treated with immediate defibrillation. If the patient is stable, with short bursts of ventricular tachycardia, pharmacologic management is preferred. Should be differentiated from supraventricular tachycardia with aberrancy (SVT-A). Compensatory pause and atrioventricular dissociation suggest a PVC. P waves and SR' (V_1) and slowing to vagal stimulus also suggest SVT-A.

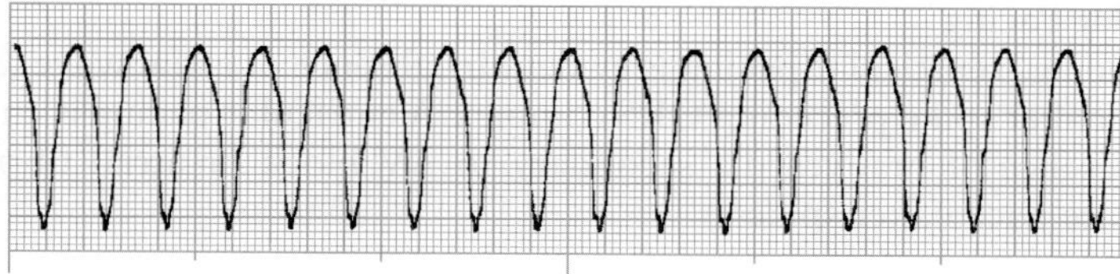

Wolff-Parkinson-White Syndrome (WPW)
Rate: <100 beats/min
Rhythm: Regular
PR interval: P wave normal; PR interval short (<0.12 seconds)
QT interval: Duration (>0.10 seconds) with slurred QRS complex (delta wave). Type A has delta wave, RBBB, with upright QRS complex V_1. Type B has delta wave and downward QRS-V_1. ST-segment and T wave usually normal.

Note: Digoxin should be avoided in the presence of WPW because it increases conduction through the accessory bypass tract (bundle of Kent) and decreases AV node conduction; consequently, ventricular fibrillation can occur.

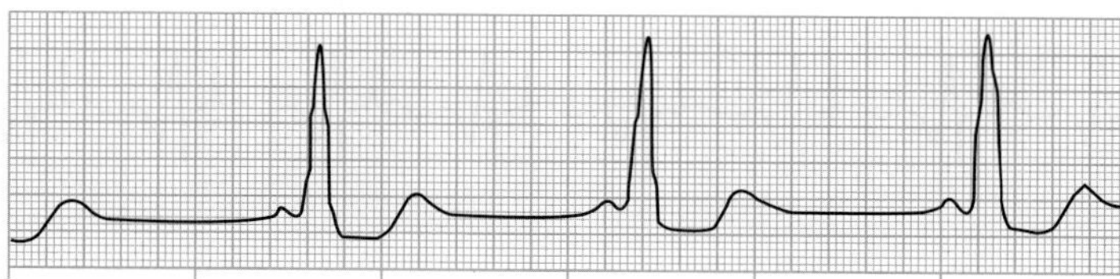

Atrial Pacing

Pacemaker Tracings

Atrial pacing as demonstrated in this figure is used when the atrial impulse can proceed through the AV node. Examples are sinus bradycardia and junctional rhythms associated with clinically significant decreases in blood pressure. (*Arrows* are pacemaker spikes.)

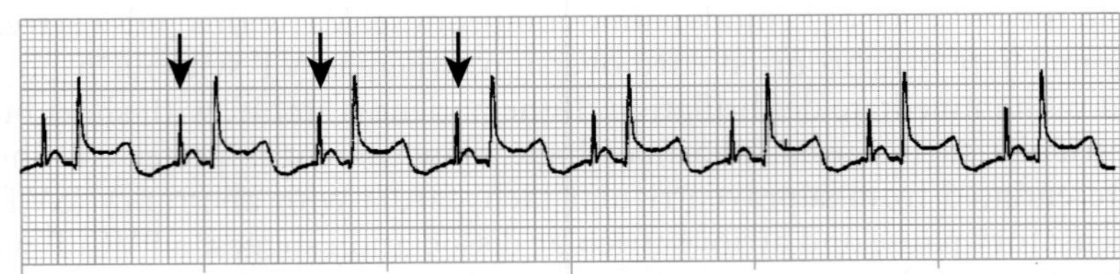

Ventricular Pacing

In this tracing, ventricular pacing is evident by absence of atrial wave (P wave) and pacemaker spike preceding QRS complex. Ventricular pacing is employed in the presence of bradycardia secondary to AV block or atrial fibrillation. (*Arrows* are pacemaker spikes.)

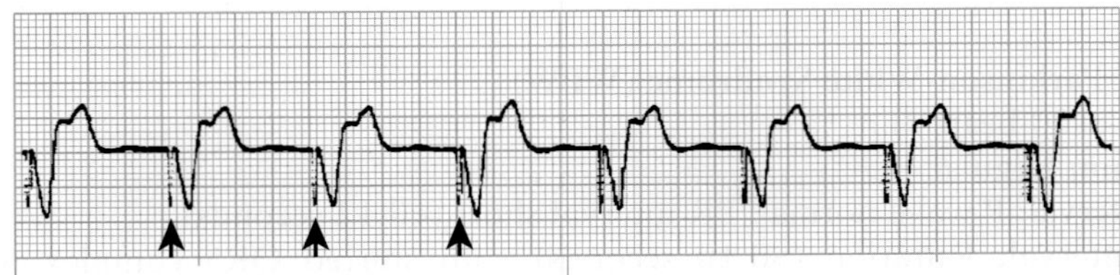

DDD Pacing

DDD pacing, one of the most commonly used pacing modes, paces and senses both the right atrium and right ventricle (A-V sequential pacing). Each atrial and the right ventricular complex are preceded by a pacemaker spike.

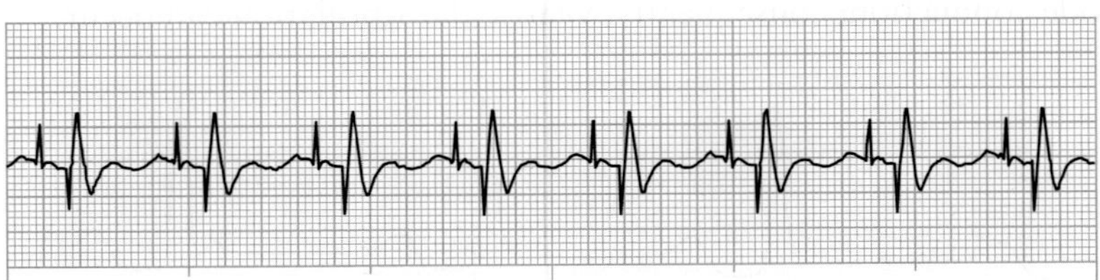

Acknowledgments

The editors of the 2nd edition gratefully acknowledge the past contributions of Gina C. Badescu, Benjamin M. Sherman, James R. Zaidan, and Paul G. Barash.

Illustrations in the atlas are derived from Aehlert B. *ECGs Made Easy*. 4th ed. Mosby/Elsevier; 2011; Goldberger AL. *Clinical Electrocardiography: A Simplified Approach*. 7th ed. Mosby/Elsevier; 2006; Groh WJ, Zipes DP. *Neurological Disorders and Cardiovascular Disease*. In: Bonow RO, Mann DL, Zipes DP, et al, eds. *Braunwald's Heart Disease: A Textbook of Cardiovascular Medicine*. 9th ed. Saunders/Elsevier; 2012; Huszar RJ. *Basic Dysrhythmias: Interpretation and Management*. 2nd ed. Mosby Lifeline; 1994; and Soltani P, Malozzi CM, Saleh BA, et al. Electrocardiogram Manifestation of Spontaneous Pneumothorax. *Am J Emerg Med*. 2009;27:750.e1-750.e5.

C Pacemaker and Implantable Cardiac Defibrillator Protocols

Cardiac implantable electronic devices (CIEDs)—pacemakers
Cardiac implantable electronic devices (CIEDs)—implantable cardiac defibrillators (ICDs)
Potential intraoperative problems with cardiac electronic implantable devices
General principles of perioperative management of patients with CIED
Risk mitigation strategies
Recommendations for postoperative follow-up of the patient with CIED
Optimization of pacing after cardiopulmonary bypass (CPB)

Cardiac Implantable Electronic Devices—Pacemakers

Pacemakers are devices that deliver electrical energy and control the patient's conduction system when necessary (**Table C.1**).

Common indications for permanent pacemaker implantation: (For a complete list of indications, please refer to the ACC/AHA/HRS 2008 guidelines for device-based therapy of cardiac rhythm abnormalities.)

1. Sinus node dysfunction:
   - Documented symptomatic bradycardia
   - Documented symptomatic chronotropic incompetence
   - Documented symptomatic bradycardia induced by essential medical therapy
   - Syncope of unexplained origin with inducible sinus bradycardia or pauses on electrophysiologic studies
   - Symptomatic patients with assumed sinus bradycardia and no other possible etiologies
2. Atrioventricular (AV) node dysfunction:
   - Third-degree AV block
   - Type II second-degree AV block
   - Symptomatic type I second-degree AV block
   - Symptomatic first-degree AV block
   - Asymptomatic first-degree AV block with coexisting disease that can impair the conduction system (ie, sarcoidosis, amyloidosis, neuromuscular diseases)
   - Drug- or medication-induced AV block that is thought to recur despite discontinuation of the drug or medication
3. Bifascicular block and:
   - Alternating bundle-branch block
   - Electrophysiologic evidence of a markedly prolonged HV interval ≥100 ms. (His bundle [H] potential and the onset of ventricular activity, also known as the HV interval, is normally 35-45 ms)
   - Concomitant neuromuscular disease (ie, myotonic muscular dystrophy, Erb dystrophy)
4. ST-segment elevation myocardial infarction (STEMI) with second- or third-degree AV block
5. Hypersensitive carotid sinus syndrome and neurocardiogenic syncope
6. Cardiac transplantation patients who develop persistent inappropriate bradycardia
7. Prevention and termination of certain arrhythmias such as the following:
   - Sustained pause-dependant VT
   - High-risk patients with congenital long-QT syndrome
   - Recurrent refractory symptomatic atrial fibrillation and SND
   - Symptomatic recurrent SVT that is reliably terminated by pacing and catheter ablation and medication management has failed
8. Hemodynamic indications:
   - Cardiac resynchronization therapy (CRT) in patients with NYHA class III or ambulatory class IV heart failure with optimal medical management and an ejection fraction (EF) ≤35% and QRS ≥120 ms
   - Hypertrophic cardiomyopathy with sinus node dysfunction (SND) or AV node dysfunction
9. Congenital heart diseases with associated bradyarrhythmias or AV block

Table C.1 Abbreviation Table

Abbrev.	Meaning
3D	Three dimensional
ASA	American Society of Anesthesiologists
ATP	Antitachycardia pacing
AV	Atrioventricular
AVB	Atrioventricular block
BPEG	British Pacing and Electrophysiology Group
bpm	Beats per minute
CAD	Coronary artery disease
CIED	Cardiac implantable electronic devices
CPB	Cardiopulmonary bypass
CRP	Current return pad
CRT	Cardiac resynchronization therapy
CRT-D	Cardiac resynchronization therapy-defibrillation
CT	Cautery tool
DCM	Dilated cardiomyopathy
ECG	Electrocardiogram
ECT	Electroconvulsive therapy
EF	Ejection fraction
EMI	Electromagnetic interference
HCM	Hypertrophic cardiomyopathy
HR	Heart rate
HRS	Heart Rhythm Society
HV	HV interval
ICD	Implantable cardiac defibrillators
LV	Left ventricle
LVOT	Left ventricular outflow tract
MRI	Magnetic resonance imaging
NASPE	North American Society of Pacing and Electrophysiology
NBG	N (NASPE), B (BPEG), G (GENERIC)
PG	Pulse generator
PP	External cardioversion-defibrillation pads or paddles
RA	Right atrium
RF	Radio frequency
R&R	Rate and rhythm
RT	Radiation therapy
RV	Right ventricle
SCD	Sudden cardiac death
SND	Sinus node dysfunction
STEMI	ST-segment elevation myocardial infarction
TUNA	Transurethral needle ablation
TURP	Transurethral resection of prostate
VT	Ventricular tachycardia
VF	Ventricular fibrillation

Cardiac Implantable Electronic Devices (CIEDs)—Implantable Cardiac Defibrillators (ICDs)

Implantable cardiac defibrillators (ICDs) are rhythm management devices that consist of a generator and a lead system. One lead is usually placed in the right atrium and the second lead in the right ventricular apex. A specific type of ICD is the biventricular pacemaker used for cardiac resynchronization therapy (CRT). This device will have a third lead placed in the coronary sinus to pace the left ventricular (LV) lateral wall in synchrony with the right ventricle (RV), in the patient with EF ≤35% and a QRS duration ≥120 ms.

Common indications for ICD implantation: (For a complete list of indications, please refer to the ACC/AHA/HRS 2008 guidelines for device-based therapy of cardiac rhythm abnormalities.)

1. Prevention of sudden cardiac death (SCD) in survivors of prior cardiac arrest due to VF or unstable VT without a reversible cause.
2. Structural heart disease with spontaneous sustained VT or syncope not otherwise specified.
3. Sustained VT with normal or near-normal LV function.
4. Syncope of undetermined origin with clinically relevant, hemodynamically significant, sustained VT or VF induced by an electrophysiologic study.
5. Unexplained syncope with significant LV dysfunction and nonischemic DCM.
6. Prior myocardial infarction (not within 40 days) and an EF ≤35%.
7. Nonischemic dilated cardiomyopathy (DCM) and an EF ≤35%.
8. Nonsustained VT due to prior MI with an EF ≤–40% and inducible VF or sustained VT on electrophysiologic study.
9. HCM with one or more risk factors for SCD.
10. Arrhythmogenic right ventricular dysplasia/cardiomyopathy with one or more risk factors for SCD. (**Table C.2**)

Table C.2 Generic Pacemaker Code: NASPE/BPEG Revised (2002)

Position I, Pacing Chamber(s)	Position II, Sensing Chamber(s)	Position III, Response(s) to Sensing	Position IV, Programmability	Position V, Multisite Pacing
0 = none	0 = none	0 = none	0 = none	0 = none
A = atrium	A = atrium	I = inhibited	R = rate modulation	A = atrium
V = ventricle	V = ventricle	T = triggered		V = ventricle
D = dual (A + V)	D = dual (A + V)	D = dual (T + I)		D = dual (A + V)

BPEG, British Pacing and Electrophysiology Group; NASPE, North American Society of Pacing and Electrophysiology, now called the Heart Rhythm Society.

Reproduced with permission from: Practice advisory for perioperative management of patients with cardiac rhythm management devices: Pacemakers and implantable cardioverter-defibrillators. A report by the American Society of Anesthesiologists Task Force on Perioperative Management of Patients with Cardiac Rhythm Management Devices. *Anesthesiology*. 2011;114:247-261. Table 1.

11. Long-QT syndrome with syncope and/or VT due to beta-blocker therapy or other risk factors for SCD.
12. Brugada syndrome with syncope or VT.
13. Catecholaminergic polymorphic VT with syncope while receiving beta-blocker therapy.
14. Diseases associated with cardiac involvement (ie, Chagas disease, giant cell myocarditis, sarcoidosis).
15. Familial cardiomyopathy associated with SCD.
16. LV noncompaction.

Potential Intraoperative Problems With Cardiac Electronic Implantable Devices

Electromagnetic interference (EMI) with a CIED is more likely when electrocautery is used above the umbilicus in a patient with the CIED implanted in the subclavicular region. Current expert opinion further states that the region 15 cm around the generator and cardiac leads are with the highest risk of EMI interference. For generators placed elsewhere (eg, abdominal site), this 15-cm rule still applies.

EMI interference leads to the following:

1. Inhibition of pacemaker by EMI
2. Inappropriate delivery of antitachycardia therapy by ICD
3. Changes in lead parameters:
   a. Atrial mode switching
   b. Inappropriate ventricular sensing
   c. Electrical reset
   d. Increase in ventricular thresholds
4. "Runaway" pacemaker
5. Conversion from VOO back to backup mode (reprogramming)
6. Transient or permanent loss of capture (**Table C.3**)

Table C.3 Generic Defibrillator Code (NBG): NASPE/BPEG

Position I, Shock Chamber(s)	Position II, Antitachycardia Pacing Chamber(s)	Position III, Tachycardia Detection	Position IV,[a] Antibradycardia Pacing Chamber(s)
O = none	O = none	E = electrogram	O = none
A = atrium	A = atrium	H = hemodynamic	A = atrium
V = ventricle	V = ventricle		V = ventricle
D = dual (A + V)	D = dual (A + V)		D = dual (A + V)

NBG: N refers to North American Society of Pacing and Electrophysiology (NASPE), now called the Heart Rhythm Society (HRS); B refers to British Pacing and Electrophysiology Group (BPEG); and G refers to generic.

[a]For robust identification, position IV is expanded into its complete NBG code. For example, a biventricular-pacing defibrillator with ventricular shock and antitachycardia pacing functionality would be identified as VVE-DDDRV, assuming that the pacing section was programmed DDDRV. Currently, no hemodynamic sensors have been approved for tachycardia detection (position III).

Reproduced with permission from: Practice advisory for perioperative management of patients with cardiac rhythm management devices: Pacemakers and implantable cardioverter-defibrillators. A report by the American Society of Anesthesiologists Task Force on Perioperative Management of Patients with Cardiac Rhythm Management Devices. *Anesthesiology.* 2011;114:247-261. Table 2.

7. Noise reversal mode
8. Pacemaker failure after direct contact with electrocautery and cardioversion
9. Myocardial burns with increased pacing thresholds if electrocautery travels through leads into the myocardium
10. Rate-adaptive pacing (interaction of minute ventilation sensor with ECG/plethysmography)
11. Oversensing and inhibition with use of lithotripsy
12. Radiofrequency ablation has a high risk of interference due to long episodes of exposure to current
13. Therapeutic ionizing radiation is especially damaging to CIEDs by damaging internal components

General Principles of Perioperative Management of Patients With CIED

- The perioperative management of the patient with a CIED is via an individualized recommendation made by the CIED team (electrophysiologist cardiologist) in collaboration with members of the surgical/anesthesia team (perioperative team). The recommendations should not be made by the industry representative without supervision by a physician who is qualified to manage these devices.
- The perioperative team should provide information to the CIED team regarding the upcoming procedure (see **Table C.4**).
- The CIED team should in turn provide information about the device and a recommendation for perioperative management of the device (see **Table C.5**).
- The patient with a pacemaker should have had an interrogation of the device in the 12 months prior to the surgical procedure, whereas the patient with an ICD should have had the device interrogated within 6 months prior to the scheduled procedure.

Table C.4 Essential Elements of the Information Given to the CIED Physician

- Type of procedure
- Anatomic location of surgical procedure
- Patient position during the procedure
- Will monopolar electrosurgery be used? (If so, anatomic location of EMI delivery.)
- Will other sources of EMI likely be present?
- Will cardioversion or defibrillation be used?
- Surgical venue (operating room, procedure suite, etc)
- Anticipated postprocedural arrangements (anticipated discharge to home <23 h, inpatient admission to critical care bed, telemetry bed)
- Unusual circumstances: Cardiothoracic or chest wall surgical procedure that could impair/damage or encroach upon the CIED leads, anticipated large blood loss, operation in close proximity to CIED

Reproduced with permission from Crossley GH, Poole JE, Rozner MA, et al. The Heart Rhythm Society (HRS)/American Society of Anesthesiologists (ASA) Expert Consensus Statement on the Perioperative Management of Patients with Implantable Defibrillators, Pacemakers, and Arrhythmia Monitors: Facilities and Patient Management. This document was developed as a joint project with the American Society of Anesthesiologists (ASA), and in collaboration with the American Heart Association (AHA), and the Society of Thoracic Surgeons (STS). *Heart Rhythm.* 2011;8(7):1114-1154.

Table C.5 Essential Elements of the Preoperative CIED Evaluation to be Provided to the Operative Team

- Date of last device interrogation
- Type of device: Pacemaker ICD, CRT-D, CRT-P, ILR, implantable hemodynamic monitor
- Manufacturer and model
- Indication for device
  - Pacemaker: Sick sinus syndrome, AV block, syncope
  - ICD: Primary or secondary prevention
  - Cardiac resynchronization therapy
- Battery longevity documented as >3 mo
- Are any of the leads <3 mo old?
- Programming
  - Pacing mode and programmed lower rate
  - ICD therapy
    - Lowest heart rate for shock delivery
    - Lowest heart rate for ATP delivery
  - Rate-responsive sensor type, if programmed on
- Is the patient pacemaker-dependent, and what is the underlying rhythm and heart rate if it can be determined?
- What is the response of this device to magnet placement?
  - Magnet pacing rate for a pacemaker
  - Pacing amplitude response to magnet function
  - Will ICD detections resume automatically with removal of the magnet? Does this device allow for magnet application function to be disabled? If so, document programming of patient's device for this feature
- Any alert status on CIED generator or lead
- Last pacing threshold: Document adequate safety margin with the date of that threshold

Reproduced with permission from Crossley GH, Poole JE, Rozner MA, et al. The Heart Rhythm Society (HRS)/American Society of Anesthesiologists (ASA) Expert Consensus Statement on the Perioperative Management of Patients with Implantable Defibrillators, Pacemakers, and Arrhythmia Monitors: Facilities and Patient Management. This document was developed as a joint project with the American Society of Anesthesiologists (ASA), and in collaboration with the American Heart Association (AHA), and the Society of Thoracic Surgeons (STS). *Heart Rhythm.* 2011;8(7):1114-1154.

- The inactivation of the ICD or programming of a pacemaker to asynchronous mode is recommended when electromagnetic interference (EMI) is likely to occur.
- In patients in whom the ICD antiarrhythmia detection is turned off, an external defibrillator should be immediately available and ready to deliver therapy.
- In cases where EMI is likely, the function of the CIED can be altered either by a ferrous magnet or by reprogramming. (see below for magnet response for ICD.)
- Magnet response: Placing a magnet over a pacemaker generator will turn the pacemaker to asynchronous mode in most models. Placing a magnet over an ICD will suspend the arrhythmia detection. It will not switch the pacemaker function to asynchronous mode; therefore, in patients who are pacemaker-dependent, the team must be aware of the risk of inhibition of the pacemaker by EMI. If EMI is likely to occur, the recommendation is

to reprogram the CIED prior to the operation by turning off the arrhythmia detection function and programming the pacemaker to asynchronous mode. Due to the fact that a minority of models do not respond to magnet application in the fashion described above, it is always recommended to contact the manufacturer and confirm the response to a magnet for the specific model one is dealing with (**Table C.6; Figure C.1**).

Table C.6 Example of a Stepwise Approach to the Perioperative Management of the Patient With a Cardiac Implantable Electronic Device

Perioperative Period	Patient/CIED Condition	Intervention
Preoperative evaluation	Patient has CIED	Focused history Focused physical examination
	Determine CIED type (PM, ICD, CRT)	Manufacturer's CIED identification card Chest x-ray (no data available) Supplemental resources[a]
	Determine if patient is CIED-dependent for pacing function	Verbal history Bradyarrhythmia symptoms Atrioventricular node ablation No spontaneous ventricular activity[b]
	Determine CIED function	Comprehensive CIED evaluation[c] Determine if pacing pulses are present and create paced beats
Preoperative preparation	EMI unlikely during procedure	If EMI is unlikely, then special precautions are not needed
	EMI likely; CIED is PM	Reprogram to asynchronous mode when indicated Suspend rate-adaptive functions[d]
	EMI likely; CIED is ICD	Suspend antitachyarrhythmia functions. If patient is dependent on pacing function, then alter pacing function as above
	EMI likely; All CIED	Use bipolar cautery; ultrasonic scalpel Temporary pacing and cardioversion-defibrillation available
	Intraoperative physiologic changes likely (eg, bradycardia, ischemia)	Plan for possible adverse CIED-patient interaction
Intraoperative management	Monitoring	Electrocardiographic monitoring per ASA standard Peripheral pulse monitoring
	Electrocautery interference	CT/CRP no current through PG/leads Avoid proximity of CT to PG/leads Short bursts at lowest possible energy Use bipolar cautery; ultrasonic scalpel
	RF catheter ablation	Avoid contact of RF catheter with PG/leads RF current path far away from PG/leads Discuss these concerns with operator
	Lithotripsy	Do not focus lithotripsy beam near PG R wave triggers lithotripsy? Disable atrial pacing

Table C.6 Example of a Stepwise Approach to the Perioperative Management of the Patient With a Cardiac Implantable Electronic Device (*Continued*)

Perioperative Period	Patient/CIED Condition	Intervention
	MRI	Generally contraindicated If required, consult ordering physician, cardiologist, radiologist, and manufacturer
	Radiation therapy	PG/leads must be outside of RT field Possible surgical relocation of PG Verify PG function during/after RT course
	ECT	Consult with ordering physician, patient's cardiologist, a CIED service, or CIED manufacturer
Emergency defibrillation-cardioversion	ICD: magnet-disabled	Terminate all EMI sources Remove magnet to reenable therapies Observe for appropriate therapies
	ICD: programming disabled	Programming to reenable therapies or proceed directly with external cardioversion/defibrillation
	ICD: either of above	Minimize current flow through PG/leads PP as far as possible from PG PP perpendicular to major axis PG/leads To extent possible, PP in anterior–posterior location
	Regardless of CIED type	Use clinically appropriate cardioversion/defibrillation energy
Postoperative management	Immediate postoperative period	Monitor cardiac R&R continuously
	Postoperative interrogation and restoration of CIED function	Back-up pacing and cardioversion/defibrillation capability Interrogation to assess function Settings appropriate?[e] Is CIED an ICD?[f] Use cardiology/PM-ICD service if needed

[a]Manufacturer's databases, pacemaker clinic records, cardiology consultation.
[b]With cardiac rhythm management device (CRMD) programmed VVI at lowest programmable rate.
[c]Ideally, CIED function assessed by interrogation, with function altered by reprogramming if required.
[d]Most times, this will be necessary; when in doubt, assume so.
[e]If necessary, reprogram appropriate setting.
[f]Restore all antitachycardia therapies.
Reproduced with permission from: Practice advisory for perioperative management of patients with cardiac rhythm management devices: Pacemakers and implantable cardioverter-defibrillators. A report by the American Society of Anesthesiologists Task Force on Perioperative Management of Patients with Cardiac Rhythm Management Devices. *Anesthesiology*. 2011;114:247-261. Table 3.

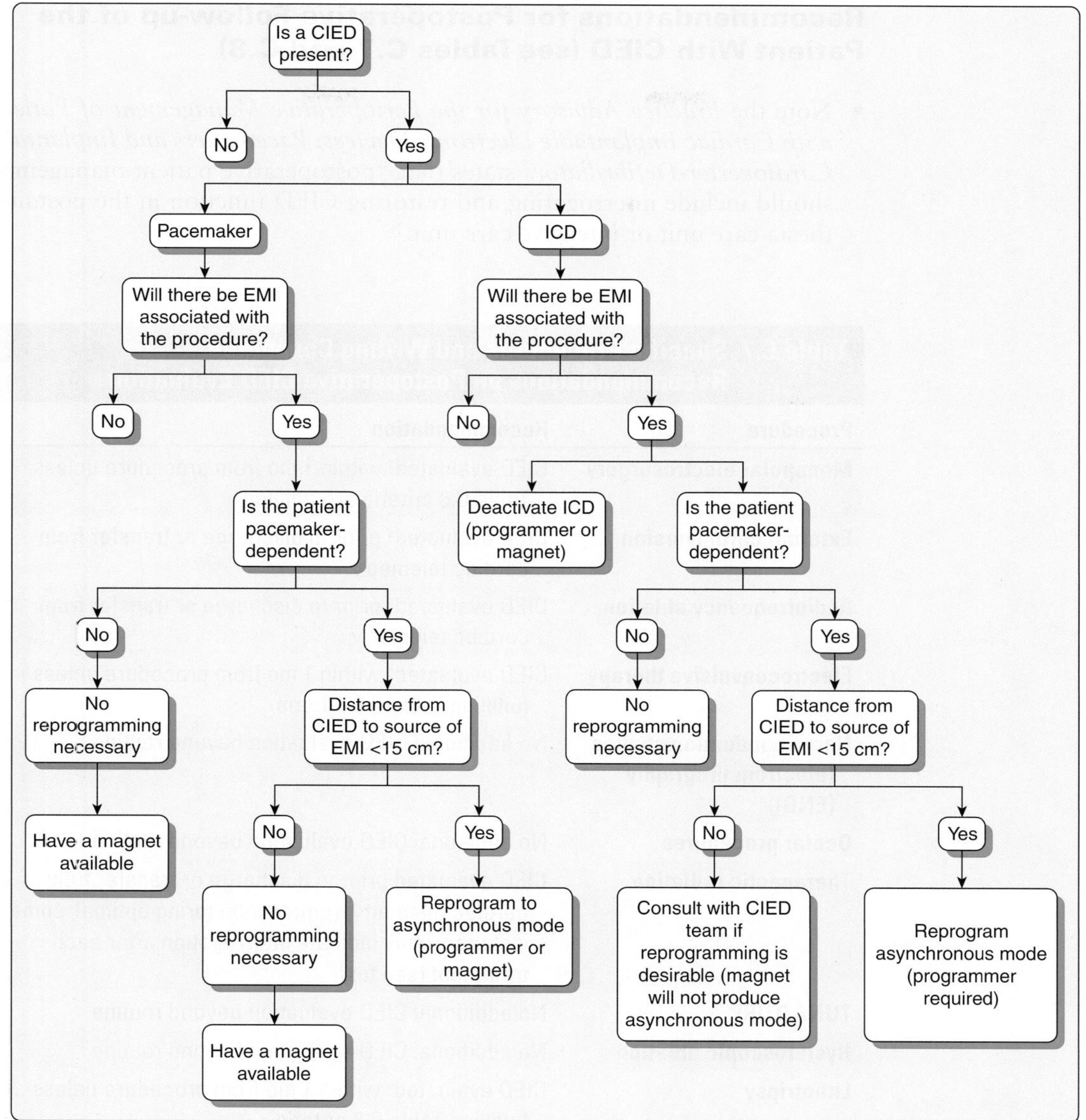

Figure C.1 Example of an algorithm for perioperative management of patients with CIED. (From Stone ME, Salter B, Fischer A. Perioperative management of patients with cardiac implantable electronic devices. *Br J Anaesth*. 2011;107(suppl 1):i16-i26. Figure 3, with permission.)

Risk Mitigation Strategies

- Have a magnet available.
- Use bipolar cautery where possible.
- Use short bursts of monopolar cautery (5 seconds or less).
- Place the return current pad in such a way to avoid current crossing the generator.
- Have rescue equipment, including external pacemaker/defibrillator, immediately available for all patients with a CIED.
- Be aware of other potential sources of EMI in addition to electrocautery.
- Be aware of dislodgement of leads during atrial fibrillation ablations, central intravenous catheter insertions, or other catheter-based procedures.

Recommendations for Postoperative Follow-up of the Patient With CIED (see Tables C.7 and C.8)

- Note the *Practice Advisory for the Perioperative Management of Patients with Cardiac Implantable Electronic Devices: Pacemakers and Implantable Cardioverter-Defibrillators* states that "postoperative patient management should include interrogating and restoring CIED function in the postanesthesia care unit or intensive care unit."

Table C.7 Specific Procedures and Writing Committee Recommendations on Postoperative CIED Evaluation

Procedure	Recommendation
Monopolar electrosurgery	CIED evaluated[a] within 1 mo from procedure unless Table C.8 criteria are fulfilled
External cardioversion	CIED evaluated[a] prior to discharge or transfer from cardiac telemetry
Radiofrequency ablation	CIED evaluated[a] prior to discharge or transfer from cardiac telemetry
Electroconvulsive therapy	CIED evaluated[a] within 1 mo from procedure unless fulfilling Table C.8 criteria
Nerve conduction studies (electroneurography [ENG])	No additional CIED evaluation beyond routine
Ocular procedures	No additional CIED evaluation beyond routine
Therapeutic radiation	CIED evaluated prior to discharge or transfer from cardiac telemetry; remote monitoring optimal; some instances may indicate interrogation after each treatment (see text)
TUNA/TURP	No additional CIED evaluation beyond routine
Hysteroscopic ablation	No additional CIED evaluation beyond routine
Lithotripsy	CIED evaluated[a] within 1 mo from procedure unless fulfilling Table C.8 criteria
Endoscopy	No additional CIED evaluation beyond routine
Iontophoresis	No additional CIED evaluation beyond routine
Photodynamic therapy	No additional CIED evaluation beyond routine
X-ray/CT scans/ mammography	No additional CIED evaluation beyond routine

CIED, cardiac implantable electronic device; CT, computed tomography; TUNA, transurethral needle ablation; TURP, transurethral resection of prostate.

[a]This evaluation is intended to reveal electrical reset. Therefore, an interrogation alone is needed. This can be accomplished in person or by remote telemetry.

Reproduced with permission from: Crossley GH, Poole JE, Rozner MA, et al. The Heart Rhythm Society (HRS)/American Society of Anesthesiologists (ASA) Expert Consensus Statement on the Perioperative Management of Patients with Implantable Defibrillators, Pacemakers, and Arrhythmia Monitors: Facilities and Patient Management. This document was developed as a joint project with the American Society of Anesthesiologists (ASA), and in collaboration with the American Heart Association (AHA), and the Society of Thoracic Surgeons (STS). *Heart Rhythm.* 2011;8(7):1114-1154.

Table C.8 Indications for the Interrogation of CIEDS Prior to Patient Discharge or Transfer from a Cardiac Telemetry Environment

- Patients with CIEDs reprogrammed prior to the procedure that left the device nonfunctional such as disabling tachycardia detection in an ICD.
- Patients with CIEDs who underwent hemodynamically challenging surgeries such as cardiac surgery or significant vascular surgery (eg, abdominal aortic aneurysmal repair).[a]
- Patients with CIEDs who experienced significant intraoperative events including cardiac arrest requiring temporary pacing or cardiopulmonary resuscitation and those who required external electrical cardioversion.
- Emergent surgery where the site of EMI exposure was above the umbilicus.
- Cardiothoracic surgery.
- Patients with CIEDs who underwent certain types of procedures (Table C.7) that emit EMI with a greater probability of affecting device function.
- Patients with CIEDs who have logistical limitations that would prevent reliable device evaluation within 1 mo from their procedure.

CIED, cardiac implantable electrical device; EMI, electromagnetic interference; ICD, implantable cardiac defibrillator.

[a]The general purpose of this interrogation is to ensure that reset did not occur. In these cases, a full evaluation including threshold evaluations is suggested.

Reproduced with permission from Crossley GH, Poole JE, Rozner MA, et al. The Heart Rhythm Society (HRS)/American Society of Anesthesiologists (ASA) Expert Consensus Statement on the Perioperative Management of Patients with Implantable Defibrillators, Pacemakers, and Arrhythmia Monitors: Facilities and Patient Management. This document was developed as a joint project with the American Society of Anesthesiologists (ASA), and in collaboration with the American Heart Association (AHA), and the Society of Thoracic Surgeons (STS). *Heart Rhythm.* 2011;8(7):1114-1154.

Optimization of Pacing After Cardiopulmonary Bypass (CPB)

During separation from CPB, it is not uncommon for a patient to develop a conduction abnormality, ranging from the more benign first-degree AV block or sinus bradycardia to the more severe interventricular delays or third-degree AV block.

Optimizing pacing:

1. **Lead placement:** Right atrial (RA) lead—place at the cephalic atrial wall, between the atrial appendages. Right ventricular lead—place at the level of the right ventricle outflow tract (RVOT). For the patient with obstructive cardiomyopathy, the RV lead is better placed in the RV apex for less dynamic obstruction of the LVOT. Biventricular pacing can be initiated for patients with intraventricular conduction lesions and dyssynchrony of contraction. The LV lead should be placed at the basal posterolateral wall, and the two ventricular leads can be connected through a Y piece to the ventricular output of the temporary pacemaker box.
2. **Rate:** Program to obtain the best improvement in cardiac output and improvement in mixed venous saturation and arterial blood pressure.
3. **AV delay:** In patients with LV dysfunction, we can maximize the contribution of the atria to the preload. Use pulse wave Doppler through the mitral valve inflow and modify the AV delay to obtain clear E and A waveforms and to ensure that the A wave ends before the onset of the

Table C.9 Treatment of Pacemaker Failure

Rate	Possible Response
Adequate to maintain blood pressure	1. Oxygen, airway control 2. Place magnet over pacemaker 3. Atropine if sinus bradycardia
Severe bradycardia and hypotension	1. Oxygen, airway control 2. Place magnet over pacemaker 3. Other types of pacing if magnet does not activate the pacemaker (transcutaneous, esophageal, or transvenous) 4. Atropine if sinus bradycardia 5. Isoproterenol to increase ventricular rate
No escape rhythm	1. Cardiopulmonary resuscitation 2. Place magnet over pacemaker 3. Other types of pacing if magnet does not activate the pacemaker (transcutaneous, esophageal, or transvenous) 4. Isoproterenol to increase ventricular rate

Dervied from Zaidan JR, Youngberg JA, Lake CL, et al, eds. *Pacemakers, Cardiac, Vascular and Thoracic Anesthesia*. Churchill Livingstone; 2000.

QRS. The closure of the mitral valve should happen at the end of the A wave but before any diastolic mitral regurgitation. If echocardiography is not available, adjust the AV interval to achieve highest cardiac output. (**Table C.9**)

4. **Pacing mode:** Three modes are explained here. In the patient with normal AV conduction, AAI mode allows for an increase in HR and a physiologic depolarization of the ventricles. If inhibition by electrocautery is a concern, use asynchronous pacing in AOO mode. For the patient with AV conduction delay, DOO or DDI should be used. DDI mode also avoids tracking of rapid atrial rates in cases of postbypass atrial fibrillation.
5. **Biventricular pacing:** In patients with EF ≤35% and QRS ≥120 ms, acute biventricular pacing improves torsion and mechanics of contraction, particularly in patients with mitral regurgitation due to papillary muscle dyssynchrony. Speckle-tracking, 3D echocardiography, M-mode definition of septal to wall motion delay, color Doppler tissue imaging, and analysis of segmental velocity are used to characterize ventricular dyssynchrony. Currently available temporary pacemakers only allow biventricular pacing through a Y connection of the two ventricular epicardial wires to the ventricular output of the box. Acute CRT leads to an increase in myocardial performance with a slight decrease in myocardial oxygen consumption.

Acknowledgments

The editors of the 2nd edition gratefully acknowledge the past contributions of Gina C. Badescu, Benjamin M. Sherman, James R. Zaidan, and Paul G. Barash.

D

American Society of Anesthesiologists Standards, Guidelines, and Statements

*This is not an ASA document but is included because of its relevance to fire safety (APSF Newsletter 2012; 26:43, www.apsf.org).

Standards for Basic Anesthetic Monitoring

Committee of Origin: Standards and Practice Parameters

(Approved by the ASA House of Delegates on October 21, 1986, and last amended on October 20, 2010, with an effective date of July 1, 2011)

These standards apply to all anesthesia care although, in emergency circumstances, appropriate life support measures take precedence. These standards may be exceeded at any time based on the judgment of the responsible anesthesiologist. They are intended to encourage quality patient care, but observing them cannot guarantee any specific patient outcome. They are subject to revision from time to time, as warranted by the evolution of technology and practice. They apply to all general anesthetics, regional anesthetics, and monitored anesthesia care. This set of standards addresses only the issue of basic anesthetic monitoring, which is one component of anesthesia care. In certain rare or unusual circumstances, (1) some of these methods of monitoring may be clinically impractical, and (2) appropriate use of the described monitoring methods may fail to detect untoward clinical developments. Brief interruptions of continual* monitoring may be unavoidable. These standards are not intended for application to the care of the obstetrical patient in labor or in the conduct of pain management.

Standard I

Qualified anesthesia personnel shall be present in the room throughout the conduct of all general anesthetics, regional anesthetics, and monitored anesthesia care.

Objective

Because of the rapid changes in patient status during anesthesia, qualified anesthesia personnel shall be continuously present to monitor the patient and provide anesthesia care. In the event there is a direct known hazard, eg, radiation, to the anesthesia personnel which might require intermittent remote observation of the patient, some provision for monitoring the patient must be made. In the event that an emergency requires the temporary absence of the person primarily responsible for the anesthetic, the best judgment of the anesthesiologist will be exercised in comparing the emergency with the anesthetized patient's condition and in the selection of the person left responsible for the anesthetic during the temporary absence.

Standard II

During all anesthetics, the patient's oxygenation, ventilation, circulation, and temperature shall be continually evaluated.

Oxygenation

Objective

To ensure adequate oxygen concentration in the inspired gas and the blood during all anesthetics.

Methods

1. Inspired gas: During every administration of general anesthesia using an anesthesia machine, the concentration of oxygen in the patient breathing

*Note that "continual" is defined as "repeated regularly and frequently in steady rapid succession," whereas "continuous" means "prolonged without any interruption at any time."

system shall be measured by an oxygen analyzer with a low oxygen concentration limit alarm in use.†

2. Blood oxygenation: During all anesthetics, a quantitative method of assessing oxygenation such as pulse oximetry shall be employed.†
3. When the pulse oximeter is utilized, the variable pitch pulse tone and the low threshold alarm shall be audible to the anesthesiologist or the anesthesia care team personnel.† Adequate illumination and exposure of the patient are necessary to assess color.†

Ventilation

Objective

To ensure adequate ventilation of the patient during all anesthetics.

Methods

1. Every patient receiving general anesthesia shall have the adequacy of ventilation continually evaluated. Qualitative clinical signs such as chest excursion, observation of the reservoir breathing bag, and auscultation of breath sounds are useful. Continual monitoring for the presence of expired carbon dioxide shall be performed unless invalidated by the nature of the patient, procedure, or equipment. Quantitative monitoring of the volume of expired gas is strongly encouraged.†
2. When an endotracheal tube or laryngeal mask is inserted, its correct positioning must be verified by clinical assessment and by identification of carbon dioxide in the expired gas. Continual end-tidal carbon dioxide analysis, in use from the time of endotracheal tube/laryngeal mask placement, until extubation/removal or initiating transfer to a postoperative care location, shall be performed using a quantitative method such as capnography, capnometry, or mass spectroscopy.† When capnography or capnometry is utilized, the end-tidal CO_2 alarm shall be audible to the anesthesiologist or the anesthesia care team personnel.†
3. When ventilation is controlled by a mechanical ventilator, there shall be in continuous use a device that is capable of detecting disconnection of components of the breathing system. The device must give an audible signal when its alarm threshold is exceeded.
4. During regional anesthesia (with no sedation) or local anesthesia (with no sedation), the adequacy of ventilation shall be evaluated by continual observation of qualitative clinical signs. During moderate or deep sedation, the adequacy of ventilation shall be evaluated by continual observation of qualitative clinical signs and monitoring for the presence of exhaled carbon dioxide unless precluded or invalidated by the nature of the patient, procedure, or equipment.

Circulation

Objective

To ensure the adequacy of the patient's circulatory function during all anesthetics.

Methods

1. Every patient receiving anesthesia shall have the electrocardiogram continuously displayed from the beginning of anesthesia until preparing to leave the anesthetizing location.†

†Under extenuating circumstances, the responsible anesthesiologist may waive the requirements marked with an dagger (†); it is recommended that when this is done, it should be so stated (including the reasons) in a note in the patient's medical record.

2. Every patient receiving anesthesia shall have arterial blood pressure and heart rate determined and evaluated at least every five minutes.[†]
3. Every patient receiving general anesthesia shall have, in addition to the above, circulatory function continually evaluated by at least one of the following: palpation of a pulse, auscultation of heart sounds, monitoring of a tracing of intra-arterial pressure, ultrasound peripheral pulse monitoring, or pulse plethysmography or oximetry.

Body Temperature

Objective

To aid in the maintenance of appropriate body temperature during all anesthetics.

Methods

Every patient receiving anesthesia shall have temperature monitored when clinically significant changes in body temperature are intended, anticipated, or suspected.

Continuum of Depth of Sedation: Definition of General Anesthesia and Levels of Sedation/Analgesia*

Committee of Origin: Quality Management and Departmental Administration

(Approved by the ASA House of Delegates on October 13, 1999, and last amended on October 15, 2014)

	Minimal Sedation (Anxiolysis)	Moderate Sedation/ Analgesia (Conscious Sedation)	Deep Sedation/ Analgesia	General Anesthesia
Responsiveness	Normal response to verbal stimulation	Purposeful[†] response to verbal or tactile stimulation	Purposeful[†] response following repeated or painful stimulation	Unarousable even with painful stimulus
Airway	Unaffected	No intervention required	Intervention may be required	Intervention often required
Spontaneous Ventilation	Unaffected	Adequate	May be inadequate	Frequently inadequate
Cardiovascular Function	Unaffected	Usually maintained	Usually maintained	May be impaired

*Monitored Anesthesia Care (MAC) does not describe the continuum of depth of sedation rather it describes "a specific anesthesia service in which an anesthesiologist has been requested to participate in the care of a patient undergoing a diagnostic or therapeutic procedure."
[†]Reflex withdrawal from a painful stimulus is NOT considered a purposeful response.

Minimal Sedation (Anxiolysis) is a drug-induced state during which patients respond normally to verbal commands. Although cognitive function and physical coordination may be impaired, airway reflexes and ventilatory and cardiovascular functions are unaffected.

Moderate Sedation/Analgesia (Conscious Sedation) is a drug-induced depression of consciousness during which patients respond purposefully[†] to verbal commands, either alone or accompanied by light tactile stimulation. No interventions are required to maintain a patent airway, and spontaneous ventilation is adequate. Cardiovascular function is usually maintained.

Deep Sedation/Analgesia is a drug-induced depression of consciousness during which patients cannot be easily aroused but respond purposefully[†] following repeated or painful stimulation. The ability to independently maintain ventilatory function may be impaired. Patients may require assistance in maintaining a patent airway, and spontaneous ventilation may be inadequate. Cardiovascular function is usually maintained.

General Anesthesia is a drug-induced loss of consciousness during which patients are not arousable, even by painful stimulation. The ability to independently maintain ventilatory function is often impaired. Patients often require assistance in maintaining a patent airway, and positive pressure ventilation may be required because of depressed spontaneous ventilation or drug-induced depression of neuromuscular function. Cardiovascular function may be impaired.

Because sedation is a continuum, it is not always possible to predict how an individual patient will respond. Hence, practitioners intending to produce a given level of sedation should be able to rescue[‡] patients whose level of sedation becomes deeper than initially intended. Individuals administering moderate sedation/analgesia (Conscious Sedation) should be able to rescue[‡] patients who enter a state of deep sedation/analgesia, while those administering deep sedation/analgesia should be able to rescue[‡] patients who enter a state of general anesthesia.

[†]Reflex withdrawal from a painful stimulus is NOT considered a purposeful response.

[‡]Rescue of a patient from a deeper level of sedation than intended is an intervention by a practitioner proficient in airway management and advanced life support. The qualified practitioner corrects adverse physiologic consequences of the deeper-than-intended level of sedation (such as hypoventilation, hypoxia, and hypotension) and returns the patient to the originally intended level of sedation. It is not appropriate to continue the procedure at an unintended level of sedation.

Basic Standards for Preanesthesia Care

Committee of Origin: Standards and Practice Parameters

(Approved by the ASA House of Delegates on October 14, 1987, and last affirmed on December 13, 2020)

These standards apply to all patients who receive anesthesia care. Under exceptional circumstances, these standards may be modified. When this is the case, the circumstances shall be documented in the patient's record.

An anesthesiologist shall be responsible for determining the medical status of the patient and developing a plan of anesthesia care.

The anesthesiologist, before the delivery of anesthesia care, is responsible for the following:

1. Reviewing the available medical record.
2. Interviewing and performing a focused examination of the patient to:
   a. Discuss the medical history, including previous anesthetic experiences and medical therapy.
   b. Assess those aspects of the patient's physical condition that might affect decisions regarding perioperative risk and management.
3. Ordering and reviewing pertinent available tests and consultations as necessary for the delivery of anesthesia care.
4. Ordering appropriate preoperative medications.
5. Ensuring that consent has been obtained for the anesthesia care.
6. Documenting in the chart that the above has been performed.

Standards for Postanesthesia Care

Committee of Origin: Standards and Practice Parameters

(Approved by the ASA House of Delegates on October 27, 2004, and last amended on October 23, 2019)

These standards apply to postanesthesia care in all locations. These standards may be exceeded based on the judgment of the responsible anesthesiologist. They are intended to encourage quality patient care but cannot guarantee any specific patient outcome. They are subject to revision from time to time as warranted by the evolution of technology and practice.

Standard I

All patients who have received general anesthesia, regional anesthesia, or monitored anesthesia care shall receive appropriate postanesthesia management.[1]

1. A postanesthesia care unit (PACU) or an area which provides equivalent postanesthesia care (eg, a surgical intensive care unit) shall be available to receive patients after anesthesia care. All patients who receive anesthesia care shall be admitted to the PACU or its equivalent **except** by specific order of the anesthesiologist responsible for the patient's care.
2. The medical aspects of care in the PACU (or equivalent area) shall be governed by policies and procedures which have been reviewed and approved by the Department of Anesthesiology.
3. The design, equipment, and staffing of the PACU shall meet requirements of the facility's accrediting and licensing bodies.

Standard II

A patient transported to the PACU shall be accompanied by a member of the anesthesia care team who is knowledgeable about the patient's condition. The patient shall be continually evaluated and treated during transport with monitoring and support appropriate to the patient's condition.

Standard III

Upon arrival in the PACU, the patient shall be reevaluated and a verbal report provided to the responsible PACU nurse by the member of the anesthesia care team who accompanies the patient.

1. The patient's status on arrival in the PACU shall be documented.
2. Information concerning the preoperative condition and the surgical/anesthetic course shall be transmitted to the PACU nurse.
3. The member of the anesthesia care team shall remain in the PACU until the PACU nurse accepts responsibility for the nursing care of the patient.

Standard IV

The patient's condition shall be evaluated continually in the PACU.

1. The patient shall be observed and monitored by methods appropriate to the patient's medical condition. Particular attention should be given to monitoring oxygenation, ventilation, circulation, level of consciousness, and temperature. During recovery from all anesthetics, a quantitative method of assessing oxygenation such as pulse oximetry shall be

[1]Refer to Perianesthesia Nursing Standards, Practice Recommendations and Interpretive Statements, published by ASPAN, for issues of nursing care.

employed in the initial phase of recovery.* This is not intended for application during the recovery of the obstetrical patient in whom regional anesthesia was used for labor and vaginal delivery.

2. An accurate written report of the PACU period shall be maintained. Use of an appropriate PACU-scoring system is encouraged for each patient on admission at appropriate intervals prior to discharge and at the time of discharge.
3. General medical supervision and coordination of patient care in the PACU should be the responsibility of an anesthesiologist.
4. There shall be a policy to assure the availability in the facility of a physician capable of managing complications and providing cardiopulmonary resuscitation for patients in the PACU.

Standard V

A physician is responsible for the discharge of the patient from the postanesthesia care unit.

1. When discharge criteria are used, they must be approved by the Department of Anesthesiology and the medical staff. They may vary depending upon whether the patient is discharged to a hospital room, to the intensive care unit, to a short-stay unit, or home.
2. In the absence of the physician responsible for the discharge, the PACU nurse shall determine that the patient meets the discharge criteria. The name of the physician accepting responsibility for discharge shall be noted on the record.

*Under extenuating circumstances, the responsible anesthesiologist may waive the requirements marked with an asterisk (*); it is recommended that when this is done, it should be so stated (including the reasons) in a note in the patient's medical record.

Practice Advisory for the Prevention and Management of Operating Room Fires (Figures D.1 and D.2)

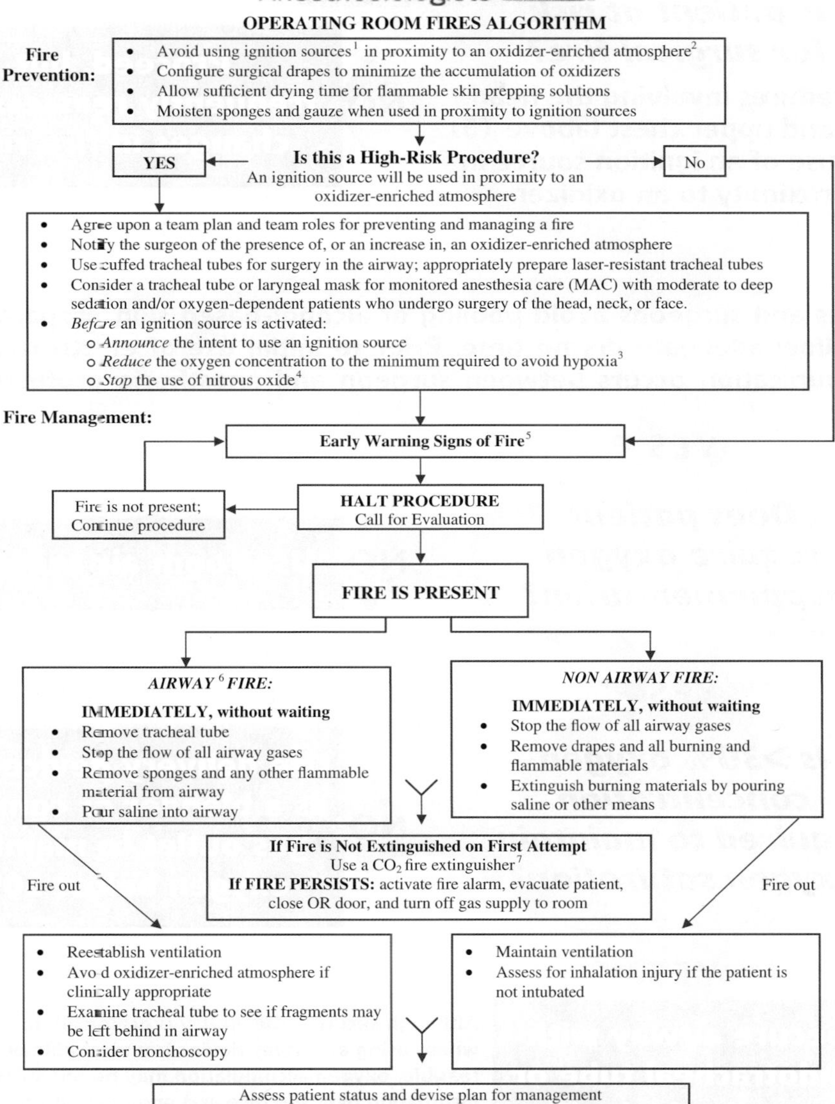

American Society of Anesthesiologists
OPERATING ROOM FIRES ALGORITHM
Fire Prevention:
• Avoid using ignition sources[1] in proximity to an oxidizer-enriched atmosphere[2]
• Configure surgical drapes to minimize the accumulation of oxidizers
• Allow sufficient drying time for flammable skin prepping solutions
• Moisten sponges and gauze when used in proximity to ignition sources
YES
Is this a High-Risk Procedure?
An ignition source will be used in proximity to an oxidizer-enriched atmosphere
No
• Agree upon a team plan and team roles for preventing and managing a fire
• Notify the surgeon of the presence of, or an increase in, an oxidizer-enriched atmosphere
• Use cuffed tracheal tubes for surgery in the airway; appropriately prepare laser-resistant tracheal tubes
• Consider a tracheal tube or laryngeal mask for monitored anesthesia care (MAC) with moderate to deep sedation and/or oxygen-dependent patients who undergo surgery of the head, neck, or face.
• Before an ignition source is activated:
o Announce the intent to use an ignition source
o Reduce the oxygen concentration to the minimum required to avoid hypoxia[3]
o Stop the use of nitrous oxide[4]
Fire Management:
Early Warning Signs of Fire[5]
Fire is not present; Continue procedure
HALT PROCEDURE
Call for Evaluation
FIRE IS PRESENT
AIRWAY[6] FIRE:
IMMEDIATELY, without waiting
• Remove tracheal tube
• Stop the flow of all airway gases
• Remove sponges and any other flammable material from airway
• Pour saline into airway
NON AIRWAY FIRE:
IMMEDIATELY, without waiting
• Stop the flow of all airway gases
• Remove drapes and all burning and flammable materials
• Extinguish burning materials by pouring saline or other means
Fire out
If Fire is Not Extinguished on First Attempt
Use a CO_2 fire extinguisher[7]
If FIRE PERSISTS: activate fire alarm, evacuate patient, close OR door, and turn off gas supply to room
Fire out
• Reestablish ventilation
• Avoid oxidizer-enriched atmosphere if clinically appropriate
• Examine tracheal tube to see if fragments may be left behind in airway
• Consider bronchoscopy
• Maintain ventilation
• Assess for inhalation injury if the patient is not intubated
Assess patient status and devise plan for management
1 Ignition sources include but are not limited to electrosurgery or electrocautery units and lasers.
2 An oxidizer-enriched atmosphere occurs when there is any increase in oxygen concentration above room air level and/or the presence of any concentration of nitrous oxide.
3 After minimizing delivered oxygen, wait a period of time (e.g., 1-3 min) before using an ignition source. For oxygen-dependent patients, reduce supplemental oxygen delivery to the minimum required to avoid hypoxia. Monitor oxygenation with pulse oximetry, and if feasible, inspired, exhaled, and/or delivered oxygen concentration.
4 After stopping the delivery of nitrous oxide, wait a period of time (e.g., 1-3 min) before using an ignition source.
5 Unexpected flash, flame, smoke or heat, unusual sounds (e.g., a "pop," snap or "foomp") or odors, unexpected movement of drapes, discoloration of drapes or breathing circuit, unexpected patient movement or complaint.
6 In this algorithm, airway fire refers to a fire in the airway or breathing circuit.
7 A CO_2 fire extinguisher may be used on the patient if necessary.

Figure D.1 Operating room fires algorithm. CO_2, carbon dioxide; OR, operating room. (From Caplan RA, Barker SJ, Connis RT, et al; American Society of Anesthesiologists Task Force on Operating Room Fires. Practice advisory for the Prevention and Management of Operating Room Fires: a report by the American Society of Anesthesiologists Task Force on Operating Room Fires. *Anesthesiology.* 2008;108:786-801. Figure 1, with permission.)

OR Fire Prevention Algorithm*

Start Here

Is patient at risk for surgical fire?

Procedures involving the head, neck and upper chest (above T5) *and* use of an ignition source in proximity to an oxidizer.

NO → **Proceed, but frequently reassess for changes in fire risk.**

Nurses and surgeons avoid pooling of alcohol-based skin preparations and allow adequate drying time. Prior to initial use of electrocautery, communication occurs between surgeon and anesthesia professional.

YES

Does patient require oxygen supplementation?

NO → **Use room air sedation.**

YES

Is >30% oxygen concentration required to maintain oxygen saturation?

NO → **Use delivery device such as a blender or common gas outlet to maintain oxygen below 30%.**

YES

Secure airway with endotracheal tube or supraglottic device.

Although securing the airway is preferred, for cases where using an airway device is undesirable or not feasible, oxygen accumulation may be minimized by air insufflation over the face and open draping to provide wide exposure of the surgical site to the atmosphere.

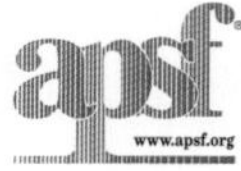

Provided as an educational resource by the **Anesthesia Patient Safety Foundation**

 www.apsf.org

The following organizations have indicated their support for APSF's efforts to increase awareness of the potential for surgical fires in at-risk patients: American Society of Anesthesiologists, American Association of Nurse Anesthetists, American Academy of Anesthesiologist Assistants, American College of Surgeons, American Society of Anesthesia Technologists and Technicians, American Society of PeriAnesthesia Nurses, Association of periOperative Registered Nurses, ECRI Institute, Food and Drug Administration Safe Use Initiative, National Patient Safety Foundation, The Joint Commission

Figure D.2 Fire Safety Algorithm. Note: This is not an ASA document but is included because of its relevance to fire safety. (From Cowles C, Ehrenwerth J. *Surgical Fire Prevention: A Review*. Anesthesia Patient Safety Foundation (APSF). Accessed June 9, 2021. https://www.apsf.org/article/surgical-fire-prevention-a-review/)

Position on Monitored Anesthesia Care

Committee of Origin: Economics

(Approved by the House of Delegates on October 25, 2005, and last amended on October 17, 2018)

Monitored anesthesia care is a specific anesthesia service performed by a qualified anesthesia provider, for a diagnostic or therapeutic procedure. Indications for monitored anesthesia care include, but are not limited to, the nature of the procedure, the patient's clinical condition and/or the need for deeper levels of analgesia and sedation than can be provided by moderate sedation (including potential conversion to a general or regional anesthetic. Unlike monitored anesthesia care, moderate sedation is a proceduralist directed service which does not include a qualified anesthesia provider's periprocedural assessment and has the inherent limitations that are policy directed for the non-anesthesia qualified provider. Moderate sedation is a proceduralist directed service that may be governed by separate institutional policies.

Monitored anesthesia care includes all aspects of anesthesia care – a preprocedure assessment and optimization, intraprocedure care and postprocedure management that is inherently provided by a qualified anesthesia provider as part of the bundled specific service. During monitored anesthesia care, the anesthesiologist provides or medically directs a number of specific services, including but not limited to:

- Preprocedural assessment and management of patient comorbidity and periprocedural risk
- Diagnosis and treatment of clinical problems that occur during the procedure
- Support of vital functions inclusive of hemodynamic stability, airway management and appropriate management of the procedure induced pathologic changes as they affect the patient's coexisting morbidities
- Administration of sedatives, analgesics, hypnotics, anesthetic agents or other medications as necessary for patient safety
- Psychological support and physical comfort
- Provision of other medical services as needed to complete the procedure safely.

Monitored anesthesia care may include varying levels of sedation, awareness, analgesia and anxiolysis as necessary. The qualified anesthesiologist provider of monitored anesthesia care must be prepared to convert to general anesthesia and respond to the pathophysiology (airway and hemodynamic changes) of procedure and position in the management in induction of general anesthesia when necessary. If the patient loses consciousness and the ability to respond purposefully, the anesthesia care is a general anesthetic, irrespective of whether airway instrumentation is required. Moderate Sedation/Analgesia on the other hand is a drug induced depression of consciousness in which the patient responds purposefully to verbal commands, either alone or accompanied by light tactile stimulation. It is not anticipated that intervention will be required to maintain a patent airway and adequate spontaneous ventilation. Similarly, it is expected that cardiovascular function will be maintained without intervention.

Monitored anesthesia care is a physician service provided to an individual patient. Whereas "Moderate Sedation/Analgesia" is a service directed by the Proceduralist who is preoccupied in focusing on successfully completing the scheduled procedure. The Proceduralist may not be cognizant of ongoing pathophysiologic effects of sedatives given or procedure/position changes. Monitored anesthesia care should be subject to the same level of payment as general or regional anesthesia. Accordingly, the ASA Relative Value Guide® provides for the use of proper base units, time and any appropriate modifier units as the basis for determining payment.

Distinguishing Monitored Anesthesia Care (MAC) From Moderate Sedation/Analgesia (Conscious Sedation)

Committee of Origin: Economics

(Approved by the ASA House of Delegates on October 27, 2004, last amended on October 21, 2009, and reaffirmed on October 17, 2018)

Moderate Sedation/Analgesia (Conscious Sedation; hereinafter known as Moderate Sedation) is a physician service recognized in the CPT procedural coding system. During Moderate Sedation, a physician supervises or personally administers sedative and/or analgesic medications that can allay patient anxiety and limit pain during a diagnostic or therapeutic procedure. During Moderate Sedation the responsible physician typically assumes the dual role of performing the procedure and supervising the sedation. Such drug-induced depression of a patient's level of consciousness to a "moderate" level of sedation, as defined in the Joint Commission (TJC) standards, is intended to facilitate the successful performance of the diagnostic or therapeutic procedure while providing patient comfort and cooperation. Physicians providing moderate sedation must be qualified to recognize "deep" sedation, manage its consequences and adjust the level of sedation to a "moderate" or lesser level. The continual appraisal of the effects of sedative or analgesic medications on the level of consciousness and on cardiac and respiratory function is an integral element of this service.

The American Society of Anesthesiologists has defined Monitored Anesthesia Care (see *Position on Monitored Anesthesia Care, updated on October 17, 2018*). This physician service can be distinguished from Moderate Sedation in several ways. An essential component of MAC is the periprocedural anesthesia assessment and understanding of the patient's coexisting medical conditions and management of the patient's actual or anticipated physiological derangements during a diagnostic or therapeutic procedure. While Monitored Anesthesia Care may include the administration of sedatives and/or analgesics often used for Moderate Sedation, the qualified anesthesia provider of MAC is focused exclusively and continuously on the patient for any attendant airway, hemodynamic and physiologic derangements. Further, the provider of MAC must be prepared and qualified to convert to general anesthesia. The proceduralist providing moderate sedation may have their attention diverted to their primary focus, the procedure. Additionally, a provider's ability to intervene to rescue a patient's airway from any sedation-induced compromise is a prerequisite to the qualifications to provide Monitored Anesthesia Care. By contrast, Moderate Sedation is not expected to induce depths of sedation that would impair the patient's respiratory function or ability to maintain the integrity of his or her airway. These components of Monitored Anesthesia Care are unique aspects of an anesthesia service that are not part of Moderate Sedation.

The administration of sedatives, hypnotics, analgesics, as well as anesthetic drugs commonly used for the induction and maintenance of general anesthesia is often, but not always, a part of Monitored Anesthesia Care. In some patients who may require only minimal sedation, MAC is often indicated because even small doses of these medications could precipitate adverse physiologic responses that would necessitate acute clinical interventions and resuscitation. The attention of the proceduralist is focused on the completion of the procedure, not physiologic alterations. If a patient's condition and/or a procedural requirement is likely to require sedation to a "deep" level or even to a transient period of general anesthesia, only a practitioner privileged to provide anesthesia services should be allowed to manage the sedation. Due to the strong likelihood that "deep" sedation may, with or without intention, transition to general anesthesia, the skills of an anesthesia provider are necessary to manage the effects of general anesthesia on the patient as well as to return the patient quickly to a state of "deep" or lesser sedation.

Like all anesthesia services, Monitored Anesthesia Care includes an array of post-procedure responsibilities beyond the expectations of practitioners providing Moderate Sedation, including assuring a return to baseline consciousness, relief of pain, management of adverse physiological responses or side effects from medications administered during the procedure, as well as the diagnosis and treatment of co-existing medical problems.

Monitored Anesthesia Care allows for the safe administration of a maximal depth of sedation in excess of that provided during Moderate Sedation. The ability to adjust the sedation level from full consciousness to general anesthesia during the course of a procedure provides maximal flexibility in matching sedation level to patient needs and procedural requirements. In situations where the procedure is more invasive or when the patient is especially fragile, optimizing sedation level is necessary to achieve ideal procedural conditions.

In summary, Monitored Anesthesia Care is a physician service that is clearly distinct from Moderate Sedation due to the expectations and qualifications of the provider who must be able to utilize all anesthesia resources to support life and to provide patient comfort and safety during a diagnostic or therapeutic procedure.

Ethical Guidelines for the Anesthesia Care of Patients With Do-Not-Resuscitate Orders or Other Directives that Limit Treatment

Committee of Origin: Ethics

(Approved by the ASA House of Delegates on October 17, 2001, and last amended on October 17, 2018)

These guidelines apply both to patients with decision-making capacity and also to patients without decision-making capacity who have previously expressed their preferences.

I. Given the diversity of published opinions and cultures within our society, an essential element of preoperative preparation and perioperative care for patients with do-not-resuscitate (DNR) orders or other directives that limit treatment is communication among involved parties. It is necessary to document relevant aspects of this communication.

II. Policies automatically suspending DNR orders or other directives that limit treatment prior to procedures involving anesthetic care may not sufficiently address a patient's rights to self-determination in a responsible and ethical manner. Such policies, if they exist, should be reviewed and revised, as necessary, to reflect the content of these guidelines.

III. The administration of anesthesia necessarily involves some practices and procedures that might be viewed as "resuscitation" in other settings. Prior to procedures requiring anesthetic care, any existing directives to limit the use of resuscitation procedures (ie, do-not-resuscitate orders and/or advance directives) should, when possible, be reviewed with the patient or designated surrogate. As a result of this review, the status of these directives should be clarified or modified based on the preferences of the patient. One of the three following alternatives may provide for a satisfactory outcome in many cases.

   A. Full Attempt at Resuscitation: The patient or designated surrogate may request the full suspension of existing directives during the anesthetic and immediate postoperative period, thereby consenting to the use of any resuscitation procedures that may be appropriate to treat clinical events that occur during this time.

   B. Limited Attempt at Resuscitation Defined With Regard to Specific Procedures: The patient or designated surrogate may elect to continue to refuse certain specific resuscitation procedures (eg, chest compressions, defibrillation, or tracheal intubation). The anesthesiologist should inform the patient or designated surrogate about which procedures are (1) essential to the success of the anesthesia and the proposed procedure, and (2) which procedures are not essential and may be refused

   C. Limited Attempt at Resuscitation Defined With Regard to the Patient's Goals and Values: The patient or designated surrogate may allow the anesthesiologist and surgical/procedural team to use clinical judgment in determining which resuscitation procedures are appropriate in the context of the situation and the patient's stated goals and values. For example, some patients may want full resuscitation procedures to be used to manage adverse clinical events that are believed to be quickly and easily reversible but to refrain from treatment for conditions that are likely to result in permanent sequelae, such as neurologic impairment or unwanted dependence upon life-sustaining technology.

IV. Any clarifications or modifications made to the patient's directive should be documented in the medical record. In cases where the patient or designated surrogate requests that the anesthesiologist use clinical judgment in determining which resuscitation procedures are appropriate, the anesthesiologist should document the discussion with particular attention to the stated goals and values of the patient.

V. Plans for postoperative/postprocedural care should indicate if or when the original, preexistent directive to limit the use of resuscitation procedures will be reinstated. This occurs when the patient leaves the postanesthesia care unit or when the patient has recovered from the acute effects of anesthesia and surgery/procedure. Consideration should be given to whether continuing to provide the patient with a time-limited or event-limited postoperative/postprocedure trial of therapy would help the patient or surrogate better evaluate whether continued therapy would be consistent with the patient's goals.

VI. It is important to discuss and document whether there are to be any exceptions to the injunction(s) against intervention should there occur a specific recognized complication of the surgery/procedure or anesthesia.

VII. Concurrence on these issues by the primary physician (if not the surgeon/proceduralist of record), the surgeon/proceduralist and the anesthesiologist is desirable. If possible, these physicians should meet together with the patient (or the patient's legal representative) when these issues are discussed. This duty of the patient's physicians is deemed to be of such importance that it should not be delegated. Other members of the healthcare team who are (or will be) directly involved with the patient's care during the planned procedure should, if feasible, be included in this process.

VIII. Should conflicts arise, the following resolution processes are recommended:

A. When an anesthesiologist finds the patient's or surgeon's/proceduralist's limitations of intervention decisions to be irreconcilable with one's own moral views, then the anesthesiologist should withdraw in a nonjudgmental fashion, providing an alternative for care in a timely fashion.

B. When an anesthesiologist finds the patient's or surgeon's/proceduralist's limitation of intervention decisions to be in conflict with generally accepted standards of care, ethical practice, or institutional policies, then the anesthesiologist should voice such concerns and present the situation to the appropriate institutional body.

C. If these alternatives are not feasible within the time frame necessary to prevent further morbidity or suffering, then in accordance with the American Medical Association's Principles of Medical Ethics, care should proceed with reasonable adherence to the patient's directives, being mindful of the patient's goals and values.

IX. A representative from the hospital's anesthesiology service should establish a liaison with surgical, procedural, and nursing services for presentation, discussion, and procedural application of these guidelines. Hospital staff should be made aware of the proceedings of these discussions and the motivations for them.

X. Modification of these guidelines may be appropriate when they conflict with local standards or policies and in those emergency situations involving patients lacking decision-making capacity whose intentions have not been previously expressed.

Practice Guidelines for Preoperative Fasting and Use of Pharmacologic Agents to Reduce Risk of Pulmonary Aspiration: Application to Healthy Patients Undergoing Elective Procedures

Committee of Origin: Ethics

(*Anesthesiology* March 2017, Vol. 126, 376–393.)

A. Fasting Recommendations*	
Ingested Material	Minimum Fasting Period†
• Clear liquids‡	2h
• Breast milk	4h
• Infant formula	6h
• Nonhuman milk§	6h
• Light meal**	6h
• Fried foods, fatty foods, or meat	Additional fasting time (e.g., 8 or more hours) may be needed
B. Pharmacologic Recommendations	
Medication Type and Common Examples	Recommendation
Gastriointestinal stimulants:	
• Metoclopramide	May be used/no routine use
Gastric acid secretion blockers:	
• Climetidine	May be used/no routine use
• Famotidine	May be used/no routine use
• Ranitidine	May be used/no routine use
• Omeprazole	May be used/no routine use
• Lansoprazole	May be used/no routine use
Antacids:	
• Sodium citrate	May be used/no routine use
• Sodium bicarbonate	May be used/no routine use
• Magnesium trisillicate	May be used/no routine use
Antiemetics:	
• Ondansetron	May be used/no routine use

Anticholinergics:	
• Atropine	No use
• Scopolamine	No use
• Glycopyrrolate	No use
Combinations of the medications above:	No routine use

*These recommendations apply to healthy patients who are undergoing elective procedures. They are not intended for women in labor. Following the guidelines does not guarantee complete gastric emptying.

†The fasting periods noted above apply to all ages.

‡Examples of clear liquids include water, fruit juices without pulp, carbonated beverages, clear tea, and black coffee.

§Since nonhuman milk is similar to solids in gastric emptying time, the amount ingested must be considered when determining an appropriate fasting period.

**A light meal typically consists of toast and clear liquids. Meals that include fried or fatty foods or meat may prolong gastric emptying time. Additional fasting time (e.g., 8 or more hours) may be needed in these cases. Both the amount and type of foods ingested must be considered when determining an appropriate fasting period.

E The Airway Approach Algorithm and Difficult Airway Algorithm

The Airway Approach (Figure E.1)

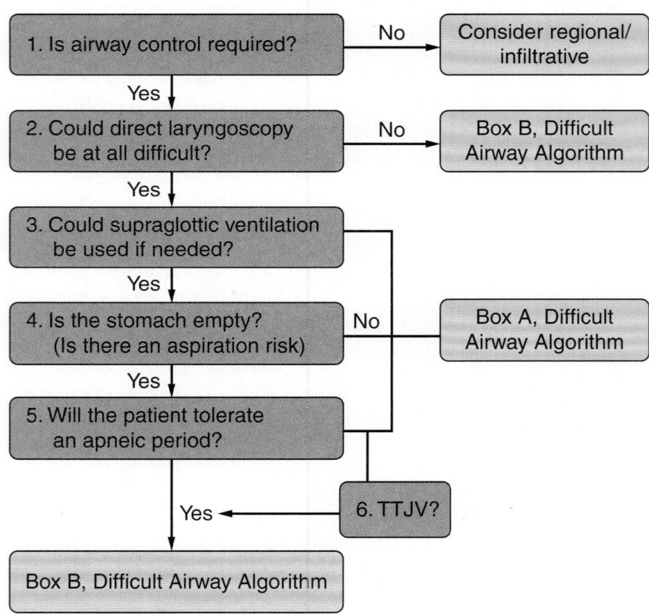

Figure E.1 The airway approach algorithm: A decision-tree approach to entry into the American Society of Anesthesiologists difficult airway algorithm. TTJV, trans-tracheal jet ventilation. (From Rosenblatt WH, Abrons RO, Sukhupragarn W. Airway management. In: Barash PG, Cahalan MK, Cullen BF, et al, eds. *Clinical Anesthesia*. 8th ed. Wolters Kluwer; 2018:767-808. Figure 28.21.)

The Difficult Airway (Figure E.2)

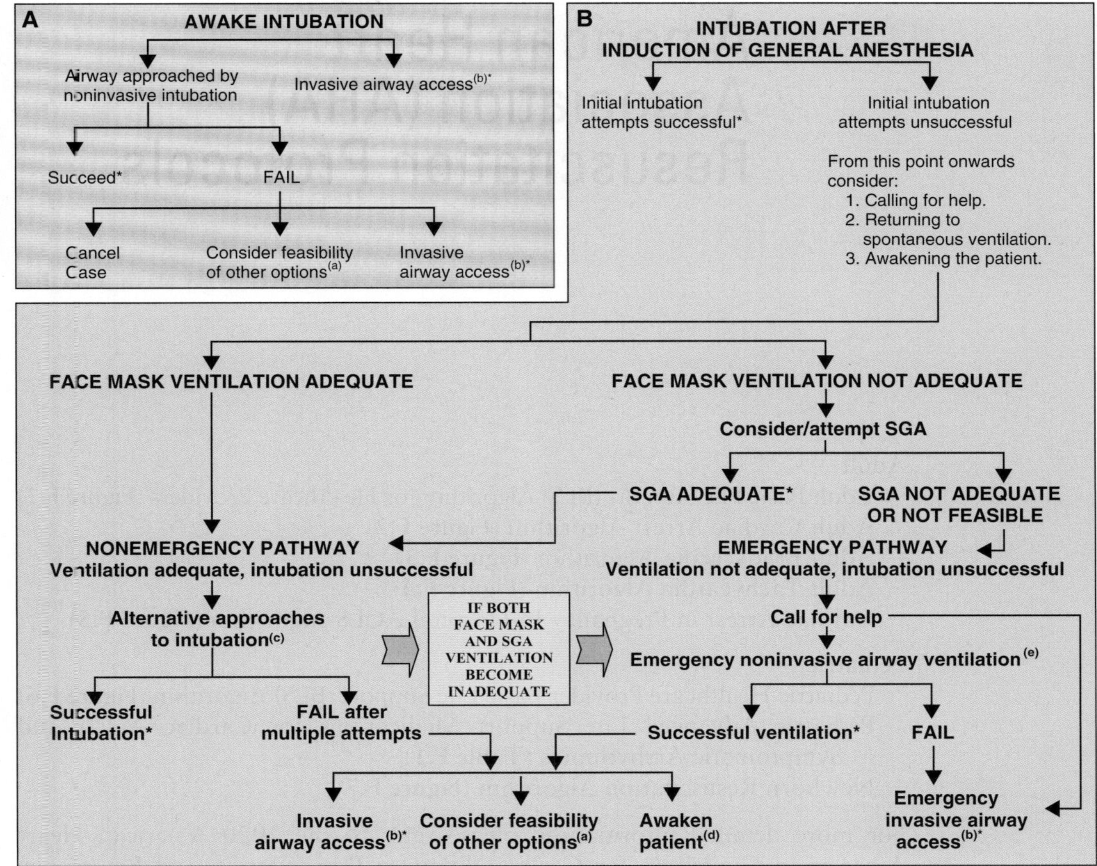

***Confirm ventilation, tracheal intubation, or SGA placement with exhaled CO_2.**

a. Other options include (but are not limited to) surgery utilizing face mask or supraglottic airway (SGA) anesthesia (eg, LMA, ILMA, laryngeal tube), local anesthesia infiltration or regional nerve blockade. Pursuit of these options usually implies that mask ventilation will not be problematic. Therefore, these options may be of limited value if this step in the algorithm has been reached via the Emergency Pathway.

b. Invasive airway access includes surgical or percutaneous airway, jet ventilation, and retrograde intubation.

c. Alternative difficult intubation approaches include (but are not limited to) video-assisted laryngoscopy, alternative laryngoscope blades, SGA (eg, LMA or ILMA) as an intubation conduit (with or without fiberoptic guidance), fiberoptic intubation, intubating stylet or tube changer, light wand, and blind oral or nasal intubation.

d. Consider repreparation of the patient for awake intubation or canceling surgery.

e. Emergency noninvasive airway ventilation consists of a SGA.

Figure E.2 The American Society of Anesthesiologists difficult airway algorithm. **A,** Awake intubation. **B,** Intubation after induction of general anesthesia. (From Apfelbaum JL, Hagberg CA, Caplan RA, et al; American Society of Anesthesiologists Task Force on Management of the Difficult Airway. Practice guidelines for management of the difficult airway: an updated report by the American Society of Anesthesiologists Task Force on Management of the Difficult Airway. *Anesthesiology.* 2013;118(2): 251-270, with permission.)

F American Heart Association (AHA) Resuscitation Protocols

Adult

Adult Basic Life Support (BLS) Algorithm for Healthcare Providers (**Figure F.1**)
Adult Cardiac Arrest Algorithm (**Figure F.2**)
Adult Bradycardia Algorithm (**Figure F.3**)
Adult Tachycardia Algorithm (**Figure F.4**)
Cardiac Arrest in Pregnancy In-Hospital ACLS Algorithm (**Figure F.5**)

Pediatric

Pediatric Healthcare Provider Basic Life Support (BLS) Algorithm (**Figure F.6**)
Pediatric Advanced Life Support Medications for Cardiac Arrest and Symptomatic Arrhythmias (**Table F.1**)
Newborn Resuscitation Algorithm (**Figure F.7**)

For more detailed information, please refer to the 2020 American Heart Association Guidelines for Cardiopulmonary Resuscitation and Emergency Cardiovascular Care.

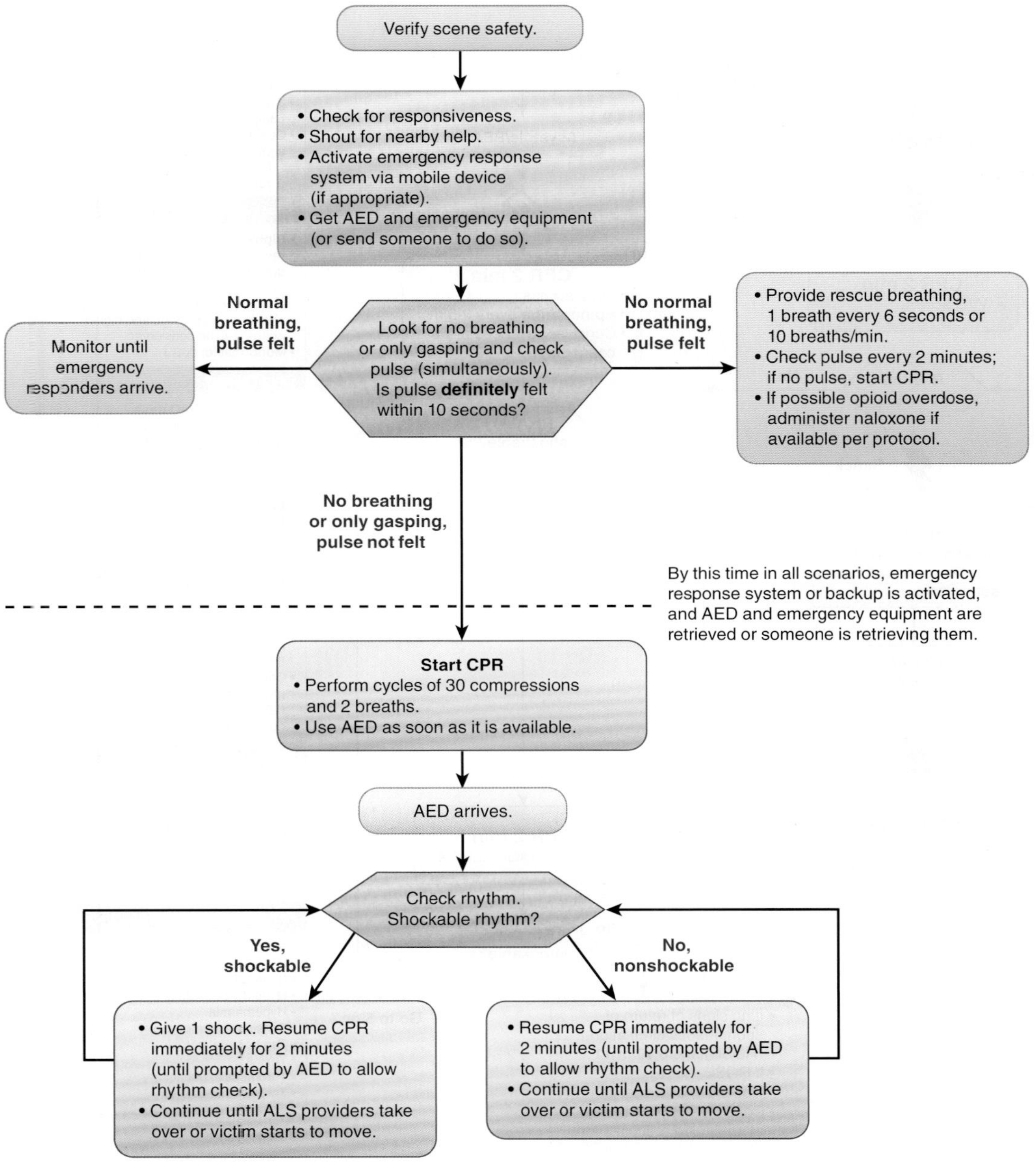

Figure F.1 Adult BLS Algorithm for Healthcare Providers. AED indicates automated external defibrillator; ALS, advanced life support; BLS, basic life support; and CPR, cardiopulmonary resuscitation. (Reprinted with permission *Circulation* 2020;142:S366-S468, ©2020 American Heart Association, Inc.)

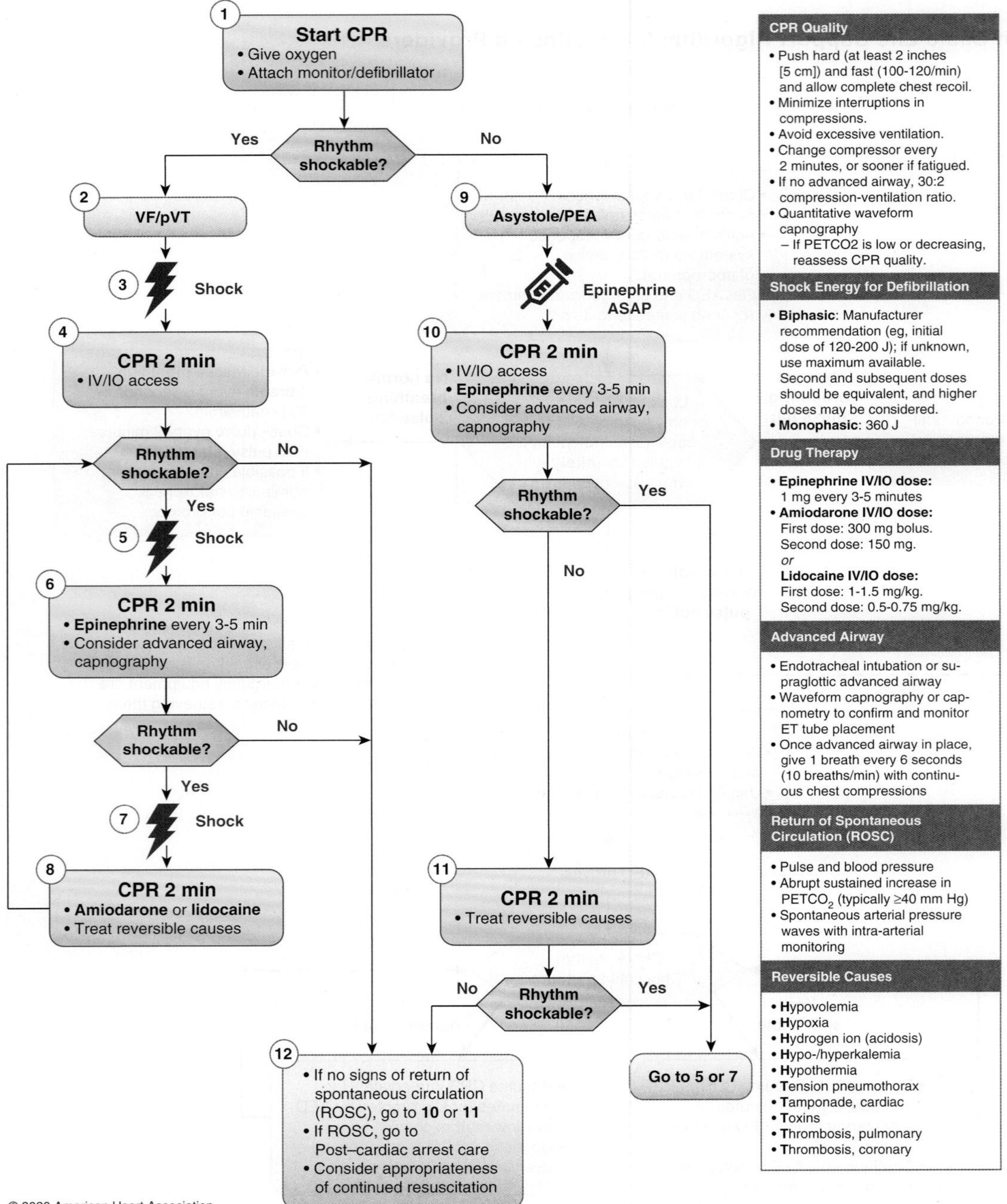

Figure F.2 Adult Cardiac Arrest Algorithm. CPR indicates cardiopulmonary resuscitation; ET, endotracheal; IO, intraosseous; IV, intravenous; PEA, pulseless electrical activity; pVT, pulseless ventricular tachycardia; and VF, ventricular fibrillation. (Reprinted with permission *Circulation* 2020;142:S366-S468, ©2020 American Heart Association, Inc.)

Adult Bradycardia Algorithm

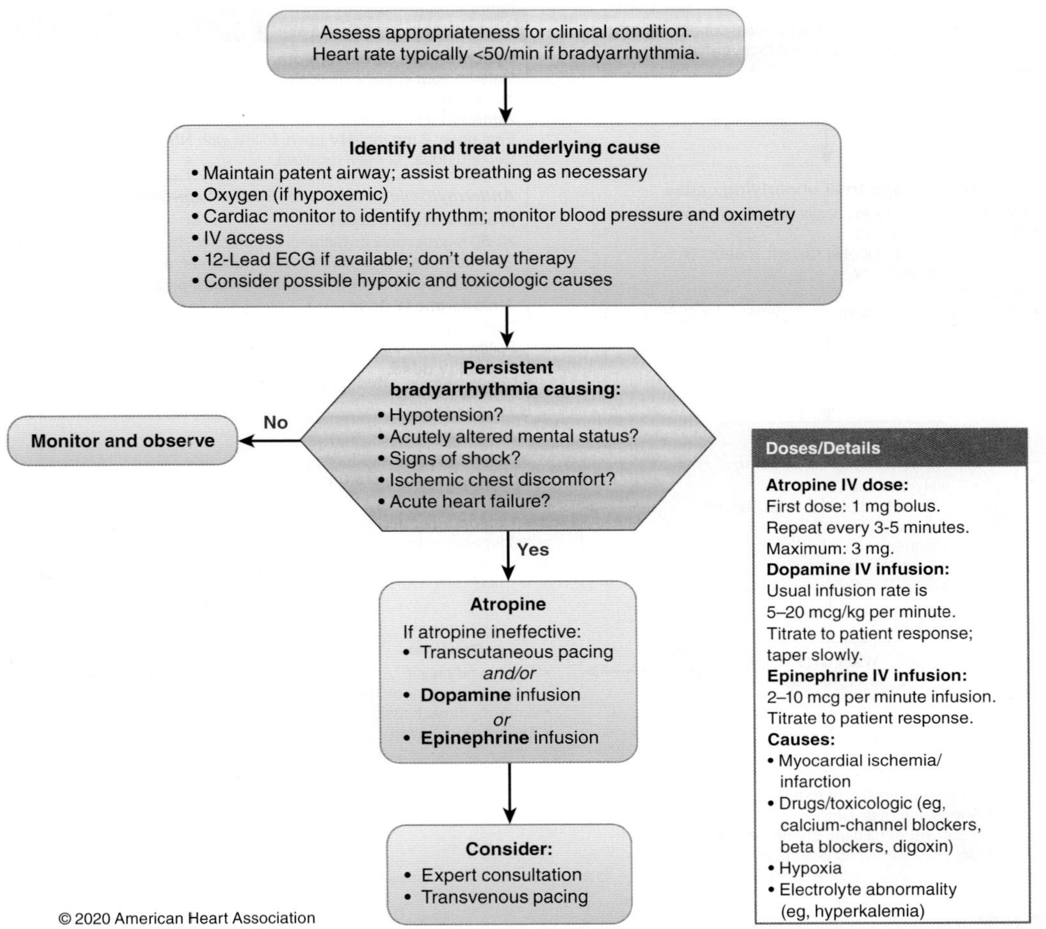

Assess appropriateness for clinical condition.
Heart rate typically <50/min if bradyarrhythmia.
Identify and treat underlying cause
• Maintain patent airway; assist breathing as necessary
• Oxygen (if hypoxemic)
• Cardiac monitor to identify rhythm; monitor blood pressure and oximetry
• IV access
• 12-Lead ECG if available; don't delay therapy
• Consider possible hypoxic and toxicologic causes
Persistent bradyarrhythmia causing:
• Hypotension?
• Acutely altered mental status?
• Signs of shock?
• Ischemic chest discomfort?
• Acute heart failure?
No
Monitor and observe
Yes
Atropine
If atropine ineffective:
• Transcutaneous pacing
and/or
• Dopamine infusion
or
• Epinephrine infusion
Consider:
• Expert consultation
• Transvenous pacing
Doses/Details
Atropine IV dose:
First dose: 1 mg bolus.
Repeat every 3-5 minutes.
Maximum: 3 mg.
Dopamine IV infusion:
Usual infusion rate is
5–20 mcg/kg per minute.
Titrate to patient response;
taper slowly.
Epinephrine IV infusion:
2–10 mcg per minute infusion.
Titrate to patient response.
Causes:
• Myocardial ischemia/infarction
• Drugs/toxicologic (eg, calcium-channel blockers, beta blockers, digoxin)
• Hypoxia
• Electrolyte abnormality (eg, hyperkalemia)
© 2020 American Heart Association

Figure F.3 Adult Bradycardia Algorithm. (Reprinted with permission Advanced Cardiovascular Life Support Provider Manual ©2020 American Heart Association, Inc.)

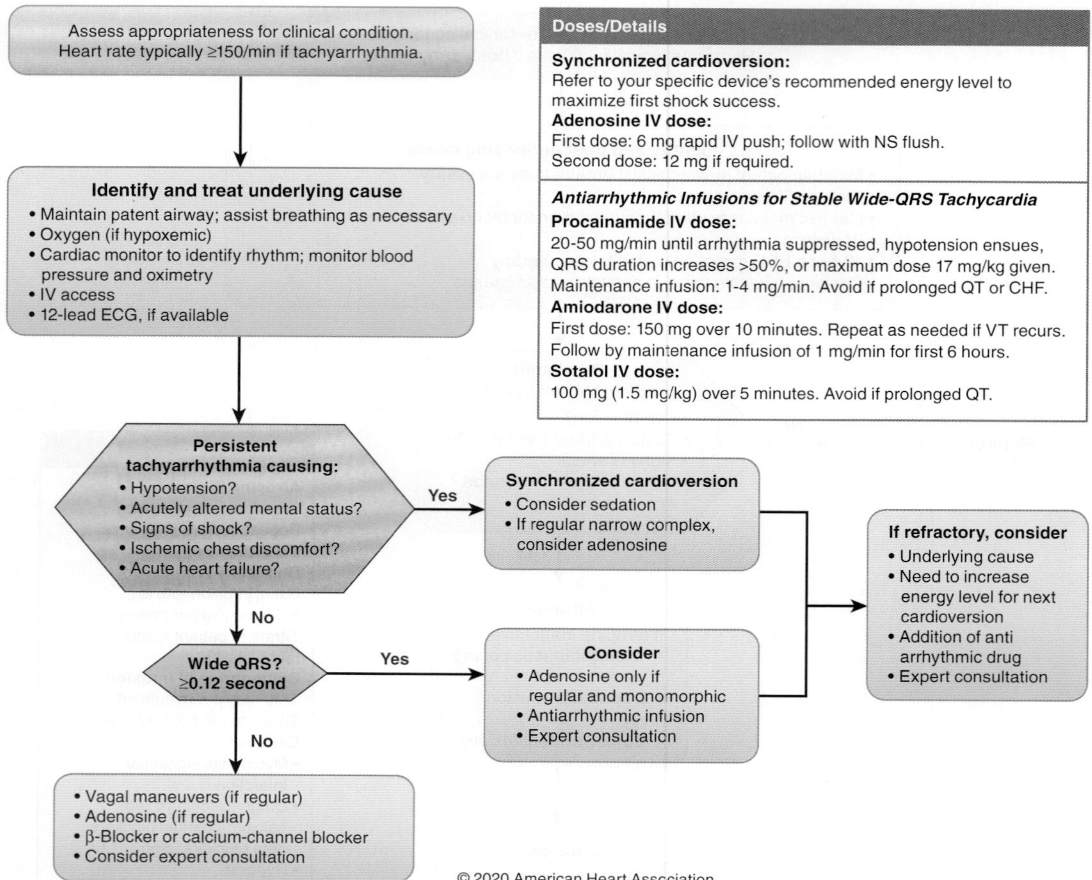

Figure F.4 Adult Tachycardia with Pulse Algorithm. (Reprinted with permission Advanced Cardiovascular Life Support Provider Manual ©2020 American Heart Association, Inc.)

Cardiac Arrest in Pregnancy In-Hospital ACLS Algorithm

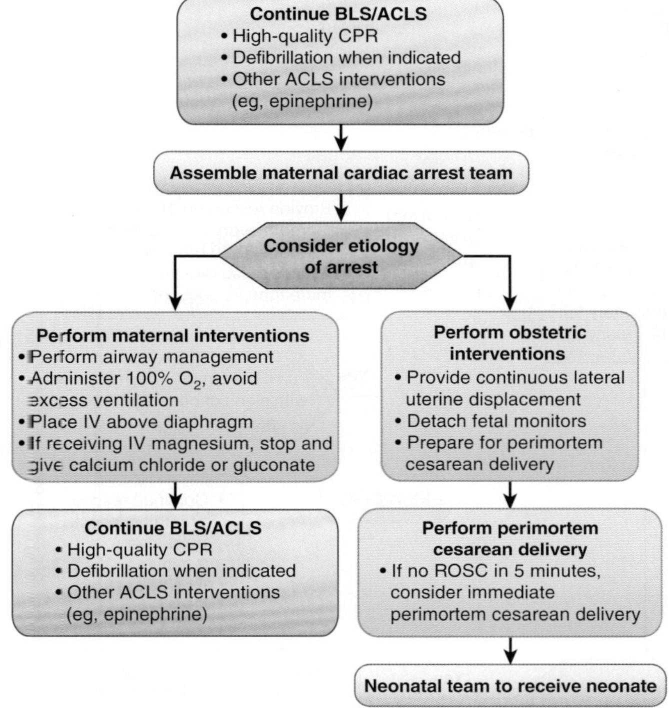

Continue BLS/ACLS
• High-quality CPR
• Defibrillation when indicated
• Other ACLS interventions (eg, epinephrine)
Assemble maternal cardiac arrest team
Consider etiology of arrest
Perform maternal interventions
• Perform airway management
• Administer 100% O_2, avoid excess ventilation
• Place IV above diaphragm
• If receiving IV magnesium, stop and give calcium chloride or gluconate
Perform obstetric interventions
• Provide continuous lateral uterine displacement
• Detach fetal monitors
• Prepare for perimortem cesarean delivery
Continue BLS/ACLS
• High-quality CPR
• Defibrillation when indicated
• Other ACLS interventions (eg, epinephrine)
Perform perimortem cesarean delivery
• If no ROSC in 5 minutes, consider immediate perimortem cesarean delivery
Neonatal team to receive neonate

Maternal Cardiac Arrest

- Team planning should be done in collaboration with the obstetric, neonatal, emergency, anesthesiology, intensive care, and cardiac arrest services.
- Priorities for pregnant women in cardiac arrest should include provision of high-quality CPR and relief of aortocaval compression with lateral uterine displacement.
- The goal of perimortem cesarean delivery is to improve maternal and fetal outcomes.
- Ideally, perform perimortem cesarean delivery in 5 minutes, depending on provider resources and skill sets.

Advanced Airway

- In pregnancy, a difficult airway is common. Use the most experienced provider.
- Provide endotracheal intubation or supraglottic advanced airway.
- Perform waveform capnography or capnometry to confirm and monitor ET tube placement.
- Once advanced airway is in place, give 1 breath every 6 seconds (10 breaths/min) with continuous chest compressions.

Potential Etiology of Maternal Cardiac Arrest

A Anesthetic complications
B Bleeding
C Cardiovascular
D Drugs
E Embolic
F Fever
G General nonobstetric causes of cardiac arrest (H's and T's)
H Hypertension

Figure F.5 Cardiac Arrest in Pregnancy In-Hospital ACLS Algorithm. (Reprinted with permission *Circulation* 2020;142:S366-S468, ©2020 American Heart Association, Inc.)

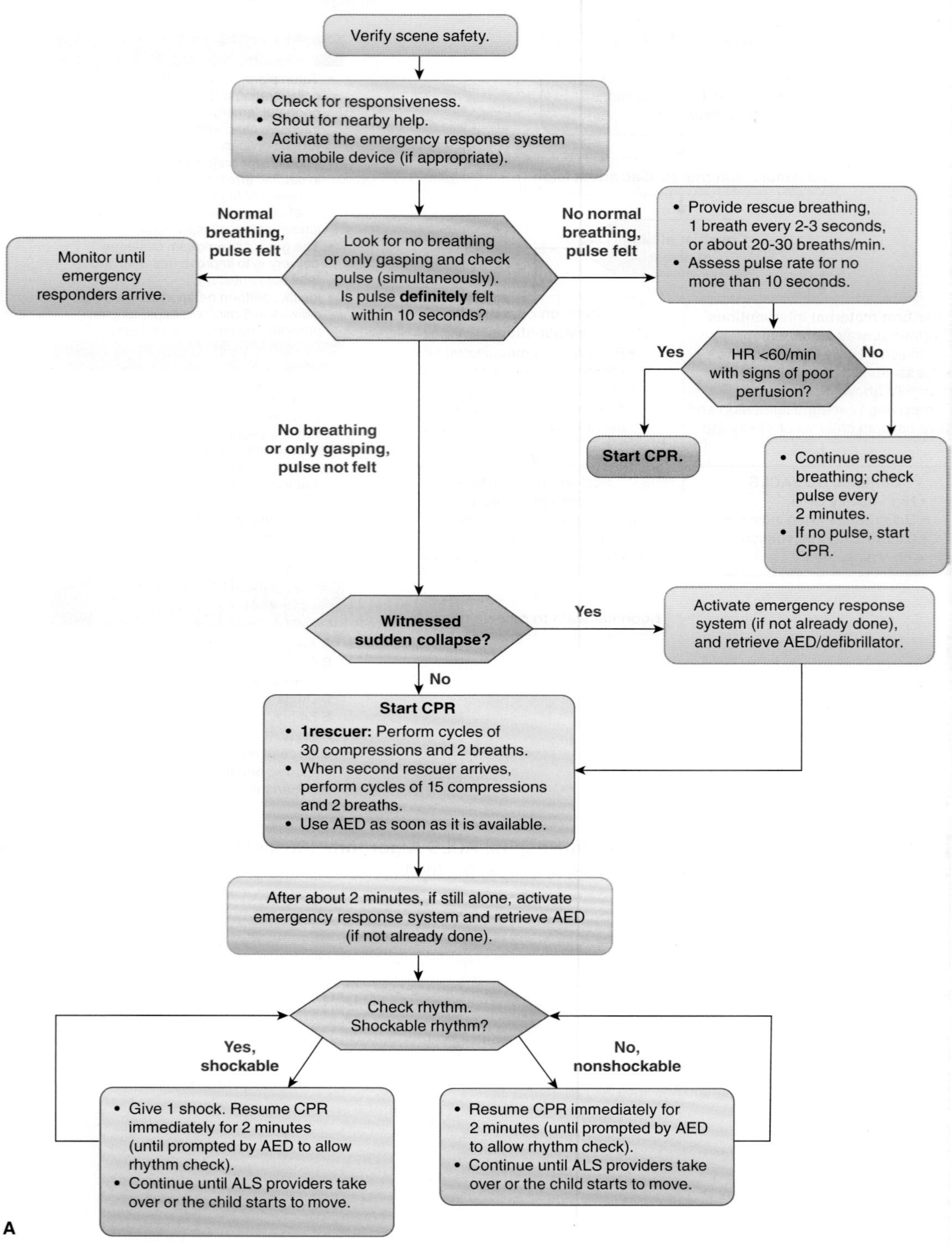

Figure F.6 A, Pediatric Basic Life Support Algorithm for Healthcare Providers—Single Rescuer. B, Pediatric Basic Life Support Algorithm for Healthcare Providers—Two or More Rescuers. AED indicates automated external defibrillator; ALS, advanced life support; CPR, cardiopulmonary resuscitation; and HR, heart rate. (A, B: Reprinted with permission *Circulation* 2020;142:S469-S523, ©2020 American Heart Association, Inc.)

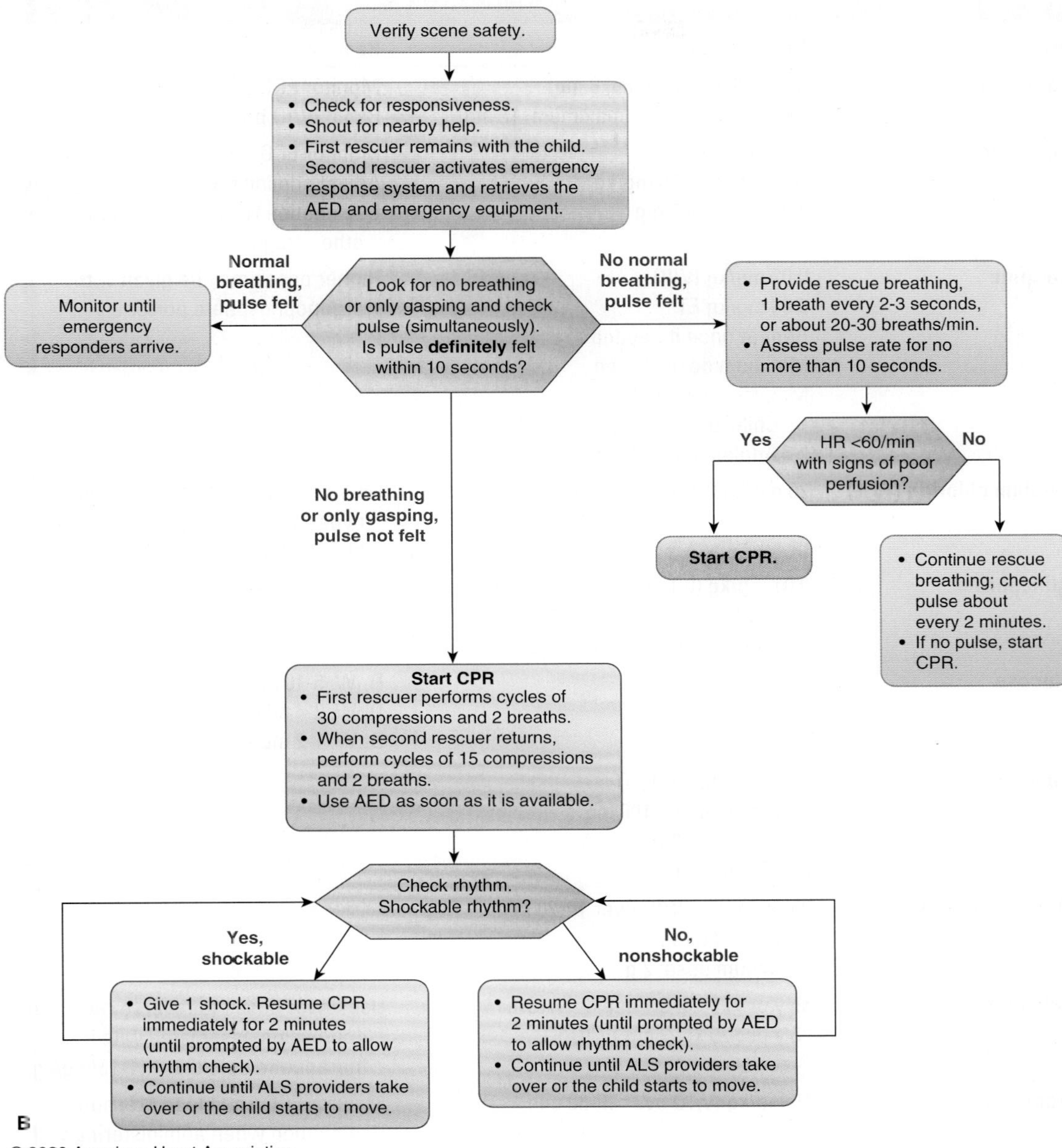

Figure F.6 Cont'd

Table F.1 Pediatric Advanced Life Support Medications for Cardiac Arrest and Symptomatic Arrhythmias

Drug	Dosage (Pediatric)	Remarks
Adenosine	0.1 mg/kg (maximum, 6 mg) Repeat: 0.2 mg/kg (maximum, 12 mg)	Monitor ECG during dose Rapid IV/IO bolus
Amiodarone	5 mg/kg IV/IO Repeat up to 15 mg/kg Maximum: 300 mg	Monitor ECG and blood pressure Adjust administration rate to urgency Use caution when administering with other drugs that prolong QT
Atropine	0.02 mg/kg IV/IO 0.03 mg/kg ET[a] Repeat once if needed Minimum dose: 0.1 mg Maximum single dose: Child, 0.5 mg Adolescent, 1.0 mg	Higher doses may be given with organophosphate poisoning
Calcium chloride (10%)	20 mg/kg IV/IO (0.2 mL/kg)	Give slow IV push for hypocalcemia, hypermagnesemia, calcium channel blocker toxicity
Epinephrine	0.01 mg/kg (0.1 mL/kg 1:10,000) IV/IO 0.1 mg/kg (0.1 mL/kg 1:1000) ET[a] Maximum dose: 1 mg IV/IO; 10 mg ET	May repeat every 3-5 min
Glucose	0.5-1.0 g/kg IV/IO	$D_{10}W$: 5-10 mL/kg $D_{25}W$: 2-4 mL/kg $D_{50}W$: 1-2 mL/kg
Lidocaine	Bolus: 1 mg/kg IV/IO Maximum dose: 100 mg Infusion: 20-50/g/kg/min ET[a]: 2-3 mg/kg	—
Magnesium sulfate	25-50 mg/kg IV/IO over 10-20 min; faster in torsades Maximum dose: 2 g	—
Naloxone	≤5 y or <20 kg: 0.1 mg/kg IV/IO/ET[a] ≥5 y or >20 kg: 2 mg IV/IO/ET[a]	Use lower doses to reverse respiratory depression associated with therapeutic opioid use (1-15/mg/kg)
Procainamide	15 mg/kg IV/IO over 30-60 min Adult dose: 20 mg/min IV infusion up to total maximum dose of 17 mg/kg	Monitor ECG and blood pressure Use caution when administering with other drugs that prolong QT
Sodium bicarbonate	1 mEq/kg IV/IO slowly	After adequate ventilation

ECG, electrocardiogram; ET, endotracheal; IO, intraosseous; IV, intravenous.

[a]Flush with 5 mL of normal saline and follow with five ventilations.

Data from ECC Committee, Subcommittees and Task Forces of the American Heart Association. 2005 American Heart Association Guidelines for cardiopulmonary resuscitation and emergency cardiovascular care. *Circulation.* 2005;112(24 suppl):IV1-203.

Neonatal Resuscitation Algorithm

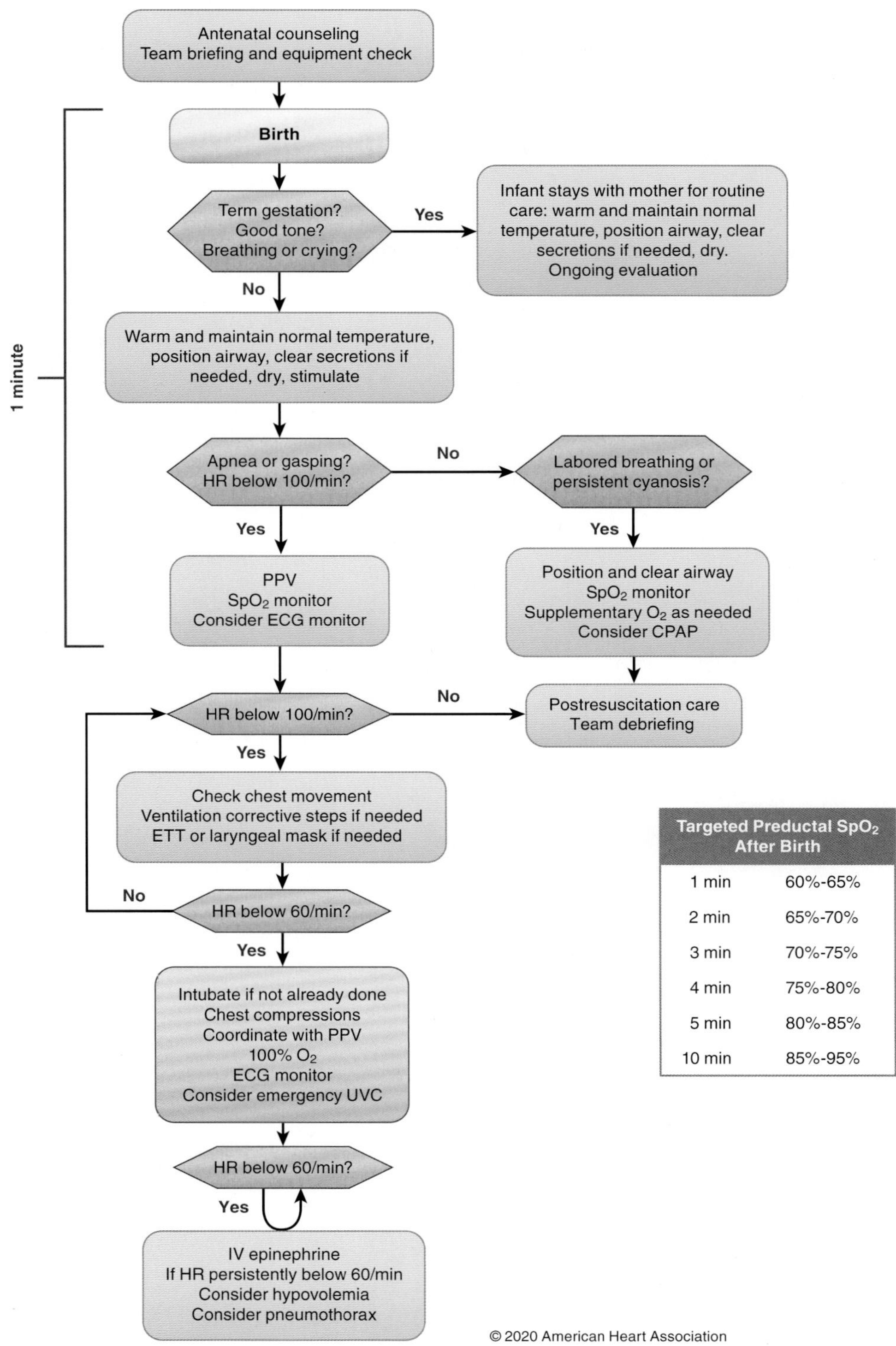

Targeted Preductal SpO_2 After Birth	
1 min	60%-65%
2 min	65%-70%
3 min	70%-75%
4 min	75%-80%
5 min	80%-85%
10 min	85%-95%

Figure F.7 Neonatal Resuscitation Algorithm. CPAP indicates continuous positive airway pressure; ECG, electrocardiogram; ETT, endotracheal tube; HR, heart rate; IV, intravenous; O_2, oxygen; Spo_2, oxygen saturation; and UVC, umbilical venous catheter. (Reprinted with permission *Circulation* 2020;142:S524-S550, ©2020 American Heart Association, Inc.)

Index

Note: Page numbers followed by "f" indicate figures and "t" indicate tables.

I

O